# HANDBOOK OF
# DISEASES

## SECOND EDITION

D0596798

SPRINGHOUSE CORPORATION
Springhouse, Pennsylvania

## STAFF

**Vice President**
Matthew Cahill

**Clinical Director**
Judith A. Schilling McCann, RN, MSN

**Art Director**
John Hubbard

**Managing Editor**
H. Nancy Holmes

**Clinical Editors**
Joanne Bartelmo, RN, MSN, CCRN (clinical project manager), Jill Curry, RN, BSN, CCRN

**Editors**
Rachel Bedard, Barbara Hodgson, Peter H. Johnson, Doris Weinstock

**Copy Editors**
Brenna Mayer (manager), Priscilla DeWitt, Mary T. Durkin, Shana Harrington, Barbara Hodgson, Jaime Stockslager, Pamela Wingrod

**Designers**
Arlene Putterman (associate art director), Linda Franklin (project manager), Donna S. Morris, Jeff Sklarow, Jarrett Zigon

**Typographers**
Diane Paluba (manager), Joyce Rossi Biletz, Valerie Molettiere

**Manufacturing**
Deborah Meiris (director), Patricia K. Dorshaw (manager), Otto Mezei (book production manager)

**Editorial Assistants**
Beverly Lane, Marcia Mills, Liz Schaeffer

**Indexer**
Barbara Hodgson

**Cover illustrations**
Top left: Transmission electron micrograph of herpes simplex virus nucleocapside, ©Jason Burns/Phototake. Top right: Electron micrograph of herpes simplex virus from a family of viruses suspected of causing chronic fatigue syndrome, ©Dr. Dennis Kunkel/Phototake. Bottom: Spiral computed tomography scan angiograph of carotid artery showing atherosclerotic plaque, ©CNRI/Phototake.

©2000 by Springhouse Corporation. All rights reserved. No part of this publication may be used or reproduced in any manner whatsoever without written permission except for brief quotations embodied in critical articles and reviews. For information, write Springhouse Corporation, 1111 Bethlehem Pike, P.O. Box 908, Springhouse, PA 19477-0908. Authorization to photocopy any items for internal or personal use, or for the internal or personal use of specific clients, is granted by Springhouse Corporation for users registered with the Copyright Clearance Center (CCC) Transactional Reporting Service, provided that the fee of $.75 per page is paid directly to CCC, 27 Congress St., Salem, MA 01970. For those organizations that have been granted a license by CCC, a separate system of payment has been arranged. The fee code for users of the Transactional Reporting Service is 0874349796/2000 $00.00 + $.75.

Printed in the United States of America.

HBD2-D

03 02 01   10 9 8 7 6 5 4

**Library of Congress Cataloging-in-Publication Data**

Handbook of diseases. — 2nd ed.
    p.cm.
Includes bibliographical references and index.
1. Diseases Handbooks, manuals, etc.
I. Springhouse Corporation.
[DNLM: 1. Disease Handbooks. 2. Diagnosis Handbooks. 3. Therapeutics Handbooks.    QZ 39 H2358 1999]
RC55.H265 1999
616—dc21
DNLM/DLC                                        99-16734
ISBN 0-87434-979-6                                  CIP

# CONTENTS

# CONTRIBUTORS

**Gerald A. Charnogursky,** MD, FACE
Medical Director
The MacNeal Diabetes Center
MacNeal Hospital
Riverside, Ill.

**JoAnn Coleman,** RN, MS, ACNP-CS, AOCN
Acute Care Nurse Practitioner, Case
    Manager GI Surgery
Johns Hopkins Hospital
Baltimore

**Rae L. Conley,** RN, MSN
Clinical Nurse Specialist
Thomas Jefferson University Hospital
Philadelphia

**Carol L. Danning,** MD
Clinical Associate
Arthritis and Rheumatism Branch
National Institute of Arthritis and
    Musculoskeletal and Skin Disease
National Institutes of Health
Bethesda, Md.

**Lori Sholders Farmer,** RN, ARNP, MS
Director of Genetic and Perinatal
    Counseling
Fayetteville (N.C.) Diagnostic Center

**Marilyn A. Folcik,** RN, MPH
Assistant Director
Department of Surgery
Hartford (Conn.) Hospital

**Arnold W. Gurevitch,** MD
Professor and Chief
Division of Dermatology
University of Southern California
School of Medicine
Los Angeles

**Karen A. Jantzi,** RN, MSN
Clinical Consultant
Doctoral Student
Temple University
Philadelphia

**Mark Johnson,** MD
Assistant Clinical Professor of
    Orthopedic Surgery
Baylor College of Medicine
Houston

**Thomas E. Lafferty,** BCHE, MD
Physician
Ocala (Fla.) Orthopaedic Group, P.A.

**Kay L. Luft,** MN, CCRN, TNCC
Assistant Professor
Saint Luke's College
Kansas City, Mo.

**Heather Boyd-Monk,** SRN, BSN, CRNO
Assistant Director of Nursing
Ophthalmic Educational Programs
Wills Eye Hospital
Philadelphia

**Teresa Murphy,** RN, BSN, CCRN
Nurse Manager of Medical ICU and
    Surgical ICU
Graduate Hospital
Philadelphia

**Iris M. Reyes,** MD
Assistant Professor of Emergency
    Medicine
Hospital of the University of
    Pennsylvania
Philadelphia

**Kristine A. Bludau Scordo**
PHD, RN
Assistant Professor
Wright State University-CONH
Dayton, Ohio

**Constance L. Seymour,** RN, BSN, CIC
Nurse Epidemiologist
Consultant
Hatboro, Pa.

**Sylvia J. Smith,** RNC, CRNP
Nurse Practitioner, Obstetrics/
    Gynecology
Rosedale Women's Care, P.C.
Pottstown, Pa.

**Warren Summer,** MD
Section Chief, Pulmonary Critical Care
Louisiana State University Medical
    Center
New Orleans

**Michele Turner,** RN, MS, CNRN, CNS
Clinical Faculty
Wright State University
College of Nursing and Health
Dayton, Ohio

**Joseph M. Vitello,** MD
Associate Professor of Surgery
University of Illinois
Chicago

# FOREWORD

There is no question that the practice of medicine is constantly changing. One need only read the medical literature from a few years ago to realize that great advances have been made in standard patient care delivery. In some cases, the very names and definitions of illnesses have changed, and modern understanding of disease mechanisms is evolving at a breathtaking rate. More efficient and sensitive diagnostic schemes are being devised, and new, effective treatments are quickly replacing older ones as the standard of care. Consequently, the health care professional is faced with the important task of keeping up to date with the latest information on a wide variety of illnesses in order to provide the most effective patient care. Even in the age of computer technology, this is a remarkably difficult and often time-consuming endeavor. Therefore, having a comprehensive, pocket-size reference book at one's fingertips can be extremely valuable.

*Handbook of Diseases,* Second Edition, is designed with the health care provider in mind. It contains concise, up-to-date information on more than 435 diseases, including many new disease entries in each specialty area, from common infections to complicated autoimmune disorders and life-threatening cardiovascular illnesses. The entries are conveniently listed in alphabetical order. Each entry includes a brief summary paragraph of the disease, a description of signs and symptoms, an overview of the cause, a listing of diagnostic testing, and an outline of treatment. Other pertinent information, such as *DSM-IV* criteria for psychiatric disorders and staging charts for different cancers, is also included.

Apart from being a handy reference book, the *Handbook* has other unique features to aid the busy clinician. Eye-catching symbols direct the reader to information about potential hazards of a particular illness and point out life-threatening disorders. New to this second edition, useful clinical tips are highlighted in the text margins for easy survey. Handy teaching checklists for patients are also readily available, and the text is supplemented with helpful illustrations and quick review charts. Furthermore, an appendix of about 150 additional diseases, some relatively uncommon, is included to provide an even more comprehensive listing of different disorders.

Clearly, this latest edition of *Handbook of Diseases* is filled with comprehensive and up-to-date yet practical and important information. Its easy-to-use format makes it a useful quick-reference book to keep in one's office, clinic, hospital ward, or home. There is no doubt that today's health care provider will find this handbook an extremely valuable tool for keeping track of the latest information in medicine.

**Carol L. Danning, MD**
Clinical Associate
Arthritis and Rheumatism Branch
National Institute of Arthritis and
    Musculoskeletal and Skin
    Diseases
National Institutes of Health
Bethesda, Md.

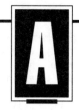

# ABDOMINAL INJURIES

Blunt and penetrating abdominal injuries may damage major blood vessels as well as internal organs. Their most immediate life-threatening consequences are hemorrhage and hypovolemic shock; later threats include infection. The prognosis depends on the extent of injury and on which organs are damaged, but it's generally improved by prompt diagnosis and surgical repair.

## Causes

Blunt (nonpenetrating) abdominal injuries usually result from motor vehicle accidents, falls from heights, or athletic injuries; penetrating abdominal injuries, from stab and gunshot wounds.

## Signs and symptoms

Depending on the degree of injury and the organs involved, symptoms vary as follows:

• Penetrating abdominal injuries cause obvious wounds. For example, gunshots often produce both entrance and exit wounds, with variable blood loss, pain, and tenderness. These injuries often cause pallor, cyanosis, tachycardia, shortness of breath, and hypotension.

• Blunt abdominal injuries cause severe pain (such pain may radiate beyond the abdomen, for instance, to the shoulders), bruises, abrasions, contusions, or distention. They may also result in tenderness, abdominal splinting or rigidity, nausea, vomiting, pallor, cyanosis, tachycardia, and shortness of breath. Rib fractures often accompany blunt injuries.

In both blunt and penetrating injuries, massive blood loss may cause hypovolemic shock. In general, damage to solid abdominal organs (liver, spleen, pancreas, and kidneys) causes hemorrhage; damage to hollow organs (stomach, intestines, gallbladder, and bladder) causes rupture and release of the organs' contents (including bacteria) into the abdomen, which, in turn, produces inflammation.

## Diagnosis

A history of abdominal trauma, clinical features, and laboratory results confirm the diagnosis and determine organ damage. Consider any upper abdominal injury a thoracicoabdominal injury until proven otherwise. Diagnostic studies vary with the patient's condition but usually include:

• *chest X-rays* (preferably done with the patient upright, to show free air)

• *examination of stool and stomach aspirate* for blood

• *blood studies* (decreased hematocrit and hemoglobin levels point to severe blood loss; coagulation studies evaluate hemostasis; white blood cell count is usually elevated but doesn't necessarily point to infection; type and crossmatch to prepare for blood transfusion)

1

- *arterial blood gas analysis* to evaluate respiratory status
- *serum amylase levels,* which often may be elevated in pancreatic injury
- *aspartate aminotransferase and alanine aminotransferase levels,* which increase with tissue injury and cell death
- *excretory urography* and *cystourethrography* to detect renal and urinary tract damage
- *angiography* to detect specific injuries, especially to the kidneys
- *peritoneal lavage,* with insertion of a lavage catheter to check for blood, urine, pus, ascitic fluid, bile, and chyle (a milky fluid absorbed by the intestinal lymph vessels during digestion). In blunt trauma with equivocal abdominal findings, this procedure helps establish the need for exploratory surgery.
- *computed tomography scan* to detect abdominal, head, or other injuries
- *exploratory laparotomy* to detect specific injuries when other clinical evidence is incomplete
- other laboratory studies to rule out associated injuries.

### Treatment

Abdominal injuries require emergency treatment to control hemorrhage and prevent hypovolemic shock, by infusion of I.V. fluids and blood components. After stabilization, most abdominal injuries require surgical repair; some patients, however, require immediate surgery. Analgesics and antibiotics increase patient comfort and prevent infection. Most patients require hospitalization; if they're asymptomatic, they may require observation for only 6 to 24 hours.

### Special considerations

- Emergency care in patients with abdominal injuries supports vital functions by maintaining airway, breathing, and circulation. At admission, immediately evaluate respiratory and circulatory status and, if possible, obtain a history.
- To maintain airway and breathing, intubate the patient and provide mechanical ventilation as necessary; otherwise, provide supplemental oxygen.
- Using a large-bore needle, start two or more I.V. lines for monitoring and rapid fluid infusion, using normal saline solution (or blood transfusions if the patient is hemodynamically unstable). Then draw a blood sample for laboratory studies. Also, insert a nasogastric tube and, if necessary, an indwelling urinary catheter; monitor stomach aspirate and urine for blood.
- Obtain vital signs for baseline data; continue to monitor them every 15 minutes.
- Apply a sterile dressing to open wounds. After assessing the patient, splint a suspected pelvic injury by tying the patient's legs together with a pillow between them. Try not to move the patient.
- Give analgesics for pain. Usually, narcotics aren't recommended; if the pain is severe, however, give narcotics in titrated I.V. doses.
- If necessary, give tetanus prophylaxis and prophylactic I.V. antibiotics.
- Prepare the patient for surgery. Remove the patient's dentures. Type and crossmatch blood. Get a consent form signed by the patient or a responsible relative.

➤ CLINICAL TIP A consent form is necessary unless surgery must be performed immediately to save the patient's life.

- If the injury was caused by a motor vehicle accident, find out whether the police were notified and, if not, notify them. If the patient suffered a gunshot or stab wound, notify the police, place all his clothes in a bag, and retain them for the police. Document the number and sites of the wounds. Contact the patient's family and offer them reassurance.

# ABORTION

Abortion is the spontaneous or induced (therapeutic) expulsion of the products of conception from the uterus before fetal viability (fetal weight < 500 g [17⅝ oz] or gestation < 20 weeks). Up to 15% of all pregnancies and approximately 30% of all first pregnancies end in spontaneous abortion (miscarriage). At least 75% of miscarriages occur during the first trimester.

### Causes

*Spontaneous abortion* may result from fetal, placental, or maternal factors. (See *Types of spontaneous abortion.*) Fetal factors, which usually cause such abortions between the 9th and 12th week of gestation, include the following:

• defective embryologic development resulting from abnormal chromosome division (most common cause of fetal death)

• faulty implantation of the fertilized ovum

• failure of the endometrium to accept the fertilized ovum.

Placental factors usually cause abortion around the 14th week of gestation, when the placenta takes over the hormone production necessary to maintain the pregnancy. These factors include:

• premature separation of the normally implanted placenta

• abnormal placental implantation.

Maternal factors usually cause abortion between the 11th and 19th week of gestation and include:

• maternal infection, severe malnutrition, and abnormalities of the repro-

---

## TYPES OF SPONTANEOUS ABORTION

• *Threatened abortion:* Bloody vaginal discharge occurs during the first half of pregnancy. Approximately 20% of pregnant women have vaginal spotting or actual bleeding early in pregnancy; of these, about 50% abort.

• *Inevitable abortion:* Membranes rupture and the cervix dilates. As labor continues, the uterus expels the products of conception.

• *Incomplete abortion:* Uterus retains part or all of the placenta. Before the 10th week of gestation, the fetus and placenta usually are expelled together; after the 10th week, separately. Because part of the placenta may adhere to the uterine wall, bleeding continues. Hemorrhage is possible because the uterus doesn't contract and seal the large vessels that fed the placenta.

• *Complete abortion:* Uterus passes all the products of conception. Minimal bleeding usually accompanies complete abortion because the uterus contracts and compresses maternal blood vessels that fed the placenta.

• *Missed abortion:* Uterus retains the products of conception for 2 months or more after the death of the fetus. Uterine growth ceases; uterine size may even seem to decrease. Prolonged retention of the dead products of conception may cause coagulation defects, such as disseminated intravascular coagulation.

• *Habitual abortion:* Spontaneous loss of three or more consecutive pregnancies constitutes habitual abortion.

• *Septic abortion:* Infection accompanies abortion. This may occur with spontaneous abortion but usually results from an illegal abortion.

ductive organs (especially an incompetent cervix, in which the cervix dilates painlessly and bloodlessly in the second trimester)

• endocrine problems, such as thyroid dysfunction or a luteal phase defect

• trauma, including any surgery that requires manipulation of the pelvic organs

• phospholipid antibody disorder

• blood group incompatibility

• drug ingestion.

The goal of *therapeutic abortion* is to preserve the mother's mental or physical health in cases of rape, unplanned pregnancy, or medical conditions, such as moderate or severe cardiac dysfunction.

### Signs and symptoms

Prodromal signs of spontaneous abortion may include a pink discharge for several days or a scant brown discharge for several weeks before the onset of cramps and increased vaginal bleeding. For a few hours, the cramps intensify and occur more frequently; then the cervix dilates to expel uterine contents. If the entire contents are expelled, cramps and bleeding subside. However, if any contents remain, cramps and bleeding continue.

### Diagnosis

Diagnosis of spontaneous abortion is based on clinical evidence of expulsion of uterine contents, pelvic examination, and laboratory studies. Human chorionic gonadotropin (HCG) in the blood or urine confirms pregnancy; decreased HCG levels suggest spontaneous abortion.

➤ CLINICAL TIP   Spontaneous abortion may result from a decrease in serum progesterone. Levels should be checked every 7 to 10 days. HCG levels should be checked every 48 hours and should be double in comparison with the previous level.

Pelvic examination determines the size of the uterus and whether this size is consistent with the length of the pregnancy. Tissue cytology indicates evidence of products of conception. Laboratory tests reflect decreased hemoglobin levels and hematocrit due to blood loss.

### Treatment

An accurate evaluation of uterine contents is necessary before a plan of treatment can be formulated. The progression of spontaneous abortion can't be prevented, except in cases caused by an incompetent cervix. The patient must be hospitalized to control severe hemorrhage. If bleeding is severe, a transfusion with packed red blood cells or whole blood is required. Initially, I.V. administration of oxytocin stimulates uterine contractions. If any remnants remain in the uterus, dilatation and curettage or dilatation and evacuation (D&E) should be performed.

D&E is also performed in first- and second-trimester therapeutic abortions. In second-trimester therapeutic abortions, the insertion of a prostaglandin vaginal suppository induces labor and the expulsion of uterine contents.

After an abortion, spontaneous or induced, an Rh-negative female with a negative indirect Coombs' test should receive $Rh_o(D)$ immune globulin (human) to prevent further Rh isoimmunization.

In a habitual aborter, spontaneous abortion can result from an incompetent cervix. Treatment involves surgical reinforcement of the cervix (McDonald or Shirodkar-Barter procedure) 12 to 14 weeks after the last menses. A few weeks before the estimated delivery date, the sutures are removed and the patient awaits the onset of labor. An alternative procedure, especially for the woman who wants to have more children, is to leave the sutures in place and to deliver the infant by cesarean section.

### Special considerations

Before possible abortion:
- Explain all procedures thoroughly.
- The patient should *not* have bathroom privileges because she may expel uterine contents without knowing it. After she uses the bedpan, inspect the contents carefully for intrauterine material.

After spontaneous or elective abortion:
- Note the amount, color, and odor of vaginal bleeding. Save all the pads the patient uses, for evaluation.
- Administer oxytocin and analgesics, as ordered.
- Give good perineal care.
- Obtain vital signs every 4 hours for 24 hours.
- Monitor urine output.

Care of the patient who has had a spontaneous abortion includes emotional support and counseling during the grieving process. Encourage the patient and her partner to express their feelings. Some couples may want to talk to a member of the clergy or, depending on their religion, may wish to have the fetus baptized.

The patient who has had a therapeutic abortion also benefits from support. Encourage her to verbalize her feelings. Remember, she may feel ambivalent about the procedure; intellectual and emotional acceptance of abortion aren't the same. Refer her for counseling if necessary.

To prepare the patient for discharge:
- Tell the patient to expect vaginal bleeding or spotting and to report excessive bright-red blood immediately or any bleeding that lasts longer than 10 days.
- Advise the patient to watch for signs of infection, such as a temperature high-er than 100.5° F (38° C) and foul-smelling vaginal discharge.
- Encourage the gradual increase of daily activities to include whatever tasks the patient feels comfortable doing, as long as these activities don't increase vaginal bleeding or cause fatigue. Most patients return to work within 1 to 4 weeks.
- Urge 1 to 2 weeks' abstinence from intercourse, and encourage use of a contraceptive when intercourse is resumed.
- Instruct the patient to avoid using tampons for 1 to 2 weeks.
- Be sure to inform the patient who desires an elective abortion of all the available alternatives. She needs to know what the procedure involves, what the risks are, and what to expect during and after the procedure, both emotionally and physically. Be sure to ascertain whether the patient is comfortable with her decision to have an elective abortion. Encourage her to verbalize her thoughts both when the procedure is performed and at a follow-up visit, usually 2 weeks later. If you identify an inappropriate coping response, refer the patient for professional counseling.
- To help prevent elective abortion, medical and nursing personnel need to make contraceptive information available. An educated population motivated to utilize contraception would have little need for elective abortion.
- Tell the patient to see her doctor in 2 to 4 weeks for a follow-up examination.

To minimize the risk of future spontaneous abortions, emphasize to the pregnant woman the importance of good nutrition and the need to avoid alcohol, cigarettes, and drugs. Most clinicians recommend that the couple wait two or three normal menstrual cycles after a spontaneous abortion has occurred before attempting conception. If the patient has a history of spontaneous abortions, suggest that she and her partner

## DEGREES OF PLACENTAL SEPARATION IN ABRUPTIO PLACENTAE

Mild separation with internal bleeding between placenta and uterine wall

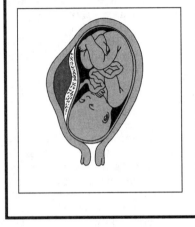

Moderate separation with external hemorrhage through the vagina

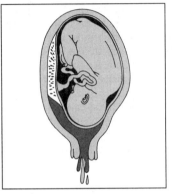

have thorough examinations. For the woman, this includes premenstrual endometrial biopsy, a hormone assessment (estrogen, progesterone, and thyroid, follicle-stimulating, and luteinizing hormones), and hysterosalpingography and laparoscopy to detect anatomic abnormalities. Genetic counseling may also be indicated.

# ABRUPTIO PLACENTAE

In abruptio placentae, also called placental abruption, the placenta separates from the uterine wall prematurely, usually after the 20th week of gestation, producing hemorrhage. Abruptio placentae occurs most often in multigravidas — usually in women over age 35 — and is a common cause of bleeding during the second half of pregnancy. Fetal prognosis depends on gestational age and amount of blood lost; maternal prognosis is good if hemorrhage can be controlled.

## Causes
The cause of abruptio placentae is unknown. Predisposing factors include trauma (such as a direct blow to the uterus resulting from abuse or accidental trauma), placental site bleeding from a needle puncture during amniocentesis, chronic or pregnancy-induced hypertension (which raises pressure on the maternal side of the placenta), multiparity more than 5, short umbilical cord, dietary deficiency, smoking, advanced maternal age, and pressure on the vena cava from an enlarged uterus.

In abruptio placentae, blood vessels at the placental bed rupture spontaneously owing to a lack of resiliency or to abnormal changes in uterine vasculature. Hypertension complicates the

Severe separation

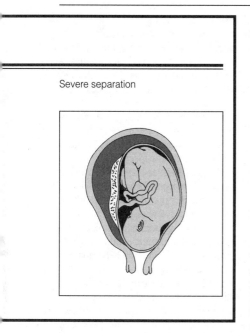

situation, as does an enlarged uterus, which can't contract sufficiently to seal off the torn vessels. Consequently, bleeding continues unchecked, possibly shearing off the placenta partially or completely. Typically, such bleeding is external or marginal (in about 80% of patients) if a peripheral portion of the placenta separates from the uterine wall; it's internal or concealed (in about 20% of patients) if the central portion of the placenta becomes detached and the still-intact peripheral portions trap the blood. As blood enters the muscle fibers, complete relaxation of the uterus becomes impossible, increasing uterine tone and irritability. If bleeding into the muscle fibers is profuse, the uterus turns blue or purple and the accumulated blood prevents its normal contractions after delivery (Couvelaire uterus, or utero-placental apoplexy).

## Signs and symptoms

Abruptio placentae produces a wide range of clinical effects, depending on the extent of placental separation and the amount of blood lost from maternal circulation. (See *Degrees of placental separation in abruptio placentae.*) Mild abruptio placentae (marginal separation) develops gradually and produces mild to moderate bleeding, vague lower abdominal discomfort, mild to moderate abdominal tenderness, and uterine irritability. Fetal heart tones remain strong and regular.

Moderate abruptio placentae (about 50% placental separation) may develop gradually or abruptly and produces continuous abdominal pain, moderate dark red vaginal bleeding, a tender uterus that remains firm between contractions, barely audible or irregular and bradycardic fetal heart tones and, possibly, signs of shock. Labor usually starts within 2 hours and often proceeds rapidly.

Severe abruptio placentae (70% placental separation) develops abruptly and causes agonizing, unremitting uterine pain (described as tearing or stabbing); a boardlike, tender uterus; moderate vaginal bleeding; rapidly progressive shock; and absence of fetal heart tones.

In addition to hemorrhage and shock, complications of abruptio placentae may include renal failure, disseminated intravascular coagulation (DIC), and maternal and fetal death.

## Diagnosis

Diagnostic measures for abruptio placentae include observations of clinical features, pelvic examination (under double setup), and ultrasonography to rule out placenta previa.

➤ CLINICAL TIP  Draw a line at the level of the fundus and check it every 30 minutes. If the level of the fundus increases, suspect abruptio placentae.

Decreased hemoglobin (Hb) levels and platelet counts support the diagnosis. Periodic assays for fibrin split products aid in monitoring the progression of abruptio placentae and detecting the development of DIC.

### Treatment

Treatment of abruptio placentae is designed to assess, control, and restore the amount of blood lost; to deliver a viable infant; and to prevent coagulation disorders. Immediate measures for abruptio placentae include starting I.V. infusion (via a large-bore catheter) of appropriate fluids (lactated Ringer's solution) to combat hypovolemia; placing a central venous line and urinary catheter to monitor fluid status; drawing a blood sample for Hb level and hematocrit determination, coagulation studies, and typing and crossmatching; initiating external electronic fetal monitoring; and monitoring maternal vital signs and vaginal bleeding.

After determination of the severity of abruption and appropriate fluid and blood replacement, prompt delivery by cesarean section is necessary if the fetus is in distress. If the fetus isn't in distress, monitoring continues; delivery is usually performed at the first sign of fetal distress. Because of possible fetal blood loss through the placenta, a pediatric team should be ready at delivery to assess and treat the newborn for shock, blood loss, and hypoxia. If placental separation is severe and there are no signs of fetal life, vaginal delivery may be performed unless uncontrolled hemorrhage or other complications contraindicate it.

Complications of abruptio placentae require appropriate treatment. For example, DIC requires immediate intervention with heparin, platelets, and whole blood to prevent exsanguination.

### Special considerations

● Check maternal blood pressure, pulse rate, respirations, central venous pressure, intake and output, and amount of vaginal bleeding every 10 to 15 minutes. Monitor fetal heart tones electronically.

● Prepare the patient and family for cesarean section. Thoroughly explain postpartum care so the patient and her family know what to expect.

● If vaginal delivery is elected, provide emotional support during labor. Because of the infant's prematurity, the mother may not receive analgesics during labor and may experience intense pain. Reassure the patient of her progress through labor, and keep her informed of the fetus's condition.

● Tactfully suggest the possibility of neonatal death. Tell the mother the infant's survival depends primarily on gestational age, blood loss, and associated hypertensive disorders. Assure her that frequent monitoring and prompt management greatly reduce the risk of fatality.

# ACHILLES TENDON CONTRACTURE

Achilles tendon contracture is a shortening of the Achilles tendon (tendon calcaneus or heel cord), which causes foot pain and strain, with limited ankle dorsiflexion.

### Causes

Achilles tendon contracture may reflect a congenital structural anomaly or a muscular reaction to chronic poor posture, especially in women who wear high-heeled shoes and joggers who land on the balls of their feet instead of their heels. Other causes include paralytic conditions of the legs, such as poliomyelitis and cerebral palsy.

### Signs and symptoms

Sharp, spasmodic pain during dorsiflexion of the foot characterizes the reflex type of Achilles tendon contracture. In footdrop (fixed equinus), contracture of the flexor foot muscle prevents placing the heel on the ground.

### Diagnosis

Physical examination and patient history suggest Achilles tendon contracture. A simple test confirms the condition: While the patient keeps his knee flexed, the examiner places the foot in dorsiflexion; gradual knee extension forces the foot into plantar flexion.

### Treatment

Achilles tendon contracture is treated conservatively by raising the inside heel of the shoe (in the reflex type); gradually lowering the heels of shoes (sudden lowering can aggravate the problem), and stretching exercises, if the cause is high heels; or using support braces or casting to prevent footdrop in a paralyzed patient. Alternative therapy includes using wedged plaster casts or stretching the tendon by manipulation. Analgesics may be given to relieve pain.

With fixed footdrop, treatment may include surgery (tenotomy), although this procedure may weaken the tendon. Tenotomy allows further stretching by cutting the tendon. After surgery, a short leg cast maintains the foot in 90-degree dorsiflexion for 6 weeks. Some surgeons allow partial weight bearing on a walking cast after 2 weeks.

### Special considerations

• After surgery to lengthen the Achilles tendon, elevate the casted foot to decrease venous pressure and edema by raising the foot of the bed or supporting the foot with pillows.

• Record the neurovascular status of the toes (temperature, color, sensation, capillary refill time, toe mobility) every hour for the first 24 hours, then every 4 hours. If any changes are detected, increase the elevation of the patient's leg and notify the surgeon immediately.

• Prepare the patient for ambulation by having him dangle his foot over the side of the bed for short periods (5 to 15 minutes) before he gets out of bed, allowing for gradual increase of venous pressure.

• Assist the patient in walking (usually within 24 hours of surgery), using crutches and a non-weight-bearing or touch-down gait.

• Protect the patient's skin with moleskin or by "petaling" the edges of the cast.

• Before discharge, teach the patient how to care for the cast, and advise him to elevate his foot regularly when sitting or whenever the foot throbs or becomes edematous.

• Make sure the patient understands how much exercise and walking are recommended after discharge.

➤ CLINICAL TIP To prevent Achilles tendon contracture in paralyzed patients, apply support braces, universal splints, casts, or high-topped sneakers. Make sure the weight of the sheets doesn't keep paralyzed feet in plantar flexion.

• For patients who aren't paralyzed, teach good foot care, and urge them to seek immediate medical care for foot problems. Warn women against wearing high heels constantly, and suggest regular foot (dorsiflexion) exercises.

# ACNE VULGARIS

An inflammatory disease of the sebaceous follicles, acne vulgaris primarily affects adolescents, although lesions can appear as early as age 8. Although acne strikes boys more often and more severely than girls, it usually occurs in girls at an earlier age and tends to last longer, sometimes into adulthood. The prognosis is good with treatment.

## Causes

Many factors may promote acne, but theories regarding dietary influences appear to be groundless. Research now centers on follicular occlusion, androgen-stimulated sebum production, and *Propionibacterium acnes* as possible primary causes.

Predisposing factors include heredity; oral contraceptives (many females experience an acne flare-up during their first few menses after starting or discontinuing oral contraceptives); androgen stimulation; certain drugs, including corticosteroids, corticotropin, androgens, iodides, bromides, trimethadione, phenytoin, isoniazid, lithium, and halothane; cobalt irradiation; and hyperalimentation.

Other precipitating factors include exposure to heavy oils, greases, or tars; trauma or rubbing from tight clothing; cosmetics; emotional stress; and unfavorable climate.

More is known about the pathogenesis of acne. Androgens stimulate sebaceous gland growth and production of sebum, which is secreted into dilated hair follicles that contain bacteria. The bacteria, usually *P. acnes* and *Staphylococcus epidermidis* — which are normal skin flora — secrete lipase. This enzyme interacts with sebum to produce free fatty acids, which provoke inflammation. Also, the hair follicles produce more keratin, which joins with the sebum to form a plug in the dilated follicle.

## Signs and symptoms

The acne plug may appear as a closed comedo, or whitehead (if it doesn't protrude from the follicle and is covered by the epidermis), or as an open comedo, or blackhead (if it does protrude and isn't covered by the epidermis). The black coloration is caused by the melanin or pigment of the follicle.

Rupture or leakage of an enlarged plug into the dermis produces inflammation and characteristic acne pustules, papules or, in severe forms, cysts or abscesses. Chronic, recurring lesions produce acne scars.

## Diagnosis

The appearance of characteristic acne lesions, especially in an adolescent patient, confirms the presence of acne vulgaris.

## Treatment

Commonly, acne is treated topically with benzoyl peroxide, clindamycin, or erythromycin antibacterial agents, alone or in combination with tretinoin (retinoic acid), a keratolytic. Benzoyl peroxide and tretinoin agents may irritate the skin.

Systemic therapy consists primarily of antibiotics, usually tetracycline, to decrease bacterial growth until the patient is in remission; then a lower dose is used for long-term maintenance. Tetracycline is contraindicated during pregnancy and childhood because it discolors developing teeth. Erythromycin is an alternative for these patients. Exacerbation of pustules or abscesses during either type of antibiotic therapy requires a culture to identify a possible secondary bacterial infection.

Oral isotretinoin combats acne by inhibiting sebaceous gland function and abnormal keratinization. Because of its severe adverse effects, the 16- to 20-week course of isotretinoin is limited to those with severe papulopustular or cystic acne who don't respond to conventional therapy. (See *Risks of isotretinoin therapy*.)

Females may benefit from taking birth control pills (such as Ortho Tri-Cyclen) or spironolactone because these drugs produce antiandrogenic effects.

Other treatments for acne vulgaris include intralesional corticosteroid injections, exposure to ultraviolet light (but never when a photosensitizing agent, such as tretinoin, is being used), cryotherapy, and acne surgery.

**Special considerations**
- Check the patient's drug history because certain medications, such as some oral contraceptives, may cause an acne flare-up.
- Try to identify predisposing factors that may be eliminated or modified.
- Explain the causes of acne to the patient and his family. Make sure they understand that the prescribed treatment is more likely to improve acne than a strict diet and fanatic scrubbing with soap and water. Provide written instructions regarding treatment.
- Instruct the patient receiving tretinoin to apply it at least 30 minutes after washing the face and at least 1 hour before bedtime. Warn against using it around the eyes or lips. After treatments, the skin should look pink and dry. If it appears red or starts to peel, the preparation may have to be weakened or applied less often.
- Advise the patient to avoid exposure to sunlight or to use a sunscreen. If the prescribed regimen includes tretinoin and benzoyl peroxide, avoid skin irritation by using one preparation in the morning and the other at night.

> **CLINICAL TIP**
>
> ## RISKS OF ISOTRETINOIN THERAPY
>
> Because isotretinoin is known to cause birth defects, the manufacturer, with approval of the Food and Drug Administration, recommends the following precautions:
>
> - pregnancy testing before dispensing
> - dispensing only a 30-day supply
> - repeat pregnancy testing throughout the treatment period
> - effective contraception during treatment
> - informed consent of the patient or parents regarding the drug's adverse effects.

- Instruct the patient to take tetracycline on an empty stomach and not to take it with antacids or milk because it interacts with their metallic ions and is then poorly absorbed.
- Tell the patient who is taking isotretinoin to avoid vitamin A supplements, which can worsen any adverse effects. Also discuss how to deal with the dry skin and mucous membranes that usually occur during treatment. Warn the female patient about the severe risk of teratogenesis. Monitor liver function and lipid levels.
- Inform the patient that acne takes a long time to clear—even years for complete resolution. Encourage continued local skin care even after acne clears. Explain the adverse effects of all drugs.
- Pay special attention to the patient's perception of his physical appearance, and offer emotional support.

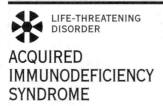

LIFE-THREATENING
DISORDER

# ACQUIRED IMMUNODEFICIENCY SYNDROME

Currently one of the most widely publicized diseases, acquired immunodeficiency syndrome (AIDS) is marked by progressive failure of the immune system. Although it's characterized by gradual destruction of cell-mediated (T-cell) immunity, it also affects humoral immunity and even autoimmunity because of the central role of the CD4$^+$ T lymphocyte in immune reactions. The resultant immunodeficiency makes the patient susceptible to opportunistic infections, unusual cancers, and other abnormalities that define AIDS.

This syndrome was first described by the Centers for Disease Control and Prevention (CDC) in 1981. Since then, the CDC has declared a case surveillance definition for AIDS and has modified it several times, most recently in 1993.

A retrovirus — the human immunodeficiency virus (HIV) type I — is the primary causative agent. Transmission of HIV occurs by contact with infected blood or body fluids and is associated with identifiable high-risk behaviors. It's therefore disproportionately represented in homosexual and bisexual men, I.V. drug users, neonates of HIV-infected women, recipients of contaminated blood or blood products (dramatically decreased since mid-1985), and heterosexual partners of persons in the former groups. Because of similar routes of transmission, AIDS shares epidemiologic patterns with hepatitis B and sexually transmitted diseases (STDs).

The natural history of AIDS infection begins with infection by the HIV retrovirus, which is detectable only by laboratory tests, and ends with the severely immunocompromised, terminal stage of this disease. Depending on individual variations and the presence of cofactors that influence progression, the time elapsed from acute HIV infection to the appearance of symptoms (mild to severe) to the diagnosis of AIDS and, eventually, to death varies greatly. Current combination antiretroviral therapy (for example, with zidovudine, ritonavir, and others) and treatment and prophylaxis of common opportunistic infections can delay the natural progression of HIV disease and prolong survival.

**Causes**
AIDS results from infection with HIV, which strikes cells bearing the CD4$^+$ antigen; the latter (normally a receptor for major histocompatibility complex molecules) serves as a receptor for the retrovirus and lets it enter the cell. HIV prefers to infect the CD4$^+$ lymphocyte or macrophage but may also infect other CD4$^+$ antigen-bearing cells of the GI tract, uterine cervical cells, and neuroglial cells. The virus gains access by binding to the CD4$^+$ molecule on the cell surface along with a coreceptor (thought to be the receptor CCR5). After invading a cell, HIV replicates, leading to cell death, or becomes latent. HIV infection leads to profound pathology, either directly, through destruction of CD4$^+$ cells, other immune cells, and neuroglial cells, or indirectly, through the secondary effects of CD4$^+$ T-cell dysfunction and resultant immunosuppression.

The infection process takes three forms:

• immunodeficiency (opportunistic infections and unusual cancers)

• autoimmunity (lymphoid interstitial pneumonia, arthritis, hypergamma-globulinemia, and production of autoimmune antibodies)

• neurologic dysfunction (AIDS dementia complex, HIV encephalopathy, and peripheral neuropathies).

### Transmission
HIV is transmitted by direct inoculation during intimate sexual contact, especially associated with the mucosal trauma of receptive rectal intercourse; transfusion of contaminated blood or blood products (a risk diminished by routine testing of all blood products); sharing of contaminated needles; or transplacental or postpartum transmission from an infected mother to the fetus (by cervical or blood contact at delivery and in breast milk).

Accumulating evidence suggests that HIV isn't transmitted by casual household or social contact. The average time between exposure to the virus and diagnosis of AIDS is 8 to 10 years, but shorter and longer incubation times have also been recorded.

### Signs and symptoms
HIV infection manifests itself in many ways.

> CLINICAL TIP After a high-risk exposure and inoculation, the infected person usually experiences a mononucleosis-like syndrome, which may be attributed to the flu or another virus, and then may remain asymptomatic for years. In this latent stage, the only sign of HIV infection is laboratory evidence of seroconversion.

When symptoms appear, they may take many forms:

• persistent generalized adenopathy

• nonspecific symptoms (weight loss, fatigue, night sweats, fevers)

• neurologic symptoms resulting from HIV encephalopathy

• opportunistic infection or cancer.

The clinical course varies slightly in children with AIDS. Apparently, their incubation time is shorter with a mean of 17 months. Signs and symptoms resemble those in adults, except for findings related to STDs. Children show virtually all of the opportunistic infections observed in adults, with a higher incidence of bacterial infections: otitis media, sepsis, chronic salivary gland enlargement, *Mycobacterium avium* complex function, and pneumonias, including *Pneumocystis carinii* and lymphoid interstitial pneumonias.

### Diagnosis
The CDC defines AIDS as an illness characterized by one or more "indicator" diseases coexisting with laboratory evidence of HIV infection and other possible causes of immunosuppression. The CDC's current AIDS surveillance case definition requires laboratory confirmation of HIV infection in people who have a $CD4^+$ T-cell count of 200 cells/$\mu$l or who have an associated clinical condition or disease.

### Antibody tests
The most commonly performed tests, antibody tests indicate HIV infection indirectly by revealing HIV antibodies. The recommended protocol requires initial screening of individuals and blood products with an enzyme-linked immunosorbent assay (ELISA). A positive ELISA should be repeated and then confirmed by an alternate method, usually the Western blot or an immunofluorescence assay. However, antibody testing isn't always reliable. Because the body takes a variable amount of time to produce a detectable level of antibodies, a "window" varying from a few weeks to as long as 35 months in one documented case allows an HIV-infected

person to test negative for HIV antibodies.

Antibody tests are also unreliable in neonates because transferred maternal antibodies persist for 6 to 10 months. To overcome these problems, direct testing is performed to detect HIV. Direct tests include antigen tests (p24 antigen), HIV cultures, nucleic acid probes of peripheral blood lymphocytes with determination of HIV-1 ribonucleic acid levels, and the polymerase chain reaction.

### Other tests

Additional tests to support the diagnosis and help evaluate the severity of immunosuppression include CD4$^+$ and CD8$^+$ T-lymphocyte subset counts, erythrocyte sedimentation rate, complete blood count, serum beta$_2$-microglobulin, p24 antigen, neopterin levels, and anergy testing. Because many opportunistic infections in AIDS patients are reactivations of previous infections, patients are also tested for syphilis, hepatitis B, tuberculosis, toxoplasmosis and, in some areas, histoplasmosis.

### Treatment

No cure has yet been found for AIDS; however, primary therapy for HIV infection includes three different types of antiretroviral agents:
• protease inhibitors (PIs), such as ritonavir, indinavir, nelfinavir, and saquinavir
• nucleoside reverse transcriptase inhibitors (NRTIs), such as zidovudine, didanosine, zalcitabine, lamivudine, and stavudine
• nonnucleoside reverse transcriptase inhibitors (NNRTIs), such as nevirapine and delavirdine.

These agents, used in various combinations, are designed to inhibit HIV viral replication. Other potential therapies include immunomodulatory agents designed to boost the weakened immune system and anti-infective and antineoplastic agents to combat opportunistic infections and associated cancers; some are used prophylactically to help patients resist opportunistic infections.

Current treatment protocols combine three agents in an effort to gain the maximum benefit with the fewest adverse reactions. Such regimens include one PI and are considered the most effective treatment. Many variations and drug interactions are under study. Combination therapy helps inhibit the production of resistant, mutant strains. Supportive treatments help maintain nutritional status and relieve pain and other distressing physical and psychological symptoms.

Many pathogens in AIDS respond to anti-infective drugs but tend to recur after treatment ends. For this reason, most patients need continuous anti-infective treatment, presumably for life or until the drug is no longer tolerated or effective.

### Zidovudine

Treatment with zidovudine has proved effective in slowing the progression of HIV infection, decreasing opportunistic infections, and prolonging survival. However, it often produces serious adverse reactions and toxicities. The drug is often combined with other agents (such as lamivudine) but has also been used as a single agent for pregnant HIV-positive women.

The current recommendation is to take 100 mg every 4 hours for a total daily dose of 600 mg, or 500 mg if the patient doesn't want to interrupt sleep. Other NRTIs, such as didanosine and zalcitabine, may also be used in combination regimens for patients who can't tolerate or no longer respond to zidovudine.

## Special considerations

● Health care workers and the public are advised to use precautions in all situations that risk exposure to blood, body fluids, and secretions. Diligently practicing standard precautions can prevent the inadvertent transmission of AIDS, hepatitis B, and other infectious diseases that are transmitted by similar routes.

> **CLINICAL TIP** Combination antiretroviral therapy aims to maximally suppress HIV replication, thereby improving survival. However, poor drug compliance may lead to resistance and treatment failure. Patients must understand that medication regimens must be followed closely and may be required for many years, if not throughout life.

● Recognize that a diagnosis of AIDS is profoundly distressing because of the disease's social impact and the discouraging prognosis. The patient may lose his job and financial security as well as the support of family and friends. Coping with an altered body image, the emotional burden of serious illness, and the threat of death may overwhelm the patient.

# ACROMEGALY AND GIGANTISM

Chronic, progressive diseases, acromegaly and gigantism are marked by hormonal dysfunction and startling skeletal overgrowth. Acromegaly occurs after epiphyseal closure, causing bone thickening and transverse growth and visceromegaly. Gigantism begins before epiphyseal closure and causes proportional overgrowth of all body tissues. Although the prognosis depends on the causative factor, these disorders usually reduce life expectancy unless treated in a timely way.

## Causes

Typically, oversecretion of human growth hormone (HGH) produces changes throughout the entire body, resulting in acromegaly and, when oversecretion occurs before puberty, gigantism. Eosinophilic or mixed-cell adenomas of the anterior pituitary gland may cause this oversecretion, but the cause of the tumors themselves remains unclear. Rarely, HGH levels are elevated in more than one family member, which suggests the possibility of a genetic cause.

The earliest clinical sign of acromegaly is soft-tissue swelling of the extremities, which causes coarsening of the facial features. This rare form of hyperpituitarism occurs equally among men and women, usually between ages 30 and 50.

In gigantism, proportional overgrowth of all body tissues starts before epiphyseal closure. This causes remarkable height increases of as much as 6″ (15 cm) a year. Gigantism affects infants and children, causing them to attain as much as three times the normal height for their age. As adults, they may ultimately reach a height of more than 80″ (203 cm).

## Signs and symptoms

Acromegaly develops slowly, whereas gigantism develops abruptly.

### Acromegaly

Acromegaly typically produces diaphoresis, oily skin, hypermetabolism, and hypertrichosis. Severe headache, central nervous system impairment, bitemporal hemianopia, loss of visual acuity, and blindness may result from the intrasellar tumor compressing the optic chiasm or nerves.

Hypersecretion of HGH produces cartilaginous and connective tissue overgrowth, resulting in a characteristic hulking appearance, with an enlarged supraorbital ridge and thickened ears and nose. Prognathism, projection of the jaw, becomes marked and may interfere with chewing. Laryngeal hypertrophy, paranasal sinus enlargement, and thickening of the tongue cause the voice to sound deep and hollow. Distal phalanges display an arrowhead appearance on X-rays, and the fingers are thickened. Irritability, hostility, and various psychological disturbances may occur.

Prolonged effects of excessive HGH secretion include bowlegs, barrel chest, arthritis, osteoporosis, kyphosis, hypertension, and arteriosclerosis. Both gigantism and acromegaly may also cause signs of glucose intolerance and clinically apparent diabetes mellitus because of the insulin-antagonistic character of HGH.

### *Gigantism*
Gigantism produces some of the same skeletal abnormalities seen in acromegaly. As the disease progresses, the pituitary tumor enlarges and invades normal tissue, resulting in the loss of other trophic hormones, such as thyroid-stimulating hormone, luteinizing hormone, follicle-stimulating hormone, and corticotropin, thus causing the target organ to stop functioning.

### Diagnosis
Plasma HGH levels measured by radioimmunoassay typically are elevated. However, because HGH secretion is pulsatile, the results of random sampling may be misleading. IGF-1 (somatomedin-C) levels offer a better screening alternative.

The glucose suppression test offers more reliable information. Glucose normally suppresses HGH secretion; therefore, a glucose infusion that doesn't suppress the hormone level to below the accepted normal value of 2 ng/ml, when combined with characteristic clinical features, strongly suggests hyperpituitarism.

In addition, skull X-rays, a computed tomography scan, arteriography, and magnetic resonance imaging determine the presence and extent of the pituitary lesion. Bone X-rays showing a thickening of the cranium (especially of frontal, occipital, and parietal bones) and of the long bones as well as osteoarthritis in the spine support this diagnosis.

### Treatment
Overproduction of HGH is curbed through removal of the underlying tumor by cranial or transsphenoidal hypophysectomy or pituitary radiation therapy. In acromegaly, surgery is mandatory when a tumor causes blindness or other severe neurologic disturbances.

Postoperative therapy often requires replacement of thyroid and gonadal hormones and cortisone. Adjunctive treatment may include administration of bromocriptine and octreotide, which inhibit HGH synthesis.

### Special considerations
• Grotesque body changes characteristic of this disorder can cause severe psychological stress. Provide emotional support to help the patient cope with an altered body image.
• Examine the patient for skeletal manifestations, such as arthritis of the hands and osteoarthritis of the spine. Administer prescribed medications. To promote maximum joint mobility, perform or assist with range-of-motion exercises.

• Evaluate muscle weakness, especially in the patient with late-stage acromegaly. Check the strength of his handclasp. If it's very weak, help with tasks such as cutting food.

• Keep the skin dry. Avoid using an oily lotion because the skin is already oily.

• Monitor serum glucose levels. Check for signs of hyperglycemia (fatigue, polyuria, polydipsia).

• Be aware that the tumor may cause visual problems. If the patient has hemianopia, stand where he can see you.

• Keep in mind that this disease can also cause inexplicable mood changes. Reassure the family that these mood changes result from the disease and can be modified with treatment.

• Before surgery, reinforce what the surgeon has told the patient, if possible, and try to allay the patient's fear with a clear and honest explanation of the scheduled operation. If the patient is a child, explain to his parents that such surgery prevents permanent soft-tissue deformities but won't correct bone changes that have already taken place. Arrange for counseling, if necessary, to help the child and parents cope with these permanent defects.

• After surgery, diligently monitor vital signs and neurologic status. Be alert for any alteration in level of consciousness, pupil equality, or visual acuity as well as vomiting, falling pulse rate, or rising blood pressure. These changes may signal an increase in intracranial pressure due to intracranial bleeding or cerebral edema.

• Check blood glucose levels often. Remember, HGH levels usually fall rapidly after surgery, removing an insulin antagonist effect in many patients and possibly precipitating hypoglycemia.

• Measure intake and output hourly, and watch for large increases. Transient diabetes insipidus, which sometimes occurs after surgery for hyperpituitarism, can cause such increases in urine output.

• If the transsphenoidal approach is used, a large nasal pack is kept in place for several days. Because the patient must breathe through his mouth, give good mouth care.

• Pay special attention to the mucous membranes — which usually become very dry — and the incision site under the upper lip, at the top of the gum line.

• The surgical site is packed with a piece of tissue generally taken from a mid-thigh donor site. Watch for cerebrospinal fluid (CSF) leaks from the packed site. Look for increased external nasal drainage or drainage into the nasopharynx. CSF leaks may necessitate additional surgery to repair the leak.

• Encourage the patient to ambulate on the 1st or 2nd day after surgery.

• If necessary, before the patient is discharged, emphasize the importance of continuing hormone replacement therapy. Make sure the patient and his family understand which hormones are to be taken and why as well as the correct times and doses. Warn against stopping the hormones suddenly.

• Advise the patient to wear a medical identification bracelet at all times and to bring his hormone replacement schedule with him whenever he returns to the facility.

• Instruct the patient to have follow-up checkups for the rest of his life because there's a slight chance that the tumor that caused his condition could recur.

➤ CLINICAL TIP   A patient with acromegaly should be periodically screened for colon polyps because the incidence of polyps increases with chronic elevated HGH levels.

**LIFE-THREATENING DISORDER**

# ACUTE RESPIRATORY FAILURE IN C.O.P.D.

In patients with essentially normal lung tissue, acute respiratory failure (ARF) usually means a partial pressure of arterial carbon dioxide ($Paco_2$) greater than 50 mm Hg and a partial pressure of arterial oxygen ($Pao_2$) less than 50 mm Hg. These limits, however, don't apply to patients with chronic obstructive pulmonary disease (COPD), who often have a consistently high $Paco_2$ and low $Pao_2$. In patients with COPD, only acute deterioration in arterial blood gas (ABG) values, with corresponding clinical deterioration, indicates ARF.

## Causes

ARF may develop in COPD patients from any condition that increases the work of breathing and decreases the respiratory drive. Such conditions include respiratory tract infection (such as bronchitis or pneumonia) — the most common precipitating factor — bronchospasm, or accumulating secretions secondary to cough suppression. Other causes of ARF in COPD include:

• *central nervous system (CNS) depression* — head trauma or injudicious use of sedatives, narcotics, tranquilizers, or oxygen

• *cardiovascular disorders* — myocardial infarction, heart failure, or pulmonary emboli

• *airway irritants* — smoke or fumes

• *endocrine and metabolic disorders* — myxedema or metabolic alkalosis

• *thoracic abnormalities* — chest trauma, pneumothorax, or thoracic or abdominal surgery.

## Signs and symptoms

In COPD patients with ARF, increased ventilation-perfusion mismatching and reduced alveolar ventilation decrease $Pao_2$ (hypoxemia) and increase $Paco_2$ (hypercapnia). This rise in carbon dioxide tension lowers the pH. The resulting hypoxemia and acidemia affect all body organs, especially the central nervous, respiratory, and cardiovascular systems. Specific symptoms vary with the underlying cause of ARF but may include the following:

• *Respiratory symptoms.* Rate may be increased, decreased, or normal, depending on the cause; respirations may be shallow or deep or alternate between the two; and air hunger may occur. Cyanosis may or may not be present, depending on the hemoglobin (Hb) level and arterial oxygenation. Auscultation of the chest may reveal crackles, rhonchi, wheezes, or diminished breath sounds.

• *CNS symptoms.* The patient shows evidence of restlessness, confusion, loss of concentration, irritability, tremulousness, diminished tendon reflexes, and papilledema; he may slip into a coma.

• *Cardiovascular symptoms.* Tachycardia, with increased cardiac output and mildly elevated blood pressure secondary to adrenal release of catecholamines, occurs early in response to a low $Pao_2$. With myocardial hypoxia, arrhythmias may develop. Pulmonary hypertension also occurs.

## Diagnosis

Progressive deterioration with ABG levels and pH, when compared with the patient's "normal" values, strongly suggests ARF in COPD. (In patients with essentially normal lung tissue, pH < 7.35 usually indicates ARF, but COPD patients display an even greater deviation from this normal value, as they do with blood $Paco_2$ and $Pao_2$.) The following findings are also supportive:

• *Bicarbonate levels* are increased, reflecting metabolic alkalosis or metabolic compensation for chronic respiratory acidosis.

• *Hematocrit and Hb levels* are abnormally low, which may be due to blood loss, indicating decreased oxygen-carrying capacity.

• *Serum electrolyte levels* may indicate hypokalemia, which may result from compensatory hyperventilation — an attempt to correct alkalosis; hypochloremia often occurs in metabolic alkalosis.

• *White blood cell count* is elevated if ARF is due to bacterial infection; Gram stain and sputum culture can identify pathogens.

• *Chest X-ray findings* identify pulmonary pathology, such as emphysema, atelectasis, lesions, pneumothorax, infiltrates, and effusions.

• *Electrocardiogram* reveals arrhythmias, which commonly suggest cor pulmonale and myocardial hypoxia.

### Treatment

ARF in COPD patients is an emergency that requires cautious oxygen therapy (using nasal prongs or a Venturi mask) to raise the patient's $Pao_2$. If significant respiratory acidosis persists, mechanical ventilation through an endotracheal or a tracheostomy tube may be necessary. High-frequency ventilation may be used if the patient doesn't respond to conventional mechanical ventilation. Treatment routinely includes antibiotics for infection, bronchodilators and, possibly, steroids.

### Special considerations

• Because most ARF patients are treated in the intensive care unit (ICU), orient them to the environment, procedures, and routines to minimize their anxiety.

• To reverse hypoxemia, administer oxygen at concentrations to maintain $Pao_2$ of at least 50 to 60 mm Hg. Patients with COPD usually require only small amounts of supplemental oxygen. Watch for a positive response, such as improvement in the patient's breathing and color and in ABG results.

• Maintain a patent airway. If the patient is retaining carbon dioxide, encourage him to cough and to breathe deeply with pursed lips. If the patient is alert, have him use an incentive spirometer; if he's intubated and lethargic, turn him every 1 to 2 hours.

• Use postural drainage and chest physiotherapy to help clear secretions.

• In an intubated patient, suction the trachea, as needed, after hyperoxygenation. Observe for a change in quantity, consistency, and color of the sputum. Provide humidification to liquefy secretions.

• Observe the patient closely for respiratory arrest. Auscultate for chest sounds. Monitor ABG values, and be alert for any changes.

• Monitor and record serum electrolyte levels carefully, and correct imbalances; monitor fluid balance by recording intake and output or daily weights.

• Check the cardiac monitor for arrhythmias.

If the patient requires mechanical ventilation:

• Check ventilator settings, cuff pressures, and ABG values often because the fraction of inspired oxygen ($Fio_2$) setting depends on ABG levels. Draw a blood sample for ABG analysis 20 to 30 minutes after every $Fio_2$ change or check ABG levels with oximetry.

• Prevent infection by using sterile technique while suctioning and by changing ventilator circuits every 24 to 48 hours.

➤ CLINICAL TIP  Because stress ulcers are common in intubated ICU patients, check gastric secretions for evidence of bleeding if the patient has a nasogastric tube or complains of epigastric tenderness, nausea, or vomiting. Monitor hemoglobin level and hematocrit, and check all stool for occult blood. Administer antacids, histamine₂-receptor antagonists, or sucralfate.

- Prevent tracheal erosion that can result from artificial airway cuff overinflation, which compresses tracheal wall vasculature. Use minimal leak technique and a cuffed tube with high residual volume (low-pressure cuff), a foam cuff, or a pressure-regulating valve on the cuff.

- To prevent nasal necrosis, keep the nasotracheal tube midline within the nostrils and provide good hygiene. Loosen tape periodically to prevent skin breakdown. Avoid excessive movement of any tubes and make sure the ventilator tubing is adequately supported.

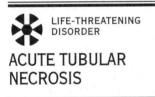

LIFE-THREATENING DISORDER

# ACUTE TUBULAR NECROSIS

Also known as acute tubulointerstitial nephritis, acute tubular necrosis (ATN) accounts for about 75% of all cases of acute renal failure. It's the most common cause of acute renal failure in critically ill patients. ATN injures the tubular segment of the nephron, causing renal failure and uremic syndrome. Mortality ranges from 40% to 70%, depending on complications from underlying diseases. Nonoliguric forms of ATN have a better prognosis.

## Causes

ATN results from ischemic or nephrotoxic injury, most commonly in debilitated patients, such as the critically ill and those who have undergone extensive surgery.

In ischemic injury, disruption of blood flow to the kidneys may result from circulatory collapse, severe hypotension, trauma, hemorrhage, dehydration, cardiogenic or septic shock, surgery, anesthetics, or reactions to transfusions. Ischemic ATN can damage the epithelial and basement membranes and can cause lesions in the renal interstitium.

In nephrotoxic injury, damage may follow ingestion of certain chemical agents or result from a hypersensitive reaction of the kidneys. Because nephrotoxic ATN doesn't damage the basement membrane of the nephron, it's potentially reversible.

ATN may result from:

- diseased tubular epithelium that allows leakage of glomerular filtrate across the membranes and reabsorption of filtrate into the blood

- obstruction of urine flow by the collection of damaged cells, casts, red blood cells (RBCs), and other cellular debris within the tubular walls

- ischemic injury to glomerular epithelial cells, resulting in cellular collapse and decreased glomerular capillary permeability

- ischemic injury to vascular endothelium, eventually resulting in cellular swelling and obstruction.

## Signs and symptoms

ATN is usually difficult to recognize in its early stages because effects of the critically ill patient's primary disease may mask the symptoms of ATN. The first recognizable effect may be decreased urine output. Generally, hyperkalemia and the characteristic uremic syndrome soon follow, with oliguria (or, rarely, anuria) and confusion, which may progress to uremic coma. Other possible complications include heart failure, uremic pericarditis, pulmonary edema, uremic lung, anemia, anorexia, intractable vomiting, and poor wound healing due to debilitation.

Fever and chills are ominous signs of infection, the leading cause of death in ATN.

### Diagnosis

ATN is hard to diagnose accurately until it has progressed to an advanced stage. The most significant laboratory clues are urinary sediment containing RBCs and casts and diluted urine with a low specific gravity (1.010), low osmolality (< 400 mOsm/kg), and high sodium level (40 to 60 mEq/L).

Blood studies reveal elevated blood urea nitrogen and serum creatinine levels, anemia, defects in platelet adherence, metabolic acidosis, and hyperkalemia. An electrocardiogram may show arrhythmias (from electrolyte imbalances) and, with hyperkalemia, a widening QRS segment, disappearing P waves, and tall, peaked T waves.

### Treatment

Vigorous supportive measures are required during the acute phase of ATN until normal kidney function resumes.

Initial treatment may include administration of diuretics and infusion of a large volume of fluids to flush tubules of cellular casts and debris and to replace fluid loss. However, this treatment carries a risk of fluid overload. Long-term fluid management requires daily replacement of projected and calculated losses (including insensible loss).

Other appropriate measures to control complications include transfusion of packed RBCs for anemia and administration of antibiotics for infection. Hyperkalemia may require emergency

I.V. administration of 50% glucose, regular insulin, and sodium bicarbonate. Sodium polystyrene sulfonate with sorbitol may be given orally or by enema to reduce extracellular potassium levels. Peritoneal dialysis or hemodialysis may be needed if the patient is catabolic.

### Special considerations

• Maintain fluid balance. Watch for fluid overload, a common complication of therapy. Accurately record intake and output, including wound drainage, nasogastric output, and peritoneal dialysis and hemodialysis balances. Weigh the patient daily.

• Monitor hemoglobin (Hb) level and hematocrit, and administer blood products as needed. Use fresh packed cells instead of whole blood to prevent fluid overload and heart failure.

• Maintain electrolyte balance. Monitor laboratory results, and be alert for evidence of imbalances. Enforce dietary restriction of foods containing sodium and potassium, such as bananas, orange juice, and baked potatoes. Check for potassium content in prescribed medications (for example, penicillin G potassium and penicillin V potassium).

• To maintain an anabolic state, provide adequate calories and essential amino acids, while restricting protein intake. Total parenteral nutrition may be indicated in the severely debilitated or catabolic patient.

• Use aseptic technique, particularly when handling catheters, because the debilitated patient is vulnerable to infection. Watch for fever, chills, delayed wound healing, or flank pain if the patient has an indwelling urinary catheter in place.

• Be alert for complications. If anemia worsens (pallor, weakness, lethargy with decreased Hb level), administer RBCs. For acidosis, give sodium bicarbonate or assist with dialysis in severe cases as needed. Watch for signs of diminishing renal perfusion (hypotension and decreased urine output). Encourage coughing and deep breathing to prevent pulmonary complications.

• Perform passive range-of-motion exercises. Provide good skin care; apply lotion or bath oil for dry skin. Help the patient to walk as soon as possible, but guard against exhaustion.

• Provide reassurance and emotional support. Encourage the patient and family to express their fears.

• Fully explain each procedure; repeat the explanation each time the procedure is done. Help the patient and family set realistic goals based on the patient's prognosis.

> ☛ CLINICAL TIP  To prevent ATN, make sure all patients are well hydrated before surgery or after X-rays that use a contrast medium. Mannitol is administered to high-risk patients before and during these procedures.

• Carefully monitor patients receiving blood transfusions to detect early signs of a transfusion reaction (fever, rash, chills), and discontinue such transfusions immediately.

# ADRENAL HYPOFUNCTION

Primary adrenal hypofunction or insufficiency (Addison's disease) originates within the adrenal gland itself and is characterized by decreased mineralocorticoid, glucocorticoid, and androgen secretion. Secondary adrenal hypofunction is due to impaired pituitary secretion of corticotropin and is characterized by decreased glucocorticoid secretion. Secretion of aldosterone, the major mineralocorticoid, is often unaffected.

Addison's disease is a relatively uncommon disorder and can occur at any age and in both sexes. Secondary adrenal hypofunction occurs when a patient abruptly stops taking long-term exogenous steroid therapy or when the pituitary is injured by a tumor or by infiltrative or autoimmune processes. With an early diagnosis and adequate replacement therapy, the prognosis for adrenal hypofunction is good.

Adrenal crisis (addisonian crisis), a critical deficiency of mineralocorticoids and glucocorticoids, generally follows acute stress, sepsis, trauma, surgery, or omission of steroid therapy in patients who have chronic adrenal insufficiency. A medical emergency, adrenal crisis necessitates immediate, vigorous treatment.

## Causes

The following are causes of primary and secondary adrenal hypofunction and adrenal crisis.

### Primary hypofunction

Addison's disease occurs when more than 90% of both adrenal glands are destroyed. Such destruction usually results from an autoimmune process in which circulating antibodies react specifically against the adrenal tissue.

Other causes include tuberculosis (once the chief cause; now responsible for less than 10% of adult cases), bilateral adrenalectomy, hemorrhage into the adrenal gland, neoplasms, and infections (histoplasmosis, cytomegalovirus). Rarely, a family history of autoimmune disease predisposes the patient to Addison's disease and other endocrinopathies.

### Secondary hypofunction

Secondary hypofunction, which results in glucocorticoid deficiency, can stem from hypopituitarism (causing decreased corticotropin secretion), abrupt withdrawal of long-term corticosteroid therapy (long-term exogenous corticosteroid stimulation suppresses pituitary corticotropin secretion and results in adrenal gland atrophy), or the removal of a corticotropin-secreting tumor.

### Adrenal crisis

Following trauma, surgery, or other physiologic stress, adrenal crisis exhausts the body's stores of glucocorticoids in a person with adrenal hypofunction.

## Signs and symptoms

Clinical features vary with the type of adrenal hypofunction.

### Primary hypofunction

Addison's disease typically produces such effects as weakness, fatigue, weight loss, nausea, vomiting, and anorexia.

The disorder also usually causes a conspicuous bronze coloration of the skin. The patient appears to be deeply suntanned, especially in the creases of the hands and over the metacarpophalangeal joints, the elbows, and the knees. He also may exhibit a darkening of scars, areas of vitiligo (absence of pigmentation), and increased pigmentation of the mucous membranes, especially the buccal mucosa. Such abnormal skin and mucous membrane coloration results from decreased secretion of cortisol (one of the glucocorticoids), which causes the pituitary gland to simultaneously secrete excessive amounts of corticotropin and melanocyte-stimulating hormone (MSH).

Associated cardiovascular abnormalities in Addison's disease include orthostatic hypotension, decreased cardiac size and output, and a weak, irregular pulse.

Other clinical effects include decreased tolerance for even minor stress,

fasting hypoglycemia (due to decreased gluconeogenesis), and a craving for salty food due to decreased mineralocorticoid secretion, which normally causes salt retention.

### Secondary hypofunction

Secondary hypofunction produces clinical effects similar to those of primary hypofunction but without hyperpigmentation because corticotropin and MSH levels are low. Because aldosterone secretion may continue at fairly normal levels in secondary adrenal hypofunction, this condition doesn't necessarily cause accompanying hypotension and electrolyte abnormalities.

### Adrenal crisis

Producing profound weakness, adrenal crisis also causes fatigue, nausea, vomiting, hypotension, dehydration and, occasionally, high fever followed by hypothermia. If untreated, this condition can ultimately lead to vascular collapse, renal shutdown, coma, and death.

## Diagnosis

Measurement of plasma cortisol levels confirms adrenal insufficiency. If secondary adrenal hypofunction is suspected, the metyrapone test is indicated.

The *metyrapone test* requires oral or I.V. administration of metyrapone, which blocks cortisol production and should stimulate the release of corticotropin from the hypothalamic-pituitary system. In Addison's disease, the hypothalamic-pituitary system responds normally, and plasma reveals high levels of corticotropin; however, because the adrenal glands are destroyed, plasma levels of cortisol precursor and urinary concentrations of 17-hydroxycorticosteroids don't rise. If either primary or secondary adrenal hypofunction is sus-

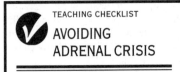

TEACHING CHECKLIST

## AVOIDING ADRENAL CRISIS

The patient with adrenal hypofunction will require lifelong steroid therapy. To help him comply with the prescribed treatment, review the following:

• Teach the patient to recognize the symptoms of too great or too little a dose.
• Tell the patient that the dose may need to be increased during times of stress (when he has a cold, for example).
• Warn that infection, injury, or profuse sweating in hot weather may precipitate adrenal crisis.
• Instruct the patient to always carry a medical identification card stating that he takes a steroid and giving the name of the drug and the dosage.
• Teach the patient how to give himself an injection of hydrocortisone.
• Advise the patient to keep an emergency kit available containing hydrocortisone in a prepared syringe for use in times of stress.
• Warn that any stress may require additional cortisone to prevent adrenal crisis.

pected, a corticotropin stimulation test is indicated.

The *corticotropin stimulation test* involves I.V. administration of corticotropin over 6 to 8 hours, after samples have been obtained to determine baseline plasma cortisol and 24-hour urine cortisol levels. In Addison's disease, plasma and urine cortisol levels fail to rise normally in response to corticotropin; in secondary hypofunction, repeated doses of corticotropin over successive days produce a gradual increase

in cortisol levels until normal values are reached.

In a patient with typical addisonian symptoms, the following laboratory findings strongly suggest acute adrenal insufficiency:

• decreased cortisol levels in plasma (< 10 μg/dl in the morning, with lower levels in the evening)
• decreased serum sodium and fasting blood glucose levels
• increased serum potassium and blood urea nitrogen levels
• elevated hematocrit and lymphocyte and eosinophil counts
• X-rays showing a small heart and adrenal calcification.

### Treatment

For all patients with primary or secondary adrenal hypofunction, lifelong corticosteroid replacement, usually with cortisone or hydrocortisone (both of which also have a mineralocorticoid effect), is the primary treatment.

Addison's disease will require treatment with oral fludrocortisone, a synthetic mineralocorticoid, to prevent dangerous dehydration, hypotension, and electrolyte disturbances with hyponatremia and hyperkalemia. (See *Avoiding adrenal crisis.*)

Adrenal crisis requires prompt I.V. bolus administration of 100 mg hydrocortisone. Later, 50- to 100-mg doses are given I.M. or are diluted with dextrose in saline solution and given I.V. until the patient's condition stabilizes; up to 300 mg/day of hydrocortisone and 3 to 5 L of I.V. saline solution may be required during the acute stage of adrenal crisis.

With proper treatment, adrenal crisis usually subsides quickly; the patient's blood pressure should stabilize, and water and sodium levels should return to normal. After the crisis, maintenance doses of hydrocortisone preserve physiologic stability.

**Special considerations**
• In adrenal crisis, monitor vital signs carefully, especially for hypotension, volume depletion, and other signs of shock (decreased level of consciousness and urine output). Watch for hyperkalemia before treatment and for hypokalemia after treatment (from excessive mineralocorticoid effect).
• If the patient also has diabetes, check the blood glucose level periodically because steroid replacement may necessitate adjustment of insulin dosage.
• Record weight and intake and output carefully because the patient may have volume depletion. Until the onset of the mineralocorticoid effect, force fluids to replace excessive fluid loss.

> CLINICAL TIP  Patients with Addison's disease who have an acute medical illness or those undergoing surgical procedures require additional steroids to cover these stressful periods.

To manage the patient receiving maintenance therapy:
• Advise the patient to watch for symptoms of adrenal crisis, and tell the patient how to provide the necessary self-care upon discharge from the facility.
• Arrange for a diet that maintains sodium and potassium balances.
• Observe the patient receiving steroids for cushingoid signs, such as fluid retention around the eyes and face. Watch for fluid and electrolyte imbalance, especially if the patient is receiving mineralocorticoids. Monitor weight and check blood pressure to assess body fluid status. Be aware that steroids administered in the late afternoon or evening may cause stimulation of the central nervous system and insomnia in some patients.

• If the patient receives glucocorticoids alone, observe for orthostatic hypotension or electrolyte abnormalities, which may indicate a need for mineralocorticoid therapy.

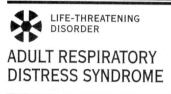

LIFE-THREATENING DISORDER

# ADULT RESPIRATORY DISTRESS SYNDROME

A form of pulmonary edema that causes acute respiratory failure, adult respiratory distress syndrome (ARDS, shock lung, stiff lung) results from increased permeability of the alveolo-capillary membrane. Fluid accumulates in the lung interstitium, alveolar spaces, and small airways, causing the lung to stiffen. Effective ventilation is thus impaired, prohibiting adequate oxygenation of pulmonary capillary blood. Severe ARDS can cause intractable and fatal hypoxemia; however, patients who recover may have little or no permanent lung damage.

**Causes**
ARDS results from a variety of respiratory and nonrespiratory insults, such as:
• aspiration of gastric contents
• sepsis (primarily gram-negative), trauma (lung contusion, head injury, long bone fracture with fat emboli), or oxygen toxicity
• viral, bacterial, or fungal pneumonia or microemboli (fat or air emboli or disseminated intravascular coagulation)
• drug overdose (barbiturates, glutethimide, narcotics) or blood transfusion
• smoke or chemical inhalation (nitrous oxide, chlorine, ammonia)

# ALCOHOLISM

A chronic disorder, alcoholism is usually described as an uncontrolled intake of alcoholic beverages that interferes with physical and mental health, social and familial relationships, and occupational responsibilities. Alcoholism cuts across all social and economic groups, involves both sexes, and occurs at all stages of the life cycle, beginning as early as elementary school age. About 13% of all adults over age 18 have suffered from alcohol abuse or dependence at some time in their lives.

Drinking is most prevalent between ages 21 and 34, but current statistics show that up to 19% of 12- to 17-year-olds have a serious drinking problem. Males are two to five times more likely to abuse alcohol than are females. According to some statistics, alcohol abuse is a factor in 60% of all motor vehicle accidents.

## Causes

Numerous biological, psychological, and sociocultural factors appear to be involved in alcohol addiction. An offspring of one alcoholic parent is seven to eight times more likely to become an alcoholic than is a peer without such a parent. Biological factors may include genetic or biochemical abnormalities, nutritional deficiencies, endocrine imbalances, and allergic responses.

Psychological factors may include the urge to drink alcohol to reduce anxiety or symptoms of mental illness; the desire to avoid responsibility in familial, social, and work relationships; and the need to bolster self-esteem.

Sociocultural factors include the availability of alcoholic beverages, group or peer pressure, an excessively stressful lifestyle, and social attitudes that approve of frequent drinking.

## Signs and symptoms

Because people with alcohol dependence may hide or deny their addiction and may temporarily manage to maintain a functional life, assessing for alcoholism can be difficult.

### Physical and psychosocial symptoms

• The patient's history may suggest a need for daily or episodic alcohol use to maintain adequate functioning, an inability to discontinue or reduce alcohol intake, episodes of anesthesia or amnesia (blackouts) during intoxication, episodes of violence during intoxication, and interference with social and familial relationships and occupational responsibilities.

• Many minor complaints may be alcohol-related. The patient may mention malaise, dyspepsia, mood swings or depression, and an increased incidence of infection. Observe the patient for poor personal hygiene and untreated injuries, such as cigarette burns, fractures, and bruises, that he can't fully explain. Note any evidence of an unusually high tolerance for sedatives and narcotics.

• Watch for secretive behavior. Suspect alcoholism if the patient uses inordinate amounts of aftershave lotion or mouthwash. When confronted, the patient may deny or rationalize the problem. Alternatively, he may be guarded or hostile in his response and may even sign out of the facility against medical advice. He also may project his anger or feelings of guilt or inadequacy onto others to avoid confronting his illness.

• Chronic alcohol abuse brings with it an array of physical complications, including malnutrition, cirrhosis of the liver, peripheral neuropathy, brain damage, and cardiomyopathy. Watch for these complications in a patient with an alcohol-related disorder.

• After abstinence or reduction of alcohol intake, signs and symptoms of withdrawal — which begin shortly after drinking has stopped and last for 5 to 7 days — may vary. The patient initially experiences anorexia, nausea, anxiety, fever, insomnia, diaphoresis, and tremor, progressing to severe tremulousness, agitation and, possibly, hallucinations and violent behavior. Major tonic-clonic seizures (known as "rum fits") can occur during withdrawal. Suspect alcoholism in any patient with unexplained seizures.

### Diagnosis
For characteristic findings in patients with alcoholism, see *Diagnosing substance dependence and related disorders,* page 297.

Clinical findings may help support the diagnosis of alcoholism. For example, laboratory tests can confirm alcohol use and complications and document recent alcohol ingestion, as follows:

• *Blood alcohol level* of 0.10% weight/volume (200 mg/dl) is accepted as the level of intoxication.

• *Blood urea nitrogen level* rises in severe hepatic disease.

• *Serum glucose level* is decreased.

• *Serum ammonia and amylase levels* are increased.

• *Urine toxicology studies* may help detect other types of drug abuse in patients with alcohol withdrawal delirium or another acute complication.

• *Liver function studies* reveal increased levels of serum cholesterol, lactate dehydrogenase, alanine aminotransferase, aspartate aminotransferase, and creatine kinase, which indicate liver damage, and elevated serum amylase and lipase levels, which point to acute pancreatitis.

• *Blood studies* may identify anemia, thrombocytopenia, increased prothrombin time, and increased partial thromboplastin time.

### Treatment
Total abstinence from alcohol is the only effective treatment. Supportive programs that offer detoxification, rehabilitation, and aftercare, including continued involvement in Alcoholics Anonymous (AA), may produce good long-term results.

Acute intoxication is treated symptomatically by supporting respiration, preventing aspiration of vomitus, replacing fluids, administering I.V. glucose to prevent hypoglycemia, correcting hypothermia or acidosis, and initiating emergency treatment for trauma, infection, or GI bleeding.

Treatment of chronic alcoholism relies on medications to treat the effects of withdrawal; psychotherapy (consisting of behavior modification techniques, group therapy, and family therapy); and appropriate measures to relieve associated physical problems.

Aversion, or deterrent, therapy involves a daily oral dose of disulfiram to prevent compulsive drinking. (See *Avoiding the risks of disulfiram therapy,* page 30.) Another form of aversion therapy attempts to induce aversion by administering alcohol with an emetic. Aversion therapy with disulfiram may only substitute one drug dependence for another, so it should be used prudently. For long-term success, the recovering individual must learn to fill the place alcohol once occupied in his life with something constructive.

Tranquilizers, particularly the benzodiazepines, occasionally are used to relieve overwhelming anxiety during rehabilitation. However, these drugs have addictive potential (substituting one substance abuse problem for an-

CLINICAL TIP

## AVOIDING THE RISKS OF DISULFIRAM THERAPY

Disulfiram acts by interfering with alcohol metabolism, which allows toxic levels of acetaldehyde to accumulate in the patient's blood.

*Disulfiram can produce immediate and potentially fatal distress if the patient consumes alcohol up to 2 weeks after taking it.*

Disulfiram is contraindicated during pregnancy and in patients with diabetes, heart disease, severe hepatic disease, or any disorder in which such a reaction could be especially dangerous.

---

other), and they can precipitate a coma or even death when combined with alcohol.

Phenothiazines and other antipsychotics are prescribed to control hyperactivity and psychosis. Anticonvulsants, antiemetics, and antidiarrheals also are used to treat symptoms of alcohol withdrawal.

Supportive counseling or individual, group, or family psychotherapy may help. Ongoing support groups are also helpful. In AA, a self-help group with more than 1 million members worldwide, the alcoholic finds emotional support from others with similar problems. About 40% of AA's members stay sober as long as 5 years, and 30% stay sober longer than 5 years.

### Special considerations

● During acute intoxication or withdrawal, carefully monitor the patient's mental status, heart rate, breath sounds, and blood pressure every 15 minutes until stable, then every hour for 6 hours. Also, closely monitor temperature until stable.

● Examine the patient for signs of inadequate nutrition and dehydration. Institute seizure precautions and administer drugs prescribed to treat the signs and symptoms of withdrawal in chronic alcohol abuse.

● During withdrawal, the patient may have hallucinations and may try to harm himself or others. Maintain a calm environment, minimizing noise and shadows to reduce the incidence of delusions and hallucinations. Avoid restraining the patient unless necessary to protect him or others.

● Approach the patient in a nonthreatening way. Limit sustained eye contact. Even if he's verbally abusive, listen attentively, and respond with empathy. Explain all procedures.

● Monitor the patient for signs of depression or an impending suicide attempt.

● In chronic alcoholism, help the patient accept his drinking problem and the necessity for abstinence. Confront him about his behavior, urging him to examine his actions more realistically.

● If the patient is taking disulfiram (or has taken it within the past 2 weeks), warn him of the effects of alcohol ingestion, which may last from 30 minutes to 3 hours or longer. The reaction includes nausea, vomiting, facial flushing, headache, shortness of breath, red eyes, blurred vision, sweating, tachycardia, hypotension, and fainting. Emphasize that even a small amount of alcohol will induce this adverse reaction and that the longer he takes the drug, the greater his sensitivity to alcohol will be. Because of this, he must avoid even medicinal sources of alcohol, such as mouthwash, cough syrups, liquid vitamins, and cold remedies.

> **CLINICAL TIP** Refer the patient to AA and offer to arrange a visit from an AA member. Stress the effectiveness of this organization.

● For individuals who have lost all contact with family and friends and who have a long history of unemployment, trouble with the law, or other problems associated with alcohol abuse, rehabilitation may involve job training, sheltered workshops, halfway houses, and other supervised facilities.

● Refer spouses of alcoholics to Al-Anon and children of alcoholics to Alateen. By participating in these self-help groups, family members learn to relinquish responsibility for the individual's drinking. Point out that family involvement in rehabilitation can reduce family tensions.

● Refer adult children of alcoholics to the National Association for Children of Alcoholics.

# ALLERGIC PURPURA

A type of nonthrombocytopenic purpura, allergic purpura is an acute or a chronic vascular inflammation affecting the skin, joints, and GI and genitourinary (GU) tracts in association with allergy symptoms. When allergic purpura primarily affects the GI tract, with accompanying joint pain, it's called Henoch-Schönlein syndrome or anaphylactoid purpura. However, the term *allergic purpura* applies to purpura associated with many other conditions, such as erythema nodosum. An acute attack of allergic purpura can last for several weeks and is potentially fatal

(usually from renal failure); however, most patients do recover.

Fully developed allergic purpura is persistent and debilitating, possibly leading to chronic glomerulonephritis (especially following a streptococcal infection). Allergic purpura affects males more often than females and is most prevalent in children ages 3 to 7. The prognosis is more favorable for children than for adults.

## Causes

The most common identifiable cause of allergic purpura is probably an autoimmune reaction directed against vascular walls, triggered by a bacterial infection (particularly streptococcal infection). Typically, an upper respiratory tract infection occurs 1 to 3 weeks before the onset of symptoms. Other possible causes include allergic reactions to some drugs and vaccines, allergic reactions to insect bites, and allergic reactions to some foods (such as wheat, eggs, milk, and chocolate).

## Signs and symptoms

Allergic purpura produces characteristic purple skin lesions that are macular, ecchymotic, and of varying size and are caused by vascular leakage into the skin and mucous membranes. The lesions usually appear in symmetrical patterns on the arms and legs and are accompanied by pruritus, paresthesia and, occasionally, angioneurotic edema. In children, skin lesions are generally urticarial and expand and become hemorrhagic. Scattered petechiae may appear on the legs, buttocks, and perineum.

Henoch-Schönlein syndrome commonly produces transient or severe colic, tenesmus (spasmodic contraction of the anal sphincter) and constipation, vomiting, and edema or hemorrhage of the mucous membranes of the bowel, resulting in GI bleeding, occult blood in the stool and, possibly, intussusception. Such GI abnormalities may *precede* overt, cutaneous signs of purpura. Musculoskeletal symptoms, such as rheumatoid pains and periarticular effusions, mostly affect the legs and feet.

In 25% to 50% of patients, allergic purpura is associated with GU symptoms: nephritis; renal hemorrhages that may cause microscopic hematuria and disturb renal function; bleeding from the mucosal surfaces of the ureters, bladder, or urethra; and, occasionally, glomerulonephritis. Also possible are moderate and irregular fever, headache, anorexia, and localized edema of the hands, feet, or scalp.

### Diagnosis

No laboratory test clearly identifies allergic purpura (although the white blood cell count and erythrocyte sedimentation rate are elevated). Diagnosis therefore requires careful clinical observation, often during the second or third attack. Except for a positive tourniquet test, coagulation and platelet function tests are usually normal. X-rays of the small bowel may reveal areas of transient edema; tests for blood in the urine and stool are often positive. Increased blood urea nitrogen and serum creatinine levels may indicate renal involvement. The diagnosis must rule out other forms of nonthrombocytopenic purpura.

### Treatment

In allergic purpura, treatment is generally aimed at relieving symptoms; for example, severe allergic purpura may require steroids to relieve edema and analgesics to relieve joint and abdominal pain. Some patients with chronic renal disease may benefit from immunosuppression with azathioprine, along with identification of the provocative

allergen. An accurate allergy history is essential.

### Special considerations

● Encourage the patient to maintain an elimination diet to help identify specific allergenic foods so that these foods can be eliminated from the patient's diet.
● Monitor skin lesions and level of pain. Provide analgesics as needed.

➤ CLINICAL TIP  Watch carefully for complications: GI and GU tract bleeding, edema, nausea, vomiting, headache, hypertension (with nephritis), abdominal rigidity and tenderness, and absence of stool (with intussusception).
● To prevent muscle atrophy in the bedridden patient, provide passive or active range-of-motion exercises.
● After the acute stage, stress the need for the patient to *immediately* tell the doctor of *any* recurrence of symptoms (recurrence is most common about 6 weeks after the initial onset) and to return for follow-up urinalysis as scheduled.

# ALLERGIC RHINITIS

An immune disorder, allergic rhinitis is a reaction to airborne (inhaled) allergens. Depending on the allergen, the resulting rhinitis and conjunctivitis may be seasonal (hay fever) or occur year-round (perennial allergic rhinitis). Allergic rhinitis is the most common atopic allergic reaction, affecting over 20 million Americans. It's most prevalent in young children and adolescents but can occur in all age-groups.

### Causes

Hay fever reflects an immunoglobulin E (IgE)-mediated, Type I hypersensitivity response to an environmental antigen (allergen) in a genetically susceptible individual. In most cases, it's induced by wind-borne pollens: in the spring by tree pollens (oak, elm, maple, alder, birch, cottonwood); in the summer by grass pollens (crabgrass, bluegrass, fescue, and ryegrass); and in the fall by weed pollens (ragweed). Occasionally, hay fever is induced by allergy to fungal spores.

In perennial allergic rhinitis, inhaled allergens provoke antigen responses that produce recurring symptoms year-round.

The major perennial allergens and irritants include dust mites, feather pillows, mold, cigarette smoke, upholstery, and animal danders. Seasonal pollen allergy may exacerbate symptoms of perennial rhinitis.

### Signs and symptoms

In seasonal allergic rhinitis, the key signs and symptoms are paroxysmal sneezing, profuse watery rhinorrhea, nasal obstruction or congestion, and pruritus of the nose and eyes, usually accompanied by pale, cyanotic, edematous nasal mucosa; red and edematous eyelids and conjunctivae; excessive lacrimation; and headache or sinus pain. Some patients also complain of itching in the throat and malaise.

In perennial allergic rhinitis, conjunctivitis and other extranasal effects are rare, but chronic nasal obstruction is common and often extends to eustachian tube obstruction, particularly in children.

In both types of allergic rhinitis, dark circles may appear under the patient's eyes ("allergic shiners") because of venous congestion in the maxillary sinuses. The severity of signs and symptoms may vary from season to season and from year to year.

Some patients may develop chronic complications, including sinusitis and nasal polyps.

### Diagnosis

Microscopic examination of sputum and nasal secretions reveals large numbers of eosinophils. Blood chemistry studies show normal or elevated IgE levels, possibly linked to seasonal overproduction of interleukin-4 and -5 (involved in the allergic inflammatory process). A firm diagnosis rests on the patient's personal and family history of allergies and on physical findings during a symptomatic phase. Skin testing, paired with tested responses to environmental stimuli, can pinpoint the responsible allergens when interpreted in light of the patient's history

To distinguish between allergic rhinitis and other disorders of the nasal mucosa, remember these differences:

• In chronic vasomotor rhinitis, eye symptoms are absent, rhinorrhea is mucoid, and seasonal variation is absent.

➤ CLINICAL TIP  In infectious rhinitis (the common cold), the nasal mucosa is beet red; nasal secretions contain polymorphonuclear, not eosinophilic, exudate; and signs and symptoms include fever and sore throat. This condition isn't a recurrent seasonal phenomenon.

• In rhinitis medicamentosa, which results from excessive use of nasal sprays or drops, nasal drainage and mucosal redness and swelling disappear when such medication is withheld.

• In children, a differential diagnosis should rule out a nasal foreign body, such as a bean or a button.

### Treatment

Symptoms are controlled by eliminating the environmental antigen, if possible, and by drug therapy and immunotherapy.

Antihistamines and nasal decongestants are useful for treating acute symptoms. These drugs block histamine effects but commonly produce anticholinergic adverse effects (sedation, dry mouth, nausea, dizziness, blurred vision, and nervousness).

Newer antihistamines, such as cetirizine and loratadine, have proved effective in clinical trials. Fexofenadine, a derivative of terfenadine, may be effective but with less sedation and a lower risk of cardiac arrhythmias than terfenadine.

Inhaled intranasal steroids produce local anti-inflammatory effects with minimal systemic adverse effects. The most commonly used intranasal steroids are flunisolide and beclomethasone. These drugs usually aren't effective for acute exacerbations but can help control chronic symptoms.

Advise the patient to use intranasal steroids regularly, as prescribed, for optimal effectiveness. Cromolyn sodium may be helpful in preventing allergic rhinitis. But this drug may take up to 4 weeks to produce a satisfactory effect and must be taken regularly during allergy season.

Long-term management includes immunotherapy or desensitization with injections of extracted allergens administered before or during allergy season or perennially. Seasonal allergies require particularly close dosage regulation. Local nasal immunotherapy is also being studied as an alternative route of allergen administration.

**Special considerations**
• When caring for the patient with allergic rhinitis, monitor his compliance with the prescribed drug treatment regimen. Also carefully note any changes in the control of his symptoms or any signs of drug misuse.
• Before giving allergen injections, assess the patient's symptom status. Afterward, watch for adverse reactions, including anaphylaxis and severe localized erythema.
• Keep epinephrine and emergency resuscitation equipment available, and observe the patient for 30 minutes after the injection.
• Instruct the patient to call the doctor if a delayed reaction should occur, and teach the patient how to reduce environmental exposures. (See *Avoiding bouts of allergic rhinitis*.)
• In severe and resistant cases, patients may have to consider drastic changes in lifestyle, such as relocation to a pollen-free area either seasonally or year-round.

# ALOPECIA

Alopecia, or hair loss, usually occurs on the scalp; hair loss elsewhere on the body is less common and less conspicuous. In the nonscarring form of this disorder (noncicatricial alopecia), the hair follicle can generally regrow hair. But scarring alopecia usually destroys the hair follicle, making hair loss irreversible.

## Causes

The most common form of nonscarring alopecia is male-pattern alopecia, which appears to be related to androgen levels and to aging. Genetic predisposition commonly influences the time of onset, degree of baldness, speed with which it spreads, and pattern of hair loss. Women may experience a similar disorder, called androgenetic alopecia, characterized by diffuse thinning over the top of the scalp.

Other forms of nonscarring alopecia include:

• *physiologic alopecia* (usually temporary): sudden hair loss in infants, loss of straight hairline in adolescents, and diffuse hair loss after childbirth

• *alopecia areata* (autoimmune disorder): generally reversible and self-limiting; occurs most frequently in young and middle-aged adults of both sexes; also occurs in children

• *trichotillomania:* compulsive pulling out of one's own hair; most common in children.

Predisposing factors of nonscarring alopecia also include radiation, many types of drug therapies and drug reactions, bacterial and fungal infections, psoriasis, seborrheic dermatitis (from scratching the affected area), and endocrine disorders, such as thyroid, parathyroid, and pituitary dysfunctions.

Scarring alopecia causes irreversible hair loss. It may result from physical or chemical trauma or chronic tension on a hair shaft, as occurs in braiding. Diseases that produce scarring alopecia include destructive skin tumors, granulomas, lupus erythematosus, scleroderma, follicular lichen planus, and severe

fungal, bacterial, or viral infections, such as kerion, deep folliculitis, and herpes zoster.

## Signs and symptoms

In male-pattern alopecia, hair loss is gradual and usually affects the thinner, shorter, and less pigmented hairs of the frontal and parietal portions of the scalp. In women, hair loss is generally more diffuse; completely bald areas are uncommon but may occur.

Alopecia areata affects small patches of the scalp but may also occur as alopecia totalis, which involves the entire scalp, or as alopecia universalis, which involves the entire body. Although mild erythema may occur initially, affected areas of scalp or skin appear normal. "Exclamation point" hairs (loose hairs with dark, rough, brushlike tips on narrow, less-pigmented shafts) occur at the periphery of new patches. Regrowth initially appears as fine, downy hair, which is replaced by normal hair. (See *Alopecia areata,* page 36.)

In trichotillomania, patchy, incomplete areas of hair loss with many broken hairs appear on the scalp but may occur on other areas, such as the eyebrows.

## Diagnosis

Physical examination is usually sufficient to confirm alopecia. In trichotillomania, an occlusive dressing can establish a diagnosis by allowing new hair to grow, revealing that the hair is being pulled out. The diagnosis must also identify any underlying disorder.

## Treatment

Topical application of minoxidil, a peripheral vasodilator more typically used as an oral antihypertensive, has had limited success in treating male-pattern alopecia. A new DNA drug, Propecia (finasteride), has been approved for use

## ALOPECIA AREATA

"Exclamation point" hairs often border new patches of alopecia areata. Not seen in any other type of alopecia, these hairs indicate that the patch is expanding.

Epidermis

Sebaceous glands

Hair follicle

Hair bulb

in men. An alternate treatment is surgical redistribution of hair follicles by autografting.

In alopecia areata, treatment may be unnecessary because spontaneous regrowth is common. Intralesional corticosteroid injections are beneficial for small patches and may produce regrowth in 4 to 6 weeks. High-potency topical steroids are less effective. Hair loss that persists for over a year has a poor prognosis for regrowth.

Treatment of other types of alopecia varies according to the underlying cause.

**Special considerations**
• Reassure a woman with female-pattern alopecia that it rarely leads to total baldness. Suggest that she try topical minoxidil or consider the use of a wig in severe cases.

• If the patient has alopecia areata, explain the disorder and give reassurance that complete regrowth is possible.

# ALZHEIMER'S DISEASE

Also known as primary degenerative dementia, Alzheimer's disease accounts for over half of all dementias. An estimated 5% of people over age 65 have a severe form of this disease, and 12% suffer from mild to moderate dementia. Because this is a primary progressive dementia, the prognosis for a patient with this disease is poor.

**Causes**
Alzheimer's disease is thought to be related to several causal factors. They include *neurochemical factors,* such as

deficiencies in acetylcholine (a neuro-transmitter), somatostatin, substance P, and norepinephrine; *environmental factors,* such as aluminum and manganese; *viral factors,* such as slow-growing central nervous system viruses; *trauma;* and *genetic immunologic factors.*

The brain tissue of patients with Alzheimer's disease has three hallmark features: neurofibrillary tangles, neuritic plaques, and granulovascular degeneration.

### Signs and symptoms

Onset is insidious. Initially, the patient experiences almost imperceptible changes, such as forgetfulness, recent memory loss, difficulty learning and remembering new information, deterioration in personal hygiene and appearance, and an inability to concentrate. Gradually, tasks that require abstract thinking and activities that require judgment become more difficult. Progressive and severe deterioration in memory, language, and motor function results in a loss of coordination and an inability to write or speak.

Personality changes (restlessness, irritability) and nocturnal awakenings are common. Eventually, the patient becomes disoriented, and emotional lability and physical and intellectual disability progress. The patient becomes very susceptible to infection and accidents. Secondary to loss of the cough reflex, pulmonary diseases such as pneumonia may result in death.

### Diagnosis

Early diagnosis of Alzheimer's disease is difficult because the patient's signs and symptoms are subtle. A positive diagnosis is based on an accurate history from a reliable family member, mental status and neurologic examinations, and psychometric testing.

A positron emission tomography scan measures the metabolic activity of the cerebral cortex and may help in reaching an early diagnosis. An EEG and a computed tomography scan may help in later diagnosis.

Currently, the disease is diagnosed by exclusion: Various tests are performed to rule out other disorders. It can't be confirmed until death, when an autopsy reveals pathologic findings.

> **CLINICAL TIP** Many researchers believe that the aluminum and silicon found in neurofibrillary tangles and neuritic plaques occurs as a result of damage and isn't a cause.

### Treatment

Cerebral vasodilators, such as ergoloid mesylates, isoxsuprine, and cyclandelate, are prescribed to enhance the brain's circulation; hyperbaric oxygen, to increase oxygenation to the brain; psychostimulators such as methylphenidate, to enhance the patient's mood; and antidepressants, if depression seems to exacerbate the patient's dementia. Tacrine, a centrally acting anticholinesterase agent, is given to treat memory deficits.

Most drug therapies currently being used are experimental. These include choline salts, lecithin, physostigmine, deanol, enkephalins, and naloxone, which may slow the disease process. Another approach to treatment includes avoiding the use of antacids containing aluminum, aluminum cooking utensils, and aluminum-containing deodorants to help decrease aluminum intake.

### Special considerations

• Focus on supporting the patient's abilities and compensating for those abilities he has lost.
• Establish an effective communication system with the patient and his family to help them adjust to the patient's altered cognitive abilities.

• Offer emotional support to the patient and his family. Teach them about the disease, and refer them to social service and community resources for legal and financial advice and support.

• Provide the patient with a safe environment. Encourage him to exercise to help maintain mobility.

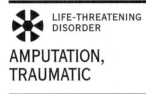

LIFE-THREATENING
DISORDER

# AMPUTATION, TRAUMATIC

Traumatic amputation involves the accidental loss of a body part, usually a finger, a toe, an arm, or a leg. In complete amputation, the member is totally severed; in partial amputation, some soft-tissue connection remains.

The prognosis has improved as a result of early improved emergency and critical care management, new surgical techniques, early rehabilitation, prosthesis fitting, and new prosthesis design. New limb reimplantation techniques have been moderately successful, but incomplete nerve regeneration remains a major limiting factor.

### Causes

Traumatic amputations usually result directly from accidents at the factory or farm, or from power tools or motor vehicle accidents.

### Assessment

Every traumatic amputee requires careful monitoring of vital signs. If amputation involves more than just a finger or a toe, assessment of airway, breathing, and circulation is also required. Because profuse bleeding is likely, watch for signs of hypovolemic shock, and draw blood for hemoglobin level, hematocrit, and typing and crossmatching. In partial amputation, check for pulses distal to the amputation. After any traumatic amputation, assess for other traumatic injuries as well.

### Treatment

Because the greatest immediate threat after traumatic amputation is blood loss and hypovolemic shock, emergency treatment consists of local measures to control bleeding, fluid replacement with normal saline solution and colloids, and blood replacement as needed.

Reimplantation remains controversial, but it's becoming more common and successful because of advances in microsurgery. If reconstruction or reimplantation is possible, surgical intervention attempts to preserve usable joints. When arm or leg amputations are done, the surgeon creates a stump to be fitted with a prosthesis. A rigid dressing permits early prosthesis fitting and rehabilitation.

### Special considerations

• During emergency treatment, monitor vital signs (especially in hypovolemic shock), clean the wound, and give tetanus prophylaxis, analgesics, and antibiotics as needed.

➤ CLINICAL TIP   After complete amputation, wrap the amputated part in a dry, sterile towel, and put it in a plastic bag. Keep the bag cool but not cold enough to damage or freeze the amputated part. Flush the wound with sterile saline solution, apply a sterile pressure dressing, and elevate the limb. Notify the reimplantation team.

• After partial amputation, position the limb in normal alignment, and drape it with towels or dressings soaked in sterile normal saline solution.

- Preoperative care includes thorough wound irrigation and debridement (using a local nerve block).
- Postoperative dressing changes using sterile technique help prevent skin infection and ensure skin graft viability.
- Help the amputee cope with his altered body image. Reinforce exercises and prevent stump trauma.

---

LIFE-THREATENING
DISORDER

# AMYOTROPHIC LATERAL SCLEROSIS

---

Commonly called Lou Gehrig's disease, after the New York Yankee first baseman who died of this disorder, amyotrophic lateral sclerosis (ALS) is the most common of the motor neuron diseases causing muscular atrophy. Other motor neuron diseases include progressive muscular atrophy and progressive bulbar palsy. Onset occurs between ages 40 and 70. A chronic, progressively debilitating disease, ALS is rapidly fatal.

## Causes

More than 30,000 Americans have ALS; about 5,000 new cases are diagnosed each year, with men affected three times more often than women. The exact cause of ALS is unknown, but about 5% to 10% of ALS cases have a genetic component. In these cases, it's an autosomal dominant trait and affects men and women equally.

ALS and other motor neuron diseases may result from:
- a slow-acting virus
- nutritional deficiency related to a disturbance in enzyme metabolism
- metabolic interference in nucleic acid production by the nerve fibers
- autoimmune disorders that affect immune complexes in the renal glomerulus and basement membrane.

Precipitating factors for acute deterioration include trauma, viral infections, and physical exhaustion.

## Signs and symptoms

Patients with ALS develop fasciculations, accompanied by atrophy and weakness, especially in the muscles of the forearms and the hands. Other signs include impaired speech; difficulty chewing, swallowing, and breathing, particularly if the brain stem is affected; and, occasionally, choking and excessive drooling.

Mental deterioration doesn't usually occur, but patients may become depressed as a reaction to the disease. Progressive bulbar palsy may cause crying spells or inappropriate laughter.

## Diagnosis

Characteristic clinical features indicate a combination of upper and lower motor neuron involvement without sensory impairment. Electromyography and a muscle biopsy help show nerve, rather than muscle, disease. The protein content of cerebrospinal fluid is increased in one-third of patients, but this finding alone doesn't confirm ALS.

Diagnosis must rule out multiple sclerosis, spinal cord neoplasm, polyarteritis, syringomyelia, myasthenia gravis, and progressive muscular dystrophy.

## Treatment

Management aims to control symptoms and provide emotional, psychological, and physical support.

> **CLINICAL TIP** A new drug, Rilutek (riluzole), may provide a treatment for ALS that increases survival time and quality of life.

### Special considerations
• Care begins with a complete neurologic assessment — a baseline for future evaluations of progressing disease.
• Implement a rehabilitation program designed to maintain independence as long as possible.
• Help the patient obtain equipment, such as a walker and a wheelchair. Arrange for a visiting nurse to monitor the patient's status, to provide support, and to teach the family about the illness.
• Depending on the patient's muscular capacity, assist with bathing, personal hygiene, and transfers from wheelchair to bed. Help establish a regular bowel and bladder routine.
• To help the patient handle increased accumulation of secretions and dysphagia, teach him to suction himself. He should have a suctioning machine handy at home to reduce his fear of choking.
• To prevent skin breakdown, provide good skin care when the patient is bedridden. Turn him often, keep his skin clean and dry, and use sheepskins or pressure-relieving devices.
• If the patient has trouble swallowing, give him soft, solid foods and position him upright during meals. Gastrostomy and nasogastric tube feedings may be necessary if he can no longer swallow. Teach the patient (if he's still able to feed himself) or family members how to administer gastrostomy feedings.
• Provide emotional support. Prepare the patient and family for his eventual death, and encourage the start of the grieving process. Patients with ALS may benefit from a hospice program.

**LIFE-THREATENING DISORDER**

# ANAPHYLAXIS

Anaphylaxis is a dramatic and widespread acute atopic reaction marked by the sudden onset of rapidly progressive urticaria and respiratory distress. A severe anaphylactic reaction may precipitate vascular collapse, leading to systemic shock and, sometimes, death.

## Causes
The source of anaphylactic reactions is ingestion of or other systemic exposure to sensitizing drugs or other substances.

### Sensitizing substances
Sensitizing substances may include serums (usually horse serum), vaccines, allergen extracts, enzymes (such as L-asparaginase), hormones, penicillin and other antibiotics, sulfonamides, local anesthetics, salicylates, polysaccharides, diagnostic chemicals (sulfobromophthalein, sodium dehydrocholate, and radiographic contrast media), foods (legumes, nuts, berries, seafoods, and egg albumin) and sulfite-containing food additives, insect venom (honeybees, wasps, hornets, yellow jackets, fire ants, mosquitoes, and certain spiders).

A common cause on cause of anaphylaxis is penicillin, which induces anaphylaxis in 1 to 4 of every 10,000 patients treated with it. Penicillin is most likely to induce anaphylaxis after parenteral administration or prolonged therapy and in atopic patients with an allergy to other drugs or foods.

### Pathophysiology
An anaphylactic reaction requires previous sensitization or exposure to the

specific antigen, resulting in the production of specific immunoglobulin E (IgE) antibodies by plasma cells. This antibody production takes place in the lymph nodes and is enhanced by helper T cells. IgE antibodies then bind to membrane receptors on mast cells (found throughout connective tissue, often near small blood vessels) and basophils.

On reexposure, the antigen binds to adjacent IgE antibodies or cross-linked IgE receptors, activating a series of cellular reactions that trigger degranulation — the release of powerful preformed chemical mediators (such as histamine, prostaglandins, and platelet activating factor) from mast cell stores. IgG or IgM enters into the reaction and activates the release of complement fractions.

This acute phase of the response occurs within minutes of exposure. Because of the systemic nature of the exposure, activation of mast cells is widespread, and the massive release of these powerful mediators near blood vessels leads to vascular collapse by stimulating contraction of certain groups of smooth muscles and by increasing vascular permeability. In turn, increased vascular permeability leads to decreased peripheral resistance and plasma leakage from the circulation to extravascular tissues (which lowers blood volume, causing hypotension, hypovolemic shock, and cardiac dysfunction).

In the later phase of this response (8 to 12 hours later), other mediators are synthesized and released, including chemokines, leukotrienes, and cytokines. These agents mediate the inflammatory response by recruiting eosinophils and lymphocytes. This delayed response may be less dramatic than the acute phase of anaphylaxis, but with a diffuse inflammatory response, further smooth muscle contraction and edema can occur and progress to grave systemic symptoms.

## Signs and symptoms

An anaphylactic reaction produces sudden physical distress within seconds or minutes after exposure to an allergen. A delayed or persistent reaction may occur up to 24 hours later. The severity of the reaction is inversely related to the interval between exposure to the allergen and the onset of symptoms. Usually, the first symptoms include a feeling of impending doom or fright, weakness, sweating, sneezing, shortness of breath, nasal pruritus, urticaria, and angioedema, followed rapidly by symptoms in one or more target organs.

### *Systemic effects*

Cardiovascular symptoms include hypotension, shock, and sometimes cardiac arrhythmias, which, if untreated, may precipitate circulatory collapse.

Respiratory symptoms can occur at any level in the respiratory tract and commonly include nasal mucosal edema, profuse watery rhinorrhea, itching, nasal congestion, and sudden sneezing attacks. Edema of the upper respiratory tract, resulting in hypopharyngeal and laryngeal obstruction (hoarseness, stridor, and dyspnea), is an early sign of acute respiratory failure, which can be fatal.

GI and genitourinary symptoms include severe stomach cramps, nausea, diarrhea, and urinary urgency and incontinence.

## Diagnosis

Anaphylaxis can be diagnosed by the rapid onset of severe respiratory or cardiovascular symptoms after ingestion or injection of a drug, vaccine, diagnostic agent, food, or food additive or after an insect sting. If these symptoms occur without a known allergic stimulus, rule out other possible causes of shock (such as acute myocardial infarction, status asthmaticus, and heart failure).

### Treatment and special considerations

• Anaphylaxis is always an emergency. It requires an *immediate* injection of epinephrine 1:1,000 aqueous solution, 0.1 to 0.5 ml, repeated every 5 to 20 minutes as necessary.
• In the early stages of anaphylaxis, when the patient hasn't yet lost consciousness and is still normotensive, give epinephrine I.M. or subcutaneously (S.C.), and help it move into the circulation faster by massaging the injection site. In severe reactions, when the patient has lost consciousness and is hypotensive, give epinephrine I.V.
• Maintain airway patency. Observe for early signs of laryngeal edema (stridor, hoarseness, and dyspnea), which will probably necessitate endotracheal tube insertion or a tracheotomy and oxygen therapy.
• In case of cardiac arrest, begin cardiopulmonary resuscitation, including closed-chest heart massage, assisted ventilation, and sodium bicarbonate; other therapy is indicated by clinical response.
• Watch for hypotension and shock, and maintain circulatory volume with volume expanders (plasma, plasma expanders, saline solution, and albumin) as needed. Stabilize blood pressure with the I.V. vasopressors norepinephrine and dopamine. Monitor blood pressure, central venous pressure, and urine output as a response index.
• After the initial emergency, administer other medications, such as S.C. epinephrine, longer-acting epinephrine, corticosteroids, and diphenhydramine I.V., for long-term management and

aminophylline I.V. over 10 to 20 minutes for bronchospasm.

*Caution:* Rapid infusion of aminophylline may cause or aggravate severe hypotension.

CLINICAL TIP   Even after the acute anaphylactic event has been controlled, patients must be counseled about the risks of delayed symptoms. Any recurrence of shortness of breath, chest tightness, sweating, angioedema, or other symptoms must be reported immediately.

• To prevent anaphylaxis, teach the patient to avoid exposure to known allergens. In a food or drug allergy, the sensitized person must learn to avoid the offending food or drug in all its forms. In an allergy to insect stings, he should avoid open fields and wooded areas during the insect season and should carry an anaphylaxis kit (containing epinephrine, an antihistamine, and a tourniquet) whenever he goes outdoors. Instruct him in the use of the kit. (See *Showing patients how to use an anaphylaxis kit.*) In addition, every patient prone to anaphylaxis should wear a medical identification bracelet identifying his allergies.
• If a patient must receive a drug to which he's allergic, prevent a severe reaction by making sure he receives careful desensitization with gradually increasing doses of the antigen or advance administration of steroids.
• A person with a known history of allergies should receive a drug with a high anaphylactic potential only after cautious pretesting for sensitivity. Closely monitor the patient during testing, and make sure you have resuscitative equipment and epinephrine ready.
• When any patient needs a drug with high anaphylactic potential (particularly parenteral drugs), make sure he receives each dose under close medical observation.

# SHOWING PATIENTS HOW TO USE AN ANAPHYLAXIS KIT

If the doctor has prescribed an anaphylaxis kit for the patient to use in an emergency, explain that the kit contains everything that he needs to treat an allergic reaction: a prefilled syringe containing two doses of epinephrine, alcohol swabs, a tourniquet, and antihistamine tablets.

Instruct the patient to notify the doctor at once if anaphylaxis occurs (or to ask someone else to call him) and to use the anaphylaxis kit as follows.

### Getting ready
• Take the prefilled syringe from the kit and remove the needle cap. Hold the syringe with the needle pointing up. Expel air from the syringe by pushing in the plunger until it stops.
• Next, clean about 4″ (10 cm) of the skin on your arm or thigh with an alcohol swab. (If you're right-handed, clean your left arm or thigh. If you're left-handed, clean your right arm or thigh.)

### Injecting the epinephrine
• Rotate the plunger one-quarter turn to the right so that it's aligned with the slot. Insert the entire needle — like a dart — into the skin.
• Push down on the plunger until it stops. It will inject 0.3 ml of the drug for persons over age 12. Withdraw the needle.
*Note.* The dose and administration for babies and for children under age 12 must be directed by a doctor.

### Removing the insect's stinger
• Quickly remove the insect's stinger if it's visible. Use a dull object, such as a fingernail or tweezers, to pull it straight out. If the stinger can't be removed quickly, stop trying. Go on to the next step.

### Applying the tourniquet
• It you were stung on an arm or a leg, apply a tourniquet between the sting site and your heart. Tighten the tourniquet by pulling the string.
• After 10 minutes, release the tourniquet by pulling on the metal ring.

### Taking the antihistamine tablets
• Chew and swallow the antihistamine tablets. (Children age 12 and younger should follow the directions supplied by the doctor or provided in the kit.)

### Following up
• Apply ice packs — if available — to the sting site. Avoid exertion, keep warm, and see a doctor or go to a hospital immediately.
• *Important:* If you don't notice an improvement within 10 minutes, give yourself a second injection by following the directions in the kit. If the syringe has a preset second dose, don't depress the plunger until you're ready to give the second injection. Proceed as before, following the injection instructions.

### Special instructions
• Keep the kit handy for emergency treatment at all times.
• Ask the pharmacist for storage guidelines.
• Periodically check the epinephrine in the preloaded syringe. A pinkish brown solution needs to be replaced.
• Note the kit's expiration date and replace the kit before that date.

• Closely monitor a patient undergoing diagnostic tests that use radiographic contrast dyes, such as cardiac catheterization, excretory urography, and angiography.

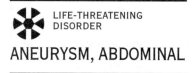
LIFE-THREATENING DISORDER

# ANEURYSM, ABDOMINAL

In abdominal aneurysm, an abnormal dilation in the arterial wall generally occurs in the aorta between the renal arteries and iliac branches. Such aneurysms are four times more common in men than in women and are most prevalent in whites ages 50 to 80. Over 50% of all people with untreated abdominal aneurysms die within 2 years of diagnosis, primarily from aneurysmal rupture; over 85%, within 5 years.

## Causes

About 95% of abdominal aortic aneurysms result from arteriosclerosis; the rest, from cystic medial necrosis, trauma, syphilis, and other infections. These aneurysms develop slowly.

First, a focal weakness in the muscular layer of the aorta (tunica media), due to degenerative changes, allows the inner layer (tunica intima) and outer layer (tunica adventitia) to stretch outward. Blood pressure within the aorta progressively weakens the vessel walls and enlarges the aneurysm.

## Signs and symptoms

Although abdominal aneurysms usually don't produce symptoms, most are evident (unless the patient is obese) as a pulsating mass in the periumbilical area, accompanied by a systolic bruit over the aorta. Some tenderness may be present on deep palpation. A large aneurysm may produce symptoms that mimic renal calculi, lumbar disk disease, and duodenal compression. Abdominal aneurysms rarely cause diminished peripheral pulses or claudication unless embolization occurs.

### *Pain, rupture, and hemorrhage*

Lumbar pain that radiates to the flank and groin from pressure on lumbar nerves may signify enlargement and imminent rupture. If the aneurysm ruptures into the peritoneal cavity, it causes severe, persistent abdominal and back pain, mimicking renal or ureteral colic.

Signs of hemorrhage — such as weakness, sweating, tachycardia, and hypotension — may be subtle because rupture into the retroperitoneal space produces a tamponade effect that prevents continued hemorrhage. Patients with such rupture may remain stable for hours before shock and death occur, although 20% die immediately.

## Diagnosis

Because an abdominal aneurysm rarely produces symptoms, its often detected accidentally as the result of an X-ray or a routine physical examination. Several tests can confirm suspected abdominal aneurysm:

• *Serial ultrasonography* allows accurate determination of aneurysm size, shape, and location.

• *Anteroposterior and lateral X-rays* of the abdomen can detect aortic calcification, which outlines the mass, at least 75% of the time.

• *Aortography* shows the condition of vessels proximal and distal to the aneurysm and the extent of the aneurysm but may underestimate the aneurysm's diameter because it visualizes only the flow channel and not the surrounding clot.

## Treatment

Usually, an abdominal aneurysm requires resection of the aneurysm and replacement of the damaged aortic section with a Dacron graft. If the aneurysm is small and produces no symptoms, surgery may be delayed; however, small aneurysms may also rupture. Beta blockers may be administered to decrease the rate of growth of the aneurysm. Regular physical examinations and ultrasound checks are necessary to detect enlargement, which may presage a rupture. In asymptomatic patients, surgery is advised when the aneurysm is 2″ to 2.3″(5 to 6 cm) in diameter. In symptomatic patients, repair is indicated regardless of size. In patients with poor distal runoff, external grafting may be done.

## Special considerations

• Monitor vital signs, and type and crossmatch blood.

• Obtain kidney function tests (blood urea nitrogen, creatinine, electrolytes), blood samples (complete blood count with differential), an electrocardiogram and cardiac evaluation, baseline pulmonary function tests, and arterial blood gas (ABG) analysis.

• Be alert for signs of rupture, which may be immediately fatal. Watch closely for any signs of acute blood loss (decreasing blood pressure; increasing pulse and respiratory rates; cool, clammy skin; restlessness; and decreased sensorium).

• If rupture does occur, the first priority is to get the patient to surgery *immediately*. A pneumatic antishock garment may be used while transporting him to surgery. Surgery allows direct compression of the aorta to control hemorrhage. Large amounts of blood may be needed during the resuscitative period to replace blood loss. In such a patient, renal failure due to ischemia is a

major postoperative complication, possibly requiring hemodialysis.

• Before elective surgery, weigh the patient, insert an indwelling urinary catheter and an I.V. line, and assist with insertion of an arterial line and a pulmonary artery catheter to monitor fluid and hemodynamic balance. Give prophylactic antibiotics.

• Explain the surgical procedure and the expected postoperative care in the intensive care unit (ICU) to patients undergoing complex abdominal surgery (I.V. lines, endotracheal [ET] and nasogastric [NG] intubation, mechanical ventilation).

• After surgery, closely monitor vital signs, intake and hourly output, neurologic status (level of consciousness, pupil size, sensation in arms and legs), and ABG levels.

• Assess the depth, rate, and character of respirations and breath sounds at least every hour.

• Watch for signs of bleeding (such as increased pulse and respiratory rates and hypotension), which may occur retro-peritoneally from the graft site. Check abdominal dressings for excessive bleeding or drainage.

• Be alert for fever and other signs of infection.

• After NG intubation for intestinal decompression, irrigate the tube frequently to ensure patency. Record the amount and type of drainage.

• Suction the ET tube often. If the patient can breathe unassisted and has good breath sounds and adequate ABG levels, tidal volume, and vital capacity 24 hours after surgery, he will be extubated and will require oxygen by mask. Weigh the patient daily to evaluate fluid balance.

• Help the patient walk as soon as he's able (generally the 2nd day after surgery).

• Provide psychological support for the patient and family. Help ease their fears about the ICU, the threat of impending rupture, and surgery by providing appropriate explanations and answering all questions.

---

**LIFE-THREATENING DISORDER**

# ANEURYSM, CEREBRAL

---

In cerebral aneurysm, localized dilation of a cerebral artery results from a weakness in the arterial wall. Its most common form is the berry aneurysm, a saclike outpouching in a cerebral artery. Cerebral aneurysms usually arise at an arterial junction in the circle of Willis, the circular anastomosis forming the major cerebral arteries at the base of the brain. Cerebral aneurysms often rupture and cause subarachnoid hemorrhage.

The prognosis is guarded. About half of all patients who suffer a subarachnoid hemorrhage die immediately; of those who survive untreated, 40% die from the effects of hemorrhage and another 20% die later from recurring hemorrhage. With new and better treatment, the prognosis is improving.

## Causes

Cerebral aneurysms may result from a congenital defect, a degenerative process, or a combination of both. For example, hypertension and atherosclerosis may disrupt blood flow and exert pressure against a congenitally weak arterial wall, stretching it like an overblown balloon and making it likely to rupture.

Such a rupture is followed by subarachnoid hemorrhage, in which blood spills into the space normally occupied by cerebrospinal fluid (CSF). Sometimes, blood also spills into brain tissue and subsequently forms a clot. This may result in potentially fatal increased intracranial pressure (ICP) and brain tissue damage.

Incidence is slightly higher in women than in men, especially those in their late 40s or early to middle 50s, but a cerebral aneurysm may occur at any age, in both women and men.

## Signs and symptoms

Occasionally, rupture of a cerebral aneurysm causes premonitory symptoms that last several days, such as headache, nuchal rigidity, stiff back and legs, and intermittent nausea. Usually, however, the rupture occurs abruptly and without warning, causing a sudden severe headache, nausea, vomiting and, depending on the severity and location of bleeding, altered level of consciousness (LOC), including a deep coma.

Bleeding causes meningeal irritation, resulting in nuchal rigidity, back and leg pain, fever, restlessness, irritability, occasional seizures, and blurred vision. Bleeding into the brain tissues causes hemiparesis, hemisensory defects, dysphagia, and visual defects. If the aneurysm is near the internal carotid artery, it compresses the oculomotor nerve and causes diplopia, ptosis, dilated pupil, and inability to rotate the eye.

### Degrees of severity

The severity of symptoms varies from patient to patient, depending on the site and amount of bleeding. To better describe their conditions, patients with ruptured cerebral aneurysms are grouped as follows:

• *Grade I: minimal bleeding.* The patient is alert with no neurologic deficit; he may have a slight headache and nuchal rigidity.

- *Grade II: mild bleeding.* The patient is alert, with a mild to severe headache, nuchal rigidity and, possibly, third-nerve palsy.
- *Grade III: moderate bleeding.* The patient is confused or drowsy, with nuchal rigidity and, possibly, a mild focal deficit.
- *Grade IV: severe bleeding.* The patient is stuporous, with nuchal rigidity and, possibly, mild to severe hemiparesis.
- *Grade V: moribund (often fatal).* If the rupture is nonfatal, the patient is in a deep coma or decerebrate.

### *Life-threatening factors*

Generally, a cerebral aneurysm poses three major threats:

- *Death from increased ICP.* Increased ICP may push the brain downward, impair brain stem function, and cut off blood supply to the part of the brain that supports vital functions.
- *Bleeding episode.* Generally, after the initial bleeding episode, a clot forms and seals the rupture, which reinforces the wall of the aneurysm for 7 to 10 days. However, after the 7th day, fibrinolysis begins to dissolve the clot and increases the risk of rebleeding. This rebleeding produces signs and symptoms similar to those accompanying the initial hemorrhage. Rebleeding episodes during the first 24 hours after the initial hemorrhage aren't uncommon, and they contribute to cerebral aneurysm's high mortality.
- *Vasospasm.* The reason for this complication isn't clearly understood. Usually, vasospasm occurs in blood vessels adjacent to the cerebral aneurysm, but it may extend to major vessels of the brain, causing ischemia and altered brain function.

Other complications of a cerebral aneurysm include acute hydrocephalus (due to abnormal accumulation of CSF

> **CLINICAL TIP**
>
> ## DANGER SIGNALS IN CEREBRAL ANEURYSM
>
> Watch for an enlarging aneurysm, rebleeding, intracranial clot, vasospasm, and other complications. These complications may be heralded by:
>
> - decreased level of consciousness
> - unilateral enlarged pupil
> - onset or worsening of hemiparesis or motor deficit
> - increased blood pressure
> - slowed pulse
> - worsening of headache or sudden onset of a headache
> - renewed or worsened nuchal rigidity
> - renewed or persistent vomiting.
>   Intermittent signs, such as restlessness, extremity weakness, and speech alterations, can also indicate increasing intracranial pressure.

within the cranial cavity because of CSF blockage by blood or adhesions) and pulmonary embolism (a possible adverse effect of deep vein thrombosis or aneurysm treatment). (See *Danger signals in cerebral aneurysm.*)

### Diagnosis

In cerebral aneurysm, diagnosis is based on the patient history; a neurologic examination; a computed tomography (CT) scan, which reveals subarachnoid or ventricular blood; and magnetic resonance imaging or magnetic resonant angiography, which can identify a cerebral aneurysm as a "flow void" or by computer reconstruction of cerebral vessels.

Cerebral angiography remains the procedure of choice for diagnosing a cerebral aneurysm. Lumbar puncture may be used to identify blood in CSF when CT is negative. However, its use is contraindicated in patients with signs of increased ICP.

Other baseline laboratory studies include a complete blood count, urinalysis, arterial blood gas (ABG) analysis, coagulation studies, serum osmolality, and electrolyte and glucose levels.

**Treatment**

The risk of vasospasm and cerebral infarction is reduced by repairing the aneurysm. Usually, surgical repair (by clipping, ligation, or wrapping the aneurysm neck with muscle) takes place 7 to 10 days after the initial hemorrhage; however, surgery performed within 1 to 2 days after the hemorrhage has also shown promise in grade I and II aneurysms.

When surgical correction is risky, when the aneurysm is in a dangerous location, or when surgery is delayed because of vasospasm, treatment includes:
• bed rest in a relaxing environment that allows patients to participate in activities that reduce stress and allow for stabilization of blood pressure (If immediate surgery isn't possible, bed rest may continue for 4 to 6 weeks.)
• avoidance of coffee, other stimulants, and aspirin
• codeine or another analgesic as needed

➤ CLINICAL TIP To avoid the constipating effect of codeine, a stool softener is crucial to prevent straining and resultant rebleeding.

• hydralazine or another antihypertensive agent if the patient is hypertensive
• calcium channel blockers to decrease spasm
• corticosteroids to reduce edema
• phenytoin or another anticonvulsant
• phenobarbital or another sedative

• aminocaproic acid, a fibrinolytic inhibitor, to minimize the risk of rebleeding by delaying blood clot lysis. However, this drug's effectiveness has been disputed.

After surgical repair, the patient's condition depends on the extent of damage from the initial hemorrhage and the degree of success of the treatment of resulting complications. Surgery can't improve the patient's neurologic condition unless it removes a hematoma or reduces the compression effect.

**Special considerations**

• During initial treatment after a hemorrhage, establish and maintain a patent airway because the patient may need supplemental oxygen. Position the patient to promote pulmonary drainage and prevent upper airway obstruction. If he's intubated, preoxygenation with 100% oxygen before suctioning to remove secretions will prevent hypoxia and vasodilation from carbon dioxide accumulation.
• Provide frequent nose and mouth care.
• Institute aneurysm precautions to minimize the risk of rebleeding and to avoid increased ICP. Such precautions include bed rest in a quiet, darkened room (keeping the head of the bed flat or under 30 degrees); limiting visitors; avoidance of caffeine, other stimulants, and strenuous physical activity; and restricted fluid intake. Be sure to explain why these restrictive measures are necessary.
• Turn the patient often. Encourage deep breathing and leg movement. Warn the patient to avoid all unnecessary physical activity. Assist with active range-of-motion (ROM) exercises (unless the doctor has forbidden them); if the patient is paralyzed, perform regular passive ROM exercises.
• Monitor ABG levels, LOC, and vital signs often, and accurately measure intake and output. Avoid taking tempera-

ture rectally because vagus nerve stimulation may cause cardiac arrest.

• Watch for ominous signs of life-threatening complications.

• Give fluids, and monitor I.V. infusions to avoid increased ICP.

• Assess the patient for dysphagia: gurgling voice, coughing, pulmonary secretion, delayed swallow, food pocketing, and cranial nerve dysfunction (V, VII, IX, X, XII).

• Initiate a speech evaluation for assessment and recommendations for maximum safety during feeding, such as positioning, food consistency, and swallow strategies. If the patient is at risk for aspiration, insert a nasogastric or gastric tube.

• If the patient can eat, provide a high-bulk diet (bran, salads, and fruit) to prevent straining during defecation, which can increase ICP.

• Administer a stool softener, such as dioctyl sodium sulfosuccinate, or a mild laxative as needed. *Don't* force fluids. Implement a bowel elimination program based on previous habits. If the patient is receiving steroids, check the stool for blood.

• With weakness of cranial nerve III (impaired lid closure), V (impaired sensation), and VII (impaired tearing), administer artificial tears or ophthalmic ointment to minimize corneal damage. An occlusive metal eye patch may also be needed.

• To minimize stress, give a sedative. Be alert for signs of oversedation. Raise the side rails to help protect the patient from injury. If possible, avoid using restraints because they can cause agitation and raise ICP.

• Administer hydralazine or another antihypertensive if necessary. Carefully monitor blood pressure and be alert for any significant change, especially a rise in systolic pressure. Be careful to avoid activities that may suddenly increase blood pressure.

• Administer aminocaproic acid I.V. in dextrose 5% in water or orally at least every 2 hours to maintain therapeutic blood levels. (Renal insufficiency may require a dosage adjustment.) Monitor the patient for adverse reactions, such as nausea and diarrhea (most common with oral administration) and phlebitis (most common with I.V. administration).

• Reduce deep vein thrombosis by applying antiembolism stockings or sequential compression sleeves.

• If the patient can't speak, establish a simple means of communication, or use cards or a slate. Try to limit conversation to topics that won't further frustrate him. Encourage his family to speak to him in a normal tone, even if he doesn't seem to respond.

• Provide emotional support, and include the patient's family in his care as much as possible. Encourage family members to adopt a realistic attitude, but don't discourage hope.

• Before discharge, refer the patient to a visiting nurse or a rehabilitation center if necessary, and teach the patient and family how to recognize signs of rebleeding.

# ANEURYSMS, FEMORAL AND POPLITEAL

Femoral and popliteal aneurysms result from progressive atherosclerotic changes occurring in the walls (medial layer) of the major peripheral arteries. Aneurysmal formations may be *fusiform* (spindle-shaped) or *saccular* (pouchlike), with fusiform occurring three times more frequently than saccular. They may be single or multiple segmental lesions, often affecting both legs, and may accompany other arterial aneurysms located in the abdominal aorta or iliac arteries.

This condition occurs most frequently in men over age 50. The clinical course is usually progressive, eventually ending in thrombosis, embolization, and gangrene. Elective surgery before complications arise greatly improves the prognosis.

### Causes

Femoral and popliteal aneurysms are usually secondary to atherosclerosis. Rarely, they result from congenital weakness in the arterial wall. They may also result from trauma (blunt or penetrating), bacterial infection, or peripheral vascular reconstructive surgery (which causes "suture line" aneurysms, whereby a blood clot forms a second lumen, also called false aneurysms).

### Signs and symptoms

Popliteal aneurysms may cause pain in the popliteal space when they're large enough to compress the medial popliteal nerve and edema and venous distention if the vein is compressed. Femoral and popliteal aneurysms can produce symptoms of severe ischemia in the leg or foot, due to acute thrombosis within the aneurysmal sac, embolization of mural thrombus fragments and, rarely, rupture.

Symptoms of acute aneurysmal thrombosis include severe pain, loss of pulse and color, coldness in the affected leg or foot, and gangrene. Distal petechial hemorrhages may develop from aneurysmal emboli.

### Diagnosis

In femoral aneurysm, the diagnosis is usually confirmed by bilateral palpation that reveals a pulsating mass above or below the inguinal ligament. When thrombosis has occurred, palpation detects a firm, nonpulsating mass.

Arteriography or ultrasonography may be indicated in doubtful situations. Arteriography may also detect associated aneurysms, especially those in the abdominal aorta and the iliac arteries. Ultrasonography may be helpful in determining the size of the popliteal or femoral aneurysm.

### Treatment

Femoral and popliteal aneurysms require surgical bypass and reconstruction of the artery, usually with an autogenous saphenous vein graft replacement. Arterial occlusion that causes severe ischemia and gangrene may require leg amputation.

### Special considerations

Before corrective surgery:
- Evaluate the patient's circulatory status, noting the location and quality of peripheral pulses in the affected arm or leg.
- Administer prophylactic antibiotics or anticoagulants as needed.
- Discuss expected postoperative procedures with the patient, and review the surgical procedure.

After arterial surgery:
- Monitor carefully for early signs of thrombosis or graft occlusion (loss of pulse, decreased skin temperature and sensation, severe pain) and infection (fever).
- Palpate distal pulses at least every hour for the first 24 hours, then as frequently as needed. Correlate these findings with preoperative circulatory assessment. Mark the sites on the patient's skin where pulses are palpable, to facilitate repeated checks.
- Help the patient walk soon after surgery, to prevent venostasis and possible thrombus formation.

To prepare the patient for discharge:

• Tell the patient to immediately inform the doctor of any recurrence of symptoms because the saphenous vein graft replacement can fail or another aneurysm may develop.

• Explain to the patient with popliteal artery resection that swelling may persist for some time. If antiembolism stockings are prescribed, make sure they fit properly, and teach the patient how to apply them. Warn against wearing constrictive apparel.

• If the patient is receiving anticoagulants, suggest measures to prevent bleeding, such as using an electric razor. Tell the patient to report any signs of bleeding immediately (bleeding gums; black, tarry stool; easy bruising).

• Explain the importance of follow-up blood studies to monitor anticoagulant therapy. Warn the patient to avoid trauma, tobacco, and aspirin.

---

LIFE-THREATENING DISORDER

# ANEURYSM, THORACIC AORTIC

---

Thoracic aortic aneurysm is characterized by an abnormal widening of the ascending, transverse, or descending part of the aorta. Aneurysm of the ascending aorta is most common and most often fatal.

The aneurysm may be *dissecting,* a hemorrhagic separation in the aortic wall, usually within the medial layer; *saccular,* an outpouching of the arterial wall, with a narrow neck; or *fusiform,* a spindle-shaped enlargement encompassing the entire aortic circumference.

Some aneurysms progress to serious and, eventually, lethal complications, such as rupture of an untreated thoracic dissecting aneurysm into the pericardium, with resulting tamponade.

## Causes
Commonly, a thoracic aortic aneurysm results from atherosclerosis, which weakens the aortic wall and gradually distends the lumen. An intimal tear in the ascending aorta initiates a dissecting aneurysm in about 60% of patients.

An ascending aortic aneurysm, the most common type, is usually seen in hypertensive men under age 60. A descending aortic aneurysm, usually found just below the origin of the subclavian artery, is most common in elderly hypertensive men. It's also seen in younger patients with a history of traumatic chest injury; less often in those with infection. A transverse aortic aneurysm is the least common.

Other causes include:
• fungal infection (mycotic aneurysms) of the aortic arch and descending segments
• congenital disorders, such as coarctation of the aorta
• trauma, usually of the descending thoracic aorta, from an accident that shears the aorta transversely (acceleration-deceleration injuries)
• syphilis, usually of the ascending aorta (uncommon because of antibiotics)
• hypertension (in dissecting aneurysm).

## Signs and symptoms
Pain most commonly accompanies a thoracic aortic aneurysm. (See *Clinical characteristics of thoracic dissection,* page 52.) In an ascending aneurysm, the pain is described as severe, boring, and ripping and extends to the neck, shoulders, lower back, and abdomen but rarely radiates to the jaw and arms. Pain is more severe on the right side.

Other signs of an ascending aneurysm may include bradycardia, aortic insufficiency, pericardial friction rub caused

# CLINICAL CHARACTERISTICS OF THORACIC DISSECTION

| ASCENDING AORTA | DESCENDING AORTA | TRANSVERSE AORTA |
|---|---|---|
| **CHARACTER OF PAIN** | | |
| Severe, boring, ripping; extending to neck, shoulders, lower back, and abdomen (rarely to jaw and arms); more severe on right side | Sudden onset, sharp, tearing; usually between the shoulder blades; may radiate to the chest; most diagnostic feature | Sudden onset, sharp, boring, tearing; radiates to shoulders |
| **OTHER SYMPTOMS AND EFFECTS** | | |
| If dissection involves carotid arteries, abrupt onset of neurologic deficit (usually intermittent); bradycardia, aortic insufficiency, and hemopericardium detected by pericardial friction rub; unequal intensity of right and left carotid pulses and radial pulses; difference in blood pressure, especially systolic, between right and left arms | Aortic insufficiency without murmur, hemopericardium, or pleural friction rub; carotid and radial pulses and blood pressure in both arms typically equal | Hoarseness, dyspnea, pain, dysphagia, and dry cough due to compression of surrounding structures |
| **DIAGNOSTIC FEATURES** | | |
| **Chest X-ray** | | |
| Best diagnostic tool; shows widening of mediastinum, enlargement of ascending aorta | Widening of mediastinum; descending aorta larger than ascending section | Shows widening of mediastinum; descending aorta larger than ascending section; widened transverse arch |
| **Aortography** | | |
| False lumen; narrowing of lumen of aorta in ascending section | False lumen; narrowing of lumen of aorta in descending section | False lumen; narrowing of lumen of aorta in transverse arch |
| **TREATMENT** | | |
| A medical emergency that requires immediate, aggressive treatment to reduce blood pressure (usually with nitroprusside or trimethaphan); surgical repair required | Surgical repair required but less urgent than for the ascending dissection; to control hypertension, nitroprusside and propranolol may be used if bradycardia and heart failure are absent | Immediate surgical repair (mortality as high as 50%); control of hypertension |

by a hemopericardium, unequal intensities of the right and left carotid pulses and radial pulses, and a difference in blood pressure between the right and left arms. If dissection involves the carotid arteries, an abrupt onset of neurologic deficits may occur.

In a descending aneurysm, pain usually starts suddenly between the shoulder blades and may radiate to the chest; it's described as sharp and tearing.

A transverse aneurysm causes sudden, sharp, tearing pain radiating to the shoulders. It may also cause hoarseness, dyspnea, dysphagia, and dry cough because of compression of surrounding structures.

### Diagnosis

The patient history, clinical features, and appropriate tests provide diagnostic information. In an asymptomatic patient, diagnosis often occurs accidentally when chest X-rays show widening of the mediastinum. The following other tests help confirm an aneurysm:

• *Aortography,* the definitive test, shows the lumen of the aneurysm, its size and location, and the false lumen in a dissecting aneurysm.

• *Electrocardiography (ECG)* helps distinguish a thoracic aneurysm from myocardial infarction.

• *Echocardiography* may help identify a dissecting aneurysm of the aortic root.

• *Hemoglobin level* may be normal or low because of blood loss from a leaking aneurysm.

• *Computed tomography scan* can confirm and locate the aneurysm and may be used to monitor its progression.

• *Magnetic resonance imaging* may aid diagnosis.

• *Transesophageal echocardiography* is used to measure the aneurysm in both the ascending and the descending aorta.

### Treatment

A dissecting aortic aneurysm is an emergency that requires prompt surgery and stabilizing measures: antihypertensives such as nitroprusside; negative inotropic agents that decrease contractility force, such as propranolol; oxygen for respiratory distress; narcotics for pain; and I.V. fluids and, possibly, whole-blood transfusions.

Surgery consists of resecting the aneurysm, restoring normal blood flow through a Dacron or Teflon graft replacement and, with aortic valve insufficiency, replacing the aortic valve.

Postoperative measures include careful monitoring and continuous assessment in the intensive care unit, antibiotics, endotracheal (ET) intubation, chest tube insertion, ECG monitoring, and pulmonary artery (PA) catheterization.

### Special considerations

• Monitor the patient's blood pressure, pulmonary artery wedge pressure (PAWP), and central venous pressure (CVP). Also evaluate pain, breathing, and carotid, radial, and femoral pulses.

• Review laboratory test results, which must include a complete blood count with differential, electrolyte levels, typing and crossmatching for whole blood, arterial blood gas analysis, and urinalysis.

• Insert an indwelling urinary catheter. Administer dextrose 5% in water or lactated Ringer's solution and antibiotics as needed. Carefully monitor nitroprusside I.V. infusion rate; use a separate I.V. line for infusion. Adjust the dose by slowly increasing the infusion rate. Meanwhile, check blood pressure every 5 minutes until it stabilizes.

• With suspected bleeding from an aneurysm, give a whole-blood transfusion.

• Explain diagnostic tests. If surgery is scheduled, explain the procedure and expected postoperative care (I.V. lines, ET and drainage tubes, cardiac monitoring, ventilation).

After repair of a thoracic aneurysm:
• Evaluate the patient's level of consciousness. Monitor vital signs; PA pressure, PAWP, and CVP; pulse rate; urine output; and pain.
• Check respiratory function. Carefully observe and record type and amount of chest tube drainage, and frequently assess heart and breath sounds.
• Monitor I.V. therapy.
• Give medications as appropriate.
• Watch for signs of infection, especially fever, and excessive wound drainage.
• Assist with range-of-motion exercises of legs to prevent thromboembolism due to venostasis during prolonged bed rest.
• After stabilization of vital signs and respiration, encourage and assist the patient in turning, coughing, and deep breathing. If necessary, provide intermittent positive pressure breathing to promote lung expansion.
• Help the patient walk as soon as he's able.
• Before discharge, ensure adherence to antihypertensive therapy by explaining the need for such drugs and the expected adverse effects. Teach the patient how to monitor his blood pressure.

> **CLINICAL TIP** Refer the patient to community agencies for continued support and assistance as needed.

• Throughout hospitalization, offer the patient and family psychological support.

**LIFE-THREATENING DISORDER**

# ANEURYSM, VENTRICULAR

Ventricular aneurysm is marked by an outpouching (almost always of the left ventricle) that produces ventricular wall dysfunction in 10% to 20% of patients after myocardial infarction (MI). A ventricular aneurysm may develop within weeks after MI, usually following anterior P wave infarctions.

An untreated ventricular aneurysm can lead to arrhythmias, systemic embolization, or heart failure and may cause sudden death. Resection improves the prognosis in heart failure and in patients with refractory ventricular arrhythmias.

## Causes

When MI destroys a large muscular section of the left ventricle, necrosis reduces the ventricular wall to a thin sheath of fibrous tissue. Under intracardiac pressure, this thin layer stretches and forms a separate noncontractile sac (aneurysm).

### Abnormal muscle wall movement

Accompanying ventricular aneurysm, abnormal muscle wall movement includes akinesia (lack of movement), dyskinesia (paradoxical movement), asynergia (decreased and inadequate movement), and asynchrony (uncoordinated movement).

During systolic ejection, the abnormal muscle wall movements associated with the aneurysm cause the remaining normally functioning myocardial fibers to increase the force of contraction in order to maintain stroke volume and cardiac output. At the same time, a portion of the stroke volume is lost to passive distention of the noncontractile sac.

## Signs and symptoms

A ventricular aneurysm may cause arrhythmias (such as premature ventricular contractions and ventricular tachycardia), palpitations, signs of cardiac dysfunction (weakness on exertion, fatigue, angina) and, occasionally, a visible or palpable systolic precordial bulge.

This condition may also lead to left ventricular dysfunction, with chronic heart failure (dyspnea, fatigue, edema, crackles, gallop rhythm, neck vein distention); pulmonary edema; systemic embolization; and, with left-sided heart failure, pulsus alternans. Ventricular aneurysms enlarge but rarely rupture.

## Diagnosis

Persistent ventricular arrhythmias, onset of heart failure, or systemic embolization in a patient with left-sided heart failure and a history of MI strongly suggests a ventricular aneurysm. Indicative tests include the following:

• *Left ventriculography* reveals left ventricular enlargement with an area of akinesia or dyskinesia (during cineangiography) and diminished cardiac function.

• *Electrocardiography* may show persistent ST-T wave elevations after MI.

• *Chest X-ray* may demonstrate an abnormal bulge distorting the heart's contour if the aneurysm is large; the X-ray may be normal if the aneurysm is small.

• *Noninvasive nuclear cardiology scan* may indicate the site of infarction and suggest the area of aneurysm.

• *Echocardiography* shows abnormal motion in the left ventricular wall.

## Treatment

Depending on the size of the aneurysm and the complications, treatment may require only routine medical examination to follow the patient's condition or aggressive measures for intractable ventricular arrhythmias, heart failure, and emboli.

Emergency treatment of ventricular arrhythmias consists of antiarrhythmics I.V. or cardioversion. Preventive treatment continues with oral antiarrhythmics, such as procainamide, quinidine, and amiodarone.

Emergency treatment for heart failure with pulmonary edema includes oxygen, digitalis glycosides I.V., furosemide I.V., morphine sulfate I.V. and, when necessary, nitroprusside I.V. and intubation. Maintenance therapy may include oral nitrates and an angiotensin-converting enzyme inhibitor such as captopril or enalapril maleate (Vasotec).

Systemic embolization requires anticoagulation therapy or embolectomy.

Refractory ventricular tachycardia, heart failure, recurrent arterial embolization, and persistent angina with coronary artery occlusion may require surgery; the most effective procedure is aneurysmectomy with myocardial revascularization.

## Special considerations

• If ventricular tachycardia occurs, monitor blood pressure and heart rate. If sustained ventricular tachycardia occurs, administer lidocaine I.V.

• If cardiac arrest develops, initiate cardiopulmonary resuscitation (CPR) and call for assistance, resuscitative equipment, and medication.

• In a patient with heart failure, closely monitor vital signs, heart sounds, intake and output, fluid and electrolyte balances, and blood urea nitrogen and creatinine levels.

• Because of the threat of systemic embolization, frequently check peripheral pulses and the color and temperature of extremities. Be alert for sudden changes in sensorium that indicate cerebral embolization and for any signs that suggest renal failure or progressive MI.

• If the patient is conscious and requires cardioversion, give diazepam I.V. as needed before cardioversion. Explain that cardioversion is a lifesaving procedure that provides brief electric shocks to the heart.

• If the patient is receiving antiarrhythmics, check appropriate laboratory tests. For instance, if the patient takes procainamide, check antinuclear antibodies because this drug may induce symptoms that mimic those of lupus erythematosus.

If the patient is scheduled to undergo resection:

• Before surgery, explain expected postoperative care in the intensive care unit (including use of such things as endotracheal tube, ventilator, hemodynamic monitoring, chest tubes, and drainage bottle).

• After surgery, monitor vital signs, intake and output, heart sounds, and pulmonary artery pressures. Watch for signs of infection, such as fever and purulent drainage.

• Teach the patient to report light-headedness or dizziness, which may indicate arrhythmia. Encourage him to follow his prescribed medication regimen — even during the night — and to watch for adverse reactions.

• Because arrhythmias can cause sudden death, refer the family to a community-based CPR training program.

• Provide psychological support for the patient and his family.

# ANKYLOSING SPONDYLITIS

A chronic, usually progressive inflammatory disease, ankylosing spondylitis (AS) primarily affects the sacroiliac, apophyseal, and costovertebral joints and adjacent soft tissue. Generally, the disease begins in the sacroiliac joints and gradually progresses to the lumbar, thoracic, and cervical regions of the spine. Deterioration of bone and cartilage can lead to fibrous tissue formation and eventual fusion of the spine or peripheral joints.

Prevalence of AS among whites is estimated at 0.5% to 1.0%, affecting five times as many males as females. Progressive disease is well recognized in men, but the diagnosis is often overlooked or missed in women, who tend to have more peripheral joint involvement. Secondary AS may be associated with reactive arthritis (Reiter's syndrome), psoriatic arthritis, or inflammatory bowel disease. These disorders, together with primary AS, are often classified as seronegative spondyloarthropathies.

## Causes
Recent evidence strongly suggests a familial tendency in AS. The presence of histocompatibility antigen HLA-B27 (positive in over 90% of patients with this disease) and circulating immune complexes suggests immunologic activity. A possible link to underlying infection is being investigated.

## Signs and symptoms
The first indication is intermittent low back pain that's usually most severe in the morning or after a period of inac-

tivity. Other symptoms depend on the disease stage and may include:

• stiffness and limited motion of the lumbar spine

➤ CLINICAL TIP To test for lumbar mobility, perform the Schober test: With the patient standing erect, make a pen mark over the lumbar spine at L5 (even with the dimples of Venus). Measure 1½″ (10 cm) upward along the spine and make a second mark. Then ask the patient to bend forward as far as he can while keeping his knees straight. Measure the distance between the two marks while the patient is flexed. In normal lumbar mobility, the distance between the marks should increase by at least 2⅜″ (15 cm).

• pain and limited expansion of the chest due to involvement of the costovertebral joints

• peripheral arthritis involving shoulders, hips, and knees

• kyphosis in advanced stages, caused by chronic stooping to relieve symptoms, and hip deformity and associated limited range of motion (ROM)

• tenderness over the site of inflammation

• pain or tenderness at tendon insertion sites (enthesitis), especially the Achilles or patellar tendon

• mild fatigue, fever, anorexia, or loss of weight; unilateral acute anterior uveitis; aortic insufficiency and cardiomegaly; upper lobe pulmonary fibrosis (mimics tuberculosis)

• severe neurologic complications, such as cauda equina syndrome and paralysis, which can occur secondary to fracture of a rigid cervical spine or C1-C2 subluxation.

These symptoms progress unpredictably, and the disease can go into remission, exacerbation, or arrest at any stage.

### Diagnosis

Typical symptoms, a family history, and the presence of HLA-B27 strongly suggest AS. However, confirmation requires these characteristic X-ray findings:

• blurring of the bony margins of joints in the early stage

• bilateral sacroiliac involvement

• patchy sclerosis with superficial bony erosions

• eventual squaring of vertebral bodies

• "bamboo spine" with complete ankylosis.

Erythrocyte sedimentation rate and alkaline phosphatase and creatine kinase levels may be slightly elevated. A negative rheumatoid factor helps rule out rheumatoid arthritis, which produces similar symptoms.

### Treatment

Because AS's progression can't be stopped, treatment aims to delay further deformity by good posture, stretching and deep-breathing exercises and, in some patients, braces and lightweight supports. Patients must understand that a long-term daily exercise program is essential to delaying loss of function. Anti-inflammatory analgesics, such as aspirin, indomethacin, sulfasalazine, and sulindac, are given to control pain and inflammation.

Severe hip involvement usually necessitates surgical hip replacement. Severe spinal involvement may require a spinal wedge osteotomy to separate and reposition the vertebrae. This surgery is performed only on selected patients because of the risk of spinal cord damage and the long convalescence involved.

### Special considerations

• AS can be an extremely painful and crippling disease, so the caregiver's main responsibility is to promote the patient's comfort while preserving as much mobility as possible. Keep in mind that his limited ROM makes simple tasks difficult. Offer support and reassurance.

• Administer medications as needed.

• Apply local heat and provide massage to relieve pain. Assess mobility and degree of discomfort frequently.

• Teach and assist with daily exercises as needed to maintain strength and function. Stress the importance of maintaining good posture.

• If treatment includes surgery, provide good postoperative care.

• Because AS is a chronic, progressively crippling condition, comprehensive treatment should also reflect counsel from a social worker, visiting nurse, and dietitian.

To minimize deformities, advise the patient to:

• avoid any physical activity that places undue stress on the back, such as lifting heavy objects

• stand upright; sit upright in a high, straight chair; and avoid leaning over a desk

• sleep in a prone position on a hard mattress and avoid using pillows under the neck or knees

• avoid prolonged walking, standing, sitting, and driving

• perform regular stretching and deep-breathing exercises and swim regularly, if possible

• have height measured every 3 to 4 months to detect any tendency toward kyphosis

• seek vocational counseling if his work requires standing or prolonged sitting at a desk

• contact the local Arthritis Foundation chapter for a support group.

# ANOREXIA NERVOSA

The key feature of anorexia nervosa is self-imposed starvation resulting from a distorted body image and an intense and irrational fear of gaining weight, even when the patient is obviously emaciated. An anorexic patient is preoccupied with her body size, describes herself as "fat," and commonly expresses dissatisfaction with a particular aspect of her physical appearance.

Although the term anorexia suggests that the patient's weight loss is associated with a loss of appetite, this is rare. Anorexia nervosa and bulimia nervosa can occur simultaneously. In anorexia nervosa, the refusal to eat may be accompanied by compulsive exercising, self-induced vomiting, or abuse of laxatives or diuretics.

Anorexia occurs in 5% to 10% of the population; about 95% of those affected are women. This disorder occurs primarily in adolescents and young adults but also may affect older women. The occurrence among males is rising.

The prognosis varies but improves if the patient is diagnosed early or if she wants to overcome the disorder and seeks help voluntarily. Mortality ranges from 5% to 15% — the highest mortality associated with a psychiatric disturbance. One-third of these deaths can be attributed to suicide.

## Causes

No one knows what causes anorexia nervosa. Researchers in neuroendocrinology are seeking a physiologic cause but have found nothing definite. Clearly, social attitudes that equate slimness with beauty play some role in provoking this disorder; family factors also are implicated. Most theorists believe that refusing to eat is a subconscious effort to exert personal control over one's life.

## Signs and symptoms

The patient's history usually reveals a 25% or greater weight loss for no organic reason, coupled with a morbid dread of being fat and a compulsion to be thin. Such a patient tends to be angry and ritualistic. She may report amenorrhea, infertility, loss of libido, fatigue, sleep alterations, intolerance to cold, and constipation.

Hypotension and bradycardia may be present. Inspection may reveal an emaciated appearance, with skeletal muscle atrophy, loss of fatty tissue, atrophy of breast tissue, blotchy or sallow skin, lanugo on the face and body, and dryness or loss of scalp hair. Calluses on the knuckles and abrasions and scars on the dorsum of the hand may result from tooth injury during self-induced vomiting. Other signs of vomiting include dental caries and oral or pharyngeal abrasions.

Palpation may disclose painless salivary gland enlargement and bowel distention. Slowed reflexes may occur on percussion. Oddly, the patient usually demonstrates hyperactivity and vigor (despite malnourishment) and may exercise avidly without apparent fatigue.

### Psychosocial assessment

During psychosocial assessment, the anorexic patient may express a morbid fear of gaining weight and an obsession with her physical appearance. Paradoxically, she also may be obsessed with food, preparing elaborate meals for others. Social regression, including poor sexual adjustment and fear of failure, is common. Like bulimia nervosa, anorexia nervosa often is associated with depression. The patient may report feel-

---

### DIAGNOSING ANOREXIA NERVOSA

A diagnosis of anorexia nervosa is made when the patient meets the following criteria from the *Diagnostic and Statistical Manual of Mental Disorders*, 4th ed.:

• refusal to maintain body weight over a minimal normal weight for age and height (for instance, weight loss leading to maintenance of body weight 15% below that expected); or failure to achieve expected weight gain during a growth period, leading to a body weight 15% below that expected
• intense fear of gaining weight or becoming fat, despite underweight status
• a distorted perception of body weight, size, or shape (that is, the person claims to feel fat even when emaciated or believes that one body area is too fat even when it's obviously underweight)
• in women, absence of at least three consecutive menses when otherwise expected to occur.

---

ings of despair, hopelessness, and worthlessness as well as suicidal thoughts.

## Diagnosis

For characteristic findings in patients with this condition, see *Diagnosing anorexia nervosa*.

In addition, laboratory tests help to identify various disorders and deficiencies and help to rule out endocrine, metabolic, and central nervous system abnormalities; cancer; malabsorption syndrome; and other disorders that cause physical wasting.

Abnormal findings that may accompany a weight loss exceeding 30% of normal body weight include:
• low hemoglobin level, platelet count, and white blood cell count

- prolonged bleeding time due to thrombocytopenia
- decreased erythrocyte sedimentation rate
- decreased levels of serum creatinine, blood urea nitrogen, uric acid, cholesterol, total protein, albumin, sodium, potassium, chloride, calcium, and fasting blood glucose (resulting from malnutrition)
- elevated levels of alanine aminotransferase and aspartate aminotransferase in severe starvation states
- elevated serum amylase levels when pancreatitis isn't present
- in females, decreased levels of serum luteinizing hormone and follicle-stimulating hormone
- decreased triiodothyronine levels resulting from a lower basal metabolic rate
- dilute urine caused by the kidneys' impaired ability to concentrate urine
- nonspecific ST interval, prolonged PR interval, and T-wave changes on the electrocardiogram. Ventricular arrhythmias also may be present.

### Treatment

Appropriate treatment aims to promote weight gain or control the patient's compulsive binge eating and purging and to correct malnutrition and the underlying psychological dysfunction. Hospitalization in a medical or psychiatric unit may be required to improve the patient's precarious physical condition. The facility stay may be as brief as 2 weeks or may stretch from a few months to 2 years or longer.

#### A team approach

The most effective treatment in anorexia combines aggressive medical management, nutritional counseling, and individual, group, or family psychotherapy or behavior modification therapy. Treatment results may be discouraging.

Many clinical centers are now developing inpatient and outpatient programs specifically aimed at managing eating disorders.

Treatment may include behavior modification (privileges depend on weight gain); curtailed activity for physical reasons (such as arrhythmias); vitamin and mineral supplements; a reasonable diet with or without liquid supplements; subclavian, peripheral, or enteral hyperalimentation (enteral and peripheral routes carry less risk of infection); and group, family, or individual psychotherapy.

All forms of psychotherapy, from psychoanalysis to hypnotherapy, have been used in treating anorexia nervosa, with varying success. To be successful, psychotherapy should address the underlying problems of low self-esteem, guilt, anxiety, feelings of hopelessness and helplessness, and depression.

### Special considerations

- During hospitalization, regularly monitor vital signs, nutritional status, and intake and output. Weigh the patient daily—before breakfast if possible. Because the patient fears being weighed, vary the weighing routine. Keep in mind that weight should increase from morning to night.
- Help the patient establish a target weight, and support her efforts to achieve this goal.
- Negotiate an adequate food intake with the patient. Make sure she understands that she'll need to comply with this contract or lose privileges. Frequently offer small portions of food or drinks if the patient wants them. Allow the patient to maintain control over the types and amounts of food she eats, if possible.
- Maintain one-on-one supervision of the patient during meals and for 1 hour afterward to ensure compliance with the

dietary treatment program. For the hospitalized anorexic patient, food is considered a medication.

• During an acute anorexic episode, nutritionally complete liquids are more acceptable than solid food because they eliminate the need to choose between foods — something the anorexic patient often finds difficult.

• If tube feedings or other special feeding measures become necessary, fully explain these measures to the patient and be ready to discuss her fears or reluctance; limit the discussion about food itself.

• Anticipate a weight gain of about 1 lb (0.5 kg) per week.

• If edema or bloating occurs after the patient has returned to normal eating behavior, reassure her that this phenomenon is temporary. She may fear that she's becoming fat and stop complying with the prescribed treatment.

• Encourage the patient to recognize and express her feelings freely. If she understands that she can be assertive, she gradually may learn that expressing her true feelings won't result in her losing control or love.

• If a patient receiving outpatient treatment must be hospitalized, maintain contact with her treatment team to facilitate a smooth return to the outpatient setting.

➤ CLINICAL TIP  Remember that the anorexic patient uses exercise, preoccupation with food, ritualism, manipulation, and lying as mechanisms to preserve the only control she thinks that she has in her life.

• Because the patient and her family may need therapy to uncover and correct dysfunctional patterns, refer them to Anorexia Nervosa and Related Eating Disorders, a national information and support organization. This organization may help them understand what anorexia is, convince them that they need help, and help them find a psychotherapist or medical doctor who is experienced in treating this disorder.

• Teach the patient how to keep a food journal, including the types of food eaten, eating frequency, and feelings associated with eating and exercise.

• Advise family members to avoid discussing food with the patient.

# ANXIETY DISORDER, GENERALIZED

Anxiety is a feeling of apprehension that some describe as an exaggerated sensation of impending doom, dread, or uneasiness. Unlike fear — a reaction to danger from a specific external source — anxiety is a reaction to an internal threat, such as an unacceptable impulse or a repressed thought that is straining to reach a conscious level.

A rational response to a real threat, occasional anxiety is a normal part of life. Overwhelming anxiety, however, can result in generalized anxiety disorder — uncontrollable, unreasonable worry that persists for at least 6 months and narrows perceptions or interferes with normal functioning. Recent evidence indicates that the incidence of generalized anxiety disorder is greater than previously thought and may be even greater than that of depression.

## Causes

Theorists share a common premise: Conflict, whether intrapsychic, sociopersonal, or interpersonal, promotes an anxiety state.

## Signs and symptoms

Generalized anxiety disorder can begin at any age but typically has an onset in the 20s and 30s. It's equally common in

## DIAGNOSING GENERALIZED ANXIETY DISORDER

When the patient's symptoms match criteria documented in the *Diagnostic and Statistical Manual of Mental Disorders,* 4th ed., the diagnosis of generalized anxiety disorder is confirmed. The criteria include the following:

• Excessive anxiety and worry about a number of events or activities occur more days than not for at least 6 months.
• The patient has difficulty in controlling the worry.
• The anxiety and worry are associated with at least three of the following six symptoms:
– restlessness or feeling keyed up or on edge
– being easily fatigued
– difficulty concentrating or mind going blank
– irritability
– muscle tension
– sleep disturbances (difficulty falling or staying asleep, or restless, unsatisfying sleep).
• The focus of the anxiety and worry isn't confined to features of an Axis I disorder.
• The anxiety, worry, or physical symptoms cause clinically significant distress or impairment in social, occupational, or other important areas of functioning.
• The disturbance is not due to the direct physiologic effects of a substance or a general medical condition and does not occur exclusively during a mood disorder, a psychotic disorder, or a pervasive developmental disorder.

toms, with unusual self-awareness and alertness to the environment. Moderate anxiety leads to selective inattention but with the ability to concentrate on a single task. Severe anxiety causes an inability to concentrate on more than scattered details of a task. A panic state with acute anxiety causes a complete loss of concentration, often with unintelligible speech.

Physical examination of the patient with generalized anxiety disorder may reveal symptoms of motor tension, including trembling, muscle aches and spasms, headaches, and an inability to relax. Autonomic signs and symptoms include shortness of breath, tachycardia, sweating, and abdominal complaints.

In addition, the patient may startle easily and complain of feeling apprehensive, fearful, or angry and of having difficulty concentrating, eating, and sleeping. The medical, psychiatric, and psychosocial histories fail to identify a specific physical or environmental cause of the anxiety.

### Diagnosis

For characteristic findings in patients with this condition, see *Diagnosing generalized anxiety disorder.*

In addition, laboratory tests must exclude organic causes of the patient's signs and symptoms, such as hyperthyroidism, pheochromocytoma, coronary artery disease, supraventricular tachycardia, and Ménière's disease. For example, an electrocardiogram can rule out myocardial ischemia in a patient who complains of chest pain. Blood tests, including a complete blood count, white blood cell count and differential, and serum lactate and calcium levels, can rule out hypocalcemia.

Because anxiety is the central feature of other mental disorders, psychiatric evaluation must rule out phobias, ob-

men and women. Psychological or physiologic symptoms of anxiety states vary with the degree of anxiety. Mild anxiety mainly causes psychological symp-

sessive-compulsive disorders, depression, and acute schizophrenia.

### Treatment

A combination of drug therapy and psychotherapy may help a patient with generalized anxiety disorder. The benzodiazepine antianxiety drugs may relieve mild anxiety and improve the patient's ability to cope. They should be used cautiously due to their addictive nature. Tricyclic antidepressants or higher doses of benzodiazepines may relieve the patient of severe anxiety and panic attacks. Buspirone, an antianxiety drug, causes the patient less sedation and poses less risk of physical and psychological dependence than the benzodiazepines.

Psychotherapy for generalized anxiety disorder has two goals: helping the patient identify and deal with the underlying emotional and psychological issues and eliminating environmental factors that precipitate an anxious reaction. In addition, the patient can learn relaxation techniques, such as deep breathing, progressive muscle relaxation, focused relaxation, and visualization.

### Special considerations

• Stay with the patient when he's anxious, and encourage him to discuss his feelings. Reduce environmental stimuli and remain calm.

**CLINICAL TIP**   Reassure the patient that he's safe and can be helped.

• Administer antianxiety drugs or tricyclic antidepressants as prescribed, and evaluate the patient's response to these drugs.

• Emphasize the need for compliance with the medication regimen. Review potential adverse reactions with the patient. (See *Preventing anxiety attacks.*)

• Teach the patient effective coping strategies and relaxation techniques.

---

**TEACHING CHECKLIST**

## PREVENTING ANXIETY ATTACKS

To help the patient avoid anxiety attacks, review the following points.

• Take any prescribed medication as ordered.
• Attend therapy sessions regularly.
• Practice relaxation exercises.
• Identify support systems, such as family and friends.

---

• Help the patient identify stressful situations that trigger his anxiety, and provide him with positive reinforcement when he uses alternative coping strategies.

# APLASTIC AND HYPOPLASTIC ANEMIAS

Aplastic and hypoplastic anemias result from injury to or destruction of stem cells in bone marrow or the bone marrow matrix, causing pancytopenia (anemia, granulocytopenia, thrombocytopenia) and bone marrow hypoplasia. Although often used interchangeably with other terms for bone marrow failure, aplastic anemias properly refer to pancytopenia resulting from the decreased functional capacity of a hypoplastic, fatty bone marrow.

These disorders generally produce fatal bleeding or infection, particularly when they're idiopathic or stem from the use of chloramphenicol or from infectious hepatitis. Mortality for aplastic anemias with severe pancytopenia is 80% to 90%.

# UNDERSTANDING BONE MARROW TRANSPLANTATION

In bone marrow transplantation, usually 500 to 700 ml of marrow are aspirated from the pelvic bones of a human leukocyte antigen (HLA)-compatible donor (allogeneic) or of the recipient himself during periods of complete remission (autologous). The aspirated marrow is filtered and then infused into the recipient in an attempt to repopulate the patient's marrow with normal cells.

This procedure has effected long-term, healthy survivals in about half of the patients with severe aplastic anemia. Bone marrow transplantation may also be effective in treating patients with acute leukemia, certain immunodeficiency diseases, and solid-tumor cancers.

Because bone marrow transplantation carries serious risks, it requires strict adherence to infection protection techniques and strict aseptic technique and a primary caregiver to provide consistent care and continuous monitoring of the patient's status.

**Before bone marrow infusion**
• Explain that the success rate depends on the stage of the disease and on finding an HLA-identical sibling match.
• After bone marrow aspiration is completed under local anesthetic, apply pressure dressings to the *donor's* aspiration sites. Observe the sites for bleeding. Relieve pain with analgesics and ice packs as needed.
• Assess the patient's understanding of bone marrow transplantation. If necessary, correct any misconceptions about this procedure, and provide additional information. Prepare the patient to expect an extended hospital stay. Explain that chemotherapy and, possibly, radiation therapy are necessary to remove cells that may cause the body to reject the transplant.
• Various treatment protocols are used. For example, I.V. cyclophosphamide may be used with additional chemotherapeutic agents or total-body irradiation and requires aggressive hydration to prevent hemorrhagic cystitis. Control nausea and vomiting with an antiemet-

## Causes

Aplastic anemias usually develop when damaged or destroyed stem cells inhibit red blood cell (RBC) production. Less commonly, they develop when damaged bone marrow microvasculature creates an unfavorable environment for cell growth and maturation. About half of such anemias result from drugs (antibiotics, anticonvulsants), toxic agents (such as benzene and chloramphenicol), or radiation. The rest may result from immunologic factors (unconfirmed), severe disease (especially hepatitis), or preleukemic and neoplastic infiltration of bone marrow. (See *Understanding bone marrow transplantation*.)

Idiopathic anemias may be congenital and account for about 50% of all confirmed occurrences. Two such forms of aplastic anemia have been identified: congenital hypoplastic anemia (Blackfan-Diamond anemia), which develops between ages 2 months and 3 months, and Fanconi's syndrome, which develops between birth and age 10.

In Fanconi's syndrome, chromosomal abnormalities are typically associated with multiple congenital anomalies — such as dwarfism and hypoplasia of the kidneys and spleen. In the absence of a consistent familial or genetic history of aplastic anemia, researchers suspect that these congenital

ic, such as ondansetron, prochlorperazine, or metoclopramide, as needed. Give allopurinol, as prescribed, to prevent hyperuricemia resulting from tumor breakdown products. Because alopecia is a common adverse effect of high-dose cyclophosphamide therapy, encourage the patient to choose a wig or scarf before treatment begins.

● Total-body irradiation (in one dose or several daily doses) follows chemotherapy, inducing total marrow aplasia. Warn the patient that cataracts, GI disturbances, and sterility are possible adverse effects.

### During bone marrow infusion
● Monitor vital signs every 15 minutes.
● Watch for complications of marrow infusion, such as pulmonary embolus and volume overload.
● Reassure the patient throughout the procedure.

### After bone marrow infusion
● Continue to monitor the patient's vital signs every 15 minutes for 2 hours after infusion, then every 4 hours. Watch for fever and chills, which may be the only signs of infection. Give prophylactic antibiotics, as prescribed. To reduce the possibility of bleeding, don't administer medications rectally or I.M.

● Administer methotrexate or cyclosporine, as prescribed, to prevent graft-versus-host (GVH) reaction, a potentially fatal complication of allogeneic transplantation. Watch for signs of GVH reaction, such as maculopapular rash, pancytopenia, jaundice, joint pain, and anasarca.

● Administer vitamins, steroids, and iron and folic acid supplements as appropriate. Administration of blood products, such as platelets and packed red blood cells, may also be indicated, depending on the results of daily blood studies.

● Provide good mouth care every 2 hours. Use hydrogen peroxide and nystatin mouthwash or oral fluconazole, for example, to prevent candidiasis and other mouth infections.

● Also provide meticulous skin care, paying special attention to pressure points and open sites, such as aspiration and I.V. sites.

---

abnormalities result from an induced change in the development of the fetus.

### Signs and symptoms
Clinical features of aplastic anemias vary with the severity of pancytopenia but often develop insidiously. Anemic symptoms include progressive weakness and fatigue, shortness of breath, headache, pallor and, ultimately, tachycardia and heart failure. Thrombocytopenia leads to ecchymosis, petechiae, and hemorrhage, especially from the mucous membranes (nose, gums, rectum, vagina) or into the retina or central nervous system. Neutropenia may lead to infection (fever, oral and rectal ulcers, sore throat) but without characteristic inflammation.

### Diagnosis
Confirmation of aplastic anemia requires a series of laboratory tests:
● *RBCs* are usually normochromic and normocytic (although macrocytosis [larger-than-normal erythrocytes] and anisocytosis [excessive variation in erythrocyte size] may exist), with a total count of $1,000,000/\mu l$ or less. *Absolute reticulocyte count* is very low.

● *Serum iron* is elevated (unless bleeding occurs), but total iron-binding capacity is normal or slightly reduced. Hemosiderin is present, and tissue iron storage is visible microscopically.

- *Platelet, neutrophil,* and *white blood cell counts* fall.
- *Coagulation tests* (bleeding time), reflecting decreased platelet count, are abnormal.
- *Bone marrow aspiration* from several sites may yield a "dry tap," and a biopsy will show severely hypocellular or aplastic marrow, with varied amounts of fat, fibrous tissue, or gelatinous replacement; absence of tagged iron (because iron is deposited in the liver rather than in bone marrow) and megakaryocytes; and depression of erythroid elements.

A differential diagnosis must rule out paroxysmal nocturnal hemoglobinuria and other diseases in which pancytopenia is common.

## Treatment

Identifiable causes must be eliminated and vigorous supportive measures must be provided, such as transfusions of packed RBCs, platelets, and experimental human leukocyte antigen-matched leukocytes. Even after elimination of the cause, recovery can take months. Bone marrow transplantation is the treatment of choice for anemia due to severe aplasia and for patients who need constant RBC transfusions.

### Preventing infection

Patients with low leukocyte counts need special measures to prevent infection. The infection itself may require specific antibiotics; however, they aren't given prophylactically because they tend to encourage resistant strains of organisms. Patients with low hemoglobin (Hb) levels may need respiratory support with oxygen, in addition to blood transfusions.

### Other treatments

Other appropriate treatments include corticosteroids to stimulate erythroid production; marrow-stimulating agents, such as androgens (which are controversial); antilymphocyte globulin (experimental); immunosuppressants (if the patient doesn't respond to other therapy); and colony-stimulating factors to encourage growth of specific cellular components.

## Special considerations

- If the platelet count is low (> 20,000/μl), prevent hemorrhage by avoiding I.M. injections, suggesting the use of an electric razor and a soft toothbrush, humidifying oxygen to prevent drying of mucous membranes, and promoting regular bowel movements through the use of a stool softener and a proper diet to prevent constipation.
- Apply pressure to venipuncture sites until bleeding stops. Detect bleeding early by checking for blood in the urine and stool and assessing the skin for petechiae.
- Help prevent infection by washing your hands thoroughly before entering the patient's room, by making sure the patient is receiving a nutritious diet (high in vitamins and proteins) to improve his resistance, and by encouraging meticulous mouth and perianal care.
- Watch for life-threatening hemorrhage, infection, adverse reactions to drug therapy, and blood transfusion reaction.
- Make sure routine throat, urine, nose, rectal, and blood cultures are done regularly and correctly to check for infection. Teach the patient to recognize signs of infection, and tell him to report them immediately.
- If the patient's Hb level is low, which causes fatigue, schedule frequent rest periods.

• Administer oxygen therapy as needed.

• If blood transfusions are necessary, be alert for a transfusion reaction by checking the patient's temperature and watching for other signs, such as rash, hives, itching, back pain, restlessness, and shaking chills.

• Reassure and support the patient and family by explaining the disease and its treatment, particularly if the patient has recurring acute episodes. Explain the purpose of all prescribed drugs, and discuss possible adverse reactions, including which ones should be reported promptly.

• Encourage the patient who doesn't require hospitalization to continue his normal lifestyle, with appropriate restrictions (such as regular rest periods), until remission occurs.

• To prevent aplastic anemia, monitor blood studies carefully in the patient receiving anemia-inducing drugs.

• Support efforts to educate the public about the hazards of toxic agents. Tell parents to keep toxic agents out of the reach of children.

• Encourage people who work with radiation to wear protective clothing and a radiation-detecting badge and to observe plant safety precautions.

**CLINICAL TIP** Those who work with the solvent benzene should know that 10 ppm is the highest safe environmental level and that a delayed reaction to benzene may develop.

# APPENDICITIS

The most common abdominal surgical disease, appendicitis is inflammation of the vermiform appendix due to an obstruction. Appendicitis may occur at any age and affects both sexes equally, usually between puberty and age 30. Since the advent of antibiotics, the incidence and the death rate of appendicitis have declined. If left untreated, gangrene and perforation develop within 36 hours.

## Causes
Appendicitis probably results from an obstruction of the intestinal lumen caused by a fecal mass, stricture, barium ingestion, or viral infection. This obstruction sets off an inflammatory process that can lead to infection, thrombosis, necrosis, and perforation. If the appendix ruptures or perforates, the infected contents spill into the abdominal cavity, causing peritonitis, the most common and most perilous complication of appendicitis.

## Signs and symptoms
Appendicitis usually begins with generalized or localized colicky periumbilical or epigastric pain, followed by anorexia, nausea, and a few episodes of vomiting. Pain eventually localizes in the lower right abdomen (McBurney's point) with abdominal "boardlike" rigidity, retractive respirations, increasing tenderness, increasingly severe abdominal spasms and, almost invariably, rebound tenderness. (Rebound tenderness on the opposite side of the abdomen suggests peritoneal inflammation.)

Later symptoms include constipation (although diarrhea is also possible), slight fever, and tachycardia. Sudden cessation of abdominal pain indicates a perforation or infarction of the appendix. The elderly patient may present with minimal, vague symptoms and mild abdominal tenderness, delaying diagnosis of appendicitis.

**CLINICAL TIP** When asked to cough, patients may be able to precisely localize a painful area. This is a sign of peritoneal irritation.

## Diagnosis

Physical findings and characteristic clinical symptoms allow diagnosis of appendicitis. Findings that support the diagnosis include a temperature of 99° to 102° F (37.2° to 38.9° C) and a moderately elevated white blood cell count (12,000 to 20,000/µl), with increased immature cells.

The diagnosis must rule out illnesses with similar symptoms: gastritis, gastroenteritis, ileitis, colitis, diverticulitis, pancreatitis, renal colic, bladder infection, and gynecologic disorders, such as ovarian cyst, acute salpingitis, and tubo-ovarian abscess.

Imaging studies aren't necessary in patients with a typical presentation of appendicitis.

## Treatment

Appendectomy is the only effective treatment. Laparoscopic appendectomies, which decrease the recovery time and the facility stay, are now performed. If peritonitis develops, treatment involves GI intubation, parenteral replacement of fluids and electrolytes, and administration of antibiotics.

## Special considerations

• Administer I.V. fluids to prevent dehydration. *Never* administer cathartics or enemas, which may rupture the appendix.
• Provide the patient with nothing by mouth.
• Administer systemic antibiotics to reduce postoperative wound infection.
• To lessen pain, place the patient in Fowler's position. *Never* apply heat to the patient's lower right abdomen; this may cause the appendix to rupture.
• Following appendectomy, monitor vital signs and intake and output.
• Teach the patient to cough, breathe deeply, and turn frequently to prevent pulmonary complications.

• Document bowel sounds, passing of flatus, and bowel movements. These signs in a patient whose nausea and abdominal rigidity have subsided indicate that the patient may resume oral fluids.
• Watch closely for possible surgical complications. Continuing pain and fever may signal an abscess. The complaint that "something gave way" may mean wound dehiscence. If an abscess or peritonitis develops, incision and drainage may be necessary Monitor wound drainage.
• Help the patient ambulate as soon as possible after surgery (within 24 hours).
• In appendicitis complicated by peritonitis, a nasogastric tube may be needed to decompress the stomach and reduce nausea and vomiting.

# ARM AND LEG FRACTURES

Fractures of the arms and legs usually result from trauma and often cause substantial muscle, nerve, and other soft-tissue damage. The prognosis varies with the extent of disablement or deformity, the amount of tissue and vascular damage, the adequacy of reduction and immobilization, and the patient's age, health, and nutritional status.

Children's bones usually heal rapidly and without deformity. Bones of adults in poor health and with impaired circulation may never heal properly. Severe open fractures, especially of the femoral shaft, may cause substantial blood loss and life-threatening hypovolemic shock.

## Causes

Most arm and leg fractures result from major trauma; for example, a fall on an outstretched arm, a skiing accident, or child abuse (shown by multiple or repeated episodes of fractures). However, in a person with a pathologic bone-weakening condition, such as osteoporosis, bone tumors, or metabolic disease, a mere cough or sneeze can also produce a fracture. Prolonged standing, walking, or running can cause stress fractures of the foot and ankle — usually in nurses, postal workers, soldiers, and joggers.

### Signs and symptoms

Arm and leg fractures may produce any or all of the "5 Ps": pain and point tenderness, pallor, pulse loss, paresthesia, and paralysis. (The last three are distal to the fracture site.) Other signs include deformity, swelling, discoloration, crepitus, and loss of limb function. Numbness and tingling, mottled cyanosis, cool skin at the end of the extremity, and loss of pulses distal to the injury indicate possible arterial compromise or nerve damage. Open fractures also produce an obvious skin wound.

Complications of arm and leg fractures include:
- permanent deformity and dysfunction if bones fail to heal (nonunion) or heal improperly (malunion)
- aseptic necrosis of bone segments from impaired circulation
- hypovolemic shock as a result of blood vessel damage (This is especially likely to develop in patients with a fractured femur.)
- muscle contractures
- renal calculi from decalcification (produced by prolonged immobility)
- fat embolism.

### Diagnosis

A history of trauma and a physical examination, including gentle palpation and a cautious attempt by the patient to move parts distal to the injury, suggest an arm or a leg fracture.

When performing the physical examination, also check for other injuries. Anteroposterior and lateral X-rays of the suspected fracture as well as X-rays of the joints above and below it confirm the diagnosis.

### Treatment

The following treatments are performed in arm and leg fractures.

CLINICAL TIP  In an emergency, the limb is splinted above and below the suspected fracture, a cold pack is applied, and the limb is elevated to reduce edema and pain.

In severe fractures that cause blood loss, direct pressure should be applied to control bleeding, and fluid replacement should be administered as soon as possible to prevent or treat hypovolemic shock.

### *Reduction*

After a fracture has been confirmed, treatment begins with reduction (which involves restoring displaced bone segments to their normal position).
- After reduction, the fractured arm or leg must be immobilized by a splint or a cast or with traction. In closed reduction (which is accomplished by manual manipulation), a local anesthetic (such as lidocaine) and an analgesic (such as morphine I.M.) help relieve pain, whereas a muscle relaxant (such as diazepam I.V.) or a sedative (such as midazolam) facilitates the muscle stretching necessary to realign the bone.
- An X-ray study is ordered to confirm that reduction has been successful and that proper bone alignment has been achieved.
- When closed reduction is impossible, open reduction during surgery reduces and immobilizes the fracture by means of rods, plates, or screws. Afterward, a plaster cast is usually applied.

**TEACHING CHECKLIST**

## CAST CARE

Instruct your patient on the following points when providing care for the patient with a cast.

- When sitting or lying down, support the cast with pillows.
- Watch for irritation around the edges of the cast.
- Check for and report foul odor or discharge.
- Report signs of impaired circulation immediately (skin coldness, numbness, tingling, discoloration).
- Don't get the cast wet.
- Don't insert foreign objects under the cast.

• When a splint or cast fails to maintain the reduction, immobilization requires skin or skeletal traction, using a series of weights and pulleys.

• In skin traction, elastic bandages and sheepskin coverings are used to attach traction devices to the patient's skin. In skeletal traction, a pin or wire inserted through the bone distal to the fracture and attached to a weight allows more prolonged traction.

*Other measures*
Treatment of open fractures also requires tetanus prophylaxis, prophylactic antibiotics, surgery to repair soft-tissue damage, and thorough debridement of the wound.

**Special considerations**
• Watch for signs of shock in the patient with a severe open fracture of a large bone, such as the femur.
• Monitor vital signs, and be especially alert for a rapid pulse, decreased blood pressure, pallor, and cool, clammy skin— all of which may indicate that the patient is in shock.
• Administer I.V. fluids as needed.
• Offer reassurance. With any fracture, the patient is likely to be frightened and in pain.
• Ease pain with analgesics as needed.
• Help the patient set realistic goals for recovery.
• If the fracture requires long-term immobilization with traction, reposition the patient often to increase comfort and prevent pressure ulcers. Assist with active range-of-motion exercises to prevent muscle atrophy. Encourage deep breathing and coughing to avoid hypostatic pneumonia.
• Urge adequate fluid intake to prevent urinary stasis and constipation. Watch for signs of renal calculi (flank pain, nausea, vomiting).
• Provide good cast care. (See *Cast care*.)
• Encourage the patient to start moving around as soon as he's able. Help him to walk. (Remember, the patient who has been bedridden for some time may be dizzy at first.) Demonstrate how to use crutches properly.
• After cast removal, refer the patient for physical therapy to restore limb mobility.

# ARTERIAL OCCLUSIVE DISEASE

In arterial occlusive disease, the obstruction or narrowing of the lumen of the aorta and its major branches causes an interruption of blood flow, usually to the legs and feet. Arterial occlusive disease may affect the carotid, vertebral, innominate, subclavian, mesenteric, and celiac arteries. Occlusions may be acute or chronic and often cause severe ischemia, skin ulceration, and gangrene.

Arterial occlusive disease is more common in males than in females. The prognosis depends on the location of the occlusion, the development of collateral circulation to counteract reduced blood flow and, in acute disease, the time elapsed between occlusion and its removal.

### Causes

Arterial occlusive disease is a frequent complication of atherosclerosis. The occlusive mechanism may be endogenous, due to embolus formation or thrombosis, or exogenous, due to trauma or fracture. Predisposing factors include smoking; aging; conditions such as hypertension, hyperlipidemia, and diabetes; and a family history of vascular disorders, myocardial infarction, or cerebrovascular accident (CVA).

### Signs and symptoms

Evidence of this disease varies widely, according to the occlusion site. (See *Clinical features of arterial occlusive disease,* page 72.)

### Diagnosis

In arterial occlusive disease, the diagnosis is usually based on the patient history and physical examination.

Pertinent supportive diagnostic tests include the following:

• *Arteriography* demonstrates the type (thrombus or embolus), location, and degree of obstruction and collateral circulation. Arteriography is particularly useful in chronic disease or for evaluating candidates for reconstructive surgery.

• *Doppler ultrasonography* and *plethysmography* are noninvasive tests that, in acute disease, show decreased blood flow distal to the occlusion.

• *Ophthalmodynamometry* helps determine the degree of obstruction in the internal carotid artery by comparing ophthalmic artery pressure with brachial artery pressure on the affected side. A more than 20% difference between pressures suggests insufficiency.

• *EEG* and a *computed tomography scan* may be necessary to rule out brain lesions.

### Treatment

Effective treatment depends on the cause, location, and size of the obstruction. For mild chronic disease, supportive measures include elimination of smoking, hypertension control, and walking exercise. For carotid artery occlusion, antiplatelet therapy may begin with aspirin. For intermittent claudication of chronic occlusive disease, pentoxifylline may improve blood flow through the capillaries, particularly for patients who are poor candidates for surgery.

Acute arterial occlusive disease usually requires surgery to restore circulation to the affected area. Possible procedures include the following:

• *Embolectomy:* A balloon-tipped catheter is used to remove thrombotic material from the artery. Embolectomy is used mainly for mesenteric, femoral, or popliteal artery occlusion.

• *Thromboendarterectomy:* The occluded artery is opened and the obstructing thrombus and the medial layer of the arterial wall are removed. This procedure is usually performed after angiography and often used with autogenous vein or Dacron bypass surgery (femoral-popliteal or aortofemoral).

• *Patch grafting:* This procedure involves removal of the thrombosed arterial segment and replacement with an autogenous vein or Dacron graft.

• *Bypass graft:* Blood flow is diverted through an anastomosed autogenous or

# CLINICAL FEATURES OF ARTERIAL OCCLUSIVE DISEASE

| SITE OF OCCLUSION | SIGNS AND SYMPTOMS |
| --- | --- |
| **Carotid arterial system**<br>• Internal carotid arteries<br>• External carotid arteries | Neurologic dysfunction (transient ischemic attacks [TIAs] due to reduced cerebral circulation produce unilateral sensory or motor dysfunction [transient monocular blindness, hemiparesis], possible aphasia or dysarthria, confusion, decreased mentation, and headache; these recurrent clinical features usually last 5 to 10 minutes but may persist up to 24 hours and may herald a stroke); absent or decreased pulsation with an auscultatory bruit over the affected vessels |
| **Vertebrobasilar system**<br>• Vertebral arteries<br>• Basilar arteries | Neurologic dysfunction (TIAs of brain stem and cerebellum produce binocular visual disturbances, vertigo, dysarthria, and "drop attacks" [falling down without loss of consciousness]); less common than carotid TIA |
| **Innominate**<br>Brachiocephalic artery | Neurologic dysfunction (signs and symptoms of vertebrobasilar occlusion); indications of ischemia (claudication) of right arm; possible bruit over right side of neck |
| **Subclavian artery** | Subclavian steal syndrome (characterized by the backflow of blood from the brain through the vertebral artery on the same side as the occlusion, into the subclavian artery distal to the occlusion); clinical effects of vertebrobasilar occlusion and exercise-induced arm claudication; possible gangrene, usually limited to the digits |
| **Mesenteric artery**<br>• Superior (most commonly affected)<br>• Celiac axis<br>• Inferior | Bowel ischemia, infarct necrosis, and gangrene; sudden, acute abdominal pain; nausea and vomiting; diarrhea; leukocytosis; and shock due to massive intraluminal fluid and plasma loss |
| **Aortic bifurcation**<br>(saddle block occlusion, an emergency associated with cardiac embolization) | Sensory and motor deficits (muscle weakness, numbness, paresthesia, paralysis) and signs of ischemia (sudden pain; cold, pale legs with decreased or absent peripheral pulses) in both legs |
| **Iliac artery**<br>(Leriche's syndrome) | Intermittent claudication of lower back, buttocks, and thighs relieved by rest; absent or reduced femoral or distal pulses; possible bruit over femoral arteries; impotence |
| **Femoral and popliteal arteries**<br>(associated with aneurysm formation) | Intermittent claudication of the calves on exertion; ischemic pain in feet; pretrophic pain (heralds necrosis and ulceration); leg pallor and coolness; blanching of feet on elevation; gangrene; no palpable pulses in ankles and feet |

Dacron graft past the thrombosed segment.

- *Thrombolytic therapy:* Any clot around or in the plaque is lysed by urokinase, streptokinase, or alteplase.
- *Atherectomy:* Plaque is excised using a drill or slicing mechanism.
- *Balloon angioplasty:* The obstruction is compressed using balloon inflation.
- *Laser angioplasty:* Excision and hot-tip lasers are used to vaporize the obstruction.
- *Stents:* A mesh of wires that stretch and mold to the arterial wall are inserted to prevent reocclusion.
- *Combined therapy:* Any of the above treatments are used concomitantly.
- *Lumbar sympathectomy:* The procedure is an adjunct to surgery, depending on the condition of the sympathetic nervous system.

Amputation becomes necessary with failure of arterial reconstructive surgery or with the development of gangrene, persistent infection, or intractable pain.

Other treatments include heparin to prevent embolus formation (for embolic occlusion) and bowel resection after restoration of blood flow (for mesenteric artery occlusion).

**Special considerations**
- Provide comprehensive patient teaching, such as proper foot care. Explain all diagnostic tests and procedures. Advise the patient to stop smoking and to follow the prescribed medical regimen.

Preoperatively (during an acute episode):
- Assess the patient's circulatory status by checking for the most distal pulses and by inspecting his skin color and temperature.
- Provide pain relief as needed.
- Administer heparin by continuous I.V. drip as needed. Use an infusion monitor or pump to ensure the proper flow rate.

- Wrap the patient's affected foot in soft cotton batting, and reposition it frequently to prevent pressure on any one area. Strictly avoid elevating or applying heat to the affected leg.
- Watch for signs of fluid and electrolyte imbalance, and monitor intake and output for signs of renal failure (urine output < 30 ml/hour).
- If the patient has a carotid, innominate, vertebral, or subclavian artery occlusion, monitor him for signs of CVA, such as numbness in an arm or a leg and intermittent blindness.

Postoperatively:
- Monitor the patient's vital signs. Continuously assess his circulatory function by inspecting skin color and temperature and by checking for distal pulses. In charting, compare earlier assessments and observations. Watch closely for signs of hemorrhage (tachycardia, hypotension), and check dressings for excessive bleeding.
- In carotid, innominate, vertebral, or subclavian artery occlusion, assess neurologic status frequently for changes in level of consciousness, muscle strength, and pupil size.
- In mesenteric artery occlusion, connect a nasogastric tube to low intermittent suction. Monitor intake and output (low urine output may indicate damage to renal arteries during surgery). Check bowel sounds for the return of peristalsis. Increasing abdominal distention and tenderness may indicate extension of bowel ischemia with resulting gangrene, necessitating further excision, or they may indicate peritonitis.
- In aortic bifurcation, also known as saddle block occlusion, check distal pulses for adequate circulation. Watch for signs of renal failure and mesenteric artery occlusion (severe abdominal pain) and for cardiac arrhythmias, which may precipitate embolus formation.

• In iliac artery occlusion, monitor urine output for signs of renal failure from decreased perfusion to the kidneys as a result of surgery. Provide meticulous catheter care.

• In both femoral and popliteal artery occlusion, assist with early ambulation, but discourage prolonged sitting.

• After amputation, check the patient's stump carefully for drainage and record its color and amount and the time. Elevate the stump, and administer adequate analgesic medication. Because phantom limb pain is common, explain this phenomenon to the patient.

• When preparing the patient for discharge, instruct him to watch for signs of recurrence (pain, pallor, numbness, paralysis, absence of pulse) that can result from graft occlusion or occlusion at another site. Warn him against wearing constrictive clothing.

# ASBESTOSIS

A form of pneumoconiosis, asbestosis is characterized by diffuse interstitial fibrosis. It can develop as long as 15 to 20 years after regular exposure to asbestos has ended. A potent cocarcinogen, it aggravates the risk of lung cancer in cigarette smokers.

## Causes

Asbestosis results from the inhalation of respirable asbestos fibers (50 microns or more in length, 0.5 micron or less in diameter), which assume a longitudinal orientation in the airway, move in the direction of airflow, and penetrate respiratory bronchioles and alveolar walls.

Sources include the mining and milling of asbestos, the construction industry (where asbestos is used in a prefabricated form), and the fireproofing and textile industries; asbestos is also used in the production of paints, plastics, and brake and clutch linings.

Asbestos-related diseases develop in families of asbestos workers as a result of exposure to fibrous dust shaken off workers' clothing at home. Such diseases develop in the general public as a result of exposure to fibrous dust or waste piles from nearby asbestos plants.

## Pathophysiology

Inhaled fibers become encased in a brown, proteinlike sheath rich in iron (ferruginous bodies or asbestos bodies), found in sputum and lung tissue. Interstitial fibrosis develops in lower lung zones, causing obliterative changes in lung parenchyma and pleurae. Raised hyaline plaques may form in parietal pleura, diaphragm, and pleura contiguous with the pericardium.

## Signs and symptoms

Clinical features may appear before chest X-ray changes. The first symptom is usually dyspnea on exertion, typically after 10 years' exposure. As fibrosis extends, dyspnea on exertion increases until, eventually, dyspnea occurs even at rest; advanced disease also causes a dry cough (may be productive in smokers), chest pain (often pleuritic), recurrent respiratory tract infections, and tachypnea.

Cardiovascular complications include pulmonary hypertension, right ventricular hypertrophy, and cor pulmonale. Finger clubbing commonly occurs.

## Diagnosis

The patient history reveals occupational, family, or neighborhood exposure to asbestos fibers. Physical examination reveals characteristic dry crackles at lung bases.

Chest X-rays show fine, irregular, and linear diffuse infiltrates; extensive fibrosis results in a "honeycomb" or "ground-glass" appearance. X-rays may also show pleural thickening and pleural calcification, with bilateral obliteration of costophrenic angles and, in later stages, an enlarged heart with a classic "shaggy" border.

Pulmonary function studies show:
• *vital capacity, forced vital capacity*, and *total lung capacity:* decreased
• *forced expiratory volume*: decreased or normal
• *diffusing capacity of the lungs for carbon monoxide:* reduced when fibrosis destroys alveolar walls and thickens alveolocapillary membrane.

Arterial blood gas analysis reveals:
• *partial pressure of oxygen:* decreased
• *partial pressure of carbon dioxide:* low because of hyperventilation.

### Treatment and special considerations

• Respiratory symptoms may be relieved by chest physiotherapy techniques, such as controlled coughing and segmental bronchial drainage, with chest percussion and vibration. Aerosol therapy, inhaled mucolytics, and increased fluid intake (at least 3 qt [3 L] daily) may also help relieve respiratory symptoms.
• Diuretics, digitalis glycoside preparations, and salt restriction may be indicated for patients with cor pulmonale.
• Hypoxia requires oxygen administration by cannula or mask (1 to 2 L/minute) or by mechanical ventilation if arterial oxygen can't be maintained above 40 mm Hg.
• Prompt administration of antibiotics is required for respiratory tract infections.
• Teach the patient to prevent infections by avoiding crowds and persons with infections and by receiving influenza and pneumococcal vaccines.

> CLINICAL TIP Improve the patient's ventilatory efficiency by encouraging physical reconditioning, energy conservation in daily activities, and relaxation techniques.

## ASCARIASIS

Also known as roundworm infection, ascariasis is caused by the parasitic worm *Ascaris lumbricoides*. It occurs worldwide but is most common in tropical areas with poor sanitation and in Asia, where farmers use human stool as fertilizer. In the United States, it's more prevalent in the South, particularly among 4- to 12-year-olds.

### Causes

*A. lumbricoides* is a large roundworm resembling an earthworm. It's transmitted to humans by ingestion of soil contaminated with human stool that harbors *A. lumbricoides* ova. Such ingestion may occur directly (by eating contaminated soil) or indirectly (by eating poorly washed raw vegetables grown in contaminated soil).

Ascariasis never passes directly from person to person. After ingestion, *A. lumbricoides* ova hatch and release larvae, which penetrate the intestinal wall and reach the lungs through the bloodstream. After about 10 days in pulmonary capillaries and alveoli, the larvae migrate to the bronchioles, bronchi, trachea, and epiglottis. There they are swallowed and return to the intestine to mature into worms.

### Signs and symptoms

Mild intestinal ascariasis may cause only vague stomach discomfort. The first clue may be vomiting a worm or passing a worm in the stool. Severe disease, however, causes stomach pain, vomiting, restlessness, disturbed sleep and, in extreme cases, intestinal obstruction. Larvae migrating by the lymphatic and the circulatory systems cause symptoms that vary; for instance, when they invade the lungs, pneumonitis may result.

### Diagnosis

Microscopic identification of ova in the stool or observation of adult worms, which may be passed rectally or by mouth, confirms the diagnosis. When migrating larvae invade the alveoli, other conclusive tests include X-rays that show characteristic bronchovascular markings: infiltrates, patchy areas of pneumonitis, and widening of hilar shadows. In a patient with ascariasis, these findings usually accompany a complete blood count that shows eosinophilia.

### Treatment

Anthelmintic drug therapy, the primary treatment, consists of pyrantel or piperazine to temporarily paralyze the worms, permitting peristalsis to expel them. Mebendazole and albendazole are also used to block helminth nutrition. These drugs are up to 95% effective, even after a single dose.

In multiple helminth infection, one of these drugs must be the first treatment; using some other anthelmintic first may stimulate *A. lumbricoides* perforation into other organs. No specific treatment exists for migratory infection because anthelmintics affect only mature worms.

In intestinal obstruction, nasogastric (NG) suctioning controls vomiting. When suctioning can be discontinued, instill piperazine and clamp the tube. If vomiting doesn't occur, give a second dose of piperazine orally 24 hours later. If this is ineffective, treatment probably requires surgery.

### Special considerations

• Isolation is unnecessary; proper disposal of stool and soiled linen, using standard precautions, should be adequate.

• If the patient is receiving NG suctioning, be sure to provide good mouth care.

• Teach the patient to prevent reinfection by washing hands thoroughly, especially before eating and after defecation, and by bathing and changing his underwear and bed linens daily.

• Inform the patient of possible drug adverse effects. Tell him that piperazine may cause stomach upset, dizziness, and urticaria.

➤ CLINICAL TIP Be aware that piperazine is contraindicated in seizure disorders. Pyrantel produces red stool and vomit and may cause stomach upset, headache, dizziness, and rash; albendazole and mebendazole may cause abdominal pain and diarrhea.

# ASPERGILLOSIS

Aspergillosis is an opportunistic, sometimes life-threatening infection caused by fungi of the genus *Aspergillus,* usually *A. fumigatus, A. flavus,* or *A. niger.* It occurs in four major forms:

• *aspergilloma,* which produces a fungus ball in the lungs (called a mycetoma)

• *allergic aspergillosis,* a hypersensitive asthmatic reaction to *Aspergillus* antigens

• *aspergillosis endophthalmitis,* an infection of the anterior and posterior chambers of the eye that can lead to blindness

• *disseminated aspergillosis,* an acute infection that produces septicemia, thrombosis, and infarction of virtually any organ but especially the heart, lungs, brain, and kidneys.

*Aspergillus* may cause infection of the ear (otomycosis), cornea (mycotic keratitis), and prosthetic heart valves (endocarditis); pneumonia (especially in persons receiving immunosuppressants, such as antineoplastic agents or high-dose steroids); sinusitis; and brain abscesses.

The prognosis varies with each form. Occasionally, aspergilloma causes fatal hemoptysis.

## Causes

*Aspergillus* is found worldwide, often in fermenting compost piles and damp hay. It's transmitted by inhalation of fungal spores or, in aspergillosis endophthalmitis, by the invasion of spores through a wound or other tissue injury. It's a common laboratory contaminant.

*Aspergillus* produces clinical infection only in persons who become especially vulnerable to it. Such vulnerability can result from excessive or prolonged use of antibiotics, glucocorticoids, or other immunosuppressants; from radiation; from such conditions as acquired immunodeficiency syndrome, Hodgkin's disease, leukemia, azotemia, alcoholism, sarcoidosis, bronchitis, or bronchiectasis; from organ transplants; and, in aspergilloma, from tuberculosis or another cavitary lung disease.

## Signs and symptoms

The incubation period in aspergillosis ranges from a few days to weeks. In aspergilloma, colonization of the bronchial tree with *Aspergillus* produces plugs and atelectasis and forms a tangled ball of hyphae (fungal filaments), fibrin, and exudate in a cavity left by a previous illness such as tuberculosis. Character-istically, aspergilloma either produces no symptoms or mimics tuberculosis, causing a productive cough and purulent or blood-tinged sputum, dyspnea, empyema, and lung abscesses.

Allergic aspergillosis causes wheezing, dyspnea, cough with some sputum production, pleural pain, and fever.

Aspergillosis endophthalmitis usually appears 2 to 3 weeks after an eye injury or surgery and accounts for half of all cases of endophthalmitis. It causes clouded vision, eye pain, and reddened conjunctivae. Eventually, *Aspergillus* infects the anterior and posterior chambers, where it produces purulent exudate.

In disseminated aspergillosis, *Aspergillus* invades blood vessels and causes thrombosis, infarctions, and the typical signs of septicemia (chills, fever, hypotension, delirium), with azotemia, hematuria, urinary tract obstruction, headaches, seizures, bone pain and tenderness, and soft-tissue swelling. This form of the disorder is rapidly fatal.

## Diagnosis

In patients with aspergilloma, a chest X-ray reveals a crescent-shaped radiolucency surrounding a circular mass, but this isn't definitive for aspergillosis. In aspergillosis endophthalmitis, a history of ocular trauma or surgery and a culture or exudate showing *Aspergillus* is diagnostic. In allergic aspergillosis, sputum examination shows eosinophils. Culture of mouth scrapings or sputum showing *Aspergillus* is inconclusive because even healthy persons harbor this fungus. In disseminated aspergillosis, culture and microscopic examination of affected tissue can confirm the diagnosis, but this form is usually diagnosed at autopsy.

## Treatment and special considerations
- Aspergillosis doesn't require isolation.
- Treatment of aspergilloma necessitates local excision of the lesion and supportive therapy, such as chest physiotherapy and coughing, to improve pulmonary function.
- Allergic aspergillosis requires desensitization and, possibly, steroids.
- Disseminated aspergillosis and aspergillosis endophthalmitis require a 2- to 3-week course of I.V. amphotericin B (as well as prompt cessation of immunosuppressive therapy). However, the disseminated form of aspergillosis often resists amphotericin B therapy and rapidly progresses to death.

 CLINICAL TIP Itraconazole may be useful in slowly progressing immunocompetent cases.

---

LIFE-THREATENING DISORDER

# ASPHYXIA

---

A condition of insufficient oxygen and accumulating carbon dioxide in the blood and tissues due to interference with respiration, asphyxia results in cardiopulmonary arrest. Without prompt treatment, it's fatal.

## Causes
Asphyxia results from any condition or substance that inhibits respiration:
- hypoventilation as a result of narcotic abuse, medullary disease or hemorrhage, pneumothorax, respiratory muscle paralysis, or cardiopulmonary arrest
- intrapulmonary obstruction, as in airway obstruction, severe asthma, foreign-body aspiration, pulmonary edema, pneumonia, and near-drowning

- extrapulmonary obstruction, as in tracheal compression from a tumor, strangulation, trauma, or suffocation
- inhalation of toxic agents, as in carbon monoxide poisoning, smoke inhalation, and excessive oxygen inhalation.

## Signs and symptoms
Depending on the duration and degree of asphyxia, common symptoms include anxiety, dyspnea, agitation and confusion leading to coma, altered respiratory rate (apnea, bradypnea, occasional tachypnea), decreased breath sounds, central and peripheral cyanosis (cherry-red mucous membranes in late-stage carbon monoxide poisoning), seizures, and fast, slow, or absent pulse.

## Diagnosis
The patient history and laboratory test results provide the diagnosis. Pulse oximetry reveals decreased hemoglobin (Hb) saturation with oxygen. Arterial blood gas analysis, the most important test, indicates decreased partial pressure of oxygen (< 60 mm Hg) and increased partial pressure of carbon dioxide (> 50 mm Hg). Chest X-rays may show a foreign body, pulmonary edema, or atelectasis. Toxicology tests may show drugs, or chemicals. Abnormal Hb may also be detected in a CBC. Pulmonary function tests may indicate respiratory muscle weakness.

## Treatment
Asphyxia requires immediate respiratory support — with cardiopulmonary resuscitation, endotracheal intubation, and supplemental oxygen as needed. The underlying cause must be remedied: bronchoscopy for extraction of a foreign body; a narcotic antagonist, such as naloxone, for narcotic overdose; gastric lavage for poisoning; and limited, graded use of supplemental oxygen for

carbon dioxide narcosis caused by excessive oxygen therapy.

**Special considerations**
- Respiratory distress is frightening, so reassure the patient during treatment.
- Give prescribed medications.
- Suction carefully, as needed, and encourage deep breathing.
- Closely monitor vital signs and laboratory test results.

> CLINICAL TIP To prevent drug-induced asphyxia, warn patients about the danger of taking alcohol with other central nervous system depressants.

# ASTHMA

A reversible lung disease, asthma is characterized by obstruction or narrowing of the airways, which are typically inflamed and hyperresponsive to a variety of stimuli. It may resolve spontaneously or with treatment. Its symptoms range from mild wheezing and dyspnea to life-threatening respiratory failure. Symptoms of bronchial airway obstruction may persist between acute episodes.

**Causes**
Although this common condition can strike at any age, half of all cases first occur in children under age 10; in this age-group, asthma affects twice as many boys as girls.

*Extrinsic and intrinsic asthma*
Asthma that results from sensitivity to specific external allergens is known as extrinsic. In cases in which the allergen isn't obvious, asthma is referred to as intrinsic. Allergens that cause extrinsic asthma include pollen, animal dander,

house dust or mold, kapok or feather pillows, food additives containing sulfites, and any other sensitizing substance.

Extrinsic (atopic) asthma usually begins in childhood and is accompanied by other manifestations of atopy (Type I, immunoglobulin E [IgE]-mediated allergy), such as eczema and allergic rhinitis.

In intrinsic (nonatopic) asthma, no extrinsic allergen can be identified. Most cases are preceded by a severe respiratory tract infection. Irritants, emotional stress, fatigue, exposure to noxious fumes, and endocrine, temperature, and humidity changes may aggravate intrinsic asthma attacks. In many asthmatics, intrinsic and extrinsic asthma coexist.

*Other asthma triggers*
Several drugs and chemicals may provoke an asthma attack without using the IgE pathway. Apparently, they trigger release of mast-cell mediators via prostaglandin inhibition. Examples of these substances include aspirin, various nonsteroidal anti-inflammatory drugs (such as indomethacin and mefenamic acid), and tartrazine, a yellow food dye.

Exercise may also provoke an asthma attack. In exercise-induced asthma, bronchospasm may follow heat and moisture loss in the upper airways.

*Two-phase allergic response*
When the patient inhales an allergenic substance, sensitized IgE antibodies trigger mast-cell degranulation in the lung interstitium, releasing histamine, cytokines, prostaglandins, thromboxanes, leukotrienes, and eosinophil chemotaxic factors. Histamine then attaches to receptor sites in the larger bronchi, causing irritation, inflammation, and edema. In the late phase, inflammatory cells

# DETERMINING AN ACUTE ASTHMA ATTACK'S SEVERITY

| MILD ASTHMA | MODERATE ASTHMA | SEVERE ASTHMA | RESPIRATORY FAILURE |
|---|---|---|---|
| **SIGNS AND SYMPTOMS DURING ACUTE PHASE** | | | |
| • Brief wheezing, coughing, dyspnea with activity<br>• Infrequent nocturnal coughing or wheezing<br>• Adequate air exchange<br>• Intermittent, brief (< 1 hour) wheezing, cough, or dyspnea once or twice a week<br>• Asymptomatic between attacks | • Respiratory distress at rest<br>• Hyperpnea<br>• Marked coughing and wheezing<br>• Air exchange normal or below normal<br>• Exacerbations that may last several days | • Marked respiratory distress<br>• Marked wheezing or absent breath sounds<br>• Pulsus paradoxus > 10 mm Hg<br>• Chest wall contractions<br>• Continuous symptoms<br>• Frequent exacerbations | • Severe respiratory distress<br>• Impaired consciousness<br>• Severe wheezing or silent chest<br>• Use of accessory muscles of respiration<br>• Prominent pulsus paradoxus (30 to 50 mm Hg) |
| **DIAGNOSTIC TEST RESULTS** | | | |
| • Forced expiratory volume in 1 second ($FEV_1$) or peak flow 80% of normal values<br>• pH normal or increased<br>• Partial pressure of arterial oxygen ($Pao_2$) normal or decreased<br>• Partial pressure of arterial carbon dioxide ($Paco_2$) normal or decreased<br>• Chest X-ray normal | • $FEV_1$ or peak flow 60% to 80% of normal values; may vary 20% to 30% with symptoms<br>• pH generally elevated<br>• $Pao_2$ increased<br>• $Paco_2$ generally decreased<br>• Chest X-ray that shows hyperinflation | • $FEV_1$ or peak flow < 60% of normal values; may normally vary 20% to 30% with routine medications and up to 50% with exacerbations<br>• pH normal or reduced<br>• $Pao_2$ decreased<br>• $Paco_2$ normal or increased<br>• Chest X-ray that may show hyperinflation | • $FEV_1$ or peak flow < 25% of normal values<br>• pH decreased<br>• $Pao_2$ < 60 mm Hg<br>• $Paco_2$ > 40 mm Hg |

## DETERMINING AN ACUTE ASTHMA ATTACK'S SEVERITY (continued)

| MILD ASTHMA | MODERATE ASTHMA | SEVERE ASTHMA | RESPIRATORY FAILURE |
|---|---|---|---|
| **OTHER ASSESSMENT FINDINGS** | | | |
| • One attack per week (or none) <br> • Positive response to bronchodilator therapy within 24 hours <br> • No signs of asthma between episodes <br> • No sleep interruption <br> • No hyperventilation <br> • Minimal evidence of airway obstruction <br> • Minimal or no increase in lung volume | • Symptoms occur more than two times weekly <br> • Coughing and wheezing between episodes <br> • Diminished exercise tolerance <br> • Possible sleep interruption <br> • Increased lung volume | • Frequent severe attacks <br> • Daily wheezing <br> • Poor exercise tolerance <br> • Frequent sleep interruption <br> • Bronchodilator therapy doesn't completely reverse airway obstruction <br> • Markedly increased lung volume | • Cyanosis <br> • Tachycardia |

flow in. The influx of eosinophils provides additional inflammatory mediators and contributes to local injury.

### Signs and symptoms

An asthma attack may begin dramatically, with simultaneous onset of many severe symptoms, or insidiously, with gradually increasing respiratory distress. It typically includes progressively worsening shortness of breath, cough, wheezing, and chest tightness or some combination of these symptoms.

During an acute attack, the cough sounds tight and dry. As the attack subsides, tenacious mucoid sputum is produced (except in young children, who don't expectorate). Characteristic wheezing may be accompanied by coarse rhonchi, but fine crackles aren't heard unless associated with a related complication. Between acute attacks, breath sounds may be normal.

The intensity of breath sounds in symptomatic asthma is typically reduced. A prolonged phase of forced expiration is typical of airflow obstruction. Evidence of lung hyperinflation (use of accessory muscles, for example) is particularly common in children. Acute attacks may be accompanied by tachycardia, tachypnea, and diaphoresis. In severe attacks, the patient may be unable to speak more than a few words without pausing for breath. Cyanosis, confusion, and lethargy indicate the onset of life-threatening status asthmaticus and respiratory failure. (See *Determining an acute asthma attack's severity*.)

## Diagnosis

Laboratory studies in patients with asthma often show these abnormalities:

• *Pulmonary function studies* reveal signs of airway obstruction (decreased peak expiratory flow rates and forced expiratory volume in 1 second [$FEV_1$]), low-normal or decreased vital capacity, and increased total lung and residual capacity. However, pulmonary function studies may be normal between attacks.

• *Pulse oximetry* may reveal decreased arterial oxygen saturation ($SaO_2$).

• *Arterial blood gas (ABG) analysis* provides the best indications of an attack's severity. In acutely severe asthma, the partial pressure of arterial oxygen is < 60 mm Hg, the partial pressure of arterial carbon dioxide ($PaCO_2$) is 40 mm Hg or more, and pH is usually decreased.

• *Complete blood count with differential* reveals an increased eosinophil count.

• *Chest X-rays* may show hyperinflation with areas of focal atelectasis or may be normal.

Before initiating tests for asthma, rule out other causes of airway obstruction and wheezing. In children, such causes include cystic fibrosis, tumors of the bronchi or mediastinum, and acute viral bronchitis; in adults, other causes include obstructive pulmonary disease, heart failure, and epiglottitis.

## Treatment

Acute asthma is treated by decreasing bronchoconstriction, reducing bronchial airway edema, and increasing pulmonary ventilation. Treatment after an acute episode includes avoiding or removing precipitating factors, such as environmental allergens or irritants.

If asthma is known to be caused by a particular antigen, it may be treated by desensitizing the patient through a series of injections of limited amounts of the antigen. The aim is to curb the patient's immune response to the antigen.

If asthma results from an infection, antibiotics are prescribed. Drug therapy, which is most effective when begun soon after the onset of signs and symptoms, usually includes:

• bronchodilators to decrease bronchoconstriction, for example, methylxanthines (theophylline and aminophylline) and beta$_2$- adrenergic agonists (albuterol and terbutaline)

• corticosteroids (hydrocortisone sodium succinate, prednisone, methylprednisolone, and beclomethasone) for their anti-inflammatory and immunosuppressive effects, which decrease inflammation and edema of the airways

• cromolyn and nedocromil to help prevent the release of the chemical mediators (histamine and leukotrienes) that cause bronchoconstriction

• anticholinergic bronchodilators (such as ipratropium), which block acetylcholine, another chemical mediator.

For the most part, medical treatment of asthma attacks must be tailored to each patient. However. the following treatments are generally used.

### Chronic mild asthma

A beta$_2$-adrenergic agonist by metered-dose inhaler is used (alone or with cromolyn) before exercise and exposure to an allergen or other stimuli to prevent symptoms. The beta$_2$-adrenergic agonist is used every 3 to 4 hours if symptoms occur.

### Chronic moderate asthma

Initial treatment may include an inhaled beta-adrenergic bronchodilator, an inhaled corticosteroid, and cromolyn. Anticholinergic bronchodilators may also be added. If symptoms persist, the inhaled corticosteroid dose may be increased, and sustained-release theophylline or an oral beta$_2$-adrenergic agonist (or both) may be added. Short courses of oral corticosteroids may also be used.

### Chronic severe asthma
Initially, around-the-clock oral bronchodilator therapy with a long-acting theophylline or a beta$_2$-adrenergic agonist may be required, supplemented with an inhaled beta$_2$-adrenergic agonist and an inhaled corticosteroid with or without cromolyn. An oral corticosteroid, such as prednisone, may be added in acute exacerbations.

### Acute asthma attack
Acute attacks that don't respond to self-treatment may require hospital care, beta$_2$-adrenergic agonists by inhalation or subcutaneous (S.C.) injection (in three doses over 60 to 90 minutes) and, possibly, oxygen for hypoxemia. If the patient responds poorly, systemic corticosteroids and, possibly, S.C. epinephrine may help. Beta$_2$-adrenergic agonist inhalation continues hourly. I.V. aminophylline may be added to the regimen and I.V. fluid therapy is started. Patients who don't respond to this treatment, whose airways remain obstructed, and who have increasing respiratory difficulty are at risk for status asthmaticus and may require mechanical ventilation.

### Status asthmaticus
Treatment consists of aggressive drug therapy: a beta$_2$-adrenergic agonist by nebulizer every 30 to 60 minutes, possibly supplemented with S.C. epinephrine, I.V. corticosteroids, I.V. aminophylline, oxygen administration, I.V. fluid therapy, and intubation and mechanical ventilation for hypercapnia respiratory failure (Paco$_2$ of 40 mm Hg or more).

### Special considerations
During an acute attack:
- First assess the severity of asthma.
- Administer the prescribed treatments and assess the patient's response.
- Place the patient in high Fowler's position. Encourage pursed-lip and diaphragmatic breathing. Help him to relax.
- Monitor the patient's vital signs. Keep in mind that developing or increasing tachypnea may indicate worsening asthma and that tachycardia may indicate worsening asthma or drug toxicity. Blood pressure readings may reveal pulsus paradoxus, indicating severe asthma. Hypertension may indicate asthma-related hypoxemia.
- Administer prescribed humidified oxygen by nasal cannula at 2 L/minute to ease breathing and to increase Sao$_2$. Later, adjust oxygen according to the patient's vital signs and ABG values.
- Anticipate intubation and mechanical ventilation if the patient fails to maintain adequate oxygenation.
- Monitor serum theophylline levels to ensure they're in the therapeutic range. Observe the patient for signs of theophylline toxicity (vomiting, diarrhea, headache) as well as for signs of subtherapeutic dosage (respiratory distress, increased wheezing).
- Observe the frequency and severity of the patient's cough, and note whether it's productive. Then auscultate his lungs, noting adventitious or absent sounds. If his cough isn't productive and rhonchi are present, teach him effective coughing techniques. If the patient can tolerate postural drainage and chest percussion, perform these procedures to clear secretions. Suction an intubated patient as needed.
- Treat dehydration with I.V. fluids until the patient can tolerate oral fluids, which will help loosen secretions.

**TEACHING CHECKLIST**

## USING A METERED-DOSE INHALER

When instructing your patient about proper metered-dose inhaler (MDI) use, include the following points:

- Shake the MDI well before use.
- Hold the MDI mouthpiece about 1½" to 2" (38 to 51 mm ) from the open mouth.
- Exhale normally, then begin slow, steady inspirations through the mouth.
- While inhaling slowly, squeeze firmly on the MDI to deliver the dose while continuing to breathe in (one deep steady breath, not several shallow ones).
- Hold the breath for 10 seconds before exhaling.
- Breathe normally for several breaths before administering a second dose.
- After using a corticosteroid MDI, rinse out the mouth with water.

  *Note:* When using an extender or a spacer device, follow the same routine as above, with the MDI mouthpiece inserted in one end of the spacer and the other end placed in the mouth. Many spacers are equipped with a small whistle that sounds if the dose is being inhaled too fast.

---

- If conservative treatment fails to improve the airway obstruction, anticipate bronchoscopy or bronchial lavage when the area of collapse is a lobe or larger.

  During long-term care:
- Monitor the patient's respiratory status to detect baseline changes, to assess response to treatment, and to prevent or detect complications.
- Auscultate the lungs frequently, noting the degree of wheezing and quality of air movement.

- Review ABG levels, pulmonary function test results, and $Sao_2$ readings.
- If the patient is taking systemic corticosteroids, observe for complications, such as elevated blood glucose levels and friable skin and bruising.
- Cushingoid effects resulting from long-term use of corticosteroids may be minimized by alternate-day dosage or use of prescribed inhaled corticosteroids.
- If the patient is taking corticosteroids by inhaler, watch for signs of candidal infection in the mouth and pharynx. Using an extender device and rinsing the mouth afterward may prevent this.

  ▶ CLINICAL TIP  For patients with moderate to severe chronic disease, regular use of an extender device may facilitate better delivery of inhaled medications.
- Observe the patient's anxiety level. Keep in mind that measures that reduce hypoxemia and breathlessness should help relieve anxiety.
- Keep the room temperature comfortable and use an air conditioner or a fan in hot, humid weather.
- Control exercise-induced asthma by instructing the patient to use a bronchodilator or cromolyn 30 minutes before exercise. Also instruct him to use pursed-lip breathing while exercising.

  For all patients:
- Teach the patient and his family to avoid known allergens and irritants.
- Describe prescribed drugs, including their names, dosages, actions, adverse effects, and special instructions.
- Teach the patient how to use a metered-dose inhaler. (See *Using a metered-dose inhaler.*) If he has difficulty using an inhaler, he may need an extender device to optimize drug delivery and lower the risk of candidal infection with orally inhaled corticosteroids.
- If the patient has moderate to severe asthma, explain how to use a peak-flow meter to measure the degree of airway

obstruction. Tell him to keep a record of peak-flow readings and to bring it to medical appointments. Explain the importance of calling the doctor at once if the peak flow drops suddenly. (A drop can signal severe respiratory problems.)

• Tell the patient to notify the doctor if he develops a temperature higher than 100° F (37.8° C), chest pain, shortness of breath without coughing or exercising, or uncontrollable coughing. An uncontrollable asthma attack requires immediate attention.

• Teach the patient diaphragmatic and pursed-lip breathing as well as effective coughing techniques.

• Urge the patient to drink at least 3 qt (3 L) of fluids daily to help loosen secretions and maintain hydration.

# ATELECTASIS

Atelectasis is marked by incomplete expansion of lobules (clusters of alveoli) or lung segments, which may result in partial or complete lung collapse. The collapsed areas are unavailable for gas exchange; unoxygenated blood passes through these areas unchanged, thereby producing hypoxia.

Atelectasis may be chronic or acute and occurs to some degree in many patients undergoing upper abdominal or thoracic surgery. The prognosis depends on prompt removal of any airway obstruction, relief of hypoxia, and reexpansion of the collapsed lung.

### Causes

Atelectasis often results from bronchial occlusion by mucus plugs and is frequently a problem in patients with chronic obstructive pulmonary disease, bronchiectasis, or cystic fibrosis and in those who smoke heavily. (Smoking increases mucus production and damages cilia.) Atelectasis may also result from occlusion by foreign bodies, bronchogenic carcinoma, and inflammatory lung disease.

Other causes include respiratory distress syndrome of the newborn (hyaline membrane disease), oxygen toxicity, and pulmonary edema, in which alveolar surfactant changes increase surface tension and permit complete alveolar deflation.

External compression, which inhibits full lung expansion, or any condition that makes deep breathing painful may also cause atelectasis. Such compression or pain may result from upper abdominal surgical incisions, rib fractures, pleuritic chest pain, tight dressings around the chest, or obesity (which elevates the diaphragm and reduces tidal volume).

Atelectasis may also result from prolonged immobility, which causes preferential ventilation of one area of the lung over another, or mechanical ventilation using constant small tidal volumes without intermittent deep breaths.

Central nervous system depression (as in drug overdose) eliminates periodic sighing and is a predisposing factor of progressive atelectasis.

### Signs and symptoms

Clinical effects vary with the cause of collapse, the degree of hypoxia, and any underlying disease but generally include some dyspnea. Atelectasis of a small area of the lung may produce only minimal symptoms that subside without specific treatment.

However, massive collapse can produce severe dyspnea, anxiety, cyanosis, diaphoresis, peripheral circulatory collapse, tachycardia, and substernal or intercostal retraction. Also, atelectasis may result in compensatory hyperinflation of unaffected areas of the lung, mediastinal shift to the affected side, and elevation of the ipsilateral hemidiaphragm.

## Diagnosis

An accurate patient history, a physical examination, and a chest X-ray provide baseline data for a diagnosis. Auscultation reveals diminished or bronchial breath sounds. When much of the lung is collapsed, percussion reveals dullness. However, extensive areas of "microatelectasis" may exist without abnormalities on the chest X-ray. In widespread atelectasis, the chest X-ray shows characteristic horizontal lines in the lower lung zones and, with segmental or lobar collapse, characteristic dense shadows often associated with hyperinflation of neighboring lung zones.

If the cause is unknown, diagnostic procedures may include bronchoscopy to rule out an obstructing neoplasm or a foreign body.

## Treatment

Appropriate treatment includes incentive spirometry, mucolytics, chest percussion, postural drainage, and frequent coughing and deep-breathing exercises. If these measures fail, bronchoscopy may help remove secretions. Humidity and bronchodilators can improve mucociliary clearance and dilate airways; they're sometimes used with a nebulizer.

Atelectasis secondary to an obstructing neoplasm may require surgery or radiation therapy. Postoperative thoracic and abdominal surgery patients require analgesics to facilitate deep breathing, which minimizes the risk of atelectasis.

## Special considerations

• To prevent atelectasis, encourage postoperative and other high-risk patients to cough and deep-breathe every 1 to 2 hours.

• To minimize pain during coughing exercises in postoperative patients, hold a pillow tightly over the incision; teach the patient this technique as well. *Gently* reposition these patients often and help them walk as soon as possible.

• Administer adequate analgesics to control pain.

• During mechanical ventilation, maintain tidal volume at 10 to 15 ml/kg of the patient's body weight to ensure adequate lung expansion. Use the sigh mechanism on the ventilator, if appropriate, to intermittently increase tidal volume at the rate of 10 to 15 sighs/hour.

• Use an incentive spirometer to encourage deep inspiration through positive reinforcement. Teach the patient how to use the spirometer and encourage him to use it every 1 to 2 hours.

• Humidify inspired air and encourage adequate fluid intake to mobilize secretions. To promote loosening and clearance of secretions, use postural drainage and chest percussion.

• If the patient is intubated or uncooperative, provide suctioning as needed. Use sedatives with discretion because they depress respirations and the cough reflex and suppress sighing.

➤ CLINICAL TIP  Know that the patient won't cooperate with treatment if he's in pain.

• Assess breath sounds and ventilatory status frequently and be alert for any changes.

• Teach the patient about respiratory care, including postural drainage, coughing, and deep breathing.

• Encourage the patient to stop smoking, to lose weight, or both, as needed. Refer him to appropriate support groups for help.

• Provide reassurance and emotional support because the patient may be frightened by his limited breathing capacity.

# ATOPIC DERMATITIS

Atopic dermatitis is characterized by superficial skin inflammation and intense itching. Although atopic dermatitis may appear at any age, it typically begins during infancy or early childhood. It may then subside spontaneously, followed by exacerbations in late childhood, adolescence, or early adulthood. Atopic dermatitis affects less than 1% of the population.

## Causes

Several theories attempt to explain the pathogenesis of this disorder, which has an unknown cause. One theory suggests an underlying metabolically or biochemically induced skin disorder that's genetically linked to elevated serum immunoglobulin E (IgE) levels; another suggests defective T-cell function.

Exacerbating factors of atopic dermatitis include irritants, infections (commonly caused by *Staphylococcus aureus*), and some allergens. Although no reliable link exists between atopic dermatitis and exposure to inhalant allergens (such as house dust and animal dander), exposure to food allergens (such as soybeans, fish, or nuts) may coincide with flare-ups of atopic dermatitis.

## Signs and symptoms

Scratching the skin causes vasoconstriction and intensifies pruritus, resulting in erythematous, weeping lesions. Eventually, the lesions become scaly and lichenified. Usually, they're located in areas of flexion and extension, such as the neck, antecubital fos-sa, and popliteal folds, and behind the ears. Patients with atopic dermatitis are prone to unusually severe viral infections, bacterial and fungal skin infections, ocular complications, and allergic contact dermatitis.

## Diagnosis

Typically, the patient has a history of atopy, such as asthma, hay fever, or urticaria; family members may have a similar history. Laboratory tests reveal eosinophilia and elevated serum IgE levels.

## Treatment

Measures to ease this chronic disorder include meticulous skin care, environmental control of offending allergens, and drug therapy.

> CLINICAL TIP Because dry skin aggravates itching, frequent application of nonirritating topical lubricants is important, especially after bathing or showering. Minimizing exposure to allergens and irritants, such as wools and harsh detergents, also helps control symptoms.

Drug therapy involves corticosteroids and antipruritics. Active dermatitis responds well to topical corticosteroids, such as fluocinolone acetonide and flurandrenolide. These drugs should be applied immediately after bathing for optimal penetration. Oral antihistamines, especially the phenothiazine derivatives, such as methdilazine and trimeprazine, help control itching. A bedtime dose of antihistamines may reduce involuntary scratching during sleep. If a secondary infection develops, antibiotics are necessary.

Because this disorder may frustrate the patient and strain family ties, counseling may play a role in treatment.

### Special considerations

● Monitor the patient's compliance with drug therapy.

● Teach the patient when and how to apply topical corticosteroids.

● Emphasize the importance of good personal hygiene.

● Be alert for signs and symptoms of secondary infection; teach the patient how to recognize them as well.

● If the patient's diet is modified to exclude food allergens, monitor his nutritional status.

● Discourage the use of laundry additives.

● Offer support to help the patient and his family cope with this chronic disorder.

# ATTENTION DEFICIT HYPERACTIVITY DISORDER

The patient with attention deficit hyperactivity disorder (ADHD) has difficulty focusing his attention or engaging in quiet, passive activities, or both. Although the disorder is present at birth, diagnosis before age 4 or 5 is difficult unless the child shows severe symptoms. Some patients, though, aren't diagnosed until adulthood. Males are three times more likely to be affected than females.

### Causes

ADHD is commonly thought to be a physiologic brain disorder with a familial tendency. Some studies indicate that it may result from disturbances in neurotransmitter levels in the brain.

### Signs and symptoms

Typically, the patient is characterized as a fidgeter and a daydreamer. Other descriptive terms include inattentive and lazy. Although the patient may be highly intelligent, his school or work performance patterns are sporadic, and he may jump from one partly completed project, thought, or task to another. Some patients have an attention deficit without hyperactivity; they're less likely to be diagnosed and treated.

In a younger child, signs and symptoms include an inability to wait in line, remain seated, wait his turn, or concentrate on one activity until its completion. An older child or an adult may be described as impulsive and easily distracted by irrelevant thoughts, sounds, or sights. He may also be characterized as emotionally labile or inattentive. His disorganization becomes apparent when he has difficulty meeting deadlines and keeping track of school or work tools and materials.

### Diagnosis

Commonly, the child with ADHD is referred for evaluation by the school. Diagnosis of this disorder usually begins by obtaining data from several sources, including the parents, teachers, and the child himself. Complete psychological, medical, and neurologic evaluations rule out other problems. Then the child undergoes tests that measure impulsiveness, attention, and the ability to sustain a task. The combined findings portray a clear picture of the disorder and of the areas of support the child will need.

For characteristic findings in patients with this condition, see *Diagnosing attention deficit hyperactivity disorder*.

### Treatment

Education represents the first step in effective treatment.

➤ CLINICAL TIP   For effective treatment, the entire treatment team (which ideally includes parents, tea-

## DIAGNOSING ATTENTION DEFICIT HYPERACTIVITY DISORDER

The *Diagnostic and Statistical Manual of Mental Disorders,* 4th ed., groups a selection of symptoms into inattention and hyperactivity-impulsivity categories. The diagnosis of attention deficit hyperactivity disorder (ADHD) is based on the person demonstrating at least six symptoms from the inattention group or at least six symptoms from the hyperactivity-impulsivity group. The symptoms must have persisted for at least 6 months to a degree that is maladaptive and inconsistent with the person's developmental level.

### Symptoms of inattention
The person manifesting inattention:
- often fails to give close attention to details or makes careless mistakes in schoolwork, work, or other activities
- often has difficulty sustaining attention in tasks or play activities
- often does not seem to listen when spoken to directly
- often does not follow through on instructions and fails to finish schoolwork, chores, or duties in the workplace (not because of oppositional behavior or failure to understand instructions)
- often has difficulty organizing tasks and activities
- often avoids, dislikes, or is reluctant to engage in tasks that require sustained mental effort (such as schoolwork or homework)
- often loses things necessary for tasks or activities (for example, toys, school assignments, pencils, books, or tools)
- often becomes distracted by extraneous stimuli

- often demonstrates forgetfulness in daily activities.

### Symptoms of hyperactivity-impulsivity
The person manifesting hyperactivity:
- often fidgets with hands or feet or squirms in seat
- often leaves his seat in the classroom or in other situations in which remaining seated is expected
- often runs about or climbs excessively in situations in which remaining seated is expected
- often has difficulty playing or engaging in leisure activities quietly
- often is characterized as "on the go" or acts as if "driven by a motor"
- often talks excessively.
  The person manifesting impulsivity:
- often blurts out answers before questions have been completed
- often has difficulty awaiting his turn
- often interrupts or intrudes on others.

### Additional features
- Some symptoms that caused impairment were evident before age 7.
- Some impairment from the symptoms is present in two or more settings.
- Clinically significant impairment in social, academic, or occupational functioning must be clearly evident.
- The symptoms do not occur exclusively during the course of a pervasive developmental disorder, schizophrenia, or another psychotic disorder and are not better accounted for by another mental disorder.

chers, and therapists as well as the patient and the doctor) must understand ADHD and its effect on the individual's functioning.

Treatment varies, depending on the severity of symptoms and their effect on the patient's ability to function. Behavior modification, coaching, external structure, use of planning and organizing systems, and supportive psychotherapy help the patient cope with the disorder.

Some patients benefit from medication to relieve symptoms. Ideally, the treatment team identifies the symptoms to be managed, selects appropriate medication, and then tracks the patient's symptoms to determine the effectiveness of the medication. Stimulants, such as methylphenidate and dextroamphetamine, are the most commonly used agents. However, other drugs, including tricyclic antidepressants (such as desipramine and nortriptyline), mood stabilizers, and beta blockers, sometimes help control symptoms.

### Special considerations

- Work with the individual to develop external structure and controls.
- Set realistic expectations and limits because the patient with an attention deficit disorder is easily frustrated (which leads to decreased self-control).
- Remain calm and consistent.
- Keep instructions short and simple.
- Provide praise, rewards, and positive feedback whenever possible.
- Refer parents to Children and Adults with Attention Deficit Disorder or other support groups.

# AUTISTIC DISORDER

A severe, pervasive developmental disorder, autistic disorder is marked by unresponsiveness to social contact, gross deficits in intelligence and language development, ritualistic and compulsive behaviors, restricted capacity for developmentally appropriate activities and interests, and bizarre responses to the environment. Autistic disorder may be complicated by epileptic seizures, depression and, during periods of stress, catatonic phenomena.

Autism usually becomes apparent before the child reaches age 30 months, but in some children, the actual onset is difficult to determine. Occasionally, autistic disorder isn't recognized until the child enters school. Autistic disorder is rare, affecting 4 to 5 children per 10,000 births. It affects three to four times more boys than girls, usually the firstborn boy. The prognosis is poor; most patients require a structured environment throughout life.

### Causes

Autistic disorder is thought to result from a combination of psychological, physiologic, and sociological factors. The parents of an autistic child may appear distant and unaffectionate. However, because autistic children are unresponsive or respond with rigid, screaming resistance to touch and attention, parental remoteness may be merely a frustrated, helpless reaction to this disorder, not its cause.

Some autistic children show abnormal but nonspecific EEG findings that suggest brain dysfunction, possibly resulting from trauma, disease, or a structural abnormality. Autistic disorder also has been associated with maternal rubella, untreated phenylketonuria, tuberous sclerosis, anoxia during birth, encephalitis, infantile spasms, and fragile X syndrome.

### Signs and symptoms

Typical features of infantile autistic disorder include unresponsiveness to people, language impairment, lack of imaginative play, bizarre behavior patterns, and abnormal reactions to sensory stimuli.

### Unresponsiveness to people

Infants with this disorder avoid eye contact, have little or no facial expression, and are indifferent to affection and physical contact. Parents may report that the child becomes rigid or flaccid when held, cries when touched, and shows little or no interest in human contact.

As the infant grows older, his smiling response is delayed or absent. He doesn't lift his arms in anticipation of being picked up or form an attachment to a specific caregiver. Nor does he show the anxiety about strangers that's typical in the 8-month-old infant.

The autistic child fails to learn the usual socialization games (peek-a-boo, pat-a-cake, or bye-bye). He's likely to relate to others only to fill a physical need and then without eye contact or speech. The end result may be mutual withdrawal between parents and child.

### Severe language impairment

The child may be mute or may use immature speech patterns. For example, he may use a single word to express a series of activities; he may say "ground" when referring to any step in using a playground slide.

His speech commonly shows echolalia (meaningless repetition of words or phrases addressed to him) and pronoun reversal ("you go walk" when he means "I want to go for a walk"). When answering a question, he may simply repeat the question to mean yes and remain silent to mean no.

### Lack of imaginative play

The child shows little imagination, seldom acting out adult roles or engaging in fantasy play. In fact, he may insist on lining up an exact number of toys in the same manner over and over or repetitively mimic the actions of someone else.

### Bizarre behavior

The autistic child shows characteristically bizarre behavior patterns, such as screaming fits, rituals, rhythmic rocking, arm flapping, crying without tears, and disturbed sleeping and eating patterns. His behavior may be self-destructive (hand biting, eye gouging, hair pulling, or head banging) or self-stimulating (playing with his own saliva, stool, and urine).

His bizarre responses to his environment include an extreme compulsion for sameness.

### Abnormal response to sensory stimuli

The autistic child may underreact or overreact to sensory stimuli; he may ignore objects — dropping those he is given or not looking at them — or he may become excessively absorbed in them — continually watching the objects or the movement of his own fingers over the objects. He commonly responds to stimuli by head banging, rocking, whirling, and hand flapping. He tends to avoid using sight and hearing to interact with the environment.

### Other behavioral abnormalities

Other characteristics of an autistic child may include:

• cognitive impairment (most have a measured IQ of 35 to 49; assessment of their true level of intelligence is difficult due to their poor social and verbal skills)

• eating, drinking, and sleeping problems, for example, limiting his diet to just a few foods, excessive drinking, or repeatedly waking during the night and rocking

• mood disorders, including labile mood, giggling or crying without reason, lack of emotional responses, no fear of real danger but excessive fear of

# DIAGNOSING AUTISTIC DISORDER

Autism is diagnosed when the patient meets the criteria in the *Diagnostic and Statistical Manual of Mental Disorders*, 4th ed. At least six characteristics from the following three categories must be present, including at least two from the social interaction category and one each from the communication and patterns categories.

## Social interaction
Impairment in social interaction, as shown by at least two of the following:
- marked impairment in the use of multiple nonverbal behaviors, such as eye-to-eye gaze, facial expression, body postures, and gestures to regulate social interaction
- failure to develop peer relationships appropriate to developmental level
- no spontaneous sharing of enjoyment, interests, or achievements with others
- lack of social or emotional reciprocity
- gross impairment in ability to make peer friendships.

## Communication
Impairment in communication, as shown by at least one of the following:
- delay in or total lack of spoken language development
- in individuals with adequate speech, marked impairment in initiating or sustaining a conversation with others
- stereotyped and repetitive use of language or idiosyncratic language
- lack of varied, spontaneous make-believe play or social imitative play appropriate to developmental level.

## Patterns
Restricted, repetitive, and stereotyped patterns of behavior, interests, and activities, as manifested by at least one of the following:
- encompassing preoccupation with one or more stereotyped and restricted patterns of interest that is abnormal either in intensity or focus
- apparently inflexible adherence to specific nonfunctional routines or rituals
- stereotyped and repetitive motor mannerisms
- persistent preoccupation with parts of objects.

## Additional criteria
Delays or abnormal functioning in at least one of the following before age 3:
- social interaction
- language as used in social communication
- symbolic or imaginative play.

The disturbance is not better accounted for by Rett's syndrome or childhood disintegrative disorder.

harmless objects, and generalized anxiety.

## Diagnosis
For characteristic findings in patients with this condition, see *Diagnosing autistic disorder*.

## Treatment
The difficult and prolonged treatment of autistic disorder must begin early, continue for years (through adolescence), and coordinate efforts to encourage social adjustment and speech development and to reduce self-destructive behavior.

Behavioral techniques are used to decrease symptoms and increase the child's ability to respond. Positive reinforcement, using food and other rewards, can enhance language and social skills. Providing pleasurable sensory and motor stimulation (jogging, playing with a ball) encourages appropriate behavior and helps eliminate inappropriate behavior. Drug therapy with an agent such as haloperidol may be helpful.

Treatment may take place in a psychiatric facility, in a specialized school, or in a day-care program, but the current trend is toward home treatment. Because family members tend to feel inadequate and guilty, they may need counseling. Until the causes of infantile autism are known, prevention isn't possible.

**Special considerations**
• Reduce self-destructive behaviors. Physically stop the child from harming himself, while firmly saying "no." When he responds to your voice, first give a primary reward (such as food); later, substitute verbal or physical reinforcement (such as saying "good" or giving the child a hug or a pat on the back).
• Foster appropriate use of language. Provide positive reinforcement when the child indicates his needs correctly. Give verbal reinforcement at first (such as "good" or "great"); later, give physical reinforcement (such as a hug or a pat on the hand or shoulder).
• Encourage development of self-esteem. Show the child that he's acceptable as a person.
• Encourage self-care. For example, place a brush in the child's hand and guide his hand to brush his hair. Similarly, teach him to wash his hands and face.
• Encourage acceptance of minor environmental changes. Prepare the child for the change by telling him about it. Make the change minor; for example, change the color of his bedspread or the placement of food on his plate. When he has accepted minor changes, move on to bigger ones.

➤ CLINICAL TIP    Provide emotional support to the parents, and refer them to the Autism Society of America. Emphasize that they aren't responsible for the child's condition.
• Teach the parents how to physically care for the child's needs.
• Teach the parents how to identify signs of excessive stress and the coping skills to use under these circumstances. Emphasize that they'll be ineffective caregivers if they don't take the time to meet their own needs in addition to those of their child.

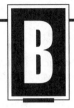

# BASAL CELL EPITHELIOMA

A slow-growing, destructive skin tumor, basal cell epithelioma or carcinoma usually occurs in persons over age 40; it's more prevalent in blond, fair-skinned males and is the most common malignant tumor affecting whites.

## Causes

Prolonged sun exposure is the most common cause of basal cell epithelioma, but arsenic ingestion, radiation exposure, burns, immunosuppression and, rarely, vaccinations are other possible causes.

Although the pathogenesis of basal cell epithelioma is uncertain, some experts now hypothesize that it originates when, under certain conditions, undifferentiated basal cells become carcinomatous instead of differentiating into sweat glands, sebum, and hair.

## Signs and symptoms

Three types of basal cell epithelioma occur:

• *Noduloulcerative lesions* occur most often on the face, particularly the forehead, eyelid margins, and nasolabial folds. In early stages, these lesions are small, smooth, pinkish, and translucent papules. Telangiectatic vessels cross the surface, and the lesions are occasionally pigmented. As the lesions enlarge, their centers become depressed and their borders become firm and elevated. Ulceration and local invasion eventually occur. These ulcerated tumors, known as "rodent ulcers," rarely metastasize; however, if untreated, they can spread to vital areas and become infected. If they invade large blood vessels, they can cause massive hemorrhage.

• *Superficial basal cell epitheliomas* are often numerous and commonly occur on the chest and back. They're oval or irregularly shaped, lightly pigmented plaques, with sharply defined, slightly elevated threadlike borders. Because of superficial erosion, these lesions appear scaly and have small, atrophic areas in the center that resemble psoriasis or eczema. They're usually chronic and don't tend to invade other areas. Superficial basal cell epitheliomas are related to ingestion of or exposure to arsenic-containing compounds.

• *Sclerosing basal cell epitheliomas (morphealike epitheliomas)* are waxy, sclerotic, yellow to white plaques without distinct borders. Occurring on the head and neck, sclerosing basal cell epitheliomas often look like small patches of scleroderma.

## Diagnosis

All types of basal cell epitheliomas are diagnosed by clinical appearance, an incisional or excisional biopsy, and histologic study.

## Treatment

Depending on the size, location, and depth of the lesion, treatment may include curettage and electrodesiccation, chemotherapy, surgical excision, irradiation, cryotherapy, or chemosurgery.

• Curettage and electrodesiccation offer good cosmetic results for small lesions.

**>** CLINICAL TIP   Topical fluorouracil is often used for superficial lesions. This medication produces marked local irritation or inflammation in the involved tissue but no systemic effects.

• Microscopically controlled surgical excision carefully removes recurrent lesions until a tumor-free plane is achieved. After removal of large lesions, skin grafting may be required.

• Irradiation is used if the tumor location requires it and for elderly or debilitated patients who might not withstand surgery.

• Cryotherapy with liquid nitrogen freezes and kills the cells.

• Chemosurgery is often necessary for persistent or recurrent lesions. Chemosurgery consists of periodic applications of a fixative paste (such as zinc chloride) and subsequent removal of fixed pathologic tissue. Treatment continues until tumor removal is complete.

## Special considerations

• Instruct the patient to eat frequent small meals that are high in protein. Suggest eggnog, pureed foods, or liquid protein supplements if the lesion has invaded the oral cavity and caused eating problems.

• Tell the patient that to prevent disease recurrence, he needs to avoid excessive sun exposure and use a strong sunscreen or sunshade to protect his skin from damage by ultraviolet rays.

• Advise the patient to relieve local inflammation from topical fluorouracil with cool compresses or corticosteroid ointment.

• Instruct the patient with noduloulcerative basal cell epithelioma to wash his face gently when ulcerations and crusting occur; scrubbing too vigorously may cause bleeding.

# BELL'S PALSY

This neurologic disorder affects the seventh cranial (facial) nerve, producing unilateral facial weakness or paralysis. Onset is rapid. While it affects all age-groups, it occurs most often in persons under age 60. In 80% to 90% of patients, it subsides spontaneously, with complete recovery in 1 to 8 weeks; however, recovery may be delayed in older adults. If recovery is partial, contractures may develop on the paralyzed side of the face. Bell's palsy may recur on the same or opposite side of the face.

## Causes

The seventh cranial nerve is responsible for motor innervation of the facial muscles. In Bell's palsy, the nerve is blocked by an inflammatory reaction around the nerve (usually at the internal auditory meatus). This is often associated with infections and can result from hemorrhage, tumor, meningitis, or local trauma.

## Signs and symptoms

Bell's palsy usually produces unilateral facial weakness, occasionally with aching pain around the angle of the jaw or behind the ear. On the weak side, the mouth droops (causing the patient to drool saliva from the corner of his mouth), and taste perception is distorted over the affected anterior portion of the tongue. In addition, the forehead appears smooth, and the patient's ability to close his eye on the weak side is markedly impaired. When he tries to close this eye, it rolls upward (Bell's phenomenon) and shows excessive tearing.

Although Bell's phenomenon occurs in normal persons, it's not apparent because the eye closes completely and covers this eye motion. In Bell's palsy, incomplete eye closure makes this upward motion obvious.

### Diagnosis

Clinical presentation in Bell's palsy includes distorted facial appearance and inability to raise the eyebrow, close the eyelid, smile, show the teeth, or puff out the cheek. After 10 days, electromyography helps predict the level of expected recovery by distinguishing temporary conduction defects from a pathologic interruption of nerve fibers.

### Treatment

In Bell's palsy, treatment consists of prednisone, an oral corticosteroid that reduces facial nerve edema and improves nerve conduction and blood flow. After the 14th day of prednisone therapy, electrotherapy may help prevent atrophy of facial muscles.

### Special considerations

● During treatment with prednisone, watch for adverse reactions, especially GI distress and fluid retention. If GI distress is troublesome, a concomitant antacid usually provides relief. If the patient has diabetes, prednisone must be used with caution and necessitates frequent monitoring of serum glucose levels.

● To reduce pain, apply moist heat to the affected side of the face, taking care not to burn the skin.

● To help maintain muscle tone, massage the patient's face with a gentle up-ward motion two to three times daily for 5 to 10 minutes, or have him massage his face himself. When he's ready for active exercises, teach him to exercise by grimacing in front of a mirror.

● Advise the patient to protect his eye by covering it with an eye patch, especially when outdoors. Tell him to keep warm and avoid exposure to dust and wind. When exposure is unavoidable, instruct him to cover his face.

▶ CLINICAL TIP   To prevent complications related to swallowing difficulty (aspiration and weight loss), instruct the patient to always sit up straight when eating, chew on the unaffected side, take small bites, and eat nutritionally balanced meals while avoiding foods that are hard to chew.

● Arrange for privacy at mealtimes to reduce embarrassment.

● Apply a facial sling to improve lip alignment.

● Give the patient frequent and complete mouth care, being careful to remove residual food that collects between the cheeks and gums.

● Offer psychological support. Give reassurance that recovery is likely within 1 to 8 weeks.

# BENIGN PROSTATIC HYPERPLASIA

Although most men over age 50 have some prostatic enlargement, in benign prostatic hyperplasia or hypertrophy (BPH), the prostate gland enlarges sufficiently to compress the urethra and cause some overt urinary obstruction. Depending on the size of the enlarged prostate, the age and health of the patient, and the extent of obstruction, BPH is treated symptomatically or surgically.

## Causes

Recent evidence suggests a link between BPH and hormonal activity. As men age, production of androgenic hormones decreases, causing an imbalance in androgen and estrogen levels and high levels of dihydrotestosterone, the main prostatic intracellular androgen. Other theoretical causes include neoplasm, arteriosclerosis, inflammation, and metabolic or nutritional disturbances.

Whatever the cause, BPH begins with changes in periurethral glandular tissue. As the prostate enlarges, it may extend into the bladder and obstruct urinary outflow by compressing or distorting the prostatic urethra. BPH may also cause a pouch to form in the bladder that retains urine when the rest of the bladder empties. This retained urine may lead to calculus formation or cystitis.

## Signs and symptoms

Clinical features of BPH depend on the extent of prostatic enlargement and the lobes affected.

### Urinary symptoms

Characteristically, the condition starts with a group of symptoms known as *prostatism:* reduced urinary stream caliber and force, difficulty starting micturition (straining), feeling of incomplete voiding and, occasionally, urine retention. As obstruction increases, urination becomes more frequent, with nocturia, incontinence and, possibly, hematuria.

Physical examination reveals a visible midline mass (distended bladder) that represents an incompletely emptied bladder; rectal palpation discloses an enlarged prostate. The examination may also detect secondary anemia and, possibly, renal insufficiency secondary to obstruction.

### Later effects

As BPH worsens, complete urinary obstruction may follow infection or ingestion of decongestants, tranquilizers, alcohol, antidepressants, or anticholinergics. Possible complications include infection, renal insufficiency, hemorrhage, and shock.

## Diagnosis

Clinical features and a rectal examination are usually sufficient for a diagnosis. Other test findings help to confirm it.

- *Excretory urography* may indicate urinary tract obstruction, hydronephrosis, calculi or tumors, and filling and emptying defects in the bladder.
- *Elevated blood urea nitrogen and serum creatinine levels* suggest impaired renal function.
- *Urinalysis* and *urine culture* show hematuria, pyuria and, when the bacterial count exceeds 100,000/µl, urinary tract infection.

In severe symptoms, a cystourethroscopy is definitive, but this test is performed only immediately before surgery to help determine the best procedure. It can show prostate enlargement, bladder wall changes, and a raised bladder.

## Treatment

Conservative therapy includes prostate massages, sitz baths, fluid restriction for bladder distention, and antimicrobials for infection. Regular ejaculation may help relieve prostatic congestion.

Urine flow rates can be improved with alpha$_1$-adrenergic blockers, such as terazosin and prazosin. These drugs relieve bladder outlet obstruction by preventing contractions of the prostatic capsule and bladder neck. Finasteride may also reduce the size of the prostate in some patients.

> CLINICAL TIP
>
> # COMBATING SEPTIC SHOCK IN PROSTATE SURGERY
>
> If the postsurgical patient develops severe chills, sudden fever, tachycardia, hypotension, or other signs of shock, do the following immediately:
>
> - Notify other care team members.
> - Start rapid infusion of I.V. antibiotics as needed.
> - Watch for pulmonary embolism, heart failure, and renal shutdown.
> - Monitor vital signs, central venous pressure, and arterial pressure continuously.
>
> The patient may need supportive care in the intensive care unit.

Surgery is the only effective therapy to relieve acute urine retention, hydronephrosis, severe hematuria, recurrent urinary tract infections, and other intolerable symptoms. (See *Combating septic shock in prostate surgery.*)

A transurethral resection may be performed if the prostate weighs less than 2 oz (56.7 g). In this procedure, a resectoscope removes tissue with a wire loop and electric current. In high-risk patients, continuous drainage with an indwelling urinary catheter alleviates urine retention.

Alternatively, very large prostates can be removed by one of two surgical approaches:

- *suprapubic (transvesical) resection:* most common and useful when prostatic enlargement remains within the bladder

- *retropubic (extravesical) resection:* allows direct visualization; potency and continence are usually maintained.

Balloon dilatation of the prostate isn't effective. Transurethral microwaves (heat therapy) are now being used in some patients. Their efficacy lies between that of the use of alpha$_1$-adrenergic blockers and surgery.

## Special considerations

- Monitor and record the patient's vital signs, intake and output, and daily weight. Watch closely for signs of postobstructive diuresis (such as increased urine output and hypotension), which may lead to serious dehydration, lowered blood volume, shock, electrolyte loss, and anuria.

- Administer antibiotics, as needed, for urinary tract infection, urethral instrumentation, and cystoscopy.

- If urine retention is present, insert an indwelling urinary catheter (usually difficult in a patient with BPH). If the catheter can't be passed transurethrally, assist with suprapubic cystostomy (under local anesthetic). Watch for rapid bladder decompression.

After prostate surgery:

- Maintain patient comfort, and watch for and prevent postoperative complications.

- Observe for immediate dangers of prostatic bleeding (shock and hemorrhage). Check the catheter frequently (every 15 minutes for the first 2 to 3 hours) for patency and urine color; check the dressings for bleeding.

- Many urologists insert a three-way catheter and establish continuous bladder irrigation. Keep the catheter open at a rate sufficient to maintain returns that are clear and light pink.

- Watch for fluid overload from absorption of the irrigating fluid into systemic circulation. If a regular catheter is being used, observe it closely. If drainage stops because of clots, irrigate the catheter, usually with 80 to 100 ml of normal saline solution, while maintaining strict aseptic technique.

- Also watch for septic shock, the most serious complication of prostate surgery.
- Administer belladonna and opium suppositories or other anticholinergics, as needed, to relieve painful bladder spasms that often occur after transurethral resection.
- After an open procedure, provide suppositories (except after perineal prostatectomy), analgesics to control incisional pain, and frequent dressing changes.
- Continue infusing fluids I.V. until the patient can drink a sufficient amount (2 to 3 qt [2 to 3 L] a day) to maintain adequate hydration.
- Administer stool softeners and laxatives, as required, to prevent straining. *Do not* check for fecal impaction; a rectal examination could precipitate bleeding.
- After the catheter is removed, the patient may experience frequency, dribbling, and occasional hematuria. Reassure him that he will gradually regain urinary control. Explain this to the patient's family so that they can also reassure the patient.
- Reinforce prescribed limits on activity. Warn the patient against lifting, strenuous exercise, and long automobile rides because these increase bleeding tendency. Also caution him to restrict sexual activity for at least several weeks after discharge.
- Instruct the patient to follow the prescribed oral antibiotic drug regimen, and tell him the indications for using gentle laxatives. Urge him to seek medical care immediately if he can't void, if he passes bloody urine, or if he develops a fever.

# BERYLLIOSIS

A form of pneumoconiosis, berylliosis, or beryllium poisoning, is a systemic granulomatous disorder with dominant pulmonary manifestations. It occurs in two forms: acute nonspecific pneumonitis and chronic noncaseating granulomatous disease with interstitial fibrosis, which may cause death from respiratory failure and cor pulmonale. Most patients with chronic interstitial disease become only slightly to moderately disabled by impaired lung function and other symptoms, but with each acute exacerbation, the prognosis worsens.

## Causes

Berylliosis results from inhalation of beryllium or from its absorption through the skin. Its severity varies with the amount inhaled. The mechanism by which beryllium exerts its toxic effect is unknown.

This disease occurs among beryllium alloy workers, cathode ray tube makers, gas mantle makers, fluorescent light workers, missile technicians, and nuclear reactor workers; it's generally associated with the milling and use of beryllium and, less commonly, with the mining of beryl ore. Families of beryllium workers and people who live near plants where beryllium alloy is used are also at risk for berylliosis.

## Signs and symptoms

Absorption of beryllium through broken skin produces an itchy rash that usually subsides within 2 weeks after exposure. A "beryllium ulcer" results from accidental implantation of beryllium metal in the skin.

### Respiratory features

Respiratory signs and symptoms of acute berylliosis include swelling and ulceration of nasal mucosa, which may progress to septal perforation, tracheitis, and bronchitis (dry cough). Acute pulmonary disease may develop rapidly (within 3 days) or weeks later, producing a progressive dry cough, tightness in the chest, substernal pain, tachycardia, and signs of bronchitis. This form of the disease has a significant mortality related to respiratory failure.

About 10% of patients with acute berylliosis develop chronic disease 10 to 15 years after exposure. The chronic form causes increasing dyspnea that becomes progressively unremitting, along with mild chest pain, dry unproductive cough, and tachypnea. Pneumothorax may occur, with pulmonary scarring and bleb formation.

➤ CLINICAL TIP   Cardiovascular complications of berylliosis include pulmonary hypertension, right ventricular hypertrophy, and cor pulmonale. Other clinical features include hepatosplenomegaly, renal calculi, lymphadenopathy, anorexia, and fatigue.

### Diagnosis

The patient history reveals occupational, family, or neighborhood exposure to beryllium dust, fumes, or mist. In *acute berylliosis,* chest X-rays may suggest pulmonary edema, showing acute miliary process or a patchy acinus filling, and diffuse infiltrates with prominent peribronchial markings. In *chronic berylliosis,* X-rays show reticulonodular infiltrates, hilar adenopathy, and large coalescent infiltrates in both lungs.

Pulmonary function studies show decreased vital capacity, forced vital capacity, residual volume and total lung capacity, and diffusing capacity of the lungs for carbon monoxide as well as decreased compliance as the lungs stiffen from fibrosis. Arterial blood gas analysis shows decreased partial pressure of arterial oxygen ($Pao_2$) and partial pressure of arterial carbon dioxide.

The following additional tests may be performed:

● *In vitro lymphoblast transformation test* diagnoses berylliosis and monitors workers for occupational exposure to beryllium.

● *Beryllium patch test* establishes only hypersensitivity to beryllium, not the presence of disease.

● *Tissue biopsy* and *spectrographic analysis* are positive for most exposed workers but not absolutely diagnostic.

● *Urinalysis* may show beryllium in urine, but this only indicates exposure.

Differential diagnosis must rule out sarcoidosis and granulomatous infections.

### Treatment

● Beryllium ulcer requires excision or curettage. Acute berylliosis requires prompt corticosteroid therapy.

● Hypoxia may require oxygen administration by nasal cannula or mask (1 to 2 L/minute). Severe respiratory failure requires mechanical ventilation if $Pao_2$ can't be maintained above 40 mm Hg.

● Chronic berylliosis is usually treated with corticosteroids, although it's not certain that steroids alter the progression of the disease. Lifelong maintenance therapy may be necessary.

● Respiratory symptoms may be treated with bronchodilators, increased fluid intake (at least 3 qt [3 L] daily), and chest physiotherapy techniques. Diuretics, digitalis glycosides, and salt restriction may be useful in patients with cor pulmonale.

### Special considerations

● Teach the patient to prevent infection by avoiding crowds and persons with infection and by receiving influenza and pneumococcal vaccines.

• Encourage the patient to practice physical reconditioning, energy conservation in daily activities, and relaxation techniques.

# BIPOLAR DISORDERS

Marked by severe pathologic mood swings from hyperactivity and euphoria to sadness and depression, bipolar disorders involve various symptom combinations:

• Type I bipolar disorder is characterized by alternating episodes of mania and depression.

• Type II is characterized by recurrent depressive episodes and occasional manic episodes.

• In some patients, bipolar disorder assumes a seasonal pattern, marked by a cyclic relation between the onset of the mood episode and a particular 60-day period of the year.

*Incidence*
The American Psychiatric Association estimates that 0.4% to 1.2% of adults experience bipolar disorder. This disorder affects women and men equally, is more common in higher socioeconomic groups, and is associated with high levels of creativity. It can begin at any time after adolescence, but onset usually occurs between ages 20 and 35; about 35% of patients experience onset between ages 35 and 60.

Before the onset of overt symptoms, many patients with bipolar disorder have an energetic and outgoing personality with a history of wide mood swings. A related but less severe form of illness, called cyclothymic disorder, common-

## CYCLOTHYMIC DISORDER

A chronic mood disturbance of at least 2 years' duration, cyclothymic disorder involves numerous episodes of hypomania or depression that aren't of sufficient severity or duration to qualify as a major depressive episode or a bipolar disorder.

Cyclothymia commonly starts in adolescence or early adulthood. Beginning insidiously, this disorder leads to persistent social and occupational dysfunction.

**Signs and symptoms**
In the hypomanic phase, the patient may experience insomnia; hyperactivity; inflated self-esteem; increased productivity and creativity; overinvolvement in pleasurable activities, including an increased sexual drive; physical restlessness; and rapid speech. Depressive symptoms may include insomnia, feelings of inadequacy, decreased productivity, social withdrawal, loss of libido, loss of interest in pleasurable activities, lethargy, slow speech, and crying.

**Diagnosis**
A number of medical disorders (for example, cerebrovascular accident, brain tumors, head trauma, and endocrinopathies such as Cushing's disease) and a drug overdose can produce a similar pattern of mood alteration. These organic causes must be ruled out before making a diagnosis of cyclothymic disorder.

ly precedes a bipolar disorder. (See *Cyclothymic disorder.*)

Bipolar disorder recurs in some patients; as they grow older, the episodes recur more frequently and last longer.

This illness is associated with a significant mortality; about 20% of patients commit suicide, many just as the depression lifts.

## Causes

The origins of bipolar disorder are unclear, but hereditary, biological, and psychological factors may play a part.

### Hereditary factors

The incidence of bipolar disorder among relatives of affected patients is higher than in the general population and highest among maternal relatives. The closer the relationship, the greater the susceptibility. A child with one affected parent has a 25% chance of developing bipolar disorder; a child with two affected parents, a 50% chance. The incidence of this illness in siblings is 20% to 25%; in identical twins, the incidence is 66% to 96%.

### Biological factors

Although certain biochemical changes accompany mood swings, it's not clear whether these changes cause the mood swings or result from them. In both mania and depression, intracellular sodium concentration increases during illness and returns to normal with recovery.

Patients with mood disorders have a defect in the way the brain handles certain neurotransmitters — chemical messengers that shuttle nerve impulses between neurons. Low levels of the chemicals dopamine and norepinephrine, for example, have been linked to depression, whereas excessively high levels of these chemicals are associated with mania.

Changes in the concentration of acetylcholine and serotonin also may play a role. Although neurobiologists have yet to prove that these chemical shifts cause bipolar disorder, it's widely assumed that most antidepressant medications work by modifying these neurotransmitter systems.

New data suggest that changes in the circadian rhythms that control hormone secretion, body temperature, and appetite may contribute to the development of bipolar disorder.

### Emotional and physical factors

Emotional or physical trauma, such as bereavement, disruption of an important relationship, or a serious accidental injury, may precede the onset of bipolar disorder; however, bipolar disorder often appears without identifiable predisposing factors.

Manic episodes may follow a stressful event, but they're also associated with antidepressant therapy and childbirth. Major depressive episodes may be precipitated by chronic physical illness, psychoactive drug dependence, psychosocial stressors, and childbirth. Other familial influences, especially the early loss of a parent, parental depression, incest, or abuse, may predispose a person to depressive illness.

## Signs and symptoms

Clinical presentation varies widely, depending on whether the patient is experiencing a manic or a depressive episode.

### Manic features

The *manic* patient typically appears euphoric, expansive, or irritable with little control over his activities and responses. He may describe hyperactive or excessive behavior, including elaborate plans for numerous social events, efforts to renew old acquaintances by telephoning friends at all hours of the night, buying sprees, or promiscuous sexual activity. He seldom hesitates to start projects for which he has little aptitude.

The patient's activities may have a bizarre quality, such as dressing in colorful or strange garments, wearing excessive makeup, or giving advice to passing strangers. He often expresses an inflated sense of self-esteem, ranging from uncritical self-confidence to marked grandiosity, which may be delusional. Common features of the manic phase are accelerated speech, frequent changes of topic, and flight of ideas. The patient is easily distracted and responds rapidly to external stimuli, such as background noise or a ringing telephone.

Physical examination of the manic patient may reveal signs of malnutrition and poor personal hygiene. He may report sleeping and eating less than usual.

*Hypomania,* more common than acute mania, can be recognized during the assessment interview by three classic symptoms: elated but unstable mood, pressured speech, and increased motor activity. The hypomanic patient may appear elated, hyperactive, easily distracted, talkative, irritable, impatient, impulsive, and full of energy but seldom exhibits flight of ideas, delusions, or an absence of discretion and self-control.

### Depressive features

The patient who experiences a *depressive episode* may report a loss of self-esteem, overwhelming inertia, social withdrawal, and feelings of hopelessness, apathy, or self-reproach. He may believe that he's wicked and deserves to be punished. His growing sadness, guilt, negativity, and fatigue place extraordinary burdens on his family.

During the assessment interview, the depressed patient may speak and respond slowly. He may complain of difficulty concentrating or thinking clear-

ly but usually isn't obviously disoriented or intellectually impaired.

Physical examination may reveal reduced psychomotor activity, lethargy, low muscle tonus, weight loss, slowed gait, and constipation. The patient also may report sleep disturbances (falling asleep, staying asleep, or early morning awakening), sexual dysfunction, headaches, chest pains, and a heaviness in the limbs. Typically, symptoms are worse in the morning and gradually subside as the day goes on.

His concerns about his health may become hypochondriacal: He may worry excessively about having cancer or some other serious illness. In an elderly patient, physical symptoms may be the only clues to depression.

Suicide is an ever-present risk, especially as the depression begins to lift. At that point, a rising energy level may strengthen the patient's resolve to carry out suicidal plans.

The suicidal patient may also harbor homicidal ideas, for example, thinking of killing his family either in anger or to spare them pain and disgrace.

### Diagnosis

For characteristic findings in patients with this condition, see *Diagnosing bipolar disorders,* pages 104 and 105.

Physical examination and laboratory tests, such as endocrine function studies, rule out medical causes of the mood disturbances, including intra-abdominal neoplasm, hypothyroidism, heart failure, cerebral arteriosclerosis, parkinsonism, psychoactive drug abuse, brain tumor, and uremia. Moreover, a review of the medications prescribed for other disorders may point to drug-induced depression or mania.

### Treatment

Widely used to treat bipolar disorder, lithium has proved to be highly effec-

*(Text continues on page 106.)*

# DIAGNOSING BIPOLAR DISORDERS

The diagnosis of bipolar disorder is confirmed when the patient meets the criteria documented in the *Diagnostic and Statistical Manual of Mental Disorders,* 4th ed.

## For a manic episode
• A distinct period of abnormally and persistently elevated, expansive, or irritable mood lasting at least 1 week (or any duration if hospitalization is needed)
• During the mood disturbance period, at least three of the following symptoms must have persisted (four, if the mood is only irritable) and have been present to a significant degree:
– inflated self-esteem or grandiosity
– decreased need for sleep
– more talkative than usual or pressured to keep talking
– flight of ideas or subjective experience that thoughts are racing
– distractibility
– increased goal-directed activity or psychomotor agitation
– excessive involvement in pleasurable activities that have a high potential for painful consequences.
• The symptoms do not meet the criteria for a mixed episode.
• The mood disturbance is sufficiently severe to cause one of the following to occur:
– marked impairment in occupational functioning or in usual social activities or relationships with others
– hospitalization to prevent harm to self or others
– evidence of psychotic features.
• The symptoms are not due to the direct physiologic effects of a substance or a general medical condition.

## For a hypomanic episode
• A distinct period of abnormally and persistently elevated, expansive, or irritable mood lasting at least 4 days that's clearly different from the usual nondepressed mood

• During the mood disturbance period, at least three of the following symptoms must have persisted (four, if the mood is only irritable) and have been present to a significant degree:
– inflated self-esteem or grandiosity
– decreased need for sleep
– more talkative than usual or pressured to keep talking
– flight of ideas or subjective experience that thoughts are racing
– distractibility
– increased goal-directed activity or psychomotor agitation
– excessive involvement in pleasurable activities that have a high potential for painful consequences.
• The episode is associated with an unequivocal change in functioning that's uncharacteristic of the person when he's not symptomatic.
• Others can recognize the disturbance in mood and the change in functioning.
• The episode is not severe enough to markedly impair social or occupational functioning or to necessitate hospitalization to prevent harm to self or others, and no psychotic features are evident.
• The symptoms are not due to the direct physiologic effects of a substance or a general medical condition.

## For a bipolar I single manic episode
• Presence of only one manic episode and no past major depressive episodes
• The manic episode is not better accounted for by schizoaffective disorder and is not superimposed on schiozophrenia, schizophreniform disorder, delusional disorder, or psychotic disorder not otherwise specified.

## For a bipolar I disorder, most recent episode hypomanic
• Currently (or most recently) in a hypomanic episode

## DIAGNOSING BIPOLAR DISORDERS *(continued)*

• The person previously had at least one manic episode or mixed episode.
• The mood symptoms cause clinically significant distress or impairment in social, occupational, or other important areas of functioning.
• The first two exacerbations of the mood episode (above) are not better accounted for by schizoaffective disorder and are not superimposed on schizophrenia, schizophreniform disorder, delusional disorder, or psychotic disorder not otherwise specified.

### For a bipolar I disorder, most recent episode manic

• Currently (or most recently) in a manic episode
• The person previously had at least one major depressive episode, manic episode, or mixed episode.
• The first two exacerbations of mood episode (above) are not better accounted for by schizoaffective disorder and are not superimposed on schizophrenia, schizophreniform disorder, delusional disorder, or psychotic disorder not otherwise specified.

### For a bipolar I disorder, most recent episode mixed

• Currently (or most recently) in a mixed episode
• The person previously had at least one major depressive episode, manic episode, or mixed episode.
• The first two exacerbations of mood episode (above) are not better accounted for by schizoaffective disorder and are not superimposed on schizophrenia, schizophreniform disorder, delusional disorder, or psychotic disorder not otherwise specified.

### For a bipolar I disorder, most recent episode depressed

• Currently (or most recently) in a major depressive episode
• The person previously had at least one manic episode or mixed episode.

• The first two exacerbations of mood episode (above) aren't better accounted for by schizoaffective disorder and aren't superimposed on schizophrenia, schizophreniform disorder, delusional disorder, or psychotic disorder not otherwise specified.

### For a bipolar I disorder, most recent episode unspecified

• Criteria, except for duration, are currently (or most recently) met for a manic, hypomanic, mixed, or major depressive episode.
• The person previously had at least one manic episode or mixed episode.
• The mood symptoms cause clinically significant distress or impairment in social, occupational, or other important areas of functioning.
• The first two exacerbations of mood episode (above) are not better accounted for by schizoaffective disorder and are not superimposed on schizophrenia, schizophreniform disorder, delusional disorder, or psychotic disorder not otherwise specified.
• The first two exacerbations of mood episode (above) are not due to the direct physiologic effects of a substance or a general medical condition.

### For a bipolar II disorder

• Presence (or history) of one or more major depressive episodes
• Presence (or history) of at least one hypomanic episode
• The patient has never had a manic episode or a mixed episode.
• The first two exacerbations of mood episode (above) are not better accounted for by schizoaffective disorder and are not superimposed on schizophrenia, schizophreniform disorder, delusional disorder, or psychotic disorder not otherwise specified.
• The symptoms cause clinically significant distress or impairment in social, occupational, or other important areas of functioning.

## PREVENTING COMPLICATIONS OF LITHIUM THERAPY

When teaching your patient about taking lithium, include the following points:

• Take the medication exactly as prescribed.
• Have blood tests regularly as ordered.
• Report any of the following signs to the doctor:
– ataxia
– severe tremors
– impaired motor coordination
– blurred vision
– slurred speech
– lethargy
– diarrhea.
*Note:* Vomiting, diarrhea, or excessive sweating can raise lithium levels.

Anticonvulsants, such as carbamazepine, valproic acid, and clonazepam, are used either alone or with lithium to treat mood disorders. (See *Preventing complications of lithium therapy.*) Carbamazepine, a potent antimanic drug, is effective in many lithium-resistant patients.

Antidepressants are used to treat depressive symptoms, but they may trigger a manic episode.

**Special considerations**

For the manic patient:

• Attend to the manic patient's physical needs. Give small, frequent meals, including finger foods, that can be eaten while pacing.
• As the patient's symptoms subside, encourage him to assume responsibility for personal care.

➤ CLINICAL TIP  Provide emotional support, maintain a calm environment, and set realistic goals for behavior.

• Provide diversional activities suited to a short attention span; firmly discourage the patient if he tries to overextend himself.
• When necessary, reorient the patient to reality, and tactfully divert conversations when they become intimately concerned with other patients or staff members.
• Set limits in a calm, clear, and self-confident manner for the manic patient's demanding, hyperactive, manipulative, and acting-out behaviors. Setting limits tells the patient you'll provide security and protection by refusing inappropriate and possibly harmful requests.
• Listen to requests attentively and with a neutral attitude, but avoid power struggles if a patient tries to put you on the spot for an immediate answer. Explain that you'll seriously consider the request and will respond later.

tive in relieving and preventing manic episodes. It curbs the accelerated thought processes and hyperactive behavior without producing the sedating effect of antipsychotic drugs. In addition, it may prevent the recurrence of depressive episodes; however, it's ineffective in treating acute depression.

Because lithium has a narrow therapeutic range, treatment must be initiated cautiously and the dosage adjusted slowly. Therapeutic blood levels must be maintained for 7 to 10 days before the drug's beneficial effects appear; for this reason, antipsychotic drugs commonly are used in the interim to provide sedation and symptomatic relief. Because lithium is excreted by the kidneys, any renal impairment necessitates withdrawal of the drug.

- Collaborate with other staff members to provide consistent responses to the patient's manipulative or acting-out behaviors.

- Watch for early signs of frustration (when the patient's anger escalates from verbal threats to hitting an object). Tell the patient firmly that threats and hitting are unacceptable and that these behaviors show that he needs help to control his behavior. Then tell him that the staff will help him move to a quiet area and will help him control his behavior so he won't hurt himself or others. Staff members who have practiced as a team can work effectively to prevent acting-out behavior or to remove and confine a patient.

- Alert the staff team promptly when acting-out behavior escalates. It's safer to have help available before you need it than to try controlling an anxious or frightened patient by yourself.

- Once the incident is over and the patient is calm and in control, discuss his feelings with him and offer suggestions on how to prevent a recurrence.

- If the patient is taking lithium, tell him and his family to discontinue the drug and notify the doctor if signs of toxicity, such as diarrhea, abdominal cramps, vomiting, unsteadiness, drowsiness, muscle weakness, polyuria, and tremors, occur.

For the depressed patient:

- The depressed patient needs continual positive reinforcement to improve his self-esteem. Provide a structured routine, including activities to boost his self-confidence and promote interaction with others (for instance, group therapy), and keep reassuring him that his depression will lift.

- Encourage the patient to talk or to write down his feelings if he's having trouble expressing them. Listen attentively and respectfully, and allow him time to formulate his thoughts if he

seems sluggish. Record your observations and conversations.

- To prevent possible self-injury or suicide, remove harmful objects (glass, belts, rope, bobby pins) from the patient's environment, observe him closely, and strictly supervise his medications. Institute suicide precautions as dictated by your facility's policy.

- Attend to the patient's physical needs. If he's too depressed to take care of himself, help him with personal hygiene measures. Encourage him to eat, or feed him if necessary. If he's constipated, add high-fiber foods to his diet; offer small, frequent meals; and encourage physical activity. To help him sleep, give him back rubs or warm milk at bedtime.

- If the patient is taking an antidepressant, watch for signs of mania.

# BLADDER CANCER

Bladder tumors can develop on the surface of the bladder wall (benign or malignant papillomas) or grow within the bladder wall (generally more virulent) and quickly invade underlying muscles. Most bladder tumors (90%) are transitional cell carcinomas, arising from the transitional epithelium of mucous membranes. Less common are adenocarcinomas, epidermoid carcinomas, squamous cell carcinomas, sarcomas, tumors in bladder diverticula, and carcinoma in situ. Bladder tumors are most prevalent in men over age 50 and are more common in densely populated industrial areas.

## Causes

Certain environmental carcinogens, such as 2-naphthylamine, benzidine, tobacco, and nitrates, predispose people to transitional cell tumors. Thus, workers in certain industries — rubber workers, weavers, leather finishers, aniline dye workers, hairdressers, petroleum workers, and spray painters — are at high risk for such tumors. The period between exposure to the carcinogen and development of symptoms is about 18 years.

Squamous cell carcinoma of the bladder is most common in geographic areas where schistosomiasis is endemic. It's also associated with chronic bladder irritation and infection (for example, from kidney stones, indwelling urinary catheters, and cystitis caused by cyclophosphamide).

### Signs and symptoms

In early stages, approximately 25% of patients with bladder tumors have no symptoms. Commonly, the first sign is gross, painless, intermittent hematuria (often with clots in the urine). Patients with invasive lesions often have suprapubic pain after voiding. Other symptoms include bladder irritability, urinary frequency, nocturia, and dribbling.

### Diagnosis

Only cystoscopy and a biopsy can confirm bladder cancer. Cystoscopy should be performed when hematuria first appears. When it's performed under anesthesia, a bimanual examination is usually done to determine if the bladder is fixed to the pelvic wall. A thorough history and physical examination may help determine whether the tumor has invaded the prostate or the lymph nodes. (See *Comparing staging systems for bladder cancer*.)

The following tests can provide essential information about the tumor:

• *Urinalysis* can detect blood in the urine and malignant cytology.

• *Excretory urography* can identify a large, early-stage tumor or an infiltrating tumor, delineate functional problems in the upper urinary tract, assess hydronephrosis, and detect rigid deformity of the bladder wall.

• *Retrograde cystography* evaluates bladder structure and integrity. Test results help to confirm the diagnosis.

• *Pelvic arteriography* can reveal tumor invasion into the bladder wall.

• *Computed tomography scan* reveals the thickness of the involved bladder wall and detects enlarged retroperitoneal lymph nodes.

• *Ultrasonography* can detect metastasis beyond the bladder and can distinguish a bladder cyst from a tumor.

### Treatment

Appropriate treatment for bladder cancer varies.

#### Superficial bladder tumors

Superficial bladder tumors are removed by transurethral (cystoscopic) resection and fulguration (electrical destruction). This procedure is adequate when the tumor hasn't invaded the muscle.

Intravesicular chemotherapy is also used for superficial tumors (especially those that occur in many sites) and to prevent tumor recurrence. This treatment involves washing the bladder directly with antineoplastic drugs — most commonly, thiotepa, doxorubicin, mitomycin, or bacille Calmette-Guérin.

If additional tumors develop, fulguration may have to be repeated every 3 months for years. However, if the tumors penetrate the muscle layer or recur frequently, cystoscopy with fulguration is no longer appropriate.

Tumors too large to be treated through a cystoscope require segmental bladder resection to remove a full-thickness section of the bladder. This procedure is feasible only if the tumor isn't near the bladder neck or ureteral orifices. Bladder instillations of thiotepa after transurethral resection may also help control such tumors.

# COMPARING STAGING SYSTEMS FOR BLADDER CANCER

Staging helps determine the most appropriate treatment for bladder cancer. One of two staging systems may be used: the TNM (tumor, node, metastasis) system or the JSM (Jewett-Strong-Marshall) system. The JSM system grades cancers 0 and A through D. Both systems distinguish superficial bladder cancers from invasive bladder cancers, which penetrate bladder muscle and may spread to other sites.

| TNM | STAGE | JSM |
|---|---|---|
| **SUPERFICIAL TUMOR** | | |
| TX | Primary tumor can't be assessed | — |
| T0 | No tumor | 0 |
| Tis | Carcinoma in situ | 0 |
| Ta | Noninvasive papillary tumor | 0 |
| **INVASIVE TUMOR** | | |
| T1 | Tumor invades subepithelial connective tissue | – |
| T2 | Tumor invades superficial muscle (inner half) | B1 |
| T3a | Tumor invades deep muscle | B2 |
| T3b | Tumor invades perivesical fat | C |
| T4 | Tumor invades prostate, uterus, vagina, pelvic wall, or abdominal wall | D1 |
| NX | Regional lymph nodes can't be assessed | – |
| N0 | No evidence of lymph node involvement | – |
| N1 | Metastasis in a single lymph node, 2 cm or less in greatest dimension | D1 |
| N2 | Metastasis in a single lymph node, between 2 and 5 cm in greatest dimension, or metastases in several lymph nodes, none greater than 5 cm in greatest dimension | – |
| N3 | Metastasis in a lymph node more than 5 cm in greatest dimension | – |
| MX | Distant metastasis can't be assessed | – |
| M0 | No evidence of distant metastasis | – |
| M | Distant metastasis | D2 |

TEACHING CHECKLIST

## CARING FOR A URINARY STOMA

If your patient has a urinary stoma, give him these instructions:
• First, show the patient how to prepare and apply the pouch, which may be reusable or disposable. If he chooses the reusable type, he'll need at least two.
• To select the right pouch size, teach the patient to measure the stoma and order a pouch with an opening that clears the stoma with a 1/8" margin. Instruct him to remeasure the stoma after he goes home, in case the size changes. The pouch should have a drainage valve at the bottom. Tell him to empty the pouch when it's one-third full or every 2 to 3 hours.
• To ensure a good skin seal, advise the patient to select a skin barrier that contains synthetics and little or no karaya (which urine tends to destroy). Check the pouch frequently to make sure that the skin seal remains intact. A good skin seal with a skin barrier may last for 3 to 6 days, so change the pouch only that often. Tell the patient that he can wear a loose-fitting elastic belt to help secure the pouch.
• The ileal conduit stoma reaches its permanent size 2 to 4 months after surgery. Because the intestine normally produces mucus, tell the patient not to be alarmed by mucus that appears in the draining urine.
• Instruct the patient to keep the skin around the stoma clean and free of irritation, as follows:
– After removing the pouch, wash the skin with water and mild soap. Rinse well with clear water to remove soap residue, and then gently pat the skin dry; don't rub.
– Place a gauze sponge soaked with vinegar-water (1 part : 3 parts) over the stoma for a few minutes to prevent uric acid crystal buildup. While preparing the skin, place a rolled-up dry sponge over the stoma to collect draining urine.
– Coat the skin with a silicone skin protector, and cover with the collection pouch. If skin irritation or breakdown occurs, apply a layer of antacid precipitate to the clean, dry skin before coating with the skin protector.
• Advise the patient that he can level uneven surfaces on his abdomen, such as gullies, scars, or wedges, with a variety of specially prepared products or skin barriers.

### Infiltrating bladder tumors

Radical cystectomy is the treatment of choice for infiltrating bladder tumors. The week before cystectomy, treatment may include external beam therapy to the bladder. Surgery involves removal of the bladder with perivesical fat, lymph nodes, urethra, the prostate and seminal vesicles (in males), and the uterus and adnexa (in females). The surgeon forms a urinary diversion, usually an ileal conduit. The patient must then wear an external pouch continuously. (See *Caring for a urinary stoma.*) Other diversions include ureterostomy, nephrostomy, vesicostomy, ileal bladder, ileal loop, and sigmoid conduit.

Males are impotent following radical cystectomy and urethrectomy because these procedures damage the sympathetic and parasympathetic nerves that control erection and ejaculation. At a later date, the patient may desire a penile implant to make sexual intercourse (without ejaculation) possible.

### Advanced bladder cancer

For patients with advanced bladder cancer, treatment includes cystectomy to remove the tumor, radiation therapy, and systemic chemotherapy with such drugs as cyclophosphamide, fluorouracil, doxorubicin, and cisplatin. This combination sometimes is successful in arresting bladder cancer.

Cisplatin is the most effective single agent.

### Investigational treatments

Such treatments include photodynamic therapy and intravesicular administration of interferon alfa and tumor necrosis factor. Photodynamic therapy involves I.V. injection of a photosensitizing agent such as hematoporphyrin ether, which malignant cells readily absorb. Then a cystoscopic laser device introduces laser energy into the bladder, exposing the malignant cells to laser light, which kills them. Because this treatment also produces photosensitivity in normal cells, the patient must totally avoid sunlight for about 30 days.

### Special considerations

• Before surgery, assist in selecting a stoma site that the patient can see (usually in the rectus muscle to minimize the risk of herniation). Do so by assessing the abdomen in various positions.

• After surgery, encourage the patient to look at the stoma. Provide a mirror to make viewing easier.

• To obtain a specimen for culture and sensitivity testing, catheterize the patient using sterile technique. Insert the lubricated tip of the catheter into the stoma about 2″ (5 cm). In many facilities, a double telescope-type catheter is available for ileal conduit catheterization.

• Advise the patient with a urinary stoma that he may participate in most activities, except for heavy lifting and contact sports.

CLINICAL TIP When a patient with a urinary diversion is discharged, arrange for follow-up home health care or refer him to an enterostomal therapist, who will help coordinate the patient's care.

• Teach the patient about his urinary stoma. Encourage his spouse, a friend, or a relative to attend the teaching session. Advise this person beforehand that a negative reaction to the stoma can impede the patient's adjustment.

• All high-risk people — for example, chemical workers and people with a history of benign bladder tumors or persistent cystitis — should have periodic cytologic examinations and learn about the dangers of disease-causing agents.

• Refer ostomates to such resources as the American Cancer Society and the United Ostomy Association.

# BLASTOMYCOSIS

Also called Gilchrist's disease, blastomycosis is caused by the yeastlike fungus *Blastomyces dermatitidis,* which usually infects the lungs and produces bronchopneumonia. Less frequently, this fungus may disseminate through the blood and cause osteomyelitis and central nervous system (CNS), skin, and genital disorders.

Untreated blastomycosis is slowly progressive and usually fatal; however, spontaneous remissions occasionally occur. With antifungal drug therapy and supportive treatment, the prognosis for patients with blastomycosis is good.

### Causes

Blastomycosis is generally found in North America (where *B. dermatitidis* normally inhabits the soil) and is endemic to the southeastern United States.

Sporadic cases have also been reported in Africa. Blastomycosis usually infects men ages 30 to 50, but no occupational link has been found. *B. dermatitidis* is probably inhaled by people who are in close contact with the soil. The incubation period may range from weeks to months.

## Signs and symptoms

Initial clinical indicators of pulmonary blastomycosis mimic those of a viral upper respiratory tract infection. These findings typically include a dry, hacking, or productive cough (occasionally hemoptysis), pleuritic chest pain, fever, shaking, chills, night sweats, malaise, anorexia, and weight loss.

● Cutaneous blastomycosis causes small, painless, nonpruritic, and nondistinctive macules or papules on exposed body parts. These lesions become raised and reddened and occasionally progress to draining skin abscesses or fistulas.

● Skeletal involvement causes soft-tissue swelling, tenderness, and warmth over bony lesions, which generally occur in the thoracic, lumbar, and sacral regions; long bones of the legs; and, in children, the skull.

● Genital involvement produces painful swelling of the testes, the epididymis, or the prostate; deep perineal pain; pyuria; and hematuria.

● CNS involvement causes meningitis or cerebral abscesses, resulting in a decreased level of consciousness (LOC), lethargy, and change in mood or affect.

Other dissemination may result in Addison's disease (adrenal insufficiency), pericarditis, and arthritis.

## Diagnosis

Various tests may be ordered to diagnose blastomycosis, including:

● *culture* of *B. dermatitidis* from skin lesions, pus, sputum, or pulmonary secretions

● *biopsy* of tissue from the skin or lungs or of bronchial washings, sputum, or pus, as the doctor finds appropriate.

● *complement fixation testing.* Although such testing isn't conclusive, a high titer in extrapulmonary disease is a poor prognostic sign.

● *immunodiffusion testing.* This specific study detects antibodies for the A and B antigen of blastomycosis.

In addition, suspected pulmonary blastomycosis requires a chest X-ray, which may show pulmonary infiltrates. Other abnormal laboratory findings include an increased white blood cell count and erythrocyte sedimentation rate, slightly increased serum globulin levels, mild normochromic anemia and, with bone lesions, an increased alkaline phosphatase level.

## Treatment

All forms of blastomycosis respond to amphotericin B. Ketoconazole and fluconazole may be used as alternatives. Patient care is mainly supportive.

## Special considerations

● In severe pulmonary blastomycosis, check for hemoptysis. If the patient is febrile, provide a cool room and give tepid sponge baths.

● If blastomycosis causes joint pain or swelling, elevate the joint and apply heat.

● In CNS infection, watch the patient carefully for decreasing LOC and unequal pupillary response.

● In men with disseminated disease, watch for hematuria.

➤ CLINICAL TIP  Infuse I.V. amphotericin B slowly (a too-rapid infusion may cause circulatory collapse). During the infusion, monitor vital signs. (Temperature may rise but should subside within 1 to 2 hours.) Watch for decreased urine output and monitor laboratory results for increased blood urea nitrogen and serum creatinine levels and hypokalemia, which may indicate renal toxicity. Report any hearing loss, tinnitus, or dizziness immediately.

• To relieve adverse effects of amphotericin B, give antiemetics and antipyretics as needed.

# BLEPHARITIS

A common inflammation, blepharitis produces a red-rimmed appearance of the margins of the eyelids. It's frequently chronic and bilateral and can affect both upper and lower lids. *Seborrheic blepharitis* is characterized by waxy scales and is common in older adults and in persons with red hair. *Staphylococcal (ulcerative) blepharitis* is characterized by tiny ulcerated areas along the lid margins. Both types may coexist.

Blepharitis tends to recur and become chronic. It can be controlled if treatment begins before the onset of ocular involvement.

## Causes

Seborrheic blepharitis generally results from seborrhea of the scalp, eyebrows, and ears; ulcerative blepharitis, from *Staphylococcus aureus* infection. (People with this infection may also tend to develop chalazions and styes.)

## Signs and symptoms

Clinical features of blepharitis include itching, burning, foreign-body sensation, and sticky, crusted eyelids on waking. This constant irritation results in unconscious rubbing of the eyes (causing reddened rims) or continual blinking. Other signs include waxy scales in seborrheic blepharitis; flaky scales on lashes, loss of lashes, and ulcerated ar-

eas on lid margins in ulcerative blepharitis.

## Diagnosis

In blepharitis, diagnosis depends on the patient history and characteristic symptoms. In ulcerative blepharitis, a culture of the ulcerated lid margin shows *S. aureus*.

## Treatment

Early treatment is essential to prevent recurrence or complications. In addition to warm compresses, treatment depends on the type of blepharitis:

• *seborrheic blepharitis:* daily shampooing of eyelashes (using a mild shampoo on a damp applicator stick or a washcloth) to remove scales from the lid margins; also, frequent shampooing of the scalp and eyebrows

• *ulcerative blepharitis:* warm compresses may be applied and an appropriate antibiotic, such as erythromycin or bacitracin, may be used at bedtime; additionally, a combination antibiotic and steroid, such as prednisolone (sulfa and steroid; Vasocidin or Blephamide), may be used

• *blepharitis resulting from pediculosis:* removal of nits (with forceps) or application of ophthalmic physostigmine or other ointment as an insecticide. (This may cause pupil constriction and, possibly, headache, conjunctival irritation, and blurred vision from the film of ointment on the cornea.)

## Special considerations

• Instruct the patient to gently remove scales from the lid margins daily with an applicator stick or a clean washcloth.

• Teach the patient the following method for applying warm compresses: First, run warm water into a clean bowl. Then immerse a clean cloth in the water and wring it out. Place the warm cloth against the closed eyelid. (Be careful not to burn the skin.) Hold the compress in place until it cools. Continue this procedure for 15 minutes.

• Antibiotic ophthalmic ointment should be applied after a 15-minute application of warm compresses.

• Treatment of seborrheic blepharitis also requires attention to the face and scalp.

# BONE TUMORS, PRIMARY MALIGNANT

A rare type of bone cancer, primary malignant bone tumors (sarcomas of the bone) constitute less than 1% of all malignant tumors. Most malignant bone tumors are secondary, caused by seeding from a primary site. Primary malignant bone tumors are more common in males, especially in children and adolescents, although some types do occur in people between ages 35 and 60.

The tumors may originate in osseous or nonosseous tissue. Osseous bone tumors arise from the bony structure itself and include osteogenic sarcoma (the most common), parosteal osteogenic sarcoma, chondrosarcoma, and malignant giant cell tumor. Together they make up 60% of all malignant bone tumors. Nonosseous tumors arise from hematopoietic, vascular, and neural tissues and include Ewing's sarcoma, fibrosarcoma, and chordoma. Osteogenic and Ewing's sarcomas are the most common bone tumors in childhood. (See *Types of primary malignant bone tumors,* pages 116 and 117.)

## Causes

Although some cases of osteosarcoma are associated with genetic abnormalities (Li-Fraumeni, retinoblastoma, Rothmund-Thomson) or exposure to carcinogens (such as ingested radium in watch dial painters), most cases have no immediately apparent cause. Ewing's sarcoma cells demonstrate a characteristic translocation of genetic material from chromosome 22 to chromosome 11. Additional theories point to heredity, trauma, and excessive radiation therapy.

## Signs and symptoms

Bone pain is the most common indication of primary malignant bone tumors. It's often more intense at night and isn't usually associated with mobility. The pain is dull and usually localized, although it may be referred from the hip or spine and result in weakness or a limp. Another common sign is the presence of a mass or tumor.

The tumor site may be tender and swell; the tumor itself is often palpable. Pathologic fractures are common. In late stages, the patient may be cachectic, with fever and impaired mobility.

## Diagnosis

A biopsy (by incision or by aspiration) is essential for confirming primary malignant bone tumors. Bone X-rays and radioisotope bone and computed tomography (CT) scans show tumor size. Serum alkaline phosphatase is usually elevated in patients with sarcoma.

➤ CLINICAL TIP Bone X-rays, CT scans, and magnetic resonance imaging are all useful in assessing tumor size. Bone scans and CT scans of the lungs are important in checking for metastatic disease.

## Treatment

• Excision of the tumor along with a 3″ (7.6 cm) margin is the treatment of choice. It may be combined with preoperative chemotherapy.

• In some patients, radical surgery (such as hemipelvectomy or interscapulothoracic amputation) is necessary. However, surgical resection of the tumor (often with preoperative *and* postoperative chemotherapy) has saved limbs from amputation.

• Intensive chemotherapy includes administration of doxorubicin, vincristine, cyclophosphamide, cisplatin, and dacarbazine. Chemotherapy may be infused intra-arterially into the long bones of the legs.

**Special considerations**

• Be sensitive to the emotional strain caused by the threat of amputation. Encourage communication and help the patient set realistic goals.

• If the surgery will affect the patient's lower extremities, have a physical therapist teach him how to use assistive devices (such as a walker) preoperatively.

• Teach the patient how to readjust his body weight so that he can get into and out of the bed and wheelchair.

• Before surgery, start I.V. infusions to maintain fluid and electrolyte balance and to have an open vein available if blood or plasma is needed during surgery.

• After surgery, check vital signs every hour for the first 4 hours, every 2 hours for the next 4 hours, and then every 4 hours if the patient is stable.

• Check the dressing periodically for oozing.

• Elevate the foot of the bed or place the stump on a pillow for the first 24 hours. (Be careful not to leave the stump elevated for more than 48 hours because this may lead to contractures.)

• To ease the patient's anxiety, administer analgesics for pain before morning care. If necessary, brace him with pillows, keeping the affected part at rest.

• Urge the patient to eat foods high in protein and vitamins and to get plenty of rest and sleep to promote recovery.

**CLINICAL TIP**   Dietary folate should be avoided in patients receiving methotrexate.

• Encourage some physical exercise. Administer laxatives, if necessary, to maintain proper elimination.

• Encourage fluids to prevent dehydration. Record intake and output accurately. After a hemipelvectomy, insert a nasogastric tube to prevent abdominal distention. Continue low gastric suction for 2 days after surgery or until the patient can tolerate a liquid diet. Administer antibiotics to prevent infection. Give transfusions if necessary, and administer medication to control pain. Keep drains in place to facilitate wound drainage and prevent infection. Use an indwelling urinary catheter until the patient can void voluntarily.

• Keep in mind that rehabilitation programs after limb salvage surgery will vary, depending on the patient, the body part affected, and the type of surgery performed. For example, one patient may have a surgically implanted prosthesis (for example, after joint surgery), whereas another may have reconstructive surgery requiring an allograft (such as bone from a bone bank) or an autograft (bone from the patient's own body).

Encourage early rehabilitation for amputees as follows:

• Start physical therapy 24 hours postoperatively. Pain usually isn't severe after amputation. If it is, watch for a wound complication, such as hematoma, excessive stump edema, or infection.

• Be aware of the "phantom limb" syndrome, in which the patient "feels" an itch or tingling in an amputated extremity. This can last for several hours or persist for years. Explain that this sensation is normal and usually subsides.

• To avoid contractures and ensure the best conditions for wound healing, warn the patient not to hang the stump over

# TYPES OF PRIMARY MALIGNANT BONE TUMORS

| TYPE | CLINICAL FEATURES |
|---|---|
| **OSSEOUS ORIGIN** | |
| Osteogenic sarcoma | • Osteoid tumor present in specimen<br>• Tumor arises from bone-forming osteoblast<br>• Occurs most often in the femur but also in the tibia and the humerus and, occasionally, the fistula, ileum, vertebra, or mandible<br>• Usually occurs in males ages 10 to 30<br>• May metastasize to the lungs |
| Parosteal osteogenic sarcoma | • Develops on surface of bone instead of interior<br>• Progresses slowly<br>• Occurs most often in the distal femur but also in the tibia, humerus, and ulna<br>• Usually occurs in females ages 30 to 40 |
| Chondro-sarcoma | • Develops from cartilage<br>• Painless; grows slowly but is locally recurrent and invasive<br>• Occurs most often in the pelvis, proximal femur, ribs, and shoulder girdle<br>• Usually occurs in males ages 30 to 50 |
| Malignant giant cell tumor | • Arises from benign giant cell tumor<br>• Found most often in long bones, especially in knee area<br>• Usually occurs in females ages 18 to 50 |
| **NONOSSEOUS ORIGIN** | |
| Ewing's sarcoma | • Originates in bone marrow and invades shafts of long and flat bones<br>• Usually affects lower extremities, most often the femur, innominate bones, ribs, tibia, humerus, vertebra, and fibula; may metastasize to the lungs<br>• Patients may present with systemic symptoms suggesting infection (fever, local tenderness, warmth, swelling)<br>• Pain increasingly severe and persistent<br>• Usually occurs in males ages 10 to 20<br>• Prognosis has improved dramatically with effective chemotherapy |
| Fibrosarcoma | • Relatively rare<br>• Originates in fibrous tissue of bone<br>• Invades long or flat bones (femur, tibia, mandible) but also involves the periosteum and overlying muscle<br>• Usually occurs in males ages 30 to 40 |
| Chordoma | • Derived from embryonic remnants of notochord<br>• Progresses slowly<br>• Usually found at end of vertebral column and in sphenooccipital, sacrococcygeal, and vertebral areas<br>• Characterized by constipation and visual disturbances<br>• Usually occurs in males ages 50 to 60 |

## TREATMENT

- Preoperative chemotherapy
- Surgery (wide resection or amputation)
- Postoperative chemotherapy

- Surgery (tumor resection, possible amputation, interscapulothoracic surgery, hemipelvectomy)

- Wide surgical resection if possible; amputation if necessary

- Total excision
- Radiation for recurrent disease
- Chemotherapy

- High-voltage radiation (tumor is very radiosensitive.)
- Chemotherapy to slow growth
- Amputation only if there's no evidence of metastasis

- Amputation
- Radiation
- Chemotherapy
- Bone grafts (with low-grade fibrosarcoma)

- Surgical resectioning (often resulting in neural defects)
- Radiation (palliative, or when surgery isn't applicable, as in occipital area)

the edge of the bed; sit in a wheelchair with the stump flexed; place a pillow under his hip, knee, or back or between his thighs; lie with knees flexed; rest an above-the-knee stump on the crutch handle; or abduct an above-the-knee stump.

- Wash the stump, massage it gently, and keep it dry until it heals. Make sure the bandage is firm and worn day and night. Know how to reapply the bandage to shape the stump for a prosthesis.

- To help the patient select a prosthesis, consider his needs and the types of prostheses available. The rehabilitation staff will help him make the final decision, but because most patients are uninformed about choosing a prosthesis, give some guidelines. Keep in mind the patient's age and possible vision problems. Generally, children need relatively simple devices, whereas older adults may need prostheses that provide more stability. Consider finances too. Children outgrow prostheses, so advise parents to plan accordingly.

- The same points are applicable for an interscapulothoracic amputee, but losing an arm causes a greater cosmetic problem. Consult an occupational therapist, who can teach the patient how to perform daily activities with one arm.

- Try to instill a positive attitude toward recovery. Urge the patient to resume an independent lifestyle. Refer older patients to community health services if necessary. Suggest tutoring for children to help them keep up with schoolwork.

- Urge patients to report any new pain or masses immediately.

- Patients with large bone grafts or prosthetic implants require antibiotic prophylaxis when undergoing dental procedures.

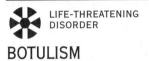

## LIFE-THREATENING DISORDER

# BOTULISM

A paralytic illness, botulism results from an exotoxin produced by the gram-positive, anaerobic bacillus *Clostridium botulinum.* It occurs as botulism food poisoning, wound botulism, and infant botulism. Mortality from botulism is about 25%, with death most often caused by respiratory failure during the first week of illness.

## Causes

Botulism is usually the result of ingesting inadequately cooked contaminated foods, especially those with low acid content, such as home-canned fruits and vegetables, sausages, and smoked or preserved fish or meat. Honey and corn syrup may contain *C. botulinum* spores and shouldn't be fed to infants. Rarely, botulism results from wound infection with *C. botulinum.*

Botulism occurs worldwide and affects adults more often than children. Recently, findings have shown that an infant's GI tract can become colonized with *C. botulinum* from some unknown source, and then the exotoxin is produced within the infant's intestine. Incidence had been declining, but the current trend toward home canning has resulted in an upswing (approximately 250 cases per year in the United States) in recent years.

## Signs and symptoms

The disease usually presents within 12 to 36 hours (range is 6 hours to 8 days) after the ingestion of contaminated food. The severity varies with the amount of toxin ingested and the patient's degree of immunocompetence. Generally, early onset (within 24 hours) signals critical and potentially fatal illness. Initial symptoms include dry mouth, sore throat, weakness, vomiting, and diarrhea.

The cardinal sign of botulism, though, is acute symmetrical cranial nerve impairment (ptosis, diplopia, dysarthria), followed by descending weakness or paralysis of muscles in the extremities or trunk and dyspnea from respiratory muscle paralysis. Such impairment doesn't affect mental or sensory processes and isn't associated with fever.

### Infant botulism

Usually afflicting infants ages 3 to 20 weeks, infant botulism can produce hypotonic (floppy) infant syndrome. Symptoms are constipation, feeble cry, depressed gag reflex, and inability to suck. Cranial nerve deficits also occur in infants and are manifested by a flaccid facial expression, ptosis, and ophthalmoplegia. Infants also develop generalized muscle weakness, hypotonia, and areflexia. Loss of head control may be striking. Respiratory arrest is likely.

## Diagnosis

Identification of the offending toxin in the patient's serum, stool, or gastric content or in the suspected food confirms the diagnosis. An electromyogram showing diminished muscle action potential after a single supramaximal nerve stimulus is also diagnostic.

Diagnosis also must rule out other diseases often confused with botulism, such as Guillain-Barré syndrome, myasthenia gravis, cerebrovascular accident, staphylococcal food poisoning, tick paralysis, chemical intoxications, carbon monoxide poisoning, fish poisoning, trichinosis, and diphtheria.

## Treatment

I.V. or I.M. administration of botulinum antitoxin (available through the Centers for Disease Control and Prevention) is the treatment of choice.

> CLINICAL TIP Antibiotics and aminoglycosides shouldn't be administered due to the risk of neuromuscular blockade. They should be used only to treat secondary infections.

## Special considerations

If you suspect ingestion of contaminated food:

• Obtain a careful history of the patient's food intake for the past several days. Check to see if other family members exhibit similar symptoms and share a common food history.

• Observe carefully for abnormal neurologic signs. If the patient returns home, tell his family to watch for signs of weakness, blurred vision, and slurred speech and to return the patient to the facility immediately if such signs appear.

• If ingestion has occurred within several hours, induce vomiting, begin gastric lavage, and give a high enema to purge any unabsorbed toxin from the bowel.

If clinical signs of botulism appear:

• Bring the patient to the intensive care unit, and monitor cardiac and respiratory function carefully.

• Administer botulinum antitoxin, as required, to neutralize any circulating toxin. Before giving antitoxin, obtain an accurate patient history of allergies, especially to horses, and perform a skin test.

> CLINICAL TIP Serum samples should be collected to identify the toxin before antitoxin is administered.

• After administration of antitoxin, watch for anaphylaxis or other hypersensitivity and serum sickness. Keep epinephrine 1:1,000 (for subcutaneous administration) and emergency airway equipment available.

• Closely observe and accurately record neurologic function, including bilateral motor status (reflexes, ability to move arms and legs).

• Give I.V. fluids as needed. Turn the patient often, and encourage deep-breathing exercises. Assisted respiration may be required. Isolation isn't required.

• Because botulism is sometimes fatal, keep the patient and his family informed about the course of the disease.

• Immediately notify local public health authorities of all cases of botulism.

To help prevent botulism, encourage patients to observe proper techniques in processing and preserving foods. Warn them to avoid even *tasting* food from a bulging can or one with a peculiar odor and to sterilize by boiling any utensil that comes in contact with suspected food. Ingestion of even a small amount of food contaminated with botulism toxin can prove fatal.

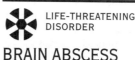
LIFE-THREATENING DISORDER

# BRAIN ABSCESS

Brain abscess is a free or encapsulated collection of pus that usually occurs in the temporal lobe, cerebellum, or frontal lobes. It can vary in size and may present singly or multilocularly. Brain abscess has a relatively low occurrence. Although it can occur at any age, it's most common in people ages 10 to 35 and is rare in older adults.

An untreated brain abscess is usually fatal; with treatment, the prognosis is only fair. About 30% of patients develop focal seizures. Multiple metastatic abscesses secondary to systemic or other infections have the poorest prognosis.

## Causes

A brain abscess usually occurs secondary to some other infection, especially otitis media, sinusitis, dental abscess, and mastoiditis. Other causes include subdural empyema; bacterial endocarditis; human immunodeficiency virus infection; bacteremia; pulmonary or pleural infection; pelvic, abdominal, and skin infections; and cranial trauma, such as a penetrating head wound or compound skull fracture.

This condition also occurs in about 2% of children with congenital heart disease, possibly because the hypoxic brain is a good culture medium for bacteria. Common infecting organisms are pyogenic bacteria, such as *Staphylococcus aureus* and *Streptococcus viridans*. Penetrating head trauma or bacteremia usually leads to staphylococcal infection; pulmonary disease, to streptococcal infection.

### Pathophysiology

A brain abscess usually begins with localized inflammatory necrosis and edema, septic thrombosis of vessels, and suppurative encephalitis. This is followed by thick encapsulation of accumulated pus, and adjacent meningeal infiltration by neutrophils, lymphocytes, and plasma cells.

### Signs and symptoms

Onset varies according to cause and location. Early symptoms are characteristic of a bacterial infection and include headache, chills, fever, malaise, confusion, and drowsiness. The white blood cell count is elevated with a differential indicating infection. As the lesion enlarges, it produces clinical effects similar to those of a brain tumor. At this time, symptoms correlate with a disturbance of function in the invaded lobe. Other features differ with the site of the abscess:

- *temporal lobe abscess:* auditory-receptive dysphasia, central facial weakness, hemiparesis
- *cerebellar abscess:* dizziness, coarse nystagmus, gaze weakness on the lesion side, tremor, ataxia
- *frontal lobe abscess:* expressive dysphasia, hemiparesis with unilateral motor seizure, drowsiness, inattention, mental function impairment, seizures.

### Diagnosis

A history of infection—especially of the middle ear, mastoid, nasal sinuses, heart, or lungs—or a history of congenital heart disease, along with a physical examination showing such characteristic clinical features as increased intracranial pressure (ICP), points to a brain abscess. An enhanced computed tomography (CT) scan and, occasionally, arteriography (which highlights the abscess by a halo) help locate the site.

Examination of cerebrospinal fluid can help confirm infection, but lumbar puncture is too risky because it can release the increased ICP and provoke cerebral herniation. A CT-guided stereotactic biopsy may be performed to drain and culture the abscess. Other tests include culture and sensitivity of drainage to identify the causative organism, skull X-rays, and a radioisotope scan.

### Treatment

Therapy consists of antibiotics to combat the underlying infection and surgical aspiration or drainage of the abscess. However, surgery is delayed until the abscess becomes encapsulated (a CT scan helps determine this) and is contraindicated in patients with congenital heart disease or another debilitating cardiac condition. Administration of a penicillinase-resistant antibiotic, such as nafcillin or methicillin, for at least 2 weeks before surgery can reduce the risk of spreading infection.

Other treatments during the acute phase are palliative and supportive; they include mechanical ventilation and administration of I.V. fluids with diuretics (urea, mannitol) and glucocorticoids (dexamethasone) to combat increased ICP and cerebral edema. Anticonvulsants, such as phenytoin and phenobarbital, help prevent seizures.

### Special considerations

• The patient with an acute brain abscess requires intensive care monitoring.

• Frequently assess neurologic status, especially cognition and mentation, speech, and sensorimotor and cranial nerve function.

➤ CLINICAL TIP  Early increases in ICP can be detected by using such diagnostic tools as the mini-mental status examination, Glasgow Coma Scale, and National Institutes of Health Stroke Scale. These highly sensitive tools facilitate recognition of early neurologic changes and may assist in retarding the increase of ICP. Once increased ICP results in abnormal pupils, depressed respirations, widened pulse pressure, and tachycardia or bradycardia, the cycle of increased ICP may not be reversible.

• Assess and record vital signs at least every hour.

• Monitor fluid intake and output carefully because fluid overload could contribute to cerebral edema.

• If surgery is necessary, explain the procedure to the patient and answer his questions.

• After surgery, continue frequent neurologic assessment. Monitor vital signs and intake and output.

• Watch for signs of meningitis (nuchal rigidity, headaches, chills, sweats), an ever-present threat.

• Change a damp dressing often. *Never allow bandages to remain damp.* Reinforce the dressing or change it as ordered. To promote drainage and prevent reaccumulation of the abscess, position the patient on the operative side. Measure drainage from Jackson-Pratt or other types of drains as instructed by the surgeon.

• If the patient remains stuporous or comatose for an extended period, give meticulous skin care to prevent pressure ulcers, and position him to preserve function and prevent contractures.

• If the patient requires isolation because of postoperative drainage, make sure he and his family understand why.

• Ambulate the patient as soon as possible to prevent immobility and encourage independence.

• To prevent brain abscess, stress the need for treatment of otitis media, mastoiditis, dental abscess, and other infections. Give prophylactic antibiotics as needed after a compound skull fracture or penetrating head wound.

# BRAIN TUMORS, MALIGNANT

With an incidence of 4.5 per 100,000, malignant brain tumors (gliomas, meningiomas, and schwannomas) are common (slightly more so in men than in women).

Tumors may occur at any age. In adults, incidence is generally highest between ages 40 and 60. The most common tumor types in adults are gliomas and meningiomas; these tumors are usually supratentorial (above the covering of the cerebellum).

In children, incidence is generally highest before age 1 and then again between ages 2 and 12. The most common tumors in children are astrocytomas, medulloblastomas, ependymomas, and brain stem gliomas. In children, brain tumors are one of the most common causes of death from cancer.

## Causes
The cause of brain tumors is unknown.

## Signs and symptoms
Brain tumors cause central nervous system changes by invading and destroying tissues and by secondary effect — mainly compression of the brain, cranial nerves, and cerebral vessels; cerebral edema; and increased intracranial pressure (ICP). Generally, clinical features result from increased ICP; these features vary with the type of tumor, its location, and the degree of invasion. The onset of symptoms is usually insidious, and brain tumors are commonly misdiagnosed. (See *Clinical features of malignant brain tumors.*)

## Diagnosis
In many cases, a definitive diagnosis follows a tissue biopsy performed by stereotactic surgery. In this procedure, a head ring is affixed to the skull, and an excisional device is guided to the lesion by a computed tomography (CT) scan or magnetic resonance imaging (MRI).

Other diagnostic tools include a patient history, a neurologic assessment, skull X-rays, a brain scan, a CT scan, MRI, and cerebral angiography. Lumbar puncture shows increased pressure and protein levels, decreased glucose levels and, occasionally, tumor cells in cerebrospinal fluid (CSF).

## Treatment
Remedial approaches include removing a resectable tumor; reducing a nonresectable tumor; relieving cerebral edema, increased ICP, and other symptoms; and preventing further neurologic damage.

The mode of therapy depends on the tumor's histologic type, radiosensitivity, and location and may include surgery, radiation, chemotherapy, or decompression of increased ICP with diuretics, corticosteroids or, possibly, ventriculoatrial or ventriculoperitoneal shunting of CSF.

● *Gliomas.* Treatment usually requires resection by craniotomy, followed by radiation therapy and chemotherapy. The combination of nitrosoureas (carmustine [BCNU], lomustine [CCNU, or procarbazine) and postoperative radiation is more effective than radiation alone.

● *Astrocytomas.* Surgical resection of low-grade cystic cerebellar astrocytomas brings long-term survival. Treatment of other astrocytomas includes repeated surgery, radiation therapy, and shunting of fluid from obstructed CSF pathways. Some astrocytomas are highly radiosensitive, but others are radioresistant.

● *Oligodendrogliomas* and *ependymomas.* Treatment includes resection and radiation therapy.

● *Medulloblastomas.* Treatment involves resection and, possibly, intrathecal infusion of methotrexate or another antineoplastic drug.

● *Meningiomas.* Treatment requires resection, including dura mater and bone (operative mortality may reach 10% because of large tumor size).

● *Schwannomas.* Microsurgical technique allows complete resection of the tumor and preservation of facial nerves. Although schwannomas are moderately radioresistant, postoperative radiation therapy is necessary.

Chemotherapy for malignant brain tumors includes the nitrosoureas that help break down the blood-brain barri-

*(Text continues on page 125.)*

# CLINICAL FEATURES OF MALIGNANT BRAIN TUMORS

| TUMOR | CLINICAL FEATURES |
|---|---|
| **Glioblastoma multiforme**<br>*(spongioblastoma multiforme)*<br>• Peak incidence between ages 50 and 60; twice as common in males; most common glioma<br>• Unencapsulated, highly malignant; grows rapidly and infiltrates the brain extensively; may become enormous before diagnosed<br>• Occurs most often in cerebral hemispheres, especially frontal and temporal lobes (rarely in brain stem and cerebellum)<br>• Occupies more than one lobe of affected hemisphere; may spread to opposite hemisphere by corpus callosum; may metastasize into cerebrospinal fluid (CSF), producing tumors in distant parts of the central nervous system (CNS) | *General*<br>• Increased intracranial pressure (ICP), causing nausea, vomiting, headache, papilledema<br>• Mental and behavioral changes<br>• Altered vital signs (increased systolic pressure, widened pulse pressure, respiratory changes)<br>• Speech and sensory disturbances<br>• In children, irritability, projectile vomiting<br>*Localized*<br>• Midline: headache (bifrontal or biooccipital); worse in morning; intensified by coughing, straining, or sudden head movements<br>• Temporal lobe: psychomotor seizures<br>• Central region: focal seizures<br>• Optic and oculomotor nerves: visual defects<br>• Frontal lobe: abnormal reflexes, motor responses |
| **Astrocytoma**<br>• Second most common malignant glioma (approximately 30% of all gliomas)<br>• Occurs at any age; incidence higher in males<br>• Occurs most often in white matter of cerebral hemispheres; may originate in any part of the CNS<br>• Cerebellar astrocytomas usually confined to one hemisphere | *General*<br>• Headache; mental activity changes<br>• Decreased motor strength and coordination<br>• Seizures; scanning speech<br>• Altered vital signs<br>*Localized*<br>• Third ventricle: changes in mental activity and level of consciousness, nausea, pupillary dilation and sluggish light reflex; later—paresis or ataxia<br>• Brain stem and pons: early—ipsilateral trigeminal, abducens, and facial nerve palsies; later—cerebellar ataxia, tremors, other cranial nerve deficits<br>• Third or fourth ventricle or aqueduct of Sylvius: secondary hydrocephalus<br>• Thalamus or hypothalamus: variety of endocrine, metabolic, autonomic, and behavioral changes |

*(continued)*

CLINICAL FEATURES OF MALIGNANT BRAIN TUMORS *(continued)*

| TUMOR | CLINICAL FEATURES |
|---|---|
| **Oligodendroglioma**<br>• Third most common glioma<br>• Occurs in middle adult years; more common in women<br>• Slow-growing | *General*<br>• Mental and behavioral changes<br>• Decreased visual acuity and other visual disturbances<br>• Increased ICP<br>*Localized*<br>• Temporal lobe: hallucinations, psychomotor seizures<br>• Central region: seizures (confined to one muscle group or unilateral)<br>• Midbrain or third ventricle: pyramidal tract symptoms (dizziness, ataxia, paresthesia of the face)<br>• Brain stem and cerebrum: nystagmus, hearing loss, dizziness, ataxia, paresthesia of face, cranial nerve palsies, hemiparesis, suboccipital tenderness, loss of balance |
| **Ependymoma**<br>• Rare glioma<br>• Most common in children and young adults<br>• Locates most often in fourth and lateral ventricles | *General*<br>• Similar to oligodendrioglioma<br>• Increased ICP and obstructive hydrocephalus, depending on tumor size |
| **Medulloblastoma**<br>• Rare glioma<br>• Incidence highest in children ages 4 to 6<br>• Affects males more than females<br>• Frequently metastasizes via CSF | *General*<br>• Increased ICP<br>*Localized*<br>• Brain stem and cerebrum: papilledema, nystagmus, hearing loss, flashing lights, dizziness, ataxia, paresthesia of face, cranial nerve palsies (V, VI, VII, IX, X, primarily sensory), hemiparesis, suboccipital tenderness; compression of supratentorial area produces other general and focal symptoms |

## CLINICAL FEATURES OF MALIGNANT BRAIN TUMORS *(continued)*

| TUMOR | CLINICAL FEATURES |
|---|---|
| **Meningioma**<br>• Most common nongliomatous brain tumor (15% of primary brain tumors)<br>• Peak incidence among 50-year-olds; rare in children; more common in females than in males (ratio 3:2)<br>• Arises from the meninges<br>• Common locations include parasagittal area, sphenoidal ridge, anterior part of the skull, cerebellopontile angle, spinal canal<br>• Benign, well-circumscribed, highly vascular tumors that compress underlying brain tissue by invading overlying skull | *General*<br>• Headache<br>• Seizures (in two-thirds of patients)<br>• Vomiting<br>• Changes in mental activity<br>• Similar to schwannomas<br>*Localized*<br>• Skull changes (bony bulge) over tumor<br>• Sphenoidal ridge, indenting optic nerve: unilateral visual changes and papilledema<br>• Prefrontal parasagittal: personality and behavioral changes<br>• Motor cortex: contralateral motor changes<br>• Anterior fossa compressing both optic nerves and frontal lobes: headaches and bilateral vision loss<br>• Pressure on cranial nerves causes varying symptoms |
| **Schwannoma**<br>(acoustic neurinoma, neurilemoma, cerebellopontile angle tumor)<br>• Accounts for approximately 10% of all intracranial tumors<br>• Higher incidence in women<br>• Onset of symptoms between ages 30 and 60<br>• Affects the craniospinal nerve sheath, usually cranial nerve VIII; also V and VII and, to a lesser extent, VI and X on the same side as the tumor<br>• Benign but often classified as malignant because of its growth patterns; slow-growing — may be present for years before symptoms occur | *General*<br>• Stiff neck and suboccipital discomfort<br>• Secondary hydrocephalus<br>• Ataxia and uncoordinated movements of one or both arms due to pressure on brain stem and cerebellum<br>*Localized*<br>• V: early — facial hypoesthesia or paresthesia on side of hearing loss; unilateral loss of corneal reflex<br>• VI: diplopia or double vision<br>• VII: paresis progressing to paralysis (Bell's palsy)<br>• VIII: Unilateral hearing loss with or without tinnitus<br>• X: weakness of palate, tongue, and nerve muscles on same side as tumor |

er and allow other chemotherapeutic drugs to go through as well. Intrathecal and intra-arterial administration of drugs maximizes drug actions.

Palliative measures for gliomas, astrocytomas, oligodendrogliomas, and ependymomas include dexamethasone for cerebral edema and antacids and histamine-receptor antagonists for stress ulcers. These tumors and schwannomas may also require anticonvulsants.

## Special considerations

• Perform a comprehensive assessment (including a complete neurologic evaluation) to provide baseline data and guide subsequent care. Obtain a thorough health history concerning onset of symptoms.

• Assist the patient and his family in coping with the treatment, potential disabilities, and changes in lifestyle resulting from his tumor.

Throughout hospitalization:

• Carefully document seizure activity (occurrence, nature, and duration).

• Maintain airway patency.

• Monitor patient safety.

• Administer anticonvulsants as required.

• Check continuously for changes in neurologic status, and watch for an increase in ICP.

• Watch for and immediately report sudden unilateral pupillary dilation with loss of light reflex; this ominous change indicates imminent transtentorial herniation.

• Monitor respiratory changes carefully.

➤ CLINICAL TIP Abnormal respiratory rate and depth may point to rising ICP or herniation of the cerebellar tonsils from an expanding infratentorial mass.

• Monitor temperature carefully. Fever commonly follows hypothalamic anoxia but might also indicate meningitis. Use hypothermia blankets preoperatively and postoperatively to keep the patient's temperature down and minimize cerebral metabolic demands.

• Administer steroids and osmotic diuretics, such as mannitol, as needed, to reduce cerebral edema. Fluids may be restricted to 1,500 ml/24 hours. Monitor fluid and electrolyte balance to avoid dehydration.

• Observe for signs of stress ulcers: abdominal distention, pain, vomiting, and black, tarry stool. Administer antacids as needed.

Surgery requires additional patient care. After craniotomy:

• Continue to monitor general neurologic status and watch for signs of increased ICP, such as an elevated bone flap and typical neurologic changes. To reduce the risk of increased ICP, restrict fluids to 1,500 ml/24 hours.

• To promote venous drainage and reduce cerebral edema after supratentorial craniotomy, elevate the head of the patient's bed about 30 degrees. Position him on his side to allow drainage of secretions and prevent aspiration.

• As appropriate, instruct the patient to avoid Valsalva's maneuver or isometric muscle contractions when moving or sitting up in bed; they can increase intrathoracic pressure and thereby increase ICP.

• Withhold oral fluids, which may provoke vomiting and, consequently, raise ICP.

• After infratentorial craniotomy, keep the patient flat for 48 hours, but logroll him every 2 hours to minimize complications of immobilization. Prevent other complications by paying careful attention to ventilatory status and to cardiovascular, GI, and musculoskeletal function.

• Radiation therapy is usually delayed until after the surgical wound heals, but it can induce wound breakdown even then. Observe the wound carefully for infection and sinus formation.

• Because radiation may cause brain inflammation, watch for signs of rising ICP.

• Because the nitrosoureas — carmustine (BCNU), lomustine (CCNU), and procarbazine — used as adjuncts to radiotherapy and surgery can cause delayed bone marrow depression, tell the patient to watch for and immediately report any signs of infection or bleeding that appear within 4 weeks after the start of chemotherapy.

• Before chemotherapy, give prochlor-perazine or another antiemetic, as needed, to minimize nausea and vomiting.

• Teach the patient signs of recurrence; urge compliance with the treatment regimen.

• Because brain tumors may cause residual neurologic deficits that handicap the patient physically or mentally, begin rehabilitation early.

• Consult with occupational and physical therapists to encourage independence in daily activities.

• As necessary, provide aids for self-care and mobilization, such as bathroom rails for wheelchair patients.

• If the patient is aphasic, arrange for consultation with a speech pathologist.

# BREAST CANCER

Breast cancer is the most common cancer affecting women and is the number two killer (after lung cancer) of women ages 35 to 54. It occurs in men but rarely. The overall breast cancer death rate for American women has fallen from 27.5 cases per 100,000 women in 1989 to 25.9 cases per 100,000 women in 1993. Lymph node involvement is the most valuable prognostic predictor. With adjuvant therapy, 70% to 75% of women with negative nodes will survive 10 years or more, compared with 20% to 25% of women with positive nodes.

Although breast cancer may develop anytime after puberty, it's most common after age 50.

## Causes

The cause of breast cancer isn't known, but its high incidence in women implicates estrogen. Certain predisposing factors are clear; women at *high risk* include those who:

• have a family history of breast cancer

• have long menses; began menses early or menopause late

• have never been pregnant

• were first pregnant after age 31

• have had unilateral breast cancer

• have had endometrial or ovarian cancer

• were exposed to low-level ionizing radiation.

Many other possible predisposing factors have been investigated, including estrogen therapy, antihypertensives, high-fat diet, obesity, and fibrocystic disease of the breasts.

Women at *lower risk* include those who:

• were pregnant before age 20

• have had multiple pregnancies

• are Indian or Asian.

### Pathophysiology

Breast cancer occurs more often in the left breast than in the right and more often in the upper outer quadrant. Growth rates vary. Theoretically, slow-growing breast cancer may take up to 8 years to become palpable at ⅜" (1 cm) in size. It spreads by way of the lymphatic system and the bloodstream, through the right heart to the lungs and, eventually, to the other breast, the chest wall, liver, bone, and brain.

Many refer to the estimated growth rate of breast cancer as "doubling time," or the time it takes the malignant cells to double in number. Survival time for breast cancer is based on tumor size and spread; the number of involved nodes is the single most important factor in predicting survival time.

Classified by histologic appearance and location of the lesion, breast cancer may be:

• *adenocarcinoma* — arising from the epithelium

• *intraductal* — developing within the ducts (includes Paget's disease)

• *infiltrating* — occurring in parenchymal tissue of the breast

• *inflammatory (rare)* — reflecting rapid tumor growth, in which the overlying skin becomes edematous, inflamed, and indurated

• *lobular carcinoma in situ* — reflecting tumor growth involving lobes of glandular tissue

• *medullary or circumscribed* — a large tumor with a rapid growth rate.

These histologic classifications should be coupled with a staging or nodal status classification system for a clearer understanding of the extent of the cancer. The most commonly used system for staging cancer, both before and after surgery, is the tumor-node-metastasis (TNM) system. (See *Staging breast cancer*.)

**Signs and symptoms**

Warning signals of possible breast cancer include:

• a lump or mass in the breast (a hard, stony mass is usually malignant)

• a change in symmetry or size of the breast

• a change in breast skin (thickening, scaly skin around the nipple, dimpling, edema [peau d'orange], or ulceration)

• a change in skin temperature (a warm, hot, or pink area; suspect cancer in a nonlactating woman past childbearing age until proven otherwise)

• unusual drainage or discharge (a spontaneous discharge of any kind in a non-breast-feeding, nonlactating woman warrants thorough investigation; so does any discharge produced by breast manipulation [greenish black, white,

creamy, serous, or bloody]). If a breast-feeding infant rejects one breast, this may suggest possible breast cancer.

• a change in the nipple, such as itching, burning, erosion, or retraction

• pain (not usually a symptom of breast cancer unless the tumor is advanced, but it should be investigated)

• bone metastasis, pathologic bone fractures, and hypercalcemia

• edema of the arm.

**Diagnosis**

Diagnostic measures in breast cancer include the following.

***Breast self-examination***

The most reliable method of detecting breast cancer is the monthly breast self-examination, followed by immediate evaluation of any abnormality.

***Mammography and biopsies***

Other diagnostic measures include mammography, a needle biopsy, and a surgical biopsy. Mammography is indicated for any woman whose physical examination might suggest breast cancer. It should be done as a baseline on women ages 35 to 39; every 1 to 2 years for ages 40 to 49; and annually on women over age 50, women who have a family history of breast cancer, and women who have had unilateral breast cancer, to check for new disease. However, the value of mammography is questionable for women under age 35 (because of the density of the breasts), except those who are strongly suspected of having breast cancer.

False-negative results can occur in as many as 30% of all tests. Consequently, with a suspicious mass, a negative mammogram should be disregarded, and a fine-needle aspiration or surgical biopsy should be done. Ultrasonography, which can distinguish a fluid-filled

# STAGING BREAST CANCER

Cancer staging helps form a prognosis and a treatment plan. For breast cancer, most clinicians use the TNM (tumor, node, metastasis) system developed by the American Joint Committee on Cancer.

### Primary tumor

*TX*—primary tumor can't be assessed

*TO*—no evidence of primary tumor

*Tis*—carcinoma in situ: intraductal carcinoma, lobular carcinoma in situ, or Paget's disease of the nipple with no tumor

*T1*—tumor 2 cm or less in greatest dimension

*T1a*—tumor 0.5 cm or less in greatest dimension

*T1b*—tumor more than 0.5 cm but not more than 1 cm in greatest dimension

*T1c*—tumor more than 1 cm but not more than 2 cm in greatest dimension

*T2*—tumor more than 2 cm but not more than 5 cm in greatest dimension

*T3*—tumor more than 5 cm in greatest dimension

*T4*—tumor at any size that extends to the chest wall or skin

*T4a*—tumor extends to the chest wall

*T4b*—tumor accompanied by edema, ulcerated breast skin, or satellite skin nodules on the same breast

*T4c*—both T4a and T4b

*T4d*—inflammatory carcinoma

### Regional lymph nodes

*NX*—regional lymph nodes can't be assessed

*NO*—no evidence of nodal involvement

*N1*—movable ipsilateral axillary nodal involvement

*N2*—ipsilateral axillary nodal involvement with nodes fixed to one another or to other structures

*N3*—ipsilateral internal mammary nodal involvement

### Distant metastasis

*MX*—distant metastasis can't be assessed

*MO*—no evidence of distant metastasis

*M1*—distant metastasis (including metastasis to ipsilateral supraclavicular nodes)

### Staging categories

Breast cancer progresses from mild to severe as follows:

*Stage 0*—Tis, N0, M0

*Stage I*—T1, N0, M0

*Stage IIA*—T0, N1, M0; T1, N1, M0; T2, N0, M0

*Stage IIB*—T2, N1, M0, T3, N0, M0

*Stage IIIA*—T0, N2, M0; T1, N2, M0; T2, N2, M0; T3, N1 or N2, M0

*Stage IIIB*—T4, any N, M0; any T, N3, M0

*Stage IV*—any T, any N, M1

---

cyst from a tumor, can also be used instead of an invasive surgical biopsy.

*Other tests*

Bone scan, computed tomography scan, measurement of alkaline phosphatase levels, liver function studies, and a liver biopsy can detect distant metastasis. A hormonal receptor assay done on the tumor can determine if the tumor is estrogen- or progesterone-dependent.

(This test guides decisions to use therapy that blocks the action of the estrogen hormone that supports tumor growth.)

**Treatment**

Much controversy exists over breast cancer treatments. In choosing therapy, the patient and doctor should consider the stage of the disease, the woman's age and menopausal status, and the disfiguring effects of the surgery. Treatment for breast cancer may include one or any combination of the following.

### Surgery

In breast cancer, surgery involves either mastectomy or lumpectomy. A *lumpectomy* may be done on an outpatient basis and may be the only surgery needed, especially if the tumor is small and there's no evidence of axillary node involvement. Radiation therapy is often combined with this surgery.

A two-stage procedure, in which the surgeon removes the lump, confirms that it's malignant, and discusses treatment options with the patient, is desirable because it allows the patient to participate in her treatment plan. Sometimes, if the tumor is diagnosed as clinically malignant, such planning can be done before surgery. In *lumpectomy and dissection of the axillary lymph nodes,* the tumor and the axillary lymph nodes are removed, leaving the breast intact.

A *simple mastectomy* removes the breast but not the lymph nodes or pectoral muscles. A *modified radical mastectomy* removes the breast and the axillary lymph nodes. A *radical mastectomy,* the performance of which has declined, removes the breast, pectoralis major and minor, and the axillary lymph nodes.

After a mastectomy, reconstructive surgery can create a breast mound if the patient desires it and doesn't have evidence of advanced disease.

### Chemotherapy, tamoxifen, and peripheral stem cell therapy

Various cytotoxic drug combinations are used as either adjuvant or primary therapy, depending on several factors, including the TNM staging and estrogen receptor status. The most commonly used antineoplastic drugs are cyclophosphamide, fluorouracil, methotrexate, doxorubicin, vincristine, paclitaxel, and prednisone. A common drug combination used in both premenopausal and postmenopausal women is cyclophosphamide, methotrexate, and fluorouracil.

Tamoxifen, an estrogen antagonist, is the adjuvant treatment of choice for postmenopausal patients with positive estrogen receptor status.

Peripheral stem cell therapy may be used for advanced breast cancer.

### Primary radiation therapy

Used before or after tumor removal, primary radiation therapy is effective for small tumors in early stages with no evidence of distant metastasis; it's also used to prevent or treat local recurrence. Presurgical radiation to the breast in inflammatory breast cancer helps make tumors more surgically manageable.

### Other drug therapy

Breast cancer patients may also receive estrogen, progesterone, androgen, or antiandrogen aminoglutethimide therapy. The success of these drug therapies with growing evidence that breast cancer is a systemic, not local, disease has led to a decline in ablative surgery.

### Special considerations

● To provide good care for a breast cancer patient, begin with a history; assess the patient's feelings about her illness, and determine what she knows about it and what she expects.

Preoperative care:

Be sure you know what kind of surgery is scheduled, so you can prepare the patient. If a mastectomy is scheduled, in addition to the usual preoperative preparation (for example, skin preparations and allowing nothing by mouth), provide the following information:

• Teach the patient how to deep-breathe and cough to prevent pulmonary complications and how to rotate her ankles to help prevent thromboembolism.

• Tell the patient she can ease her pain by lying on the affected side or by placing a hand or pillow on the incision. Show her where the incision will be. Inform her that she'll receive pain medication and that she needn't fear addiction.

• Explain that after mastectomy, an incisional drain or suction device (Hemovac) will be used to remove accumulated serous or sanguineous fluid and to keep the tension off the suture line, promoting healing.

Postoperative care:

• Inspect the dressing anteriorly and posteriorly. Be alert for bleeding.

• Measure and record the amount and note the color of drainage. Expect drainage to be bloody during the first 4 hours and afterward become serous.

• Check circulatory status (blood pressure, pulse, respirations, and bleeding).

• Monitor intake and output for at least 48 hours after general anesthesia.

• Be aware that adequate pain relief encourages coughing and turning and promotes general well-being. Positioning a small pillow under the patient's arm provides comfort.

• Encourage the patient to get out of bed as soon as possible (even as soon as the anesthesia wears off or the first evening after surgery).

• Prevent lymphedema of the arm, which may be an early complication of any breast cancer treatment that involves lymph node dissection. Help the patient prevent lymphedema by instructing her to exercise her hand and arm regularly and to avoid activities that might cause infection in this hand or arm (infection increases the chance of developing lymphedema). Such prevention is important because lymphedema can't be treated effectively.

• Inspect the incision. Encourage the patient and her partner to look at her incision as soon as feasible, perhaps when the first dressing is removed.

• Advise the patient to ask her doctor about reconstructive surgery or to call the local or state medical society for the names of plastic reconstructive surgeons who regularly perform surgery to create breast mounds. In many cases, reconstructive surgery may be planned prior to the mastectomy.

• Instruct the patient about breast prostheses. The American Cancer Society's Reach to Recovery group can provide instruction, emotional support and counseling, and a list of area stores that sell prostheses.

• Give psychological and emotional support. Many patients fear cancer and possible disfigurement and worry about loss of sexual function. Explain that breast surgery doesn't interfere with sexual function and that the patient may resume sexual activity as soon as she desires after surgery

➤ CLINICAL TIP Explain to the patient that she may experience "phantom breast syndrome" (a phenomenon in which a tingling or a pins-and-needles sensation is felt in the area of the amputated breast tissue) or depression following mastectomy. Listen to the patient's concerns, offer support, and refer her to an appropriate organization, such as the American Cancer Society's Reach to Recovery, which offers caring and sharing groups to help breast cancer patients in the facility and at home.

# BRONCHIECTASIS

A condition marked by chronic abnormal dilation of bronchi and destruction of bronchial walls, bronchiectasis can occur throughout the tracheobronchial tree or can be confined to one segment or lobe. However, it's usually bilateral and involves the basilar segments of the lower lobes. This disease has three forms: cylindrical (fusiform), varicose, and saccular (cystic).

It affects people of both sexes and all ages. Because of the availability of antibiotics to treat acute respiratory tract infections, the incidence of bronchiectasis has dramatically decreased in the past 20 years. Its incidence is highest among the Inuit of the Arctic and the Maoris of New Zealand. Bronchiectasis is irreversible once established.

## Causes

The different forms of bronchiectasis may occur separately or simultaneously. In *cylindrical bronchiectasis,* the bronchi expand unevenly, with little change in diameter, and end suddenly in a squared-off fashion. In *varicose bronchiectasis,* abnormal, irregular dilation and narrowing of the bronchi give the appearance of varicose veins. In *saccular bronchiectasis,* many large dilations end in sacs.

This disease results from conditions associated with repeated damage to bronchial walls and abnormal mucociliary clearance, which cause a breakdown of supporting tissue adjacent to airways. Such conditions include:
• mucoviscidosis (cystic fibrosis)
• immunologic disorders (agammaglobulinemia, for example)
• recurrent, inadequately treated bacterial respiratory tract infections, such

as tuberculosis, and complications of measles, pneumonia, pertussis, or influenza
• obstruction (by a foreign body, tumor, or stenosis) in association with recurrent infection
• inhalation of corrosive gas or repeated aspiration of gastric juices into the lungs
• congenital anomalies (uncommon), such as bronchomalacia, congenital bronchiectasis, immotile-cilia syndrome (ICS), and Kartagener's syndrome, a variant of ICS characterized by situs inversus, bronchiectasis, and either nasal polyps or sinusitis.
• In bronchiectasis, hyperplastic squamous epithelium denuded of cilia replaces ulcerated columnar epithelium. Abscess formation involving all layers of the bronchial wall produces inflammatory cells and fibrous tissue, resulting in both dilation and narrowing of the airways. Mucus or fibrous tissue obliterates smaller bronchioles, while peribronchial lymphoid tissue becomes hyperplastic. Extensive vascular proliferation of bronchial circulation occurs and produces frequent hemoptysis.

## Signs and symptoms

Initially, bronchiectasis may be asymptomatic. When symptoms do arise, they're often attributed to other illnesses. The patient usually complains of frequent bouts of pneumonia or hemoptysis. The classic symptom, however, is a chronic cough that produces copious, foul-smelling, mucopurulent secretions, possibly totaling several cupfuls daily. Characteristic findings include coarse crackles during inspiration over involved lobes or segments, occasional wheezes, dyspnea, sinusitis, weight loss, anemia, malaise, clubbing, recurrent fever, chills, and other signs of infection.

Advanced bronchiectasis may produce chronic malnutrition and amyloidosis as well as right-sided heart failure and cor pulmonale due to hypoxic pulmonary vasoconstriction.

## Diagnosis

A history of recurrent bronchial infections, pneumonia, and hemoptysis in a patient whose chest X-rays show peribronchial thickening, areas of atelectasis, and scattered cystic changes suggests bronchiectasis.

In recent years, computed tomography scanning has supplanted bronchography as the most useful diagnostic test for bronchiectasis. It's sometimes used with high-resolution techniques to better determine anatomic changes. Bronchoscopy doesn't establish the diagnosis of bronchiectasis, but it does help to identify the source of secretions. Bronchoscopy can also be instrumental in pinpointing the site of bleeding in hemoptysis.

Other helpful laboratory tests include:
- *sputum culture* and *Gram stain* to identify predominant organisms
- *complete blood count* to detect anemia and leukocytosis
- *pulmonary function studies* to detect decreased vital capacity, expiratory flow, and hypoxemia; these tests also help determine the physiologic severity of the disease and the effects of therapy and help evaluate patients for surgery.

Evaluation may also include urinalysis and an electrocardiogram. (The latter is normal unless cor pulmonale develops.) When cystic fibrosis is suspected as the underlying cause of bronchiectasis, a sweat electrolyte test is useful.

## Treatment

Typically, antibiotics are given orally or I.V. for 7 to 10 days or until sputum production decreases. Bronchodilators,

TEACHING CHECKLIST

## TEACHING ABOUT BRONCHIECTASIS

Review the following points with the patient and his family:

- Instruct the patient to perform coughing and deep-breathing exercises.
- Advise the patient to stop smoking.
- Encourage as much rest as possible.
- Encourage balanced, high-protein meals and fluids.
- Teach postural drainage, percussion, and mouth care.
- Teach proper disposal of secretions.
- Tell the patient to avoid air pollutants and people who have upper respiratory tract infections.

combined with postural drainage and chest percussion, help remove secretions if the patient has bronchospasm and thick, tenacious sputum. Bronchoscopy may be used to help mobilize secretions.

Hypoxia requires oxygen therapy; severe hemoptysis often requires lobectomy, segmental resection, or bronchial artery embolization if pulmonary function is poor.

## Special considerations

- Provide supportive care and help the patient adjust to the permanent changes in lifestyle that irreversible lung damage necessitates. Thorough teaching is vital.
- Administer antibiotics as needed, and explain all diagnostic tests.
- Perform chest physiotherapy, including postural drainage and chest percussion designed for involved lobes, several times a day. The best times to do

this are early morning and just before bedtime. Instruct the patient to maintain each position for 10 minutes; then perform percussion and tell him to cough.

• Review patient teaching guidelines. (See *Teaching about bronchiectasis*, page 133.)

➤ CLINICAL TIP To help prevent bronchiectasis, treat bacterial pneumonia vigorously and stress the need for immunization to prevent childhood diseases.

# BRONCHIOLITIS OBLITERANS WITH ORGANIZING PNEUMONIA, IDIOPATHIC

Idiopathic bronchiolitis obliterans with organizing pneumonia (BOOP), also known as cryptogenic organizing pneumonia, is one of several types of bronchiolitis obliterans. "Bronchiolitis obliterans" is a generic term used to describe an inflammatory disease of the small airways. "Organizing pneumonia" refers to unresolved pneumonia, in which inflammatory alveolar exudate persists and eventually undergoes fibrosis.

Although BOOP was first described in 1901, confusing terminology and pathology that overlapped other diseases of the small airways kept it from being sufficiently recognized until the mid-1980s, when it was classified as a distinct clinical entity. Since that time, BOOP has been diagnosed with increasing frequency, although much debate still exists about the various pathologies and classifications of bronchiolitis obliterans.

Most patients with BOOP are between ages 50 and 60. Incidence is equally divided between men and women. A smoking history doesn't seem to increase the risk of developing BOOP.

## Causes

BOOP has no known cause. However, other forms of bronchiolitis obliterans and organizing pneumonia may be associated with specific diseases or situations, such as bone marrow, heart, or heart-lung transplantation; collagen vascular diseases, such as rheumatoid arthritis and systemic lupus erythematosus; inflammatory diseases, such as Crohn's disease, ulcerative colitis, and polyarteritis nodosa; bacterial, viral, or mycoplasmal respiratory infections; inhalation of toxic gases; and drug therapy with amiodarone, bleomycin, penicillamine, or lomustine.

## Signs and symptoms

The presenting symptoms of BOOP are usually subacute, with a flulike syndrome of fever, persistent and nonproductive cough, dyspnea (especially on exertion), malaise, anorexia, and weight loss lasting from several weeks to several months. Physical assessment findings may reveal dry crackles as the only abnormality. Less common symptoms include a productive cough, hemoptysis, chest pain, generalized aching, and night sweats.

## Diagnosis

Diagnosis begins with a thorough patient history meant to exclude any known cause of bronchiolitis obliterans or diseases with a pathology that includes an organizing pneumonia pattern.

• *Chest X-ray* usually shows patchy, diffuse airspace opacities with a ground-glass appearance that may migrate from one location to another. High-resolution computed tomography scans show areas of consolidation. Except for the migrating opacities, these findings are nonspecific and present in many other respiratory disorders.

• *Pulmonary function tests* may be normal or show reduced capacities. The diffusing capacity for carbon monoxide ($DL_{CO}$) is generally low.

• *Arterial blood gas analysis* usually shows mild to moderate hypoxemia at rest, which worsens with exercise.

• *Blood tests* reveal an increased erythrocyte sedimentation rate, increased C-reactive protein level, and increased white blood cell count with a somewhat increased proportion of neutrophils and a minor rise in eosinophils. Immunoglobulin (Ig) G and IgM levels are normal or slightly increased, and the IgE level is normal.

• *Bronchoscopy* reveals normal or slightly inflamed airways. Bronchoalveolar lavage fluid obtained during bronchoscopy shows a moderate elevation in lymphocytes and, sometimes, elevated neutrophil and eosinophil levels. Foamy-looking alveolar macrophages may also be found.

Lung biopsy, thoracoscopy, or bronchoscopy is required to confirm the diagnosis of BOOP. Pathologic changes in lung tissue include plugs of connective tissue in the lumen of the bronchioles, alveolar ducts, and alveolar spaces.

These changes may occur in other types of bronchiolitis and in other diseases that cause organizing pneumonia. They also differentiate BOOP from constrictive bronchiolitis, characterized by inflammation and fibrosis that surround and may narrow or completely obliterate the bronchiolar airways. Although the pathologic findings in proliferative and constrictive bronchiolitis are different, the causes and presentations may overlap. Any known cause of bronchiolitis obliterans or organizing pneumonia must be ruled out before the diagnosis of BOOP is made.

**Treatment**

Corticosteroids are the current treatment for BOOP, although the ideal dosage and duration of treatment remain topics of discussion. In most cases, treatment begins with 1 mg/kg/day of prednisone for at least several days to several weeks; the dosage is then gradually reduced over several months to a year, depending on the patient's response. Relapse is common when steroids are tapered off or stopped but usually can be reversed when steroids are increased or resumed. Occasionally, a patient may need to continue corticosteroids indefinitely.

Immunosuppressant-cytotoxic drugs, such as cyclophosphamide, have been used in the few cases in which the patient couldn't tolerate or was unresponsive to corticosteroids.

Oxygen is used to correct hypoxemia. The patient may need either no oxygen or a small amount of oxygen at rest and a greater amount when he exercises.

Other treatments vary, depending on the patient's symptoms, and may include inhaled bronchodilators, cough suppressants, and bronchial hygiene therapies.

BOOP is responsive to treatment and usually can be completely reversed with corticosteroid therapy. However, a few deaths have been reported, particularly in patients who had more widespread pathologic changes in the lungs or patients who developed opportunistic infections or other complications related to steroid therapy.

**Special considerations**

• Explain all diagnostic tests. The patient may experience anxiety and frustration because of the length of time and number of tests needed to establish the diagnosis.

• Explain the diagnosis to the patient and his family. This uncommon diagnosis may cause confusion and anxiety.

• Monitor the patient for adverse effects of corticosteroid therapy: weight gain, "moon face," glucose intolerance, fluid and electrolyte imbalance, mood swings, cataracts, peptic ulcer disease, opportunistic infections, and osteoporosis leading to bone fractures. These effects may leave many patients unable to tolerate the treatment. Teach the patient and family about these adverse effects, emphasizing which reactions they should report to the doctor.

• Teach measures that may help prevent complications related to treatment, such as infection control and improved nutrition.

• Teach breathing, relaxation, and energy conservation techniques to help the patient manage symptoms.

• Monitor oxygenation, both at rest and with exertion. The doctor will probably prescribe an oxygen flow rate for use when the patient is at rest and a higher one for exertion. Teach the patient how to increase the oxygen flow rate to the appropriate level for exercise.

➤ CLINICAL TIP   If the patient needs oxygen at home, ensure continuity of care by making appropriate referrals to discharge planners, respiratory care practitioners, and home equipment vendors.

# BUERGER'S DISEASE

Buerger's disease, also known as thromboangiitis obliterans, is an inflammatory, nonatheromatous occlusive condition that causes segmental lesions and subsequent thrombus formation in the small and medium arteries (and sometimes the veins), resulting in decreased blood flow to the feet and legs. It may produce ulceration and, eventually, gangrene.

## Causes
Although the cause of Buerger's disease is unknown, a definite link exists to smoking, suggesting a hypersensitivity reaction to nicotine. Incidence is highest among men of Jewish ancestry, ages 20 to 40, who smoke heavily.

## Signs and symptoms
Buerger's disease typically produces intermittent claudication of the instep, which is aggravated by exercise and relieved by rest. During exposure to low temperatures, the feet initially become cold, cyanotic, and numb; later, they redden, become hot, and tingle. Occasionally, Buerger's disease also affects the hands, possibly resulting in painful fingertip ulcerations.

Associated signs and symptoms may include impaired peripheral pulses, migratory superficial thrombophlebitis and, in later stages, ulceration, muscle atrophy, and gangrene.

## Diagnosis
Patient history and physical examination strongly suggest Buerger's disease. Supportive diagnostic tests include:

• *Doppler ultrasonography* to show diminished circulation in the peripheral vessels

• *plethysmography* to help detect decreased circulation in the peripheral vessels

• *arteriography* to locate lesions and rule out atherosclerosis.

## Treatment

Therapy may include an exercise program that uses gravity to fill and drain the blood vessels or, in severe disease, a lumbar sympathectomy to increase blood supply to the skin. Amputation may be necessary for nonhealing ulcers, intractable pain, or gangrene.

## Special considerations

▶ CLINICAL TIP  Strongly urge the patient to discontinue smoking permanently to enhance the effectiveness of treatment. If necessary, refer him to a self-help group to stop smoking.

• Warn the patient to avoid precipitating factors, such as emotional stress, exposure to extreme temperatures, and trauma.

• Teach proper foot care, especially the importance of wearing well-fitting shoes and cotton or wool socks. Show the patient how to inspect his feet daily for cuts, abrasions, and signs of skin breakdown, such as redness and soreness. Remind him to seek medical attention immediately after any trauma.

• If the patient has ulcers and gangrene, enforce bed rest and use a padded footboard or bed cradle to prevent pressure from bed linens. Protect the feet with soft padding. Wash them gently with a mild soap and tepid water, rinse thoroughly, and pat dry with a soft towel.

• Provide emotional support. If necessary, refer the patient for psychological counseling to help him cope with restrictions imposed by this chronic disease.

• If the patient has undergone amputation, assess rehabilitative needs, especially regarding changes in body image. Refer him to physical therapists, occupational therapists, and social service agencies as needed.

# BULIMIA NERVOSA

The essential features of bulimia nervosa include eating binges followed by feelings of guilt, humiliation, and self-deprecation. These feelings cause the patient to engage in self-induced vomiting, use laxatives or diuretics, follow a strict diet, or fast to overcome the effects of the binges.

Unless the patient spends an excessive amount of time bingeing and purging, bulimia nervosa seldom is incapacitating. However, electrolyte imbalances (metabolic alkalosis, hypochloremia, and hypokalemia) and dehydration can occur, increasing the risk of physical complications.

Bulimia nervosa usually begins in adolescence or early adulthood and can occur simultaneously with anorexia nervosa. It affects nine women for every man affected. Nearly 2% of adult women meet the diagnostic criteria for bulimia nervosa; 5% to 15% have some symptoms of the disorder.

## Causes

Bulimia nervosa has no known cause, but psychosocial factors may contribute to its development, including family disturbance or conflict, sexual abuse, maladaptive learned behavior, struggle for control or self-identity, cultural overemphasis on physical appearance, and parental obesity.

▶ CLINICAL TIP  Bulimia nervosa is also associated with depression.

## Signs and symptoms

The history of a patient with bulimia nervosa is marked by episodes of binge eating that may occur up to several times a day. The patient commonly reports a binge-eating episode during which she

## DIAGNOSING BULIMIA NERVOSA

The diagnosis of bulimia nervosa is made when the patient meets criteria put forth in the *Diagnostic and Statistical Manual of Mental Disorders,* 4th ed. Both of the behaviors listed below must occur at least twice a week for 3 months:

• recurrent episodes of binge eating (rapid consumption of a large amount of food in a discrete period of time and a feeling of lack of control over eating behavior during the eating binges)
• recurrent inappropriate compensatory behavior to prevent weight gain (self-induced vomiting; misuse of laxatives, diuretics, enemas or other medications; fasting; excessive exercise).

continues eating until abdominal pain, sleep, or the presence of another person interrupts it. The preferred food usually is sweet, soft, and high in calories and carbohydrate content.

The bulimic patient may appear thin and emaciated. Typically, however, although her weight frequently fluctuates, it usually stays within normal limits through the use of diuretics, laxatives, vomiting, and exercise. So, unlike the anorexic patient, the bulimic patient can usually hide her eating disorder.

Overt clues to this disorder include hyperactivity, peculiar eating habits or rituals, frequent weighing, and a distorted body image.

The patient may complain of abdominal and epigastric pain caused by acute gastric dilation. She may also have amenorrhea. Repetitive vomiting may cause painless swelling of the salivary glands, hoarseness, throat irritation or lacerations, and dental erosion. The patient may also exhibit calluses on the knuckles or abrasions and scars on the dorsum of the hand, resulting from tooth injury during self-induced vomiting.

### Psychosocial factors

A bulimic patient commonly is perceived by others as a "perfect" student, mother, or career woman; an adolescent may be distinguished for participation in competitive activities such as sports. However, the patient's psychosocial history may reveal an exaggerated sense of guilt, symptoms of depression, childhood trauma (especially sexual abuse), parental obesity, or a history of unsatisfactory sexual relationships.

### Diagnosis

For characteristic findings in this condition, see *Diagnosing bulimia nervosa.*

Additional diagnostic tools include the Beck Depression Inventory, which may identify coexisting depression, and laboratory tests to help determine the presence and severity of complications. Serum electrolyte studies may show elevated bicarbonate, decreased potassium, and decreased sodium levels.

A baseline electrocardiogram may be done if tricyclic antidepressants will be prescribed for the patient.

### Treatment

Interrelated physical and psychological symptoms must be treated simultaneously. Therapy may continue for several years. Merely promoting weight gain isn't sufficient to guarantee long-term recovery. A patient whose physical status is severely compromised by inadequate or chaotic eating patterns is difficult to engage in the psychotherapeutic process.

Psychotherapy concentrates on interrupting the binge-purge cycle and helping the patient regain control over her eating behavior. Treatment may be provided in either an inpatient or an outpatient setting and includes behavior modification therapy, which may take place in highly structured psychoeducational group meetings.

Individual psychotherapy and family therapy, which address the eating disorder as a symptom of unresolved conflict, may help the patient understand the basis of her behavior and teach her self-control strategies. Antidepressant drugs may be used as an adjunct to psychotherapy.

The patient also may benefit from participation in self-help groups, such as Overeaters Anonymous, or in a drug rehabilitation program if she has a concurrent substance abuse problem.

**Special considerations**
● Supervise the patient during mealtimes and for a specified period after meals (usually 1 hour). Set a time limit for each meal. Provide a pleasant, relaxed environment for eating.
● Using behavior modification techniques, reward the patient for satisfactory weight gain.
● Establish a contract with the patient, specifying the amount and type of food to be eaten at each meal.
● Encourage the patient to recognize and express her feelings about her eating behavior. Maintain an accepting and nonjudgmental attitude, controlling your reactions to her behavior and feelings.
● Encourage the patient to talk about stressful issues, such as achievement, independence, socialization, sexuality, family problems, and control.
● Identify the patient's elimination patterns.
● Assess her suicide potential.

● Refer the patient and her family to the American Anorexia/Bulimia Association and to Anorexia Nervosa and Related Eating Disorders for additional information and support.
● Teach the patient how to keep a food journal to monitor her treatment progress.
● Outline the risks of laxative, emetic, and diuretic abuse for the patient.
● Provide assertiveness training to help the patient gain control over her behavior and achieve a realistic and positive self-image.
● If the patient is taking a prescribed tricyclic antidepressant, instruct her to take the drug with food. Warn her to avoid consuming alcoholic beverages; exposing herself to sunlight, heat lamps, or tanning salons; and discontinuing the medication unless she has notified the doctor.

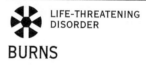 LIFE-THREATENING DISORDER

## BURNS

A major burn is a horrifying injury, necessitating painful treatment and a long period of rehabilitation. It's often fatal or permanently disfiguring and incapacitating (both emotionally and physically). In the United States, about 2 million persons annually suffer burns. Of these, 300,000 are burned seriously and over 6,000 are fatalities, making burns this nation's third-leading cause of accidental death.

**Causes**
*Thermal burns,* the most common type, are frequently the result of residential fires, motor vehicle accidents, playing with matches, improperly stored gasoline, space heater or electrical mal-

## DEPTH OF BURN

This illustration shows the depth of tissue damage in partial- and full-thickness burns. A partial-thickness burn damages the epidermis and part of the dermis, whereas a full-thickness burn affects the epidermis, dermis, and subcutaneous tissue.

Epidermis

Dermis

Subcutaneous tissue

Muscle

Damaged tissue

Dead tissue

Normal skin

Partial thickness

Full thickness

functions, or arson. Other causes include improper handling of firecrackers, scalding accidents, and kitchen accidents (such as a child climbing on top of a stove or grabbing a hot iron). Burns in children are sometimes traced to parental abuse.

*Chemical burns* result from the contact, ingestion, inhalation, or injection of acids, alkalis, or vesicants. *Electrical burns* usually occur after contact with faulty electrical wiring or high-voltage power lines or when electric cords are chewed (by young children). *Friction or abrasion burns* happen when the skin is rubbed harshly against a coarse surface. *Sunburn,* of course, follows excessive exposure to sunlight.

### Assessment
The depth of damage to the skin and tissue and the size of the burn are importance factors in burn assessment.

### *Depth of skin and tissue damage*
A traditional method gauges burn depth by degrees, although most burns are a combination of different degrees and thicknesses. (See *Depth of burn.*)
● *First-degree*—Damage is limited to the epidermis, causing erythema and pain.

• *Second-degree* — The epidermis and part of the dermis are damaged, producing blisters and mild to moderate edema and pain.

• *Third-degree* — The epidermis and the dermis are damaged. No blisters appear, but white, brown, or black leathery tissue and thrombosed vessels are visible.

• *Fourth-degree* — Damage extends through deeply charred subcutaneous tissue to muscle and bone.

### Burn size

The size is usually expressed as the percentage of body surface area (BSA) covered by the burn. The Rule of Nines chart most commonly provides this estimate, although the Lund-Browder chart is more accurate because it allows for BSA changes with age. A correlation of the burn's depth and size permits an estimate of its severity.

• *Major* — third-degree burns on more than 10% of BSA; second-degree burns on more than 25% of adult BSA (more than 20% in children); burns of hands, face, feet, or genitalia; burns complicated by fractures or respiratory damage; electrical burns; all burns in poor-risk patients

• *Moderate* — third-degree burns on 2% to 10% of BSA; second-degree burns on 15% to 25% of adult BSA (10% to 20% in children)

• *Minor* — third-degree burns on less than 2% of BSA; second-degree burns on less than 15% of adult BSA (10% in children).

### Other considerations

• *Location* — Burns on the face, hands, feet, and genitalia are the most serious because of possible loss of function.

• *Configuration* — Circumferential burns can cause total occlusion of circulation in an extremity as a result of edema. Burns on the neck can produce airway obstruction, whereas burns on the chest can lead to restricted respiratory expansion.

• *History of complicating medical problems* — Note disorders that impair peripheral circulation, especially diabetes, peripheral vascular disease, and chronic alcohol abuse.

• *Other injuries* sustained at the time of the burn.

• *Patient age* — Victims under age 4 or over age 60 have a higher incidence of complications and, consequently, a higher mortality.

• *Pulmonary injury* — Smoke inhalation can cause pulmonary injury.

## Treatment and special considerations

• Immediate, aggressive burn treatment increases the patient's chance for survival. Later, supportive measures and strict aseptic technique can minimize infection. Meticulous, comprehensive burn care can make the difference between life and death. (See *Fluid replacement: The first 24 hours after a burn,* page 142.)

• If the patient's burns are minor, immerse the burned area in cool water (55° F [12.8° C]) or apply cool compresses. Give him pain medication as needed.

> CLINICAL TIP  Don't apply ice directly to the wound.

• Debride the devitalized tissue, taking care not to break any blisters. Cover the wound with an antimicrobial agent and a nonstick bulky dressing, and administer tetanus prophylaxis as needed.

• Provide thorough teaching and complete aftercare instructions for the patient. Stress the importance of keeping the dressing dry and clean, elevating the burned extremity for the first 24 hours, taking prescribed analgesics, and returning for a wound check in 1 to 2 days.

## FLUID REPLACEMENT: THE FIRST 24 HOURS AFTER A BURN

Use one of these two formulas as a general guideline for the amount of fluid replacement, but vary the specific infusions according to the patient's response, especially urine output.

### Parkland formula
Administer 4 ml/kg of crystalloid × % body surface area (BSA) burn (up to 50%)

### Galveston formula (for pediatric patients)
Based on BSA rather than weight. Administer 5,000 ml/m² lactated Ringer's solution × % BSA burn + 2,000 ml/m² over 24 hours of maintenance. Give half the total fluid over the first 8 hours and the balance over the next 16 hours.

---

● In moderate and major burns, immediately assess the patient's airway, breathing, and circulation. Be especially alert for signs of smoke inhalation and pulmonary damage: singed nasal hairs, mucosal burns, voice changes, coughing, wheezing, soot in the mouth or nose, and darkened sputum. Assist with endotracheal intubation and administer 100% oxygen.

● Control bleeding, and remove smoldering clothing, rings, and other constricting items.

➤ CLINICAL TIP  If clothing is stuck to the patient's skin, soak it first in saline solution.

● Be sure to cover burns with a clean, dry, sterile bed sheet. *(Never* cover large burns with saline-soaked dressings because they can drastically lower body temperature.)

● Begin I.V. therapy immediately to prevent hypovolemic shock and maintain cardiac output. Use lactated Ringer's solution or a fluid replacement formula.

● Once the patient is stable, take a brief history of the burn.

● Draw blood samples for a complete blood count; electrolyte, glucose, blood urea nitrogen, and creatinine levels; arterial blood gas analysis; and typing and crossmatching.

● Closely monitor intake and output, and frequently check vital signs. Although it may make you nervous, don't be afraid to take the patient's blood pressure because of burned limbs. An arterial line may be inserted if blood pressure is unobtainable with a cuff.

● In the facility, a central venous pressure line, additional I.V. lines (using venous cutdown if necessary), and an indwelling urinary catheter may be inserted.

● To combat fluid evaporation through the burn and the release of fluid into interstitial spaces (possibly resulting in hypovolemic shock), continue fluid therapy as needed.

Send a urine specimen to the laboratory to check for myoglobinuria and hemoglobinuria.

● Insert a nasogastric tube to decompress the stomach and avoid aspiration of stomach contents.

● Electrical and chemical burns demand special attention. Tissue damage from electrical burns is difficult to assess because internal destruction along the conduction pathway is usually greater than the surface burn would indicate. Electrical burns that ignite the patient's clothes may cause thermal burns as well. If the electric shock caused ventricular fibrillation and cardiac and respiratory arrest, begin cardiopulmonary resuscitation at once. Get an estimate of the voltage.

● In a chemical burn, irrigate the wound with copious amounts of water or normal saline solution.

▶ CLINICAL TIP  Using a weak base (such as sodium bicarbonate) to neutralize hydrofluoric acid, hydrochloric acid, or sulfuric acid on skin or mucous membrane is contraindicated because the neutralizing agent can actually produce more heat and tissue damage.

● If the chemical entered the patient's eyes, flush them with large amounts of water or saline solution for at least 30 minutes; in an alkali burn, irrigate until the pH of the cul-de-sacs returns to 7. Have the patient close his eyes, and cover them with a dry, sterile dressing. Note the type of chemical causing the burn and the presence of any noxious fumes. The patient will need an emergency ophthalmologic examination.

● Don't treat the burn wound itself in the emergency department if the patient is to be transferred to a specialized burn care unit within 4 hours after the burn. Instead, prepare the patient for transport by wrapping him in a sterile sheet and a blanket for warmth and elevating the burned extremity to decrease edema. Then, transport the patient immediately. Once at the burn unit, the patient will receive specialized treatments, including skin grafts of various types.

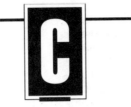

# CALCIUM IMBALANCE

Calcium plays an indispensable role in cell permeability, formation of bones and teeth, blood coagulation, transmission of nerve impulses, and normal muscle contraction. Nearly all (99%) of the body's calcium is found in the bones. The remaining 1% exists in ionized form in serum, and it's the maintenance of the 1% of ionized calcium in the serum that's critical to healthy neurologic function.

The parathyroid glands regulate ionized calcium and determine its resorption into bone, absorption from the GI mucosa, and excretion in urine and stool. Severe calcium imbalance requires emergency treatment because a deficiency (hypocalcemia) can lead to tetany and seizures; an excess (hypercalcemia), to cardiac arrhythmias and coma.

## Causes
Several factors can cause calcium imbalance.

### Hypocalcemia
- *Inadequate intake of calcium and vitamin D* results in inhibited intestinal absorption of calcium.
- *Hypoparathyroidism* as a result of injury, disease, or surgery decreases or eliminates secretion of parathyroid hormone (PTH), which is necessary for calcium absorption and normal serum calcium levels.
- *Malabsorption or loss of calcium from the GI tract* can result from increased intestinal motility from severe diarrhea or laxative abuse. Malabsorption of calcium from the GI tract can also result from inadequate levels of vitamin D or PTH or a reduction in gastric acidity, which decreases the solubility of calcium salts.
- *Severe infections or burns* can lead to diseased and burned tissue trapping calcium from the extracellular fluid.
- *Overcorrection of acidosis* can lead to alkalosis, which causes decreased ionized calcium and induces symptoms of hypocalcemia.
- *Pancreatic insufficiency* may cause malabsorption of calcium and subsequent calcium loss in stool. In pancreatitis, participation of calcium ions in saponification contributes to calcium loss.
- *Renal failure* results in excessive excretion of calcium secondary to increased retention of phosphate. Renal failure also results in loss of the active metabolite of vitamin D, which impairs calcium absorption.
- *Hypomagnesemia* causes decreased PTH secretion and blocks the peripheral action of that hormone.

### Hypercalcemia
- *Hyperparathyroidism* increases serum calcium levels by promoting calcium absorption from the intestine, resorp-

## SIGNS AND SYMPTOMS OF CALCIUM IMBALANCE

| DYSFUNCTION | HYPOCALCEMIA | HYPERCALCEMIA |
|---|---|---|
| Central nervous system | • Anxiety, irritability, twitching around mouth, laryngospasm, seizures, Chvostek's sign, Trousseau's sign | • Drowsiness, lethargy, headaches, depression or apathy, irritability, confusion, coma |
| Musculoskeletal | • Paresthesia (tingling and numbness of the fingers), tetany or painful tonic muscle spasms, facial spasms, abdominal cramps, muscle cramps, spasmodic contractions | • Weakness, muscle flaccidity, bone pain, pathologic fractures |
| Cardiovascular | • Arrhythmias, hypotension | • Signs of heart block, cardiac arrest in systole, hypertension |
| GI | • Increased GI motility, diarrhea | • Anorexia, nausea, vomiting, constipation, dehydration, polydipsia |
| Other | • Blood clotting abnormalities (rare) | • Renal polyuria, flank pain, kidney stones and, eventually, azotemia |

tion from bone, and reabsorption from the kidneys.

• *Hypervitaminosis D* can promote increased absorption of calcium from the intestine.

• *Tumors* raise serum calcium levels by destroying bone or by releasing PTH or a PTH-like substance, osteoclast-activating factor, prostaglandins and, perhaps, a vitamin D–like sterol.

• *Multiple fractures and prolonged immobilization* release bone calcium and raise the serum calcium level.

• *Multiple myeloma* promotes loss of calcium from bone.

Other causes include milk-alkali syndrome, sarcoidosis, hyperthyroidism, adrenal insufficiency, and thiazide diuretics.

### Signs and symptoms

Indications of calcium imbalance depend on the type of imbalance. (See *Signs and symptoms of calcium imbalance.*)

### *Hypocalcemia*

A lack of calcium causes nerve fiber irritability and repetitive muscle spasms. Consequently, characteristic symptoms of hypocalcemia include perioral paresthesia, twitching, carpopedal spasm, tetany, seizures and, possibly, cardiac arrhythmias. Although Chvostek's sign and Trousseau's sign are reliable indicators of hypocalcemia, they're not specific.

### Hypercalcemia

Clinical effects of hypercalcemia include muscle weakness, decreased muscle tone, lethargy, anorexia, constipation, nausea, vomiting, dehydration, polydipsia, and polyuria. Severe hypercalcemia (serum levels that exceed 5.7 mEq/L) may produce cardiac arrhythmias and, eventually, coma.

### Diagnosis

A serum calcium level less than 4.5 mEq/L confirms hypocalcemia; a level above 5.5 mEq/L confirms hypercalcemia. (However, because approximately one-half of serum calcium is bound to albumin, changes in serum protein must be considered when interpreting serum calcium levels.)

The Sulkowitch urine test shows increased urine calcium precipitation in hypercalcemia. In hypocalcemia, an electrocardiogram (ECG) reveals a lengthened QT interval, a prolonged ST segment, and arrhythmias; in hypercalcemia, a shortened QT interval and heart block.

### Treatment

An acute imbalance requires immediate correction, followed by maintenance therapy and correction of the underlying cause.

### Hypocalcemia

A mild calcium deficit may require nothing more than an adjustment in diet to allow adequate intake of calcium, vitamin D, and protein, possibly with oral calcium supplements. Acute hypocalcemia is an emergency that needs immediate correction by I.V. administration of calcium gluconate or calcium chloride.

Chronic hypocalcemia also requires vitamin D supplements to facilitate GI absorption of calcium. To correct mild deficiency states, the amounts of vitamin D in most multivitamin preparations are adequate. For severe deficiency, vitamin D is used in four forms: ergocalciferol (vitamin $D_2$), cholecalciferol (vitamin $D_3$), calcitriol, and dihydrotachysterol, a synthetic form of vitamin $D_2$.

### Hypercalcemia

Treatment of hypercalcemia primarily eliminates excess serum calcium through hydration with normal saline solution, which promotes calcium excretion in urine. Loop diuretics, such as ethacrynic acid and furosemide, also promote calcium excretion. (Thiazide diuretics are contraindicated in hypercalcemia because they inhibit calcium excretion.)

Corticosteroids, such as prednisone and hydrocortisone, are helpful in treating sarcoidosis, hypervitaminosis D, and certain tumors. Mithramycin can also lower the serum calcium level and is especially effective against hypercalcemia secondary to certain tumors. Calcitonin may also be helpful in certain instances.

Sodium phosphate solution administered by mouth or by retention enema promotes calcium deposits in bone and inhibits its absorption from the GI tract.

### Special considerations

CLINICAL TIP  Watch for hypocalcemia in patients receiving massive transfusions of citrated blood and in those with chronic diarrhea, severe infections, and insufficient dietary intake of calcium and protein (especially elderly patients).

If the patient has hypocalcemia:
• Monitor serum calcium levels every 12 to 24 hours; a calcium level below 4.5 mEq/L requires immediate atten-

tion. When giving calcium supplements, frequently check the pH level; an alkalotic state that exceeds 7.45 pH inhibits calcium ionization. Check for Trousseau's and Chvostek's signs.

• Administer calcium gluconate slow I.V. in dextrose 5% in water *(never* in saline solution, which encourages renal calcium loss). Don't add calcium gluconate I.V. to solutions containing bicarbonate; it will precipitate.

• When administering calcium solutions, watch for anorexia, nausea, and vomiting; they are possible signs of overcorrection to hypercalcemia.

• If the patient is receiving calcium chloride, watch for abdominal discomfort.

• Monitor the patient closely for a possible drug interaction if he's receiving digitalis glycosides with large doses of oral calcium supplements; watch for signs of digitalis toxicity (anorexia, nausea, vomiting, yellow vision, and cardiac arrhythmias). Administer oral calcium supplements 1 to 1½ hours after meals or with milk.

• Provide a quiet, stress-free environment for the patient with tetany. Observe seizure precautions for patients with severe hypocalcemia that may lead to seizures.

• To prevent hypocalcemia, advise all patients (especially the elderly ones) to eat foods rich in calcium, vitamin D, and protein, such as fortified milk and cheese. Explain how important calcium is for normal bone formation and blood coagulation. Discourage chronic use of laxatives. Also, warn hypocalcemic patients not to overuse antacids because they may aggravate the condition.

If the patient has hypercalcemia:

• Monitor serum calcium levels frequently. Watch for cardiac arrhythmias if the serum calcium level exceeds 5.7 mEq/L. Increase fluid intake to dilute calcium in serum and urine and to prevent renal damage and dehydration.

• Watch for signs of heart failure in patients receiving normal saline solution diuresis therapy.

• Administer loop diuretics (not thiazide diuretics). Monitor intake and output, and check the urine for renal calculi and acidity. Provide acid-ash drinks, such as cranberry or prune juice, because calcium salts are more soluble in acid than in alkali.

• Check the patient's ECG and vital signs frequently. In the patient receiving digitalis glycosides, watch for signs of toxicity, such as anorexia, nausea, vomiting, and bradycardia (often with arrhythmia).

• Help the patient walk as soon as possible. Handle the patient with chronic hypercalcemia *gently* to prevent pathologic fractures.

• If the patient is bedridden, reposition him frequently, and encourage range-of-motion exercises to promote circulation and prevent urinary stasis and calcium loss from bone.

• To prevent recurrence, suggest a low-calcium diet and increased fluid intake.

# CANDIDIASIS

Also called candidosis and moniliasis, candidiasis is usually a mild, superficial fungal infection caused by the *Candida* genus. Most often, it infects the nails (onychomycosis), skin (diaper rash), or mucous membranes, especially the oropharynx (thrush), vagina (moniliasis), esophagus, and GI tract.

Rarely, these fungi enter the bloodstream and invade the kidneys, lungs, endocardium, brain, or other structures, causing serious infections. Such systemic infection is most prevalent among

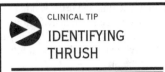

CLINICAL TIP

## IDENTIFYING THRUSH

Candidiasis of the oropharyngeal mucosa (thrush) causes cream-colored or bluish white pseudomembranous patches on the tongue, mouth, or pharynx. Fungal invasion may extend to circumoral tissues.

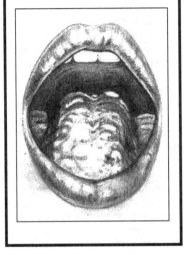

drug abusers and patients already hospitalized, particularly diabetics and immunosuppressed patients. The prognosis varies, depending on the patient's resistance.

### Causes

Most cases of *Candida* infection result from *C. albicans.* Other infective strains include *C. parapsilosis, C. tropicalis,* and *C. guillermondii.*

These fungi are part of the normal flora of the GI tract, mouth, vagina, and skin. They cause infection when some change in the body permits their sudden proliferation — rising glucose levels from diabetes mellitus; lowered resistance from a disease (such as can-

cer), an immunosuppressant drug, radiation, aging, or human immunodeficiency virus (HIV) infection; or when they're introduced systemically by I.V. or urinary catheters, drug abuse, hyperalimentation, or surgery.

However, the most common predisposing factor remains the use of broad-spectrum antibiotics, which decrease the number of normal flora and permit an increasing number of candidal organisms to proliferate. The infant of a mother with vaginal moniliasis can contract oral thrush while passing through the birth canal.

The incidence of candidiasis is rising because of wider use of I.V. therapy and a greater number of immunocompromised patients, especially those with HIV infection.

### Signs and symptoms

Superficial candidiasis produces symptoms that correspond to the following sites of infection:
- skin: scaly, erythematous, papular rash, sometimes covered with exudate, appearing below the breast, between the fingers, and at the axillae, groin, and umbilicus (In diaper rash, papules appear at the edges of the rash.)
- nails: red, swollen, darkened nailbed; occasionally, purulent discharge and the separation of a pruritic nail from the nailbed
- oropharyngeal mucosa (thrush): cream-colored or bluish white patches of exudate on the tongue, mouth, or pharynx that reveal bloody engorgement when scraped. They may swell, causing respiratory distress in infants. They're only occasionally painful but cause a burning sensation in the throats and mouths of adults. (See *Identifying thrush.*)
- esophageal mucosa: dysphagia, retrosternal pain, regurgitation and, occasionally, scales in the mouth and throat

- vaginal mucosa: white or yellow discharge, with pruritus and local excoriation; white or gray raised patches on vaginal walls, with local inflammation; dyspareunia.

Systemic infection produces chills; high, spiking fever; hypotension; prostration; and occasional rash. Specific symptoms depend on the site of infection, as follows:

- pulmonary system: hemoptysis, fever, cough
- renal system: fever, flank pain, dysuria, hematuria, pyuria
- brain: headache, nuchal rigidity, seizures, focal neurologic deficits
- endocardium: systolic or diastolic murmur, fever, chest pain, embolic phenomena
- eye: endophthalmitis, blurred vision, orbital or periorbital pain, scotoma, exudate.

### Diagnosis

Identification of superficial candidiasis depends on evidence of *Candida* on a Gram stain of skin, vaginal scrapings, pus, or sputum or on skin scrapings prepared in potassium hydroxide solution. Systemic infections require obtaining a sample for blood or tissue culture.

### Treatment

The first aim of treatment is to improve the underlying condition that predisposes the patient to candidiasis, such as controlling diabetes or discontinuing antibiotic therapy and catheterization, if possible.

Nystatin is an effective antifungal for superficial candidiasis. Clotrimazole, fluconazole, ketoconazole, and miconazole are effective in mucous membrane and vaginal *Candida* infections. Ketoconazole or fluconazole is the treatment of choice for chronic candidiasis of the mucous membranes. Treatment for systemic infection consists of I.V. amphotericin B with or without 5-fluorocytosine.

### Special considerations

- Instruct a patient using nystatin solution to swish it around in his mouth for several minutes before he swallows the solution.
- Swab nystatin on the oral mucosa of an infant with thrush.
- Provide the patient with a nonirritating mouthwash to loosen tenacious secretions and a soft toothbrush to avoid irritation.
- Relieve the patient's mouth discomfort with a topical anesthetic, such as lidocaine, at least 1 hour before meals. (It may suppress the gag reflex and cause aspiration.)
- Provide a soft diet for the patient with severe dysphagia. Tell the patient with mild dysphagia to chew food thoroughly, and make sure he doesn't choke.
- Use cornstarch or dry padding in intertriginous areas of obese patients to prevent irritation.
- Note dates of insertion of I.V. catheters, and replace them according to your facility's policy to prevent phlebitis.
- Assess the patient with candidiasis for underlying causes, such as diabetes mellitus. If the patient is receiving amphotericin B for systemic candidiasis, he may have severe chills, fever, anorexia, nausea, and vomiting. Premedicate with acetaminophen, antihistamines, or antiemetics to help reduce adverse reactions.
- Frequently check vital signs of patients with systemic infections. Provide appropriate supportive care.
- In patients with renal involvement, carefully monitor intake and output and urine for blood and protein.
- Check high-risk patients daily, especially those receiving antibiotics, for patchy areas, irritation, sore throat, bleeding of mouth or gums, or other

signs of superinfection. Check for vaginal discharge; record the color and amount.

● Encourage women in their third trimester of pregnancy to be examined for vaginal candidiasis to protect their infants from infection at birth.

---

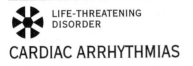

LIFE-THREATENING DISORDER

# CARDIAC ARRHYTHMIAS

---

Abnormal electrical conduction or automaticity changes heart rate and rhythm in cardiac arrhythmias, also called cardiac dysrhythmias. (See *Types of cardiac arrhythmias.*)

Arrhythmias vary in severity, from those that are mild, asymptomatic, and require no treatment (such as sinus arrhythmia, in which the heart rate increases and decreases with respirations) to catastrophic ventricular fibrillation, which necessitates immediate resuscitation.

Arrhythmias are generally classified according to their origin (ventricular or supraventricular). Their effect on cardiac output and blood pressure, partially influenced by the site of origin, determines their clinical significance.

## Causes

Arrhythmias may be congenital or they may result from one of several factors, including myocardial ischemia, myocardial infarction, and organic heart disease. Drug toxicity or degeneration of the conductive tissue necessary to maintain normal heart rhythm (sick sinus syndrome) sometimes can also precipitate arrhythmias.

## Special considerations

● Assess an unmonitored patient for rhythm disturbances.

● If the patient's pulse is abnormally rapid, slow, or irregular, watch for signs of hypoperfusion, such as hypotension and diminished urine output.

● Document any arrhythmias in a monitored patient, and assess for possible causes and effects.

● When life-threatening arrhythmias develop, rapidly assess the level of consciousness, respirations, and pulse.

● Initiate cardiopulmonary resuscitation, if indicated.

● Evaluate the patient for altered cardiac output resulting from arrhythmias.

● Administered medications as needed, and prepare for medical procedures (for example, cardioversion) if indicated.

● Monitor for predisposing factors — such as fluid and electrolyte imbalance — and signs of drug toxicity, especially with digoxin. Drug toxicity may require withholding the next dose.

● To prevent arrhythmias in a postoperative cardiac patient, provide adequate oxygen and reduce the heart's workload, while carefully maintaining metabolic, neurologic, respiratory, and hemodynamic status.

● To avoid temporary pacemaker malfunction, install a fresh battery before each insertion. Carefully secure the external catheter wires and the pacemaker box. Assess the threshold daily. Watch closely for premature contractions, a sign of myocardial irritation.

● To avert permanent pacemaker malfunction, restrict the patient's activity after insertion. Monitor the pulse rate regularly, and watch for signs of decreased cardiac output.

● If the patient has a permanent pacemaker, warn him about environmental hazards, as indicated by the pacemaker manufacturer.

*(Text continues on page 159.)*

# TYPES OF CARDIAC ARRHYTHMIAS

This chart reviews many common cardiac arrhythmias and outlines their features, causes, and treatments. Use a normal electrocardiogram strip, if available, to compare normal cardiac rhythm configurations with the rhythm strips below. Characteristics of normal rhythm include:

- ventricular and atrial rates of 60 to 100 beats/minute
- regular and uniform QRS complexes and P waves
- PR interval of 0.12 to 0.2 second
- QRS duration < 0.12 second
- identical atrial and ventricular rates, with constant PR interval.

| ARRHYTHMIA AND FEATURES | CAUSES | TREATMENT |
|---|---|---|
| **Sinus arrhythmia** • Irregular atrial and ventricular rhythms • Normal P wave preceding each QRS complex | • A normal variation of normal sinus rhythm in athletes, children, and elderly people • Also seen in digitalis toxicity and inferior wall myocardial infarction (MI) | • Atropine if rate decreases below 40 beats/minute and the patient is symptomatic |
| **Sinus tachycardia** • Atrial and ventricular rates regular • Rate > 100 beats/minute; rarely, > 160 beats/minute • Normal P wave preceding each QRS complex | • Normal physiologic response to fever, exercise, anxiety, pain, dehydration; may also accompany shock, left-sided heart failure, cardiac tamponade, hyperthyroidism, anemia, hypovolemia, pulmonary embolism, and anterior wall MI • May also occur with atropine, epinephrine, isoproterenol, quinidine, caffeine, alcohol, and nicotine use | • Correction of underlying cause • Propranolol for symptomatic patients |

*(continued)*

## TYPES OF CARDIAC ARRHYTHMIAS *(continued)*

| ARRHYTHMIA AND FEATURES | CAUSES | TREATMENT |
|---|---|---|
| **Sinus bradycardia**<br>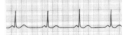<br>• Regular atrial and ventricular rates<br>• Rate < 60 beats/minute<br>• Normal P waves preceding each QRS complex | • Normal, in well-conditioned heart, as in an athlete<br>• Increased intracranial pressure; increased vagal tone due to straining during defecation, vomiting, intubation, mechanical ventilation; sick sinus syndrome, hypothyroidism; inferior wall MI<br>• May also occur with anticholinesterase, beta blocker, digoxin, and morphine use | • For low cardiac output, dizziness, weakness, altered level of consciousness, or low blood pressure; advanced cardiac life support (ACLS) protocol for administration of atropine<br>• Temporary pacemaker or isoproterenol if atropine fails; may need permanent pacemaker |
| **Sinoatrial arrest or block** (sinus arrest)<br>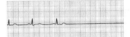<br>• Atrial and ventricular rhythms normal except for missing complex<br>• Normal P waves preceding each QRS complex<br>• Pause not equal to a multiple of the previous sinus rhythm | • Acute infection<br>• Coronary artery disease, degenerative heart disease, acute inferior wall MI<br>• Vagal stimulation, Valsalva's maneuver, carotid sinus massage<br>• Digitalis, quinidine, or salicylate toxicity<br>• Pesticide poisoning<br>• Pharyngeal irritation caused by endotracheal (ET) intubation<br>• Sick sinus syndrome | • Treat symptoms with atropine I.V.<br>• Temporary or permanent pacemaker for repeated episodes |
| **Wandering atrial pacemaker**<br>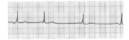<br>• Atrial and ventricular rates vary slightly<br>• Irregular PR interval<br>• P waves irregular with changing configuration, indicating that they're not all from sinoatrial (SA) node or single atrial focus; may appear after the QRS complex<br>• QRS complexes uniform in shape but irregular in rhythm | • Rheumatic carditis due to inflammation involving the SA node<br>• Digitalis toxicity<br>• Sick sinus syndrome | • No treatment if patient is asymptomatic<br>• Treatment of underlying cause if patient is symptomatic |

# TYPES OF CARDIAC ARRHYTHMIAS *(continued)*

| ARRHYTHMIA AND FEATURES | CAUSES | TREATMENT |
|---|---|---|
| **Premature atrial contraction (PAC)**<br><br>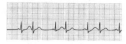<br><br>• Premature, abnormal-looking P waves that differ in configuration from normal P waves<br>• QRS complexes after P waves, except in very early or blocked PACs<br>• P wave often buried in the preceding T wave or identified in the preceding T wave | • Coronary or valvular heart disease, atrial ischemia, coronary atherosclerosis, heart failure, acute respiratory failure, chronic obstructive pulmonary disease (COPD), electrolyte imbalance, and hypoxia<br>• Digitalis toxicity; use of aminophylline, adrenergics, or caffeine<br>• Anxiety | • If occurring more than six times per minute or increasing in frequency, digoxin, quinidine, verapamil, or propranolol; after revascularization surgery, propranolol<br>• Treatment of underlying cause |
| **Paroxysmal supraventricular tachycardia**<br><br>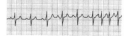<br><br>• Atrial and ventricular rates regular<br>• Heart rate > 160 beats/minute; rarely exceeds 250 beats/minute<br>• P waves regular but aberrant; difficult to differentiate from preceding T wave<br>• P wave preceding each QRS complex<br>• Sudden onset and termination of arrhythmia | • Intrinsic abnormality of atrioventricular (AV) conduction system<br>• Physical or psychological stress, hypoxia, hypokalemia, cardiomyopathy, congenital heart disease, MI, valvular disease, Wolff-Parkinson-White syndrome, cor pulmonale, hyperthyroidism, and systemic hypertension<br>• Digitalis toxicity; use of caffeine, marijuana, or central nervous system stimulants | • If patient is unstable, prepare for immediate cardioversion.<br>• If patient is stable, vagal stimulation, Valsalva's maneuver, carotid sinus massage<br>• Adenosine by rapid I.V. bolus injection to rapidly convert arrhythmia<br>• If patient is stable, determine QRS complex width. For wide complex width, follow ACLS protocol for lidocaine and procainamide. For narrow complex width and normal or elevated blood pressure, follow ACLS protocol for verapamil and consider digoxin, beta blockers, and diltiazem. For narrow complex width with low or unstable blood pressure (and for ineffective drug response for others), use synchronized cardioversion. |

*(continued)*

## TYPES OF CARDIAC ARRHYTHMIAS *(continued)*

| ARRHYTHMIA AND FEATURES | CAUSES | TREATMENT |
|---|---|---|
| **Atrial flutter**<br>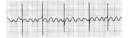<br>• Atrial rhythm at regular rate; 250 to 400 beats/minute<br>• Ventricular rate variable, depending on degree of AV block (usually 60 to 100 beats/minute)<br>• Sawtooth P-wave configuration possible (F waves)<br>• QRS complexes uniform in shape but often irregular in rate | • Heart failure, tricuspid or mitral valve disease, pulmonary embolism, cor pulmonale, inferior wall MI, and carditis<br>• Digitalis toxicity | • If patient is unstable with a ventricular rate > 150 beats/minute, prepare for immediate cardioversion.<br>• If patient is stable, drug therapy may include diltiazem, beta blockers, verapamil, digoxin, procainamide, or quinidine. |
| **Atrial fibrillation**<br>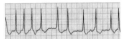<br>• Atrial rhythm grossly irregular; rate > 400 beats/minute<br>• Ventricular rate grossly irregular<br>• QRS complexes of uniform configuration and duration<br>• PR interval indiscernible<br>• No P waves, or P waves that appear as erratic, irregular, baseline fibrillatory waves | • Heart failure, COPD, thyrotoxicosis, constrictive pericarditis, ischemic heart disease, sepsis, pulmonary embolus, rheumatic heart disease, hypertension, mitral stenosis, atrial irritation, complication of coronary bypass or valve replacement surgery<br>• Nifedipine and digoxin use | • If patient is unstable with a ventricular rate > 150 beats/minute, prepare for immediate cardioversion.<br>• If patient is stable, drug therapy may include diltiazem, beta blockers, verapamil, digoxin, procainamide, or covert, given I.V. |

## TYPES OF CARDIAC ARRHYTHMIAS *(continued)*

| ARRHYTHMIA AND FEATURES | CAUSES | TREATMENT |
|---|---|---|
| **Junctional rhythm**<br>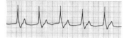<br>• Atrial and ventricular rates regular; atrial rate 40 to 60 beats/minute; ventricular rate usually 40 to 60 beats/minute (60 to 100 beats/minute is accelerated junctional rhythm)<br>• P waves preceding, hidden within (absent), or after QRS complex; inverted if visible<br>• PR interval (when present) < 0.12 second<br>• QRS complex configuration and duration normal, except in aberrant conduction | • Inferior wall MI or ischemia, hypoxia, vagal stimulation, sick sinus syndrome<br>• Acute rheumatic fever<br>• Valve surgery<br>• Digitalis toxicity | • Atropine for symptomatic slow rate<br>• Pacemaker insertion if patient doesn't respond to drugs<br>• Discontinuation of digoxin if appropriate |
| **Premature junctional contractions** (junctional premature beats)<br>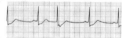<br>• Atrial and ventricular rhythms irregular<br>• P waves inverted; may precede, be hidden within, or follow QRS complex<br>• PR interval < 0.12 second if P wave precedes QRS complex<br>• QRS complex configuration and duration normal | • MI or ischemia<br>• Digitalis toxicity and excessive caffeine or amphetamine use | • Correction of underlying cause<br>• Atropine<br>• Discontinuation of digoxin if appropriate<br>• May require pacemaker |
| **First-degree AV block**<br>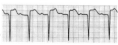<br>• Atrial and ventricular rates regular<br>• PR interval > 0.20 second<br>• P wave precedes QRS complex<br>• QRS complex normal | • May be seen in a healthy person<br>• Inferior wall MI or ischemia, hypothyroidism, hypokalemia, hyperkalemia<br>• Digitalis toxicity; use of quinidine, procainamide, or propranolol | • Cautious use of digoxin<br>• Correction of underlying cause<br>• Possibly atropine if PR interval exceeds 0.26 second or bradycardia develops |

*(continued)*

## TYPES OF CARDIAC ARRHYTHMIAS *(continued)*

| ARRHYTHMIA AND FEATURES | CAUSES | TREATMENT |
|---|---|---|
| **Second-degree AV block**<br>Mobitz I (Wenckebach)<br>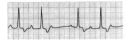<br>● Atrial rhythm regular<br>● Ventricular rhythm irregular<br>● Atrial rate exceeds ventricular rate<br>● PR interval progressively but only slightly longer with each cycle until QRS complex disappears (dropped beat); PR interval shorter after dropped beat | ● Inferior wall MI, cardiac surgery, acute rheumatic fever, and vagal stimulation<br>● Digitalis toxicity; use of propranolol, quinidine, or procainamide | ● Treatment of underlying cause<br>● Atropine or temporary pacemaker for symptomatic bradycardia<br>● Discontinuation of digoxin if appropriate |
| **Second-degree AV block**<br>Mobitz II<br>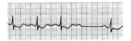<br>● Atrial rate regular<br>● Ventricular rhythm regular or irregular, with varying degree of block<br>● P-P interval constant<br>● QRS complexes periodically absent | ● Severe coronary artery disease, anterior wall MI, acute myocarditis<br>● Digitalis toxicity | ● Isoproterenol for symptomatic bradycardia<br>● Temporary or permanent pacemaker<br>● Discontinuation of digoxin if appropriate |
| **Third-degree AV block**<br>(complete heart block)<br>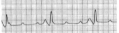<br>● Atrial rate regular<br>● Ventricular rate slow and regular<br>● No relation between P waves and QRS complexes<br>● No constant PR interval<br>● QRS interval normal (nodal pacemaker) or wide and bizarre (ventricular pacemaker) rates regular<br>● PR interval > 0.20 second<br>● P wave precedes QRS complex<br>● QRS complex normal | ● Inferior or anterior wall MI, congenital abnormality, rheumatic fever, hypoxia, postoperative complication of mitral valve replacement, Lev's disease (fibrosis and calcification that spreads from cardiac structures to the conductive tissue), Lenegre's disease (conductive tissue fibrosis)<br>● Digitalis toxicity | ● Atropine or isoproterenol for symptomatic bradycardia<br>● Temporary or permanent pacemaker |

# TYPES OF CARDIAC ARRHYTHMIAS *(continued)*

| ARRHYTHMIA AND FEATURES | CAUSES | TREATMENT |
|---|---|---|
| **Junctional tachycardia**<br>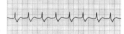<br>• Atrial rate > 100 beats/minute; however, P waves may be absent, hidden in QRS complex, or preceding T wave<br>• Ventricular rate > 100 beats/minute<br>• P wave inverted; may occur before or after QRS complex, may be hidden in QRS complex, or may be absent<br>• QRS complex configuration and duration normal<br>• onset of rhythm often sudden, occurring in bursts | • Myocarditis, cardiomyopathy, inferior wall MI or ischemia, acute rheumatic fever, complication of valve replacement surgery<br>• Digitalis toxicity | • Temporary atrial pacemaker to override the rhythm<br>• Carotid sinus massage, elective cardioversion<br>• Propranolol, verapamil, or edrophonium<br>• Discontinuation of digoxin if appropriate |
| **Premature ventricular contraction (PVC)**<br>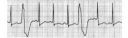<br>• Atrial rate regular<br>• Ventricular rate irregular<br>• QRS complex premature, usually followed by a complete compensatory pause<br>• QRS complex wide and distorted, usually > 0.14 second<br>• Premature QRS complexes occurring singly, in pairs, or in threes, alternating with normal beats; focus from one or more sites<br>• Ominous when clustered, multifocal, with R wave on T pattern | • Heart failure; old or acute MI, ischemia, or contusion; myocardial irritation by ventricular catheter or a pacemaker; hypercapnia; hypokalemia; hypocalcemia<br>• Drug toxicity (digitalis glycosides, aminophylline, tricyclic antidepressants, beta-adrenergics [isoproterenol or dopamine])<br>• Caffeine, tobacco, or alcohol use<br>• Psychological stress, anxiety, pain, exercise | • If warranted, lidocaine, procainamide, or bretylium I.V.<br>• Treatment of underlying cause<br>• Discontinuation of drug causing toxicity<br>• Potassium chloride I.V. if PVC induced by hypokalemia |

*(continued)*

## TYPES OF CARDIAC ARRHYTHMIAS *(continued)*

| ARRHYTHMIA AND FEATURES | CAUSES | TREATMENT |
|---|---|---|
| **Ventricular tachycardia**<br>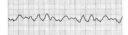<br>• Ventricular rate 140 to 220 beats/minute, regular or irregular<br>• QRS complexes wide, bizarre, and independent of P waves<br>• P waves not discernible<br>• May start and stop suddenly | • Myocardial ischemia, infarction, or aneurysm; coronary artery disease; rheumatic heart disease; mitral valve prolapse; heart failure; cardiomyopathy; ventricular catheters; hypokalemia; hypercalcemia; pulmonary embolism<br>• Digitalis, procainamide, epinephrine, or quinidine toxicity<br>• Anxiety | • With pulse: If hemodynamically stable with ventricular rate < 150 beats/minute, follow ACLS protocol for administration of lidocaine, procainamide, or bretylium; if drugs are ineffective, initiate synchronized cardioversion.<br>• If ventricular rate > 150 beats/minute, follow ACLS protocol for immediate synchronized cardioversion, followed by antiarrhythmic agents.<br>• Pulseless: Initiate cardiopulmonary resuscitation (CPR); follow ACLS protocol for defibrillation, ET intubation, and administration of epinephrine, lidocaine, bretylium, magnesium sulfate, or procainamide. |
| **Ventricular fibrillation**<br>• Ventricular rhythm rapid and chaotic<br>• QRS complexes wide and irregular; no visible P waves | • Myocardial ischemia or infarction, untreated ventricular tachycardia, R-on-T phenomenon, hypokalemia, hyperkalemia, hypercalcemia, alkalosis, electric shock, hypothermia<br>• Digitalis, epinephrine, or quinidine toxicity | • Pulseless: Initiate CPR; follow ACLS protocol for defibrillation, ET intubation, and administration of epinephrine, lidocaine, bretylium, magnesium sulfate, or procainamide. |

## TYPES OF CARDIAC ARRHYTHMIAS *(continued)*

| ARRHYTHMIA AND FEATURES | CAUSES | TREATMENT |
| --- | --- | --- |
| **Asystole**<br>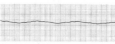<br>• No atrial or ventricular rate or rhythm<br>• No discernible P waves, QRS complexes, or T waves | • Myocardial ischemia or infarction, aortic valve disease, heart failure, hypoxia, hypokalemia, severe acidosis, electric shock, ventricular arrhythmia, AV block, pulmonary embolism, heart rupture, cardiac tamponade, hyperkalemia, electromechanical dissociation<br>• Cocaine overdose | • Continue CPR, follow ACLS protocol for ET intubation, administration of epinephrine and atropine and possibly, transcutaneous pacing |

> **CLINICAL TIP** Although, hazards may not present a problem, 24-hour Holter monitoring may be helpful in doubtful situations.
• Tell the patient to report light-headedness or syncope, and stress the importance of regular checkups.

**LIFE-THREATENING DISORDER**

# CARDIAC TAMPONADE

In cardiac tamponade, a rapid, unchecked rise in intrapericardial pressure impairs diastolic filling of the heart. The rise in pressure usually results from blood or fluid accumulation in the pericardial sac.

If fluid accumulates rapidly, this condition is commonly fatal and necessitates emergency lifesaving measures. Slow accumulation and rise in pressure, as in pericardial effusion associated with cancer, may not produce immediate symptoms because the fibrous wall of the pericardial sac can gradually stretch to accommodate 1 to 2 L of fluid.

## Causes

Increased intrapericardial pressure and cardiac tamponade may be idiopathic (Dressler's syndrome) or may result from the following conditions:
• effusion (in cancer, bacterial infections, tuberculosis and, rarely, acute rheumatic fever)
• hemorrhage from trauma (such as gunshot or stab wounds of the chest and perforation by a catheter during cardiac or central venous catheterization or after cardiac surgery)
• hemorrhage from nontraumatic causes (such as rupture of the heart or great vessels or anticoagulant therapy in a patient with pericarditis)
• acute myocardial infarction (MI)
• uremia.

## Signs and symptoms

Cardiac tamponade classically produces increased venous pressure with neck vein distention, reduced arterial blood pressure, muffled heart sounds on auscultation, and pulsus paradoxus (an abnormal inspiratory drop in systemic blood pressure > 15 mm Hg). These classic symptoms represent failure of physiologic compensatory mechanisms to override the effects of rapidly rising pericardial pressure, which limits diastolic filling of the ventricles and reduces stroke volume to a critically low level.

Generally, ventricular end-systolic volume may drop because of inadequate preload. The increasing pericardial pressure is transmitted equally across the heart cavities, producing a matching rise in intracardiac pressure, especially atrial and end-diastolic ventricular pressures.

Cardiac tamponade may also cause dyspnea, diaphoresis, pallor or cyanosis, anxiety, tachycardia, narrow pulse pressure, restlessness, and hepatomegaly, but the lung fields are clear. The patient typically sits upright and leans forward.

### Diagnosis

Classic clinical features may include the following:
• *Chest X-ray* shows slightly widened mediastinum and cardiomegaly.
• *Electrocardiography (ECG)* may reveal changes produced by acute pericarditis. This test rarely reveals tamponade but is useful to rule out other cardiac disorders.
• *Pulmonary artery catheterization* detects increased right atrial pressure, right ventricular diastolic pressure, and central venous pressure (CVP).
• *Echocardiography* records pericardial effusion with signs of right ventricular and atrial compression.

### Treatment

The goal of treatment is to relieve intrapericardial pressure and cardiac compression by removing accumulated blood or fluid. Pericardiocentesis (needle aspiration of the pericardial cavity) or surgical creation of an opening dra-

matically improves systemic arterial pressure and cardiac output with aspiration of as little as 25 ml of fluid. Such treatment necessitates continuous hemodynamic and ECG monitoring in the intensive care unit.

Trial volume loading with temporary I.V. normal saline solution with albumin and perhaps an inotropic drug, such as isoproterenol or dopamine, is necessary to maintain cardiac output in the hypotensive patient.

➤ CLINICAL TIP  Although inotropic drugs normally improve myocardial function, they may further compromise an ischemic myocardium after MI.

Depending on the cause of tamponade, additional treatment may include:
• *in traumatic injury:* blood transfusion or a thoracotomy to drain reaccumulating fluid or to repair bleeding sites
• *in heparin-induced tamponade:* the heparin antagonist protamine sulfate
• *in warfarin-induced tamponade:* vitamin K.

### Special considerations

If the patient needs pericardiocentesis:
• Explain the procedure to the patient.
• Keep a pericardial aspiration needle attached to a 50-ml syringe by a three-way stopcock, an ECG machine, and an emergency cart with a defibrillator at the bedside. Make sure the equipment is turned on and ready for immediate use.
• Position the patient at a 45- to 60-degree angle. Connect the precordial ECG lead to the hub of the aspiration needle with an alligator clamp and connecting wire. When the needle touches the myocardium during fluid aspiration, an ST-segment elevation or premature ventricular contraction is seen.
• Monitor blood pressure and CVP during and after pericardiocentesis.

• Infuse I.V. solutions to maintain blood pressure. Watch for a decrease in CVP and a concomitant rise in blood pressure, which indicate relief of cardiac compression.

• Watch for complications of pericardiocentesis, such as ventricular fibrillation, vasovagal response, or coronary artery or cardiac chamber puncture.

• Closely monitor ECG changes, blood pressure, pulse rate, level of consciousness, and urine output.

If the patient needs thoracotomy:

• Explain the procedure to him. Tell him what to expect postoperatively (chest tubes, drainage bottles, administration of oxygen). Teach him how to turn, deep-breathe, and cough.

• Give antibiotics, protamine sulfate, or vitamin K as needed.

• Postoperatively, monitor critical parameters, such as vital signs and arterial blood gas levels, and assess heart and breath sounds.

• Give pain medication as needed.

• Maintain the chest drainage system and be alert for complications, such as hemorrhage and arrhythmias.

---

**LIFE-THREATENING DISORDER**

# CARDIOGENIC SHOCK

---

Sometimes called pump failure, cardiogenic shock is a condition of diminished cardiac output that severely impairs tissue perfusion. It reflects severe left-sided heart failure and occurs as a serious complication in nearly 15% of all patients hospitalized with acute myocardial infarction (AMI).

Cardiogenic shock typically affects patients whose area of infarction exceeds 40% of muscle mass; in such patients, the fatality rate may exceed 85%.

Most patients with cardiogenic shock die within 24 hours of onset. The prognosis for those who survive is extremely poor.

## Causes
Cardiogenic shock can result from any condition that causes significant left ventricular dysfunction with reduced cardiac output, such as MI (most common), myocardial ischemia, papillary muscle dysfunction, and end-stage cardiomyopathy.

### Compensatory mechanisms
Regardless of the underlying cause, left ventricular dysfunction sets into motion a series of compensatory mechanisms that attempt to increase cardiac output and, in turn, maintain vital organ function.

As cardiac output falls in left ventricular dysfunction, aortic and carotid baroreceptors initiate sympathetic nervous responses. These responses, in turn, increase heart rate, left ventricular filling pressure, and peripheral resistance to flow to enhance venous return to the heart.

These compensatory responses initially stabilize the patient but later cause deterioration with rising oxygen demands of the already compromised myocardium. These events comprise a vicious circle of low cardiac output, sympathetic compensation, myocardial ischemia, and even lower cardiac output.

## Signs and symptoms
Cardiogenic shock produces signs of poor tissue perfusion: cold, pale, clammy skin; a drop in systolic blood pressure to 30 mm Hg below baseline or a sustained reading below 80 mm Hg not attributable to medication; tachycardia; rapid, shallow respirations; oliguria (< 20 ml of urine/hour); restlessness,

mental confusion and obtundation; narrowing pulse pressure; and cyanosis.

Although many of these clinical features also occur in heart failure and other shock syndromes, they're usually more profound in cardiogenic shock.

## Diagnosis

• *Auscultation* detects gallop rhythm, faint heart sounds and, possibly, if the shock results from rupture of the ventricular septum or papillary muscles, a holosystolic murmur.

• *Pulmonary artery pressure monitoring* reveals increased pulmonary artery pressure (PAP) and increased pulmonary artery wedge pressure (PAWP), reflecting a rise in left ventricular end-diastolic pressure (preload) and increased resistance to left ventricular emptying (afterload) resulting from ineffective pumping and increased peripheral vascular resistance. Thermodilution technique measures decreased cardiac output.

• *Invasive arterial pressure monitoring* shows hypotension from impaired ventricular ejection.

• *Arterial blood gas (ABG) levels* may show metabolic acidosis and hypoxia.

• *Electrocardiography* may reveal evidence of AMI, myocardial ischemia, or ventricular aneurysm.

• *Enzyme levels* show elevated creatine kinase (CK-MB, troponin T or troponin I), lactate dehydrogenase (LD), aspartate aminotransferase, and alanine aminotransferase, which point to MI or myocardial ischemia and suggest heart failure or shock. CK-MB and LD isoenzyme values may confirm AMI.

• *Echocardiography* (color flow Doppler) shows left ventricular function, valvular disease, aneurysmal dilation, and ventricular septal defects.

Additional tests determine other conditions that can lead to pump dysfunction and failure, such as cardiac arrhythmias, cardiac tamponade, papillary muscle infarct or rupture, ventricular septal rupture, pulmonary embolus, venous pooling (associated with venodilators and continuous intermittent positive-pressure breathing), and hypovolemia.

## Treatment

The aim of treatment is to enhance cardiovascular status by increasing cardiac output, improving myocardial perfusion, and decreasing cardiac workload. Treatment combines various cardiovascular drugs and mechanical-assist techniques.

### Cardiovascular drugs

Drug therapy may include I.V. dopamine, a vasopressor that increases cardiac output, blood pressure, and renal blood flow, and I.V. amrinone or dobutamine, inotropic agents that increase myocardial contractility. When a more potent vasoconstrictor is necessary, norepinephrine is used.

I.V. nitroprusside, a vasodilator, may be used with a vasopressor to further improve cardiac output by decreasing peripheral vascular resistance (afterload) and reducing left ventricular end-diastolic pressure (preload). However, the patient's blood pressure must be adequate to support nitroprusside therapy and must be monitored closely.

### Mechanical-assist techniques

The intra-aortic balloon pump (IABP) is a mechanical-assist device that attempts to improve coronary artery perfusion and decrease cardiac workload. The inflatable balloon pump is surgically inserted through the femoral artery into the descending thoracic aorta.

Once in place, the balloon inflates during diastole to increase coronary artery perfusion pressure and deflates before systole (before the aortic valve opens) to reduce resistance to ejection (afterload) and therefore lessen cardiac workload. Improved ventricular ejection, which significantly improves cardiac output, and a subsequent vasodilation in the peripheral vasculature lead to lower preload volume.

When drug therapy and IABP insertion fail, treatment may require an experimental device—the ventricular assist pump or the artificial heart.

**Special considerations**

● At the first sign of cardiogenic shock, check the patient's blood pressure and heart rate.

CLINICAL TIP  If the patient is hypotensive or is having difficulty breathing, ensure a patent I.V. line and a patent airway, and provide oxygen to promote tissue oxygenation.

● Monitor ABG levels to measure oxygenation and detect acidosis from poor tissue perfusion. Increase oxygen flow as indicated by blood gas measurements. Check complete blood count and electrolyte levels.

● After diagnosis, monitor cardiac rhythm continuously. Assess skin color and temperature and other vital signs often. Watch for a drop in systolic blood pressure to less than 80 mm Hg (usually compromising cardiac output further).

● Insert an indwelling urinary catheter to measure output. Watch for an output below 30 ml/hour.

● Using a pulmonary artery catheter, closely monitor PAP, PAWP and, if equipment is available, cardiac output. High PAWP indicates heart failure and requires an immediate response.

● When a patient is on the IABP, reposition him often and perform passive range-of-motion exercises to prevent skin breakdown. However, don't flex the patient's "ballooned" leg at the hip

because this may displace or fracture the catheter.

● Assess pedal pulses and skin temperature and color to make sure circulation to the leg is adequate. Check the dressing on the insertion site frequently for bleeding, and change it according to facility protocol.

● Check the insertion site for hematoma or signs of infection, and culture any drainage.

● After the patient has become hemodynamically stable, the frequency of balloon inflation is gradually reduced to wean him from the IABP. During weaning, carefully watch for monitor changes, chest pain, and other signs of recurring cardiac ischemia and shock.

● Provide psychological support. The patient and his family may be anxious about the intensive care unit, IABP, and other tubes and devices, so offer reassurance.

● To ease emotional stress, allow frequent rest periods, and provide for as much privacy as possible.

LIFE-THREATENING
DISORDER

# CARDIOMYOPATHY, DILATED

Resulting from extensively damaged myocardial muscle fibers, dilated cardiomyopathy interferes with myocardial metabolism and grossly dilates all four chambers of the heart. This gives the heart a globular appearance. In this disorder, hypertrophy may be present.

Dilated cardiomyopathy leads to intractable heart failure, arrhythmias, and emboli. The prognosis of dilated cardiomyopathy without clinical evidence of heart failure is variable, with some patients remaining stable, some gradually deteriorating, and others rapidly declining. Once heart failure is manifest, the natural history is similar to that of other causes of heart failure.

## Causes

The origin of most cardiomyopathies is unknown. Occasionally, dilated cardiomyopathy results from myocardial destruction by toxic, infectious, or metabolic agents, such as certain viruses, endocrine and electrolyte disorders, and nutritional deficiencies. Other causes include muscle disorders (myasthenia gravis, progressive muscular dystrophy, myotonic dystrophy), infiltrative disorders (hemochromatosis, amyloidosis), and sarcoidosis.

Cardiomyopathy may be a complication of alcoholism. The condition may improve with abstinence from alcohol but recurs when the patient resumes drinking.

How viruses induce cardiomyopathy is unclear, but investigators suspect a link between viral myocarditis and subsequent dilated cardiomyopathy, especially after infection with poliovirus, coxsackievirus B, influenza virus, or human immunodeficiency virus.

Metabolic cardiomyopathies are related to endocrine and electrolyte disorders and nutritional deficiencies. Thus, dilated cardiomyopathy may develop in patients with hyperthyroidism, pheochromocytoma, beriberi (thiamine deficiency), and kwashiorkor (protein deficiency). Cardiomyopathy may also result from rheumatic fever, especially among children with myocarditis.

Antepartal or postpartal cardiomyopathy may develop during the last trimester or within months after delivery. Its cause is unknown, but it occurs most frequently in multiparous women over age 30, particularly those with malnutrition or preeclampsia. In these pa-

tients, cardiomegaly and heart failure may reverse with treatment, allowing a subsequent normal pregnancy. If cardiomegaly persists despite treatment, the prognosis is extremely poor.

> **CLINICAL TIP** Dilated cardiomyopathy has a 50% mortality rate after 5 years; 50% of patients improve to normal within the first few months of delivery.

## Signs and symptoms

In dilated cardiomyopathy, the heart ejects blood less efficiently than usual. Consequently, a large volume of blood remains in the left ventricle after systole, causing signs of heart failure—both left-sided (shortness of breath, orthopnea, dyspnea on exertion, paroxysmal nocturnal dyspnea, fatigue, and an irritating dry cough at night) and right-sided (edema, liver engorgement, and jugular vein distention).

Physical examination reveals cardiomegaly, an $S_3$ gallop rhythm and, often, a murmur resulting from functional mitral insufficiency.

## Diagnosis

- *Echocardiography* confirms the presence of dilated cardiomyopathy.
- *Exercise thallium-201 scintigraphy* may suggest possible underlying coronary artery disease.
- *Electrocardiography (ECG)* and *angiography* rule out ischemic heart disease; ECG may also show biventricular hypertrophy, sinus tachycardia, atrial enlargement and, in 20% of patients, atrial fibrillation and bundle-branch heart block.
- *Chest X-ray* demonstrates cardiomegaly—usually affecting all heart chambers—and may demonstrate pulmonary congestion, pleural or pericardial effusion, or pulmonary hypertension.

## Treatment

Therapeutic goals include correcting the underlying causes and improving the heart's pumping ability with digoxin, diuretics, oxygen, and a sodium-restricted diet. Other options may involve bed rest and steroids. (See *Discharge instructions*.)

Vasodilators reduce preload and afterload, thereby decreasing congestion and increasing cardiac output. Acute heart failure requires vasodilation with nitroprusside or nitroglycerin I.V. Long-term treatment may include hydralazine, isosorbide dinitrate, angiotensin-converting enzyme inhibitors, and anticoagulants.

When these treatments fail, therapy may require heart transplantation for carefully selected patients. Cardiomyoplasty, which wraps the latissimus dorsi muscle around the ventricles, assists the ventricle to effectively pump blood. A cardiomyostimulator delivers bursts of electrical impulses during systole, to contract the muscle.

## Special considerations

• In the patient with acute failure, monitor for signs of progressive failure (bilateral crackles, increased neck vein distention) and compromised renal perfusion (oliguria, increased blood urea nitrogen and creatinine levels, electrolyte imbalances). Weigh the patient daily.
• If the patient is receiving vasodilators, frequently check his blood pressure and heart rate. If he becomes hypotensive, stop the infusion and place him in a supine position, with his legs elevated to increase venous return and to ensure cerebral blood flow.
• If the patient is receiving diuretics, monitor for signs of resolving congestion (decreased crackles and dyspnea) or too vigorous diuresis. Check his serum potassium level for hypokalemia, and check renal function for increased

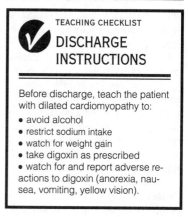

**TEACHING CHECKLIST**

## DISCHARGE INSTRUCTIONS

Before discharge, teach the patient with dilated cardiomyopathy to:
• avoid alcohol
• restrict sodium intake
• watch for weight gain
• take digoxin as prescribed
• watch for and report adverse reactions to digoxin (anorexia, nausea, vomiting, yellow vision).

creatinine level, especially if therapy includes digoxin.
• Before discharge, teach the patient about his illness and its treatment.

**> CLINICAL TIP**  Therapeutic restrictions and an uncertain prognosis usually cause profound anxiety and depression, so offer support and let the patient express his feelings. Be flexible with visiting hours.
• Encourage the patient's family members to learn cardiopulmonary resuscitation.

**LIFE-THREATENING DISORDER**

# CARDIOMYOPATHY, HYPERTROPHIC

A primary disease of the cardiac muscle, hypertrophic cardiomyopathy is characterized by disproportionate, asymmetric thickening of the interventricular septum in relation to the free wall of the left ventricle (3:1 ratio). In hypertrophic cardiomyopathy — previously known as idiopathic hypertrophic subaortic stenosis — cardiac output may be low, normal, or high, depending on whether stenosis is obstructive or nonobstructive.

The natural history of hypertrophic cardiomyopathy is highly variable. Some patients may remain asymptomatic for years. The dyspnea that results is primarily due to markedly impaired diastolic compliance rather than systolic dysfunction. Sudden death, especially during exercise, may be the initial event, as has occurred in athletes.

## Causes

Despite being designated as idiopathic, in almost all cases, hypertrophic cardiomyopathy may be inherited as a nonsex-linked autosomal dominant trait. Most patients have obstructive disease, resulting from effects of ventricular septal hypertrophy and the movement of the anterior mitral valve leaflet into the outflow tract during systole. Eventually, left ventricular dysfunction, from rigidity and decreased diastolic compliance, causes pump failure.

## Signs and symptoms

Clinical features of the disorder may not appear until it's well advanced, when atrial dilation and, possibly, atrial fibrillation abruptly reduce blood flow to the left ventricle. Reduced inflow and subsequent low output may produce angina pectoris, arrhythmias, dyspnea, orthopnea, syncope, heart failure, and death.

CLINICAL TIP  The most frequent symptoms of hypertrophic cardiomyopathy are dyspnea and chest pain. Syncope is also common, usually occurring after exertion.

Auscultation reveals a medium-pitched systolic ejection murmur along the left sternal border and at the apex. This murmur increases with Valsalva's maneuver and decreases with squatting. Palpation reveals a peripheral pulse with a characteristic double impulse (pulsus biferiens) and, with atrial fibrillation, an irregular pulse and loud $S_4$ sound.

## Diagnosis

Along with typical clinical findings, the diagnosis depends on the following test results:

● *Echocardiography* (most useful) shows increased thickness of the intraventricular septum and abnormal motion of the anterior mitral leaflet during systole, occluding left ventricular outflow in obstructive disease.

● *Cardiac catheterization* reveals elevated left ventricular end-diastolic pressure and, possibly, mitral insufficiency.

● *Electrocardiography* usually demonstrates left ventricular hypertrophy, T wave inversion, left anterior hemiblock, Q waves in precordial and inferior leads, ventricular arrhythmias and, possibly, atrial fibrillation.

## Treatment

The goals of treatment are to relax the ventricle and to relieve outflow tract obstruction. Propranolol, a beta-adrenergic blocking agent, slows heart rate and increases ventricular filling by relaxing the obstructing muscle, thereby reducing angina, syncope, dyspnea, and arrhythmias. However, propranolol may aggravate symptoms of cardiac decompensation. Atrial fibrillation necessitates cardioversion to treat the arrhythmia and, because of the high risk of systemic embolism, anticoagulant therapy. Calcium channel blockers (such as verapamil) may improve diastolic dysfunction until fibrillation subsides.

### Contraindicated drugs

Vasodilators, such as nitroglycerin, reduce venous return by permitting pooling of blood in the periphery, decreasing ventricular volume and chamber size, and may cause further obstruction.

They're contraindicated in patients with hypertrophic cardiomyopathy. Also contraindicated is digoxin as well as sympathetic stimulators, such as isoproterenol, which enhance cardiac contractility and myocardial demands for oxygen, intensifying the obstruction.

### Surgical alternatives

If drug therapy fails, surgery may be indicated. Ventricular myotomy (resection of the hypertrophied septum) alone or combined with mitral valve replacement may ease outflow tract obstruction and relieve symptoms. However, ventricular myotomy may cause complications, such as complete heart block and ventricular septal defect, and is experimental.

Dual-chamber pacing may prevent progression of hypertrophy and obstruction. Implantable defibrillators may be used in patients with malignant ventricular arrhythmias.

### Special considerations

● Because syncope or sudden death may follow well-tolerated exercise, warn such patients against any strenuous physical activity, such as running and weight lifting.

● Administer medication as needed. *Caution:* Avoid nitroglycerin, digoxin, and diuretics because they can worsen obstruction.

● Before dental work or surgery, administer prophylaxis for subacute bacterial endocarditis.

● Provide psychological support. If the patient is hospitalized for a long time, be flexible with visiting hours.

● Refer the patient for psychosocial counseling to help him and his family accept his restricted lifestyle and the poor prognosis.

● If the patient is a child, have his parents arrange for him to continue his studies in the facility.

● Because sudden cardiac arrest is possible, urge the patient's family to learn cardiopulmonary resuscitation.

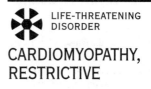

LIFE-THREATENING DISORDER

# CARDIOMYOPATHY, RESTRICTIVE

A disorder of the myocardial musculature, restrictive cardiomyopathy is characterized by restricted ventricular filling (the result of left ventricular hypertrophy) and endocardial fibrosis and thickening. If severe, it's irreversible.

### Causes

Primary restrictive cardiomyopathy is an extremely rare disorder of unknown cause. However, restrictive cardiomyopathy syndrome, a manifestation of amyloidosis, results from infiltration of amyloid into the intracellular spaces in the myocardium, endocardium, and subendocardium.

In both forms of restrictive cardiomyopathy, the myocardium becomes rigid, with poor distention during diastole, inhibiting complete ventricular filling. It fails to contract completely during systole, resulting in low cardiac output.

### Signs and symptoms

Because it lowers cardiac output and leads to heart failure, restrictive cardiomyopathy produces fatigue, dyspnea, orthopnea, chest pain, generalized edema, liver engorgement, peripheral cyanosis, pallor, $S_3$ or $S_4$ gallop rhythms, and systolic murmurs of mitral and tricuspid insufficiency.

**Diagnosis**

• *Chest X-ray* shows massive cardiomegaly in advanced stages of this disease, affecting all four chambers of the heart; pericardial effusion; and pulmonary congestion.

• *Echocardiography* rules out constrictive pericarditis as the cause of restricted filling by detecting increased left ventricular muscle mass and differences in end-diastolic pressures between the ventricles.

• *Electrocardiography* may show low-voltage complexes, hypertrophy, atrioventricular conduction defects, or arrhythmias.

• *Arterial pulsation* reveals blunt carotid upstroke with small volume.

• *Cardiac catheterization* demonstrates increased left ventricular end-diastolic pressure and rules out constrictive pericarditis as the cause of restricted filling.

**Treatment**

Although no therapy currently exists for restricted ventricular filling, digitalis glycosides, diuretics, and a restricted sodium diet ease the symptoms of heart failure.

Oral vasodilators — such as isosorbide dinitrate, prazosin, and hydralazine — may control intractable heart failure. Anticoagulant therapy may be necessary to prevent thrombophlebitis in the patient on prolonged bed rest.

**Special considerations**

• In the acute phase, monitor heart rate and rhythm, blood pressure, urine output, and pulmonary artery pressure readings to help guide treatment.

• Give psychological support. Provide appropriate diversionary activities for the patient restricted to prolonged bed rest.

• Because a poor prognosis may cause profound anxiety and depression, be especially supportive and understanding, and encourage the patient to express his fears.

> CLINICAL TIP  Refer the patient for psychosocial counseling, as necessary, for assistance in coping with his restricted lifestyle. Be flexible with visiting hours whenever possible.

• Before discharge, teach the patient to watch for and report signs of digoxin toxicity (anorexia, nausea, vomiting, yellow vision), to record and report weight gain and, if sodium restriction is ordered, to avoid canned foods, pickles, smoked meats, and use of table salt.

# CARDIOVASCULAR DISEASE IN PREGNANCY

Cardiovascular disease ranks fourth (after infection, toxemia, and hemorrhage) among the leading causes of maternal death. The physiologic stress of pregnancy and delivery is often more than a compromised heart can tolerate and often leads to maternal and fetal death.

Approximately 1% to 2% of pregnant women have cardiac disease, but the incidence is rising because medical treatment today allows more females with rheumatic heart disease and congenital defects to reach childbearing age.

With careful management, the prognosis for the pregnant patient with cardiovascular disease is good. Decompensation is the leading cause of maternal death. Infant mortality increases with decompensation because uterine congestion, insufficient oxygenation, and the elevated carbon dioxide content of the blood not only compromise the fetus but also frequently cause premature labor and delivery.

## Causes

Rheumatic heart disease is present in more than 80% of patients who develop cardiovascular complications. In the rest, these complications stem from congenital defects (10% to 15%) and coronary artery disease (2%).

The diseased heart is sometimes unable to meet the normal demands of pregnancy: a 25% increase in cardiac output, a 40% to 50% increase in plasma volume, increased oxygen requirements, retention of salt and water, weight gain, and alterations in hemodynamics during delivery. This physiologic stress often leads to the heart's failure to maintain adequate circulation (decompensation).

The degree of decompensation depends on the patient's age, the duration of cardiac disease, and the functional capacity of the heart at the outset of pregnancy.

## Signs and symptoms

Typical clinical features of cardiovascular disease in pregnancy include distended neck veins, diastolic murmurs, moist basilar pulmonary crackles, cardiac enlargement (discernible on percussion or as a cardiac shadow on a chest X-ray), and cardiac arrhythmias (other than sinus or paroxysmal atrial tachycardia). Other characteristic abnormalities may include cyanosis, pericardial friction rub, pulse delay, and pulsus alternans.

➤ CLINICAL TIP Mitral valve prolapse (MVP) probably occurs most commonly. Its accompanying symptoms include rapid heart rate, palpitations, and mitral insufficiency or murmur. Echocardiography confirms the condition.

Decompensation may develop suddenly or gradually, with persistent crackles at the lung bases. As it progresses, edema, increasing dyspnea on exertion,

palpitations, a smothering sensation, and hemoptysis may occur.

## Diagnosis

A diastolic murmur, cardiac enlargement, a systolic murmur of grade III/IV intensity, and severe arrhythmia suggest cardiovascular disease.

Determination of the extent and cause of the disease may necessitate electrocardiography, echocardiography (for valvular disorders such as rheumatic heart disease), or phonocardiography. X-rays show cardiac enlargement and pulmonary congestion. Cardiac catheterization should be postponed until after delivery, unless surgery is necessary.

## Treatment

Specific treatments vary before, during, and after delivery.

### Before delivery

The goal of antepartum management is to prevent complications and minimize the strain on the mother's heart, primarily through rest. This may require periodic hospitalization for patients with moderate cardiac dysfunction or with symptoms of decompensation, toxemia, or infection. Older women or those with previous decompensation may require hospitalization and bed rest throughout the pregnancy.

Drug therapy is often necessary and should always include the safest possible drug in the lowest possible dose to minimize harmful effects to the fetus. Diuretics and drugs that increase blood pressure, blood volume, or cardiac output should be used with extreme caution.

If an anticoagulant is needed, heparin is the drug of choice. Digitalis glycosides and common antiarrhythmics, such as quinidine and procainamide, are often required. The prophylactic use of antibiotics is reserved for patients who are susceptible to endocarditis.

A therapeutic abortion may be considered for patients with severe cardiac dysfunction, especially if decompensation occurs during the first trimester. Patients hospitalized with heart failure usually follow a regimen of digitalis glycosides, oxygen, rest, sedation, diuretics, and restricted intake of sodium and fluids. Patients whose symptoms of heart failure don't improve after treatment with bed rest and digitalis glycosides may require cardiac surgery, such as valvotomy and commissurotomy.

### During delivery

The patient in labor may require oxygen and an analgesic, such as meperidine or morphine, for relief of pain and apprehension without undue depression of the fetus or herself. Depending on which procedure promises to be less stressful for the patient's heart, delivery may be vaginal or by cesarean section.

### After delivery

Bed rest and medications already instituted should continue for at least 1 week after delivery because of a high incidence of decompensation, cardiovascular collapse, and maternal death during the early puerperal period. These complications may result from the sudden release of intra-abdominal pressure at delivery and the mobilization of extracellular fluid for excretion, which increase the strain on the heart, especially if excessive interstitial fluid has accumulated.

Breast-feeding is undesirable for patients with severely compromised cardiac dysfunction, because it increases fluid and metabolic demands on the heart.

### Special considerations

• During pregnancy, stress the importance of rest and weight control to decrease the strain on the heart. Suggest a diet of limited fluid and sodium intake to prevent vascular congestion.

• Encourage the patient to take supplementary folic acid and iron to prevent anemia.

• During labor, watch for signs of decompensation, such as dyspnea and palpitations. Monitor pulse rate, respirations, and blood pressure. Auscultate for crackles every 30 minutes during the first phase of labor and every 10 minutes during the active and transition phases. Check carefully for edema and cyanosis, and assess intake and output. Administer oxygen for respiratory difficulty.

• Use electronic fetal monitoring to watch for the earliest signs of fetal distress.

• Keep the patient in a semirecumbent position. Limit her efforts to bear down during labor, which significantly raise blood pressure and stress the heart.

• After delivery, provide reassurance, and encourage the patient to adhere to her program of treatment. Emphasize the need to rest during her hospital stay.

# CARPAL TUNNEL SYNDROME

The most common of the nerve entrapment syndromes, carpal tunnel syndrome results from compression of the median nerve at the wrist, within the carpal tunnel. This nerve passes through, along with blood vessels and flexor tendons, to the fingers and thumb. The compression neuropathy causes sensory and motor changes in the median distribution of the hand.

Carpal tunnel syndrome usually occurs in women between ages 30 and 60 and poses a serious occupational health problem. Assembly-line workers and packers, secretary-typists, and persons who repeatedly use poorly designed tools are most likely to develop this disorder. Any strenuous use of the hands — sustained grasping, twisting, or flexing — aggravates this condition.

**Causes**

The carpal tunnel is formed by the carpal bones and the transverse carpal ligament. (See *Viewing the carpal tunnel.*) Inflammation or fibrosis of the tendon sheaths that pass through the carpal tunnel often causes edema and compression of the median nerve.

Many conditions can cause the contents or structure of the carpal tunnel to swell and press the median nerve against the transverse carpal ligament.

Such conditions include rheumatoid arthritis, flexor tenosynovitis (often associated with rheumatic disease), nerve compression, pregnancy, renal failure, menopause, diabetes mellitus, acromegaly, edema following Colles' fracture, hypothyroidism, amyloidosis, myxedema, benign tumors, tuberculosis, and other granulomatous diseases. Another source of damage to the median nerve is dislocation or acute sprain of the wrist.

**Signs and symptoms**

The patient with carpal tunnel syndrome usually complains of weakness, pain, burning, numbness, or tingling in one or both hands. This paresthesia affects the thumb, forefinger, middle finger, and half of the fourth finger. The patient is unable to clench his hand into a fist. The nails may be atrophic; the skin, dry and shiny.

Because of vasodilatation and venous stasis, symptoms are often worse at night

## VIEWING THE CARPAL TUNNEL

The carpal tunnel is clearly visible in this palmar view and cross section of a right hand. Note the median nerve, flexor tendons of fingers, and blood vessels passing through the tunnel on their way from the forearm to the hand.

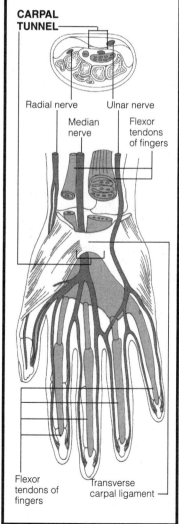

**CARPAL TUNNEL**

Radial nerve

Ulnar nerve

Median nerve

Flexor tendons of fingers

Flexor tendons of fingers

Transverse carpal ligament

and in the morning. The pain may spread to the forearm and, in severe cases, as far as the shoulder. The patient can usually relieve such pain by shaking his hands vigorously or dangling his arms at his side.

### Diagnosis

Physical examination reveals decreased sensation to light touch or pinpricks in the affected fingers. Thenar muscle atrophy occurs in about half of all cases of carpal tunnel syndrome.

The patient exhibits a positive Tinel's sign (tingling over the median nerve on light percussion). He also responds positively to Phalen's wrist-flexion test (holding the forearms vertically and allowing both hands to drop into complete flexion at the wrists for 1 minute reproduces symptoms of carpal tunnel syndrome).

A compression test supports this diagnosis: A blood pressure cuff inflated above systolic pressure on the forearm for 1 to 2 minutes provokes pain and paresthesia along the distribution of the median nerve.

Electromyography detects a median nerve motor conduction delay of more than 5 msec. Other laboratory tests may identify underlying disease.

### Treatment

Conservative treatment should be tried first, including resting the hands by splinting the wrist in neutral extension for 1 to 2 weeks. If a definite link has been established between the patient's occupation and the development of carpal tunnel syndrome, he may have to seek other work. Effective treatment may also require correction of an underlying disorder.

When conservative treatment fails, the only alternative is surgical decompression of the nerve by resecting the entire transverse carpal tunnel ligament or by using endoscopic surgical techniques. Neurolysis (freeing of the nerve fibers) may also be necessary.

### Special considerations

● Administer mild analgesics as needed.

● Encourage the patient to use his hands as much as possible. If his dominant hand has been impaired, you may have to help with eating and bathing.

● Teach the patient how to apply a splint. Tell him not to make it too tight. Show him how to remove the splint to perform gentle range-of-motion exercises, which should be done daily. Make sure the patient knows how to do these exercises before he's discharged.

● After surgery, monitor vital signs, and regularly check the color, sensation, and motion of the affected hand.

● Advise the patient who is about to be discharged to occasionally exercise his hands. If the arm is in a sling, tell him to remove the sling several times a day to do exercises for his elbow and shoulder.

● Suggest occupational counseling for the patient who has to change jobs because of carpal tunnel syndrome.

> CLINICAL TIP For those patients who must remain in their current occupation, suggest an ergonomic assessment of the work situation.

# CATARACT

A common cause of vision loss, a cataract is a gradually developing opacity of the lens or lens capsule of the eye. Cataracts commonly occur bilaterally, with each progressing independently. Exceptions are traumatic cataracts, which are usually unilateral, and congenital cataracts, which may remain stationary.

Cataracts are most prevalent in persons over age 70, as part of aging. Surgical intervention improves vision in 95% of affected people.

## Causes

Cataracts have various causes:

• *Senile cataracts* develop in elderly patients, probably because of degenerative changes in the chemical state of lens proteins.

• *Congenital cataracts* occur in neonates as genetic defects or as a sequela of maternal rubella during the first trimester.

• *Traumatic cataracts* develop after a foreign body injures the lens with sufficient force to allow aqueous or vitreous humor to enter the lens capsule.

• *Complicated cataracts* develop as secondary effects in a patient with uveitis, glaucoma, retinitis pigmentosa, or a detached retina or in the course of a systemic disease, such as diabetes, hypoparathyroidism, or atopic dermatitis. They can also result from exposure to ionizing radiation or infrared rays.

• *Toxic cataracts* result from prolonged exposure to drug or chemical toxicity with prednisone, ergot alkaloids, naphthalene, or phenothiazines; they also result from excessive exposure to sunlight.

## Signs and symptoms

Characteristically, a patient with a cataract experiences painless, gradual blurring and loss of vision. As the cataract progresses, the normally black pupil turns milky white (in extreme cases). Otherwise, lens opacity is revealed during a slit-lamp examination.

Some patients complain of blinding glare from headlights when they drive at night; others report an inability to recognize people or things at a distance.

Patients with central opacities report better vision in dim light than in bright light because the cataract is nuclear and, as the pupils dilate, patients can see around the lens opacity.

## Diagnosis

When shining a penlight on the pupil, observation of a white area behind the pupil suggests an advanced cataract. Ophthalmoscopy or a slit-lamp examination confirms the diagnosis by revealing a dark area in the normally homogeneous red reflex.

## Treatment

Cataracts require surgical extraction of the opaque lens and intraoperative correction of visual deficits with a lens implant (intraocular lens) for best visual results. This procedure is most frequently performed as same-day surgery.

### Surgical procedures

The following procedures are used to correct cataracts:

• *Extracapsular cataract extraction* removes the anterior lens capsule and cortex, leaving the posterior capsule intact. Typically, this is done using phacoemulsification equipment, which fragments the lens with ultrasound. The fragments are then removed by irrigation and aspiration. With this procedure, a posterior chamber intraocular lens (IOL) is implanted where the patient's own lens used to be. (A posterior chamber IOL is currently the most common type used in the United States.) This procedure can be used with patients of all ages.

Some patients who have an extracapsular cataract extraction develop a secondary membrane in the posterior lens capsule (which has been left intact) that causes decreased visual acuity. But this membrane can be removed by the Nd:YAG laser, which cuts an area out

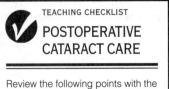

of the center of the membrane, thereby restoring vision. However, laser therapy alone can't be used to remove a cataract.

• *Intracapsular cataract extraction* removes the entire lens within the intact capsule by cryoextraction (the moist lens sticks to an extremely cold metal probe for easy and safe removal with gentle traction).

Possible complications of surgery include the loss of vitreous (during surgery), wound dehiscence from loosening of sutures and flat anterior chamber or iris prolapse into the wound, hyphema, pupillary block glaucoma, retinal detachment, and infection.

### Correction of visual deficits

A patient with an IOL implant may experience improved vision almost immediately if the retina is intact. The IOL implant usually only corrects for distance. To protect the eye postoperatively, some patients wear an eye patch for 6 to 8 hours, while others may have a collagen shield (similar to a contact lens) that dissolves in 24 hours. The patient will then need either corrective reading glasses or a corrective contact lens, which will be fitted 4 to 8 weeks after surgery.

If no IOL has been implanted, the patient may be given temporary aphakic cataract glasses; in about 4 to 8 weeks, he'll be refracted for his own glasses.

### Special considerations

• After surgery, the patient is discharged once he recovers from local anesthesia.

▸ CLINICAL TIP Remind the patient to return for a checkup the next day, and warn him to avoid activities that increase intraocular pressure, such as straining.

• Urge the patient to protect his eye from accidental injury by wearing his glasses during the day and an eye shield at night.

• Administer antibiotic ointment or drops to prevent infection and steroids to reduce inflammation, or combination steroid-antibiotic eyedrops.

• Watch for the development of complications, such as a sharp pain in the eye, indicative of increased intraocular pressure, or early signs of infection (such as hyphema or hypopion).

• Before discharge, review postoperative care points with the patient. (See *Postoperative cataract care*.)

✷ LIFE-THREATENING DISORDER

# CEREBRAL CONTUSION

A severe blow to the head can cause cerebral contusion, or bruising of the brain tissue. More serious than a concussion, contusion disrupts normal nerve functions in the bruised area and may cause loss of consciousness, hemorrhage, edema, and even death.

### Causes

Cerebral contusion results from acceleration-deceleration or coup-contrecoup injuries. Such injuries can occur directly beneath the site of impact when the brain rebounds against the skull from the force of a blow (a beating with a blunt instrument, for example), when the force of the blow drives the brain against the opposite side of the skull, or when the head is hurled forward and stopped abruptly (as in an automobile accident when a driver's head strikes the windshield).

When these injuries occur, the brain continues moving and slaps against the skull (acceleration), then rebounds (deceleration). These injuries can also cause the brain to strike against bony prominences inside the skull (especially the sphenoidal ridges), causing intracranial hemorrhage or hematoma that may result in tentorial herniation.

### Signs and symptoms

With cerebral contusion, the patient may have severe scalp wounds and labored respirations. He may lose consciousness for a few minutes or longer. If conscious, he may be drowsy, confused, disoriented, agitated, or even violent. He may display hemiparesis, decorticate or decerebrate posturing, and unequal pupillary response.

Eventually, he should return to a relatively alert state, perhaps with temporary aphasia, slight hemiparesis, or unilateral numbness. A lucid period followed by rapid deterioration suggests epidural hematoma.

### Diagnosis

An accurate history of the trauma and a neurologic examination are the principal diagnostic tools. A computed tomography scan shows ischemic tissue, hematomas, and fractures. Intracranial hemorrhage contraindicates lumbar puncture.

### Treatment and special considerations

- Establish a patent airway. The patient may also need endotracheal intubation or a tracheotomy.
- Perform a neurologic examination, focusing on level of consciousness (LOC), motor responses, and intracranial pressure.
- Start I.V. fluids with lactated Ringer's solution or normal saline solution. Mannitol I.V. may be given in consultation with a neurosurgeon to reduce cerebral edema. Dexamethasone I.V. or I.M. may be given for several days to control cerebral edema.
- Restrict total fluid intake to 1,200 to 1,500 ml/day to reduce volume and intracerebral swelling.
- If spinal injury is ruled out, elevate the head of the bed 30 degrees. Enforce bed rest.
- If the patient is intubated, hyperventilate him to a partial pressure of carbon dioxide level of 26 to 28 mm Hg.
- Type and crossmatch blood for a patient suspected of having intracerebral hemorrhage. A blood transfusion may be needed and possibly a craniotomy to control bleeding and to aspirate blood.
- Insert an indwelling urinary catheter. Monitor intake and output. With unconscious patients, insert a nasogastric tube to prevent aspiration.
- Observe carefully for leakage of cerebrospinal fluid (CSF) from the nostrils and ear canals.

CLINICAL TIP   If blood is in the ear canal and it's unclear whether CSF is mixed in, place a drop on a white sheet and check for a central spot of blood surrounded by a lighter ring (halo sign).
- If CSF leakage develops, raise the head of the bed 30 degrees. If you detect CSF leaking from the nose, place a gauze pad under the nostrils. Be sure to tell the patient not to blow his nose

but to wipe it instead. If CSF leaks from the ear, position the patient so that the ear drains naturally, and don't pack the ear or nose.

• Monitor respirations and other vital signs regularly (usually every 15 minutes). Abnormal respirations could indicate a breakdown in the respiratory center in the brain stem and a possible impending tentorial herniation— a neurologic emergency.

• Perform frequent checks of neurologic status. Assess for restlessness, LOC, and orientation.

• After the patient is stabilized, clean and dress any superficial scalp wounds. (If the skin has been broken, tetanus prophylaxis may be in order.) The wounds may need to be sutured.

# CEREBRAL PALSY

The most common cause of crippling in children, cerebral palsy comprises a group of neuromuscular disorders resulting from prenatal, perinatal, or postnatal central nervous system (CNS) damage. Although nonprogressive, these disorders may become more obvious as an affected infant grows older.

Three major types of cerebral palsy occur—*spastic, athetoid,* and *ataxic*— sometimes in mixed forms. Motor impairment may be minimal (sometimes apparent only during physical activities such as running) or severely disabling. Associated defects, such as seizures, speech disorders, and mental retardation, are common.

The prognosis varies. In mild impairment, proper treatment may make a near-normal life possible.

Cerebral palsy occurs in an estimated 1.5 to 5 per 1,000 live births every year. Incidence is highest in premature infants (anoxia plays the greatest role in contributing to cerebral palsy) and in those who are small for their gestational age. Cerebral palsy is slightly more common in males than in females and occurs often in whites.

## Causes

Conditions that result in cerebral anoxia, hemorrhage, or other CNS damage are probably responsible for cerebral palsy.

### Prenatal causes

Prenatal causes include maternal infection (especially rubella), radiation, anoxia, toxemia, maternal diabetes, abnormal placental attachment, malnutrition, and isoimmunization.

### Perinatal and birth difficulties

Examples of these causes include forceps delivery, breech presentation, placenta previa, abruptio placentae, depressed maternal vital signs from general or spinal anesthetic, and prolapsed cord with delay in the delivery of the head. Premature birth, prolonged or unusually rapid labor, and multiple birth (especially infants born last in a multiple birth) may also cause cerebral palsy.

### Infection or trauma during infancy

Cerebral palsy may follow kernicterus resulting from erythroblastosis fetalis, brain infection, head trauma, prolonged anoxia, brain tumor, cerebral circulatory anomalies causing blood vessel rupture, and systemic disease resulting in cerebral thrombosis or embolus.

## Signs and symptoms

Each type of cerebral palsy typically produces a distinctive set of clinical features, although some children display a mixed form of the disease.

### Spastic cerebral palsy

This form of the disease predominates, affecting about 70% of patients. Spastic cerebral palsy is characterized by hyperactive deep tendon reflexes, increased stretch reflexes, rapid alternating muscle contraction and relaxation, muscle weakness, underdevelopment of affected limbs, muscle contraction in response to manipulation, and a tendency toward contractures. Typically, a child with spastic cerebral palsy walks on his toes with a scissors gait, crossing one foot in front of the other.

### Athetoid cerebral palsy

Affecting about 20% of patients, this form causes involuntary movements — grimacing, wormlike writhing, dystonia, and sharp jerks — that impair voluntary movement. Usually, these involuntary movements affect the arms more severely than the legs; involuntary facial movements may make speech difficult. These athetoid movements become more severe during stress, decrease with relaxation, and disappear entirely during sleep.

### Ataxic cerebral palsy

Roughly 10% of patients have this form of the disease. Its characteristics include disturbed balance, incoordination (especially of the arms), hypoactive reflexes, nystagmus, muscle weakness, tremor, lack of leg movement during infancy, and a wide gait as the child begins to walk. Ataxia makes sudden or fine movements almost impossible.

### Mixed form

Some children with cerebral palsy display a combination of these signs and symptoms. In most, impaired motor function makes eating, especially swallowing, difficult and retards growth and development. Up to 40% of these children are mentally retarded, about 25%

have seizure disorders, and about 80% have impaired speech. Many also have dental abnormalities, vision and hearing defects, and reading disabilities.

## Diagnosis

An early diagnosis is essential for effective treatment and requires careful clinical observation during infancy and precise neurologic assessment. Suspect cerebral palsy whenever an infant:

• has difficulty sucking or keeping the nipple or food in his mouth

• seldom moves voluntarily or has arm or leg tremors with voluntary movement

• crosses his legs when lifted from behind rather than pulling them up or "bicycling" like a normal infant

• has legs that are hard to separate, making diaper changing difficult

• persistently uses only one hand or, as he gets older, uses his hands well but not his legs.

Infants at particular risk include those with low birth weight, low Apgar scores at 5 minutes, seizures, and metabolic disturbances. However, all infants should have a screening test for cerebral palsy as a regular part of their 6-month checkup.

## Treatment

Cerebral palsy can't be cured, but proper treatment can help affected children reach their full potential within the limits set by this disorder. Such treatment requires a comprehensive and cooperative effort involving doctors, nurses, teachers, psychologists, the child's family, and occupational, physical, and speech therapists. Home care is often possible. Treatment usually includes:

• braces or splints and special appliances, such as adapted eating utensils and a low toilet seat with arms, to help these children perform activities independently

• an artificial urinary sphincter for the incontinent child who can use the hand controls

• range-of-motion exercises to minimize contractures

• orthopedic surgery to correct contractures

• phenytoin, phenobarbital, or another anticonvulsant to control seizures

• sometimes muscle relaxants or neurosurgery to decrease spasticity.

Children with milder forms of cerebral palsy should attend regular school; severely afflicted children need special education classes.

**Special considerations**
• Speak slowly and distinctly to the child hospitalized for orthopedic surgery or treatment of complications. Encourage him to ask for things he wants. Listen patiently and don't rush him.

• Provide an adequate diet to meet the child's high-energy needs.

• During meals, maintain a quiet, unhurried atmosphere with as few distractions as possible. The child may need special utensils and a chair with a solid footrest. Teach him to place food far back in his mouth to facilitate swallowing.

• Encourage the child to chew food thoroughly, drink through a straw, and suck on lollipops to develop the muscle control needed to minimize drooling.

• Allow the child to wash and dress independently, assisting only as needed. The child may need clothing modifications.

• Give all care in an unhurried manner; otherwise, muscle spasticity may increase.

• Encourage the child and his family to participate in the patient's care so they can continue it at home.

• Care for associated hearing or visual disturbances as necessary.

• Give frequent mouth care and dental care as necessary.

• Reduce muscle spasms that increase postoperative pain by moving and turning the child carefully after surgery.

➤ CLINICAL TIP When spasticity occurs, gently rotate the limb inward toward the spasticity and then rotate it outward. Repeating this motion helps relax the spastic extremity. Pressure on the tendons located in the joint socket while rotating increases relaxation. Open a spastic hand by gently grabbing the lateral aspects and moving inward and out.

• When positioning, elongate the down side, making sure the down shoulder is slightly pulled out and that all limbs are well supported.

• Hand and foot orthotics may be helpful in maintaining mobility.

After orthopedic surgery:
• Give good cast care. Wash and dry the skin at the edge of the cast frequently, and rub it with alcohol to toughen the skin and prevent breakdown.

• Reposition the child often, check for foul odor, and ventilate under the cast with a cool-air blow-dryer. Use a flashlight to check for skin breakdown beneath the cast.

• Help the child relax, perhaps by giving a warm bath, before reapplying a bivalved cast.

Help parents deal with their child's handicap:
• Set realistic individual goals.

• Assist in planning crafts and other activities.

• Stress the child's need to develop peer relationships; warn the parents against being overprotective.

• Identify and deal with family stress. Parents may feel unreasonable guilt about their child's handicap and may need psychological counseling.

• Refer parents to supportive community organizations. For more information, tell parents to contact the United Cerebral Palsy Association, Inc., or their local cerebral palsy agency.

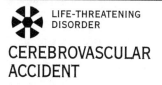

LIFE-THREATENING DISORDER

# CEREBROVASCULAR ACCIDENT

Commonly called a stroke, cerebrovascular accident (CVA) is a sudden impairment of cerebral circulation in one or more of the blood vessels supplying the brain. CVA interrupts or diminishes oxygen supply and often causes serious damage or necrosis in brain tissues.

The sooner circulation returns to normal after CVA, the better chances are for complete recovery. However, about half of those who survive a CVA remain permanently disabled and experience a recurrence within weeks, months, or years.

CVA is the third most common cause of death in the United States today and the most common cause of neurologic disability. It strikes 500,000 persons each year; half of them die as a result.

## Causes

Factors that increase the risk of CVA include history of transient ischemic attacks (TIAs), atherosclerosis, hypertension, electrocardiogram changes, arrhythmias, rheumatic heart disease, diabetes mellitus, gout, postural hypotension, cardiac or myocardial enlargement, high serum triglyceride levels, lack of exercise, use of oral contraceptives, cigarette smoking, and family history of CVA.

The major causes of CVA are thrombosis, embolism, and hemorrhage.

### *Thrombosis*

In middle-aged and elderly people, among whom there's a higher incidence of atherosclerosis, diabetes, and hypertension, thrombosis is the most common cause of CVA. Obstruction of a blood vessel causes the CVA. Typically, the main site of the obstruction is in extracerebral vessels, but sometimes it's intracerebral.

Thrombosis causes ischemia in brain tissue supplied by the affected vessel as well as congestion and edema. The latter may produce more clinical effects than thrombosis itself, but these symptoms subside with the edema.

Thrombosis may develop while the patient sleeps or shortly after he awakens; it can also occur during surgery or after a myocardial infarction. The risk increases with obesity, smoking, or the use of oral contraceptives. Cocaine-induced ischemic stroke is now being seen in younger patients.

### *Embolism*

The second most common cause of CVA, embolism is an occlusion of a blood vessel caused by a fragmented clot, a tumor, fat, bacteria, or air. It can occur at any age, especially among patients with a history of rheumatic heart disease, endocarditis, posttraumatic valvular disease, or myocardial fibrillation and other cardiac arrhythmias or after open-heart surgery.

The embolus usually develops rapidly — in 10 to 20 seconds — and without warning. When it reaches the cerebral vasculature, it cuts off circulation by lodging in a narrow portion of an artery, most often the middle cerebral artery, causing necrosis and edema.

If the embolus is septic and infection extends beyond the vessel wall, an abscess or encephalitis may develop. If the infection is within the vessel wall, an aneurysm may form, which could lead to cerebral hemorrhage.

### Hemorrhage

The third most common cause of CVA is hemorrhage. Like embolism, it may occur suddenly, at any age. Such hemorrhage results from chronic hypertension or aneurysms, which cause sudden rupture of a cerebral artery. The rupture diminishes blood supply to the area served by this artery. In addition, blood accumulates deep within the brain, further compressing neural tissue and causing even greater damage.

### CVA classification

CVAs are classified according to their course of progression. The least severe is the TIA, or "little stroke," which results from a temporary interruption of blood flow, most often in the carotid and vertebrobasilar arteries. A progressive stroke, or stroke-in-evolution (thrombus-in-evolution), begins with slight neurologic deficit and worsens in a day or two. In a completed stroke, neurologic deficits are maximal right at onset.

### Signs and symptoms

Clinical features of CVA vary with the artery affected (and, consequently, the portion of the brain it supplies), the severity of damage, and the extent of collateral circulation that develops to help the brain compensate for decreased blood supply.

If the CVA occurs in the left hemisphere, it produces symptoms on the right side; if in the right hemisphere, symptoms are on the left side. However, a CVA that causes cranial nerve damage produces signs of cranial nerve dysfunction on the same side as the hemorrhage.

Symptoms are usually classified according to the artery affected:

- *middle cerebral artery:* aphasia, dysphasia, visual field cuts, and hemiparesis on the affected side (more severe in the face and arm than in the leg)
- *carotid artery:* weakness, paralysis, numbness, sensory changes, and visual disturbances on the affected side; altered level of consciousness, bruits, headaches, aphasia, and ptosis
- *vertebrobasilar artery:* weakness on the affected side, numbness around the lips and mouth, visual field cuts, diplopia, poor coordination, dysphagia, slurred speech, dizziness, amnesia, and ataxia
- *anterior cerebral artery:* confusion, weakness and numbness (especially in the leg) on the affected side, incontinence, loss of coordination, impaired motor and sensory functions, and personality changes
- *posterior cerebral arteries:* visual field cuts, sensory impairment, dyslexia, coma, and cortical blindness. Usually, paralysis is absent.

Symptoms can also be classified as premonitory, generalized, and focal. Premonitory symptoms, such as drowsiness, dizziness, headache, and mental confusion, are rare. Generalized symptoms, such as headache, vomiting, mental impairment, seizures, coma, nuchal rigidity, fever, and disorientation, are typical. Focal symptoms, such as sensory and reflex changes, reflect the site of hemorrhage or infarction and may worsen.

### Diagnosis

Confirmation of CVA is based on observation of clinical features, a history of risk factors, and the results of diagnostic tests.

- *Computed tomography scan* shows evidence of hemorrhagic stroke immediately but may not show evidence of thrombotic infarction for 48 to 72 hours.

• *Magnetic resonance imaging* may help identify ischemic or infarcted areas and cerebral swelling.

• *Brain scan* shows ischemic areas but may not be positive for up to 2 weeks after the CVA.

• *Lumbar puncture* reveals bloody cerebrospinal fluid in hemorrhagic stroke.

• *Ophthalmoscopy* may show signs of hypertension and atherosclerotic changes in retinal arteries.

• A*ngiography* outlines blood vessels and pinpoints occlusion or rupture site.

• *EEG* helps to localize the damaged area.

Other baseline laboratory studies include urinalysis, coagulation studies, complete blood count, serum osmolality, and electrolyte, glucose, triglyceride, creatinine, and blood urea nitrogen levels.

**Treatment**

Treatment options vary, depending on the type of CVA the patient experiences. Early medical diagnosis of the type of CVA coupled with new drug treatments can greatly reduce the long-term disability secondary to ischemia.

Surgery performed to improve cerebral circulation for patients with thrombotic or embolic CVA includes an endarterectomy (the removal of atherosclerotic plaque from the inner arterial wall) or a microvascular bypass (the surgical anastomosis of an extracranial vessel to an intracranial vessel).

Medications useful in treating CVA include:

• alteplase (recombinant tissue plasminogen activator, tPA), effective in emergency treatment of embolic CVA (See *Restoring ischemic brain tissue with alteplase*.) Patients with embolic or thrombotic CVA who aren't candidates for alteplase (3 to 6 hours post-CVA) should receive aspirin or heparin.

---

## RESTORING ISCHEMIC BRAIN TISSUE WITH ALTEPLASE

The phrase "time is brain" highlights the need to treat cerebrovascular accident (CVA) as an emergency. Brain tissue can't tolerate loss of blood supply for long. During this critical time, a thrombolytic enzyme, alteplase (recombinant tissue plasminogen activator; tPA), can be effective in restoring blood flow.

When blood flow stops, an infarct occurs almost immediately. However, cells in the ischemic area (the "penumbra" surrounding the infarct) can maintain metabolism for 3 to 6 hours post-CVA, creating a "therapeutic window." Interventions such as alteplase indirectly interrupt the ischemic cascade (a complex process involving protein synthesis, deranged glucose utilization, loss of intercellular calcium, increased intracellular sodium, cellular swelling [edema], and death) to help maintain cell function and minimize the extent of permanent damage.

Research into the use of neuroprotective agents that directly protect the penumbra is under way. It appears that calcium channel blockers may also act to protect ischemic brain tissue.

---

• long-term use of aspirin or ticlopidine, used as antiplatelet agents to prevent recurrent CVA

• anticoagulants (heparin, warfarin), which may be required to treat crescendo TIAs not responsive to antiplatelet agents

• antihypertensives, antiarrhythmics, and antidiabetic agents, which may be used to treat risk factors associated with recurrent CVA.

## Special considerations
### Early supportive therapy
• Maintain homeostasis.
• Frequently assess neurologic status, using the NIH Stroke Scale to determine deficits. (See *Using the NIH Stroke Scale.*)
• Monitor for signs of hemorrhage following alteplase treatment.
• Monitor blood pressure frequently; give labetalol for severe hypertension.

CLINICAL TIP  Remember that because autoregulation is disrupted in CVA, it's necessary to maintain perfusion higher than the usual blood pressure.

• Avoid I.V. solutions containing glucose because they may worsen the CVA.
• Use acetaminophen and hypothermia blankets to control fever.
• Maintain a patent airway and oxygenation status; intubate and ventilate the patient as needed.
• Monitor blood glucose levels.
• Monitor electrocardiogram, and treat arrhythmias as early as possible.

### Ongoing care
• Watch for signs of pulmonary emboli, such as chest pains, shortness of breath, dusky color, tachycardia, fever, and changed sensorium. If the patient is unresponsive, monitor his blood gas levels often, looking for increased partial pressure of carbon dioxide or decreased partial pressure of oxygen.
• Watch for signs of other complications, such as infection, cerebral edema, hydrocephalus, seizures, aspiration pneumonia, deep vein thrombosis, pressure ulcers, urinary tract infections, contractures, and subluxation.
• Offer the urinal or bedpan every 2 hours. If the patient is incontinent, he may need an indwelling urinary catheter, but this should be avoided, if possible, because of the risk of infection.

• Ensure adequate nutrition. Check the patient's gag reflex before offering small oral feedings of semisolid foods. (A speech pathologist should assess the patient to determine his needs and specific feeding strategies for dysphagia.) Place the food tray within the patient's visual field. If oral feedings aren't possible, insert a nasogastric tube.
• To prevent aspiration pneumonia, position the patient in an upright, lateral position to allow secretions to drain. Turn the patient frequently.
• Position the patient, and align his extremities correctly to prevent external rotation. Use high-topped sneakers to prevent footdrop when the patient is sitting up and feet are on the floor.
• Provide range-of-motion exercises throughout the day; consult a physical therapist for additional positioning and transfer strategies and splinting devices.
• Consult physical therapy, occupational therapy, and speech therapy for short- and long-term rehabilitative care. A multidisciplinary approach is necessary to assist in minimizing long-term disability. Deficits can include motor weakness, coordination and balance problems, diminished corneal reflex, visual field deficits, dysarthria, dysphasia, impaired memory and concentration, and pain.
• Establish and maintain communication with the patient. If he's aphasic, set up a simple method of communicating basic needs. Remember to phrase your questions so he'll be able to answer using this system. Repeat yourself quietly and calmly (remember, he isn't deaf!) and use gestures if necessary to help him understand. Even the unresponsive patient can hear, so don't say anything in his presence you wouldn't want him to hear and remember.
• Provide psychological support. Set realistic short-term goals. Involve the pa-

# USING THE N.I.H. STROKE SCALE

| CATEGORY | DESCRIPTION | SCORE | BASELINE DATE/TIME | DATE/ TIME |
|---|---|---|---|---|
| 1a. Level of con-sciousness (LOC) | Alert<br>Drowsy<br>Stuporous<br>Coma | 0<br>1<br>2<br>3 | 7/15/99<br>1100<br>1 | |
| 1b. LOC questions (Month, age) | Answers both correctly<br>Answers one correctly<br>Incorrect | 0<br>1<br>2 | 0 | |
| 1c. LOC commands (Open/close eyes, make fist, let go) | Obeys both correctly<br>Obeys one correctly<br>Incorrect | 0<br>1<br>2 | 1 | |
| 2. Best gaze (Eyes open — patient follows ex-aminer's finger or face.) | Normal<br>Partial gaze palsy<br>Forced deviation | 0<br>1<br>2 | 0 | |
| 3. Visual (Introduce visual stimulus/threat to patient's visual field quadrants.) | No visual loss<br>Partial hemianopia<br>Complete hemianopia<br>Bilateral hemianopia | 0<br>1<br>2<br>3 | 1 | |
| 4. Facial palsy (Show teeth, raise eyebrows, and squeeze eyes shut.) | Normal<br>Minor<br>Partial<br>Complete | 0<br>1<br>2<br>3 | 2 | |
| 5a. Motor arm — left (Elevate extremity to 90 degrees and score drift/move-ment.) | No drift<br>Drift<br>Can't resist gravity<br>No effort against gravity<br>No movement<br>Amputation, joint fusion (explain) | 0<br>1<br>2<br>3<br>4<br>9 | 4 | |
| 5b. Motor arm — right (Elevate extremity to 90 degrees and score drift/move-ment.) | No drift<br>Drift<br>Can't resist gravity<br>No effort against gravity<br>No movement<br>Amputation, joint fusion (explain) | 0<br>1<br>2<br>3<br>4<br>9 | 0 | |

*(continued)*

## USING THE N.I.H. STROKE SCALE *(continued)*

| CATEGORY | DESCRIPTION | SCORE | BASELINE DATE/TIME | DATE/TIME |
|---|---|---|---|---|
| 6a. Motor leg — left (Elevate extremity to 30 degrees and score drift/movement.) | No drift<br>Drift<br>Can't resist gravity<br>No effort against gravity<br>No movement<br>Amputation, joint fusion (explain) | 0<br>1<br>2<br>3<br>4<br>9 | 4 | |
| 6b. Motor leg — right (Elevate extremity to 30 degrees and score drift/movement.) | No drift<br>Drift<br>Can't resist gravity<br>No effort against gravity<br>No movement<br>Amputation, joint fusion (explain) | 0<br>1<br>2<br>3<br>4<br>9 | 0 | |
| 7. Limb ataxia (Finger-nose, heel down shin) | Absent<br>Present in one limb<br>Present in two limbs | 0<br>1<br>2 | | |

| CATEGORY | DESCRIPTION | SCORE | BASELINE DATE/TIME | | DATE/TIME | |
|---|---|---|---|---|---|---|
| | | | R | L | R | L |
| 8. Sensory (Pinprick to face, arm, trunk, and leg — compare side to side.) | Normal<br>Partial loss<br>Severe loss | 0<br>1<br>2 | 0 | 2 | | |

| CATEGORY | DESCRIPTION | SCORE | BASELINE DATE/TIME | DATE/TIME |
|---|---|---|---|---|
| 9. Best language (Name items; describe a picture and read sentences.) | No aphasia<br>Mild to moderate aphasia<br>Severe aphasia<br>Mute | 0<br>1<br>2<br>3 | 1 | |
| 10. Dysarthria (Evaluate speech clarity by patient repeating listed words.) | Normal articulation<br>Mild to moderate dysarthria<br>Near to unintelligible or worse<br>Intubated or other physical barrier | 0<br>1<br>2<br>9 | 1 | |
| 11. Extinction and inattention (Use information from prior testing to identify neglect or double simultaneous stimuli testing.) | No neglect<br>Partial neglect<br>Complete neglect | 0<br>1<br>2 | 0 | |
| | | **Total** | 17 | |

Individual Administering Scale: *H. Hareson, RN*

tient's family in his care when possible, and explain his deficits and strengths.
• Establish rapport with the patient. Spend time with him, and provide a means of communication. Simplify your language, asking questions that can be answered yes or no whenever possible. Don't correct his speech or treat him like a child. Remember that building rapport may be difficult because of the mood changes that may result from brain damage or as a reaction to being dependent.
• If necessary, teach the patient to comb his hair, dress, and wash. With the aid of a physical therapist and an occupational therapist, obtain appliances, such as walking frames, hand bars by the toilet, and ramps as needed.
• If speech therapy is indicated, encourage the patient to begin as soon as possible and follow through with the speech pathologist's suggestions.
• To reinforce teaching, involve the patient's family in all aspects of rehabilitation. With their cooperation and support, devise realistic discharge goals, and let them help decide when the patient can return home.
• Before discharge, warn the patient or his family to report any premonitory signs of a CVA, such as severe headache, drowsiness, confusion, and dizziness. Emphasize the importance of regular follow-up visits.
• If aspirin has been prescribed to minimize the risk of embolic stroke, tell the patient to watch for possible GI bleeding related to ulcer formation. Make sure the patient realizes that he can't substitute acetaminophen for aspirin.

# CERVICAL CANCER

The third most common cancer of the female reproductive system, cervical cancer is classified as either preinvasive or invasive.

Preinvasive carcinoma ranges from minimal cervical dysplasia, in which the lower third of the epithelium contains abnormal cells, to carcinoma in situ, in which the full thickness of epithelium contains abnormally proliferating cells (also known as cervical intraepithelial neoplasia).

Preinvasive cancer is curable 75% to 90% of the time with early detection and proper treatment. If untreated (and depending on the form in which it appears), it may progress to invasive cervical cancer.

In invasive carcinoma, cancer cells penetrate the basement membrane and can spread directly to contiguous pelvic structures or disseminate to distant sites by lymphatic routes. Invasive carcinoma of the uterine cervix is responsible for 8,000 deaths annually in the United States alone.

In almost all cases (95%), the histologic type is squamous cell carcinoma, which varies from well-differentiated cells to highly anaplastic spindle cells. Only 5% are adenocarcinomas. Usually, invasive carcinoma occurs between ages 30 and 50; rarely, under age 20.

## Causes

Although the cause is unknown, several predisposing factors have been related to the development of cervical cancer: intercourse at a young age (under age 16), multiple sexual partners, multiple pregnancies, and herpesvirus II and other bacterial or viral venereal infections.

## STAGING CERVICAL CANCER

Cervical cancer treatment decisions depend on accurate staging. The International Federation of Gynecology and Obstetrics defines cervical cancer stages as follows.

**Stage 0** carcinoma in situ, intraepithelial carcinoma

**Stage I** cancer confined to the cervix (extension to the corpus should be disregarded)

**Stage IA** – clinical malignant lesions of the cervix (diagnosed only microscopically)

**Stage IA1** minimal microscopically evident stromal invasion

**Stage IA2** lesions detected microscopically, measuring 5 mm or less from the base of the epithelium, either surface or glandular, from which it originates; lesion width shouldn't exceed 7 mm

**Stage IB** lesions measuring more than 5 mm deep and 7 mm wide, whether seen clinically or not (preformed space involvement shouldn't alter the staging but should be recorded for future treatment decisions)

**Stage II** extension beyond the cervix but not to the pelvic wall; the cancer involves the vagina but hasn't spread to the lower third

**Stage IIA** no obvious parametrial involvement

**Stage IIB** obvious parametrial involvement

**Stage III** extension to the pelvic wall; on rectal examination, no cancer-free space exists between the tumor and the pelvic wall; the tumor involves the lower third of the vagina; this includes all cases with hydronephrosis or nonfunctioning kidney

**Stage IIIA** no extension to the pelvic wall

**Stage IIIB** extension to the pelvic wall and hydronephrosis or nonfunctioning kidney, or both

**Stage IV** extension beyond the true pelvis or involvement of the bladder or the rectal mucosa

**Stage IVA** spread to adjacent organs

**Stage IVB** spread to distant organs

### Signs and symptoms

Preinvasive cervical cancer produces no symptoms or other clinically apparent changes. Early invasive cervical cancer causes abnormal vaginal bleeding, persistent vaginal discharge, and postcoital pain and bleeding. In advanced stages, it causes pelvic pain, vaginal leakage of urine and stool from a fistula, anorexia, weight loss, and anemia.

### Diagnosis

A cytologic examination (Papanicolaou [Pap] test) can detect cervical cancer before clinical evidence appears. (Systems of Pap test classification may vary from facility to facility.) Abnormal cervical cytology routinely calls for colposcopy, which can detect the presence and extent of preclinical lesions requiring a biopsy and histologic examination.

Staining with Lugol's solution (strong iodine) or Schiller's solution (iodine, potassium iodide, and purified water) may identify areas for a biopsy when the smear shows abnormal cells but there's no obvious lesion. Although the tests are nonspecific, they do distinguish between normal and abnormal tissues: Normal tissues absorb the iodine and turn brown; abnormal tissues are devoid of glycogen and won't change color.

Additional studies, such as lymphangiography, cystography, and scans, can detect metastasis. (See *Staging cervical cancer.*)

## Treatment

Appropriate treatment depends on accurate clinical staging. Preinvasive lesions may be treated with a total excisional biopsy, cryosurgery, laser destruction, conization (and frequent Pap test follow-up) or, rarely, hysterectomy. Therapy for invasive squamous cell carcinoma may include radical hysterectomy and radiation therapy (internal, external, or both).

## Special considerations

• If the patient needs a biopsy, drape and prepare her as for a routine Pap test and pelvic examination. Have a container of formaldehyde ready to preserve the specimen during transfer to the pathology laboratory. Explain to the patient that she may feel pressure, minor abdominal cramps, or a pinch from the punch forceps. Reassure her that pain will be minimal because the cervix has few nerve endings.

• If the patient is having cryosurgery, drape and prepare her as for a routine Pap test and pelvic examination. Explain that the procedure takes approximately 15 minutes, during which time refrigerant will be used to freeze the cervix. Warn the patient that she may experience abdominal cramps, headache, and sweating, but reassure her that she'll feel little, if any, pain.

• If the patient needs laser therapy, drape and prepare her as for a routine Pap test and pelvic examination. Explain that the procedure takes approximately 30 minutes and may cause abdominal cramps.

• Tell the patient to expect a discharge or spotting for about 1 week after an excisional biopsy, cryosurgery, or laser therapy, and advise her not to douche, use tampons, or engage in sexual intercourse during this time. Tell her to watch for and report signs of infection. Stress the need for a follow-up Pap test and a pelvic examination within 3 to 4 months after these procedures and periodically thereafter.

• Tell the patient what to expect postoperatively if she'll have a hysterectomy.

• After surgery, monitor vital signs every 4 hours.

• Watch for signs and symptoms of complications, such as bleeding, abdominal distention, severe pain, and breathing difficulties.

• Administer analgesics, prophylactic antibiotics, and subcutaneous heparin as needed.

• Encourage the patient to perform deep-breathing and coughing exercises.

• Find out whether the patient is to have internal or external radiation therapy, or both. Usually, internal radiation therapy is the first procedure.

• Explain the internal radiation procedure, and answer the patient's questions. Internal radiation requires a 2- to 3-day facility stay, bowel preparation, a povidone-iodine vaginal douche, a clear liquid diet, and nothing by mouth the night before the implantation; it also requires an indwelling urinary catheter.

• Tell the patient that the internal radiation procedure is performed in the operating room under general anesthesia and that an applicator containing radioactive material (such as radium or cesium) will be implanted.

➤ CLINICAL TIP Remember that safety precautions — time, distance, and shielding — begin as soon as the radioactive source is in place. Inform the patient that she'll require a private room.

• Encourage the patient to lie flat and limit movement while the implant is in

## IDENTIFYING A CHALAZION

A chalazion is a nontender granulomatous inflammation of a meibomian gland on the eyelid.

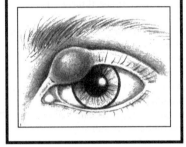

place. If she prefers, elevate the head of the bed slightly.

• Check vital signs every 4 hours; watch for skin reaction, vaginal bleeding, abdominal discomfort, or evidence of dehydration. Make sure the patient can reach everything she needs without stretching or straining.

• Assist the patient in range-of-motion *arm* exercises (leg exercises and other body movements could dislodge the implant). If needed, administer a tranquilizer to help the patient relax and remain still. Organize the time you spend with the patient to minimize your exposure to radiation.

• Inform visitors of safety precautions, and hang a sign listing these precautions on the patient's door.

• Explain that external radiation therapy, when necessary, continues for 4 to 6 weeks on an outpatient basis.

• Teach the patient to watch for and report uncomfortable effects. Because radiation therapy may increase susceptibility to infection by lowering the white blood cell count, warn the patient to avoid persons with obvious infections during therapy.

• Teach the patient to use a vaginal dilator to prevent vaginal stenosis and to facilitate vaginal examinations and sexual intercourse.

• Reassure the patient that this disease and its treatment shouldn't radically alter her lifestyle or prohibit sexual intimacy.

# CHALAZION

A common eye disorder, a chalazion is a granulomatous inflammation of a meibomian gland in the upper or lower eyelid. This disorder is characterized by localized swelling and usually develops slowly over several weeks.

A chalazion may become large enough to press on the eyeball, producing astigmatism; a large chalazion seldom subsides spontaneously and may have to be incised and curetted surgically. A person susceptible to developing chalazia may have more than one because the upper and lower eyelids contain many meibomian glands. If a chalazion becomes persistent and chronic, a neoplasm should be ruled out by biopsy.

### Causes
Obstruction of the meibomian (sebaceous) gland duct causes a chalazion.

### Signs and symptoms
A chalazion occurs as a painless, hard lump that usually *points toward* the conjunctival side of the eyelid. Eversion of the lid reveals a red elevated area on the conjunctival surface. (See *Identifying a chalazion.*)

### Diagnosis
Visual examination and palpation of the eyelid reveal a small bump or nodule.

Persistently recurrent chalazia, especially in an adult, necessitate a biopsy to rule out meibomian cancer.

### Treatment
Initial treatment consists of the application of warm compresses to open the lumen of the gland and, occasionally, instillation of sulfonamide eyedrops. If such therapy fails or if the chalazion presses on the eyeball or causes a severe cosmetic problem, steroid injection or incision and curettage under local anesthetic may be necessary.

After such surgery, a pressure eye patch applied for 8 to 24 hours controls bleeding and swelling. After removal of the patch, treatment again consists of warm compresses applied for 10 to 15 minutes, two to four times daily, and antimicrobial eyedrops or ointment to prevent secondary infection.

### Special considerations
• Instruct the patient how to properly apply *warm* compresses: Tell him to take special care to avoid burning the skin, to always use a clean cloth, and to discard used compresses.

**CLINICAL TIP** Tell the patient to start applying warm compresses at the first sign of lid irritation to increase the blood supply and keep the lumen open.

LIFE-THREATENING
DISORDER

# CHEST INJURIES, BLUNT

One-fourth of all trauma deaths in the United States result from chest injuries. Many are blunt chest injuries, which include myocardial contusion and rib and sternal fractures that may be simple, multiple, displaced, or jagged. Such fractures may cause potentially fatal complications, such as hemothorax, pneumothorax, hemorrhagic shock, and diaphragmatic rupture.

### Causes
Most blunt chest injuries result from motor vehicle accidents. Other common causes include sports and blast injuries.

### Signs and symptoms
Rib fractures produce tenderness, slight edema over the fracture site, and pain that worsens with deep breathing and movement; this painful breathing causes the patient to display shallow, splinted respirations that may lead to hypoventilation.

Sternal fractures, which are usually transverse and located in the middle or upper sternum, produce persistent chest pain, even at rest. If a fractured rib tears the pleura and punctures a lung, it causes pneumothorax, which usually produces severe dyspnea, cyanosis, agitation, extreme pain and, when air escapes into chest tissue, subcutaneous emphysema.

### Effects of multiple fractures
Multiple rib fractures may cause flail chest: a portion of the chest wall "caves" in, which causes a loss of chest wall integrity and prevents adequate lung inflation. Bruised skin, extreme pain caused by rib fracture and disfigurement, paradoxical chest movements, and rapid, shallow respirations are all signs of flail chest, as are tachycardia, hypotension, respiratory acidosis, and cyanosis.

Flail chest can also cause tension pneumothorax, a condition in which air enters the chest but can't be ejected during exhalation; life-threatening thoracic pressure buildup causes lung collapse and subsequent mediastinal shift. The cardinal symptoms of tension pneumothorax include tracheal deviation (away from the affected side), cyanosis, severe dyspnea, absent breath sounds (on the affected side), agitation, distended jugular veins, and shock.

### Hemothorax

When a rib lacerates lung tissue or an intercostal artery, hemothorax occurs, causing blood to collect in the pleural cavity, thereby compressing the lung and limiting respiratory capacity. It can also result from rupture of large or small pulmonary vessels.

Massive hemothorax is the most common cause of shock following chest trauma. Although slight bleeding occurs even with mild pneumothorax, such bleeding resolves very quickly, usually without changing the patient's condition.

Rib fractures may also cause pulmonary contusion (resulting in hemoptysis, hypoxia, dyspnea and, possibly, obstruction), large myocardial tears (which can be rapidly fatal), and small myocardial tears (which can cause pericardial effusion).

### Further complications

Myocardial contusions produce electrocardiogram (ECG) abnormalities. Laceration or rupture of the aorta is nearly always immediately fatal. Rarely, aortic laceration may develop 24 hours after blunt injury, so patient observation is critical.

Diaphragmatic rupture (usually on the left side) causes severe respiratory distress. Unless treated early, abdominal viscera may herniate through the rupture into the thorax, compromising both circulation and the lungs' vital capacity.

Other complications of blunt chest trauma may include cardiac tamponade, pulmonary artery tears, ventricular rupture, and bronchial, tracheal, or esophageal tears or rupture.

### Diagnosis

A history of trauma with dyspnea, chest pain, and other typical clinical features suggest a blunt chest injury. A physical examination and diagnostic tests determine the extent of injury.

- *Percussion* reveals dullness in hemothorax and tympany in tension pneumothorax.
- *Auscultation* may reveal a change in position of the loudest heart sound in tension pneumothorax.
- *Chest X-rays* may confirm rib and sternal fractures, pneumothorax, flail chest, pulmonary contusions, lacerated or ruptured aorta, tension pneumothorax, diaphragmatic rupture, lung compression, or atelectasis with hemothorax.
- *ECG* may show abnormalities with cardiac damage, including multiple premature ventricular contractions, unexplained tachycardias, atrial fibrillation, bundle-branch heart block (usually right), and ST-segment changes.
- *Serial aspartate aminotransferase, alanine aminotransferase, lactate dehydrogenase, creatine kinase (CK),* and *CK-MB* levels are elevated.
- *Retrograde aortography* and *transesophageal echocardiography* reveal aortic laceration or rupture.
- *Contrast studies* and *liver* and *spleen scans* detect diaphragmatic rupture.
- *Echocardiography, computed tomography scans,* and *cardiac* and *lung scans* show the injury's extent.

### Treatment and special considerations

> CLINICAL TIP  Blunt chest injuries call for immediate physical assessment, control of bleeding, maintenance of a patent airway, adequate ventilation, and fluid and electrolyte balance.

- Check all pulses and level of consciousness. Also evaluate color and temperature of skin, depth of respiration, use of accessory muscles, and length of inhalation compared with exhalation.

• Check pulse oximetry values for adequate oxygenation.

• Observe tracheal position. Look for distended jugular veins and paradoxical chest motion. Listen to heart and breath sounds carefully; palpate for subcutaneous emphysema (crepitation) or a lack of structural integrity of the ribs.

• Obtain a history of the injury. Unless severe dyspnea is present, ask the patient to locate the pain, and ask if he's having trouble breathing. Obtain an order for laboratory studies (arterial blood gas analysis, cardiac enzyme studies, complete blood count, and typing and crossmatching).

• For simple rib fractures, give mild analgesics, encourage bed rest, and apply heat. To prevent atelectasis, instruct the patient on incentive spirometry and deep breathing, coughing, and splinting. Don't strap or tape the chest.

• For more severe fractures, intercostal nerve blocks may be needed. Obtain X-rays before and after the nerve blocks to rule out pneumothorax.

• Intubate the patient with excessive bleeding or hemopneumothorax. Chest tubes may be inserted to treat hemothorax and to assess the need for thoracotomy. To prevent atelectasis, turn the patient frequently and encourage coughing and deep breathing.

• For pneumothorax, the patient may need a chest tube placed anterior to the midaxillary line at the fifth intercostal space to aspirate as much air as possible from the pleural cavity and to reexpand the lungs. Insert chest tubes attached to water-seal drainage and suction.

• For flail chest, place the patient in semi-Fowler's position. Reexpansion of the lung is the first definitive care measure. Administer oxygen at a high flow rate under positive pressure. Suction the patient frequently, as completely as pos-

sible. Observe carefully for signs of tension pneumothorax.

• Start I.V. therapy for the patient with flail chest. Use lactated Ringer's solution or normal saline solution. Beware of both excessive and insufficient fluid resuscitation.

• For hemothorax, treat shock with I.V. infusions of lactated Ringer's solution or normal saline solution. Administer packed red blood cells for blood losses greater than 1,500 ml or circulating blood volume losses exceeding 30%. Autotransfusion is an option. Administer oxygen.

• The patient with hemothorax will also need insertion of chest tubes in the fifth or sixth intercostal space anterior to the midaxillary line to remove blood. Monitor and document vital signs and blood loss. Watch for falling blood pressure, rising pulse rate, and hemorrhage—all require thoracotomy to stop bleeding.

• For pulmonary contusions, give limited amounts of colloids (for example, salt-poor albumin, whole blood, or plasma) to replace volume and maintain oncotic pressure. Give analgesics, diuretics and, if necessary, corticosteroids as needed. Monitor blood gas values to ensure adequate ventilation; provide oxygen therapy, mechanical ventilation, and chest tube care.

• For suspected cardiac damage, close intensive care or telemetry may detect arrhythmias and prevent cardiogenic shock. Impose bed rest in semi-Fowler's position (unless the patient requires shock position); as needed, administer oxygen, analgesics, and supportive drugs to control heart failure or supraventricular arrhythmia.

• Watch for cardiac tamponade, which calls for pericardiocentesis. Essentially, provide the same care as for a patient who has suffered myocardial infarction.

• For myocardial rupture, septal perforations, and other cardiac lacerations, immediate surgical repair is mandatory; less severe ventricular wounds require use of a digital or balloon catheter; atrial wounds require a clamp or balloon catheter.

• For the few patients with aortic rupture or laceration who reach the facility alive, immediate surgery is mandatory, using synthetic grafts or anastomosis to repair the damage. Give large volumes of I.V. fluids (lactated Ringer's or normal saline solution) and whole blood, along with oxygen at very high flow rates; then transport the patient promptly to the operating room.

• For tension pneumothorax, the patient will need insertion of a spinal or 14G to 16G needle into the second intercostal space at the midclavicular line, to release pressure in the chest. Following this, insert a chest tube to normalize pressure and reexpand the lung. Administer oxygen under positive pressure, along with I.V. fluids.

• For a diaphragmatic rupture, insert a nasogastric tube to temporarily decompress the stomach, and prepare the patient for surgical repair.

---

LIFE-THREATENING
DISORDER

# CHEST WOUNDS, PENETRATING

---

Depending on their size, penetrating chest wounds may cause varying degrees of damage to bones, soft tissue, blood vessels, and nerves. Mortality and morbidity from a chest wound depend on the size and severity of the wound.

Gunshot wounds are usually more serious than stab wounds, both because they cause more severe lacerations and cause rapid blood loss and because ricochet often damages large areas and multiple organs. With prompt, aggressive treatment, up to 90% of patients with penetrating chest wounds recover.

## Causes
Stab wounds from a knife or ice pick are the most common penetrating chest wounds; gunshot wounds are a close second. Wartime explosions or firearms fired at close range are the usual source of large, gaping wounds.

## Signs and symptoms
In addition to the obvious chest injuries, penetrating chest wounds can also cause the following:

• A sucking sound occurs as the diaphragm contracts and air enters the chest cavity through the opening in the chest wall.

• Level of consciousness varies, depending on the extent of the injury. If the patient is awake and alert, he may be in severe pain, which will make him splint his respirations, thereby reducing his vital capacity.

• Tachycardia stems from anxiety and blood loss.

• A weak, thready pulse results from massive blood loss and hypovolemic shock.

Penetrating chest wounds may also cause lung lacerations (bleeding and substantial air leakage through the chest tube), arterial lacerations (loss of more than 100 ml of blood/hour through the chest tube), and exsanguination. Pneumothorax (air in the pleural space causing loss of negative intrathoracic pressure and lung collapse), tension pneumothorax (intrapleural air accumulation causing potentially fatal mediastinal shift), and hemothorax can also result.

Other effects may include arrhythmias, cardiac tamponade, mediastinitis, subcutaneous emphysema, esophageal perforation, and bronchopleural fistula. Tracheobronchial, abdominal, or diaphragmatic injuries can also occur.

### Diagnosis

An obvious chest wound and a sucking sound during breathing confirm the diagnosis. Consider any lower thoracic chest injury a thoracicoabdominal injury until proven otherwise.

Further tests to provide baseline data include:

• *pulse oximetry* and *arterial blood gas analysis* to assess respiratory status

• *chest X-rays* before and after chest tube placement to evaluate the injury and tube placement (In an emergency, don't wait for chest X-ray results before inserting the chest tube.)

• *complete blood count,* including hemoglobin (Hb) level, hematocrit, and differential (Low Hb level and hematocrit reflect severe blood loss; in early blood loss, these values may be normal.)

• *palpation* and *auscultation* of the chest and abdomen to evaluate damage to adjacent organs and structures.

### Treatment and special considerations

> CLINICAL TIP Penetrating chest wounds require immediate support of respiration and circulation, prompt surgical repair, and measures to prevent complications.

• Immediately assess airway, breathing, and circulation. Establish a patent airway, support ventilation, and monitor pulses frequently.

• Place an occlusive dressing over the sucking wound. Monitor for signs of tension pneumothorax (tracheal shift, respiratory distress, tachycardia, tachypnea, diminished or absent breath sounds on the affected side); if tension pneumothorax develops, temporarily remove the occlusive dressing to create a simple pneumothorax.

• Control blood loss (also remember to look *under* the patient to estimate loss),

type and crossmatch blood, and replace blood and fluids as necessary.

• Prepare the patient for chest X-rays and placement of chest tubes (using water-seal drainage) to reestablish intrathoracic pressure and to drain blood in hemothorax. A second X-ray will evaluate the position of tubes and their functions.

• Emergency surgery may be needed to repair the damage caused by the wound.

• Throughout treatment, monitor central venous pressure and blood pressure to detect hypovolemia, and assess vital signs. Provide analgesics as appropriate. Tetanus and antibiotic prophylaxis may be necessary.

• Reassure the patient, especially if he's been the victim of a violent crime. Report the incident to the police in accordance with local laws. Help contact the patient's family, and offer them reassurance as well.

# CHLAMYDIAL INFECTIONS

Urethritis in men and urethritis and cervicitis in women compose a group of infections that are linked to one organism: *Chlamydia trachomatis*. These chlamydial infections are the most common sexually transmitted diseases in the United States, affecting an estimated 4 million Americans each year.

Trachoma inclusion conjunctivitis, a chlamydial infection that occurs rarely in the United States, is a leading cause of blindness in Third World countries. Lymphogranuloma venereum, a rare disease in the United States, is also caused by *C. trachomatis.*

Untreated, chlamydial infections can lead to such complications as acute epididymitis, salpingitis, pelvic inflammatory disease and, eventually, sterility. Some studies show that chlamydial infections in pregnant women are associated with spontaneous abortion and premature delivery. Other studies haven't confirmed these findings.

## Causes

Transmission of *C. trachomatis* primarily follows vaginal or rectal intercourse or oral-genital contact with an infected person. Because signs and symptoms of chlamydial infections commonly appear late in the course of the disease, sexual transmission of the organism typically occurs unknowingly.

Children born of mothers who have chlamydial infections may contract associated conjunctivitis, otitis media, and pneumonia during passage through the birth canal.

## Signs and symptoms

Both men and women with chlamydial infections may be asymptomatic or may show signs of infection on physical examination. Individual signs and symptoms vary with the specific type of chlamydial infection and are determined by the organism's route of transmission to susceptible tissue.

### Clinical features in women

Women who have *cervicitis* may develop cervical erosion, mucopurulent discharge, pelvic pain, and dyspareunia.

Women who have *endometritis* or *salpingitis* may experience signs of pelvic inflammatory disease, such as pain and tenderness of the abdomen, cervix, uterus, and lymph nodes; chills; fever; breakthrough bleeding; bleeding after intercourse; and vaginal discharge. They may also have dysuria.

Women with *urethral syndrome* may experience dysuria, pyuria, and urinary frequency.

### Clinical features in men

Men who have *urethritis* may experience dysuria, erythema, tenderness of the urethral meatus, urinary frequency, pruritus, and urethral discharge. In urethritis, such discharge may be copious and purulent or scant and clear or mucoid.

Men with *epididymitis* may experience painful scrotal swelling and urethral discharge.

Men who have *prostatitis* may have lower back pain, urinary frequency, dysuria, nocturia, and painful ejaculation.

In *proctitis*, patients may have diarrhea, tenesmus, pruritus, bloody or mucopurulent discharge, and diffuse or discrete ulceration in the rectosigmoid colon.

## Diagnosis

The following laboratory tests provide a definitive diagnosis of chlamydial infections:

- A *swab* from the site of infection (urethra, cervix, or rectum) establishes a diagnosis of urethritis, cervicitis, salpingitis, endometritis, or proctitis.
- A *culture* of aspirated material establishes a diagnosis of epididymitis.
- Antigen detection methods, including the *enzyme-linked immunosorbent assay* and the *direct fluorescent antibody test,* are the diagnostic tests of choice for identifying chlamydial infection, although tissue cell cultures are more sensitive and specific.
- Newer *nucleic acid probes* using polymerase chain reactions are also commercially available.

## Treatment

The recommended first-line treatment for adults and adolescents who have chlamydial infections is drug therapy with oral doxycycline for 7 days or oral azithromycin in a single dose. (See *What your patient needs to know about chlamydia.*)

For pregnant women with chlamydial infections, azithromycin (Zithromax), in a single 1-g dose for both the male and female partners, is the treatment of choice.

**Special considerations**

• Practice standard precautions when caring for a patient with a chlamydial infection.

• Teach the patient what he needs to know before discharge.

• Make sure that the patient fully understands the dosage requirements of any prescribed medications for this infection.

• If required in your state, report all cases of chlamydial infection to the appropriate local public health authorities, who will then conduct follow-up notification of the patient's sexual contacts.

• Suggest that the patient and his sexual partners receive testing for human immunodeficiency virus.

• Check newborns of infected mothers for signs of chlamydial infection. Obtain appropriate specimens for diagnostic testing.

---

# CHLORIDE IMBALANCE

Hypochloremia and hyperchloremia are, respectively, conditions of deficient or excessive serum levels of the anion chloride. A predominantly extracellular anion, chloride accounts for two-thirds of all serum anions.

Secreted by stomach mucosa as hydrochloric acid, chloride provides an acid medium conducive to digestion and activation of enzymes. It also participates in maintaining acid-base and body water balances, influences the osmolality or tonicity of extracellular fluid, plays a role in the exchange of oxygen

---

TEACHING CHECKLIST

### WHAT YOUR PATIENT NEEDS TO KNOW ABOUT CHLAMYDIA

Before discharge, teach the patient with a chlamydial infection to:

• complete drug therapy, even after symptoms subside
• follow meticulous personal hygiene
• avoid touching the discharge
• wash and dry his hands before touching his eyes
• abstain from intercourse until he and his partner are cured
• inform sexual contacts of his infection
• return for follow-up testing.

---

and carbon dioxide in red blood cells, and helps activate salivary amylase (which, in turn, activates the digestive process).

**Causes**

Chloride imbalance can stem from a variety of causes.

*Hypochloremia*

Insufficient serum chloride levels can result from decreased chloride intake or absorption, as in low dietary sodium intake, sodium deficiency, potassium deficiency, and metabolic alkalosis. Administration of dextrose I.V. without electrolytes can also interfere with chloride absorption.

Excessive chloride loss can result from prolonged diarrhea or diaphoresis as well as loss of hydrochloric acid in gastric secretions from vomiting, gastric suctioning, or gastric surgery.

## Hyperchloremia

Excessive chloride intake or absorption — as in hyperingestion of ammonium chloride or ureterointestinal anastomosis — can lead to hyperchloremia by allowing reabsorption of chloride by the bowel.

> **CLINICAL TIP**   Excessive chloride intake can also result from administering normal saline solution I.V. or by another route, such as orally or by nasogastric tube, saline enema, or irrigation.

Hemoconcentration from dehydration can also lead to excess serum chloride.

Compensatory mechanisms for other metabolic abnormalities can also cause hyperchloremia. These abnormalities include metabolic acidosis, brain stem injury causing neurogenic hyperventilation, and hyperparathyroidism.

### Signs and symptoms

Because of the natural affinity of sodium and chloride ions, chloride imbalance frequently produces signs and symptoms also associated with sodium imbalance.

## Hypochloremia

Indications of hypochloremia include the characteristic muscle weakness and twitching that mark hyponatremia because renal chloride loss always accompanies sodium loss, and sodium reabsorption isn't possible without chloride.

However, if chloride depletion results from metabolic alkalosis secondary to loss of gastric secretions, chloride is lost independently from sodium. Typical symptoms include muscle hypertonicity, tetany, and shallow, depressed breathing.

## Hyperchloremia

The clinical effects of hyperchloremia typically match those of hypernatremia and resulting extracellular fluid volume excess: agitation, tachycardia, hypertension, pitting edema, and dyspnea. Hyperchloremia associated with metabolic acidosis results from excretion of base bicarbonate by the kidneys and induces deep, rapid breathing; weakness; diminished cognitive ability; and, ultimately, coma.

### Diagnosis

A serum chloride level that's less than 98 mEq/L confirms hypochloremia; supportive values with metabolic alkalosis include a serum pH greater than 7.45 and a serum carbon dioxide level greater than 32 mEq/L.

A serum chloride level greater than 108 mEq/L confirms hyperchloremia; with metabolic acidosis, serum pH is less than 7.35 and the serum carbon dioxide level is less than 22 mEq/L.

### Treatment

In either kind of chloride imbalance, treatment must correct the underlying disorder.

## Hypochloremia

In addtion to correcting the condition that caused excessive chloride loss, treatment can include giving oral replacement such as salty broth. When oral therapy isn't possible or when emergency measures are necessary, treatment may include normal saline solution I.V. (if hypovolemia is present); chloride-containing drugs, such as ammonium chloride, to increase serum chloride levels; and potassium chloride for metabolic alkalosis.

## Hyperchloremia

For severe hyperchloremic acidosis, treatment consists of sodium bicarbonate I.V. to raise serum bicarbonate level and permit renal excretion of the chloride anion because bicarbonate and chloride compete for combination with sodium. For mild hyperchloremia, lactated Ringer's solution is administered; it converts to bicarbonate in the liver, thus increasing base bicarbonate to correct acidosis.

### Special considerations
Watch for signs of hyperchloremia or hypochloremia. Be alert for respiratory difficulty.

For hypochloremia:
• Monitor serum chloride levels frequently, particularly during I.V. therapy.
• To prevent hypochloremia, monitor laboratory results (serum electrolyte levels and arterial blood gas values) and fluid intake and output of patients who are vulnerable to chloride imbalance, particularly those recovering from gastric surgery.
• Watch for excessive or continuous loss of gastric secretions as well as prolonged infusion of dextrose in water without saline.

For hyperchloremia:
• Check serum electrolyte levels every 3 to 6 hours. If the patient is receiving high doses of sodium bicarbonate, watch for signs of overcorrection (metabolic alkalosis, respiratory depression) or lingering signs of hyperchloremia, which indicate inadequate treatment.
• To prevent hyperchloremia, check laboratory results for elevated serum chloride levels or potassium imbalance if the patient is receiving I.V. solutions containing sodium chloride, and monitor fluid intake and output.

> **CLINICAL TIP** Watch for signs of metabolic acidosis. When administering I.V. fluids containing lactated Ringer's solution, monitor flow rate according to the patient's age, physical

condition, and bicarbonate level, watching for irregularities.

# CHOLELITHIASIS, CHOLECYSTITIS, AND RELATED DISORDERS

Diseases of the gallbladder and biliary tract are common and often painful conditions that usually require surgery and may be life-threatening. They're often associated with deposition of calculi and inflammation. (See *Common sites of calculus formation,* page 198.)

In most cases, gallbladder and bile duct diseases occur during middle age. Between ages 20 and 50, they're six times more common in women, but the incidence in men and women becomes equal after age 50. After that, incidence rises with each succeeding decade.

### Causes
The origin and frequency of gallbladder and biliary tract disease vary with the particular disorder.

#### Cholelithiasis
The presence of stones or calculi (gallstones) in the gallbladder results from changes in bile components. Gallstones are made of cholesterol, calcium bilirubinate, or a mixture of cholesterol and bilirubin pigment. They arise during periods of sluggishness in the gallbladder resulting from pregnancy, oral contraceptives, diabetes mellitus, Crohn's disease, cirrhosis of the liver, pancreatitis, obesity, and rapid weight loss.

Cholelithiasis is the fifth leading cause of hospitalization among adults and accounts for 90% of all gallbladder and duct diseases. The prognosis is usually good with treatment unless infection occurs, in which case the progno-

## COMMON SITES OF CALCULUS FORMATION

Stones vary in size; small stones may travel.

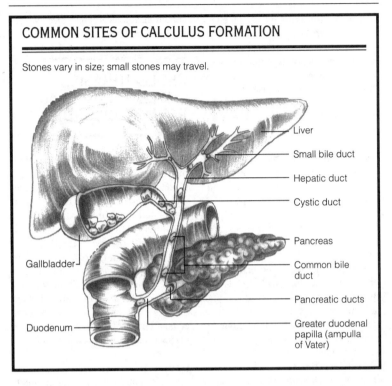

Liver

Small bile duct

Hepatic duct

Cystic duct

Pancreas

Common bile duct

Pancreatic ducts

Greater duodenal papilla (ampulla of Vater)

Gallbladder

Duodenum

---

sis depends on the infection's severity and response to antibiotics.

### Choledocholithiasis
One out of every 10 patients with gallstones develops choledocholithiasis, or gallstones in the common bile duct (sometimes called common duct stones). This occurs when stones passed out of the gallbladder lodge in the hepatic and common bile ducts and obstruct the flow of bile into the duodenum. The prognosis is good unless infection occurs.

### Cholangitis
An infection of the bile duct, cholangitis is often associated with choledocholithiasis and may follow percutaneous transhepatic cholangiography. Predisposing factors may include bacterial or metabolic alteration of bile acids. Widespread inflammation may cause fibrosis and stenosis of the common bile duct. The prognosis for this rare condition is poor without stenting or surgery.

### Cholecystitis
Cholecystitis, an acute or chronic inflammation of the gallbladder, is usually associated with a gallstone impacted in the cystic duct; the inflammation develops behind the obstruction. Cholecystitis accounts for 10% to 25% of all patients requiring gallbladder surgery.

The acute form is most common during middle age; the chronic form, among elderly people. The prognosis is good with treatment.

### Cholesterolosis

Cholesterol polyps or cholesterol crystal deposits in the gallbladder's submucosa may result from bile secretions containing high concentrations of cholesterol and insufficient bile salts. The polyps may be localized or may speckle the entire gallbladder. Cholesterolosis, the most common pseudotumor, isn't related to widespread inflammation of the mucosa or lining of the gallbladder. The prognosis is good with surgery.

### Biliary cirrhosis

Primary biliary cirrhosis is a chronic, progressive disease of the liver characterized by autoimmune destruction of the intrahepatic bile ducts and cholestasis. This condition usually leads to obstructive jaundice and pruritus and involves the portal and periportal spaces of the liver. It strikes women ages 40 to 60 nine times more often than men. The prognosis is poor without liver transplantation.

### Gallstone ileus

Gallstone ileus results from a gallstone lodging in the terminal ileum. It is more common in elderly people. The prognosis is good with surgery.

### Postcholecystectomy syndrome

Postcholecystectomy syndrome commonly results from retained or recurrent common bile duct stones, spasm of the sphincter of Oddi, functional bowel disorder, technical errors, or mistaken diagnoses. It occurs in 1% to 5% of all patients whose gallbladders have been surgically removed and may produce right upper quadrant abdominal pain, biliary colic, fatty food intolerance, dyspepsia, and indigestion. The prognosis is good with selected radiologic procedures, endoscopic procedures, or surgery.

### Complications

Each of these disorders produces its own set of complications. Cholelithiasis may lead to any of the disorders associated with gallstone formation: cholangitis, cholecystitis, choledocholithiasis, and gallstone ileus.

Cholecystitis can progress to gallbladder complications, such as empyema, hydrops or mucocele, or gangrene. Gangrene may lead to perforation, resulting in peritonitis, fistula formation, pancreatitis, limy bile, and porcelain gallbladder. Other complications include chronic cholecystitis and cholangitis.

Choledocholithiasis may lead to cholangitis, obstructive jaundice, pancreatitis, and secondary biliary cirrhosis. Cholangitis, especially in the suppurative form, may progress to septic shock and death. Gallstone ileus may cause bowel obstruction, which can lead to intestinal perforation, peritonitis, septicemia, secondary infection, and septic shock.

### Signs and symptoms

Although gallbladder disease may produce no symptoms, acute cholelithiasis, acute cholecystitis, choledocholithiasis, and cholesterolosis produce the symptoms of a classic gallbladder attack. Such attacks often follow meals rich in fats or may occur at night, suddenly awakening the patient.

A gallbladder attack may begin with acute abdominal pain in the right upper quadrant that may radiate to the back, between the shoulders, or to the front of the chest. The pain may be so severe that the patient seeks emergency department care.

Other features may include recurring fat intolerance, biliary colic, belching, flatulence, indigestion, diaphoresis, nausea, vomiting, chills, low-grade fever, jaundice (if a stone obstructs the common bile duct), and clay-colored stool (with choledocholithiasis).

Clinical features of cholangitis include a rise in eosinophils, jaundice, abdominal pain, high fever, and chills. Biliary cirrhosis may produce jaundice, related itching, weakness, fatigue, slight weight loss, and abdominal pain. Gallstone ileus produces signs of small-bowel obstruction — nausea, vomiting, abdominal distention, and absent bowel sounds if the bowel is completely obstructed. Its most telling sign is intermittent recurrence of colicky pain over several days.

## Diagnosis

Ultrasonography and X-rays detect gallstones. Specific procedures include the following:

• *Ultrasonography* reflects stones in the gallbladder with 96% accuracy.

• *Percutaneous transhepatic cholangiography* allows imaging under fluoroscopic control that distinguishes between gallbladder or bile duct disease and cancer of the pancreatic head in patients with jaundice.

• *Endoscopic retrograde cholangiopancreatography* visualizes the biliary tree after insertion of an endoscope down the esophagus into the duodenum, cannulation of the common bile and pancreatic ducts, and injection of contrast medium.

• *HIDA scan* of the gallbladder detects obstruction of the cystic duct.

• *Computed tomography scan,* although not used routinely, helps distinguish between obstructive and nonobstructive jaundice.

• *Plain abdominal X-rays* identify calcified but not cholesterol stones with 15% accuracy.

• *Oral cholecystography* shows stones in the gallbladder and biliary duct obstruction.

Elevated icteric index and elevated total bilirubin, urine bilirubin, and alkaline phosphatase levels support the diagnosis. White blood cell count is slightly elevated during a cholecystitis attack.

Differential diagnosis is essential because gallbladder disease can mimic other diseases (myocardial infarction, angina, pancreatitis, pancreatic head cancer, pneumonia, peptic ulcer, hiatal hernia, esophagitis, and gastritis). Serum amylase distinguishes gallbladder disease from pancreatitis. With suspected heart disease, serial enzyme tests and an electrocardiogram should precede gallbladder and upper GI diagnostic tests.

## Treatment

Surgery, usually elective, is the treatment of choice for gallbladder and bile duct diseases. Surgery may include open or laparoscopic cholecystectomy, cholecystectomy with operative cholangiography and, possibly, exploration of the common bile duct.

Other treatment includes a low-fat diet to prevent attacks and vitamin K for itching, jaundice, and bleeding tendencies resulting from vitamin K deficiency. Treatment during an acute attack may include insertion of a nasogastric tube and an I.V. line and, possibly, antibiotic administration.

A nonsurgical treatment for choledocholithiasis involves insertion of a flexible catheter, formed around a biliary tube (T tube), through a sinus tract into the common bile duct. Guided by fluoroscopy, the catheter is directed toward the stone. A Dormia basket is threaded through the catheter, opened, twirled to entrap the stone, closed, and withdrawn.

## Special considerations

• Before surgery, teach the patient to deep-breathe, cough, expectorate, and perform leg exercises that are necessary after surgery. Also teach splinting, repositioning, and ambulation techniques. Explain the perioperative procedures to help ease the patient's anxiety and ensure his cooperation.

• After surgery, monitor vital signs for indications of bleeding, infection, or atelectasis.

• If a T tube is surgically placed, maintain tube patency and secure placement. Measure and record bile drainage daily (200 to 300 ml is normal).

• Teach patients who will be discharged with a T tube how to perform dressing changes and routine skin care.

• Patients who have had a laparoscopic cholecystectomy may be discharged the same day or within 48 hours after surgery. These patients should have minimal pain, be able to tolerate a regular diet within 24 hours after surgery, and be able to return to normal activity within a few days to a week.

• Encourage the patient to perform deep-breathing and leg exercises every hour. The patient should ambulate after surgery. Provide antiembolism stockings to support leg muscles and promote venous blood flow to prevent stasis and clot formation.

• Assess the location, duration, and character of any pain. Administer analgesics to relieve pain.

• At discharge (usually the day of surgery or 1 to 2 days afterward), teach the patient that food restrictions are unnecessary unless he has an intolerance to a specific food or some underlying condition (such as diabetes, atherosclerosis, or obesity) that requires such restriction.

# CHRONIC CONSTIPATION

Also known as lazy colon, colonic stasis, colonic inertia, and atonic constipation, chronic constipation may lead to fecal impaction if left untreated. It's common in elderly and disabled people because of their inactivity and is often relieved with diet and exercise.

## Causes

Chronic constipation usually results from some deficiency in the three elements necessary for normal bowel activity: dietary bulk, fluid intake, and exercise. Other possible causes can include habitual disregard of the impulse to defecate, emotional conflicts, chronic use of laxatives, or prolonged dependence on enemas, which dull rectal sensitivity to the presence of stool.

➤ CLINICAL TIP   Anal fissure can also precipitate chronic constipation.

## Signs and symptoms

The patient often strains to produce dry, hard stool accompanied by mild abdominal discomfort. Straining can aggravate other rectal conditions, such as hemorrhoids.

## Diagnosis

A patient history of dry, hard stool and infrequent bowel movements suggests chronic constipation due to inactive colon. A digital rectal examination reveals stool in the lower portion of the rectum and a palpable colon. Analoscopy may show an unusually small colon lumen, prominent veins, and an abnormal amount of mucus. Diagnostic tests to rule out other causes include an upper GI series, barium enema, and examination of stool for occult blood from neoplasms.

---

TEACHING CHECKLIST

# ✓ BREAKING THE CONSTIPATION HABIT

Patient education can often help break the constipation habit. Advise the patient to follow these guidelines:

• Drink at least 8 to 10 glasses (at least 2 qt [2 L]) of liquid every day because fluids help keep the intestinal contents in a semisolid state for easier passage. This is particularly important for an older patient.

• Stimulate the bowel with a drink of hot coffee, warm lemonade, iced liquids — plain or with lemon — or prune juice before breakfast or in the evening.

• Add fiber to the diet with foods such as whole-grain cereals (rolled oats, bran, shredded wheat, brown rice, whole-wheat bread, oatmeal) to contribute to bulk and induce peristalsis. However, too much bran can create an irritable bowel, so check labels on foods for fiber content (low fiber — 0.3 to 1 g; moderate fiber — 1.1 to 2 g; high fiber — 2.1 to 4.2 g).

• Increase the fiber content of the diet slowly to prevent flatulence, which is sometimes a transient effect of a high-fiber diet. Include fresh fruits, with skins, in the diet for additional bulk. Also include raw and coarse vegetables (broccoli, brussels sprouts, cabbage, cauliflower, cucumbers, lettuce, and turnips).

• Consume fat-containing foods, such as bacon, butter, cream, and oil, in moderation; they will help to soften intestinal contents but sometimes cause diarrhea.

• Avoid highly refined foods, such as white rice, cream of wheat, farina, white bread, pie or cake, macaroni, spaghetti, noodles, candy, cookies, and ice cream.

• Rest at least 6 hours every night.

• Incorporate moderate exercise, such as walking, into the daily routine.

• Avoid overuse of laxatives, and maintain a regular time for bowel movements (usually after breakfast).

---

Colonoscopy may be performed for inactive colon. Manometric studies may also be done to exclude Hirschsprung's disease as well as evaluation of internal and external sphincters.

**Treatment**

Effective treatment varies with the patient's age and condition. A diet higher in fiber, sufficient exercise, and increased fluid intake often relieve constipation. (See *Breaking the constipation habit.*)

Treatment for severe constipation may include bulk-forming laxatives, such as psyllium, or well-lubricated glycerin suppositories; for fecal impaction, manual removal of stool is necessary. Administration of an oil-retention enema usually precedes stool removal; an enema is also necessary afterward. For lasting relief of constipation, the patient with inactive colon must modify his bowel habits.

**Special considerations**

• Autosuggestion, relaxation, and use of a small footstool to promote thigh flexion while sitting on the toilet may be helpful. To help the patient relax, suggest that he bring pleasant reading material.

• Tell the patient to respond promptly to the urge to defecate. If he worries about constipation, assure him that a 2- to 3-day interval between bowel movements can be normal.

• Advise the patient to take bulk-forming laxatives, such as psyllium, with at least 8 oz (240 ml) of liquid. Juices, soft drinks, or other pleasant-tasting liquids help mask this drug's grittiness.

If the patient with inactive colon is hospitalized:

• Assist the elderly patient with inactive colon to a bedside commode for a bowel movement because using a bedpan causes additional strain.

▶ CLINICAL TIP  If the patient has a history of arteriosclerosis, heart failure, or hypertension, constipation and straining may induce a "bathroom coronary" or a cerebrovascular accident.

• If the patient must use a bedpan, have him sit in Fowler's position or on the pan at the side of his bed to facilitate elimination.

• Occasional digital rectal stimulation or abdominal massage near the sigmoid area may help stimulate a bowel movement.

• If the patient requires enemas, avoid using a sodium biphosphate enema too often. Its hypertonic solution can absorb as much as 10% of the colon's sodium content or draw intestinal fluids into the colon, causing dehydration. Also, don't use other types of enemas frequently.

# CHRONIC FATIGUE AND IMMUNE DYSFUNCTION SYNDROME

Chronic fatigue and immune dysfunction syndrome (CFIDS, chronic fatigue syndrome, chronic Epstein-Barr virus [EBV], benign myalgic encephalomyelitis, "Yuppie flu") is typically marked by debilitating fatigue, neurologic abnormalities, and persistent symptoms that suggest chronic mononucleosis. It commonly occurs in adults under age 45, and its incidence is highest in women.

## Causes

Although the cause of CFIDS is unknown, researchers suspect that it may be found in human herpesvirus-6 or in other herpesviruses, enteroviruses, or retroviruses. Rising levels of antibodies to EBV, once thought to implicate EBV infection as the cause of CFIDS, are now considered a result of this disease.

CFIDS may be associated with a reaction to viral illness that's complicated by dysfunctional immune response and by other factors that may include gender, age, genetic disposition, prior illness, stress, and environment.

## Signs and symptoms

The characteristic symptom of CFIDS is prolonged, often overwhelming fatigue that's commonly associated with a varying complex of other symptoms. To aid identification of the disease, the Centers for Disease Control and Prevention (CDC) uses a "working case definition" to group symptoms and severity. (See *CDC criteria for diagnosing CFIDS,* page 204.)

## Diagnosis

The cause and nature of CFIDS are still unknown, and no single test unequivocally confirms its presence. Therefore, the diagnosis is based on the patient's history and the CDC criteria. Because the CDC criteria are admittedly a working concept that may not include all forms of this disease and are based on symptoms that can result from other diseases, a diagnosis is difficult and uncertain. Considerable overlap exists between CFIDS and fibromyalgia syndrome, with patients often having features of both.

## C.D.C. CRITERIA FOR DIAGNOSING C.F.I.D.S.

To meet the case definition by the Centers for Disease Control and Prevention (CDC) for chronic fatigue and immune dysfunction syndrome (CFIDS), a patient must fulfill the major criteria plus either 8 of the symptom criteria, or 6 of the "symptom criteria" and 2 of the physical criteria.

### Major criteria
• New onset of persistent or relapsing debilitating fatigue in a person without a history of similar symptoms; fatigue doesn't resolve with bed rest and is severe enough to reduce or impair average daily activity by 50% for 6 months.
• Exclusion of other disorders after evaluation through history, physical examination, and laboratory findings.

### Symptom criteria
The symptom criteria include the initial development of the main symptom complex over a few hours or days and the following other symptoms:
• profound or prolonged fatigue, especially after exercise levels that were easily tolerated before

• complaints of painful lymph nodes
• muscle weakness
• sleep disturbances (insomnia or hypersomnia)
• migratory arthralgia without joint swelling or redness
• photophobia, forgetfulness, irritability, confusion, depression, transient visual scotoma, difficulty thinking, and inability to concentrate.

### Physical criteria
These criteria must be recorded on at least two occasions at least 1 month apart:
• low-grade fever
• nonexudative pharyngitis
• palpable or tender nodes.

## Treatment

No therapy is known to cure CFIDS. Experimental treatments include the antiviral acyclovir and selected immunomodulating agents, such as I.V. gamma globulin, ampligen, and transfer factor.

Treatment of symptoms may include tricyclic antidepressants (doxepin), histamine$_2$-blocking agents (cimetidine), and antianxiety agents (alprazolam). In some patients, avoidance of environmental irritants and certain foods may help to relieve symptoms.

## Special considerations

> CLINICAL TIP  Refer the patient to the CFIDS Association for information as well as to local support groups; supportive contact with others

who share this disease may benefit the patient.

• If appropriate, suggest psychological counseling.

# CHRONIC GRANULOMATOUS DISEASE

In chronic granulomatous disease (CGD), abnormal neutrophil metabolism impairs phagocytosis—one of the body's chief defense mechanisms—resulting in increased susceptibility to low-virulent or nonpathogenic organisms, such as *Staphylococcus epidermidis, Escherichia coli, Aspergillus,* and *Nocardia.* Phagocytes attracted to sites of infection can engulf these invading organisms but are unable to destroy them. Patients with CGD may develop granulomatous inflammation, which leads to ischemic tissue damage.

## Causes
CGD is usually inherited as an X-linked trait, although a variant form — probably autosomal recessive — also exists. The genetic defect may be linked to deficiency of the enzymes NADH, NADPH oxidase, or NADH reductase, which renders the phagocytes unable to generate sufficient superoxide radicals to kill the bacteria.

## Signs and symptoms
Usually, the patient with CGD displays signs and symptoms by age 2, associated with infections of the skin, lymph nodes, lungs, liver, and bone. Skin infection is characterized by small, well-localized areas of tenderness. Seborrheic dermatitis of the scalp and axilla is also common. Lymph node infection typically causes marked lymphadenopathy with draining lymph nodes and hepatosplenomegaly.

Many patients develop liver abscess, which may be recurrent and multiple. Abdominal tenderness, fever, anorexia, and nausea point to abscess formation. Other common infections include osteomyelitis, which causes localized pain and fever; pneumonia; and gingivitis with severe periodontal disease.

## Diagnosis
Clinical features of osteomyelitis, pneumonia, liver abscess, or chronic lymphadenopathy in a young child provide the first clues to a diagnosis of CGD.

An important tool for confirming this diagnosis is the nitroblue tetrazolium (NBT) test. A clear yellow dye, NBT is normally reduced by neutrophil metabolism, resulting in a color change from yellow to blue. Quantifying this color change estimates the degree of neutrophil metabolism. Patients with CGD show impaired NBT reduction, indicating abnormal neutrophil metabolism. Another test measures the rate of intracellular killing by neutrophils. In CGD, killing is delayed or absent.

Other laboratory values may support the diagnosis or help monitor disease activity. Osteomyelitis typically causes an elevated white blood cell count and erythrocyte sedimentation rate; bone scans help locate and measure such infections. Recurrent liver or lung infection may eventually cause abnormal function studies. Cell-mediated and humoral immunity are usually normal in CGD, although some patients have hypergammaglobulinemia.

## Treatment
Early, aggressive treatment of infection is the chief goal in caring for a patient with CGD. Areas of suspected infection should be biopsied or cultured, with broad-spectrum antibiotics usually started immediately — without waiting for the results of cultures. Confirmed abscesses may be drained or surgically removed.

Many patients with CGD receive a combination of I.V. antibiotics, often extended beyond the usual 10- to 14-day course. However, for fungal infections with *Aspergillus* or *Nocardia*, treatment involves amphotericin B in gradually increasing doses to achieve a maximum cumulative dose.

To help treat life-threatening or antibiotic-resistant infection or to help localize infection, the patient may receive granulocyte transfusions — usually once daily until the crisis has passed. Transfusions shouldn't be given for 6 hours before or after amphotericin B to avoid severe pulmonary edema and, possibly, respiratory arrest.

Interferon is an experimental but promising treatment in CGD.

**Special considerations**

• If prophylactic antibiotics are ordered, teach the patient and his family how to administer them and how to recognize adverse reactions. Advise them to promptly report any signs or symptoms of infection. Stress the importance of good nutrition and hygiene, especially meticulous skin and mouth care.

• During hospitalizations, encourage the patient to continue his activities of daily living as much as possible. Try to arrange for a tutor to help the child keep up with his schoolwork.

• Provide meticulous wound care after drainage or removal of an abscess, including irrigation or packing.

• During I.V. drug therapy, monitor vital signs frequently and rotate the I.V. site every 48 to 72 hours.

• During granulocyte transfusions, watch for fever and chills.

➤ CLINICAL TIP Transfusion-related fever and chills can sometimes be prevented by premedication with acetaminophen.

# CHRONIC OBSTRUCTIVE PULMONARY DISEASE

Chronic obstructive pulmonary disease (COPD) — also called chronic obstructive lung disease — results from emphysema, chronic bronchitis, asthma, or any combination of these disorders. Usually, more than one of these underlying conditions coexist; most often, bronchitis and emphysema occur together. (See *Understanding chronic obstructive pulmonary disease,* pages 208 to 211.)

The most common chronic lung disease, COPD affects an estimated 17 million Americans, and its incidence is rising. It affects men more often than women, probably because, until recently, men were more likely to smoke heavily. It doesn't always produce symptoms and causes only minimal disability in many patients. However, COPD tends to worsen with time.

**Causes**

Predisposing factors include cigarette smoking, recurrent or chronic respiratory tract infections, air pollution, and allergies. Familial and hereditary factors (for example, deficiency of alpha$_1$-antitrypsin) may also predispose a person to COPD.

Smoking is by far the most important of these factors; it impairs ciliary action and macrophage function and causes inflammation in airways, increased mucus production, destruction of alveolar septae, and peribronchiolar fibrosis. Early inflammatory changes may reverse if the patient stops smoking before lung destruction is extensive.

**Signs and symptoms**

The typical patient, a long-term cigarette smoker, has no symptoms until middle age, when his ability to exercise or do strenuous work gradually starts to decline and he begins to develop a productive cough. While subtle at first, these signs become more pronounced as the patient grows older and the disease progresses.

Eventually the patient develops dyspnea on minimal exertion, frequent respiratory tract infections, intermittent or continuous hypoxemia, and grossly abnormal pulmonary function studies. In its advanced form, COPD may cause thoracic deformities, overwhelming disability, cor pulmonale, severe respiratory failure, and death.

## Treatment

The main goal of treatment is to relieve symptoms and prevent complications. Bronchodilators can help alleviate bronchospasm and enhance mucociliary clearance of secretions. Effective coughing, postural drainage, and chest physiotherapy can help mobilize secretions.

Administration of low concentrations of oxygen helps relieve symptoms; arterial blood gas analysis determines oxygen need and helps avoid carbon dioxide narcosis.

Antibiotics allow treatment of respiratory tract infections. Pneumococcal vaccination and annual influenza vaccinations are important preventive measures.

## Special considerations

• Most COPD patients receive outpatient treatment, so provide comprehensive patient teaching to help them comply with therapy and understand the nature of this chronic, progressive disease. (See *Living with COPD.*)

• If the patient is to continue oxygen therapy at home, teach him how to use the equipment correctly. Patients with COPD rarely require more than 3 L/minute to maintain adequate oxygenation. Higher flow rates will further increase the partial pressure of arterial oxygen, but patients whose ventilatory drive is largely based on hypoxemia often develop a markedly increased partial pressure of arterial carbon dioxide. In such patients, chemoreceptors in the brain are relatively insensitive to the increase in carbon dioxide.

CLINICAL TIP Teach the patient and his family that excessive oxygen therapy may eliminate the hypoxic respiratory drive, causing confusion and drowsiness, which are signs of carbon dioxide narcosis.

• Help the patient and his family adjust their lifestyles to accommodate the lim-

---

TEACHING CHECKLIST

### LIVING WITH C.O.P.D.

Review the following points with your patient and his family:

• Encourage the patient to enroll in available pulmonary rehabilitation programs.
• Urge the patient to stop smoking.
• Encourage the patient to avoid respiratory irritants and install an air conditioner with an air filter in the home.
• Review the use of any bronchodilators and antibiotics the patient is taking.
• Review signs of infection and warn the patient to avoid contact with persons who have respiratory tract infections.
• Review deep breathing, coughing, and chest physiotherapy.
• Encourage fluids and the use of a humidifier to thin secretions.
• Emphasize the importance of a balanced diet; small, frequent meals; and the use of nasal oxygen while eating.

---

itations imposed by this debilitating chronic disease. Instruct the patient to allow for daily rest periods and to exercise daily as directed.

• To help prevent COPD, advise all people, especially those with a family history of COPD or those in its early stages, not to smoke.

• Assist in the early detection of COPD by urging persons to have periodic physical examinations, including spirometry and medical evaluation of a chronic cough, and to seek treatment for recurring respiratory tract infections promptly.

*(Text continues on page 210.)*

# UNDERSTANDING CHRONIC OBSTRUCTIVE PULMONARY DISEASE

| DISEASE | CAUSES AND PATHOPHYSIOLOGY | CLINICAL FEATURES |
|---|---|---|
| **Emphysema**<br>• Abnormal irreversible enlargement of air spaces distal to terminal bronchioles due to destruction of alveolar walls, resulting in decreased elastic recoil properties of lungs<br>• Most common cause of death from respiratory disease in the United States | • Cigarette smoking, deficiency of alpha$_1$-antitrypsin<br>• Recurrent inflammation associated with release of proteolytic enzymes from cells in lungs causes bronchiolar and alveolar wall damage and, ultimately, destruction. Loss of lung-supporting structure results in decreased elastic recoil and airway collapse on expiration. Destruction of alveolar walls decreases surface area for gas exchange. | • Insidious onset, with dyspnea the predominant symptom<br>• *Other signs and symptoms of long-term disease:* chronic cough, anorexia, weight loss, malaise, barrel chest, use of accessory muscles of respiration, prolonged expiratory period with grunting, pursed-lip breathing and tachypnea, and peripheral cyanosis<br>• *Complications* include recurrent respiratory tract infections, cor pulmonale, and respiratory failure. |
| **Chronic bronchitis**<br>• Excessive mucus production with productive cough for at least 3 months/year for 2 successive years<br>• Only a minority of patients with the clinical syndrome of chronic bronchitis develop significant airway obstruction. | • Severity of disease related to amount and duration of smoking; respiratory tract infection exacerbates symptoms.<br>• Hypertrophy and hyperplasia of bronchial mucous glands, increased goblet cells, damage to cilia, squamous metaplasia of columnar epithelium, and chronic leukocytic and lymphocytic infiltration of bronchial walls; widespread inflammation, distortion, narrowing of airways, and mucus within the airways produce resistance to small airways and cause ventilation-perfusion imbalance. | • Insidious onset, with productive cough and exertional dyspnea as predominant symptoms<br>• *Other signs and symptoms:* colds associated with increased sputum production and worsening dyspnea that takes progressively longer to resolve; copious sputum (gray, white, or yellow); weight gain due to edema; cyanosis; tachypnea; wheezing; prolonged expiratory time; use of accessory muscles of respiration |

## CONFIRMING DIAGNOSTIC MEASURES

- *Physical examination:* hyperresonance on percussion, decreased breath sounds, expiratory prolongation, quiet heart sounds
- *Chest X-ray:* in advanced disease, flattened diaphragm, reduced vascular markings at lung periphery, overaeration of lungs, vertical heart, enlarged anteroposterior chest diameter, large retrosternal air space
- *Pulmonary function tests:* increased residual volume, total lung capacity, and compliance; decreased vital capacity, diffusing capacity, and expiratory volumes
- *Arterial blood gases (ABG) analysis:* reduced partial pressure of arterial oxygen ($Pao_2$) with normal partial pressure of arterial carbon dioxide ($Paco_2$)
- *Electrocardiography (ECG):* tall, symmetrical P waves in leads II, III, and $aV_F$; vertical QRS axis; signs of right ventricular hypertrophy late in disease
- *Red blood cells:* increased hemoglobin level late in disease when persistent severe hypoxia is present

## MANAGEMENT

- Bronchodilators, such as beta-adrenergics and theophylline, to reverse bronchospasm and promote mucociliary clearance
- Antibiotics to treat respiratory tract infection; flu vaccine to prevent influenza; Pneumovax to prevent pneumococcal pneumonia; and mucolytics
- Adequate fluid intake and, in selected patients, chest physiotherapy to mobilize secretions
- Oxygen at low-flow settings to treat hypoxia
- Avoidance of smoking and air pollutants
- Aerosolized or systemic corticosteroids

---

- *Physical examination:* rhonchi and wheezing on auscultation, expiratory prolongation, neck vein distention, pedal edema
- *Chest X-ray:* may show hyperinflation and increased bronchovascular markings
- *Pulmonary function tests:* increased residual volume, decreased vital capacity and forced expiratory volumes, normal static compliance and diffusing capacity
- *ABGs:* decreased $Pao_2$, normal or increased $Paco2$
- *Sputum:* contains evidence of infection
- *ECG:* may show atrial arrhythmias; peaked P waves in leads II, III, and aVF; and, occasionally, right ventricular hypertrophy

- Antibiotics for infections
- Avoidance of smoking and air pollutants
- Bronchodilators to relieve bronchospasm and facilitate mucociliary clearance
- Adequate fluid intake and chest physiotherapy to mobilize secretions
- Ultrasonic or mechanical nebulizer treatments to loosen secretions and aid in mobilization
- Occasionally, corticosteroids
- Diuretics for edema
- Oxygen for hypoxia

*(continued)*

## UNDERSTANDING CHRONIC OBSTRUCTIVE PULMONARY DISEASE *(continued)*

| DISEASE | CAUSES AND PATHOPHYSIOLOGY | CLINICAL FEATURES |
|---------|---------------------------|-------------------|
| **Asthma**<br>• Increased bronchial reactivity to a variety of stimuli, which produces episodic bronchospasm and airway obstruction in conjunction with airway inflammation<br>• Onset in adulthood: often without distinct allergies; onset in childhood: often associated with definite allergens. Status asthmaticus is an acute asthma attack with severe bronchospasm that fails to clear with bronchodilator therapy.<br>• Prognosis: More than half of asthmatic children become asymptomatic as adults; more than half of asthmatics with onset after age 15 have persistent disease with occasional severe attacks. | • Possible mechanisms include allergy (family tendency, seasonal occurrence); allergic reaction results in release of mast cell vasoactive and bronchospastic mediators.<br>• Upper airway infection, exercise, anxiety and, rarely, coughing or laughing can precipitate an asthma attack; nocturnal flare-ups are common.<br>• Paroxysmal airway obstruction associated with nasal polyps may be seen in response to aspirin or indomethacin ingestion.<br>• Airway obstruction from spasm of bronchial smooth muscle narrows airways; inflammatory edema of the bronchial wall and inspissation of tenacious mucoid secretions are also important, particularly in status asthmaticus. | • History of intermittent attacks of dyspnea and wheezing<br>• Mild wheezing progresses to severe dyspnea, audible wheezing, chest tightness (a feeling of being unable to breathe), and a cough that produces thick mucus.<br>• *Other signs:* Prolonged expiration, intercostal and supraclavicular retraction on inspiration, use of accessory muscles of respiration, flaring nostrils, tachypnea, tachycardia, perspiration, and flushing; patients often have symptoms of eczema and allergic rhinitis (hay fever).<br>• Status asthmaticus, unless treated promptly, can progress to respiratory failure. |

# CIRRHOSIS

A chronic hepatic disease, cirrhosis is characterized by diffuse destruction and fibrotic regeneration of hepatic cells. As necrotic tissue yields to fibrosis, cirrhosis alters liver structure and normal vasculature, impairs blood and lymph flow and, ultimately, causes hepatic insufficiency. (See *Circulation in portal hypertension,* page 212.)

Cirrhosis is a serious, irreversible disease that's the 11th largest cause of death in the United States. The prognosis is better in noncirrhotic forms of hepatic fibrosis, which cause minimal hepatic dysfunction and don't destroy liver cells.

## Causes

The following clinical types of cirrhosis reflect its diverse causes:

### Hepatocellular disease

*Postnecrotic cirrhosis* accounts for 10% to 30% of patients and stems from

| CONFIRMING DIAGNOSTIC MEASURES | MANAGEMENT |
|---|---|
| • *Physical examination:* usually normal between attacks; auscultation shows rhonchi and wheezing throughout lung fields on expiration and, at times, inspiration; absent or diminished breath sounds during severe obstruction. Loud bilateral wheezes may be grossly audible; chest is hyperinflated.<br>• *Chest X-ray:* hyperinflated lungs with air trapping during attack; normal during remission<br>• *Sputum:* presence of Curschmann's spirals (casts of airways), Charcot-Leyden crystals, and eosinophils<br>• *Pulmonary function tests:* during attacks, decreased forced expiratory volumes that improve significantly after inhaled bronchodilator; increased residual volume and, occasionally, total lung capacity; may be normal between attacks<br>• *ABGs:* decreased $Pao_2$; decreased, normal or increased $Paco_2$ (in severe attack)<br>• *ECG:* sinus tachycardia during an attack; severe attack may produce signs of cor pulmonale (right axis deviation, peaked P wave) that resolve after the attack.<br>• *Skin tests:* may identify allergens | • Aerosol containing beta-adrenergic agents, such as metaproterenol or albuterol; also oral beta-adrenergic agents (terbutaline) and oral methylxanthines (theophylline). Many patients require inhaled, oral, or I.V. corticosteroids.<br>• *Emergency treatment:* Oxygen therapy, corticosteroids, and bronchodilators, such as S.C. epinephrine, I.V theophylline, and inhaled agents (such as metaproterenol, albuterol, or ipratropium bromide).<br>• Monitor for deteriorating respiratory status and note sputum characteristics; provide adequate fluid intake and oxygen.<br>• *Prevention:* Tell the patient to avoid possible allergens and to use antihistamines, decongestants, cromolyn powder by inhalation, and oral or aerosol bronchodilators as needed. Explain the influence of stress and anxiety on asthma as well as its frequent association with exercise (particularly running), cold air, and nighttime flare-ups. |

various types of hepatitis (such as types A, B, C, D viral hepatitis) or toxic exposures.

*Laënnec's cirrhosis,* also called *portal, nutritional, or alcoholic cirrhosis,* is the most common type and is primarily caused by hepatitis C. Liver damage results from malnutrition (especially dietary protein) and chronic alcohol ingestion. Fibrous tissue forms in portal areas and around central veins.

*Autoimmune disease,* such as sarcoidosis and chronic inflammatory bowel disease, may result in cirrhosis.

*Cholestatic diseases*

This group includes diseases of the biliary tree (biliary cirrhosis resulting from bile duct diseases suppressing bile flow) and sclerosing cholangitis.

*Metabolic diseases*

This group includes disorders such as Wilson's disease, alpha$_1$-antitrypsin deficiency, and hemochromatosis (pigment cirrhosis).

## CIRCULATION IN PORTAL HYPERTENSION

As portal pressure rises, blood backs up into the spleen and flows through collateral channels to the venous system, bypassing the liver and causing esophageal varices.

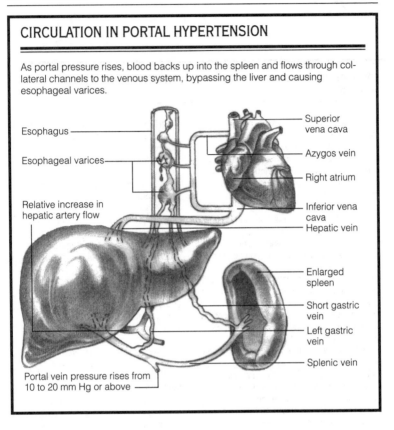

Esophagus

Esophageal varices

Relative increase in hepatic artery flow

Superior vena cava

Azygos vein

Right atrium

Inferior vena cava

Hepatic vein

Enlarged spleen

Short gastric vein

Left gastric vein

Splenic vein

Portal vein pressure rises from 10 to 20 mm Hg or above

### Other types of cirrhosis

Other types of cirrhosis include Budd-Chiari syndrome, cardiac cirrhosis, and cryptogenic cirrhosis. Cardiac cirrhosis is rare; the liver damage results from right-sided heart failure. *Cryptogenic* refers to cirrhosis of unknown cause.

### Signs and symptoms

Clinical manifestations of cirrhosis and fibrosis are similar for all types, regardless of cause. Early indications are insidious and vague but usually include weakness, fatigue, muscle cramps, weight loss, GI symptoms (anorexia, indigestion, nausea, vomiting, constipation, diarrhea), and abdominal pain (which may be attributed to an enlarged liver).

Major and late symptoms develop as a result of hepatic insufficiency and portal hypertension and include the following:

• *respiratory* — pleural effusion and limited thoracic expansion because of abdominal ascites, interfering with efficient gas exchange and leading to hypoxia

• *central nervous system* — progressive symptoms of hepatic encephalopathy: lethargy, mental changes, slurred speech, asterixis (flapping tremor), peripheral neuritis, paranoia, hallucinations, extreme obtundation, and coma

- *hematologic* — bleeding tendencies (nosebleeds, easy bruising, bleeding gums), anemia, and hematemesis
- *endocrine* — testicular atrophy, menstrual irregularities, gynecomastia, loss of chest and axillary hair, loss of libido, and sterility
- *skin* — severe pruritus, extreme dryness, poor tissue turgor, abnormal pigmentation, spider nevi (on upper half of body), palmar erythema, jaundice, and peripheral edema
- *hepatic* — jaundice, hepatomegaly, ascites, edema of the legs, hepatic encephalopathy, and hepatorenal syndrome constitute the other major effects of full-fledged cirrhosis
- *miscellaneous* — musty breath, enlarged superficial abdominal veins, muscle atrophy, pain in the right upper abdominal quadrant that worsens when the patient sits up or leans forward, splenomegaly, and wasting appearance of chronic illness. Fever may be present and usually associated with portal hepatitis, spontaneous bacterial peritonitis, or cholangitis. Bleeding from esophageal and rectal varices results from portal hypertension.

## Diagnosis

A liver biopsy, the definitive test for cirrhosis, detects destruction and fibrosis of hepatic tissue. A liver scan shows abnormal thickening and, possibly, a liver mass.

Plain films of the abdomen may reveal hepatic or splenic enlargement. Ultrasonography can assess liver size and detect ascites or hepatic enlargement. Doppler ultrasonography is used to evaluate patency of the splenic, portal, and hepatic veins. Computed tomography with I.V. contrast or magnetic resonance imaging with serum alpha-fetoprotein levels can further assess liver nodules. Suspicious liver nodules or masses can be biopsied to assess for cancer. Esophagogastroscopy can detect causes of bleeding in the esophagus, stomach, and proximal duodenum to confirm the presence of varices.

The following laboratory findings are characteristic of cirrhosis:

- decreased platelet count and hematocrit and decreased levels of hemoglobin, albumin, electrolytes (sodium, potassium, chloride, and magnesium), and folate.
- elevated levels of globulin, serum ammonia, total bilirubin, alkaline phosphatase, serum aspartate aminotransferase, serum alanine aminotransferase, and lactate dehydrogenase and increased thymol turbidity
- coagulation abnormalities characterized by prolonged prothrombin and partial thromboplastin times.

> **CLINICAL TIP** The best indications of hepatic function are prothrombin time cholesterol and albumin.

## Treatment

The goals of treatment include removing or alleviating the underlying cause of cirrhosis or fibrosis, preventing further liver damage, and preventing or treating complications.

### Dietary measures

The patient may benefit from a high-calorie and moderate- to high-protein diet, but developing hepatic encephalopathy mandates restricted protein intake. In addition, sodium is usually restricted to 400 to 800 mg/day, fluids to 1,000 to 1,500 ml/day.

If the patient's condition continues to deteriorate, he may need tube feedings or hyperalimentation. Other supportive measures include supplemental vitamins — A, B complex, D, and K — to compensate for the liver's inability to store them and vitamin B, folic acid, and thiamine for deficiency anemia. Rest, moderate exercise, and avoidance of exposure to infections and toxic agents are essential.

### Drug therapy

In cirrhosis, drug therapy requires special caution because the cirrhotic liver can't detoxify harmful substances efficiently. Alcohol is prohibited; sedatives should be avoided or prescribed with great care. Acetaminophen (Tylenol) is especially hepatotoxic, particularly when combined with alcohol.

When absolutely necessary, antiemetics, such as trimethobenzamide or benzquinamide, may be given for nausea; vasopressin, for esophageal varices; and diuretics, such as furosemide or spironolactone, for edema. However, diuretics require careful monitoring; fluid and electrolyte imbalance may precipitate hepatic encephalopathy.

Vitamin K may be given for bleeding tendencies due to hypoprothrombinemia. Transfusion of blood and fresh frozen plasma may also be necessary.

Beta blockers may be given to decrease pressure from varices.

Lactulose may be given orally or rectally for high ammonia levels.

### Other treatment

Paracentesis and infusions of salt-poor albumin may alleviate ascites. Surgical procedures include ligation of varices, splenectomy, esophagogastric resection, and splenorenal or portacaval anastomosis to relieve portal hypertension.

> CLINICAL TIP  Transjugular intrahepatic portosystemic shunt is an alternative to surgical shunting in patients with variceal bleeding refractory to standard therapy. It's helpful in severe ascites. The technique involves insertion of an expandable metal shunt between a branch of the hepatic vein and portal vein over a catheter inserted via the jugular vein. This is usually a bridging mechanism to control variceal bleeding or ascites until liver transplantation can be performed.

Hepatorenal and hepatopulmonary syndromes may occur. Treatment is ineffective except in patients who are acceptable candidates for liver transplantation.

### Special considerations

● Check skin, gums, stool, and emesis regularly for bleeding. Apply pressure to injection sites to prevent bleeding. Warn the patient against taking aspirin, straining during defecation, and blowing his nose or sneezing too vigorously. Suggest using an electric razor and a soft toothbrush.

> CLINICAL TIP  Assess the patient for internal bleeding as well as for overt signs of external bleeding.

● Observe the patient closely for signs of behavioral or personality changes — especially increasing stupor, lethargy, hallucinations, and neuromuscular dysfunction — which may indicate increasing ammonia levels. Arouse the patient periodically to determine his level of consciousness. Watch for asterixis, a sign of developing hepatic encephalopathy.

● Monitor ammonia levels to determine effectiveness of lactulose therapy.

● To assess fluid retention, weigh the patient and measure his abdominal girth daily, inspect the ankles and sacrum for dependent edema, and accurately record intake and output. Carefully evaluate the patient before, during, and after paracentesis; this drastic loss of fluid may induce shock.

● To prevent skin breakdown associated with edema and pruritus, avoid using soap when bathing the patient; instead, use lubricating lotion or moisturizing agents. Handle the patient gently, and turn and reposition him often to keep skin intact.

• Tell the patient that rest and good nutrition will conserve energy and decrease metabolic demands on the liver. Encourage frequent, small meals. Stress the need to avoid infections and abstain from alcohol.

• Support the family during this difficult time, and refer the patient to support groups and Alcoholics Anonymous as indicated.

# CLEFT LIP AND CLEFT PALATE

Cleft lip and cleft palate — an opening in the lip or palate — may occur separately or in combination. These deformities originate in the 2nd month of pregnancy, when the front and sides of the face and the palatine shelves fuse imperfectly. Cleft deformities usually occur unilaterally or bilaterally, rarely midline. Only the lip may be involved, or the defect may extend into the upper jaw or nasal cavity.

Cleft lip and cleft palate occur in twice as many males as females; isolated cleft palate is more common in females.

## Causes

Cleft lip or palate can occur as part of another chromosomal or mendelian abnormality (over 150 have been identified); however, exposure to teratogens during fetal development or a combination of genetic and environmental factors may also produce these defects.

Cleft lip with or without cleft palate occurs in approximately 1 in 1,000 births among Whites; the incidence is higher in Asians (1.7 in 1,000) and Native Americans (over 3.6 in 1,000) but lower in Blacks (1 in 2,500). Children with a family history of cleft defects have an increased incidence.

## Signs and symptoms

Congenital defects of the face occur most often in the upper lip. They range from a simple notch to a complete cleft from the lip edge through the floor of the nostril, on either side of the midline, but rarely along the midline itself.

A cleft palate may be partial or complete. A complete cleft includes the soft palate, the bones of the maxilla, and the alveolus on one or both sides of the premaxilla. A double cleft runs from the soft palate forward to either side of the nose, separating the maxilla and premaxilla into freely moving segments. The tongue and other muscles can displace these segments, enlarging the cleft. In Pierre Robin syndrome, micrognathia and glossoptosis coexist with cleft palate.

Isolated cleft palate is more often associated with other congenital defects than isolated cleft lip or cleft lip and cleft palate.

## Diagnosis

A typical clinical picture confirms the diagnosis. Cleft lip with or without cleft palate is obvious at birth; occasionally, more severe defects may be seen with diagnostic prenatal ultrasonography. Isolated cleft palate may not be detected until a mouth examination is done or until feeding difficulties develop. (See *Cleft lip and cleft palate,* page 216.)

## Treatment

Treatment consists of surgical correction, but the timing of surgery varies. Some plastic surgeons repair cleft lips within the first few days of life to make feeding the baby easier. However, many surgeons delay lip repairs for 8 to 10 weeks (sometimes as long as 6 to 8 months) to allow time for maternal

## CLEFT LIP AND CLEFT PALATE

The illustration below shows the four variations of cleft lip and cleft palate.

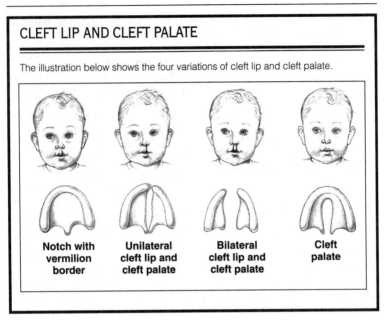

| Notch with vermilion border | Unilateral cleft lip and cleft palate | Bilateral cleft lip and cleft palate | Cleft palate |

bonding and, most important, to rule out associated congenital anomalies.

Cleft palate repair is usually completed by the 12th to 18th month. Still other surgeons repair cleft palates in two steps, repairing the soft palate between ages 6 and 18 months and the hard palate as late as age 5 years. In any case, surgery is performed only after the infant is gaining weight and is infection-free.

Surgery must be coupled with speech therapy. Because the palate is essential to speech formation, structural changes, even in a repaired cleft, can permanently affect speech patterns. To compound the problem, children with cleft palates often have hearing difficulties because of middle ear damage or infections.

### Special considerations

CLINICAL TIP   Recent research has indicated that ingestion of 0.4 mg of folic acid daily before conception decreases the risk of isolated cleft lip or palate by up to 25%. Therefore, all women of childbearing age should be encouraged to take a daily multivitamin containing folic acid until menopause or until they're no longer fertile.

● Although most infants with a cleft palate can sleep on their backs without difficulty, an infant with Pierre Robin syndrome risks having the tongue fall back and obstruct the airway if placed in this position.

● Maintain adequate nutrition to ensure normal growth and development. Experiment with feeding devices. A baby with a cleft palate has an excellent appetite but often has trouble feeding because of air leaks around the cleft and nasal regurgitation.

● Teach the mother how best to feed her infant. Advise her to hold the infant in a near-sitting position, with the flow directed to the side or back of the baby's tongue. Tell her to burp the baby frequently because he tends to swallow a lot of air. If the underside of the nasal septum becomes ulcerated and the child refuses to suck because of the pain, instruct the mother to give the mucosa time to heal. Tell her to gently clean the palatal cleft with a cotton-tipped applicator dipped in half-strength hydrogen peroxide or water after each feeding.

• Encourage the mother of a baby with cleft lip to breast-feed if the cleft does not prevent effective sucking. Breast-feeding an infant with a cleft palate or one who has just had corrective surgery is usually not possible. (Postoperatively, the infant can't suck for up to 6 weeks.) However, if the mother desires, suggest that she use a breast pump to express breast milk and then feed it to her baby from a bottle.

• Following surgery, record intake and output and maintain good nutrition. To prevent atelectasis and pneumonia, the doctor may gently suction the nasopharynx (this may be necessary before surgery too).

• Elbow restraints allow the baby to move his hands while keeping them away from his mouth. When necessary, use an infant seat to keep the child in a comfortable sitting position.

• Help the parents deal with their feelings about the child's deformity. Start by telling them about it and showing them their baby as soon as possible. Because society places undue importance on physical appearance, many parents feel shock, disappointment, and guilt when they see the child. Help them by being calm and providing positive information.

• Direct the parents' attention to their child's assets. Stress the fact that surgical repairs can be made. Include the parents in the care and feeding of the child right from the start to encourage normal bonding. Provide the instructions, emotional support, and reassurance that the parents will need to take proper care of the child at home.

• Refer them to a social worker who can guide them to community resources if needed and to a genetic counselor to determine the recurrence risk.

# CLOSTRIDIUM DIFFICILE INFECTION

*Clostridium difficile* is a gram-positive anaerobic bacterium most often associated with antibiotic-associated diarrhea. Symptoms may range from asymptomatic carrier states to severe pseudomembranous colitis and are caused by exotoxins produced by the organism: toxin A (an enterotoxin) and toxin B (a cytotoxin).

## Causes

Although *C. difficile* infection can be caused by almost any antibiotic that disrupts the intestinal flora, it's classically associated with clindamycin use. Patients at high risk for this disorder include those taking many kinds of antibiotics or antineoplastic agents that have antibiotic activity; candidates for abdominal surgery; immunocompromised individuals; pediatric patients (infections are common in day-care centers); and those in nursing homes.

Additional factors that alter normal intestinal flora include enemas and intestinal stimulants. *C. difficile* may be transmitted directly from patient to patient via contaminated hands of facility personnel (most common) or indirectly through contaminated equipment — such as bedpans, urinals, call bells, rectal thermometers, and nasogastric tubes — and surfaces — such as bed rails, floors, and toilet seats.

➤ CLINICAL TIP   Because spores of *C. difficile* are resistant to most commonly used facility disinfectants, the patient's room may be contaminated even after the patient is discharged. The immediate environment must be thoroughly cleaned and disinfected with 0.5% sodium hypochlorite.

## Signs and symptoms

Risk of *C. difficile* infection begins 1 to 2 days after antibiotic therapy is started and persists for as long as 2 to 3 months after the last dose. The patient may be asymptomatic or may present any of the following symptoms: soft, unformed stool or watery diarrhea (more than three evacuations in 24 hours) that may be foul-smelling or grossly bloody; abdominal pain, cramping, or tenderness; and fever. White blood cell count may be elevated to 20,000/μl. In severe cases, toxic megacolon, colonic perforation, and peritonitis may develop. Complications include electrolyte abnormalities, hypovolemic shock, anasarca (caused by hypoalbuminemia), sepsis, and hemorrhage. In rare cases, death may result.

## Diagnosis

*C. difficile* infection is confirmed by identification of toxins, using one of the following methods:
- *cell cytotoxin test* — highly sensitive and specific for toxins A and B of *C. difficile;* results available in 2 days
- *enzyme immunoassays* — slightly less sensitive than the cell cytotoxin test, but results are obtained in a few hours; specificity is excellent
- *stool culture* — most sensitive, with 2-day turnaround. Non–toxin-producing strains of *C. difficile* can be easily identified using three separate stool samples to test for the presence of the toxin
- *endoscopy (flexible sigmoidoscopy)* — may be used in patients who present with an acute abdomen but no diarrhea, making it difficult to obtain a stool sample. If pseudomembranes are seen, treatment for *C. difficile* is usually initiated.

## Treatment

Withdrawing the causative antibiotic (if possible) resolves symptoms in patients who are mildly symptomatic. This is usually the only treatment required.

For more severe cases, metronidazole 250 mg by mouth (P.O.) four times daily or 500 mg P.O. three times daily, or vancomycin 125 mg P.O. four times daily for 10 days are effective therapies, with metronidazole being the preferred treatment. Retesting for *C. difficile* is unnecessary if symptoms resolve.

In 10% to 20% of patients, *C. difficile* may recur within 14 to 30 days of treatment. Beyond 30 days, it's questionable whether the recurrence is a relapse or reinfection with *C. difficile*. If metronidazole was the initial treatment, low-dose vancomycin, given 125 mg P.O. four times daily for 21 days, may be effective. Alternatively, give vancomycin (125 mg P.O. four times daily) in combination with rifampin (600 mg P.O. twice daily) for 10 days.

There is no evidence to support the use of yogurt or *Lactobacillus* in these infections. Other experimental treatments include giving the yeast *Saccharomyces boulardii* with metronidazole or vancomycin and giving biological vaccines to restore normal intestinal flora.

## Special considerations

- Patients with known or suspect *C. difficile* diarrhea who are unable to practice good hygiene should be placed in a single room or with other patients with similar status.
- Standard precautions for contact with blood and body fluids should be used for all direct patient contact and contact with the patient's immediate environment. Use good hand-washing tech-

nique with antiseptic soap after direct contact with the patient or the immediate environment.

• Patients who are asymptomatic without diarrhea or fecal incontinence for 72 hours and who are able to practice good hygiene may be transferred out of single rooms.

• Reusable equipment must be disinfected before use on another patient.

• Preventive strategies include careful selection of antibiotic therapy, use of single antibiotics when possible, avoidance of antibiotics when they're not absolutely necessary, and limited duration of the antibiotic treatment regimen.

# CLUBFOOT

The most common congenital disorder of the lower extremities, clubfoot, or talipes, is marked primarily by a deformed talus and shortened Achilles tendon, which give the foot a characteristic clublike appearance. In talipes equinovarus, the foot points downward (equinus) and turns inward (varus), while the front of the foot curls toward the heel (forefoot adduction).

Clubfoot, which has an incidence of approximately 1 per 1,000 live births, usually occurs bilaterally and is twice as common in boys as in girls. It may be associated with other birth defects, such as myelomeningocele, spina bifida, and arthrogryposis. Clubfoot is correctable with prompt treatment.

## Causes
A combination of genetic and environmental factors in utero appears to cause clubfoot. Heredity is a definite factor in some cases, although the mechanism of transmission is undetermined. If a child is born with clubfoot, his sibling has a 1 in 35 chance of being born with the same anomaly. Children of a parent with clubfoot have 1 chance in 10.

In children without a family history of clubfoot, this anomaly seems linked to arrested development during the 9th and 10th weeks of embryonic life, when the feet are formed. Researchers also suspect muscle abnormalities, leading to variations in length and tendon insertions, as possible causes of clubfoot.

## Signs and symptoms
Talipes equinovarus varies in severity. Deformity may be so extreme that the toes touch the inside of the ankle, or it may be only vaguely apparent.

In every case, the talus is deformed, the Achilles tendon shortened, and the calcaneus somewhat shortened and flattened. Depending on the degree of the varus deformity, the calf muscles are shortened and underdeveloped, with soft-tissue contractures at the site of the deformity. The foot is tight in its deformed position and resists manual efforts to push it back into normal position.

Clubfoot is painless, except in older, arthritic patients. In older children, clubfoot may be secondary to paralysis, poliomyelitis, or cerebral palsy, in which case treatment must include management of the underlying disease.

## Diagnosis
An early diagnosis of clubfoot is usually no problem because the deformity is obvious. In subtle deformity, however, true clubfoot must be distinguished from apparent clubfoot (metatarsus varus or pigeon toe).

Apparent clubfoot results when a fetus maintains a position in utero that gives his feet a clubfoot appearance at birth. This can usually be corrected manually.

Another form of apparent clubfoot is inversion of the feet, resulting from the peroneal type of progressive muscular atrophy and progressive muscular dystrophy. In true clubfoot, X-rays show superimposition of the talus and the calcaneus and a ladderlike appearance of the metatarsals.

## Treatment

Appropriate treatment for clubfoot is administered in three stages:
• correcting the deformity
• maintaining the correction until the foot regains normal muscle balance
• observing the foot closely for several years to prevent the deformity from recurring.

In newborns, corrective treatment for true clubfoot should begin at once. An infant's foot contains large amounts of cartilage; the muscles, ligaments, and tendons are supple. The ideal time to begin treatment is during the first few days and weeks of life — when the foot is most malleable.

### Sequential correction

Clubfoot deformities are usually corrected in sequential order: forefoot adduction first, then varus (or inversion), then equinus (or plantar flexion). Trying to correct all three deformities at once only results in a misshapen, rocker-bottomed foot.

Forefoot adduction is corrected by uncurling the front of the foot away from the heel (forefoot abduction); the varus deformity is corrected by turning the foot so the sole faces outward (eversion); and finally, equinus is corrected by casting the foot with the toes pointing up (dorsiflexion). This last correction may have to be supplemented with a subcutaneous tenotomy of the Achilles tendon and posterior capsulotomy of the ankle joint.

### Treatment methods

Several therapeutic methods have been tested and found effective in correcting clubfoot. The first is simple manipulation and casting, whereby the foot is gently manipulated into a partially corrected position, then held there in a cast for several days or weeks. (The skin should be painted with a nonirritating adhesive liquid beforehand to prevent the cast from slipping.)

After the cast is removed, the foot is manipulated into an even better position and casted again. This procedure is repeated as many times as necessary In some cases, the shape of the cast can be transformed through a series of wedging maneuvers, instead of changing the cast each time.

After correction of clubfoot, proper foot alignment should be maintained through exercise, night splints, and orthopedic shoes. With manipulating and casting, correction usually takes about 3 months. The Denis Browne splint, a device that consists of two padded, metal footplates connected by a flat, horizontal bar, is sometimes used as a follow-up measure to help promote bilateral correction and strengthen the foot muscles.

Resistant clubfoot may require surgery. Older children, for example, with recurrent or neglected clubfoot usually need surgery.

Tenotomy, tendon transfer, stripping of the plantar fascia, and capsulotomy are some of the surgical procedures that may be used. In severe cases, bone surgery (wedge resections, osteotomy, or astragalectomy) may be appropriate. After surgery, a cast is applied to preserve the correction.

Whenever clubfoot is severe enough to require surgery, it's rarely totally correctable. However, surgery can usually ameliorate the deformity.

## Special considerations

• Look for any exaggerated attitudes in an infant's feet. Make sure you can recognize the difference between true clubfoot and apparent clubfoot. Don't use excessive force in trying to manipulate a clubfoot. The foot with apparent clubfoot moves easily.

• Stress the importance of prompt treatment to parents. Make sure they understand that clubfoot demands immediate therapy and orthopedic supervision until growth is completed.

• After casting, elevate the child's feet with pillows. Check the toes every 1 to 2 hours for temperature, color, sensation, motion, and capillary refill time; watch for edema. Before a child in a clubfoot cast is discharged, teach parents to recognize circulatory impairment.

• Insert plastic petals over the top edges of a new cast while it's still wet to keep urine from soaking and softening the cast. When the cast is dry, "petal" the edges with adhesive tape to keep out plaster crumbs and prevent skin irritation.

• Perform good skin care under the cast edges every 4 hours. After washing and drying the skin, rub it with alcohol. (Don't use oils or powders; they tend to macerate the skin.)

• Warn parents of an older child not to let the foot part of the cast get soft and thin from wear. If it does, much of the correction may be lost.

• When the wedging method is being used, check circulatory status frequently; it may be impaired because of increased pressure on tissues and blood vessels. The equinus correction especially places considerable strain on ligaments, blood vessels, and tendons.

• After surgery, elevate the child's feet with pillows to decrease swelling and pain. Watch for signs of discomfort or pain. Try to locate the source of pain —

it may result from cast pressure, not the incision. If bleeding occurs under the cast, circle the location and mark the time on the cast. Watch for indications that the bleeding is spreading.

• Explain to the older child and his parents that surgery can improve clubfoot with good function but can't totally correct it; the affected calf muscle will remain slightly underdeveloped.

• Emphasize the need for long-term orthopedic care to maintain correction. Teach the parents the prescribed exercises that their child can do at home.

• Urge the parents to be sure their child wears corrective shoes as ordered and splints during naps and at night.

➤ CLINICAL TIP    Make sure parents understand that treatment for clubfoot continues during the entire growth period. Correcting this defect permanently takes time and patience.

# COAL WORKER'S PNEUMOCONIOSIS

Coal worker's pneumoconiosis (CWP), a progressive nodular pulmonary disease, occurs in two forms. This disease goes by several names, including black lung disease, coal miner's disease, miner's asthma, and anthracosis.

Simple CWP is characterized by small lung opacities. In complicated CWP, also known as progressive massive fibrosis, masses of fibrous tissue occasionally develop in the lungs of patients with simple CWP.

The risk of developing CWP depends on the duration of exposure to coal dust (usually 15 years or longer), intensity of exposure (dust count, particle size), location of the mine, silica content of the coal (anthracite coal has the highest silica content), and the worker's susceptibility. Incidence of CWP is highest among anthracite coal miners in the eastern United States.

The prognosis varies. Simple asymptomatic disease is self-limiting, although progression to complicated CWP is more likely if CWP begins after a relatively short period of exposure. Complicated CWP may be disabling, resulting in severe ventilatory failure and right-sided heart failure secondary to pulmonary hypertension.

### Causes

CWP is caused by the inhalation and prolonged retention of respirable coal dust particles (< 5 microns in diameter). Simple CWP results in the formation of macules (accumulations of macrophages laden with coal dust) around the terminal and respiratory bronchioles, surrounded by a halo of dilated alveoli. Macule formation leads to atrophy of supporting tissue, causing permanent dilation of small airways (focal emphysema).

Simple CWP may progress to the more complicated form if the disease involves one or both lungs. If this happens, fibrous tissue masses enlarge and coalesce, causing gross distortion of pulmonary structures (destruction of vasculature, alveoli, and airways).

### Signs and symptoms

Simple CWP is asymptomatic, especially in nonsmokers. Symptoms appear if complicated CWP develops; they include exertional dyspnea and a cough that occasionally produces inky-black sputum when fibrotic changes undergo avascular necrosis and their centers cavitate.

Other clinical features of CWP include increasing dyspnea and a cough that produces milky, gray, clear, or coal-flecked sputum. Recurrent bronchial and pulmonary infections produce thick yellow or green sputum.

Complications include pulmonary hypertension, right ventricular hypertrophy and cor pulmonale, and pulmonary tuberculosis. In cigarette smokers, chronic bronchitis and emphysema may also complicate the disease.

### Diagnosis

The patient history reveals exposure to coal dust. Physical examination shows a barrel chest, hyperresonant lungs with areas of dullness, diminished breath sounds, crackles, rhonchi, and wheezes.

In simple CWP, chest X-rays show small opacities (< 10 mm in diameter), which may be present in all lung zones but are more prominent in the upper lung zones. In complicated CWP, one or more large opacities (1 to 5 cm in diameter), possibly exhibiting cavitation, are seen.

The results of pulmonary function studies include the following:

● *Vital capacity* is normal in simple CWP but decreased with complicated CWP.

● *Forced vital capacity* is decreased in complicated CWP.

● *Residual volume and total lung capacity* remains normal in simple CWP but is decreased in complicated CWP.

● *Diffusing capacity of the lungs for carbon monoxide* is significantly decreased in complicated CWP because alveolar septae are destroyed and pulmonary capillaries are obliterated.

Arterial blood gas analysis shows the following:

● *Partial pressure of oxygen* is normal in simple CWP but decreased in complicated CWP.

● *Partial pressure of carbon dioxide* usually remains normal in simple CWP but may decrease because of hyperventilation. It may also increase if the patient is hypoxic and has severe impairment of alveolar ventilation.

## Treatment

The goal of treatment is to relieve respiratory symptoms, to manage hypoxia and cor pulmonale, and to avoid respiratory tract irritants and infection. If tuberculosis develops, the patient will need antitubercular therapy.

Respiratory symptoms may be relieved through bronchodilator therapy with theophylline or aminophylline (if bronchospasm is reversible), oral or inhaled sympathomimetic amines (metaproterenol), corticosteroids (oral prednisone or an aerosol form of a corticosteroid), or cromolyn sodium aerosol. Chest physiotherapy techniques, such as controlled coughing and segmental bronchial drainage, combined with chest percussion and vibration help remove secretions.

Other measures include increased fluid intake (at least 3 qt [3 L] daily) and respiratory therapy techniques, such as aerosol therapy, inhaled mucolytics, and intermittent positive-pressure breathing. Diuretics, digitalis glycosides, and salt restriction may be indicated in cor pulmonale.

In severe cases, oxygen may be administered by cannula or mask (1 to 2 L/minute) if the patient has chronic hypoxia or by mechanical ventilation if arterial oxygen can't be maintained above 40 mm Hg. Respiratory infections require prompt administration of antibiotics.

## Special considerations

• Watch for signs of developing tuberculosis.

• Teach the patient to prevent infections by avoiding crowds and persons with respiratory tract infections and by receiving influenza and pneumococcal vaccines.

• Encourage the patient to stay active to avoid a deterioration in his physical condition but to pace his activities and practice relaxation techniques.

# COCCIDIOIDOMYCOSIS

Also known as valley fever and San Joaquin Valley fever, coccidioidomycosis is caused by the fungus *Coccidioides immitis.* It occurs primarily as a respiratory tract infection, although generalized dissemination may occur.

The primary pulmonary form is usually self-limiting and rarely fatal. The rare secondary (progressive, disseminated) form produces abscesses throughout the body and carries a mortality of up to 60%, even with treatment. Such dissemination is more common in dark-skinned men, pregnant women, and patients who are receiving immunosuppressants.

## Causes

Coccidioidomycosis is endemic to the southwestern United States, especially between the San Joaquin Valley in California and southwestern Texas. It's also found in Mexico, Guatemala, Honduras, Venezuela, Colombia, Argentina, and Paraguay.

It may result from inhalation of *C. immitis* spores found in the soil in these areas or from inhalation of spores from dressings or plaster casts of infected persons. It's most prevalent during warm, dry months.

Because of population distribution and an occupational link (it's common in migrant farm laborers), coccidioidomycosis generally strikes Filipino Americans, Mexican Americans, Native Americans, and Blacks. In primary infection, the incubation period is from 1 to 4 weeks.

## Signs and symptoms

Chronic pulmonary cavitation can occur in both the primary and the disseminated forms of coccidioidomycosis, causing hemoptysis with or without chest pain. Other signs and symptoms vary with the form of the disease.

### Primary coccidioidomycosis

Acute or subacute respiratory symptoms (dry cough, pleuritic chest pain, pleural effusion), fever, sore throat, chills, malaise, headache, and an itchy macular rash usually accompany the primary form of the disease. Occasionally, the sole symptom is a fever that persists for weeks. From 3 days to several weeks after onset, some patients, particularly white women, may develop tender red nodules (erythema nodosum) on their legs, especially the shins, with joint pain in the knees and ankles. Generally, the primary form heals spontaneously within a few weeks.

### Disseminated coccidioidomycosis

In rare cases, coccidioidomycosis spreads to other organs several weeks or months after the primary infection. Disseminated coccidioidomycosis causes fever and abscesses throughout the body, especially in skeletal, central nervous system (CNS), splenic, hepatic, renal, and subcutaneous tissues. Depending on the location of these abscesses, disseminated coccidioidomycosis may cause bone pain and meningitis.

## Diagnosis

Typical clinical features and skin and serologic studies confirm the diagnosis. The primary form—and sometimes the disseminated form—produces a positive coccidioidin skin test. In the first week of illness, complement fixation for immunoglobulin G antibodies or, in the first month, positive serum precipitins (immunoglobulins) also establish this diagnosis.

Examination or, more recently, immunodiffusion testing of sputum, pus from lesions, and a tissue biopsy may show *C. immitis* spores. The presence of antibodies in pleural and joint fluid and a rising serum or body fluid antibody titer indicate dissemination.

Other abnormal laboratory results include an increased white blood cell (WBC) count, eosinophilia, increased erythrocyte sedimentation rate, and a chest X-ray showing bilateral diffuse infiltrates.

In coccidioidal meningitis, examination of cerebrospinal fluid shows the WBC count increased to more than $500/\mu l$ (primarily because of mononuclear leukocytes) and increased protein and decreased glucose levels. Ventricular fluid obtained from the brain may contain complement fixation antibodies.

After the diagnosis has been reached, the results of serial skin tests, blood cultures, and serologic testing may document the effectiveness of therapy.

## Treatment

Usually, mild primary coccidioidomycosis requires only bed rest and relief of symptoms. Severe primary disease and dissemination, however, also require long-term I.V. infusion or, in CNS dissemination, intrathecal administration of amphotericin B and, possibly, excision or drainage of lesions. Severe pulmonary lesions may require lobectomy. Miconazole and ketoconazole suppress *C. immitis* but don't eradicate it.

## Special considerations

• Don't wash off the circle marked on the skin for serial skin tests; this aids in reading test results.

• In mild primary disease, encourage bed rest and adequate fluid intake. Record the amount and color of sputum. Watch for shortness of breath that may point to pleural effusion. In patients with arthralgia, provide analgesics.

• Coccidioidomycosis requires strict secretion precautions if the patient has draining lesions. A "no-touch" dressing technique and careful hand washing are essential. No specific isolation precautions are required.

• In CNS dissemination, monitor the patient carefully for a decreased level of consciousness or a change in mood or affect.

• Before intrathecal administration of amphotericin B, explain the procedure to the patient, and reassure him that he'll receive analgesics before a lumbar puncture.

➤ CLINICAL TIP  If the patient is to receive I.V. amphotericin B, infuse it slowly; rapid infusion may cause circulatory collapse. During infusion, monitor his vital signs. (His temperature may rise but should return to normal within 1 to 2 hours.)

• In patients receiving amphotericin B, watch for decreased urine output, and monitor laboratory results for elevated blood urea nitrogen and creatinine levels and hypokalemia. Tell patients to immediately report hearing loss, tinnitus, dizziness, and all signs of toxicity. To ease adverse reactions, give antiemetics and antipyretics.

# COLD INJURIES

Overexposure to cold air or water causes cold injuries. They occur in two major forms: localized injuries (such as frostbite) and systemic injuries (such as hypothermia). Untreated or improperly treated frostbite can lead to gangrene and may necessitate amputation; severe hypothermia can be fatal.

The risk of serious cold injuries, especially hypothermia, is increased by youth, lack of insulating body fat, wet or inadequate clothing, old age, drug abuse, cardiac disease, smoking, fatigue, hunger and depletion of caloric reserves, and excessive alcohol intake (which draws blood into the capillaries and away from body organs).

## Causes
The specific causes of frostbite and hypothermia vary.

### Frostbite
Localized cold injuries occur when ice crystals form in the tissues and expand extracellular spaces. With compression of the tissue cell, the cell membrane ruptures, interrupting enzymatic and metabolic activities. Increased capillary permeability accompanies the release of histamine, resulting in aggregation of red blood cells and microvascular occlusion. Frostbite results from prolonged exposure to dry temperatures far below freezing.

### Hypothermia
Chemical changes result from hypothermia that slow the functions of most major organ systems, such as decreased renal blood flow and decreased glomerular filtration. Hypothermia results from cold-water near-drowning and prolonged exposure to cold temperatures.

## Signs and symptoms
Both frostbite and hypothermia produce distinctive clinical features.

### Frostbite
Two types of frostbite can occur: superficial or deep. Superficial frostbite

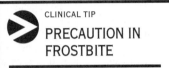

CLINICAL TIP

## PRECAUTION IN FROSTBITE

When treating a patient with frostbite, never rub the injured area. This aggravates tissue damage. Also, be careful not to rupture any blebs.

affects skin and subcutaneous tissue, especially of the face, ears, extremities, and other exposed body areas. Although it may go unnoticed at first, upon returning to a warm place, frostbite produces burning, tingling, numbness, swelling, and a mottled, blue-gray skin color.

Deep frostbite extends beyond subcutaneous tissue and usually affects the hands or feet. The skin becomes white until it's thawed; then it turns purplish blue. Deep frostbite also produces pain, skin blisters, tissue necrosis, and gangrene.

### *Hypothermia*

Indications of hypothermia (a core body temperature below 95° F [35° C]) vary with severity.

• *Mild hypothermia* produces a temperature of 89.6° to 95° F (32° to 35° C), severe shivering, slurred speech, and amnesia.

• *Moderate hypothermia* results in a temperature of 86° to 89.6° F (30° to 32° C), unresponsiveness or confusion, muscle rigidity, peripheral cyanosis and, with improper rewarming, signs of shock.

• In *severe hypothermia,* core temperature drops to 77° to 86° F (25° to 30° C), with loss of deep tendon reflexes and ventricular fibrillation. The patient may appear dead, with no palpable pulse or

audible heart sounds. His pupils may dilate, and he'll appear to be in a state of rigor mortis. A temperature drop below 77° F (25° C) causes cardiopulmonary arrest and death.

### Diagnosis

A history of severe and prolonged exposure to cold may make this diagnosis obvious. Nevertheless, hypothermia can be overlooked if outdoor temperatures are above freezing or if the patient is comatose.

### Treatment

In a localized cold injury, treatment consists of rewarming the injured part, supportive measures and, sometimes (in severe cases), a fasciotomy to increase circulation by lowering edematous tissue pressure. However, if gangrene occurs, amputation may be necessary.

In hypothermia, therapy consists of immediate resuscitative measures, careful monitoring, and gradual rewarming of the body.

### *Frostbite*

• Remove constrictive clothing and jewelry. Slowly rewarm the affected part in tepid water (about 100° to 108° F [37.8° to 42.2° C]). Give the patient warm fluids to drink.

• When the affected part begins to rewarm, the patient will feel pain, so give analgesics. Check for a pulse. If the injury is on the foot, place cotton or gauze sponges between the toes to prevent maceration. (See *Precaution in frostbite.)* Instruct the patient not to walk.

• If the injury has caused an open skin wound, give antibiotics and tetanus prophylaxis.

• Early surgical intervention isn't indicated unless wet gangrene or severe infection of the eschar develops.

CLINICAL TIP Prevent refreezing of thawed tissues because significant tissue damage may occur. Also, it's impossible to assess the depth of frostbite injury in the early stages.

### Hypothermia

• If the patient has no pulse or respiration, begin cardiopulmonary resuscitation (CPR) immediately and, if necessary, continue it for 2 to 3 hours. *(Remember:* Hypothermia helps protect the brain from anoxia, which normally accompanies prolonged cardiopulmonary arrest. Therefore, even after the patient has been unresponsive for a long time, resuscitation may be possible, especially after cold-water near-drownings.) Perform CPR until the patient is adequately rewarmed.

• Move the patient to a warm area, remove wet clothing, and keep him dry. If he's conscious, give warm fluids with high sugar content, such as tea with sugar. If the patient's core temperature is above 89.6° F (32° C), use external warming techniques. Bathe him in water that's 104° F (40° C), cover him with a heating blanket set at 97.9° to 99.9° F (36.6° to 37.7° C), and cautiously apply hot water bottles at 104° F (40° C) to groin and axillae, guarding against burns.

• If the patient's core temperature is below 89.6° F (32° C), use internal and external warming methods. Rewarm his body core and surface 1° to 2° F (0.5° to 1.1° C) per hour concurrently. (If you rewarm the surface first, rewarming shock could cause potentially fatal ventricular fibrillation.)

• To warm inhalations, provide oxygen heated to 107.6° to 114.8° F (42° to 46° C). Infuse I.V. solutions that have been warmed to 98.6° F (37° C), and perform nasogastric lavage with normal saline solution that has been warmed to the same temperature.

• The patient may need peritoneal lavage, using normal saline solution (full or half strength) warmed to 104° to 113° F (40° to 45° C); in severe hypothermia, the patient may need heart and lung bypass at controlled temperatures and thoracotomy with a direct cardiac warm-saline bath. Avoid using central venous catheters in patients with severe hypothermia to prevent arrhythmias.

> CLINICAL TIP  Consider administering antibodies if sepsis is the suspected cause of the hypothermia. Consider steroid use only if adrenal suppression or insufficiency is suspected to be the precipitating cause of the hypothermia.

### Special considerations

• Before discharging the patient with frostbite, tell him about possible long-term effects: increased sensitivity to cold, burning and tingling, and increased sweating. Warn against smoking; this causes vasoconstriction and slows healing.

• During treatment for hypothermia, monitor arterial blood gas values, intake and output, central venous pressure, temperature, and cardiac and neurologic status every half hour. Monitor laboratory results, such as complete blood count, blood urea nitrogen and electrolyte levels, and prothrombin and partial thromboplastin times.

• If the patient is a child, suspect neglect or abuse; make sure a thorough patient history is performed.

• If the patient developed a cold injury because of inadequate clothing or housing, refer him to a community social service agency.

• To help prevent future cold injuries, tell the patient to wear mittens (not gloves); windproof, water-resistant, many-layered clothing; two pairs of socks (cotton next to the skin, then wool); and a scarf and a hat that cover

## STAGING COLORECTAL CANCER

Named for pathologist Cuthbert Dukes, the Dukes Cancer Classification System assigns tumors to four stages. These stages (with substages) reflect the extent of bowel mucosa and bowel wall infiltration, lymph node involvement, and metastasis.

### Stage A
Malignant cells are confined to the bowel mucosa, and the lymph nodes contain no cancer cells. Treated promptly, about 80% of these patients remain disease-free 5 years later.

### Stage B
Malignant cells extend through the bowel mucosa but remain within the bowel wall. The lymph nodes are normal. In substage $B_2$, all bowel wall layers and immediately adjacent structures contain malignant cells, but the lymph nodes remain normal. About 50% of patients with substage $B_2$ survive for 5 or more years.

### Stage C
Malignant cells extend into the bowel wall and the lymph nodes. In substage $C_2$, malignant cells extend through the entire thickness of the bowel wall and into the lymph nodes. The 5-year survival rate for patients with stage C disease is about 25%.

### Stage D
Metastasized to distant organs by way of the lymph nodes and mesenteric vessels, malignant cells typically lodge in the lungs and liver. Only 5% of patients with stage D cancer survive 5 or more years.

the ears (to avoid substantial heat loss through the head).
• Advise the patient not to drink alcohol or smoke and to get adequate food and rest before prolonged exposure.
• Caution the patient to find shelter early or increase physical activity if caught in a severe snowstorm.

# COLORECTAL CANCER

In the United States and Europe, colorectal cancer is the second most common visceral neoplasm. Incidence is equally distributed between men and women.

Colorectal malignant tumors are almost always adenocarcinomas. About half of these are sessile lesions of the rectosigmoid area; the rest are polypoid lesions.

Colorectal cancer tends to progress slowly and remains localized for a long time. Consequently, it's potentially curable in 75% of patients if an early diagnosis allows resection before nodal involvement. With early diagnosis, the overall 5-year survival rate is nearing 50%. (See *Staging colorectal cancer.*)

## Causes
The exact cause of colorectal cancer is unknown, but studies showing concentration in areas of higher economic development suggest a relation to diet (excess animal fat, particularly beef, and low fiber). Other factors that magnify the risk of developing colorectal cancer include:
• other diseases of the digestive tract
• age (over 40)
• history of ulcerative colitis (the average interval before onset of cancer is 11 to 17 years)

- familial polyposis (cancer almost always develops by age 50).

### Signs and symptoms

Manifestations of colorectal cancer result from local obstruction and, in later stages, from direct extension to adjacent organs (bladder, prostate, ureters, vagina, sacrum) and distant metastasis (usually to the liver).

In the early stages, signs and symptoms are typically vague and depend on the anatomical location and function of the bowel segment containing the tumor. Later, they generally include pallor, cachexia, ascites, hepatomegaly, or lymphangiectasis.

#### *Cancer on the right side*

On the right side of the colon (which absorbs water and electrolytes), early tumor growth causes no signs of obstruction because the tumor tends to grow along the bowel rather than surround the lumen, and the fecal content in this area is normally liquid. It may, however, cause black, tarry stool; anemia; and abdominal aching, pressure, or dull cramps.

As the disease progresses, the patient develops weakness, fatigue, exertional dyspnea, vertigo and, eventually, diarrhea, obstipation, anorexia, weight loss, vomiting, and other signs and symptoms of intestinal obstruction. In addition, a tumor on the right side may be palpable.

#### *Cancer on the left side*

On the left side, a tumor causes signs and symptoms of an obstruction even in early stages because in this area, stool is of a formed consistency. It commonly causes rectal bleeding (often ascribed to hemorrhoids), intermittent abdominal fullness or cramping, and rectal pressure.

As the disease progresses, the patient develops obstipation, diarrhea, or "ribbon" or pencil-shaped stool. Typically, he notices that passage of stool or flatus relieves the pain. At this stage, bleeding from the colon becomes obvious, with dark or bright red blood in the stool and mucus in or on the stool.

#### *Rectal tumor signs*

With a rectal tumor, the first symptom is a change in bowel habits, often beginning with an urgent need to defecate on arising ("morning diarrhea") or obstipation alternating with diarrhea. Other indications include blood or mucus in stool and a sense of incomplete evacuation.

Late in the disease, pain begins as a feeling of rectal fullness that later becomes a dull and sometimes constant ache confined to the rectum or sacral region.

### Diagnosis

Only a tumor biopsy can verify colorectal cancer, but the following tests help detect it:

- *Digital examination* can detect almost 15% of colorectal cancers.
- *Hemoccult test* (guaiac) can detect blood in stool.
- *Proctoscopy* or *sigmoidoscopy* can detect up to 66% of colorectal cancers.
- *Colonoscopy* permits visual inspection (and photographs) of the colon up to the ileocecal valve and gives access for polypectomies and biopsies of suspected lesions.
- *Computed tomography scan* helps to detect areas affected by metastasis.
- *Barium X-ray,* utilizing a dual contrast with air, can locate lesions that are undetectable manually or visually. Barium examination should *follow* endoscopy or excretory urography because the barium sulfate interferes with these tests.

• *Carcinoembryonic antigen,* although not specific or sensitive enough for an early diagnosis, is helpful in monitoring patients before and after treatment to detect metastasis or recurrence.

## Treatment

The most effective treatment for colorectal cancer is surgery to remove the malignant tumor and adjacent tissues as well as any lymph nodes that may contain cancer cells. The type of surgery depends on the location of the tumor:

• *Cecum and ascending colon:* A right hemicolectomy (for advanced disease) is performed. It may include resection of the terminal segment of the ileum, cecum, ascending colon, and the right half of the transverse colon with corresponding mesentery.

• *Proximal and middle transverse colon:* A right colectomy is performed that includes the transverse colon and mesentery corresponding to midcolic vessels or segmental resection of the transverse colon and associated midcolic vessels.

• *Sigmoid colon:* Surgery is typically limited to the sigmoid colon and mesentery.

• *Upper rectum:* Anterior or low anterior resection is performed. A newer method, using a stapler, allows for resections much lower than were previously possible.

• *Lower rectum:* Abdominoperineal resection and permanent sigmoid colostomy is performed.

Chemotherapy is indicated for patients with metastasis, residual disease, or a recurrent inoperable tumor. Drugs used in such treatment commonly include fluorouracil with levamisole, leucovorin, methotrexate, or streptozocin. Patients whose tumor has extended to regional lymph nodes may receive fluorouracil and levamisole for 1 year postoperatively.

Radiation therapy induces tumor regression and may be used before or after surgery or combined with chemotherapy, especially fluorouracil.

## Special considerations

Before surgery:

• Monitor the patient's diet modifications, laxatives, enemas, and antibiotics—all are used to clean the bowel and to decrease abdominal and perineal cavity contamination during surgery.

• If the patient is having a colostomy, teach him and his family about the procedure.

• Emphasize that the stoma will be red, moist, and swollen and that postoperative swelling will eventually subside.

• Show them a diagram of the intestine before and after surgery, stressing how much of the bowel will remain intact. Supplement your teaching with instructional aids. Arrange a postsurgical visit from a recovered ostomate.

• Prepare the patient for postoperative I.V. infusions, a nasogastric tube, and an indwelling urinary catheter.

• Discuss the importance of cooperating during deep-breathing and coughing exercises.

After surgery:

• Explain to the patient's family the importance of their positive reactions to the patient's adjustment. Consult with an enterostomal therapist, if available, to help set up a regimen for the patient.

• Encourage the patient to look at the stoma and participate in its care as soon as possible. Teach good hygiene and skin care. Allow him to shower or bathe as soon as the incision heals.

• If appropriate, instruct the patient with a sigmoid colostomy to do his own irrigation as soon as he can after surgery. Advise him to schedule irrigation for the time of day when he normally evacuated before surgery. Many patients find that irrigating every 1 to 3 days is necessary for regularity.

• If flatus, diarrhea, or constipation occurs, eliminate suspected causative foods from the patient's diet. He may reintroduce them later.

• After several months, many ostomates establish control with irrigation and no longer need to wear a pouch. A stoma cap or gauze sponge placed over the stoma protects it and absorbs mucoid secretions.

• Before achieving such control, the patient can resume physical activities, including sports, but he should avoid injury to the stoma or surrounding abdominal muscles.

• Inform the patient that a structured, gradually progressive exercise program to strengthen abdominal muscles may be instituted under medical supervision.

• Instruct the patient to avoid heavy lifting because herniation or prolapse may occur through weakened muscles in the abdominal wall.

• If appropriate, refer the patient to a home health agency for follow-up care and counseling. Suggest sexual counseling for male patients; most are impotent after an abdominoperineal resection.

➤ CLINICAL TIP  Anyone who's had colorectal cancer is at increased risk for another primary cancer. Instruct the patient to have yearly screening and testing and to maintain a high-fiber diet.

# COMMON COLD

The common cold—an acute, usually afebrile viral infection—causes inflammation of the upper respiratory tract. It accounts for more time lost from school or work than any other cause and is the most common infectious disease.

Although it's benign and self-limiting, it can lead to secondary bacterial infections.

## Causes

The common cold is more prevalent in children than in adults; in adolescent boys than in girls; and in women than in men. In temperate zones, it occurs more often in the colder months; in the tropics, during the rainy season.

About 90% of colds stem from a viral infection of the upper respiratory passages and consequent mucous membrane inflammation; occasionally, colds result from *Mycoplasma*.

Over a hundred viruses can cause the common cold. Major offenders include rhinoviruses, coronaviruses, myxoviruses, adenoviruses, coxsackieviruses, and echoviruses.

Transmission occurs through airborne respiratory droplets, contact with contaminated objects, and hand-to-hand transmission. Children acquire new strains from their schoolmates and pass them on to family members. Fatigue or drafts don't increase susceptibility.

## Signs and symptoms

After a 1- to 4-day incubation period, the common cold produces pharyngitis, nasal congestion, rhinitis, headache, and burning, watery eyes; there may be fever (in children), chills, myalgia, arthralgia, malaise, lethargy, and a hacking, nonproductive, or nocturnal cough.

As the cold progresses, clinical features develop more fully. After a day, symptoms include a feeling of fullness with a copious nasal discharge that often irritates the nose, adding to discomfort. About 3 days after onset, major signs diminish, but the "stuffed-up" feeling often persists for a week.

Reinfection (with productive cough) is common, but complications (sinusitis, otitis media, pharyngitis, lower respiratory tract infection) are rare. A cold is communicable for 2 to 3 days after the onset of symptoms.

## Diagnosis

No explicit diagnostic test exists to isolate the specific organisms responsible for the common cold. Consequently, the diagnosis rests on a cold's typically mild, localized, and afebrile upper respiratory symptoms. Despite infection, white blood cell count and differential are within normal limits.

A diagnosis must rule out allergic rhinitis, measles, rubella, and other disorders that produce similar early symptoms. A temperature higher than 100° F (37.8 C), severe malaise, anorexia, tachycardia, exudate on the tonsils or throat, petechiae, and tender lymph glands may point to more serious disorders and require additional diagnostic tests.

## Treatment

The primary treatment—aspirin or acetaminophen, fluids, and rest—is purely symptomatic because the common cold has no cure. Aspirin eases myalgia and headache; fluids help loosen accumulated respiratory secretions and maintain hydration; and rest combats fatigue and weakness. In a child with a fever, acetaminophen is the drug of choice.

Decongestants can relieve congestion. Throat lozenges relieve soreness. Steam encourages expectoration. In infants, saline nose drops and mucus aspiration with a bulb syringe may be beneficial.

Nasal douching, sinus drainage, and antibiotics aren't necessary except in complications or chronic illness. Pure antitussives relieve severe coughs but are contraindicated with productive coughs, when cough suppression is harmful. The role of vitamin C and zinc remain controversial.

Currently, no known measure can prevent the common cold. Vitamin therapy, interferon administration, and ultraviolet irradiation are under investigation.

## Special considerations

● Emphasize that antibiotics don't cure the common cold.

● Tell the patient to maintain bed rest during the first few days, use a lubricant on his nostrils to decrease irritation, relieve throat irritation with hard candy or cough drops, increase his fluid intake, and eat light meals.

● Inform the patient that warm baths or heating pads can reduce aches and pains but won't hasten a cure. Suggest hot or cold steam vaporizers. Commercial expectorants are available, but their effectiveness is questionable.

➤ CLINICAL TIP Advise the patient against overuse of nose drops or sprays; they may cause rebound congestion.

● To help prevent colds, warn the patient to minimize contact with people who have colds.

● To avoid spreading colds, teach the patient to wash his hands often, to cover coughs and sneezes, and to avoid sharing towels and drinking glasses.

# COMMON VARIABLE IMMUNODEFICIENCY

Also called acquired hypogammaglobulinemia and agammaglobulinemia with immunoglobulin-bearing B cells, common variable immunodeficiency is characterized by progressive deterioration of B-cell (humoral) immunity. This results in increased susceptibility to infection.

Unlike X-linked hypogammaglobulinemia (which is seen in very early childhood), this disorder usually causes symptoms after infancy and childhood, between ages 25 and 40. It affects men and women equally and usually doesn't interfere with normal life span or with normal pregnancy and offspring.

## Causes

Exactly what causes common variable immunodeficiency isn't known. Most patients have a normal circulating B-cell count but defective synthesis or release of immunoglobulins. Many also exhibit progressive deterioration of T-cell (cell-mediated) immunity, which is revealed by delayed hypersensitivity skin testing.

## Signs and symptoms

In common variable immunodeficiency, pyogenic bacterial infections are characteristic but tend to be chronic rather than acute (as in X-linked hypogammaglobulinemia). Recurrent sinopulmonary infections, chronic bacterial conjunctivitis, and malabsorption (often associated with infestation by *Giardia lamblia*) are usually the first clues to immunodeficiency.

Common variable immunodeficiency may be associated with autoimmune diseases, such as systemic lupus erythematosus, rheumatoid arthritis, hemolytic anemia, and pernicious anemia, as well as with cancers, such as leukemia and lymphoma.

CLINICAL TIP Patients with common variable immunodeficiency can develop a nonseptic inflammatory arthritis similar to rheumatoid arthritis. However, because septic arthritis has also been reported, a search for an infecting organism should be undertaken in patients with new joint pain and inflammation, particularly if only one or two joints are affected.

## Diagnosis

Characteristic diagnostic markers in this disorder include decreased serum immunoglobulin M (IgM), IgA, and IgG detected by immunoelectrophoresis, along with a normal circulating B-cell count. Antigenic stimulation confirms an inability to produce specific antibodies; cell-mediated immunity may be intact or delayed. X-rays usually show signs of chronic lung disease or sinusitis.

## Treatment

Patients with common variable immunodeficiency need essentially the same treatment as patients with X-linked hypogammaglobulinemia.

Injection of immune globulin (usually weekly to monthly) helps maintain immune response. Because immune globulin is composed primarily of IgG, the patient may also need fresh frozen plasma infusions to provide IgA and IgM.

Antibiotics are the mainstay for combating infection. Regular X-rays and pulmonary function studies help monitor infection in the lungs; chest physiotherapy may forestall or help clear such infection.

## Special considerations

● Because immune globulin injections are very painful, give them deep into a large muscle mass, such as the gluteal or thigh muscles, and massage well. If the dose is more than 1.5 ml, divide the dose and inject it into more than one site; for frequent injections, rotate the injection sites.

● To help prevent severe infection, teach the patient and his family how to recognize its early signs. Warn them to avoid crowds and persons who have active infections.

● Stress the importance of good nutrition and regular follow-up care.

# COMPLEMENT DEFICIENCIES

A series of circulating enzymatic serum proteins with nine functional components make up complement. Components of complement are labeled C1 through C9. The first four complement components are numbered out of sequence (in order of their discovery) — C1, C4, C2, and C3 — but the remaining five are numbered sequentially.

When immunoglobulin G (IgG) or IgM reacts with antigens as part of an immune response, they activate C1, which then combines with C4, initiating the classic complement pathway, or cascade. (An alternative complement pathway involves the direct activation of C3 by the serum protein properdin, bypassing the initial components [C1, C4, C2] of the classic pathway.)

Complement then combines with the antigen-antibody complex and undergoes a sequence of reactions that amplify the immune response against the antigen. This complex process is called complement fixation.

Complement deficiency or dysfunction may increase susceptibility to infection due to defective phagocytosis of bacteria, for example. There may also be a relation to certain autoimmune disorders. Theoretically, any complement component may be deficient or dysfunctional, and many such disorders are under investigation.

Primary complement deficiencies are rare. The most common ones are C2, C4, C6, and C8 deficiencies and C5 familial dysfunction.

More common secondary complement abnormalities have been confirmed in patients with lupus erythematosus, in some with dermatomyositis, in one with scleroderma (and in his family), and in a few with gonococcal and meningococcal infections. The prognosis varies with the abnormality and the severity of associated diseases.

**Causes**
Primary complement deficiencies are inherited as autosomal recessive traits, except for deficiency of C1 esterase inhibitor, which is autosomal dominant. Secondary deficiencies may follow complement-fixing (complement-consuming) immunologic reactions, such as drug-induced serum sickness, acute streptococcal glomerulonephritis, and acute active systemic lupus erythematosus.

**Signs and symptoms**
Clinical effects vary with the specific deficiency as follows:
• C2 and C3 deficiencies and C5 familial dysfunction increase susceptibility to bacterial infection (which may involve several body systems simultaneously).
• C2 and C4 deficiencies are also associated with collagen vascular disease, such as lupus erythematosus, and with chronic renal failure.
• C5 dysfunction, a familial defect in infants, causes failure to thrive, diarrhea, and seborrheic dermatitis.
• Defects in latter components of the complement cascade (C5 to C9) may lead to increased susceptibility to infections with *Neisseria* species.
• C1 esterase inhibitor deficiency (hereditary angioedema) may cause periodic swelling in the face, hands, abdomen, or throat, with potentially fatal laryngeal edema.

**Diagnosis**
Careful interpretation of both clinical features and laboratory results helps to make this difficult diagnosis. Total

serum complement level (CH50) is low in various complement deficiencies.

In addition, specific assays may be done to confirm deficiency of specific complement components. For example, detection of complement components and IgG by immunofluorescent examination of glomerular tissues in glomerulonephritis strongly suggests complement deficiency.

### Treatment

Primary complement deficiencies have no known cure. Associated infection, collagen vascular disease, or renal disease requires prompt, appropriate treatment.

Transfusion of fresh frozen plasma to provide replacement of complement components is controversial because replacement therapy doesn't cure complement deficiencies and any beneficial effects are transient. Bone marrow transplantation may be helpful but can cause a potentially fatal graft-versus-host (GVH) reaction. Anabolic steroids, such as danazol, and antifibrinolytic agents are often used to reduce acute swelling in patients with hereditary angioedema.

### Special considerations

• Teach the patient (or his family, if he's a child) the importance of avoiding infection, how to recognize its early signs and symptoms, and the need for prompt treatment if it occurs.

• After bone marrow transplantation, monitor the patient closely for signs of transfusion reaction and GVH reaction.

• Provide meticulous patient care to help speed recovery and prevent complications. A patient with renal infection, for example, will need careful monitoring of intake and output, tests for serum electrolytes and acid-base balance, and observation for signs of renal failure.

➤ CLINICAL TIP  When caring for a patient with hereditary angioedema, be prepared for emergency management of laryngeal edema; keep airway equipment on hand. Also, consider giving the patient a medical identification bracelet.

# CONCUSSION

By far the most common head injury, concussion results from a blow to the head — a blow hard enough to jostle the brain and make it hit against the skull, causing temporary neural dysfunction, but not hard enough to cause a cerebral contusion. Most concussion victims recover completely within 24 to 48 hours. Repeated concussions, however, exact a cumulative toll on the brain.

### Causes

The blow that causes a concussion is usually sudden and forceful — a fall to the ground, a punch to the head, a motor vehicle accident. Also, such a blow sometimes results from child abuse. Whatever the cause, the resulting injury is mild compared with the damage done by cerebral contusions or lacerations.

### Signs and symptoms

Concussion may produce a short-term loss of consciousness, vomiting, and both anterograde and retrograde amnesia, in which the patient not only can't recall what happened immediately after the injury but also has difficulty recalling events that led up to the traumatic incident. The presence of anterograde amnesia and the duration of retrograde amnesia reliably correlate with the severity of the injury.

The injury often causes adults to be irritable or lethargic, to behave out of character, and to complain of dizziness, nausea, or severe headache. Some children have no apparent ill effects, but many grow lethargic and somnolent in a few hours.

> CLINICAL TIP Although all of the above signs occur normally with a concussion, they may also result from more serious head injuries. Medical evaluation is necessary to rule out serious injury to the brain.

Postconcussion syndrome — characterized by headache, dizziness, vertigo, anxiety, and fatigue — may persist for several weeks after the injury.

### Diagnosis

Differentiating between concussion and more serious head injuries requires a thorough history of the trauma and a neurologic examination. Such an examination must evaluate the patient's level of consciousness (LOC), mental status, cranial nerve and motor function, deep tendon reflexes, and orientation to time, place, and person.

If no abnormalities are found and if severe head injury appears unlikely, the patient should be observed for signs of more severe cerebral trauma. Observation provides a baseline for gauging any deterioration in the patient's condition.

Computed tomography (CT) scans may rule out fractures and more serious injuries; obtain them whenever you suspect severe head injuries. Skull X-rays remain controversial and are, in any case, being supplanted by CT scans.

### Treatment and special considerations

• Obtain a thorough history of the trauma from the patient (if he's not suffering from amnesia), his family, eyewitnesses, or ambulance personnel. Ask whether the patient lost consciousness.

• Monitor vital signs and check for additional injuries. Palpate the skull for tenderness or hematomas.

• If the patient has an altered LOC or if a neurologic examination reveals abnormalities, the injury may be more severe than a concussion; in such a case, the patient should undergo a CT scan and a neurosurgeon should be consulted immediately.

• If a neurologic examination reveals no abnormalities, observe the patient in the emergency department. Check his vital signs, LOC, and pupil size every 15 minutes. The patient who's stable after 4 or more hours of observation can be discharged (with a head injury instruction sheet) in the care of a responsible adult.

# CONJUNCTIVITIS

Hyperemia of the conjunctiva from infection, allergy, or chemical reactions characterizes conjunctivitis. Bacterial and viral conjunctivitis are highly contagious but are also self-limiting after two weeks' duration. Chronic conjunctivitis may result in degenerative changes to the eyelids. In the Western hemisphere, conjunctivitis is probably the most common eye disorder.

### Causes

The most common causative organisms are the following:

• *bacterial: Staphylococcus aureus, Streptococcus pneumoniae, Neisseria gonorrhoeae, Neisseria meningitidis*
• *chlamydial: Chlamydia trachomatis* (inclusion conjunctivitis)
• *viral:* adenovirus types 3, 7, and 8; herpes simplex virus type 1.

Other causes include allergic reactions to pollen, grass, topical medications, air pollutants, and smoke; occupational irritants (acids and alkalies); rickettsial diseases (Rocky Mountain spotted fever); parasitic diseases caused by *Phthirus pubis* and *Schistosoma haematobium;* and, rarely, fungal infections.

Vernal conjunctivitis (also called seasonal or warm-weather conjunctivitis) results from allergy to an unidentified allergen. This form of conjunctivitis is bilateral; it usually begins before puberty and persists for about 10 years. Sometimes it's associated with other signs and symptoms of allergy commonly related to grass or pollen sensitivity.

An idiopathic form of conjunctivitis may be associated with certain systemic diseases, such as erythema multiforme, chronic follicular conjunctivitis (orphan's conjunctivitis), thyroid disease, and Stevens-Johnson syndrome. Conjunctivitis may be secondary to pneumococcal dacryocystitis or canaliculitis from candidal infection.

### Signs and symptoms

Conjunctivitis commonly produces hyperemia of the conjunctiva, sometimes accompanied by discharge and tearing. It generally doesn't affect vision unless there's corneal involvement, which also causes pain and photophobia. Conjunctivitis usually begins in one eye and rapidly spreads to the other by contamination of towels and washcloths or by the patient's own hands.

### *Acute bacterial form*

In acute bacterial conjunctivitis (pinkeye), the infection usually lasts only 2 weeks. The patient typically complains of itching, burning, and the sensation of a foreign body in his eye. The eyelids show a crust of sticky, mucopurulent discharge. If the disorder stems from

*N. gonorrhoeae,* however, the patient exhibits a profuse, purulent discharge.

### *Viral form*

Viral conjunctivitis produces copious tearing with minimal exudate and enlargement of the preauricular lymph node. Some viruses follow a chronic course and produce severe disabling disease; others last 2 to 3 weeks.

### Diagnosis

Physical examination reveals injection of the bulbar conjunctival vessels. In children, possible systemic symptoms include sore throat and fever.

Monocytes are predominant in stained smears of conjunctival scrapings if conjunctivitis is caused by a virus. Polymorphonuclear cells (neutrophils) predominate if conjunctivitis stems from bacteria; eosinophils, if it's allergy-related. Culture and sensitivity tests identify the causative bacterial organism and indicate appropriate antibiotic therapy.

### Treatment

The cause of conjunctivitis dictates the treatment. Bacterial conjunctivitis requires topical application of the appropriate antibiotic or sulfonamide.

Although viral conjunctivitis resists treatment, broad-spectrum antibiotic eyedrops may prevent secondary infection.

Herpes simplex infection generally responds to treatment with trifluridine drops, vidarabine ointment, or oral acyclovir, but the infection may persist for 2 to 3 weeks. Treatment of vernal (allergic) conjunctivitis includes administration of corticosteroid drops followed by lodoxamide tromethamine (Alomide), a histamine$_1$-antagonist, cold compresses to relieve itching and, occasionally, oral antihistamines.

Instillation of a one-time dose of erythromycin into the eyes of newborns prevents gonococcal and chlamydial conjunctivitis.

**Special considerations**
• Teach proper hand-washing technique because some forms of conjunctivitis are highly contagious. Stress the risk of spreading infection to family members by sharing washcloths, towels, and pillows. Warn against rubbing the infected eye, which can spread the infection to the other eye and to other persons.
• Apply warm compresses and therapeutic ointment or drops. Don't irrigate the eye; this will only spread infection. Have the patient wash his hands before he uses the medication, and use clean washcloths or towels frequently so he doesn't infect his other eye.
• Teach the patient to instill eyedrops and ointments correctly—without touching the bottle tip to his eye or lashes.
• Stress the importance of safety glasses for the patient who works near chemical irritants.
• Notify public health authorities if cultures show *N. gonorrhoeae.*

➤ CLINICAL TIP If ointments are prescribed, remind the patient that ointment blurs vision.

# COR PULMONALE

The World Health Organization defines chronic cor pulmonale as "hypertrophy of the right ventricle resulting from diseases affecting the function and/or the structure of the lungs, except when these pulmonary alterations are the result of diseases that primarily affect the left side of the heart or of congenital heart disease."

Invariably, cor pulmonale follows some disorder of the lungs, pulmonary vessels, chest wall, or respiratory control center. For instance, chronic obstructive pulmonary disease (COPD) produces pulmonary hypertension, which leads to right ventricular hypertrophy and right-sided heart failure. Because cor pulmonale generally occurs late during the course of COPD and other irreversible diseases, the prognosis is generally poor.

**Causes**
Approximately 85% of patients with cor pulmonale have COPD, and 25% of patients with COPD eventually develop cor pulmonale.

Other respiratory disorders that produce cor pulmonale include:
• obstructive lung diseases — for example, bronchiectasis and cystic fibrosis
• restrictive lung diseases — for example, pneumoconiosis, interstitial pneumonitis, scleroderma, and sarcoidosis
• loss of lung tissue after extensive lung surgery
• pulmonary vascular diseases, such as recurrent thromboembolism, primary pulmonary hypertension, schistosomiasis, and pulmonary vasculitis
• respiratory insufficiency without pulmonary disease as seen in chest wall disorders, such as kyphoscoliosis, neuromuscular incompetence resulting from muscular dystrophy and amyotrophic lateral sclerosis, polymyositis, and spinal cord lesions above C6
• obesity hypoventilation syndrome (pickwickian syndrome) and upper airway obstruction
• living at high altitudes (chronic mountain sickness).

*Pathophysiology*
Pulmonary capillary destruction and pulmonary vasoconstriction (usually secondary to hypoxia) reduce the cross-sectional area of the pulmonary vascu-

lar bed. This increases pulmonary vascular resistance and causes pulmonary hypertension.

To compensate for the extra work needed to force blood through the lungs, the right ventricle dilates and hypertrophies. In response to low oxygen content, the bone marrow produces more red blood cells, causing erythrocytosis. When the hematocrit exceeds 55%, blood viscosity increases, which further aggravates pulmonary hypertension and increases the hemodynamic load on the right ventricle. Right-sided heart failure is the result.

### Incidence

Cor pulmonale accounts for about 25% of all types of heart failure. It's most common in areas of the world where the incidence of cigarette smoking and COPD is high.

Cor pulmonale affects middle-aged to elderly men more often than women, but its incidence in women is increasing. In children, cor pulmonale may be a complication of cystic fibrosis, hemosiderosis, upper airway obstruction, scleroderma, extensive bronchiectasis, neurologic diseases affecting respiratory muscles, or abnormalities of the respiratory control center.

### Signs and symptoms

As long as the heart can compensate for the increased pulmonary vascular resistance, clinical features reflect the underlying disorder and occur mostly in the respiratory system. They include chronic productive cough, exertional dyspnea, wheezing respirations, fatigue, and weakness.

Progression of cor pulmonale is associated with dyspnea (even at rest) that worsens on exertion, tachypnea, orthopnea, edema, weakness, and right upper quadrant discomfort. Chest examination reveals findings characteristic of the underlying lung disease.

Signs of cor pulmonale and right-sided heart failure include dependent edema; distended neck veins; enlarged, tender liver; prominent parasternal or epigastric cardiac impulse; hepatojugular reflux; and tachycardia.

Decreased cardiac output may cause a weak pulse and hypotension.

### Thoracic assessment

Chest examination yields various findings, depending on the underlying cause of cor pulmonale. In COPD, auscultation reveals wheezing, rhonchi, and diminished breath sounds. When the disease is secondary to upper airway obstruction or damage to central nervous system respiratory centers, chest findings may be normal except for a right ventricular lift, gallop rhythm, and loud pulmonic component of $S_2$.

Tricuspid insufficiency produces a pansystolic murmur heard at the lower left sternal border; its intensity increases on inspiration, distinguishing it from a murmur caused by mitral valve disease. A right ventricular early murmur that increases on inspiration can be heard at the left sternal border or over the epigastrium. A systolic pulmonic ejection click may also be heard.

Drowsiness and alterations in consciousness may occur.

### Diagnosis

Pulmonary artery pressure (PAP) measurements show increased right ventricular and PAPs as a result of increased pulmonary vascular resistance. Right ventricular systolic and pulmonary artery (PA) systolic pressures will exceed 30 mm Hg. PA diastolic pressure will exceed 15 mm Hg.

● *Echocardiography* or *angiography* indicates right ventricular enlargement, and echocardiography can estimate PAP.

• *Chest X-ray* shows large central pulmonary arteries and suggests right ventricular enlargement by rightward enlargement of cardiac silhouette on an anterior chest film.

• *Arterial blood gas (ABG) analysis* shows decreased partial pressure of arterial oxygen ($PaO_2$) < 70 mm Hg.

• *Electrocardiography* frequently shows arrhythmias, such as premature atrial and ventricular contractions and atrial fibrillation during severe hypoxia; it may also show right bundle-branch heart block, right axis deviation, prominent P waves and an inverted T wave in right precordial leads, and right ventricular hypertrophy.

• *Pulmonary function tests* show results consistent with the underlying pulmonary disease.

• *Hematocrit* is often greater than 50%.

## Treatment

The goals of treatment include reducing hypoxemia, increasing the patient's exercise tolerance and, when possible, correcting the underlying condition. In addition to bed rest, treatment may include administration of:

• *digitalis glycosides* (digoxin)

➤ CLINICAL TIP Digitalis glycosides (digoxin) are of questionable value and may increase the risk of toxicity.

• *antibiotics* when respiratory tract infection is present (a culture and sensitivity of a sputum specimen aids in the selection of antibiotics)

• *potent PA vasodilators* (such as diazoxide, nitroprusside, hydralazine, angiotensin-converting enzyme inhibitors, calcium channel blockers, and prostaglandins) in primary pulmonary hypertension

• *oxygen* by mask or cannula in concentrations ranging from 24% to 40%, depending on $PaO_2$, as necessary; in acute cases, therapy may also include

mechanical ventilation; patients with underlying COPD generally shouldn't receive high concentrations of oxygen because of possible subsequent respiratory depression

• *low-sodium diet, restricted fluid intake*, and *diuretics,* such as furosemide, to reduce edema

• *anticoagulation* with small doses of heparin to reduce the risk of thromboembolism.

Depending on the underlying cause, some variations in treatment may be necessary. For example, a tracheotomy may be necessary if the patient has an upper airway obstruction, and steroids may be used in patients with a vasculitis autoimmune phenomenon or acute exacerbations of COPD.

## Special considerations

• The patient will need a diet carefully planned in consultation with the staff dietitian. Because the patient may lack energy and tire easily when eating, provide small, frequent feedings rather than three heavy meals.

• Prevent fluid retention by limiting the patient's fluid intake to 1,000 to 2,000 ml/day and providing a low-sodium diet.

• Monitor serum potassium levels closely if the patient is receiving diuretics. Low serum potassium levels can potentiate the risk of arrhythmias associated with digitalis glycosides.

• Watch the patient for signs of digitalis toxicity, such as complaints of anorexia, nausea, vomiting, and yellow halos around visual images; monitor for cardiac arrhythmias.

• Teach the patient to check his radial pulse before taking digoxin or any digitalis glycoside and to report any changes in pulse rate.

• Reposition bedridden patients often to prevent atelectasis.

• Provide meticulous respiratory care, including oxygen therapy and, for

COPD patients, pursed-lip breathing exercises.

• Periodically measure ABG values and watch for signs of respiratory failure, such as a change in pulse rate; deep, labored respirations; and increased fatigue produced by exertion.

Before discharge:

• Provide the patient with information about the disorder. (See *Living with cor pulmonale*.)

• If the patient needs suctioning or supplemental oxygen therapy at home, refer him to a social service agency that can help him obtain the necessary equipment, and, as necessary, arrange for follow-up examinations.

# CORNEAL ABRASION

Often caused by a foreign body, a corneal abrasion is a scratch on the surface epithelium of the cornea. An abrasion or foreign body in the eye is the most common eye injury. With treatment, the prognosis is usually good.

## Causes

A corneal abrasion usually results from a foreign body, such as a cinder or a piece of dust, dirt, or grit, that becomes embedded under the eyelid. Even if the foreign body is washed out by tears, it may still injure the cornea.

A small piece of metal that gets in the eyes of workers who don't wear protective glasses quickly forms an abrasion and then forms a rust ring on the cornea. Such abrasions also commonly occur in the eyes of people who fall asleep wearing hard contact lenses.

A corneal scratch produced by a fingernail, a piece of paper, or another organic substance may cause a persistent lesion. The epithelium doesn't always

---

> **TEACHING CHECKLIST**
>
> ## ✔ LIVING WITH COR PULMONALE
>
> Make sure your patient understands:
>
> • importance of low-sodium diet
> • need to weigh self daily
> • how to detect edema and report it immediately
> • need for frequent rest periods
> • need to perform breathing exercises daily
> • how to detect and report early signs of pulmonary infection (increased sputum production, change in sputum color, increased coughing or wheezing, chest pain, fever, tightness in chest)
> • to avoid crowds and persons with respiratory tract infections, especially during flu season
> • to avoid nonprescribed medications, such as sedatives, which may depress ventilation time.

---

heal properly, and a recurrent corneal erosion may develop, with delayed effects more severe than those of the original injury.

## Signs and symptoms

Typically, corneal abrasions produce redness, increased tearing, a sensation of "something in the eye" and, because the cornea is richly endowed with nerve endings from the trigeminal nerve (cranial nerve V), pain disproportionate to the size of the injury. A corneal abrasion may affect visual acuity, depending on the size and location of the injury.

## Diagnosis

A history of eye trauma or prolonged wearing of contact lenses as well as typical symptoms suggest corneal abrasion. Staining the cornea with fluorescein stain confirms the diagnosis: The injured area appears green when examined with a flashlight. Slit-lamp examination discloses the depth of the abrasion.

Examining the eye with a flashlight may reveal a foreign body on the cornea; the eyelid must be everted to check for a foreign body embedded under the lid.

Before beginning treatment, a test to determine visual acuity provides a medical baseline and a legal safeguard.

### Treatment

The first steps in treatment include examining the eye and checking visual acuity. If the foreign object is visible, the eye can be irrigated with normal saline solution.

Removal of a deeply embedded foreign body is done with a foreign-body spud, using a topical anesthetic. A rust ring on the cornea must be removed at the slit-lamp examination with an ophthalmic burr, after applying a topical anesthetic. When only partial removal is possible, reepithelialization lifts the ring again to the surface and allows complete removal the next day.

Treatment also includes instillation of a cycloplegic eyedrop and broad-spectrum antibiotic eyedrops in the affected eye every 3 to 4 hours.

➤ CLINICAL TIP A pressure patch may be applied in some cases, but it's never used if the abrasion was caused by contact lens use.

### Special considerations

• Tell the patient with an eye patch to leave the patch in place for 6 to 8 hours, then to begin the antibiotic drug regimen. Wearing a patch alters depth perception, so advise caution in everyday activities, such as climbing stairs or stepping off a curb.

• Reassure the patient that the corneal epithelium usually heals in 24 to 48 hours.

• Stress the importance of instilling prescribed antibiotic eyedrops because an untreated corneal infection can lead to ulceration and permanent loss of vision. Teach the patient the proper way to instill eye medications.

• Emphasize the importance of safety glasses to protect workers' eyes from flying fragments. Also review instructions for wearing and caring for contact lenses.

# CORNEAL ULCERS

A major cause of blindness worldwide, corneal ulcers produce corneal scarring or perforation. They occur in the central or marginal areas of the cornea, vary in shape and size, and may be singular or multiple. Marginal ulcers, caused by a sensitivity to *Staphylococcus aureus,* are the most common form. Prompt treatment (within hours of onset) can prevent visual impairment.

### Causes

Corneal ulcers generally result from bacterial, protozoan, viral, or fungal infections. Common bacterial sources include *Staphylococcus aureus, Pseudomonas aeruginosa, Streptococcus viridans, Streptococcus (Diplococcus) pneumoniae,* and *Moraxella liquefaciens;* viral sources, herpes simplex type 1, and varicella-zoster viruses; and common fungi, such as *Candida, Fusarium,* and *Cephalosporium.*

Other causes include trauma, exposure, reactions to bacterial infections, toxins, and allergens. Tuberculoprotein causes a classic phlyctenular keratoconjunctivitis; vitamin A deficiency results in xerophthalmia; and fifth cranial nerve lesions, in neurotropic ulcers.

### Signs and symptoms
Typically, corneal ulceration begins with pain (aggravated by blinking) and photophobia, followed by increased tearing. Eventually, central corneal ulceration produces pronounced visual blurring. The eye may appear injected (red). If a bacterial ulcer is present, purulent discharge is possible.

### Diagnosis
A history of trauma or use of contact lenses and a flashlight examination that reveals an irregular corneal surface suggest corneal ulcer. Exudate may be present on the cornea, and a hypopion (accumulation of white cells in the anterior chamber) may appear as a half-moon.

Fluorescein dye, instilled in the conjunctival sac, delineates the outline of the ulcer. Culture and sensitivity testing of corneal scrapings, which may identify the causative bacteria or fungus, indicate appropriate antibiotic or antifungal therapy.

### Treatment
Prompt treatment is essential for all forms of corneal ulcer to prevent complications and permanent visual impairment. Treatment aims to eliminate the underlying cause of the ulcer and to relieve pain.

Until culture results identify the causative organism, treatment consists of topical broad-spectrum antibiotics. Once the causative agent is identified, specific treatments vary.

● *P. aeruginosa infection* is treated with ciprofloxacin (Ciloxan), gentamicin, or tobramycin, administered topically. This type of corneal ulcer can cause corneal perforation and loss of the eye very rapidly if left untreated. Immediate treatment and isolation of hospitalized patients are required.

A corneal ulcer should never be patched because patching creates the dark, warm, moist environment ideal for bacterial growth. However, it should be protected with a perforated shield.

● *Herpes simplex type I virus* is treated with hourly topical applications of idoxuridine or vidarabine. Corneal ulcers resulting from this viral infection often recur. Trifluridine is the treatment of choice.

● *Fungi* are treated with topical instillation of natamycin for *Fusarium, Cephalosporium,* and *Candida.*

● *Hypovitaminosis A* requires correction of dietary deficiency or GI malabsorption of vitamin A.

● *Neurotropic ulcers* or *exposure keratitis* is treated with frequent instillation of artificial tears or lubricating ointments and use of a plastic bubble eye shield or by a tarsorrhaphy (suturing the eyelids together).

### Special considerations
● Because corneal ulcers are quite painful, give analgesics as needed.

➤ CLINICAL TIP Because an associated iridocyclitis occurs when the cornea is involved, cycloplegic eyedrops are given to reduce ciliary body spasms.
● Watch for signs of secondary glaucoma (transient vision loss and halos around lights).
● The patient may be more comfortable in a darkened room or when wearing dark glasses.

# CORNS AND CALLUSES

Usually located on areas of repeated trauma (most often the feet), corns and calluses are acquired skin conditions marked by hyperkeratosis of the stratum corneum. The prognosis is good with proper foot care.

## Causes and incidence

A corn is a hyperkeratotic area that usually results from external pressure such as that from ill-fitting shoes. Less commonly, it results from internal pressure such as that caused by an underlying congenital or acquired bone deformity (from arthritis, for example).

A callus is an area of thickened skin, generally found on the foot or hand, produced by external pressure or friction. Persons whose activities produce repeated trauma (for example, manual laborers or guitarists) commonly develop calluses.

The severity of a corn or callus depends on the degree and duration of trauma.

## Signs and symptoms

Both corns and calluses cause pain through pressure on underlying tissue by localized thickened skin.

### Corns

Containing a central keratinous core, corns are smaller and more clearly defined than calluses and are usually more painful. The pain they cause may be dull and constant or sharp when pressure is applied.

Soft corns are caused by the pressure of a bony prominence. They appear as whitish thickenings and are commonly found between the toes, most often in the fourth interdigital web. Hard corns are sharply delineated and conical and appear most frequently over the dorsolateral aspect of the fifth toe.

### Calluses

Often quite large, calluses have indefinite borders. They may be asymptomatic or produce dull pain on pressure, rather than constant pain. Calluses are distinguished from plantar warts by the presence of normal skin markings.

## Diagnosis

Careful physical examination of the affected area and a patient history revealing chronic trauma or pressure lead to a diagnosis.

## Treatment

Surgical debridement may be performed to remove the nucleus of a corn, usually under a local anesthetic.

In intermittent debridement, keratolytics — usually 40% salicylic acid plasters — are applied to affected areas. Injections of corticosteroids beneath the corn may be necessary to relieve pain.

However, the simplest and best treatment is essentially preventive avoidance of trauma. Corns and calluses disappear after the source of trauma has been removed. Metatarsal pads may redistribute the weight-bearing areas of the foot; corn pads may prevent painful pressure.

Patients with persistent corns or calluses require referral to a podiatrist or dermatologist; those with corns or calluses caused by a bony malformation, as in arthritis, require orthopedic consultation.

## Special considerations

● Teach the patient how to apply salicylic acid plasters. Make sure the plaster is large enough to cover the affected area. Place the sticky side down on the foot, then cover the plaster with adhesive tape.

● Plasters are usually taken off after an overnight application but may be left in place for as long as 7 days. After removing the plaster, instruct the patient to soak the area in water and abrade the soft, macerated skin with a towel or pumice stone. Instruct the patient how to reapply the plaster and to repeat the entire procedure until all the hyperkeratotic skin has been removed.

• Warn the patient against removing corns or calluses with a sharp instrument, such as a razor blade.

• Advise the patient to wear properly fitted shoes. Suggest the use of metatarsal or corn pads to relieve pressure. Refer the patient to a podiatrist, dermatologist, or orthopedist, if necessary.

• Assure the patient that good foot care can correct this condition.

---

LIFE-THREATENING
DISORDER

# CORONARY ARTERY DISEASE

---

The dominant effect of coronary artery disease (CAD) is the loss of oxygen and nutrients to myocardial tissue because of diminished coronary blood flow. This disease is near epidemic in the Western world.

CAD occurs more often in men than in women, in whites, and in middle-aged and elderly people. In the past, this disorder rarely affected women who were premenopausal; however, that's no longer the case, perhaps because many women now take oral contraceptives, smoke cigarettes, and are employed in stressful jobs that used to be held exclusively by men.

## Causes

Atherosclerosis is the usual cause of CAD. In this form of arteriosclerosis, fatty, fibrous plaques narrow the lumen of the coronary arteries, reduce the volume of blood that can flow through them, and lead to myocardial ischemia. Plaque formation also predisposes to thrombosis, which can provoke myocardial infarction (MI).

Atherosclerosis usually develops in high-flow, high-pressure arteries, such as those in the heart, brain, kidneys, and aorta, especially at bifurcation points. It has been linked to many risk factors: family history, hypertension, obesity, smoking, diabetes mellitus, stress, a sedentary lifestyle, and high serum cholesterol and triglyceride levels.

Uncommon causes of reduced coronary artery blood flow include dissecting aneurysms, infectious vasculitis, syphilis, and congenital defects in the coronary vascular system. Coronary artery spasms may also impede blood flow. (See *Coronary artery spasm,* page 246.)

## Signs and symptoms

The classic symptom of CAD is angina, the direct result of inadequate flow of oxygen to the myocardium. It's usually described as a burning, squeezing, or tight feeling in the substernal or precordial chest that may radiate to the left arm, neck, jaw, or shoulder blade.

Typically, the patient clenches his fist over his chest or rubs his left arm when describing the pain, which may be accompanied by nausea, vomiting, fainting, sweating, and cool extremities. Anginal episodes most often follow physical exertion but may also follow emotional excitement, exposure to cold, or a large meal.

Angina has three major forms:

• *Stable* angina causes pain that's predictable in frequency and duration and can be relieved with nitrates and rest.

• *Unstable* angina causes pain that increases in frequency and duration. It's more easily induced.

• *Prinzmetal's* angina causes unpredictable coronary artery spasm.

Severe and prolonged anginal pain generally suggests MI, with potential-

# CORONARY ARTERY SPASM

A spontaneous, sustained contraction of one or more coronary arteries causes ischemia and dysfunction of the heart muscle in coronary artery spasm. This disorder also causes Prinzmetal's angina and even myocardial infarction in patients with unoccluded coronary arteries.

### Cause

Although the cause of coronary artery spasm is unknown, possible contributing factors include:
- intimal hemorrhage into the medial layer of the blood vessel
- hyperventilation
- elevated catecholamine levels
- fatty buildup in the lumen
- cocaine use.

### Signs and symptoms

Angina is the major symptom of coronary artery spasm. But unlike classic angina, this pain often occurs spontaneously and may not be related to physical exertion or emotional stress; it's also more severe, usually lasts longer, and may be cyclic, frequently recurring every day at the same time.

These ischemic episodes may cause arrhythmias, altered heart rate, lower blood pressure and, occasionally, fainting from diminished cardiac output. Spasm in the left coronary artery may result in mitral insufficiency, producing a loud systolic murmur and, possibly, pulmonary edema, with dyspnea, crackles, hemoptysis, or sudden death.

### Diagnosis and treatment

Coronary angiography and electrocardiography (ECG) allow a diagnosis. If significant lesions are not seen, ergonovine may be given I.V. to precipitate vasospasm. The patient may receive calcium channel blockers (verapamil, nifedipine, or diltiazem) to reduce coronary artery spasm and vascular resistance as well as nitrates (nitroglycerin or isosorbide dinitrate) to relieve chest pain.

### Special considerations

- When caring for a patient with coronary artery spasm, explain all necessary procedures and teach him how to take his medications safely.
- For calcium antagonist therapy, monitor blood pressure, pulse rate, and ECG patterns to detect arrhythmias.
- For nifedipine and verapamil therapy, monitor digoxin levels and check for signs of digitalis toxicity. (These drugs interfere with the excretion of digoxin.) Because nifedipine may cause peripheral and periorbital edema, watch for fluid retention.
- Because coronary artery spasm is sometimes associated with atherosclerotic disease, advise the patient to stop smoking, avoid overeating, use alcohol sparingly, and maintain a balance between exercise and rest.

---

ly fatal arrhythmias and mechanical failure.

### Diagnosis

The patient history—including the frequency and duration of angina and the presence of associated risk factors—is crucial in evaluating CAD. Additional diagnostic measures include the following:

- *Electrocardiography (ECG)* during angina may show ischemia or may be normal; it may also show arrhythmias, such as premature ventricular contractions. The ECG is apt to be normal when the patient is pain-free.

• *Treadmill* or *bicycle exercise test* may provoke chest pain and ECG signs of myocardial ischemia (ST-segment depression).

• *Coronary angiography* reveals narrowing or occlusion of the coronary artery, with possible collateral circulation.

• *Myocardial perfusion imaging* with thallium-201 or cardiolite during treadmill exercise detects ischemic areas of the myocardium, visualized as "cold spots."

### Treatment

The goal of treatment in patients with angina is to either reduce myocardial oxygen demand or increase oxygen supply. Therapy consists primarily of nitrates, such as nitroglycerin (given sublingually, orally, transdermally, or topically in ointment form), isosorbide dinitrate (given sublingually or orally), beta-adrenergic blockers (given orally), or calcium channel blockers (given orally). Obstructive lesions may necessitate coronary artery bypass surgery and the use of vein grafts.

Angioplasty may be performed during cardiac catheterization to compress fatty deposits and relieve occlusion in patients with no calcification and partial occlusion. (See *Relieving occlusions with angioplasty,* page 248.) A certain risk is associated with this procedure, but its morbidity is lower than that for surgery. Percutaneous transluminal coronary angioplasty may be done in combination with coronary stenting. Stents provide a framework to hold an artery open by securing flaps of tunica media and intima against the artery wall.

### Prevention

Because CAD is so widespread, prevention is of incalculable importance. Dietary restrictions aimed at reducing intake of calories (in obesity) and of dietary fats and cholesterol serve to minimize the risk, especially when supplemented with regular exercise. Abstention from smoking and reduction of stress are also beneficial.

Other preventive actions include control of hypertension (with sympathetic blocking agents, such as methyldopa and propranolol, or diuretics, such as hydrochlorothiazide), control of elevated serum cholesterol or triglyceride levels (with antilipemics, such as HMG-reductase inhibitors like cerivastatin sodium (Baycol), atorvastatin calcium (Lipitor), pravastatin sodium (Pravachol), or simvastatin (Zocor), and measures to minimize platelet aggregation and the danger of blood clots (with aspirin).

### Special considerations

• During anginal episodes, monitor blood pressure and heart rate. Take an ECG during anginal episodes and before administering nitroglycerin or other nitrates. Record the duration of pain, amount of medication required to relieve it, and accompanying symptoms.

• Keep nitroglycerin available for immediate use. Instruct the patient to call immediately whenever he feels chest, arm, or neck pain.

• Before cardiac catheterization, explain the procedure to the patient. Make sure he knows why it's necessary, understands the risks, and realizes that it may indicate a need for surgery.

• After catheterization, review the expected course of treatment with the patient and family. Monitor the catheter site for bleeding. Also, check for distal pulses. To counter the diuretic effect of the dye, make sure the patient drinks plenty of fluids. Maintain bed rest.

➤ CLINICAL TIP  A collagen substance (Vasoseal, Dengroseal) may be used at the femoral arterial puncture site. Tell the patient to expect to feel a hard bump the size of a large pea.

# RELIEVING OCCLUSIONS WITH ANGIOPLASTY

For a patient with an occluded coronary artery, percutaneous transluminal coronary angioplasty can open the artery without opening the chest — an important advantage over bypass surgery.

First, coronary angiography must confirm the presence and location of the arterial occlusion. Then, a guide catheter is threaded through the patient's femoral artery into the coronary artery under fluoroscopic guidance, as shown on the right.

When angiography shows the guide catheter positioned at the occlusion site, a smaller double-lumen balloon catheter is carefully inserted through the guide catheter and the balloon is directed through the occlusion (lower left). A marked pressure gradient will be obvious.

The balloon is alternately inflated and deflated until an angiogram verifies successful arterial dilation (lower right) and that the pressure gradient has decreased.

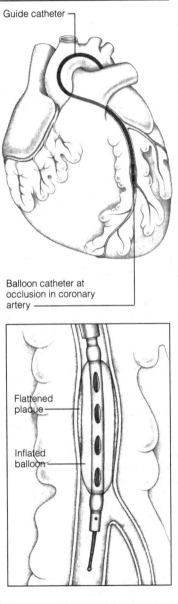

Guide catheter

Balloon catheter at occlusion in coronary artery

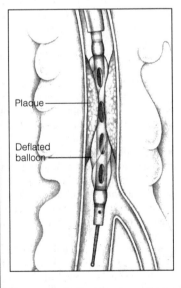

Plaque

Deflated balloon

Flattened plaque

Inflated balloon

- If the patient is scheduled for surgery, explain the procedure to the patient and family. Give them a tour of the intensive care unit, and introduce them to the staff.

- After surgery, monitor blood pressure, intake and output, breath sounds, chest tube drainage, and ECG, watching for signs of ischemia and arrhythmias. Also, observe for and treat chest pain and possible dye reactions. Give vigorous chest physiotherapy and guide the patient in coughing and deep-breathing exercises.

- Before discharge, stress the need to follow the prescribed drug regimen (antihypertensives, nitrates, and antilipemics, for example), exercise program, and diet. Encourage regular, moderate exercise. Refer the patient to a self-help program to stop smoking.

# CROHN'S DISEASE

Crohn's disease is an inflammation of the alimentary tract. It can affect any portion of the tract from the mouth to the anus. In 50% of cases, the disease involves the colon and small bowel. About 33% of cases involve the terminal ileum, and 10% to 20% of cases involve only the colon. The disease can extend through all layers of the intestinal wall and may also involve regional lymph nodes and the mesentery.

Crohn's disease is most prevalent in adults ages 20 to 40. It's two to three times more common in people of Jewish ancestry and least common in blacks.

## Causes

Although the exact cause of Crohn's disease is unknown, possible causes include allergies and other immune disorders and infection. However, no infecting organism has been isolated.

Several factors also implicate a genetic cause: Crohn's disease sometimes occurs in monozygotic twins, and up to 20% of patients with Crohn's disease have one or more affected relatives. However, no simple pattern of mendelian inheritance has been identified.

Whatever the cause of Crohn's disease, lacteal blockage in the intestinal wall leads to edema and, eventually, to mucosal inflammation, ulceration, stricturing, and fistula and abscess formation.

## Signs and symptoms

Clinical effects vary according to the location and extent of the inflammation.

### Acute disease

Acute inflammatory signs and symptoms mimic appendicitis and include steady, colicky, pain in the right lower quadrant; cramping; tenderness; flatulence; nausea; fever; and diarrhea. Bleeding may occur and, although usually mild, may be massive. Bloody stool may also occur.

### Chronic disease

Chronic symptoms are more typical of the disease, with complaints of abdominal distention and crampy abdominal pain. Symptoms may include a low-grade fever, weight loss, fatigue, and weakness. Diarrhea is usually nonbloody and intermittent, with right lower quadrant or periumbilical pain.

Fistulizing disease results from sinus tracts that can develop and penetrate through the bowel. Fistulas in the mesentery may be asymptomatic or may result in fever, chills, tender abdomen, and leukocytosis. Fistulas from the colon to small intestine can manifest with symptoms of diarrhea, weight loss, and malnutrition.

## Complications

Crohn's disease may lead to intestinal obstruction, fistula formation between the small bowel and the bladder, perianal and perirectal abscesses and fistulas, intra-abdominal abscesses, and perforation.

## Diagnosis

Upper GI series with small-bowel follow-through may demonstrate ulcerations, stricture, and fistulas.

Laboratory findings often indicate increased white blood cell count and erythrocyte sedimentation rate, hypokalemia, hypocalcemia, hypomagnesemia, and decreased hemoglobin level related to anemia from chronic inflammation, blood loss from the mucosa, and iron deficiency. Leukocytosis can be related to corticosteroid therapies, inflammation, or abscess formation. Sedimentation rate is increased in patients with active inflammation. Hypoglobulinemia may result from intestinal protein loss. A barium enema showing the string sign (segments of stricture separated by normal bowel) supports the diagnosis.

Flexible sigmoidoscopy and colonoscopy may show patchy areas of inflammation, ulcers, strictures, and granulomas, thus helping to rule out ulcerative colitis. However, a definitive diagnosis is possible only after a biopsy.

## Treatment

No cure for Crohn's disease exists; treatment is symptomatic. In debilitated patients, therapy includes I.V. hyperalimentation to maintain nutrition while resting the bowel.

Drug therapy may include antiinflammatory corticosteroids; immunosuppressive agents, such as azathioprine and mercaptopurine; and antibacterial agents, such as sulfasalazine. Antispasmodics, such as propantheline and dicyclomine, are used for abdominal cramping. Antidiarrheals used for chronic diarrhea include loperamide, diphenoxylate with atropine, and tincture of opium. Opium tincture and diphenoxylate may help combat diarrhea but are contraindicated in patients with significant intestinal obstruction. Metronidazole has proved to be effective in some patients.

Effective treatment requires important changes in lifestyle: physical rest, low-residue diet, and elimination of dairy products for lactose intolerance.

Surgery may be necessary on poor response to medical therapy to correct bowel perforation, massive hemorrhage, intra-abdominal abscess, stricture, fistulas, or acute intestinal obstruction. Colectomy with ileostomy is often necessary in patients with extensive disease of the large intestine and rectum.

## Special considerations

• Record fluid intake and output (including the amount of stool), and weigh the patient daily. Watch for dehydration and maintain fluid and electrolyte balance.

• Be alert for signs of intestinal bleeding (bloody stool); check stool daily for occult blood.

• If the patient is receiving steroids, watch for adverse reactions, such as GI bleeding. Remember that steroids can mask signs of infection.

• Check hemoglobin level and hematocrit regularly. Give iron supplements and blood transfusions as needed.

• Give analgesics as needed.

• Provide good patient hygiene and meticulous mouth care if the patient is restricted to nothing by mouth.

• After each bowel movement, give good skin care. Always keep a clean, covered bedpan within the patient's reach. Ventilate the room to eliminate odors.

- Observe the patient for fever and pain or pneumaturia, which may signal bladder fistula. Abdominal pain and distention and fever may indicate intestinal obstruction. Watch for stool from the vagina and an enterovaginal fistula.

- Before ileostomy, arrange for a visit by an enterostomal therapist for preoperative education and stoma marking.

- After surgery, frequently check the nasogastric tube for proper functioning. Monitor vital signs and fluid intake and output. Watch for wound infection.

- Provide meticulous stoma care, and teach it to the patient and family.

- Realize that ileostomy changes the patient's body image, so offer reassurance and emotional support.

> CLINICAL TIP Educate the patient regarding stress management techniques. Refer the patient to a support group if necessary.

# CROUP

A severe inflammation and obstruction of the upper airway. croup can occur as acute laryngotracheobronchitis (most common), laryngitis, and acute spasmodic laryngitis. It must always be distinguished from epiglottitis.

Croup is a childhood disease affecting boys more often than girls (typically between ages 3 months and 3 years) that usually occurs during the winter. Up to 15% of patients have a strong family history of croup. Recovery is usually complete.

## Causes
Croup usually results from a viral infection. Parainfluenza viruses cause two-thirds of such infections; adenoviruses, respiratory syncytial virus (RSV), influenza and measles viruses, and bacteria (pertussis and diphtheria) account for the rest.

## Signs and symptoms
The onset of croup usually follows an upper respiratory tract infection. Clinical features include inspiratory stridor, hoarse or muffled vocal sounds, varying degrees of laryngeal obstruction and respiratory distress, and a characteristic sharp, barklike cough. These symptoms may last only a few hours or persist for 1 to 2 days.

As croup progresses, it causes inflammatory edema and, possibly, spasm, which can obstruct the upper airway and severely compromise ventilation. Each form of croup has additional characteristics.

### Laryngotracheobronchitis
The symptoms of this form of croup seem to worsen at night. Inflammation causes edema of the bronchi and bronchioles and increasingly difficult expiration, which frightens the child. Other characteristic features include fever, diffusely decreased breath sounds, expiratory rhonchi, and scattered crackles.

### Laryngitis
Resulting from vocal cord edema, laryngitis is usually mild and produces no respiratory distress except in infants. Early indications include a sore throat and cough that, rarely, may progress to marked hoarseness, suprasternal and intercostal retractions, inspiratory stridor, dyspnea, diminished breath sounds, and restlessness. In later stages, severe dyspnea and exhaustion may result.

### Acute spasmodic laryngitis
This form of croup affects children between ages 1 and 3, particularly those with allergies and a family history of

croup. It typically begins with mild to moderate hoarseness and nasal discharge, followed by the characteristic cough and noisy inspiration (which often awaken the child at night), labored breathing with retractions, rapid pulse, and clammy skin.

The child understandably becomes anxious, which may lead to increasing dyspnea and transient cyanosis. These severe symptoms diminish after several hours but reappear in a milder form on the next night or two.

### Diagnosis

When bacterial infection is the cause, throat cultures may identify organisms and their sensitivity to antibiotics as well as rule out diphtheria. A neck X-ray may show areas of upper airway narrowing and edema in subglottic folds; laryngoscopy may reveal inflammation and obstruction in epiglottal and laryngeal areas.

In evaluating the patient, consider foreign-body obstruction (a common cause of croupy cough in young children) as well as masses and cysts.

### Treatment

For most children with croup, home care with rest, cool humidification during sleep, and antipyretics, such as acetaminophen, relieve symptoms. However, respiratory distress that interferes with oral hydration requires hospitalization and parenteral fluid replacement to prevent dehydration.

If bacterial infection is the cause, antibiotic therapy is necessary. Oxygen therapy may also be required.

### Special considerations

• Monitor and support respiration, and control fever. Because croup is so frightening to the child and his family, also provide support and reassurance.

• Carefully monitor cough and breath sounds, hoarseness, severity of retractions, inspiratory stridor, cyanosis, respiratory rate and character (especially prolonged and labored respirations), restlessness, fever, and cardiac rate.

• Keep the child as quiet as possible, but avoid sedation, which can depress respiration.

• If the patient is an infant, position him in an infant seat or prop him up with a pillow.

• Place an older child in high Fowler's position. If an older child requires a cool-mist tent to help him breathe, explain why it's needed.

• Isolate patients suspected of having RSV and parainfluenza infections, if possible. Wash your hands carefully before leaving the room to avoid transmission to other children, particularly infants. Instruct parents and others involved in the care of these children to take similar precautions.

• Control fever with sponge baths and antipyretics. Keep a hypothermia blanket on hand for temperatures above 102° F (38.9° C). Watch for seizures in infants and young children with high fevers. Give I.V. antibiotics as necessary.

➤ CLINICAL TIP Relieve sore throat with soothing, water-based ices, such as fruit sherbet and ice pops. Avoid thicker, milk-based fluids if the child is producing heavy mucus or has great difficulty swallowing.

• Apply petroleum jelly or another ointment around the nose and lips to soothe irritation from nasal discharge and mouth breathing.

• Maintain a calm, quiet environment and offer reassurance. Explain all procedures and answer any questions.

• To relieve croupy spells, tell parents to carry the child into the bathroom, shut the door, and turn on the hot water. Breathing in warm, moist air quickly eases an acute spell of croup. Suggest the use of a cool-mist humidifier (vaporizer).

• Warn parents that ear infections and pneumonia are complications of croup, which may appear about 5 days after recovery. Stress the importance of reporting earache, productive cough, high fever, or increased shortness of breath immediately.

# CRYPTOCOCCOSIS

The fungus *Cryptococcus neoformans* causes cryptococcosis, also called torulosis and European blastomycosis. Cryptococcosis usually begins as an asymptomatic pulmonary infection but disseminates to extrapulmonary sites, usually to the central nervous system (CNS) but also to the skin, bones, prostate gland, liver, or kidneys.

Cryptococcosis is most prevalent in men, usually those between ages 30 and 60, and is rare in children. It's especially likely to develop in immunocompromised patients, such as those with Hodgkin's disease, sarcoidosis, leukemia, or lymphoma and those who are receiving immunosuppressive agents. Currently, patients with acquired immunodeficiency syndrome (AIDS) are by far the most commonly affected group.

With appropriate treatment, the prognosis in pulmonary cryptococcosis is good. CNS infection, however, can be fatal, but treatment dramatically reduces mortality.

## Causes
Transmission is through inhalation of *C. neoformans* in particles of dust contaminated by pigeon stool that harbor this organism. Therefore, cryptococcosis is primarily an urban infection.

## Signs and symptoms
Typically, pulmonary cryptococcosis is asymptomatic. Onset of CNS involvement is gradual (cryptococcal meningitis) and causes progressively severe frontal and temporal headache, diplopia, blurred vision, dizziness, ataxia, aphasia, vomiting, tinnitus, memory changes, inappropriate behavior, irritability, psychotic symptoms, seizures, and fever.

If untreated, symptoms progress to coma and death, usually a result of cerebral edema or hydrocephalus. Complications include optic atrophy, ataxia, hydrocephalus, deafness, paralysis, chronic brain syndrome, and personality changes.

Skin involvement produces red facial papules and other skin abscesses, with or without ulcerations; bone involvement produces painful osseous lesions of the long bones, skull, spine, and joints.

## Diagnosis
A routine chest X-ray showing a pulmonary lesion may point to pulmonary cryptococcosis. However, this infection usually escapes diagnosis until it disseminates.

A firm diagnosis requires identification of *C. neoformans* by culture of sputum, urine, prostatic secretions, bone marrow aspirate or biopsy, or pleural biopsy; and, in CNS infection, by an India ink preparation of cerebrospinal fluid (CSF) and culture. Blood cultures are positive only in severe infection.

Supportive values include an increased antigen titer in serum and CSF in disseminated infection; increased CSF pressure, protein, and white blood cell count in CNS infection; and moderately decreased CSF glucose in about half of these patients. The diagnosis must rule out cancer and tuberculosis.

### Treatment
The patient with pulmonary cryptococcosis will require close medical observation for 1 year after diagnosis. Treatment is unnecessary unless extrapulmonary lesions develop or pulmonary lesions progress.

Treatment of disseminated infection calls for I.V. amphotericin B or fluconazole. Patients with AIDS will also need long-term therapy, usually with oral fluconazole.

### Special considerations
• Cryptococcosis doesn't require isolation.
• Check the patient's vital functions, and note any changes in mental status, orientation, pupillary response, and motor function.
• Watch for headache, vomiting, and nuchal rigidity.
• Before giving I.V. amphotericin B, check for phlebitis. Infuse slowly and dilute — rapid infusion may cause circulatory collapse.

> **CLINICAL TIP** Before therapy, draw blood for a serum electrolyte analysis to determine baseline renal status.

• During drug therapy, watch for decreased urine output, elevated blood urea nitrogen and creatinine levels, and hypokalemia.
• Monitor results of complete blood count, urinalysis, magnesium and potassium levels, and liver function tests. Ask the patient to report hearing loss, tinnitus, or dizziness.
• Give analgesics, antihistamines, and antiemetics for fever, chills, nausea, and vomiting.
• Provide psychological support to help the patient cope with long-term hospitalization.

# CUSHING'S SYNDROME

A cluster of clinical abnormalities characterize Cushing's syndrome. These abnormalities result from excessive levels of adrenocortical hormones (particularly cortisol) or related corticosteroids and, to a lesser extent, androgens and aldosterone. Its unmistakable signs include adiposity of the face (moon face), neck, and trunk and purple striae on the skin.

Cushing's syndrome is most common in women. The prognosis depends on the underlying cause; it is poor in untreated persons and in those with untreatable ectopic corticotropin-producing carcinoma.

### Causes
In approximately 80% of patients, Cushing's syndrome results from excess production of corticotropin and consequent hyperplasia of the adrenal cortex. Overproduction of corticotropin may stem from pituitary hypersecretion (Cushing's disease) or corticotropin-producing tumor in another organ (particularly bronchogenic or pancreatic carcinoma). Excessive administration of exogenous glucocorticoids can also cause Cushing's syndrome.

In the remaining 20% of patients, Cushing's syndrome results from a cortisol-secreting adrenal tumor that's usually benign. In infants, the usual cause of Cushing's syndrome is adrenal adenoma or carcinoma.

### Signs and symptoms
Like other endocrine disorders, Cushing's syndrome induces changes in multiple body systems, depending on the adrenocortical hormone involved. Spe-

cific clinical effects vary with the system affected.

• *Endocrine and metabolic systems:* diabetes mellitus, with decreased glucose tolerance, fasting hyperglycemia, and glucosuria

• *Musculoskeletal system:* muscle weakness resulting from hypokalemia or loss of muscle mass from increased catabolism, pathologic fractures from decreased bone mineral, and skeletal growth retardation in children

• *Skin:* purplish striae; fat pads above the clavicles, over the upper back (buffalo hump), on the face (moon face), and throughout the trunk, with slender arms and legs; little or no scar formation; poor wound healing; acne and hirsutism in women

• *GI system:* peptic ulcer, resulting from increased gastric secretions and pepsin production, and decreased gastric mucus

• *Central nervous system (CNS):* irritability and emotional lability, ranging from euphoric behavior to depression or psychosis; insomnia

• *Cardiovascular system:* hypertension resulting from sodium and water retention; left ventricular hypertrophy; capillary weakness from protein loss, which leads to bleeding and ecchymosis

• *Immunologic system:* increased susceptibility to infection because of decreased lymphocyte production and suppressed antibody formation; decreased resistance to stress; suppressed inflammatory response may mask even a severe infection

• *Renal and urologic systems:* sodium and secondary fluid retention; increased potassium excretion; inhibited secretion of antidiuretic hormone; ureteral calculi from increased bone demineralization with hypercalciuria

• *Reproductive system:* increased androgen production, with clitoral hypertrophy, mild virilism, and amenorrhea or oligomenorrhea in women; sexual dysfunction also occurs.

**Diagnosis**

Initially, the diagnosis of Cushing's syndrome requires determination of plasma steroid levels. In persons with normal hormone balance, plasma cortisol levels are higher in the morning and decrease gradually through the day (diurnal variation). In patients with Cushing's syndrome, cortisol levels don't fluctuate and typically remain consistently elevated; a 24-hour urine sample demonstrates elevated free cortisol levels.

***Suppression test***

A low-dose dexamethasone suppression test confirms the diagnosis of Cushing's syndrome. A high-dose dexamethasone suppression test can determine whether Cushing's syndrome results from pituitary dysfunction (Cushing's disease) or from adenoma of the adrenal gland or ectopic corticotropin secretion.

In this test, dexamethasone suppresses plasma cortisol levels, and urinary 17-hydroxycorticosteroids (17-OHCS) and 17-ketogenic steroids fall to 50% or less of basal levels. Failure to suppress these levels indicates that the syndrome results from an adrenal tumor or a nonendocrine, corticotropin-secreting tumor. This test can produce false-positive results.

***Stimulation test***

In a stimulation test, administration of metyrapone, which blocks cortisol production by the adrenal glands, tests the ability of the pituitary gland and the hypothalamus to detect and correct low levels of plasma cortisol by increasing corticotropin production. The patient with Cushing's syndrome reacts to this stimulus by secreting an excess of plasma corticotropin as measured by levels of urinary 17-OHCS.

If the patient has an adrenal or a nonendocrine corticotropin-secreting tumor, the pituitary gland — which is suppressed by the high cortisol levels — can't respond normally, so steroid levels remain stable or fall. The corticotropin-releasing hormone tests can also be used to help differentiate pituitary Cushing's and ectopic corticotropin syndrome.

### Other tests
Ultrasonography, a computed tomography (CT) scan, magnetic resonance imaging (MRI), or angiography localizes adrenal tumors; a CT scan and MRI of the head identify pituitary tumors.

### Treatment
Radiation, drug therapy, and surgery are among the treatments used to restore hormone balance and reverse Cushing's syndrome. For example, pituitary-dependent Cushing's syndrome with adrenal hyperplasia and severe cushingoid symptoms — such as psychosis, poorly controlled diabetes mellitus, osteoporosis, and severe pathologic fractures — may require adenectomy or pituitary irradiation. If the patient fails to respond, bilateral adrenalectomy may be performed.

Nonendocrine corticotropin-producing tumors require excision of the tumor. Drug therapy follows (for example, with mitotane, metyrapone, or aminoglutethimide) to decrease cortisol levels if symptoms persist.

Aminoglutethimide and ketoconazole decrease cortisol levels and have been beneficial for many cushingoid patients. Aminoglutethimide alone or in combination with metyrapone may also be useful in metastatic adrenal carcinoma.

Before surgery, the patient with cushingoid symptoms should have special management to control hypertension, edema, diabetes, and cardiovascular manifestations and to prevent infection. Glucocorticoid administration on the morning of surgery can help prevent acute adrenal insufficiency during surgery.

Cortisol therapy is essential during and after surgery to help the patient tolerate the physiologic stress imposed by removal of the pituitary or adrenals. If normal cortisol production resumes, steroid therapy may be gradually tapered and eventually discontinued. However, bilateral adrenalectomy or total hypophysectomy mandates lifelong steroid replacement therapy to correct hormonal deficiencies. (See *Dealing with lifelong treatment.*)

### Special considerations
- Frequently monitor vital signs, especially blood pressure. Carefully observe the hypertensive patient who also has cardiac disease.
- Check laboratory reports for hypernatremia, hypokalemia, hyperglycemia, and glycosuria.
- Because the cushingoid patient is likely to retain sodium and water, check for edema, and monitor daily weight and intake and output carefully.
- To minimize weight gain, edema, and hypertension, ask the dietary department to provide a diet that's high in protein and potassium but low in calories, carbohydrates, and sodium.
- Watch for infection — a particular problem in Cushing's syndrome.
- If the patient has osteoporosis and is bedridden, perform passive range-of-motion exercises carefully because of the severe risk for pathologic fractures.

**CLINICAL TIP** Cushing's syndrome produces emotional lability. Record incidents that upset the patient, and try to prevent such situations from occurring, if possible. Help him get the physical and mental rest he needs — by sedation if necessary.

• Offer support to the emotionally labile patient throughout the difficult testing period.

After surgery:

• Watch carefully for wound drainage or temperature elevation. Use strict aseptic technique in changing the patient's dressings.

• Administer analgesics and replacement steroids as necessary.

• Monitor urine output and check vital signs carefully, watching for signs of shock (decreased blood pressure, increased pulse rate, pallor, and cold, clammy skin).

• If shock develops, give vasopressors and increase the rate of I.V. fluids. Because mitotane, aminoglutethimide, and metyrapone decrease mental alertness and produce physical weakness, assess neurologic and behavioral status, and warn the patient of adverse CNS effects.

• Watch for severe nausea, vomiting, and diarrhea.

• Check laboratory reports for hypoglycemia from removal of the source of cortisol, a hormone that maintains blood glucose levels.

• Check for abdominal distention and return of bowel sounds following adrenalectomy.

• Check regularly for signs of adrenal hypofunction — orthostatic hypotension, apathy, weakness, fatigue — indicators that steroid replacement is inadequate.

• In the patient undergoing pituitary surgery, be alert for signs of increased intracranial pressure (confusion, agitation, changes in level of consciousness,

---

**TEACHING CHECKLIST**

## DEALING WITH LIFELONG TREATMENT

The patient who has been treated for Cushing's syndrome with hypophysectomy or adrenalectomy needs careful instruction to help him cope with lifelong steroid replacement. Make sure you teach him to:

• take replacement steroids with antacids or meals to minimize gastric irritation — two-thirds in the morning and the remaining third in the early afternoon to mimic diurnal adrenal secretion

• carry a medical identification card

• immediately report physiologically stressful situations, such as infections, so his steroid dose can be increased

• watch closely for fatigue, weakness, and dizziness — symptoms of inadequate steroid dose — as well as severe swelling and weight gain — signs of overdose

• take his steroids exactly as prescribed; abrupt discontinuation could produce a fatal adrenal crisis.

---

nausea, and vomiting). Also watch for hypopituitarism.

# CYSTIC FIBROSIS

Sometimes called mucoviscidosis, cystic fibrosis is a generalized dysfunction of the exocrine glands that affects multiple organ systems. Transmitted as an autosomal recessive trait, it's the most common fatal genetic disease of white children.

Cystic fibrosis is a chronic disease; however, recent improvements in treatments have increased the average life expectancy from age 16 to age 28 and older.

Incidence of cystic fibrosis is highest (1 in 2,000 live births) in Whites of northern European ancestry and lowest in Blacks (1 in 17,000 live births), Native Americans, and people of Asian ancestry. The disease occurs equally in both sexes.

## Causes

The recently identified gene responsible for cystic fibrosis encodes a protein that involves chloride transport across epithelial membranes. To date, over 100 specific mutations of this gene have been identified.

The immediate causes of symptoms are increased viscosity of bronchial, pancreatic, and other mucous gland secretions and consequent obstruction of glandular ducts. Cystic fibrosis accounts for almost all cases of pancreatic enzyme deficiency in children.

## Signs and symptoms

The clinical effects of cystic fibrosis may become apparent soon after birth or may take years to develop. They include major aberrations in sweat gland, respiratory, and GI functions.

### Sweat gland dysfunction

In cystic fibrosis, sweat gland dysfunction is the most consistent abnormality. Increased concentrations of sodium and chloride in the sweat lead to hyponatremia and hypochloremia and can eventually induce fatal shock and arrhythmias, especially in hot weather.

### Respiratory symptoms

Such symptoms reflect obstructive changes in the lungs: wheezy respirations; a dry, nonproductive, paroxysmal cough; dyspnea; and tachypnea. These changes stem from thick, tenacious secretions in the bronchioles and alveoli and eventually lead to severe atelectasis and emphysema.

Children with cystic fibrosis display a barrel chest, cyanosis, and clubbing of the fingers and toes. They suffer recurring bronchitis and pneumonia and associated nasal polyps and sinusitis. Death typically results from pneumonia, emphysema, or atelectasis.

### GI symptoms

The GI effects of cystic fibrosis occur mainly in the intestines, pancreas, and liver. One early symptom is meconium ileus; the newborn with cystic fibrosis doesn't excrete meconium, a dark green mucilaginous material found in the intestine at birth. He develops symptoms of intestinal obstruction, such as abdominal distention, vomiting, constipation, dehydration, and electrolyte imbalance.

Eventually, obstruction of the pancreatic ducts and resulting deficiency of trypsin, amylase, and lipase prevent the conversion and absorption of fat and protein in the intestinal tract. The undigested food is then excreted in frequent, bulky, foul-smelling, and pale stool with a high fat content.

This malabsorption induces poor weight gain, poor growth, ravenous appetite, distended abdomen, thin extremities, and sallow skin with poor turgor. The inability to absorb fats produces deficiency of fat-soluble vitamins (A, D, E, and K), leading to clotting problems, retarded bone growth, and delayed sexual development. Males may experience azoospermia and sterility;

females may experience secondary amenorrhea but can reproduce.

A common complication in infants and children is rectal prolapse. This stems from malnutrition and wasting of perirectal supporting tissues.

In the pancreas, fibrotic tissue, multiple cysts, thick mucus and, eventually, fat replace the acini (small saclike swellings normally found in this gland). This results in signs of pancreatic insufficiency: insufficient insulin production, abnormal glucose tolerance, and glycosuria.

About 15% of patients are pancreatic sufficient, having adequate pancreatic exocrine function for normal digestion. These patients have a better prognosis.

Biliary obstruction and fibrosis may prolong neonatal jaundice. In some patients, cirrhosis and portal hypertension may lead to esophageal varices, episodes of hematemesis and, occasionally, hepatomegaly.

### Diagnosis

The Cystic Fibrosis Foundation sets the following standards for a definitive diagnosis:

• Two *sweat tests* using a pilocarpine solution (a sweat inducer) are clearly positive; the patient also has either an obstructive pulmonary disease, confirmed pancreatic insufficiency or failure to thrive, or a family history of cystic fibrosis.

• *Chest X-rays* indicate early signs of obstructive lung disease.

• *Stool specimen analysis* indicates the absence of trypsin, suggesting pancreatic insufficiency.

The following test results may support the diagnosis:

• *Deoxyribonucleic acid testing* can now locate the presence of the Delta F 508 deletion (found in about 70% of cystic fibrosis patients, although the disease can cause more than 100 other mutations). This test can also be used for carrier detection and a prenatal diagnosis in families with a previously affected child.

• *Pulmonary function tests* reveal decreased vital capacity, elevated residual volume from air entrapments, and decreased forced expiratory volume in 1 second. This test is used if pulmonary exacerbation already exists.

• *Liver enzyme test* may reveal hepatic insufficiency.

• *Sputum culture* reveals organisms that cystic fibrosis patients typically and chronically colonize, such as *Staphylococcus* and *Pseudomonas*.

• *Serum albumin levels* help assess nutritional status.

• *Electrolyte analysis* assesses dehydration and glucose levels.

### Treatment

The aim of treatment is to help the child lead as normal a life as possible. Specific treatment depends on the organ systems involved.

• To combat sweat electrolyte losses, treatment includes generous salting of foods and, during hot weather, administration of sodium supplements.

• To offset pancreatic enzyme deficiencies, treatment includes oral pancreatic enzymes with meals and snacks. The child's diet should be low in fat but high in protein and calories, and it should include supplements of water-miscible, fat-soluble vitamins (A, D, E, and K).

• Management of pulmonary dysfunction includes chest physiotherapy, postural drainage and breathing exercises several times daily to aid removal of secretions from lungs. Antihistamines are contraindicated; they have a drying effect on mucous membranes, making expectoration of mucus difficult or impossible.

Aerosol therapy includes intermittent nebulizer treatments before postural drainage to loosen secretions. Dornase alfa, a genetically engineered pulmonary enzyme given by aerosol nebulizer, helps thin airway mucus, improving lung function and reducing the risk of pulmonary infection.

A patient with pulmonary infection will need mucopurulent secretions loosened and removed, using an intermittent nebulizer and postural drainage to relieve obstruction. Use of a mist tent is controversial because mist particles may become trapped in the esophagus and stomach and never even reach the lungs. Broad-spectrum antimicrobials help combat infection. Oxygen therapy is used as needed.

Recently, some patients have undergone lung transplantation to reduce the effects of the disease. Also, clinical trials of aerosol gene therapy show promise in reducing pulmonary symptoms.

**Special considerations**

● Suggest the use of air conditioners and humidifiers to help decrease vulnerability to respiratory tract infections. Emphasize keeping these units clean to prevent accumulation of organisms that increase the risk of infection.

● Throughout this illness, teach the patient and his family about the disease and its treatment.

● Provide emotional support, and refer the patient and his family for genetic counseling and to the Cystic Fibrosis Foundation.

◆ CLINICAL TIP    Recent research indicates that the genetic defect responsible for cystic fibrosis has also been identified in individuals experiencing some forms of unexplained pancreatitis. In addition, males with oligospermia or azoospermia have been identified as at an increased risk for carrying the cystic fibrosis mutation. These populations should also be offered cerebrospinal fluid testing.

# CYTOMEGALOVIRUS INFECTION

Also called generalized salivary gland disease and cytomegalic inclusion disease, cytomegalovirus (CMV) infection is caused by the cytomegalovirus, which is a deoxyribonucleic acid, ether-sensitive virus belonging to the herpes family. The disease occurs worldwide and is transmitted by human contact.

About four out of five persons over age 35 have been infected with CMV, usually during childhood or early adulthood. In most of these people, the disease is so mild that it's overlooked.

◆ CLINICAL TIP    Be aware that CMV infection during pregnancy can be hazardous to the fetus, possibly leading to stillbirth, brain damage, and other birth defects or to severe neonatal illness.

**Causes**

CMV has been found in the saliva, urine, semen, breast milk, stool, blood, and vaginal and cervical secretions of infected persons. Transmission usually happens through contact with these infected secretions, which harbor the virus for months or even years.

The virus may be transmitted by sexual contact and can travel across the placenta of a pregnant woman, causing a congenital infection. Immunosuppressed patients, especially those who have received transplanted organs, run a 90% chance of contracting CMV infection. Recipients of blood transfusions from donors with positive CMV antibodies are at some risk.

## Signs and symptoms

CMV probably spreads through the body in lymphocytes or mononuclear cells to the lungs, liver, GI tract, eyes, and central nervous system, where it often produces inflammatory reactions.

Most patients with CMV infection have mild, nonspecific complaints, or none at all, even though antibody titers indicate infection. In these patients, the disease usually runs a self-limiting course.

Immunodeficient patients, such as those with acquired immunodeficiency syndrome (AIDS), and those receiving immunosuppressants may develop pneumonia or other secondary infections. AIDS patients may also develop disseminated CMV infection, which may cause chorioretinitis (resulting in blindness), colitis, or encephalitis.

Infected infants ages 3 to 6 months usually appear asymptomatic but may develop hepatic dysfunction, hepatosplenomegaly, spider angiomas, pneumonitis, and lymphadenopathy.

Congenital CMV infection is seldom apparent at birth, although the infant's urine contains CMV. About 1% of all newborns have CMV.

The virus can cause brain damage that may not show up for months after birth. Occasionally, it produces a rapidly fatal neonatal illness characterized by jaundice, petechial rash, hepatosplenomegaly, thrombocytopenia, hemolytic anemia, microcephaly, psychomotor retardation, mental deficiency, and hearing loss.

In some adults, CMV may cause cytomegalovirus mononucleosis, with 3 weeks or more of irregular, high fever.

Other findings may include a normal or elevated white blood cell (WBC) count, lymphocytosis, and increased atypical lymphocytes.

## Diagnosis

Although virus isolation in urine is the most sensitive laboratory method, a diagnosis can also rest on virus isolation from saliva, throat, cervix, WBC, and biopsy specimens.

Other laboratory tests support the diagnosis, including complement fixation studies, hemagglutination inhibition antibody tests and, for congenital infections, indirect immunofluorescent tests for CMV immunoglobulin M antibody.

## Treatment

Because CMV infection is usually self-limiting, treatment aims to relieve symptoms and prevent complications. In the immunosuppressed patient, however, CMV is treated with acyclovir, ganciclovir, and foscarnet, combined with anti-CMV immune globulin for pneumonitis and possible GI disease.

## Special considerations

● Provide parents of children with severe congenital CMV infection with counseling to help them cope with the possibility of brain damage or death.

● To help prevent CMV infection, warn immunosuppressed patients and pregnant women to avoid exposure to confirmed or suspected CMV infection. Tell pregnant patients that maternal CMV infection can cause serious fetal abnormalities.

● Urge patients with CMV infection — especially young children — to wash their hands thoroughly to prevent spreading it.

● Observe standard precautions when handling body secretions.

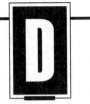

# DELUSIONAL DISORDERS

According to the *Diagnostic and Statistical Manual of Mental Disorders,* 4th edition *(DSM-IV),* delusional disorders are marked by false beliefs with a plausible basis in reality. Formerly referred to as paranoid disorders, delusional disorders involve erotomanic, grandiose, jealous, somatic, or persecutory themes. Some patients experience several types of delusions, whereas others experience unspecified delusions with no dominant theme.

Delusional disorders commonly begin in middle or late adulthood, usually between ages 40 and 55, but they can occur at a younger age. These uncommon illnesses affect less than 1% of the population; the incidence is about equal in men and women.

Typically chronic, these disorders often interfere with social and marital relationships but seldom impair intellectual or occupational functioning significantly.

## Causes

Delusional disorders of later life strongly suggest a hereditary predisposition. At least one study has linked the development of delusional disorders to inferiority feelings in the family.

Some researchers suggest that delusional disorders are the product of specific early childhood experiences with an authoritarian family structure. Others hold that anyone with a sensitive personality is particularly vulnerable to developing a delusional disorder.

Certain medical conditions — head injury, chronic alcoholism, and deafness — and aging are known to increase the risk for delusional disorders. Predisposing factors linked to aging include isolation, lack of stimulating interpersonal relationships, physical illness, and impaired hearing and vision.

Severe stress (such as a move to a foreign country) may also precipitate a delusional disorder.

## Signs and symptoms

Aside from behavior related to the patient's delusions, the psychiatric history of a delusional patient may be unremarkable. This helps distinguish it from disorders that result in behavior more dissociated from reality such as paranoid schizophrenia. (See *Delusional disorder or paranoid schizophrenia?*)

The delusional patient is likely to report problems with social and marital relationships, including depression or sexual dysfunction. He may describe a life marked by social isolation or hostility. He may deny feeling lonely, relentlessly criticizing, or placing unreasonable demands on others.

Gathering accurate information from a delusional patient may prove difficult. He may deny his feelings, disregard the circumstances that led to his hospitalization, and refuse treatment.

However, his responses and behavior during the assessment interview provide clues that can help to identify his disorder. Family members may confirm observations — for example, by reporting that the patient is chronically jealous or suspicious.

### Assessment clue: Communication

The patient's ability to communicate can be another indicator. He may be evasive or reluctant to answer questions. Or he may be overly talkative, explaining events in great detail and emphasizing what he has achieved, prominent people he knows, or places he has traveled.

The patient may make statements that at first seem logical but later prove irrelevant. Some of his answers may be contradictory, jumbled, or irrational.

A delusional patient may make expressions of denial, projection, and rationalization. Once delusions become firmly entrenched, the patient will no longer seek to justify his beliefs. However, if he's still struggling to maintain his delusional defenses, he may make statements that reveal his condition, such as "People at work won't talk to me because I'm smarter than they are."

Accusatory statements are also characteristic of the delusional patient. Pervasive delusional themes (for example, grandiose or persecutory) may become apparent.

The patient may also display nonverbal cues, such as excessive vigilance or obvious apprehension on entering the room. During questions, he may listen intently, reacting defensively to imagined slights or insults. He may sit at the edge of his seat or fold his arms as if to shield himself. If he carries papers or money, he may clutch them firmly.

### Diagnosis

The *DSM-IV* describes a characteristic set of behaviors that mark the patient

---

## DELUSIONAL DISORDER OR PARANOID SCHIZOPHRENIA?

To distinguish between these two disorders, consider the following characteristics.

### Delusional disorder

In a delusional disorder the patient's delusions reflect reality and are arranged into a coherent system. They're based on misinterpretations of, or elaborations on, reality.

The patient doesn't experience hallucinations, and his affect and behavior are normal.

### Paranoid schizophrenia

In paranoid schizophrenia, the patient's delusions are scattered, illogical, and incoherently arranged with no relation to reality.

The patient may have hallucinations, his affect is inappropriate and inconsistent, and his behavior is bizarre.

---

with delusional disorder. (See *Diagnosing delusional disorder* page 264.)

In addition, blood and urine tests, psychological tests, and neurologic evaluation can rule out organic causes of the delusions, such as amphetamine-induced psychoses and Alzheimer's disease. Endocrine function tests rule out hyperadrenalism, pernicious anemia, and thyroid disorders such as "myxedema madness."

### Treatment

Effective treatment of delusional disorders, consisting of a combination of drug therapy and psychotherapy, must correct the behavior and mood disturbances that result from the patient's mistaken belief system. Treatment also may

## DIAGNOSING DELUSIONAL DISORDER

In an individual with a suspected delusional disorder, psychiatric examination confirms the diagnosis. The examiner bases the diagnosis on the following criteria set forth in the *Diagnostic and Statistical Manual of Mental Disorders,* 4th edition:

• Nonbizzare delusions of at least 1 month's duration are present, involving real-life situations, such as being followed, poisoned, infected, loved at a distance, or deceived by one's spouse or lover.
• The patient's symptoms have never met the criteria known as characteristic symptoms of schizophrenia. However, tactile and olfactory hallucinations may be present if they're related to a delusional theme.
• Apart from being affected by the delusion or its ramifications, the patient isn't markedly impaired functionally nor is his behavior obviously odd or bizarre.
• If mood disturbances have occurred concurrently with delusions, their total duration has been brief relative to the duration of the delusional disturbance.
• The disturbance doesn't result from the direct physiologic effects of a substance or a general medical condition.

include mobilizing a support system for the isolated elderly patient.

### Antipsychotic drug therapy

Drug treatment with antipsychotic agents is similar to that used in schizophrenic disorders. Antipsychotics appear to work by blocking postsynaptic dopamine receptors. These drugs reduce the incidence of psychotic symptoms, such as hallucinations and delusions, and relieve anxiety and agitation.

Other psychiatric drugs, such as antidepressants and anxiolytics, may be prescribed to control associated symptoms.

High-potency antipsychotics include fluphenazine, haloperidol, thiothixene, and trifluoperazine. Loxapine, molindone, and perphenazine are intermediate in potency, and chlorpromazine and thioridazine are low-potency agents.

Haloperidol decanoate, fluphenazine decanoate, and fluphenazine enanthate are depot formulations that are implanted I.M. They release the drug gradually over a 30-day period, improving compliance.

Clozapine, which differs chemically from other antipsychotic drugs, may be prescribed for severely ill patients who fail to respond to standard treatment. This agent effectively controls a wider range of psychotic symptoms without the usual adverse effects.

However, clozapine can cause drowsiness, sedation, excessive salivation, tachycardia, dizziness, and seizures as well as agranulocytosis, a potentially fatal blood disorder characterized by a low white blood cell count and pronounced neutropenia.

Routine blood monitoring is essential to detect the estimated 1% to 2% of all patients taking clozapine who develop agranulocytosis. If caught in the early stages, this disorder is reversible.

### Special considerations

• In dealing with the delusional patient, be direct, straightforward, and dependable. Whenever possible, elicit his feedback. Move slowly, in a matter-of-fact manner, and respond without anger or defensiveness to his hostile remarks.

➤ CLINICAL TIP   Accept the patient's delusional system. Do not attempt to argue with him about what is "real."
• Respect the patient's privacy and space needs. Don't touch him unnecessarily.

• Take steps to reduce social isolation, if the patient allows. Gradually increase social contacts after he has become comfortable with the staff.

• Watch for refusal of medication or food, resulting from the patient's irrational fear of poisoning.

• Monitor the patient carefully for adverse effects of antipsychotic drugs: drug-induced parkinsonism, acute dystonia, akathisia, tardive dyskinesia, and malignant neuroleptic syndrome.

• If the patient is taking clozapine, stress the importance of returning weekly to the hospital or an outpatient setting to have his blood monitored.

• Involve the family in treatment. Teach them how to recognize signs of an impending relapse — tension, nervousness, insomnia, decreased concentration ability, and apathy — and suggest ways to manage them.

---

# DEPRESSION, MAJOR

Also known as unipolar disorder, major depression is a syndrome of persistently sad, dysphoric mood accompanied by disturbances in sleep and appetite, lethargy, and an inability to experience pleasure (anhedonia). Major depression occurs in up to 17% of adults, affecting all racial, ethnic, and socioeconomic groups. It affects both sexes but is more common in women.

About half of all depressed patients experience a single episode and recover completely; the rest have at least one recurrence. Major depression can profoundly alter social, family, and occupational functioning.

However, suicide is the most serious complication of major depression, resulting when the patient's feelings of worthlessness, guilt, and hopelessness are so overwhelming that he no longer considers life worth living. Nearly twice as many women as men attempt suicide, but men are far more likely to succeed.

## Causes

The multiple causes of depression are not completely understood. Current research suggests possible genetic, familial, biochemical, physical, psychological, and social causes.

### Psychological factors

Such causes may include feelings of helplessness and vulnerability, anger, hopelessness and pessimism, and low self-esteem; they may be related to abnormal character and behavior patterns and troubled personal relationships.

In many patients, the history identifies a specific personal loss or severe stressor that probably interacts with the person's predisposition to provoke major depression.

### Medical conditions

Depression may be secondary to a specific medical condition — for example, metabolic disturbances, such as hypoxia and hypercalcemia; endocrine disorders, such as diabetes and Cushing's disease; neurologic diseases, such as Parkinson's and Alzheimer's disease; and cancer, especially of the pancreas.

Other medical conditions that may underlie depression include viral and bacterial infections, such as influenza and pneumonia; cardiovascular disorders such as heart failure; pulmonary disorders such as chronic obstructive pulmonary disease; musculoskeletal disorders such as degenerative arthritis; GI disorders such as irritable bowel syndrome; genitourinary problems such as incontinence; collagen vascular diseases such as lupus; and anemias.

## DYSTHYMIC DISORDER: A CHRONIC AFFECTIVE DISORDER

This disorder is characterized by a chronic dysphoric mood (irritable mood in children) persisting at least 2 years in adults and 1 year in children and adolescents.

### Signs and symptoms
During periods of depression, the patient also may experience poor appetite or overeating, insomnia or hypersomnia, low energy or fatigue, low self-esteem, poor concentration or difficulty making decisions, and feelings of hopelessness.

### Diagnosis
Dysthymic disorder is confirmed when the patient exhibits at least two of the symptoms listed above nearly every day, with intervening normal moods lasting no more than 2 months during a 2-year period.

The disorder typically begins in childhood, adolescence, or early adulthood and causes only mild social or occupational impairment. In adults, it's more common in women; in children and adolescents, it's equally common in both sexes.

### *Drugs*
Drugs prescribed for medical and psychiatric conditions, as well as many commonly abused substances, can also cause depression. Examples include antihypertensives, psychotropics, narcotic and nonnarcotic analgesics, antiparkinsonian drugs, numerous cardiovascular medications, oral antidiabetics, antimicrobials, steroids, chemotherapeutic agents, cimetidine, and alcohol.

### Signs and symptoms
The primary features of major depression are a predominantly sad mood and a loss of interest or pleasure in daily activities. Symptoms tend to be more severe than those caused by dysthymic disorder, which is a milder, chronic form of depression. (See *Dysthymic disorder: A chronic affective disorder.*)

The depressive patient may complain of feeling "down in the dumps," express doubts about his self-worth or ability to cope, or simply appear unhappy and apathetic. He also may report feeling angry or anxious.

Other common signs include difficulty concentrating or thinking clearly, distractibility, and indecisiveness. Take special note if the patient reveals suicidal thoughts, a preoccupation with death, or previous suicide attempts.

The psychosocial history may reveal life problems or losses that can account for the depression. Alternatively, the patient's medical history may implicate a physical disorder or the use of prescription, nonprescription, or illegal drugs that can cause depression.

The patient may report an increase or a decrease in appetite, sleep disturbances (for example, insomnia or early awakening), a lack of interest in sexual activity, constipation, or diarrhea. Other signs that you may note during a physical examination include agitation (such as hand wringing or restlessness) and reduced psychomotor activity (for example, slowed speech).

### Diagnosis
The *DSM-IV* describes specific characteristics of patients with this condition. (See *Diagnosing major depression.*)

The diagnosis of major depression is supported by psychological tests, such as the Beck Depression Inventory, which may help determine the onset, severity, duration, and progression of depressive symptoms.

# DIAGNOSING MAJOR DEPRESSION

A patient is diagnosed with major depression when he fulfills the following criteria for a single major depressive episode from the *Diagnostic and Statistical Manual of Mental Disorders,* 4th edition:

• At least five of the following symptoms must have been present during the same 2-week period and must represent a change from previous functioning; one of these symptoms must be either depressed mood or loss of interest in previously pleasurable activities:

– depressed mood (irritable mood in children and adolescents) most of the day, nearly every day, as indicated by either subjective account or observation by others

– markedly diminished interest or pleasure in all, or almost all, activities most of the day, nearly every day

– significant weight loss or weight gain when not dieting or decrease or increase in appetite nearly every day (in children, consider failure to make expected weight gains)

– insomnia or hypersomnia nearly every day

– psychomotor agitation or retardation nearly every day

– fatigue or loss of energy nearly every day

– feelings of worthlessness or excessive or inappropriate guilt nearly every day

– diminished ability to think or concentrate, or indecisiveness, nearly every day

– recurrent thoughts of death, recurrent suicidal ideation without a specific plan, a suicide attempt, or a specific plan for committing suicide.

• The symptoms do not meet criteria for a mixed episode.

• The symptoms cause clinically significant distress or impairment in social, occupational, or other important areas of functioning.

• The symptoms are not due to the direct physiologic effects of a substance or a general medical condition.

• The symptoms are not better accounted for by bereavement, the symptoms persist for longer than 2 months, or the symptoms are characterized by marked functional impairment, morbid preoccupation with worthlessness, suicidal ideation, psychotic symptoms, or psychomotor retardation.

A toxicology screening may suggest drug-induced depression.

## Treatment

Depression is difficult to treat, especially in children, adolescents, elderly patients, and those with a history of chronic disease. The primary treatment methods are drug therapy, electroconvulsive therapy (ECT), and psychotherapy.

### Drug therapy

In depression, drug therapy includes tricyclic antidepressants (TCAs) such as amitriptyline, serotonin reuptake in-

hibitors such as fluoxetine, and monoamine oxidase (MAO) inhibitors, such as isocarboxazid, maprotiline, and trazodone.

• The most widely used class of antidepressant drugs, TCAs prevent the reuptake of norepinephrine or serotonin (or both) into the presynaptic nerve endings, resulting in increased synaptic concentrations of these neurotransmitters. They also cause a gradual loss in the number of beta-adrenergic receptors.

• After resolution of the acute episode, patients with a history of recurrent depression may be maintained on low doses of antidepressants as a preventive measure.

• Selective serotonin reuptake inhibitors, including fluoxetine, paroxetine, and sertraline, are increasingly becoming the drugs of choice. They are effective and produce fewer adverse effects than the TCAs; however, they're associated with sleep and GI problems and alterations in sexual desire and function.

• MAO inhibitors block the enzymatic degradation of norepinephrine and serotonin. These agents often are prescribed for patients with atypical depression (for example, depression marked by an increased appetite and need for sleep, rather than anorexia and insomnia) and for some patients who fail to respond to TCAs.

MAO inhibitors are associated with a high risk of toxicity; patients treated with one of these drugs must be able to comply with the necessary dietary restrictions. Conservative doses of an MAO inhibitor may be combined with a TCA for patients refractory to either drug alone.

Maprotiline is a potent blocker of norepinephrine uptake, whereas trazodone is a selective serotonin uptake blocker. The mechanism of action of bupropion is unknown.

### *ECT*

When a depressed patient is incapacitated, suicidal, or psychotically depressed, or when antidepressants are contraindicated or ineffective, ECT often is the treatment of choice. Six to 12 treatments usually are needed, although improvement often is evident after only a few treatments. Researchers hypothesize that ECT affects the same receptor sites as antidepressants.

### *Psychotherapy*

Short-term psychotherapy also is effective in treating major depression. Many psychiatrists believe that the best results are achieved with a combination of individual, family, or group psychotherapy and medication. Therapeutic interventions focus on identifying the patient's negative thoughts and interpretations and substituting adaptive responses.

### Special considerations

• Share your observations of the patient's behavior with him. For instance, you might say, "You're sitting all by yourself, looking very sad. Is that how you feel?" Because the patient may think and react sluggishly, speak slowly and allow ample time for him to respond.

• Avoid feigned cheerfulness. However, don't hesitate to laugh with the patient and point out the value of humor.

• Show the patient that he's important by listening attentively and respectfully, preventing interruptions, and avoiding judgmental responses.

• Provide a structured routine, including noncompetitive activities, to build the patient's self-confidence and encourage interaction with others. Urge him to join group activities and to socialize.

• Inform the patient that he can help ease depression by expressing his feelings, participating in pleasurable activities, and improving grooming and hygiene.

• Ask the patient if he thinks of death or suicide. Such thoughts signal an immediate need for consultation and assessment. Failure to detect suicidal thoughts early may encourage the patient to attempt suicide.

➤ CLINICAL TIP   The risk of suicide increases as the depression lifts.

• While tending to the patient's psychological needs, don't forget his physical needs. If he's too depressed to take care of himself, help him with personal hygiene. Encourage him to eat, or feed him if necessary. If he's constipated, add high-fiber foods to his diet; offer small, frequent meals; and encourage physical activity and fluid intake. Offer warm milk or back rubs at bedtime to improve sleep.

• If the patient is taking an antidepressant, monitor him for evidence of seizures. Some antidepressants significantly lower the seizure threshold. (See *Guidelines for antidepressant therapy.*)

• Teach the patient about depression. Emphasize that effective methods are available to relieve his symptoms. Help him to recognize distorted perceptions that may contribute to his depression. Once the patient learns to recognize depressive thought patterns, he can consciously begin to substitute self-affirming thoughts.

• Instruct the patient about prescribed medications. Stress the need for compliance and review adverse effects. For drugs that produce strong anticholinergic effects, such as amitriptyline and amoxapine, suggest sugarless gum or hard candy to relieve dry mouth.

• Many antidepressants are sedating (for example, amitriptyline and trazodone); warn the patient taking one of these drugs to avoid activities that require alertness, including driving and operating mechanical equipment, until the central nervous system (CNS) effects of the drug are known.

• Caution the patient taking a TCA to avoid drinking alcoholic beverages or taking other CNS depressants during therapy.

• If the patient is taking an MAO inhibitor, emphasize that he must avoid foods that contain tyramine, caffeine, or tryptophan. The ingestion of tyramine can cause a hypertensive crisis. Examples of foods that contain these substances are cheese, sour cream, pickled herring, liver, canned figs, raisins, bananas, avocados, chocolate, soy sauce, fava beans, yeast extracts, meat tenderizers, coffee, colas, and beer, chianti, and sherry.

---

TEACHING CHECKLIST

## GUIDELINES FOR ANTIDEPRESSANT THERAPY

Review the following teaching points with your patient who is undergoing antidepressant therapy.

• Inform the patient that it can take up to 4 weeks to feel the full benefit of the medication.

• Tell him to take the medication exactly as prescribed.

• Because there are many different types of antidepressants, several may need to be tried before finding the one that works best.

• Alcoholic beverages can increase depression.

• Review the adverse effects of the particular medication and when to call the doctor.

---

# DERMATITIS

An inflammation of the skin, dermatitis occurs in several forms: atopic (discussed here), seborrheic, nummular, contact, chronic, localized neurodermatitis (lichen simplex chronicus), exfoliative, and stasis. (See *Types of dermatitis,* pages 270 to 273.)

Atopic dermatitis (atopic or infantile eczema) is a chronic or recurrent inflammatory response often associated with other atopic diseases, such as bronchial asthma and allergic rhinitis. It usually develops in infants and toddlers between ages 1 month and 1 year, commonly in those with strong family histories of atopic disease. These children often acquire other atopic disorders as they grow older.

*(Text continues on page 272.)*

## TYPES OF DERMATITIS

| TYPE | CAUSES | SIGNS AND SYMPTOMS |
|------|--------|---------------------|
| **Seborrheic dermatitis** A subacute skin disease that affects the scalp, face, and occasionally other areas and is characterized by lesions covered with yellow or brownish gray scales | • Unknown; stress, immunodeficiency, and neurologic conditions may be predisposing factors; related to the yeast *Pityrosporum ovale* (normal flora) | • Eruptions in areas with many sebaceous glands (usually scalp, face, chest, axillae, and groin) and in skin folds • Itching, redness, and inflammation of affected areas; lesions may appear greasy; fissures may occur • Indistinct, occasionally yellowish, scaly patches from excess stratum corneum (Dandruff may be a mild seborrheic dermatitis.) |
| **Nummular dermatitis** A subacute form of dermatitis characterized by inflammation in coin-shaped, scaling, or vesicular patches, usually quite pruritic | • Possibly precipitated by stress, skin dryness, irritants, or scratching | • Round, nummular (coin-shaped), red lesions, usually on arms and legs, with distinct borders of crusts and scales • Possible oozing and severe itching • Summertime remissions common, with wintertime recurrence |
| **Contact dermatitis** Often sharply demarcated inflammation of the skin resulting from contact with an irritating chemical or atopic allergen (a substance producing an allergic reaction in the skin) and irritation of the skin resulting from contact with concentrated substances to which the skin is sensitive, such as perfumes, soaps, or chemicals | • Mild irritants: chronic exposure to detergents or solvents • Strong irritants: damage on contact with acids or alkalis • Allergens: sensitization after repeated exposure | • Mild irritants and allergens: erythema and small vesicles that ooze, scale, and itch • Strong irritants: blisters and ulcerations • Classic allergic response: clearly defined lesions, with straight lines following points of contact • Severe allergic reaction: marked erythema, blistering, and edema of affected areas |
| **Hand or foot dermatitis** A skin disease characterized by inflammatory eruptions of the hands or feet | • In many cases, unknown but may result from irritant or allergic contact • Excessive skin dryness often a contributing factor • 50% of patients are atopic | • Redness and scaling of the palms or soles • May produce painful fissures • Some cases present with blisters (dyshidrotic eczema) |

| DIAGNOSIS | TREATMENT AND INTERVENTIONS |
|---|---|
| • Patient history and physical findings, especially distribution of lesions in sebaceous gland areas, confirm seborrheic dermatitis.<br>• Diagnosis must rule out psoriasis. | • Removal of scales with frequent washing and shampooing with selenium sulfide suspension (most effective), zinc pyrithione, or tar and salicylic acid shampoo<br>• Application of topical corticosteroids and antifungals to involved area |
| • Physical findings and patient history confirm nummular dermatitis.<br>• Diagnosis must rule out fungal infections, atopic or contact dermatitis, and psoriasis. | • Elimination of known irritants<br>• Measures to relieve dry skin: increased humidification, limited frequency of baths and use of bland soap and bath oils, and application of emollients<br>• Application of wet dressings in acute phase<br>• Topical corticosteroids (occlusive dressings or intralesional injections) for persistent lesions<br>• Tar preparations and antihistamines to control itching<br>• Antibiotics for secondary infection<br>• Same as for atopic dermatitis |
| • Patient history, patch testing to identify allergens, and shape and distribution of lesions suggest contact dermatitis. | • Elimination of known allergens and decreased exposure to irritants; wearing protective clothing, such as gloves; and washing immediately after contact with irritants or allergens<br>• Topical anti-inflammatory agents (including corticosteroids), systemic corticosteroids for edema and bullae, antihistamines, and local applications of Burow's solution (for blisters)<br>• Same as for atopic dermatitis |
| • Patient history and physical findings (distribution of eruption on palms and soles) confirm diagnosis. | • Same as for nummular dermatitis<br>• Severe cases may require systemic steroids. |

*(continued)*

## TYPES OF DERMATITIS *(continued)*

| TYPE | CAUSES | SIGNS AND SYMPTOMS |
|---|---|---|
| **Localized neurodermatitis (lichen simplex chronicus, essential pruritus)** Superficial inflammation of the skin characterized by itching and papular eruptions that appear on thickened, hyperpigmented skin | • Chronic scratching or rubbing of a primary lesion or insect bite, or other skin irritation<br>• May be psychogenic | • Intense, sometimes continual scratching<br>• Thick, sharp-bordered, possibly dry, scaly lesions with raised papules and accentuated skin lines (lichenification)<br>• Usually affects easily reached areas, such as ankles, lower legs, anogenital area, back of neck, and ears<br>• One or a few lesions may be present; asymmetric distribution |
| **Exfoliative dermatitis** Severe skin inflammation characterized by redness and widespread erythema and scaling, covering virtually the entire skin surface | • Preexisting skin lesions progressing to exfoliative stage, such as in contact dermatitis, drug reaction, lymphoma, leukemia, or atopic dermatitis<br>• May be idiopathic | • Generalized dermatitis, with acute loss of stratum corneum, and erythema and scaling<br>• Sensation of tight skin<br>• Hair loss<br>• Possible fever, sensitivity to cold, shivering, gynecomastia, and lymphadenopathy |
| **Stasis dermatitis** A condition usually caused by impaired circulation and characterized by eczema of the legs with edema, hyperpigmentation, and persistent inflammation | • Secondary to peripheral vascular diseases affecting legs, such as recurrent thrombophlebitis and resultant chronic venous insufficiency | • Varicosities and edema common, but obvious vascular insufficiency not always present<br>• Usually affects the lower leg, just above internal malleolus, or sites of trauma or irritation<br>• Early signs: dusky red deposits of hemosiderin in skin, with itching and dimpling of subcutaneous tissue<br>• Later signs: edema, redness, and scaling of large areas of legs<br>• Possible fissures, crusts, and ulcers |

Typically, this form of dermatitis flares and subsides repeatedly before finally resolving during adolescence. However, it can persist into adulthood. Atopic dermatitis affects about 9 out of every 1,000 persons.

**Causes**

The cause of atopic dermatitis is unknown, but there is a genetic predisposition exacerbated by such factors as food allergies, infections, irritating chemicals, temperature and humidity,

| DIAGNOSIS | TREATMENT AND INTERVENTIONS |
|---|---|
| • Physical findings confirm diagnosis. | • Scratching must stop; then lesions will disappear in about 2 weeks.<br>• Fixed dressings or Unna's boot to cover affected areas<br>• Topical corticosteroids under occlusion or by intralesional injection<br>• Antihistamines and open wet dressings<br>• Emollients<br>• Patient informed about underlying cause |
| • Diagnosis requires identification of the underlying cause. | • Hospitalization, with protective isolation and hygienic measures to prevent secondary bacterial infection<br>• Open wet dressings, with colloidal baths<br>• Bland lotions over topical corticosteroids<br>• Maintenance of constant environmental temperature to prevent chilling or overheating<br>• Careful monitoring of renal and cardiac status<br>• Systemic antibiotics and steroids<br>• Same as for atopic dermatitis |
| • Diagnosis requires positive history of venous insufficiency and physical findings, such as varicosities. | • Measures to prevent venous stasis: avoidance of prolonged sitting or standing, use of support stockings, weight reduction in obesity, and leg elevation<br>• Corrective surgery for underlying cause<br>• After ulcer develops, encourage rest periods, with legs elevated; open wet dressings; Unna's boot (zinc gelatin dressing provides continuous pressure to affected areas); and antibiotics for secondary infection after wound culture. |

and emotions. Approximately 10% of childhood cases are caused by allergy to certain foods, particularly eggs, peanuts, milk, and wheat.

Atopic dermatitis tends to flare up in response to extremes in temperature and humidity. Other causes of flare-ups are sweating and psychological stress.

An important secondary cause of atopic dermatitis is irritation, which seems to change the epidermal structure, allowing immunoglobulin E (IgE) activity to increase. Consequently, chronic skin irritation usually continues even after exposure to the allergen has ended or after the irritation has been systemically controlled.

### Signs and symptoms

Atopic skin lesions generally begin as erythematous areas on excessively dry skin. In children, such lesions typically appear on the forehead, cheeks, and extensor surfaces of the arms and legs; in adults, at flexion points (antecubital fossa, popliteal area, and neck).

During flare-ups, pruritus and scratching cause edema, crusting, and scaling. Eventually, chronic atopic lesions lead to multiple areas of dry, scaly skin, with white dermatographia, blanching, and lichenification.

Common secondary conditions associated with atopic dermatitis include viral, fungal, or bacterial infections and ocular disorders.

Because of intense pruritus, the upper eyelid is commonly hyperpigmented and swollen, and a double fold occurs under the lower lid (Morgan's, Dennie's, or Mongolian fold). Atopic cataracts are unusual but may develop between ages 20 and 40.

Kaposi's varicelliform eruption (eczema herpeticum), a potentially serious widespread cutaneous viral infection, may develop if the patient comes in contact with a person who's infected with herpes simplex.

### Diagnosis

A family history of atopic disorders is helpful in the diagnosis of atopic dermatitis.

Typical distribution of skin lesions and course rule out other inflammatory skin lesions, such as diaper rash (lesions confined to the diapered area), seborrheic dermatitis, and chronic contact dermatitis (lesions affect hands and forearms, sparing antecubital and popliteal areas). Serum IgE levels are often elevated but are not diagnostic.

### Treatment

Effective treatment of atopic lesions consists of eliminating allergens and avoiding irritants (strong soaps, cleansers, and other chemicals), extreme temperature changes, and other precipitating factors. Local and systemic measures relieve itching and inflammation.

> **CLINICAL TIP** Prevention of excessive dryness of the skin is critical to successful therapy.

Topical application of a corticosteroid ointment, especially after bathing, often alleviates inflammation. Between steroid doses, application of a moisturizing cream can help retain moisture. Systemic corticosteroid therapy should be used only during extreme exacerbations.

Weak tar preparations and ultraviolet B light therapy are used to increase the thickness of the stratum corneum. Antibiotics are appropriate if a bacterial agent has been cultured.

### Special considerations

● Warn that drowsiness is possible with the use of antihistamines to relieve daytime itching. If nocturnal itching interferes with sleep, suggest methods for inducing natural sleep such as drinking a glass of warm milk to prevent overuse of sedatives. Antihistamines may also be useful at bedtime.

● Help the patient set up an individual schedule and plan for daily skin care.

● Instruct the patient to bathe in plain water. (He may have to limit bathing, according to the severity of the lesions.) Tell him to bathe with a special nonfatty soap and tepid water (96° F [35.6° C]), to avoid using any soap when lesions are acutely inflamed, and to limit baths or showers to 5 to 7 minutes.

• For scalp involvement, advise the patient to shampoo frequently and apply corticosteroid solution to the scalp afterward.

• Keep fingernails short to limit excoriation and secondary infections caused by scratching.

• Lubricate the skin after a shower or bath.

• To help clear lichenified skin, apply occlusive dressings (such as plastic film) over a corticosteroid cream intermittently as necessary.

• Inform the patient that irritants, such as detergents and wool, and emotional stress exacerbate atopic dermatitis.

• Be careful not to show any anxiety or revulsion when touching the lesions during treatment. Help the patient accept his altered body image, and encourage him to verbalize his feelings. Remember, coping with disfigurement is extremely difficult, especially for children and adolescents.

• Arrange for counseling, if necessary, to help the patient deal with his distressing condition more effectively.

# DERMATOPHYTOSIS

Also called tinea or ringworm, dermatophytosis is a disease that can affect the scalp (tinea capitis), body (tinea corporis), nails (tinea unguium), feet (tinea pedis), groin (tinea cruris), and bearded skin (tinea barbae).

Tinea infections are quite prevalent in the United States and are usually more common in males than in females. With effective treatment, the cure rate is very high, although about 20% of persons with infected feet or nails develop chronic conditions.

## Causes

Tinea infections (except for tinea versicolor) result from dermatophytes (fungi) of the genera *Trichophyton, Microsporum,* and *Epidermophyton.*

Transmission can occur directly (through contact with infected lesions) or indirectly (through contact with contaminated articles, such as shoes, towels, or shower stalls). Some cases come from animals or soil.

### Signs and symptoms

Lesions vary in appearance and duration with the type of infection:

• *Tinea capitis,* which mainly affects children, is characterized by round erythematous patches on the scalp, causing hair loss with scaling. In some children, a hypersensitivity reaction develops, leading to boggy, inflamed, often pus-filled lesions (kerions).

• *Tinea corporis* produces flat lesions on the skin at any site except the scalp, bearded skin, groin, palms, or soles. These lesions may be dry and scaly or moist and crusty; as they enlarge, their centers heal, causing the classic ring-shaped appearance.

• *Tinea unguium* (onychomycosis) infection typically starts at the tip of one or more toenails (fingernail infection is less common) and produces gradual thickening, discoloration, and crumbling of the nail, with accumulation of subungual debris. Eventually, the nail may be destroyed completely.

• *Tinea pedis* causes scaling and blisters between the toes. Severe infection may result in inflammation, with severe itching and pain on walking. A dry, squamous inflammation may affect the entire sole.

• *Tinea cruris* (jock itch) produces red, raised, sharply defined, itchy lesions in the groin that may extend to the buttocks, inner thighs, and the external genitalia. Warm weather and tight clothing encourage fungus growth.

• *Tinea barbae* is an uncommon infection that affects the bearded facial area of men.

### Diagnosis

Microscopic examination of lesion scrapings prepared in potassium hydroxide solution usually confirms tinea infection. Other diagnostic procedures include Wood's light examination (which is useful in only about 5% of cases of tinea capitis) and culture of the infecting organism.

### Treatment

Tinea infections usually respond to topical agents such as imidazole cream or to oral griseofulvin, which is especially effective in tinea infections of the skin and hair. Oral terbinafine or itraconazole is helpful in nail infections.

However, topical therapy is ineffective for tinea capitis; oral griseofulvin for 1 to 3 months is the treatment of choice.

➤ CLINICAL TIP  Griseofulvin is contraindicated in the patient with porphyria, and it may necessitate an increase in dosage during anticoagulant (warfarin) therapy.

In addition to imidazole, other antifungals include naftifine, ciclopirox, terbinafine, haloprogin, and tolnaftate. Topical treatments should continue for 2 weeks after lesions resolve.

Supportive measures include open wet dressings, removal of scabs and scales, and application of keratolytics such as salicylic acid to soften and remove hyperkeratotic lesions of the heels or soles.

### Special considerations

• For all tinea infections except those of the hair and nails, apply topical agents, watch for sensitivity reactions and secondary bacterial infections, and provide patient teaching.

• Monitor liver function of patients on long-term griseofulvin therapy.

• For tinea capitis, use good hand-washing technique, and teach the patient to do the same. To prevent spreading infection to others, advise washing towels, bedclothes, and combs frequently in hot water and to avoid sharing them. Suggest that family members be checked for tinea capitis.

• For tinea corporis, use abdominal pads between skin folds for the patient with excessive abdominal girth; change pads frequently. Check the patient daily for excoriated, newly denuded areas of skin. If the involved area is moist, apply open wet dressings two or three times daily to decrease inflammation and help remove scales.

• For tinea unguium, keep the patient's nails short and straight. Gently remove debris under the nails with an emery board.

• For tinea pedis, encourage the patient to expose feet to air whenever possible and to wear sandals or leather shoes and clean cotton socks. Instruct the patient to wash the feet twice daily and, after drying them thoroughly, to apply the antifungal cream followed by antifungal powder to absorb perspiration and prevent excoriation.

• For tinea cruris, instruct the patient to dry the affected area thoroughly after bathing and to evenly apply antifungal powder after applying the topical antifungal agent. Advise wearing loose-fitting clothing, which should be changed frequently and washed in hot water.

• For tinea barbae, suggest that the patient let his beard grow. (Whiskers should be trimmed with scissors, not a razor.) If the patient insists that he must shave, advise him to use an electric razor instead of a blade.

# DIABETES INSIPIDUS

A disorder of water metabolism, diabetes insipidus results from a deficiency of circulating vasopressin (also called antidiuretic hormone) or from renal resistance to this hormone. Pituitary diabetes insipidus is caused by deficiency of vasopressin, whereas nephrogenic diabetes insipidus is caused by renal tubular resistance to the action of vasopressin. Diabetes insipidus is characterized by excessive fluid intake and hypotonic polyuria.

The disorder may start in childhood or early adulthood (median age of onset is 21) and is more common in men than in women. Incidence is slightly higher today than in the past.

In uncomplicated diabetes insipidus, the prognosis is good with adequate water replacement, and patients usually lead normal lives.

## Causes
Pituitary diabetes insipidus results from intracranial neoplastic or metastatic lesions, hypophysectomy or other neurosurgery, a skull fracture, or head trauma that damages the neurohypophyseal structures. It can also result from infection, granulomatous disease, and vascular lesions; it may be idiopathic and, rarely, familial.

The hypothalamus synthesizes vasopressin. The posterior pituitary gland (or neurohypophysis) stores vasopressin and releases it into the general circulation, where it causes the kidneys to reabsorb water by making the distal tubules and collecting duct cells water-permeable.

In diabetes insipidus, the absence of vasopressin allows the filtered water to be excreted in the urine instead of being reabsorbed.

## Signs and symptoms
The patient's history typically shows an abrupt onset of extreme polyuria (usually 4 to 16 L/day of dilute urine, but sometimes as much as 30 L/day). As a result, the patient is extremely thirsty and drinks great quantities of water to compensate for the body's water loss. This disorder may also result in nocturia.

If the patient is unable to obtain adequate quantities of water, features of diabetes insipidus include signs and symptoms of dehydration (poor tissue turgor, dry mucous membranes, constipation, muscle weakness, dizziness, and hypotension). Polyuria usually begins abruptly, commonly appearing within 1 to 2 days after a basal skull fracture, a cerebrovascular accident, or surgery.

Relieving cerebral edema or increased intracranial pressure may cause all of these symptoms to subside just as rapidly as they began.

## Diagnosis
Urinalysis reveals almost colorless urine of low osmolality (50 to 200 mOsm/kg, less than that of plasma) and low specific gravity (< 1.005). However, a diagnosis requires the water deprivation test to provide evidence of vasopressin deficiency, resulting in the kidneys' inability to concentrate urine.

### Water deprivation test
In this test, after baseline vital signs, weight, and urine and plasma osmolalities are obtained, the patient is deprived of fluids and observed to make sure he doesn't drink anything surreptitiously. Hourly measurements then record the total volume of urine output, body weight, urine osmolality or specific gravity, and plasma osmolality. Throughout the test, blood pressure and pulse rate

must be monitored for signs of orthostatic hypotension.

Fluid deprivation continues until the patient loses 3% of his body weight (indicating severe dehydration). When urine osmolality stops increasing in three consecutive hourly specimens, the patient receives 5 units of aqueous vasopressin subcutaneously (S.C.).

Hourly measurements of urine volume and specific gravity continue after S.C. injection of aqueous vasopressin. Patients with pituitary diabetes insipidus respond to exogenous vasopressin with decreased urine output and increased specific gravity. Patients with nephrogenic diabetes insipidus show no response to vasopressin.

### Treatment

Until the cause of diabetes insipidus can be identified and eliminated, administration of various forms of vasopressin can control fluid balance and prevent dehydration.

#### Vasopressin injection

This aqueous preparation is administered S.C. or I.M. several times a day because it's effective for only 2 to 6 hours. This form of the drug is used as a diagnostic agent and, rarely, in acute disease.

#### Desmopressin acetate

This drug can be given orally, by nasal spray that's absorbed through the mucous membranes, or by S.C. or I.V. injection. Desmopressin acetate is effective for 8 to 20 hours, depending on the dosage.

### Special considerations

● Record fluid intake and output carefully. Maintain fluid intake that's adequate to prevent severe dehydration.
● Watch for signs of hypovolemic shock, and monitor blood pressure and heart

and respiratory rates regularly, especially during the water deprivation test. Check the patient's weight daily.
● If the patient is dizzy or has muscle weakness, institute safety precautions, including keeping the side rails up. Assist him with walking.
● Monitor urine specific gravity between doses. Watch for a decrease in specific gravity accompanied by increasing urine output, indicating the recurrence of polyuria and necessitating administration of the next dose of medication or a dosage increase.
● Provide meticulous skin and mouth care; apply petroleum jelly, as needed, to cracked or sore lips.
● Before discharge, teach the patient how to monitor intake and output.

▶ CLINICAL TIP Teach the patient the signs and symptoms of water intoxication, an adverse effect of excessive doses of desmopressin.
● Teach the patient that recurrence of polyuria, as reflected on the intake and output sheet, indicates that the dosage is too low.
● Advise the patient to wear a medical identification bracelet and to carry his medication with him at all times.
● Teach the parents of a child with diabetes insipidus about normal growth and development.
● Refer patients with diabetes insipidus and their families for counseling and psychosocial adjustment or coping and support groups, if necessary.

# DIABETES MELLITUS

A chronic disease of absolute or relative insulin deficiency or resistance, diabetes mellitus is characterized by disturbances in carbohydrate, protein, and fat metabolism.

This condition occurs in two forms: type 1, characterized by absolute insulin insufficiency, and type 2, characterized by insulin resistance with varying degrees of insulin secretory defects.

Onset of type 1 usually occurs before age 30 (although it may occur at any age); the patient is usually thin and requires exogenous insulin and dietary management to achieve control. Conversely, type 2 usually occurs in obese adults after age 40, although it's commonly seen in North American youths. It's most often treated with diet and exercise (in combination with antidiabetic drugs), although treatment may include insulin therapy.

Diabetes mellitus is estimated to affect nearly 8% of the population of the United States (16 million people), about half of whom are undiagnosed. Incidence is equal in men and women and rises with age.

Nearly two-thirds of people with diabetes will die of cardiovascular disease. It's also the leading cause of renal failure and new blindness.

## Causes

The effects of diabetes mellitus result from insulin deficiency. Insulin transports glucose into the cell for use as energy and storage as glycogen. It also stimulates protein synthesis and free fatty acid storage. Insulin deficiency compromises the body tissues' access to essential nutrients for fuel and storage.

The etiology of both type 1 and type 2 diabetes remains unknown. Genetic factors may play a part in development of all types; autoimmune disease and viral infections may be risk factors in type 1.

Other risk factors include the following:

• Obesity contributes to the resistance to endogenous insulin.

• Physiologic or emotional stress can cause prolonged elevation of stress hormone levels (cortisol, epinephrine, glucagon, and growth hormone). This raises blood glucose levels, which, in turn, places increased demands on the pancreas.

• Pregnancy causes weight gain and increases levels of estrogen and placental hormones, which antagonize insulin.

• Some medications can antagonize the effects of insulin, including thiazide diuretics, adrenal corticosteroids, and oral contraceptives.

## Signs and symptoms

Diabetes may begin dramatically with ketoacidosis in type 1 or insidiously. Its most common symptom is fatigue, from energy deficiency and a catabolic state. However, many patients with type 2 diabetes may be asymptomatic.

Insulin deficiency causes hyperglycemia, which pulls fluid from body tissues, causing osmotic diuresis, polyuria, dehydration, polydipsia, dry mucous membranes, and poor skin turgor. In ketoacidosis and hyperglycemic hyperosmolar nonketotic state, dehydration may cause hypovolemia and shock. Wasting of glucose in the urine usually produces weight loss and hunger in uncontrolled type 1 diabetes, even if the patient eats voraciously.

### Long-term effects

In diabetes, long-term effects may include retinopathy, nephropathy, atherosclerosis, and peripheral and autonomic neuropathy.

Peripheral neuropathy usually affects the hands and feet and may cause numbness or pain. Autonomic neuropathy may manifest itself in several ways, including gastroparesis (leading to delayed gastric emptying and a feeling of nausea and fullness after meals), nocturnal diarrhea, impotence, and postural hypotension.

Because hyperglycemia impairs the patient's resistance to infection, diabetes may result in skin and urinary tract infections and vaginitis. Glucose content of the epidermis and urine encourages bacterial growth.

## Diagnosis

In nonpregnant adults, diabetes mellitus is diagnosed with:
- at least two occasions of a fasting plasma glucose level ≥ 126 mg/dl
- typical symptoms of uncontrolled diabetes and a random blood glucose level ≥ 200 mg/dl
- a blood glucose level ≥ 200 mg/dl at 2 hours after ingestion of 75 grams of oral dextrose.

Two tests are required for diagnosis; they can be the same two tests or any combination and may be separated by more than 24 hours.

An ophthalmologic examination may show diabetic retinopathy. Other diagnostic and monitoring tests include urinalysis for acetone and blood testing for glycosylated hemoglobin, which reflects glucose control over the past 2 to 3 months.

## Treatment

Effective treatment for both types of diabetes normalizes blood glucose and decreases complications.

### Type 1 diabetes

Treatment includes insulin replacement, diet, and exercise. Current forms of insulin replacement include single-dose, mixed-dose, split-mixed dose, and multiple-dose regimens. The multiple-dose regimens may use an insulin pump.

Human insulin may be rapid-acting (Regular), intermediate-acting (NPH or Lente), long-acting (Ultralente), or a combination of rapid-acting and intermediate-acting (70/30 or 50/50 of NPH and Regular) mixed together.

> **CLINICAL TIP** Insulin Lispro may be used in place of Regular insulin. It is rapid in onset (15 minutes) and makes waiting to eat after injection unnecessary. It has a short duration of action (4 hours), which decreases between-meal and nocturnal hypoglycemia.

Pancreas transplantation is available and requires chronic immunosuppression.

### Type 2 diabetes

Patients may require oral antidiabetic drugs to stimulate endogenous insulin production, increase insulin sensitivity at the cellular level, suppress hepatic gluconeogenesis, and delay GI absorption of carbohydrates.

### Both types

Treatment of both types of diabetes requires a diet planned to meet nutritional needs, to control blood glucose levels, and to reach and maintain appropriate body weight.

For the obese patient with type 2 diabetes, weight reduction is a goal. In type 1, the calorie allotment may be high, depending on growth stage and activity level. For success, the diet must be followed consistently and meals eaten at regular times.

### Complications

Treatment of long-term diabetic complications may include transplantation or dialysis for renal failure, photocoagulation for retinopathy, and vascular surgery for large-vessel disease. Meticulous blood glucose control is essential.

The Diabetes Control and Complications Trial has proved that intensive insulin therapy that focuses on keeping glucose at near-normal levels for 5 years or more reduces both the onset and progression of retinopathy (up to 63%), nephropathy (up to 54%), and neuropathy (up to 60%).

## Special considerations

• Stress that compliance with the prescribed program is essential. Emphasize the effect of blood glucose control on long-term health. (See *Controlling diabetes mellitus.*)

• Watch for acute complications of diabetic therapy, especially hypoglycemia (vagueness, slow cerebration, dizziness, weakness, pallor, tachycardia, diaphoresis, seizures, and coma). Immediately give carbohydrates in the form of fruit juice, hard candy, or honey; if the patient is unconscious, subcutaneous, I.M., or I.V. glucagon or I.V. dextrose may be given.

• Be alert for signs and symptoms of ketoacidosis (acetone breath, dehydration, weak and rapid pulse, Kussmaul's respirations) and hyperosmolar coma (polyuria, thirst, neurologic abnormalities, stupor). These hyperglycemic crises require I.V. fluids, insulin and, usually, potassium replacement.

• Monitor diabetic control by testing urine for acetone and obtaining blood glucose levels.

• Watch for diabetic effects on the cardiovascular system, such as cerebrovascular, coronary artery, and peripheral vascular impairment, and on the peripheral and autonomic nervous systems.

• Treat all injuries, cuts, and blisters (particularly on the legs or feet) meticulously.

• Be alert for signs of urinary tract infection and renal disease.

• Urge regular ophthalmologic examinations to detect diabetic retinopathy.

• Assess for signs of diabetic neuropathy (numbness or pain in the hands and feet, footdrop, neurogenic bladder). Stress the need for personal safety precautions; explain that decreased sensation can mask injuries. Minimize complications by maintaining strict blood glucose control.

---

TEACHING CHECKLIST

## ✔ CONTROLING DIABETES MELLITUS

The patient with diabetes mellitus will need careful teaching. Tailor your instruction to the patient's needs, abilities, and developmental stage. Make sure you teach your patient to:

• follow dietary guidelines closely
• understand the purpose and goals of treatment
• correctly administer his medications
• recognize and report adverse reactions to medication
• maintain an exercise program
• follow procedures to monitor his condition
• maintain meticulous hygiene
• watch for and immediately report symptoms of hypoglycemia and hyperglycemia.

---

• Teach the patient to care for his feet by washing them daily, drying carefully between the toes, and inspecting for corns, calluses, redness, swelling, bruises, and breaks in the skin. Urge him to report any changes. Advise him to wear nonconstricting shoes and to avoid walking barefoot.

• Teach the patient how to manage his diabetes when he has a minor illness such as a cold, flu, or upset stomach.

CLINICAL TIP Screening should be done for diabetes mellitus on those with risk factors, including family history of the disease, obesity, ethinicity (Hispanics, Native Americans, Asian Americans, and African Americans are at higher risk), age 45 and older, history of impaired glucose tolerance or impaired fasting glucose, hypertension, hyperlipidemia, history of gestational diabetes mellitus, or women giving birth to a baby weighing more than 9 lb (4 kg).

● To delay the clinical onset of diabetes, teach persons at high risk to have good weight control and exercise regularly. Advise genetic counseling for young adult diabetics who are planning families.

● For further information, consult the Juvenile Diabetes Foundation, the American Diabetes Association, and the American Association of Diabetes Educators.

# DIABETIC COMPLICATIONS DURING PREGNANCY

Pregnancy places special demands on carbohydrate metabolism and causes the insulin requirement to increase, even in a healthy woman. Consequently, pregnancy may lead to a prediabetic state, to the conversion of an asymptomatic subclinical diabetic state to a clinical one (gestational diabetes occurs in about 1% to 2% of all pregnancies), or to complications in a previously stable diabetic state.

Prevalence of diabetes mellitus increases with age. Maternal and fetal prognoses can be equivalent to those in nondiabetic women if maternal blood glucose is well controlled and ketosis and other complications are prevented. Infant morbidity and mortality depend on recognizing and successfully controlling hypoglycemia, which may develop within hours after delivery.

## Causes

In diabetes mellitus, glucose is inadequately used either because insulin isn't synthesized (as in Type 1, insulin-dependent diabetes) or because tissues are resistant to the hormonal action of endogenous insulin (as in Type 2, non-insulin-dependent diabetes).

### Protective mechanisms

During pregnancy, the fetus relies on maternal glucose as a primary fuel source. Pregnancy triggers protective mechanisms that have anti-insulin effects: increased hormone production (placental lactogen, estrogen, and progesterone), which antagonizes the effects of insulin; degradation of insulin by the placenta; and prolonged elevation of stress hormones (cortisol, epinephrine, and glucagon), which raise blood glucose levels.

In a normal pregnancy, an increase in anti-insulin factors is counterbalanced by an increase in insulin production to maintain normal blood glucose levels. However, women who are prediabetic or diabetic can't produce sufficient insulin to overcome the insulin antagonist mechanisms of pregnancy, or their tissues are insulin-resistant.

As insulin requirements rise toward term, the patient who is prediabetic may develop gestational diabetes, necessitating dietary management and, possibly, exogenous insulin to achieve glycemic control. The insulin-dependent patient may need increased insulin dosage.

## Signs and symptoms

Indications for diagnostic screening for maternal diabetes mellitus during pregnancy include obesity, excessive weight gain, excessive hunger or thirst, polyuria, recurrent monilial infections, glycosuria, previous delivery of a large infant, polyhydramnios, maternal hypertension, and a family history of diabetes.

Uncontrolled diabetes in a pregnant woman can cause stillbirth, fetal anomalies, premature delivery, and birth of an infant who is large or small for gestational age. Such infants are predisposed to severe episodes of hypoglycemia shortly after birth. These infants may also develop hypocalcemia, hyperbilirubinemia, and respiratory distress syndrome.

## Diagnosis
The prevalence of gestational diabetes makes careful screening for hyperglycemia appropriate in all pregnancies in each trimester. Abnormal fasting or postprandial blood glucose levels and clinical signs and history suggest diabetes in patients not previously diabetic. A 3-hour glucose tolerance test confirms diabetes mellitus when two or more values are above normal.

### Diagnosis of fetal status
Procedures to assess fetal status include stress and nonstress tests, ultrasonography to determine fetal age and growth, measurement of urinary or serum estriols and of phosphatidylglycerol, and determination of the lecithin-sphingomyelin ratio from amniotic fluid to predict pulmonary maturity.

➤ CLINICAL TIP  Nonstress tests must be done from 30 to 38 weeks' gestation because the placenta tends to degenerate faster in gestational diabetes.

## Treatment
Both the newly diagnosed and the established diabetic need dietary management and insulin administration to maintain blood glucose levels within acceptable limits. Most women with overt diabetes mellitus require hospitalization at the beginning of pregnancy to assess physical status, check for cardiac and renal disease, and regulate diabetes.

For pregnant patients with diabetes, therapy includes:
• bimonthly visits to the obstetrician and the internist during the first 6 months of pregnancy; weekly visits may be necessary during the third trimester
• maintenance of blood glucose levels at or below 100 mg/dl during the third trimester
• frequent monitoring for glycosuria and ketonuria (Ketosis presents a grave threat to the fetal central nervous system.)
• weight control (Gain shouldn't exceed 3½ lb [1.6 kg]/month during the last 6 months of pregnancy.)
• a high-protein diet of 2 g/day/kg of body weight (a minimum of 80 g/day during the second half of pregnancy), a daily calorie intake of 30 to 40 calories/kg of body weight, a daily carbohydrate intake of 200 g, and enough fat to provide 36% of total calories (However, vigorous calorie restriction can cause starvation ketosis.)
• exogenous insulin if diet doesn't control blood glucose levels. Oral antidiabetic agents are contraindicated during pregnancy because they may cause fetal hypoglycemia and congenital anomalies.

### Delivery
Generally, the optimal time for delivery is between 37 and 39 weeks' gestation. The insulin-dependent diabetic requires hospitalization before delivery because bed rest promotes uteroplacental circulation and myometrial tone. In addition, hospitalization permits frequent monitoring of blood glucose levels and prompt intervention if complications develop.

Depending on fetal status and maternal history, labor may be induced or a cesarean section performed. During labor and delivery, the patient with diabetes should receive a continuous I.V. infusion of dextrose with regular insulin in water. Maternal and fetal status must be monitored closely throughout labor.

The patient may benefit from half her prepregnancy dosage of insulin before a cesarean delivery. Her insulin requirement will fall markedly after delivery.

### Special considerations
● Be alert for changes in insulin requirements from one trimester to the next and immediately postpartum.
● Teach the newly diagnosed patient about diabetes, including dietary management, insulin administration, home monitoring of blood glucose or urine testing for glucose and ketones, and skin and foot care. Instruct her to report ketonuria immediately.
● Evaluate the diabetic patient's knowledge about this disease, and provide supplementary patient teaching as she requires. Inform the patient that frequent monitoring and adjustment of insulin dosage are necessary throughout the course of her pregnancy.
● Give reassurance that strict compliance to prescribed therapy should ensure a favorable outcome.
● Refer the patient to an appropriate social service agency if financial assistance is necessary because of prolonged hospitalization.
● Encourage medical counseling regarding the prognosis of future pregnancies.

# DISLOCATIONS AND SUBLUXATIONS

In a dislocation, joint bones are displaced so that their articulating surfaces totally lose contact. Subluxations partially displace the articulating surfaces.

Dislocations and subluxations occur at the joints of the shoulders, elbows, wrists, digits, hips, knees, ankles, and feet; the injury may accompany fractures of these joints or result in deposition of fracture fragments between joint surfaces. Prompt reduction can limit the resulting damage to soft tissue, nerves, and blood vessels.

### Causes
A dislocation or subluxation may be congenital (as in congenital dislocation of the hip), or it may follow trauma or disease of surrounding joint tissues (for example, Paget's disease).

### Signs and symptoms
Dislocations and subluxations produce deformity around the joint, change the length of the involved extremity, impair joint mobility, and cause point tenderness.

When the injury results from trauma, it's extremely painful and often accompanies joint surface fractures. Even in the absence of concomitant fracture, the displaced bone may damage surrounding muscles, ligaments, nerves, and blood vessels and may cause bone necrosis, especially if reduction is delayed.

### Diagnosis
Patient history, X-rays, and clinical examination rule out or confirm fracture.

### Treatment
Immediate reduction (before tissue edema and muscle spasm make reduction difficult) can prevent additional tissue damage and vascular impairment.

Closed reduction consists of manual traction under general anesthesia (or local anesthesia and sedatives). During such reduction, I.V. morphine controls pain; I.V. midazolam controls muscle spasm and facilitates muscle stretching during traction.

Some injuries require open reduction under regional block or general anesthesia. Such surgery may include wire fixation of the joint, skeletal traction, and ligament repair.

After reduction, a splint, cast, or traction immobilizes the joint. Generally, immobilizing the digits for 2 weeks, hips for 6 to 8 weeks, and other dislocated joints for 3 to 6 weeks allows surrounding ligaments to heal.

**Special considerations**
• Until reduction immobilizes the dislocated joint, don't attempt manipulation. Apply ice to ease pain and edema. Splint the extremity "as it lies," even if the angle is awkward, unless there is loss of blood flow (no pulse, presence of pallor or cyanosis) distal to the injury.

> CLINICAL TIP  Check for signs of vascular compromise; if present, emergency reduction is necessary. Signs include pallor, pain, loss of pulses, paralysis, and paresthesia.
• When a patient receives narcotics or benzodiazepines I.V., he may develop respiratory depression or arrest. Keep an airway and a hand-held resuscitation bag in the room, and monitor respirations and pulse rate closely.
• To avoid injury from a dressing that's too tight, instruct the patient to report numbness, pain, cyanosis, or coldness of the extremity below the cast or splint.
• To avoid skin damage, watch for signs of pressure injury (pressure, pain, or soreness) both inside and outside the dressing.
• After removal of the cast or splint, inform the patient that he may gradually return to normal joint activity
• A dislocated hip needs immediate reduction. At discharge, stress the need for follow-up visits to detect aseptic femoral head necrosis from vascular damage.

# DISSEMINATED INTRAVASCULAR COAGULATION

Also called consumption coagulopathy and defibrination syndrome, disseminated intravascular coagulation (DIC) occurs as a complication of diseases and conditions that accelerate clotting. This accelerated clotting process causes small blood vessel occlusion, organ necrosis, depletion of circulating clotting factors and platelets, and activation of the fibrinolytic system — which, in turn, can provoke severe hemorrhage. (See *Three mechanisms of DIC,* page 286.)

Clotting in the microcirculation usually affects the kidneys and extremities but may occur in the brain, lungs, pituitary and adrenal glands, and GI mucosa. Other conditions, such as vitamin K deficiency, hepatic disease, and anticoagulant therapy, may cause a similar hemorrhage.

DIC is generally an acute condition but may be chronic in cancer patients. The prognosis depends on early detection and treatment, the severity of the hemorrhage, and treatment of the underlying disease or condition.

**Causes**
DIC may result from:
• *infection* (the most common cause of DIC), including gram-negative or gram-positive septicemia; viral, fungal, or rickettsial infection; and protozoal infection (falciparum malaria)
• *obstetric complications,* such as abruptio placentae, amniotic fluid embolism, and retained dead fetus
• *neoplastic disease,* including acute leukemia and metastatic carcinoma
• *disorders that produce necrosis,* such as extensive burns and trauma, brain tis-

## THREE MECHANISMS OF D.I.C.

However disseminated intravascular coagulation (DIC) begins, accelerated clotting (characteristic of DIC) usually results in excess thrombin, which in turn causes fibrinolysis with excess fibrin formation and fibrin degradation products (FDP), activation of fibrin-stabilizing factor (factor XIII), consumption of platelet and clotting factors and, eventually, hemorrhage.

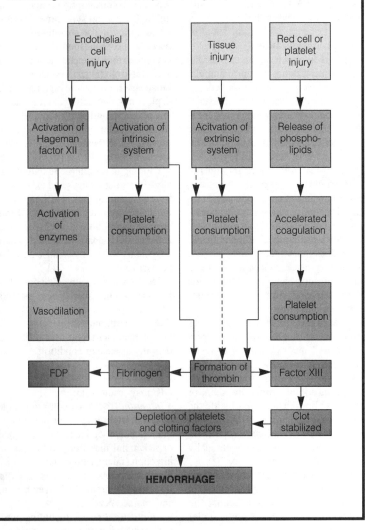

sue destruction, transplant rejection, and hepatic necrosis.

Other causes include heatstroke, shock, poisonous snakebite, cirrhosis, fat embolism, incompatible blood transfusion, cardiac arrest, surgery necessitating cardiopulmonary bypass, giant hemangioma, severe venous thrombosis, and purpura fulminans.

It's not clear why such disorders lead to DIC; nor is it certain that they lead to it through a common mechanism. In many patients, the triggering mechanisms may be the entrance of foreign protein into the circulation and vascular endothelial injury.

### Results of accelerated clotting

Regardless of how DIC begins, the typical accelerated clotting results in generalized activation of prothrombin and a consequent excess of thrombin. Excess thrombin converts fibrinogen to fibrin, producing fibrin clots in the microcirculation.

This process consumes exorbitant amounts of coagulation factors (especially fibrinogen, prothrombin, platelets, and factor V and factor VIII), causing hypofibrinogenemia, hypoprothrombinemia, thrombocytopenia, and deficiencies in factor V and factor VIII. Circulating thrombin activates the fibrinolytic system, which lyses fibrin clots into fibrin degradation products.

The hemorrhage that occurs may largely be the result of the anticoagulant activity of fibrin degradation products as well as depletion of plasma coagulation factors.

### Signs and symptoms

The most significant clinical feature of DIC is abnormal bleeding, *without* an accompanying history of a serious hemorrhagic disorder.

Principal signs of such bleeding include cutaneous oozing, petechiae, ec-

chymoses, and hematomas caused by bleeding into the skin. Bleeding from sites of surgical or invasive procedures (such as incisions or I.V. sites) and from the GI tract are equally significant indications, as are acrocyanosis and signs of acute tubular necrosis.

Related symptoms and other possible effects include nausea, vomiting, dyspnea, oliguria, seizures, coma, shock, failure of major organ systems, and severe muscle, back, and abdominal pain.

### Diagnosis

Abnormal bleeding in the absence of a known hematologic disorder suggests DIC. Initial laboratory findings supporting a tentative diagnosis of DIC include:

• *prolonged prothrombin time (PT):* > 15 seconds

• *prolonged partial thromboplastin time (PTT):* > 60 to 80 seconds

• *decreased fibrinogen levels:* < 150 mg/dl

• *decreased platelets:* < 100,000/µl

• *increased fibrin degradation products (FDP):* often > 100 µg/ml.

• *positive D-dimer test:* specific for DIC.

Other supportive data include positive fibrin monomers, diminished levels of factors V and VIII, fragmentation of red blood cells (RBCs), and decreased hemoglobin (< 10 g/dl). Assessment of renal status demonstrates a reduction in urine output (< 30 ml/hour) and elevated blood urea nitrogen (> 25 mg/dl) and serum creatinine (> 1.3 mg/dl) levels.

Final confirmation of the diagnosis may be difficult because many of these test results also occur in other disorders (primary fibrinolysis, for example). Additional diagnostic measures determine the underlying disorder.

### Treatment

Successful management of DIC necessitates prompt recognition and adequate treatment of the underlying disorder. Treatment may be supportive (when the underlying disorder is self-limiting, for example) or highly specific.

If the patient isn't actively bleeding, supportive care alone may reverse DIC. However, active bleeding may require I.V. heparin and administration of blood, fresh frozen plasma, platelets, or packed RBCs to support hemostasis.

> CLINICAL TIP Be aware of investigational drugs being tested for the treatment of DIC. Antithrombin III has been approved for use in the United States, and gabexate mesylate is being considered for use as an antithrombin to inhibit the clotting cascade.

**Special considerations**
• To prevent clots from dislodging and causing fresh bleeding, do not scrub bleeding areas. Use pressure, cold compresses, and topical hemostatic agents to control bleeding.
• Protect the patient from injury. Enforce complete bed rest during bleeding episodes. If the patient is very agitated, pad the side rails.
• Check all I.V. and venipuncture sites frequently for bleeding. Apply pressure to injection sites for at least 10 minutes. Alert other personnel to the patient's tendency to hemorrhage.
• Monitor intake and output hourly in acute DIC, especially when administering blood products.
• Watch for transfusion reactions and signs of fluid overload. To measure the amount of blood lost, weigh dressings and linen and record drainage. Weigh the patient daily, particularly in renal involvement.
• Watch for bleeding from the GI and genitourinary tracts. If you suspect intra-abdominal bleeding, measure the patient's abdominal girth at least every 4 hours, and monitor closely for signs of shock.

• Monitor the results of serial blood studies (particularly hematocrit, hemoglobin, and coagulation times).
• Inform the family of the patient's progress. Prepare them for his appearance (I.V. lines, nasogastric tubes, bruises, dried blood). Provide emotional support for the patient and family. As needed, enlist the aid of a social worker, chaplain, and other members of the health care team in providing such support.

# DIVERTICULAR DISEASE

Diverticular disease is an outpouching of the colon, usually the sigmoid. It develops from the musculature in the colon working against increased intraluminal pressures to move hard stools through. Other typical sites are the duodenum, near the pancreatic border or the ampulla of Vater, and the jejunum. Diverticular disease of the stomach is rare and is often a precursor of peptic or neoplastic disease. Diverticular disease of the ileum (Meckel's diverticulum) is the most common congenital anomaly of the GI tract.

Diverticular disease has two clinical forms. In *diverticulosis,* diverticula are present but usually the patient is asymptomatic or the symptoms (abdominal pain, fluctuating bowel habits, constipation) are questionable because they may be related to underlying irritable bowel syndrome. In *diverticulitis,* diverticula are inflamed and may cause potentially fatal obstruction, infection, or hemorrhage.

**Causes**
Diverticular disease is most prevalent in men over age 40. Diverticula probably result from high intraluminal pressure on areas of weakness in the GI wall, where blood vessels enter.

Diet may also be a contributing factor because lack of roughage reduces fecal residue, narrows the bowel lumen, and leads to higher intra-abdominal pressure during defecation. The fact that diverticulosis is most prevalent in Western industrialized nations, where processing removes much of the roughage from foods, supports this theory. Diverticulosis is less common in nations where the diet contains more natural bulk and fiber.

In diverticulitis, retained undigested food mixed with bacteria accumulates in the diverticular sac, forming a hard mass (fecalith). This substance cuts off the blood supply to the thin walls of the sac, making them more susceptible to attack by colonic bacteria.

Inflammation follows, possibly leading to perforation, abscess, peritonitis, obstruction, or hemorrhage. Occasionally, the inflamed colon segment may produce a fistula by adhering to the bladder or other organs.

## Signs and symptoms

The two forms of diverticular disease produce different clinical effects.

### *Diverticulosis*

Although diverticulosis usually produces no symptoms, it may cause recurrent left lower quadrant pain. Such pain, often accompanied by alternating constipation and diarrhea, is relieved by defecation or the passage of flatus. Symptoms resemble irritable bowel syndrome and suggest that both disorders may coexist.

In older patients, a rare complication of diverticulosis (without diverticulitis) is hemorrhage from colonic diverticula, usually in the right colon. Such hemorrhage is usually mild to moderate and easily controlled but may occasionally be life-threatening.

### *Diverticulitis*

Mild diverticulitis produces moderate left lower abdominal pain, mild nausea, flatus, irregular bowel habits, low-grade fever, and leukocytosis. Constipation or loose stools and nausea and vomiting are usually present.

In severe diverticulitis, the diverticula can perforate and produce abscesses or peritonitis. Perforation occurs in up to 20% of such patients; its symptoms include peritoneal signs of abdominal rigidity and left lower quadrant pain.

Peritonitis follows release of fecal material from the perforation site and causes signs of sepsis and shock (high fever, chills, hypotension). Perforation of diverticulum near a vessel may cause microscopic or massive hemorrhage, depending on the vessel's size.

Chronic diverticulitis may cause fibrosis and adhesions that narrow the bowel's lumen and lead to bowel obstruction. Signs and symptoms of partial obstruction include constipation, thin-caliber stools, intermittent diarrhea, and abdominal distention. Complete obstruction symptoms include abdominal rigidity and pain, diminishing or absent bowel sounds, nausea, and vomiting.

## Diagnosis

Diverticular disease frequently produces no symptoms and is often found incidental to an upper GI barium X-ray series. An upper GI series confirms diverticulosis of the esophagus and small bowel. Plain films are usually obtained to look for evidence of free abdominal air, ileus, or small- or large-bowel obstruction.

A barium enema confirms diverticulosis of the large bowel and can also identify a stricture or mass. Barium-filled diverticula can be single, multiple, or clustered like grapes and may have a wide or narrow mouth. Barium outlines, but doesn't fill, diverticula blocked by impacted feces. In patients with acute diverticulitis, a barium enema may rupture the bowel; therefore, this procedure, as well as flexible sigmoidoscopy, should not be performed during the acute stage. A colonoscopic exam can rule out malignancy. A computed tomography scan should be performed 2 to 3 days after initiation of antibiotics to evaluate for abscess.

A biopsy will confirm cancer; however, colonoscopic biopsy isn't recommended during acute diverticular disease because of the risk of perforation. Blood studies may show an elevated erythrocyte sedimentation rate in diverticulitis, especially if the diverticula are infected.

## Treatment
The two forms of the disease call for different treatment regimens.

### *Diverticulosis*
Asymptomatic diverticulosis generally doesn't require treatment. Diverticulosis with pain, nausea, or constipation may respond to a liquid or low-residue diet, stool softeners, and occasional doses of mineral oil. These measures relieve symptoms, minimize irritation, and lessen the risk of progression to diverticulitis.

After pain subsides, patients also benefit from a low-residue diet and bulk medication such as psyllium (1 teaspoon twice a day) and increased water consumption (8 glasses per day).

### *Diverticulitis*
Treatment of mild diverticulitis without signs of perforation aims to prevent constipation and combat infection. This includes bed rest, a liquid diet, stool softeners or bulking agents, a broad-spectrum antibiotic (such as

metronidazole and ciprofloxacin or co-trimoxazole), meperidine to control pain and relax smooth muscle, and an antispasmodic such as propantheline to control muscle spasms.

Diverticulitis that doesn't respond to medical treatment requires a colon resection to remove the involved segment.

➤ CLINICAL TIP Surgical consultation should be obtained if the patient fails to improve after being medically managed for 72 hours.

Perforation, peritonitis, obstruction, or a fistula that accompanies diverticulitis may require a temporary colostomy to drain abscesses and rest the colon, 6 to 8 weeks after inflammation or infection subside. The colon can be reconnected.

Complications of diverticulitis include formation of fistulas involving any of the following: bladder, ureters, bowel, and abdominal wall. Diverticulitis can also cause colon stricture, which may result in partial or complete obstruction.

Patients who hemorrhage need blood replacement and careful monitoring of fluid and electrolyte balance. Such bleeding usually stops spontaneously.

If bleeding continues, angiography may be performed to guide catheter placement for infusing vasopressin into the bleeding vessel.

## Special considerations
If the patient has diverticulosis:
● Teach the patient about diverticular disease and about how diverticula form.
● Make sure the patient understands the importance of a low-residue diet and the harmful effects of constipation and straining during defecation. Encourage increased intake of foods high in undigestible fiber, including fresh fruits and vegetables, whole grain bread, and wheat or bran cereals. Warn that a high-fiber diet may temporarily cause flatulence and discomfort.

• Advise the patient to relieve constipation with stool softeners or bulk-forming cathartics. But caution against taking bulk-forming cathartics without plenty of water; if swallowed dry, they may absorb enough moisture in the mouth and throat to swell and obstruct the esophagus or trachea.

• If the patient with diverticulosis is hospitalized, administer medication as needed; observe stool output for frequency, color, and consistency; and monitor vital signs, including temperature and pulse, because they may signal developing inflammation or complications.

If the patient has diverticulitis:

• In mild disease, administer medications, explain diagnostic tests and preparations for such tests, observe stools carefully, and maintain accurate records of temperature, pulse, respirations, and intake and output.

• If diverticular bleeding occurs, the patient may require angiography and catheter placement for vasopressin infusion. If so, inspect the insertion site frequently for bleeding, check pedal pulses often, and keep the patient from flexing his legs at the groin.

• Watch for vasopressin-induced fluid retention (apprehension, abdominal cramps, convulsions, oliguria, and anuria) and severe hyponatremia (hypotension; rapid, thready pulse; cold, clammy skin; and cyanosis).

Following surgery:

• Watch for signs of infection.

• Provide meticulous wound care; perforation may already have infected the area.

• Check drain sites frequently for signs of infection (purulent drainage, foul odor) or fecal drainage.

• Change dressings as necessary.

• Encourage coughing and deep breathing to prevent atelectasis.

• Watch for signs of postoperative bleeding (hypotension, decreased hemoglobin and hematocrit).

• Record intake and output accurately.

• Provide ostomy care and education.

• Arrange for a visit by an enterostomal therapy nurse.

# DOWN SYNDROME

The first disorder attributed to a chromosomal aberration, Down syndrome (trisomy 21) characteristically produces mental retardation, dysmorphic facial features, and other distinctive physical abnormalities. It's commonly associated with heart defects (in approximately 60% of patients) and other congenital disorders.

Life expectancy for patients with Down syndrome has increased significantly because of improved treatment for related complications (heart defects, respiratory and other infections, acute leukemia). Nevertheless, up to 44% of such patients who have associated congenital heart defects die before age 1.

## Causes

Down syndrome usually results from trisomy 21, a spontaneous chromosomal abnormality in which chromosome 21 has three copies instead of the normal two because of faulty meiosis (nondisjunction) of the ovum or, sometimes, the sperm. This results in a karyotype of 47 chromosomes instead of the normal 46. In about 4% of patients, Down syndrome results from an unbalanced translocation (chromosomal rearrangement) in which the long arm of chromosome 21 breaks and attaches to another chromosome. The disorder may also be due to chromosomal mosaicism, a mixture of two cell types—

one with a normal number of chromosomes (46) and some with 47 (an extra chromosome 21).

Down syndrome occurs in 1 in 650 to 700 live births, but the incidence increases with advanced parental age, especially when the mother is age 34 or older at delivery or the father is older than age 42. At age 20, a woman has about 1 chance in 2,000 of having a child with Down syndrome; by age 49, she has 1 chance in 12. If a woman has had one child with Down syndrome, the risk of recurrence is 1% to 2%. This risk varies according to the type of translocation the parents carry, and genetic counseling should be discussed.

**Signs and symptoms**
The physical signs of Down syndrome (especially hypotonia) as well as some dysmorphic facial features and heart defects may be apparent at birth. The degree of mental retardation may not become apparent until the infant grows older. People with Down syndrome typically have craniofacial anomalies, such as slanting, almond-shaped eyes with epicanthic folds; a flat face; a protruding tongue; a small mouth and chin; a single transverse palmar crease (simian crease); small white spots (Brushfield spots) on the iris; strabismus; a small skull; a flat bridge across the nose; slow dental development, with abnormal or absent teeth; small ears; a short neck; and cataracts.

Other physical effects may include dry, sensitive skin with decreased elasticity; umbilical hernia; short stature; short extremities, with broad, flat, squarish hands and feet; clinodactyly (small little finger that curves inward); a wide space between the first and second toe; and abnormal fingerprints and footprints. Hypotonic limb muscles impair reflex development, posture, coordination, and balance.

Congenital heart disease (septal defects or pulmonary or aortic stenosis), duodenal atresia, megacolon, and pelvic bone abnormalities are common. The incidence of leukemia and thyroid disorders may be increased. Frequent upper respiratory infections can be a serious problem. Genitalia may be poorly developed and puberty delayed. Females may menstruate and be fertile. Males are infertile with low serum testosterone levels; many have undescended testes.

Down syndrome patients may have an IQ between 30 and 70; however, social performance is usually beyond that expected for mental age. The level of intellectual function depends greatly on the environment and the amount of early stimulation received in addition to the IQ.

**Diagnosis**
Physical findings at birth, especially hypotonia, may suggest this diagnosis, but no physical feature is diagnostic in itself.

A karyotype showing the specific chromosomal abnormality provides a definitive diagnosis. Amniocentesis allows prenatal diagnosis and is recommended for pregnant women older than age 34, even if the family history is negative. Amniocentesis is also recommended for any pregnant woman if she or the father carries a translocated chromosome.

**Treatment**
Down syndrome has no known cure. Surgery to correct heart defects and other related congenital abnormalities and antibiotic therapy for recurrent infections have improved life expectancy considerably. Plastic surgery is occasionally done to correct the characteristic facial traits, especially the protruding tongue. Benefits beyond improved appearance may include improved speech,

reduced susceptibility to dental caries, and fewer orthodontic problems later. Most Down syndrome patients are now cared for at home and attend special education classes. As adults, some may work in a sheltered workshop or live in a group home facility.

**Special considerations**

Support for the parents of a child with Down syndrome is vital. By following the guidelines listed below, you can help them meet their child's physical and emotional needs.

● Establish a trusting relationship with the parents, and encourage communication during the difficult period soon after diagnosis. Recognize signs of grieving.

● Teach parents the importance of a balanced diet for the child. Stress the need for patience while feeding the child, who may have difficulty sucking and may be less demanding and seem less eager to eat than normal babies.

● Encourage the parents to hold and nurture their child.

➤ CLINICAL TIP  Emphasize the importance of adequate exercise and maximal environmental stimulation; refer the parents for infant stimulation classes, which may begin in the early months of life.

● Help the parents set realistic goals for their child. By the time he's 1 year old, the child's development may begin to lag behind that of other children. (See *Goal setting in Down syndrome.*)

● Refer the parents and older siblings for genetic counseling to help them evaluate future reproductive risks. Discuss options for prenatal testing.

● Encourage the parents to remember the emotional needs of other children in the family.

● Refer the parents to national or local Down syndrome organizations and support groups.

---

✔ TEACHING CHECKLIST

## GOAL SETTING IN DOWN SYNDROME

Review the following strategies with the child's parents:

● Set well-defined expectations that are measurable and predictable.
● Divide the expected tasks of the child into smaller steps, identifying those that may be more difficult.
● Repetition is key to beginning teaching for the child.
● Be persistent and patient; recognize the child's achievements in small areas.
● A positive approach with praise and enthusiasm works well.
● Give the child sufficient time to respond.
● Cues and prompts are helpful as well as physically helping the child initiate an activity.

---

# DRUG ABUSE AND DEPENDENCE

The National Institute on Drug Abuse defines drug abuse and dependence as the use of a legal or an illegal drug that causes physical, mental, emotional, or social harm. Examples of abused drugs include narcotics, stimulants, depressants, antianxiety agents, and hallucinogens.

Chronic drug abuse, especially I.V. use, can lead to life-threatening complications, such as cardiac and respiratory arrest, intracranial hemorrhage, acquired immunodeficiency syndrome, tetanus, subacute infective endocarditis, hepatitis, vasculitis, septicemia, thrombophlebitis, pulmonary emboli, gangrene, malnutrition and GI disturbances, respiratory infections, musculoskeletal dysfunction, trauma, depression, increased risk of suicide, and psychosis. Materials used to "cut" street drugs also can cause toxic or allergic reactions.

Drug abuse can occur at any age. Experimentation with drugs commonly begins in adolescence or even earlier. Drug abuse often leads to addiction, which may involve physical or psychological dependence or both. The most dangerous form of abuse occurs when users mix several drugs simultaneously — including alcohol.

## Causes

Drug abuse commonly results from a combination of low self-esteem, peer pressure, inadequate coping skills, and curiosity. There is also evidence of familial patterns of addiction.

Most people who are predisposed to drug abuse have few mental or emotional resources against stress, an overdependence on others, and a low tolerance for frustration. Taking the drug gives them pleasure by relieving tension, abolishing loneliness, allowing them to achieve a temporarily peaceful or euphoric state, or simply relieving boredom.

Drug dependence may follow experimentation with drugs in response to peer pressure. It also may follow the use of drugs to relieve physical pain, but this is uncommon.

## Signs and symptoms

Indications of acute intoxication vary, depending on the drug.

> CLINICAL TIP The drug user seldom seeks treatment specifically for his drug problem. Instead, he may seek emergency treatment for drug-related injuries or complications.

Friends, family members, or law enforcement officials may bring the patient to the hospital because of respiratory depression, unconsciousness, acute injury, or a psychiatric crisis.

### Physical examination

Examine the patient for signs and symptoms of drug use or drug-related complications as well as for clues to the type of drug ingested. For example, fever can result from stimulant or hallucinogen intoxication, from withdrawal, or from infection from I.V. drug use.

Inspect the eyes for lacrimation from opioid withdrawal, nystagmus from central nervous system (CNS) depressants or phencyclidine intoxication, and drooping eyelids from opioid or CNS depressant use. Constricted pupils occur with opioid use or withdrawal; dilated pupils, with the use of hallucinogens or amphetamines.

Examine the nose for rhinorrhea from opioid withdrawal and the oral and nasal mucosa for signs of drug-induced irritation. Drug sniffing can result in inflammation, atrophy, or perforation of the nasal mucosa. Dental conditions commonly result from the poor oral hygiene associated with chronic drug use. Also inspect under the tongue for evidence of I.V. drug injection.

Inspect the skin. Sweating, a common sign of intoxication with opioids or CNS stimulants, also accompanies most drug withdrawal syndromes. Drug use sometimes induces a sensation of bugs crawling on the skin, known as formication; as a result, the patient's skin may be excoriated from scratching.

Needle marks or tracks are an obvious sign of I.V. drug abuse. Keep in mind that the patient may attempt to conceal or disguise injection sites with tattoos or by selecting an inconspicuous site, such as under the nails.

In addition, self-injection can sometimes cause cellulitis or abscesses, especially in patients who also are chronic alcoholics. Puffy hands can be a late sign of thrombophlebitis or of fascial infection from self-injection on the hands or arms.

Auscultation may disclose bilateral crackles and rhonchi caused by smoking and inhaling drugs or by opioid overdose. Other cardiopulmonary signs of overdose include pulmonary edema, respiratory depression, aspiration pneumonia, and hypotension.

CNS stimulants and some hallucinogens may precipitate refractory acute-onset hypertension or cardiac arrhythmias. Withdrawal from opioids or CNS depressants also can provoke arrhythmias and, occasionally, hypotension.

During opioid withdrawal, the patient may report abdominal pain, nausea, or vomiting. Opioid abusers also commonly complain of hemorrhoids, a consequence of the constipating effects of these drugs. Palpation of an enlarged liver, with or without tenderness, may indicate hepatitis.

Neurologic symptoms of drug abuse include tremors, hyperreflexia, hyporeflexia, and seizures. Abrupt withdrawal may precipitate signs of CNS depression (ranging from lethargy to coma), hallucinations, or signs of overstimulation, including euphoria and violent behavior.

### Medical history

Carefully review the patient's medical history. Suspect drug abuse if he reports a painful injury or chronic illness but refuses a diagnostic workup. In his attempt to obtain drugs, the dependent patient may feign illnesses, such as migraine headaches, myocardial infarction, and renal colic; claim an allergy to over-the-counter analgesics; or even request a specific medication.

Also be alert for a previous history of overdose or a high tolerance for potentially addictive drugs. I.V. drug users may have a history of hepatitis or human immunodeficiency virus (HIV) infection from sharing dirty needles. Female drug users may report a history of amenorrhea.

A patient who abuses drugs may give you a fictitious name and address, be reluctant to discuss previous hospitalizations, or seek treatment at a medical facility across town rather than in his own neighborhood. If possible, interview family members to verify his responses.

If the patient admits to drug use, try to determine the extent to which this behavior interferes with his normal functioning. Note whether he expresses a desire to overcome his dependence on drugs.

If possible, obtain a drug history consisting of substances ingested, amount, frequency, and last dose. Expect incomplete or inaccurate responses. Drug-induced amnesia, a depressed level of consciousness, or ignorance may distort the patient's recollection of the facts; he also may deliberately fabricate answers to avoid arrest or to conceal a suicide attempt.

The hospitalized drug abuser is likely to be uncooperative, disruptive, or even violent. He may experience mood swings, anxiety, impaired memory, sleep disturbances, flashbacks, slurred speech, depression, and thought disorders.

Some patients resort to plays on sympathy, bribery, or threats to obtain drugs. They may also try to manipulate caregivers by pitting one against another.

### Diagnosis

The *DSM-IV* gives characteristic findings for patients with drug dependence. (See *Diagnosing substance dependence and related disorders.*)

Various tests can confirm drug use, determine the amount and type of drug taken, and reveal complications. For example, a serum or urine drug screen can detect recently ingested substances.

Characteristic findings in other tests include elevated serum globulin levels, hypoglycemia, leukocytosis, liver function abnormalities, positive rapid plasma reagin test results because of elevated protein fractions, elevated mean corpuscular hemoglobin levels, elevated uric acid levels, and reduced blood urea nitrogen levels.

## Treatment

The patient may first need treatment for drug intoxication, followed by long-term therapy to combat drug dependence.

### Drug intoxication

The patient with acute drug intoxication should receive symptomatic treatment based on the drug ingested. Measures include fluid replacement therapy and nutritional and vitamin supplements, if indicated, and detoxification with the same drug or a pharmacologically similar drug. (Exceptions include cocaine, hallucinogens, and marijuana, which aren't used for detoxification.)

Medications include sedatives to induce sleep; anticholinergics and antidiarrheal agents to relieve GI distress; antianxiety drugs for severe agitation, especially in cocaine abusers; and symptomatic treatment of complications.

Depending on the dosage and time elapsed before admission, additional treatments may include gastric lavage, induced emesis, activated charcoal, forced diuresis and, possibly, hemoperfusion or hemodialysis.

### Drug dependence

Treatment of drug dependence commonly involves a triad of care: detoxification, short- and long-term rehabilitation, and aftercare. The latter means a lifetime of abstinence, usually aided by participation in Narcotics Anonymous or a similar self-help group.

Detoxification, the controlled and gradual withdrawal of an abused drug, is achieved through substitution of a drug with similar action, which is then gradually decreased. Such gradual replacement of the abused drug controls the effects of withdrawal, thereby reducing the patient's discomfort and associated risks.

Depending on which drug the patient has abused, detoxification may be managed on an inpatient or outpatient basis. For example, withdrawal from CNS depressants can produce hazardous adverse reactions, such as generalized tonic-clonic seizures, status epilepticus, and hypotension.

The severity of these reactions determines whether the patient can be safely treated as an outpatient or requires hospitalization. Withdrawal from CNS depressants usually doesn't require detoxification.

Opioid withdrawal causes severe physical discomfort and can even be life-threatening. To minimize these effects, chronic opioid abusers commonly are detoxified with methadone.

To ease withdrawal from opioids, depressants, and other drugs, useful nonchemical measures may include psychotherapy, exercise, relaxation techniques, and nutritional support. Sedatives and tranquilizers may be administered temporarily to help the patient cope with insomnia, anxiety, and depression.

After withdrawal, the patient needs to participate in a rehabilitation program to prevent a recurrence of drug

# DIAGNOSING SUBSTANCE DEPENDENCE AND RELATED DISORDERS

The *DSM-IV* identifies the following diagnostic criteria for substance dependence, abuse, intoxication, and withdrawal.

### Substance dependence

A maladaptive pattern of substance use leading to clinically significant impairment or distress, as manifested by three or more of the following occurring at any time in the same 12-month period:

• Tolerance, as defined by either of the following: the need for increased amounts of the substance to achieve intoxication or desired effect, or a markedly diminished effect with continued use of the same amount of the substance

• Withdrawal, as manifested by either of the following: the characteristic withdrawal syndrome for the substance or the same, or similar, substance is taken to relieve or avoid withdrawal symptoms

• The person often takes the substance in larger amounts or over a longer period than was intended.

• The person experiences a persistent desire or unsuccessful efforts to cut down or control substance use.

• The person spends much time obtaining or using the substance or recovering from its effects.

• The person abandons or reduces social, occupational, or recreational activities due to substance use.

• The person continues using the substance despite knowing he has a physical or psychological problem that's likely to have been caused or exacerbated by the substance.

### Substance abuse

A maladaptive pattern of substance use leading to clinically significant impairment or distress, as manifested by one or more of the following, occurring within a 12-month period:

• recurrent substance use resulting in a failure to fulfill major role obligations at work, school, or home

• recurrent substance use in physically hazardous situations

• recurrent substance-related legal problems

• continued substance use despite having social or interpersonal problems caused or exacerbated by the effects of the substance

• The symptoms have never met the criteria for substance dependence for this class of substance.

### Substance intoxication

• The development of a reversible substance-specific syndrome resulting from recent ingestion of, or exposure to, a substance

• Clinically significant maladaptive behavioral or psychological changes resulting from the effect of the substance on the central nervous system and developing during or shortly after use of the substance

• Symptoms aren't caused by a general medical condition and aren't better accounted for by another mental disorder.

### Substance withdrawal

• A substance-specific syndrome develops from the cessation or reduction of heavy and prolonged substance use.

• The substance-specific syndrome causes clinically significant distress or impairment in social, occupational, or other areas of functioning.

• The symptoms aren't caused by a general medical condition and aren't better accounted for by another mental disorder.

abuse. Rehabilitation programs are available for both inpatients and outpatients; they usually last a month or longer and may include individual, group, and family psychotherapy. During and after rehabilitation, participation in a drug-oriented self-help group may be beneficial. The largest such group is Narcotics Anonymous.

### Special considerations
During an acute episode:
- Continuously monitor the patient's vital signs, and observe for complications of overdose and withdrawal, such as cardiopulmonary arrest, seizures, and aspiration.
- Based on standard facility policy, institute appropriate measures to prevent suicide attempts.
- Give medications as needed to decrease withdrawal symptoms; monitor and record their effectiveness.
- Maintain a quiet, safe environment during withdrawal from any drug because excessive noise may agitate the patient.
- Remove harmful objects from the patient's room, and use restraints only if you suspect that he might harm himself or others. Institute seizure precautions.

After an acute episode:
- Learn to control your reactions to the patient's undesirable behaviors — commonly, psychological dependency, manipulation, anger, frustration, and alienation.
- Set limits for dealing with demanding, manipulative behavior.
- Promote adequate nutrition and monitor the patient's nutritional intake.
- Administer medications carefully to prevent hoarding by the patient. Check the patient's mouth to ensure that he has swallowed the medication. Closely monitor visitors who might supply the patient with drugs.

- Refer the patient for detoxification and rehabilitation as appropriate. Give him a list of available resources.
- Encourage family members to seek help whether or not the abuser seeks it. You can suggest private therapy or community mental health clinics.

If the patient refuses to participate in a rehabilitation program:
- Teach him how to minimize the risk of drug-related complications. Review measures for preventing HIV infection and hepatitis. Stress that these infections are readily transmitted by sharing needles with other drug users and by unprotected sexual intercourse.
- Advise the patient to use a new needle for every injection or to clean needles with a solution of chlorine bleach and water.
- Emphasize the importance of using a condom during intercourse to prevent disease transmission and pregnancy. If necessary, teach the female drug abuser about other methods of birth control. Explain the devastating effects of drugs on the developing fetus.

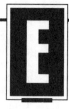

# EARDRUM PERFORATION

Perforation of the eardrum is a rupture of the tympanic membrane. Such injury may cause otitis media and hearing loss.

## Causes

The usual cause of perforated eardrum is trauma: the deliberate or accidental insertion of sharp objects (cotton swabs, bobby pins) or sudden excessive changes in pressure (explosion, a blow to the head, flying, or diving). The injury may also result from untreated otitis media and, in children, acute otitis media.

## Signs and symptoms

Sudden onset of severe earache and bleeding from the ear are the first signs of a perforated eardrum. Other symptoms include hearing loss, tinnitus, and vertigo. Purulent otorrhea within 24 to 48 hours of injury signals infection.

## Diagnosis

Severe earache and bleeding from the ear with a history of trauma strongly suggest a perforated eardrum; direct visualization of the perforated tympanic membrane with an otoscope confirms it. Additional diagnostic measures include audiometric testing and a check of voluntary facial movements to rule out facial nerve damage.

> **CLINICAL TIP** When severe force has caused the perforation, temporal lobe and skull X-ray films should be done to determine whether a fracture is also present.

## Treatment

In bleeding from the ear, use a sterile, cotton-tipped applicator to absorb the blood, and check for purulent drainage or evidence of cerebrospinal fluid leakage. A culture of the specimen may be ordered. *Irrigation of the ear is absolutely contraindicated.*

Apply a sterile dressing over the outer ear, and refer the patient to an ear specialist. Most perforations heal rapidly, and after 2 weeks, any crust remaining on the tympanic membrane may be removed under magnification to see if healing is complete.

If the perforation has not healed in 1 month, an attempt may be made to close it in the office by the Derlacki method. In this method, the margin of the perforation is stimulated and then covered with a moist cotton disk for a few weeks. If there is no response after 3 months, as evidenced by repeated discharge, surgical closure should be recommended. A large perforation with uncontrolled bleeding may require immediate surgery to approximate the ruptured edges. Additional treatment may include a mild analgesic, a sedative to decrease anxiety, and an oral antibiotic.

## Special considerations
- Find out the cause of the injury, and report suspected child abuse.
- Before discharge, tell the patient not to blow his nose or get water in his ear canal until the perforation heals.
- Welders are prone to perforations caused by hot chips of metal flying into the ear canal. Safety equipment should be used in the workplace to prevent this from occurring.
- While the tympanic membrane is healing, the ear canal should be protected from dirt and water by a cotton plug or dry dressing.

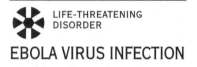
LIFE-THREATENING DISORDER

# EBOLA VIRUS INFECTION

One of the most frightening viruses to come out of the African subcontinent, the Ebola virus first appeared in 1976. More than 400 persons in Zaire (now known as Democratic Republic of Congo) and the neighboring Sudan died due to the hemorrhagic fever that the virus causes. Ebola virus has been responsible for several outbreaks since then, including one that occurred in Zaire in the summer of 1995.

An unclassified ribonucleic acid (RNA) virus, Ebola virus is morphologically similar to the Marburg virus. Both viruses cause headache, malaise, myalgia, and high fever, progressing to severe diarrhea, vomiting, and internal and external hemorrhage.

Four strains of the Ebola virus are known to exist: Ebola Zaire, Ebola Sudan, Ebola Tai, and Ebola Reston. All four types are structurally similar but have different antigenic properties. One type, Ebola Reston, affects only monkeys; the other three types affect humans.

The prognosis for Ebola virus disease is extremely poor, with a mortality rate as high as 90%. The incubation period ranges from 2 to 21 days.

## Causes
Ebola virus disease is caused by an unclassified RNA virus that is transmitted by direct contact with infected blood, body secretions, or organs. Nosocomial and community-acquired transmission can occur. Transmission through semen may occur up to 7 weeks after clinical recovery. The virus remains contagious even after the patient has died.

## Signs and symptoms
The patient's health history usually reveals contact with an infected person. However, no clear line of infection may be apparent at the beginning of an Ebola virus outbreak. The patient usually complains of flulike signs and symptoms (such as headache, malaise, myalgia, fever, cough, and sore throat), which first appear within 3 days of infection.

As the virus spreads through the body, inspection reveals bruising as capillaries rupture and dead blood cells infiltrate the skin. A maculopapular eruption appears after the 5th day of infection. The patient may also display melena, hematemesis, epistaxis, and bleeding gums. As the infection progresses, severe complications, including liver and kidney dysfunction, dehydration, and hemorrhage, may develop. In pregnant women, Ebola virus disease leads to abortion and massive hemorrhage.

In the final stages of the disease, the skin blisters and sloughs off, blood seeps from all body orifices, and the patient begins vomiting his liquefied internal organs. Death usually results during the 2nd week of illness from organ failure or hemorrhage.

## Diagnosis

Specialized laboratory tests reveal specific antigens or antibodies and may show the isolated virus. As with other types of hemorrhagic fever, tests also demonstrate neutrophil leukocytosis, hypofibrinogenemia, thrombocytopenia, and microangiopathic hemolytic anemia.

## Treatment

No cure exists for Ebola virus disease; treatment consists mainly of intensive supportive care. The administration of I.V. fluids helps offset the effects of severe dehydration. The patient may receive replacement of plasma heparin before the onset of clinical shock.

Experimental treatments include administration of plasma that contains Ebola virus–specific antibodies. Although this treatment has reduced levels of Ebola virus in the body, further evaluation is needed.

Throughout treatment, the patient should remain in isolation. If diagnostic tests indicate that the patient is free from the virus, which typically occurs 21 days after onset in those few who survive, the patient can be released.

## Special considerations

- Follow the guidelines for strict isolation precautions formulated by the Centers for Disease Control and Prevention (CDC) when assessing a patient who may have Ebola virus disease.
- Check the results of complete blood count and coagulation studies for signs of blood loss and coagulopathy.
- Assess the patient daily for petechiae, ecchymoses, and oozing blood. Note and document the size of ecchymoses at least every 24 hours.
- Protect all areas of petechiae and ecchymoses from further injury.
- Test stools, urine, and vomitus for occult blood.
- Watch for frank bleeding, including GI bleeding and, in women, menorrhagia. Note and document the amount of bleeding every 24 hours or more often.
- Monitor the patient's family and other close contacts for fever and other signs of infection.
- Provide emotional support for the patient and family during the course of this devastating disease. Encourage them to ask questions and discuss any concerns they have about the disease and its treatment.

> **CLINICAL TIP** The CDC recommends the following guidelines to help prevent the spread of this deadly disease:

- Keep the patient in isolation throughout the course of the disease.
- If possible, place the patient in a negative pressure room at the beginning of hospitalization to avoid the need for transfer as the disease progresses.
- Restrict nonessential staff members from entering the patient's room.
- Make sure that anyone who enters the patient's room wears gloves and a gown to prevent contact with any surface in the room that may have been soiled.
- Use barrier precautions to prevent skin and mucous membrane exposure to blood or other body fluids, secretions, or excretions when caring for the patient.
- If you must come within 3′ (1 m) of the patient, also wear a face shield or a surgical mask and goggles or eyeglasses with side shields.
- Don't reuse gloves or gowns unless they have been completely disinfected.
- Make sure any patient who dies of the disease is promptly buried or cremated. Precautions to avoid contact with the patient's body fluids and secretions should continue even after the patient's death.

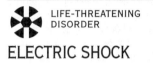

LIFE-THREATENING DISORDER

# ELECTRIC SHOCK

When an electric current passes through the body, the damage it does depends on the intensity of the current (amperes, milliamperes, or microamperes), the resistance of the tissues it passes through, the kind of current (alternating current, direct current, or mixed), and the frequency and duration of current flow.

Electric shock may cause ventricular fibrillation, respiratory paralysis, burns, and death. The prognosis depends on the site and extent of damage, the patient's state of health, and the speed and adequacy of treatment. Each year, about 1,000 persons in the United States die of electric shock.

## Causes

Electric shock usually follows accidental contact with exposed parts of electrical appliances or wiring, but it may also result from lightning or the flash of electric arcs from high-voltage power lines or machines.

The increased use of electrical medical devices in the hospital, many of which are connected directly to the patient, has raised serious concern for electrical safety and has led to the development of electrical safety standards. However, even well-designed equipment with reliable safety features can cause electric shock if it's mishandled. (See *Preventing electric shock.*)

CLINICAL TIP Electric current can cause injury in three ways: true electrical injury as the current passes through the body, arc or flash burns from current that doesn't pass through the body, and thermal surface burns caused by associated heat and flames.

## Signs and symptoms

Severe electric shock usually causes muscle contraction, followed by unconsciousness and loss of reflex control, sometimes with respiratory paralysis (by way of prolonged contraction of respiratory muscles or a direct effect on the respiratory nerve center).

After momentary shock, hyperventilation may follow muscle contraction. Passage of even the smallest electric current — if it passes through the heart — may induce ventricular fibrillation or another arrhythmia that progresses to fibrillation or myocardial infarction.

Electric shock from a high-frequency current (which generates more heat in tissues than a low-frequency current) usually causes burns as well as local tissue coagulation and necrosis. Low-frequency currents can also cause serious burns if contact with the current is concentrated in a small area — for example, when a toddler bites into an electrical cord.

Contusions, fractures, and other injuries can result from violent muscle contractions or falls during the shock; later, the patient may develop renal shutdown. Residual hearing impairment, cataracts, and vision loss may persist after severe electric shock.

## Diagnosis

Usually, the cause of electrical injuries is either obvious or suspected. An accurate history can define the voltage and length of contact.

## Treatment

Immediate emergency treatment includes carefully separating the victim from the current source, quickly assessing vital functions, and instituting emergency measures, such as cardiopulmonary resuscitation (CPR) and defibrillation.

To separate the victim from the current source, immediately turn it off or

# PREVENTING ELECTRIC SHOCK

To protect your patient from electric shock:

• Check for cuts, cracks, or frayed insulation on electric cords, call buttons (also check for warm call buttons), and electric devices attached to the bed. Keep these away from hot or wet surfaces and sharp corners.

• Don't set glasses of water, damp towels, or other wet items on electrical equipment. Wipe up accidental spills before they leak into equipment. Avoid using extension cords because they may circumvent the ground. If they're absolutely necessary, don't place them under carpeting or in areas where they'll be walked on.

• Report faulty equipment promptly to maintenance personnel. If a machine sparks, smokes, seems unusually hot, or gives you or your patient a slight shock, unplug it immediately if doing so won't endanger the patient's life.

• Check inspection labels, and report equipment overdue for inspection.

• Be especially careful when using electrical equipment near patients with pacemakers or direct cardiac lines because a cardiac catheter or pacemaker can create a direct, low-resistance path to the heart; even a small shock may cause ventricular fibrillation.

• Make sure ground connections on electrical equipment are intact. Line cord plugs should have three prongs; the prongs should be straight and firmly fixed. Check that prongs fit wall outlets properly, and that outlets aren't loose or broken. Don't use adapters on plugs.

• Remember: Dry, callused, unbroken skin offers more resistance to electric current than mucous membrane, an open wound, or thin, moist skin.

• Make sure defibrillator paddles are free of dry, caked gel before applying fresh gel because poor electrical contact can cause burns. Also, don't apply too much gel. If the gel runs over the edge of the paddle and touches your hand, you'll receive some of the defibrillator shock and the patient will lose some of the energy in the discharge.

---

unplug it. If this isn't possible, pull the victim free with a nonconductive device, such as a loop of dry cloth or rubber, a dry rope, or a leather belt.

### Emergency measures

Then begin emergency treatment as follows.

• Quickly assess vital functions. If you don't detect a pulse or breathing, start CPR at once. Continue until vital signs return or emergency help arrives with a defibrillator and other life-support equipment. Then monitor the patient's cardiac rhythm continuously and obtain a 12-lead electrocardiogram.

• Because internal tissue destruction may be much greater than indicated by skin damage, give lactated Ringer's solution I.V. to maintain a urine output of 50 to 100 ml/hour. Insert an indwelling urinary catheter, and send the first specimen to the laboratory.

• Measure intake and output hourly, and watch for tea- or port wine–colored urine, which occurs when coagulation necrosis and tissue ischemia liberate myoglobin and hemoglobin. These proteins can precipitate in the renal tubules, causing tubular necrosis and renal shutdown. To prevent this, give mannitol and furosemide.

### Special considerations

• Assess the patient's neurologic status frequently because central nervous system damage may result from ischemia or demyelination.

• Watch for sensorimotor deficits because a spinal cord injury may follow cord ischemia or a compression fracture.

• Check for neurovascular damage in the extremities by assessing peripheral pulses and capillary refill and by asking about numbness, tingling, and pain. Elevate injured extremities.

• Apply a temporary sterile dressing, and admit the patient for surgical debridement and observation as needed. Frequent debridement and the use of topical and systemic antibiotics can help reduce the risk of infection.

• Prepare the patient for grafting or, if his injuries are extreme, amputation.

• Protect patients from electric shock in the hospital.

• Tell patients how to avoid electrical hazards at home and at work. Advise parents of young children to put safety guards on all electrical outlets and keep children away from electrical devices. Warn all patients not to use electrical appliances while showering or wet.

• Warn patients *never* to touch electrical appliances while touching faucets or cold water pipes in the kitchen because these pipes often provide the ground for all circuits in the house.

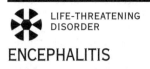

LIFE-THREATENING
DISORDER

# ENCEPHALITIS

A severe inflammation of the brain, encephalitis is usually caused by a mosquito-borne or, in some areas, a tickborne virus. Transmission by means other than arthropod bites may occur through ingestion of infected goat's milk and accidental injection or inhalation of the virus. Eastern equine encephali-

tis may produce permanent neurologic damage and is often fatal.

In encephalitis, intense lymphocytic infiltration of brain tissues and the leptomeninges causes cerebral edema, degeneration of the brain's ganglion cells, and diffuse nerve cell destruction.

## Causes
Encephalitis generally results from infection with arboviruses specific to rural areas. In urban areas, it's most frequently caused by enteroviruses (coxsackievirus, poliovirus, and echovirus).

Other causes include herpesvirus, mumps virus, human immunodeficiency virus, adenoviruses, and demyelinating diseases after measles, varicella, rubella, or vaccination.

Between World War I and the Depression, a type of encephalitis known as lethargic encephalitis, von Economo's disease, or sleeping sickness occurred with some regularity. The causative virus was never clearly identified, and the disease is rare today. Even so, the term *sleeping sickness* persists and is often mistakenly used to describe other types of encephalitis as well.

## Signs and symptoms
All viral forms of encephalitis have similar clinical features, although certain differences do occur.

Usually, the acute illness begins with sudden onset of fever, headache, and vomiting and progresses to include signs and symptoms of meningeal irritation (stiff neck and back) and neuronal damage (drowsiness, coma, paralysis, seizures, ataxia, and organic psychoses). After the acute phase of the illness, coma may persist for days or weeks.

The severity of arbovirus encephalitis may range from subclinical to rapidly fatal necrotizing disease. Herpes encephalitis also produces signs and symptoms that vary from subclinical to acute and often fatal fulminating disease. Associated effects include disturbances of taste or smell.

## Diagnosis

During an encephalitis epidemic, diagnosis is easily based on clinical findings and patient history. Sporadic cases are difficult to distinguish from other febrile illnesses, such as gastroenteritis and meningitis. When possible, identification of the virus in cerebrospinal fluid (CSF) or blood confirms the diagnosis.

The common viruses that also cause herpes, measles, and mumps are easier to identify than arboviruses. Arboviruses and herpesviruses can be isolated by inoculating young mice with specimens taken from patients. In herpes encephalitis, serologic studies may show rising titers of complement-fixing antibodies.

In all forms of encephalitis, CSF pressure is elevated, and despite inflammation, the fluid is often clear. White blood cell and protein levels in CSF are slightly elevated, but the glucose level remains normal. An EEG reveals abnormalities. Occasionally, a computed tomographic scan may be ordered to rule out cerebral hematoma.

## Treatment

The antiviral agent acyclovir is effective only against herpes encephalitis. Treatment of all other forms of encephalitis is entirely supportive.

Drug therapy includes phenytoin or another anticonvulsant, usually given I.V.; glucocorticoids to reduce cerebral inflammation and edema; furosemide or mannitol to reduce cerebral swelling; sedatives for restlessness; and aspirin or acetaminophen to relieve headache and reduce fever.

Other supportive measures include adequate fluid and electrolyte intake to prevent dehydration and antibiotics for an associated infection such as pneumonia. Isolation is unnecessary.

## Special considerations

During the acute phase of the illness:
● Assess neurologic function often. Observe the patient's mental status and cognitive abilities by performing a rapid neurologic examination. (See *Performing a rapid neurologic examination,* page 306.) If the tissue within the brain becomes edematous, changes will occur in the patient's mental status and cognitive abilities.

CLINICAL TIP Assessment should focus on early changes in intracranial dynamics. Continued swelling may result in cranial nerve compression, causing changes in pupillary reaction to light, ptosis, eyelid droop, and an eye rotating outward.
● Monitor for signs of progression of a herniation pattern (abnormal posturing movements, such as decerebration, decortication, and flaccidity, to noxious stimuli).
● Watch for cranial nerve involvement (ptosis, strabismus, diplopia), abnormal sleep patterns, and behavioral changes.
● Maintain adequate fluid intake to prevent dehydration, but avoid fluid overload, which may increase cerebral edema. Measure and record intake and output accurately.
● Give acyclovir by slow I.V. infusion only. The patient must be well hydrated and the infusion given over 1 hour to avoid kidney damage. Watch for adverse effects, such as nausea, diarrhea, pruritus, and rash, and adverse effects of other drugs. Check the infusion site often to avoid infiltration and phlebitis.
● Carefully position the patient to prevent joint stiffness and neck pain, and turn him often. Assist with range-of-motion exercises.
● Maintain adequate nutrition. It may be necessary to give the patient small,

## PERFORMING A RAPID NEUROLOGIC EXAMINATION

To assess neurologic function in the patient with encephalitis, include the following:

• Orientation: patient's knowledge of where he is, the year, season, date, day and month
• Registration and recall: patient's ability to recall three objects that you name
• Attention and calculation: patient's ability to focus on what you are saying
• Language: patient's ability to name objects, repeat words clearly, read, follow a written command
• Focus on recall of recent events: patient's ability to recall your name, what he had for breakfast, who came to visit.

As you elicit answers, be particularly concerned about the patient who requires more stimulation to provide the same responses to the above and about the restless patient.

frequent meals or to supplement these meals with nasogastric tube or parenteral feedings.
• To prevent constipation and minimize the risk of increased intracranial pressure from straining during defecation, give a mild laxative or stool softener.
• Provide good mouth care.
• Maintain a quiet environment. Darkening the room may decrease photophobia and headache. If the patient naps during the day and is restless at night, plan daytime activities to minimize napping and promote sleep at night.

• Provide emotional support and reassurance because the patient is apt to be frightened by the illness and frequent diagnostic tests.
• If the patient is delirious or confused, attempt to reorient him often. Providing a calendar or a clock in the patient's room may be helpful.
• Reassure the patient and his family that behavioral changes caused by encephalitis usually disappear. If a neurologic deficit is severe and appears permanent, refer the patient to a rehabilitation program as soon as the acute phase has passed.

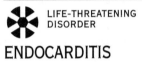 **LIFE-THREATENING DISORDER**

## ENDOCARDITIS

Also called infective endocarditis and bacterial endocarditis, endocarditis is an infection of the endocardium, heart valves, or a cardiac prosthesis, resulting from bacterial or fungal invasion. This invasion produces vegetative growths on the heart valves, the endocardial lining of a heart chamber, or the endothelium of a blood vessel that may embolize to the spleen, kidneys, central nervous system, and lungs.

In endocarditis, fibrin and platelets aggregate on the valve tissue and engulf circulating bacteria or fungi that flourish and produce friable verrucous vegetations. Such vegetations may cover the valve surfaces, causing ulceration and necrosis; they may also extend to the chordae tendineae, leading to their rupture and subsequent valvular insufficiency.

Untreated endocarditis is usually fatal, but with proper treatment, about 70% of patients recover. The prognosis is worst when endocarditis causes severe valvular damage, leading to insufficiency and heart failure, or when it involves a prosthetic valve.

## Causes

Most commonly, endocarditis occurs in I.V. drug abusers, patients with prosthetic heart valves, and those with mitral valve prolapse (especially males with a systolic murmur). These conditions have surpassed rheumatic heart disease as the leading risk factor.

Other predisposing conditions include coarctation of the aorta; tetralogy of Fallot; subaortic and valvular aortic stenosis; ventricular septal defects; pulmonary stenosis; Marfan's syndrome; degenerative heart disease, especially calcific aortic stenosis; and, rarely, syphilitic aortic valve. Some patients with endocarditis have no underlying heart disease.

### Infecting organisms

Organisms that cause infection differ among patient groups. In patients with native valve endocarditis who aren't I.V. drug abusers, causative organisms usually include, in order of frequency, streptococci (especially *Streptococcus viridans),* staphylococci, and enterococci. Although many other bacteria occasionally cause the disorder, fungal causes are rare in this group. The mitral valve is involved most commonly, followed by the aortic valve.

In patients who are I.V. drug abusers, *Staphylococcus aureus* is the most common infecting organism. Less frequently, streptococci, enterococci, gram-negative bacilli, or fungi cause the disorder. Most often the tricuspid valve is involved, followed by the aortic valve and then the mitral valve.

In patients with prosthetic valve endocarditis, "early" cases (those that develop within 60 days of valve insertion) are usually due to staphylococcal infec-

tion. Gram-negative aerobic organisms, fungi, streptococci, enterococci, or diphtheroids may also cause the disorder. The course of the infection is often fulminating and associated with a high mortality rate. "Late" cases (those that develop after 60 days) present similarly to those of native valve endocarditis.

### Signs and symptoms

Early clinical features of endocarditis are usually nonspecific and include malaise, weakness, fatigue, weight loss, anorexia, arthralgia, night sweats, chills, valvular insufficiency and, in 90% of patients, an intermittent fever that may recur for weeks. A more acute onset is associated with highly pathogenic organisms such as *S. aureus.*

Endocarditis often causes a loud, regurgitant murmur that is typical of the underlying heart lesion. A suddenly changing murmur or the discovery of a new murmur in the presence of fever is a classic physical sign of endocarditis.

In about 30% of patients, embolization from vegetating lesions or diseased valvular tissue may produce the following features of splenic, renal, cerebral, or pulmonary infarction or peripheral vascular occlusion:
- *splenic infarction:* pain in the left upper quadrant, radiating to the left shoulder; abdominal rigidity
- *renal infarction:* hematuria, pyuria, flank pain, decreased urine output
- *cerebral infarction:* hemiparesis, aphasia, or other neurologic deficits
- *pulmonary infarction* (most common in right-sided endocarditis, which usually occurs in I.V. drug abusers and after cardiac surgery): cough, pleuritic pain, pleural friction rub, dyspnea, hemoptysis
- *peripheral vascular occlusion:* numbness and tingling in an arm or a leg, finger, or toe or signs of impending peripheral gangrene.

Other signs include splenomegaly; petechiae of the skin (especially common on the upper anterior trunk) and the buccal, pharyngeal, or conjunctival mucosa; and splinter hemorrhages under the nails. Rarely, endocarditis produces Osler's nodes (tender, raised subcutaneous lesions on the fingers or toes), Roth's spots (hemorrhagic areas with white centers on the retina), and Janeway lesions (purplish macules on the palms or soles).

### Diagnosis

Three or more blood cultures in a 24- to 48-hour period identify the causative organism in up to 90% of patients. The remaining 10% may have negative blood cultures, possibly suggesting fungal infection or infections that are difficult to diagnose, such as *Haemophilus parainfluenzae.* Other abnormal but nonspecific laboratory test results include:

• normal or elevated white blood cell count

• abnormal histiocytes (macrophages)

• elevated erythrocyte sedimentation rate

• normocytic, normochromic anemia (in 70% to 90% of endocarditis cases)

• positive serum rheumatoid factor (in about one-half of all patients with endocarditis after the disease is present for 3 to 6 weeks).

Echocardiography may identify valvular damage; electrocardiography may show atrial fibrillation and other arrhythmias that accompany valvular disease.

### Treatment

The goal of treatment is to eradicate the infecting organism. Antimicrobial therapy should start promptly and continue over 4 to 6 weeks. Selection of an antibiotic is based on identification of the infecting organism and on sensitivity studies. While awaiting test results or if blood cultures are negative, empiric antimicrobial therapy is based on the likely infecting organism.

Supportive treatment includes bed rest, aspirin for fever and aches, and sufficient fluid intake. Severe valvular damage, especially aortic or mitral insufficiency, may necessitate corrective surgery if refractory heart failure develops or in cases in which an infected prosthetic valve must be replaced.

### Special considerations

• Before giving antibiotics, obtain a patient history of allergies.

CLINICAL TIP Administer antibiotics on time to maintain consistent antibiotic blood levels.

• Observe for signs of infiltration and inflammation, possible complications of long-term I.V. drug administration, at the venipuncture site. To reduce the risk of these complications, rotate venous access sites.

• Watch for signs of embolization (hematuria, pleuritic chest pain, left upper quadrant pain, and paresis), a common occurrence during the first 3 months of treatment. Tell the patient to watch for and report these signs, which may indicate impending peripheral vascular occlusion or splenic, renal, cerebral, or pulmonary infarction.

• Monitor the patient's renal status (blood urea nitrogen levels, creatinine clearance, and urine output) to check for signs of renal emboli or evidence of drug toxicity.

• Observe for signs of heart failure, such as dyspnea, tachypnea, tachycardia, crackles, neck vein distention, edema, and weight gain.

• Provide reassurance by teaching the patient and his family about this disease and the need for prolonged treatment. Tell them to watch closely for fever, anorexia, and other signs of relapse about 2 weeks after treatment stops.

Suggest quiet diversionary activities to prevent excessive physical exertion.
• Make sure a susceptible patient understands the need for prophylactic antibiotics before, during, and after dental work, childbirth, and genitourinary, GI, or gynecologic procedures.
• Teach the patient how to recognize symptoms of endocarditis, and tell him to notify the doctor immediately if they occur.

# ENDOMETRIOSIS

A diagnosis of endometriosis denotes the presence of endometrial tissue outside the lining of the uterine cavity. Such ectopic tissue is generally confined to the pelvic area, most commonly around the ovaries, uterovesical peritoneum, uterosacral ligaments, and cul-de-sac, but it can appear anywhere in the body.

This ectopic endometrial tissue responds to normal stimulation in the same way the endometrium does. During menstruation, the ectopic tissue bleeds, which causes the surrounding tissues to become inflamed. This inflammation causes fibrosis, leading to adhesions that produce pain and cause infertility.

Active endometriosis usually occurs between ages 30 and 40, especially in women who postpone childbearing; it's uncommon before age 20. Severe symptoms of endometriosis may have an abrupt onset or develop over many years. This disorder usually becomes progressively severe during the menstrual years; after menopause, it tends to subside.

## Causes
The mechanisms by which endometriosis causes symptoms, including infertility, are unknown. The main theories to explain this disorder are:

• transtubal regurgitation of endometrial cells and implantation at ectopic sites
• coelomic metaplasia (repeated inflammation may induce metaplasia of mesothelial cells to the endometrial epithelium)
• lymphatic or hematogenous spread to account for extraperitoneal disease.

## Signs and symptoms
The classic symptom of endometriosis is acquired dysmenorrhea, which may produce constant pain in the lower abdomen as well as the vagina, posterior pelvis, and back. The pain usually begins 5 to 7 days before menses, reaches its peak on days of bleeding, and lasts for 2 to 3 days. It differs from primary dysmenorrheal pain, which is more cramplike and concentrated in the abdominal midline. The severity of pain doesn't necessarily indicate the extent of the disease.

Other clinical features depend on the location of the ectopic tissue:
• *ovaries and oviducts*: infertility and profuse menses
• *ovaries or cul-de-sac:* deep-thrust dyspareunia
• *bladder:* suprapubic pain, dysuria, hematuria
• *rectovaginal septum and colon:* painful defecation, rectal bleeding with menses, pain in the coccyx or sacrum
• *small bowel and appendix:* nausea and vomiting, which worsen before menses, and abdominal cramps
• *cervix, vagina, and perineum:* bleeding from endometrial deposits in these areas during menses.

The primary complication of endometriosis is infertility.

## Diagnosis
Palpation during a pelvic examination may detect multiple tender nodules on the uterosacral ligaments or in the rectovaginal septum in one-third of pa-

tients. These nodules enlarge and become more tender during menses.

Palpation may also uncover ovarian enlargement in the presence of endometrial cysts on the ovaries or thickened, nodular adnexa (as in pelvic inflammatory disease). Laparoscopy is used to confirm the diagnosis and determine the stage of the disease before treatment is initiated.

### Treatment
The stage of the disease and the patient's age and desire to have children are treatment considerations for endometriosis. In stages I and II (mild forms with superficial endometria and filmy adhesions), conservative therapy for young women who want to have children includes androgens such as danazol, which produce a temporary remission. Progestins and oral contraceptives also relieve symptoms. Gonadotropin-releasing hormone agonists, by inducing a pseudomenopause and, thus, a "medical oophorectomy," have shown a remission of disease and are commonly used.

When ovarian masses are present (stages III and IV), surgery must rule out cancer. Conservative surgery is possible, but the treatment of choice for women who don't want to bear children and for those with extensive disease (stages III and IV) is a total abdominal hysterectomy with bilateral salpingo-oophorectomy.

### Special considerations
• Minor gynecologic procedures are contraindicated immediately before and during menstruation.
• Advise adolescents to use sanitary napkins instead of tampons; this can help prevent retrograde flow in girls with a narrow vagina or small introitus.
• Because infertility is a possible complication, advise the patient who wants children not to postpone childbearing.

> **CLINICAL TIP** Recommend to all patients that they have an annual pelvic examination and Papanicolaou test.

# EPICONDYLITIS

Also known as tennis elbow and epitrochlear bursitis, epicondylitis is inflammation of the forearm extensor supinator tendon fibers at their common attachment to the lateral humeral epicondyle. This inflammation produces acute or subacute pain.

### Causes
Epicondylitis probably begins as a partial tear and is common among tennis players and people whose activities require a forceful grasp, wrist extension against resistance, or frequent rotation of the forearm. Untreated epicondylitis may become disabling.

### Signs and symptoms
The patient's initial symptom is elbow pain that gradually worsens and often radiates to the forearm and back of the hand whenever he grasps an object or twists his elbow.

Other associated signs and symptoms include tenderness over the involved lateral or medial epicondyle or over the head of the radius and a weak grasp. In rare instances, epicondylitis may cause local heat, swelling, and restricted range of motion (ROM).

### Diagnosis
Because X-rays are almost always negative, diagnosis typically depends on clinical signs and symptoms and a patient history of playing tennis or engaging in similar activities. The pain can be reproduced by wrist extension

and supination with lateral involvement or by flexion and pronation with medial epicondyle involvement.

### Treatment

The aim of treatment is to relieve pain, usually by local injection of corticosteroid and a local anesthetic and by systemic anti-inflammatory therapy with aspirin or indomethacin.

#### *Supportive measures*

Supportive treatment includes an immobilizing splint from the distal forearm to the elbow, which generally relieves pain in 2 to 3 weeks; heat therapy, such as warm compresses, short wave diathermy, and ultrasound (alone or in combination with diathermy); and physical therapy, such as manipulation and massage to detach the tendon from the chronically inflamed periosteum.

A "tennis elbow strap" has helped many patients. This strap, which is wrapped snugly around the forearm about 1″ (2.5 cm) below the epicondyle, helps relieve the strain on affected forearm muscles and tendons.

If these measures prove ineffective, surgical release of the tendon at the epicondyle may be necessary.

### Special considerations

● Assess the patient's level of pain, ROM, and sensory function. Monitor heat therapy to prevent burns.

● Instruct the patient to rest the elbow until inflammation subsides.

● Remove the support daily, and gently move the arm to prevent stiffness and contracture.

● Instruct the patient to follow the prescribed exercise program. For example, he may stretch his arm and flex his wrist to the maximum, then press the back of his hand against a wall until he can feel a pull in his forearm, and hold this position for 1 minute.

● Advise the patient to warm up for 15 to 20 minutes before beginning any sports activity.

> **CLINICAL TIP** Suggest that the exercise equipment be assessed for proper size and weight. The playing field may also need to be reevaluated.

● Urge the patient to wear an elastic support or splint during any activity that stresses the forearm or elbow.

# EPIDIDYMITIS

This infection of the epididymis, the testicle's cordlike excretory duct, is one of the most common infections of the male reproductive tract. It usually affects adults and is rare before puberty. Epididymitis may spread to the testicle itself, causing orchitis; bilateral epididymitis may cause sterility.

### Causes

Epididymitis usually results from pyogenic organisms, such as Enterobacteriaceae and *Pseudomonas*. Epididymitis can result from an existing urinary tract infection or prostatitis and reach the epididymis through the lumen of the vas deferens.

Rarely, epididymitis is secondary to a distant infection, such as pharyngitis or tuberculosis, that spreads through the lymphatics or, less commonly, the bloodstream.

Other causes include trauma, gonorrhea, syphilis, and a chlamydial infection. Trauma may reactivate a dormant infection or initiate a new one. Epididymitis is a complication of prostatectomy and may also result from chemical irritation by extravasation of urine through the vas deferens.

## Signs and symptoms

The key symptoms are pain, extreme tenderness, and swelling in the groin and scrotum. Other clinical effects include high fever, malaise, and a characteristic waddle—an attempt to protect the groin and scrotum during walking. An acute hydrocele may also occur as a reaction to the inflammatory process.

## Diagnosis

Clinical features suggest epididymitis, but the actual diagnosis is made with the aid of the following laboratory tests:

• *Urinalysis* shows an increased white blood cell (WBC) count, indicating infection.

• *Urine culture and sensitivity tests* may identify the causative organism.

• *Serum WBC count* of more than 10,000/µl indicates infection.

• *Scrotal ultrasonography* may help differentiate acute epididymitis from other conditions such as testicular torsion, which is a surgical emergency.

## Treatment

The goal of treatment is to reduce pain and swelling and combat infection. Therapy must begin immediately, particularly in the patient with bilateral epididymitis, because sterility is always a threat.

### During the acute phase

Treatment consists of bed rest, scrotal elevation with towel rolls or adhesive strapping, broad-spectrum antibiotics, and analgesics.

An ice bag applied to the area may reduce swelling and relieve pain. (Heat is contraindicated because it may damage germinal cells, which are viable only at or below normal body temperature.) When pain and swelling subside and allow walking, an athletic supporter may prevent pain.

**CLINICAL TIP** Occasionally, corticosteroids may be prescribed to help counteract inflammation, but their use is controversial.

### Prevention

In the older patient undergoing open prostatectomy, bilateral vasectomy may be necessary to prevent epididymitis as a postoperative complication; however, antibiotic therapy alone may prevent it. When epididymitis is refractory to antibiotic therapy, epididymectomy under local anesthetic is necessary.

## Special considerations

• Watch closely for abscess formation (a localized hot, red, tender area) and extension of the infection into the testes. Closely monitor temperature, and ensure adequate fluid intake.

• Because the patient is usually uncomfortable, administer analgesics as necessary. During bed rest, check often for proper scrotum elevation.

• Before discharge, emphasize the importance of completing the prescribed antibiotic therapy, even after symptoms subside.

• If the patient faces the possibility of sterility, suggest supportive counseling as necessary.

LIFE-THREATENING DISORDER

# EPIGLOTTITIS

Acute epiglottitis is an inflammation of the epiglottis that tends to cause airway obstruction. It typically strikes children ages 2 to 8. A critical emergency, epiglottitis can prove fatal in 8% to 12% of victims unless it's recognized and treated promptly.

## Causes

Epiglottitis usually results from infection with the bacterium *Haemophilus influenzae* type B; occasionally, it results from pneumococci and group A streptococci.

## Signs and symptoms

Sometimes preceded by an upper respiratory tract infection, epiglottitis may progress to complete upper airway obstruction within 2 to 5 hours. Laryngeal obstruction results from inflammation and edema of the epiglottis. Accompanying symptoms include high fever, stridor, sore throat, dysphagia, irritability, restlessness, and drooling.

To relieve severe respiratory distress, the child with epiglottitis may hyperextend his neck, sit up, and lean forward with his mouth open, tongue protruding, and nostrils flaring as he tries to breathe. He may develop inspiratory retractions and rhonchi.

## Diagnosis

In acute epiglottitis, throat examination reveals a large, edematous, bright red epiglottis. Such examination should follow lateral neck X-rays and, generally, should not be performed if the suspected obstruction is large.

➤ CLINICAL TIP Special equipment (a laryngoscope and endotracheal [ET] tubes) should be available because a tongue depressor can cause sudden, complete airway obstruction. Trained personnel (such as an anesthesiologist) should be on hand during throat examination to secure an emergency airway.

## Treatment

A child with acute epiglottitis and airway obstruction requires emergency hospitalization; he may need emergency ET intubation or a tracheotomy and should be monitored in an intensive care unit. Respiratory distress that interferes with swallowing necessitates parenteral fluid administration to prevent dehydration.

A patient with acute epiglottitis should always receive a 10-day course of parenteral antibiotics—usually a second- or third-generation cephalosporin (if the child is allergic to penicillin, a quinolone or sulfa drug may be substituted). Oxygen therapy and arterial blood gas (ABG) monitoring may be desirable.

## Special considerations

● Keep the following equipment available in case of sudden, complete airway obstruction: a tracheotomy tray, ET tubes, a handheld resuscitation bag, oxygen equipment, and a laryngoscope with blades of various sizes. Monitor ABG levels for hypoxia and hypercapnia.
● Watch for increasing restlessness, rising heart rate, fever, dyspnea, and retractions, which may indicate the need for an emergency tracheotomy.
● After tracheotomy, anticipate the patient's needs because he won't be able to cry or call out, and provide emotional support. Reassure the patient and his family that the tracheotomy is a short-term intervention (usually from 4 to 7 days).
● Monitor the patient for rising temperature and pulse rate and for hypotension, which are signs of secondary infection.

# EPILEPSY

Seizure disorder, or epilepsy, is a condition of the brain characterized by a susceptibility to recurrent seizures (paroxysmal events associated with abnormal electrical discharges of neurons in the brain). Epilepsy is believed to affect 1% to 2% of the population. The prognosis is good if the patient with epilepsy adheres strictly to his prescribed treatment.

## Causes

In about one-half of all epilepsy cases, the cause is unknown. Possible causes include:

● birth trauma (inadequate oxygen supply to the brain, blood incompatibility, or hemorrhage)
● perinatal infection
● anoxia
● infectious diseases (meningitis, encephalitis, or brain abscess)
● ingestion of toxins (mercury, lead, or carbon monoxide)
● brain tumors
● inherited disorders or degenerative disease, such as phenylketonuria or tuberous sclerosis
● head injury or trauma
● metabolic disorders, such as hypoglycemia and hypoparathyroidism
● cerebrovascular accident (hemorrhage, thrombosis, or embolism).

## Signs and symptoms

The hallmark of epilepsy is recurring seizures, which can be classified as partial, generalized, status epilepticus, or unclassified (some patients may be affected by more than one type).

### *Partial seizures*

Arising from a localized area of the brain, partial seizures cause focal symptoms. These seizures are classified by their effect on consciousness and whether they spread throughout the motor strip, causing a generalized seizure.

A *simple partial seizure* begins locally and generally does not cause an alteration in consciousness. It is not uncommon for this type to present with sensory symptoms (lights flashing, smells, hearing hallucinations), auto-

nomic symptoms (sweating, flushing, pupil dilation), and psychic symptoms (dream states, anger, fear). The seizure lasts for a few seconds and occurs without preceding or provoking events.

A *complex partial seizure* involves impairment in consciousness. Amnesia for the events that occur during and immediately after the seizure is a differentiating characteristic. During the seizure, the patient may follow simple commands. This type of partial seizure generally lasts for 1 to 3 minutes.

### *Generalized seizures*

As the term suggests, generalized seizures cause a generalized electrical abnormality within the brain. They can be convulsive or nonconvulsive and include several types.

● *Absence seizures* occur most often in children, although they may affect adults. They usually begin with a brief change in level of consciousness, indicated by blinking or rolling of the eyes, a blank stare, and slight mouth movements. The patient retains his posture and continues preseizure activity without difficulty. Typically, each seizure lasts from 1 to 10 seconds. If not properly treated, seizures can recur as often as 100 times a day. An absence seizure is a nonconvulsive seizure, but it may progress to a generalized tonic-clonic seizure.

● *Myoclonic seizures (bilateral massive epileptic myoclonus)* are characterized by brief, involuntary muscular jerks of the body or extremities, which may occur in a rhythmic manner. Consciousness is not usually affected.

● *Generalized tonic-clonic seizures* typically begin with a loud cry, precipitated by air rushing from the lungs through the vocal cords. The patient then loses consciousness and falls to the ground. The body stiffens (tonic phase) and then alternates between episodes of muscle spasm and relaxation (clonic phase).

Tongue biting, incontinence, labored breathing, apnea, and subsequent cyanosis may also occur.

The seizure stops in 2 to 5 minutes, when abnormal electrical conduction of the neurons is completed. The patient then regains consciousness but is confused and may have difficulty talking. If he can talk, he may complain of drowsiness, fatigue, headache, muscle soreness, and arm or leg weakness. He may fall into a deep sleep after the seizure.

• *Atonic seizures* are characterized by a general loss of postural tone and a temporary loss of consciousness. They occur in young children and are sometimes called "drop attacks" because they cause the child to fall.

### Status epilepticus

Status epilepticus is a continuous seizure state that can occur in all seizure types. The most life-threatening example is generalized tonic-clonic status epilepticus, a continuous generalized tonic-clonic seizure without intervening return of consciousness.

Status epilepticus is accompanied by respiratory distress. It can result from abrupt withdrawal of anticonvulsant medications, hypoxic encephalopathy, acute head trauma, metabolic encephalopathy, or septicemia secondary to encephalitis or meningitis.

### Unclassified seizures

This category is reserved for seizures that don't fit the characteristics of partial or generalized seizures or status epilepticus. Included as unclassified are events that lack the data to make a more definitive diagnosis.

## Diagnosis

Clinically, the diagnosis of epilepsy is based on the occurrence of one or more seizures and proof or the assumption that the condition that caused them is still present.

Diagnostic information is obtained from the patient's history and description of seizure activity, family history, physical and neurologic examinations, and computed tomographic scanning or magnetic resonance imaging. These scans offer density readings of the brain and may indicate abnormalities in internal structures.

### Confirming evidence

Paroxysmal abnormalities on the EEG confirm the diagnosis by providing evidence of the continuing tendency to have seizures. A negative EEG doesn't rule out epilepsy because the paroxysmal abnormalities occur intermittently. Other tests include serum glucose and calcium studies, skull X-rays, lumbar puncture, brain scan, and cerebral angiography.

## Treatment

Generally, treatment of epilepsy consists of drug therapy specific to the type of seizure. The most commonly prescribed drugs include phenytoin, carbamazepine, phenobarbital, and primidone administered individually for generalized tonic-clonic seizures and complex partial seizures.

➤ CLINICAL TIP I.V. fosphenytoin (Cerebyx) is an alternative to phenytoin (Dilantin) that is just as effective, with a long half-life and minimal central nervous system depression. It is stable for 120 days at room temperature and compatible with many frequently used I.V. solutions. In addition, it can be administered rapidly without the adverse cardiovascular effects that occur with phenytoin.

Valproic acid, clonazepam, and ethosuximide are commonly prescribed for absence seizures. Gabapentin (Neurontin) and felbamate are other anticonvulsant drugs. A patient taking an anticonvulsant requires monitoring for signs of toxicity, such as nystagmus, ataxia, lethargy, dizziness, drowsiness, slurred speech, irritability, nausea, and vomiting.

If drug therapy fails, treatment may include surgical removal of a demonstrated focal lesion in an attempt to stop seizures.

**CLINICAL TIP** A vagus nerve stimulator implant may help reduce the incidence of focal seizure.

Emergency treatment of status epilepticus usually consists of I.V. administration of diazepam, lorazepam, phenytoin, or phenobarbital; dextrose 50% (when seizures are secondary to hypoglycemia); and thiamine (in chronic alcoholism or withdrawal).

**Special considerations**

**CLINICAL TIP** When the patient experiences a seizure, describe the seizure in detail instead of classifying it. List precipitating events, how the seizure began and progressed, its duration, all movements and activities, and level of consciousness.

• Encourage the patient and his family to express their feelings about the patient's condition. Answer their questions, and help them cope by dispelling some of the myths about epilepsy—for example, that it's contagious. Assure them that epilepsy is controllable for most patients who follow a prescribed medication regimen and that most patients maintain a normal lifestyle.
• Teach the family how to give the patient first aid when a seizure occurs. (See *Guidelines for seizures.*)
• Because drug therapy is the treatment of choice for most patients with epilepsy, information about the medications is invaluable.
• Stress the need for compliance with the prescribed drug schedule. Assure the patient that anticonvulsant drugs are safe when taken as prescribed.
• Reinforce dosage instructions, and find methods to help the patient remember to take medications. Caution him to monitor the amount of medication left so he doesn't run out of it.
• Warn against possible adverse effects, such as drowsiness, lethargy, hyperactivity, confusion, and visual and sleep disturbances, which indicate the need for dosage adjustment. Phenytoin therapy may lead to hyperplasia of the gums, which may be relieved by conscientious oral hygiene. Instruct the patient to report adverse effects immediately.
• Warn the patient against drinking alcoholic beverages.

• Emphasize the importance of having anticonvulsant blood levels checked at regular intervals, even if the seizures are under control.

• Know which social agencies in your community can help epileptic patients. Refer the patient to the Epilepsy Foundation of America for general information and to the state motor vehicle department for information about a driver's license.

# EPISTAXIS

Nosebleed, or epistaxis, may either be a primary disorder or occur secondary to another condition. Such bleeding in children generally originates in the anterior nasal septum and tends to be mild. In adults, such bleeding is most likely to originate in the posterior septum and can be severe. Epistaxis is twice as common in children as in adults.

## Causes

Epistaxis usually follows trauma from external or internal causes: a blow to the nose, nose picking, or insertion of a foreign body. Less commonly, it follows polyps; acute or chronic infections, such as sinusitis or rhinitis, that cause congestion and eventual bleeding from capillary blood vessels; or inhalation of chemicals that irritate the nasal mucosa. It may also follow sudden mechanical decompression (caisson disease) and violent exercise.

### Predisposing factors

Such factors include anticoagulant therapy, hypertension, chronic aspirin use, high altitudes and dry climates, sclerotic vessel disease, Hodgkin's disease, neoplastic disorders, scurvy, vitamin K deficiency, rheumatic fever, blood dyscrasias (hemophilia, purpura, leukemia, and anemias), and hemorrhagic telangiectasia.

## Signs and symptoms

Blood oozing from the nostrils usually originates in the anterior nose and is bright red. Blood from the back of the throat originates in the posterior area and may be dark or bright red (often mistaken for hemoptysis due to expectoration).

Epistaxis is generally unilateral, except when due to dyscrasia or severe trauma. In severe epistaxis, blood may seep behind the nasal septum; it may also appear in the middle ear and corners of the eyes.

### Associated effects

Clinical effects depend on the severity of bleeding. Moderate blood loss may produce light-headedness, dizziness, and slight respiratory difficulty; severe hemorrhage causes hypotension, rapid and bounding pulse, dyspnea, and pallor. Bleeding is considered severe if it persists longer than 10 minutes after pressure is applied. If severe, blood loss can be as great as 1 L/hour in adults.

## Diagnosis

Although simple observation confirms epistaxis, inspection with a bright light and nasal speculum is necessary to locate the site of bleeding.

Relevant laboratory values include:
• gradual reduction in hemoglobin and hematocrit (often inaccurate immediately after epistaxis due to hemoconcentration)
• decreased platelet count in a patient with blood dyscrasia
• prothrombin time and partial thromboplastin time showing a coagulation time twice the control because of a bleeding disorder or anticoagulant therapy.

Diagnosis must rule out underlying systemic causes of epistaxis, especially disseminated intravascular coagulation and rheumatic fever. Bruises or concomitant bleeding elsewhere probably indicates a hematologic disorder. A nasopharyngeal angiofibroma may present as recurrent epistaxis.

## Treatment
Different treatment measures are used for anterior and posterior bleeding. Drug therapy, transfusions, and surgery may also be necessary.

### Local measures
For anterior bleeding, treatment consists of application of a cotton ball saturated with epinephrine to the bleeding site and external pressure, followed by cauterization with electrocautery or a silver nitrate stick. If these measures don't control the bleeding, petroleum gauze nasal packing may be needed. (See *Insertion of an anterior-posterior nasal pack.*)

For posterior bleeding, treatment includes use of a nasal balloon catheter to control bleeding effectively, gauze packing inserted through the nose, or postnasal packing inserted through the mouth, depending on the bleeding site. (Gauze packing generally remains in place for 24 to 48 hours; postnasal packing remains in place for 3 to 5 days.)

### Other measures
Antibiotics may be appropriate if the packing must remain in place for longer than 24 hours. If local measures fail to control bleeding, additional treatment may include supplemental vitamin K and, for severe bleeding, blood transfusions and surgical ligation or embolization of a bleeding artery.

## Special considerations
To control epistaxis:

> CLINICAL TIP   Have the patient sit upright with his head tilted forward to minimize blood dripping into the oropharynx.

● Compress the soft portion of the nostrils against the septum continuously for 5 to 10 minutes. Apply an ice collar or cold, wet compresses to the nose. Bleeding should stop after 10 minutes.
● Administer oxygen as needed.
● Monitor vital signs and skin color; record blood loss.
● Tell the patient to breathe through his mouth and not to swallow blood, talk, or blow his nose.
● Monitor oxygen saturation levels.
● Keep vasoconstrictors such as phenylephrine handy.
● Reassure the patient and his family that epistaxis usually looks worse than it is.

To prevent a recurrence of epistaxis:
● Instruct the patient not to pick his nose or insert foreign objects into it and to avoid bending and lifting. Emphasize the need for follow-up examinations and periodic blood studies after an episode of epistaxis. Advise the patient to get prompt treatment for nasal infection or irritation.
● Suggest a humidifier for patients who live in dry climates or at high elevations or whose homes are heated with circulating hot air.
● Instruct the patient to sneeze with his mouth open.
● Caution the patient against inserting cotton or tissues into the nose on his own because these objects are difficult to remove and may further irritate the nasal mucosa.

## INSERTION OF AN ANTERIOR-POSTERIOR NASAL PACK

The first step in the insertion of an anterior-posterior nasal pack is the insertion of catheters in the nostrils. After drawing the catheters through the mouth, a suture from the pack is tied to each catheter, which positions the pack in place as the catheters are drawn back through the nostrils.

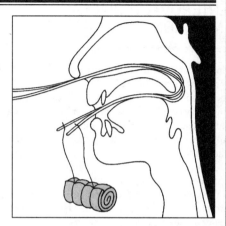

While the sutures are held tightly, packing is inserted into the anterior nose.

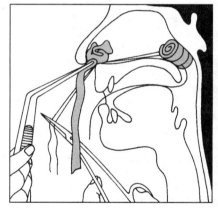

The sutures are then secured around a dental roll; the middle suture extends from the mouth and is tied to the cheek.

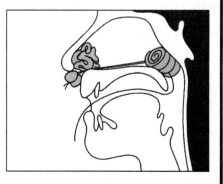

# E. COLI AND OTHER ENTEROBACTERIACEAE INFECTIONS

Enterobacteriaceae — a group of mostly aerobic gram-negative bacilli — cause local and systemic infections, including an invasive diarrhea that resembles shigella and, more often, a noninvasive toxin-mediated diarrhea that resembles cholera.

*Escherichia coli* and other Enterobacteriaceae cause most nosocomial infections. Noninvasive, enterotoxin-producing *E. coli* infections may be a major cause of diarrheal illness in children in the United States.

The prognosis in mild to moderate infection is good. Severe infection requires immediate fluid and electrolyte replacement to avoid fatal dehydration, especially among children, in whom mortality may be quite high.

## Causes

Although some strains of *E. coli* exist as part of the normal GI flora, infection usually results from certain nonindigenous strains. For example:

• Noninvasive diarrhea results from two toxins produced by strains called enterotoxic or enteropathogenic *E. coli*. These toxins interact with intestinal juices and promote excessive loss of chloride and water.

• In the invasive form, *E. coli* directly invades the intestinal mucosa without producing enterotoxins, thereby causing local irritation, inflammation, and diarrhea. Normal strains can cause infection in immunocompromised patients.

Transmission can occur directly from an infected person or indirectly by ingestion of contaminated food or water or contact with contaminated utensils. Incubation takes 12 to 72 hours.

## Incidence

The incidence of *E. coli* infection is highest among travelers returning from other countries, particularly Mexico, Southeast Asia, and South America. *E. coli* infection also induces other diseases, especially in people whose resistance is low. Another strain, *E. coli 0157:H7,* has been reported. It's associated with undercooked hamburger.

## Signs and symptoms

Effects of noninvasive diarrhea depend on the causative toxin but may include the abrupt onset of watery diarrhea with cramping abdominal pain and, in severe illness, acidosis. Invasive infection produces chills, abdominal cramps, and diarrheal stools that contain blood and pus.

Infantile diarrhea from an *E. coli* infection is usually noninvasive; it begins with loose, watery stools that change from yellow to green and contain little mucus or blood. Vomiting, listlessness, irritability, and anorexia often precede diarrhea. This condition can progress to fever, severe dehydration, acidosis, and shock. Bloody diarrhea may occur from an *E. coli 0157:H7* infection.

## Diagnosis

Because certain strains of *E. coli* normally reside in the GI tract, culturing is of little value; a working diagnosis depends on clinical observation alone.

A firm diagnosis requires sophisticated identification procedures such as bioassays that are expensive, time-consuming and, consequently, not widely available. The diagnosis must rule out salmonellosis and shigellosis, other common infections that produce similar signs and symptoms.

## Treatment

Effective treatment consists of isolation, correction of fluid and electrolyte imbalance and, in an infant, I.V. antibiotics based on the organism's drug sensitivity. For cramping and diarrhea, bismuth subsalicylate may be given.

## Special considerations

• Keep accurate intake and output records. Measure stool volume and note the presence of blood and pus. Replace fluids and electrolytes as needed, monitoring for decreased serum sodium and chloride levels and signs of gram-negative shock. Watch for signs of dehydration, such as poor skin turgor and dry mouth.

• For infants, provide isolation, give nothing by mouth, administer antibiotics, and maintain body warmth.

To prevent the spread of this infection:

• Screen all hospital personnel and visitors for diarrhea, and prevent them from making direct patient contact during epidemics.

> ► CLINICAL TIP  Report cases to the local public health authorities.

• Use proper hand-washing technique. Teach personnel, patients, and their families to do the same.

• Use standard precautions: private room, gown and gloves while handling feces, and hand washing before entering and after leaving the patient's room.

• To prevent the accumulation of these water-loving organisms, discard suction bottles, irrigating fluid, and open bottles of saline solution every 24 hours. Be sure to change I.V. tubing according to facility policy and empty the ventilator water reservoirs before refilling them with sterile water. Remember to use suction catheters only once.

• Advise travelers to foreign countries to avoid unbottled water and uncooked vegetables.

# ESOPHAGEAL CANCER

Nearly always fatal, esophageal cancer usually develops in men over age 60. This disease occurs worldwide, but incidence varies geographically. It is most common in Japan, China, the Middle East, and parts of South Africa.

## Causes

The cause of esophageal cancer is unknown, but predisposing factors include chronic irritation caused by heavy smoking and excessive use of alcohol, stasis-induced inflammation, and nutritional deficiency. Esophageal tumors are usually fungating and infiltrating. Most arise in squamous cell epithelium; a few are adenocarcinomas; fewer still are melanomas and sarcomas.

Esophageal cancer has a 5-year survival rate below 10%, and regional metastasis occurs early by way of submucosal lymphatics. Metastasis produces such serious complications as tracheoesophageal fistulas, mediastinitis, and aortic perforation. Common sites of distant metastasis include the liver and lungs. (See *Staging esophageal cancer,* page 322.)

## Signs and symptoms

Dysphagia and weight loss are the most common presenting symptoms. Dysphagia is mild and intermittent at first, but it soon becomes constant. Pain, hoarseness, coughing, and esophageal obstruction follow. Cachexia usually develops.

## Diagnosis

X-rays of the esophagus, with barium swallow and motility studies, reveal structural and filling defects and reduced peristalsis. Endoscopic examination of

# STAGING ESOPHAGEAL CANCER

The TNM (tumor, node, metastasis) staging system accepted by the American Joint Committee on Cancer classifies esophageal cancer as follows.

## Primary tumor
*TX*—primary tumor can't be assessed
*T0*—no evidence of primary tumor
*Tis*—carcinoma in situ
*T1*—tumor invades lamina propria or submucosa
*T2*—tumor invades muscularis propria
*T3*—tumor invades adventitia
*T4*—tumor invades adjacent structures

## Regional lymph nodes
*NX*—regional lymph nodes can't be assessed
*N0*—no regional lymph node metastasis
*N1*—regional lymph node metastasis

## Distant metastasis
*MX*—distant metastasis can't be assessed
*M0*—no known distant metastasis
*M1*—distant metastasis

## Staging categories
Esophageal cancer progresses from mild to severe as follows:
*Stage 0*—Tis, N0, M0
*Stage I*—T1, N0, M0
*Stage IIA*—T2, N0, M0; T3, N0, M0
*Stage IIB*—T1, N1, M0; T2, N1, M0
*Stage III*—T3, N1, M0; T4, any N, M0
*Stage IV*—any T, any N, M1

## Treatment
Whenever possible, treatment includes resection to maintain a passageway for food. This may require such radical surgery as esophagogastrectomy with jejunal or colonic bypass grafts. Palliative surgery may include a feeding gastrostomy. Other therapies consist of radiation, chemotherapy with cisplatin, and the insertion of prosthetic tubes to bridge the tumor and alleviate dysphagia.

### Treatment complications
Complications of treatment may be severe. Surgery may precipitate an anastomotic leak, a fistula, pneumonia, and empyema. Rarely, radiation may cause esophageal perforation, pneumonitis and pulmonary fibrosis, or myelitis of the spinal cord. Prosthetic tubes may dislodge and perforate the mediastinum or erode the tumor.

## Special considerations
● Before surgery, answer the patient's questions and let him know what to expect after surgery, such as gastrostomy tubes, closed chest drainage, and nasogastric suctioning.
● After surgery, monitor vital signs and watch for unexpected changes. If surgery included an esophageal anastomosis, keep the patient flat on his back to avoid tension on the suture line.
● Promote adequate nutrition, and assess the patient's nutritional and hydration status to determine the need for supplementary parenteral feedings.
● Prevent aspiration of food by placing the patient in Fowler's position for meals and allowing plenty of time to eat. Provide high-calorie, high-protein, pureed food as needed.

> CLINICAL TIP Because the patient will probably regurgitate some food, clean his mouth carefully after each meal. Keep mouthwash handy.

the esophagus, punch and brush biopsies, and an exfoliative cytologic test confirm esophageal tumors.

• If the patient has a gastrostomy tube, give food slowly, using gravity to adjust the flow rate. The prescribed amount usually ranges from 200 to 500 ml. Offer him something to chew before each feeding to promote gastric secretions and a semblance of normal eating.

• Instruct the family in gastrostomy tube care (checking tube patency before each feeding, providing skin care around the tube, and keeping the patient upright during and after feedings).

• Provide emotional support for the patient and his family; refer them to appropriate organizations such as the American Cancer Society.

# ESOPHAGEAL DIVERTICULA

An esophageal diverticulum is an epithelial-lined mucosal pouch that protrudes from the esophageal lumen. Esophageal diverticula are classified according to their location: just above the upper esophageal sphincter (Zenker's, or pulsion, diverticulum the most common type), near the midpoint of the esophagus (traction diverticulum), and just above the lower esophageal sphincter (epiphrenic diverticulum).

Generally, esophageal diverticula occur later in life, although they can affect infants and children. They are three times more common in men than in women. Zenker's diverticula occur in patients ages 30 to 50.

## Causes
Esophageal diverticula are due either to primary muscle abnormalities that may be congenital or to inflammatory processes adjacent to the esophagus.

### Zenker's diverticulum
When the pouch results from increased intraesophageal pressure, Zenker's diverticulum occurs. It is caused by developmental muscle weakness of the posterior pharynx above the border of the cricopharyngeal muscle. The pressure of swallowing aggravates this weakness, as does contraction of the pharynx before relaxation of the sphincter.

### Traction diverticulum
When the pouch is pulled out by adjacent inflamed tissue or lymph nodes, a midesophageal (traction) diverticulum occurs. It's a response to scarring and pulling on esophageal walls by an external inflammatory process such as tuberculosis. It is diagnosed as an incidental finding on a barium esophagogram and is usually asymptomatic. No specific treatment is indicated.

### Epiphrenic diverticulum
This diverticulum occurs within the distal 10 cm of the esophagus. It is a pulsion diverticulum that is caused by abnormally elevated pressure within the lumen of the esophagus.

## Signs and symptoms
Traction and epiphrenic diverticula with an associated motor disturbance (achalasia or spasm) seldom produce symptoms but may cause dysphagia, heartburn, and regurgitation from associated esophageal conditions, such as hiatal hernia, diffuse esophageal spasm, achalasia, reflux esophagitis, and cancer. Zenker's diverticulum produces distinctly staged symptoms: initially, throat irritation and, later, dysphagia and near-complete obstruction.

In early stages, regurgitation occurs soon after eating; in later stages, regurgitation after eating is delayed and may even occur during sleep, leading to food aspiration and pulmonary infection. Other symptoms include noise when liquids are swallowed, chronic cough, hoarseness, a bad taste in the mouth, and halitosis.

### Diagnosis

A barium esophagogram usually confirms the diagnosis by showing characteristic outpouching. Esophagoscopy is not performed because the scope may be passed into the diverticulum and can cause a rupture.

### Treatment

Treatment depends on the type of diverticulum. For example:

• A small, asymptomatic Zenker's diverticulum may be observed. Treatment includes a bland diet, thorough chewing, and drinking water after eating to flush out the sac. Symptomatic patients may require surgery to remove the sac or facilitate drainage. An esophagomyotomy to prevent recurrence is required in most cases.

• A midesophageal (traction) diverticulum seldom requires therapy except when esophagitis aggravates the risk of rupture. Then, treatment includes antacids and an antireflux regimen: keeping the head elevated, maintaining an upright position for 2 hours after eating, eating small meals, controlling chronic coughing, and avoiding constrictive clothing.

• Epiphrenic diverticulum requires treatment of accompanying motor disorders such as achalasia by repeated dilatations of the esophagus, of acute spasm by anticholinergic administration and diverticulum excision, and of dysphagia or severe pain by surgical excision; if there is an associated hiatal hernia or incompetent lower esophageal sphincter, an antireflux operation is performed.

• Depending on the patient's nutritional status, treatment may also include insertion of a nasogastric tube (passed carefully to prevent perforation) and tube feedings to prepare for the stress of surgery.

### Special considerations

• Carefully observe and document symptoms.

• Assess nutritional status (weight, caloric intake, appearance).

• If the patient has dysphagia, record well-tolerated foods and what circumstances ease swallowing. Provide a pureed diet with vitamin or protein supplements, and encourage thorough chewing.

• If the patient regurgitates food and mucus, protect against aspiration by elevating the patient's head in high Fowler's position.

➤ CLINICAL TIP   To prevent aspiration, tell the patient to empty any visible outpouching in the neck by massage or postural drainage before retiring.

• Teach the patient about this disorder. Explain the proposed treatment and diagnostic procedures.

# ESOPHAGITIS, CORROSIVE (CAUSTIC)

Inflammation and damage to the esophagus after ingestion of a caustic chemical is called corrosive or caustic esophagitis. Similar to a burn, this injury may be temporary or lead to permanent stricture (narrowing or stenosis) of the esophagus that requires corrective surgery.

Severe injury can quickly lead to esophageal perforation, mediastinitis, and death from infection, shock, and massive hemorrhage (due to aortic perforation).

### Causes

The most common chemical injury to the esophagus follows the ingestion of lye or other strong alkalies; less often, injury follows the ingestion of strong acids. The type and amount of chemical ingested determine the severity and location of the damage.

In children, household chemical ingestion is accidental; in adults, it's usually a suicide attempt or gesture. (See *Advice for corrosive esophagitis.*) The chemical may damage only the mucosa or submucosa, or it may damage all layers of the esophagus.

Esophageal tissue damage occurs in three phases: in the acute phase, edema and inflammation; in the latent phase, ulceration, exudation, and tissue sloughing; and in the chronic phase, diffuse scarring.

### Signs and symptoms

Effects vary from none to intense pain in the mouth and anterior chest, marked salivation, inability to swallow, and tachypnea. Bloody vomitus that contains pieces of esophageal tissue signals severe damage. Signs of esophageal perforation and mediastinitis, especially crepitation, indicate destruction of the entire esophagus. Inability to speak suggests laryngeal damage.

The acute phase subsides in 3 to 4 days, enabling the patient to eat again. Fever suggests secondary infection. Symptoms of dysphagia return if stricture develops, usually within weeks.

### Diagnosis

A history of chemical ingestion and physical examination that reveals oropharyngeal burns (including white membranes and edema of the soft palate and uvula) usually confirm the diagnosis. The type and amount of the chemical ingested must be identified; sometimes this can be done by examining empty containers of the ingested material or by calling the poison control center.

> TEACHING CHECKLIST
> ## ✔ ADVICE FOR CORROSIVE ESOPHAGITIS
>
> • The adult who has ingested a corrosive agent has usually done so with suicidal intent. Encourage and assist the patient and his family to seek psychological counseling.
> • Provide emotional support for parents whose child has ingested a chemical. They'll be distraught and may feel guilty about the accident.
> • After the emergency and without emphasizing blame, teach appropriate preventive measures, such as locking accessible cabinets and keeping all corrosive agents out of a child's reach.

Endoscopy (in the first 24 hours after ingestion) delineates the extent and location of the esophageal injury and assesses the depth of the burn. This procedure may also be performed a week after ingestion to assess stricture development.

### Treatment

Conservative treatment may be effective, or the patient may require bougienage or surgery.

#### Conservative treatment

The usual treatment for corrosive esophagitis and stricture includes monitoring the patient's condition.

#### Bougienage

This procedure involves passing a slender, flexible, cylindrical instrument called a bougie into the esophagus to dilate it and minimize stricture.

> ❯ CLINICAL TIP  Some doctors begin bougienage immediately and continue it regularly to maintain a patent lumen and prevent stricture; others delay it for a week to avoid the risk of esophageal perforation.

### Surgery
Immediate surgery may be necessary for esophageal perforation; it may also be performed later to correct stricture that is not treatable with bougienage. Corrective surgery may involve transplanting a piece of the colon to the damaged esophagus. Even after surgery, stricture may recur at the site of the anastomosis.

### Supportive treatment
Other treatment includes I.V. therapy to replace fluids and total parenteral nutrition while the patient can't swallow, gradually progressing to clear liquids and a soft diet.

### Special considerations
If you're the first health care professional to see the person who has ingested a corrosive chemical, the quality of your emergency care is critical. Follow these important guidelines.
● *Don't induce vomiting or lavage* because this exposes the esophagus and oropharynx to injury a second time.
● *Don't perform gastric lavage* because the corrosive chemical may further damage the mucous membrane of the GI lining.
● Provide vigorous support of vital functions as needed, such as oxygen therapy, mechanical ventilation, I.V. fluids, and treatment for shock, depending on the severity of the injury.
● Carefully observe and record intake and output.
● Before X-rays and endoscopy, explain the procedure to the patient to lessen

anxiety during the tests and enhance his cooperation.
● Teach patients and families how to prevent future incidents of chemical ingestion.

# EXTRAOCULAR MOTOR NERVE PALSIES

Dysfunctions of the third, fourth, and sixth cranial nerves are called extraocular motor nerve palsies. Each of these nerves innervates specific muscles.
● The oculomotor (third cranial) nerve innervates the inferior, medial, and superior rectus muscles; the inferior oblique extraocular muscles; the pupilloconstrictor muscles; and the levator palpebrae muscles.
● The trochlear (fourth cranial) nerve innervates the superior oblique muscles.
● The abducens (sixth cranial) nerve innervates the lateral rectus muscles.

The superior oblique muscles control downward rotation, intorsion, and abduction of the eye. Complete dysfunction of the third cranial nerve is called total oculomotor ophthalmoplegia and may be associated with other central nervous system abnormalities.

## Causes
The most common causes of extraocular motor nerve palsies are diabetic neuropathy and pressure from an aneurysm or brain tumor. Other causes of these disorders vary, depending on the cranial nerve involved.
● *Third-nerve (oculomotor) palsy* (acute ophthalmoplegia) may be congenital or acquired and causes diplopia. It may result from an aneurysm (particularly in the posterior communicating artery); microvascular disease, such as diabetes or hypertension; tumor; or trauma. Rare

causes include uncal herniation, cavernous sinus mass lesion, orbital disease, herpes zoster, and leukemia. In children, a cause may be ophthalmic migraine.

• *Fourth-nerve (trochlear) palsy* also results from closed head trauma (blowout fracture) or sinus surgery.

• *Sixth-nerve (abducens) palsy* more commonly results from increased intracranial pressure; vasculopathic entities, such as diabetes, hypertension, and atherosclerosis; trauma; and idiopathic thyroid disease. Less common causes include giant cell arteritis, cavernous sinus mass (meningiomas, aneurysms, or metastasis), multiple sclerosis, and cerebrovascular accident.

### Signs and symptoms

The most characteristic clinical effect of extraocular motor nerve palsies is diplopia of recent onset, which varies in different visual fields, depending on the muscles affected.

• Typically, the patient with third-nerve palsy exhibits ptosis, exotropia (in which the eye looks outward), pupil dilation, and unresponsiveness to light; the eye is unable to move and cannot accommodate.

• The patient with fourth-nerve palsy displays diplopia and an inability to rotate the eye downward or upward. The patient develops a head tilt to compensate for vertical diplopia.

• Sixth-nerve palsy causes one eye to turn; the eye cannot abduct beyond the midline. To compensate for diplopia, the patient turns his head to the unaffected side.

### Diagnosis

A complete neuro-ophthalmologic examination and thorough patient history are needed to diagnose these palsies. Differential diagnosis of third-, fourth-, or sixth-nerve palsy depends on the specific motor deficit exhibited by the patient.

For all extraocular motor nerve palsies, magnetic resonance imaging and computed tomographic scans rule out tumors. The patient is also evaluated for diabetes, and an erythrocyte sedimentation rate may be obtained to rule out giant cell arteritis.

### Treatment

Identification of the underlying cause is essential because treatment of extraocular motor nerve palsies varies accordingly. Neurosurgery is necessary if the cause is an intracranial tumor or an aneurysm. For giant cell arteritis, high-dose corticosteroids are given I.V.; this is called pulse therapy.

### Special considerations

• After treatment of the primary condition, the patient may need surgery to realign the extraocular muscles.

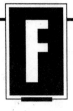

# FATTY LIVER

Steatosis, or fatty liver, is the accumulation of triglycerides and other fats in liver cells. In severe fatty liver, fat constitutes as much as 40% of the liver's weight (as opposed to 5% in a normal liver); the liver's weight may increase from 3.3 lb (1.5 kg) to as much as 11 lb (4.9 kg).

Minimal fatty changes are temporary and asymptomatic; severe or persistent changes may cause liver dysfunction. Fatty liver is usually reversible by simply eliminating the cause. (See *Reversing fatty liver.*) This disorder may result in recurrent infection or sudden death from fat emboli in the lungs.

## Causes

The most common cause of fatty liver in the United States and Europe is chronic alcoholism, with the severity of liver disease directly related to the amount of alcohol consumed. Other common, nonalcohol-related causes include acquired immunodeficiency syndrome, drug toxicity, and pregnancy.

Other causes include malnutrition (especially protein deficiency), obesity, diabetes mellitus, jejunoileal bypass surgery, Cushing's syndrome, Reye's syndrome, carbon tetrachloride intoxication, prolonged total parenteral nutrition (TPN), and DDT poisoning.

Whatever the cause, fatty infiltration of the liver probably results from mobilization of fatty acids from adipose tissues or from altered fat metabolism.

## Signs and symptoms

Clinical features of fatty liver vary with the degree of lipid infiltration, and many patients are asymptomatic. The most typical sign is a large, tender liver (hepatomegaly). Common symptoms include right upper quadrant pain (with massive or rapid infiltration), ascites, edema, jaundice, and fever (all with hepatic necrosis or biliary stasis).

Nausea, vomiting, and anorexia are less common. Splenomegaly usually accompanies cirrhosis. Rarer changes are spider angiomas, varices, transient gynecomastia, and menstrual disorders.

## Diagnosis

Typical clinical features — especially in patients with chronic alcoholism, malnutrition, poorly controlled diabetes mellitus, or obesity — suggest fatty liver. A *liver biopsy* confirms excessive fat in the liver. The following findings on liver function tests support this diagnosis:

- *albumin* — somewhat low
- *globulin* — usually elevated
- *cholesterol* — usually elevated
- *bilirubin* — elevated
- *alkaline phosphatase* — elevated

• *transaminase* — usually low (< 300 units)

• *prothrombin time* — possibly prolonged.

Other findings may include anemia, leukocytosis, albuminuria, hyperglycemia or hypoglycemia, and deficiencies of iron, folic acid, and vitamin $B_{12}$.

### Treatment

The treatment for fatty liver is essentially supportive and consists of correcting the underlying condition or eliminating its cause. Fatty liver that results from TPN may be ameliorated or prevented by giving choline.

In alcoholic fatty liver, abstinence from alcohol and a proper diet can begin to correct liver changes within 4 to 8 weeks. This requires comprehensive patient teaching.

Depending on the degree of severity, the patient may need to undergo liver transplantation.

### Special considerations

• Assess for malnutrition, especially protein deficiency, in those with chronic illness. Instruct the patient about what constitutes an adequate diet.

• Monitor an obese patient's progress in losing weight. Provide positive reinforcement for any weight loss.

• Perform comprehensive patient teaching, especially for obese, alcoholic, and diabetic patients.

---

TEACHING CHECKLIST

## REVERSING FATTY LIVER

• Suggest counseling for alcoholics, and provide emotional support for their families.

• Teach diabetic patients and their families about proper care, such as the purpose of insulin injections, diet, and exercise. Refer patients to diabetic classes to promote compliance with the treatment plan. Emphasize the need for long-term medical supervision, and urge diabetic patients to report changes in their health immediately.

• Instruct obese patients and their families about proper diet. Warn against fad diets because they may be nutritionally inadequate.

• Recommend medical supervision for patients who are more than 20% overweight.

• Encourage the patient to attend a group diet and exercise program, and if necessary, suggest a behavior modification program to correct eating habits.

• Advise patients who are receiving hepatotoxins and those who risk occupational exposure to DDT to watch for and immediately report signs of toxicity.

• Inform all patients that fatty liver is reversible *only* if they strictly follow the therapeutic program; otherwise, they risk permanent liver damage.

---

# FIBROMYALGIA SYNDROME

A diffuse pain syndrome, fibromyalgia syndrome (FMS, previously called "fibrositis") is one of the most common causes of chronic musculoskeletal pain; it's observed in up to 15% of patients seen in a general rheumatology practice and 5% of general medicine clinic patients. Symptoms of FMS include diffuse musculoskeletal pain, daily fatigue, and sleep disturbances. Multiple tender points in specific areas on examination is the characteristic feature. Women are affected much more often than men, and although FMS can affect all age-groups, its peak incidence is between ages 20 and 60. It may occur as a primary disorder or in association with an underlying disease such as systemic lupus erythematosus, rheumatoid arthritis, osteoarthritis, and sleep apnea syndromes.

FMS has also been reported in children, who tend to have more diffuse pain and sleep disturbances than adult patients. Children may have fewer tender points, and many improve over 2 to 3 years.

## Causes

The cause of FMS is unknown, but there are many theories regarding its pathophysiology. Although the pain is located primarily in muscle areas, no distinct abnormalities have been documented on microscopic evaluation of biopsies of tender points when compared with normal muscle. Other theories suggest decreased blood flow to muscle tissue (due to poor muscle aerobic conditioning versus other physiologic abnormalities); decreased blood flow in the thalamus and caudate nucleus, leading to a lowering of the pain threshold; endocrine dysfunction, such as abnormal pituitary-adrenal axis responses; and abnormal levels of the neurotransmitter serotonin in brain centers, which affect pain and sleep. Abnormal functioning of other pain-processing pathways may also be involved. Considerable overlap of symptoms with other pain syndromes, such as chronic fatigue syndrome, raises the question of an association with an infection, such as with parvovirus B19. Human immunodeficiency virus infection and Lyme disease have also been associated with FMS.

It's possible that the development of FMS is multifactorial and is influenced by stress (physical and mental), physical conditioning, and quality of sleep as well as by neuroendocrine, psychiatric and, possibly, hormonal factors (due to the female predominance).

## Signs and symptoms

The primary symptom of FMS is diffuse, dull, aching pain that is typically concentrated across the neck, shoulders, lower back, and proximal limbs. It can involve all four body quadrants — bilateral upper trunk and arms and bilateral lower trunk and legs. The pain is often worse in the morning and sometimes accompanied by stiffness. It can vary from day to day and be exacerbated by stress, lack of sleep, weather changes, and inactivity.

The sleep disturbance associated with FMS may be another factor in symptom development. Many patients with this syndrome describe a habit of being a light sleeper and experiencing frequent arousal and fragmented sleep (possibly secondary to pain in those patients who have underlying illnesses such as osteoarthritis and rheumatoid arthritis). Other patients may report feeling unrefreshed after a night's sleep. Because of this nonrestorative sleep pattern, the patient can feel fatigued a half hour to several hours after awakening and remain so for the remainder of the day.

Other clinical features associated with FMS include irritable bowel syndrome, tension headaches, "puffy hands" (sensation of hand swelling, especially in the morning), and paresthesias.

## Diagnosis

Diagnostic testing for FMS (not associated with an underlying disease) does not usually reveal significant abnormalities. For example, an examination of joints does not reveal synovitis or significant swelling; a neurologic examination is normal; and no laboratory or radiologic abnormalities are common to FMS patients. Tenderness can be elicited by applying a moderate amount of pressure to specific locations. (See *Tender points of fibromyalgia,* pages 332 and 333.) Although this examination can be fairly subjective, many FMS patients with true tender points wince or withdraw when pressure is applied to a tender point. Pressure can also be applied to nontender control points, such as the midforehead, distal forearm, and midanterior thigh, to assess for conversion reactions (psychogenic rheumatism), in which patients hurt everywhere, or for other psychosomatic illnesses.

Overall, the diagnosis of FMS is made clinically in a patient with characteristic symptoms, multiple tender points on examination, and after ruling out other illnesses that can cause similar features. A workup for arthritis, primary sleep disorders, endocrinopathies (such as hypothyroidism), infections (such as Lyme disease and human immunodeficiency virus infection), and psychiatric illness (such as major depression) should be considered in the appropriate setting.

> CLINICAL TIP FMS should not be confused with chronic myofascial pain, which is characterized by unilateral and often focal or regional pain (as opposed to FMS, in which the pain is bilateral and diffuse), minimal fatigue or stiffness, and few focal tender points (often distinguished as trigger points) that may produce a radiating pain along a muscle group or tendon (unlike in FMS, where tender points are not usually associated with radiating pain). Myofascial pain is treated with local measures, such as stretching, physical therapy, heat, and trigger point injections; the symptoms are usually temporary but may recur.

## Treatment
The most important aspect in FMS management is patient education. Patients must understand that although FMS pain can be severe and is often chronic, this syndrome is common and does not lead to deforming or life-threatening complications.

A regular, low-impact aerobic exercise program can be effective in improving muscle conditioning, energy levels, and an overall sense of well-being. The FMS patient should stretch before and after exercising to minimize injury. Any exercise program, such as walking, bicycling, and swimming, should be started at a low intensity with a slow, gradual increase as tolerated. The patient may also benefit from physical therapy, the injection of tender points with steroids or lidocaine, massage therapy, and ultrasound treatments for particularly problematic areas. A few studies have shown that acupuncture and phototherapy are also beneficial.

Drug therapy is typically used to improve the patient's quality of sleep and for pain control. A bedtime dose of a tricyclic antidepressant, such as amitriptyline, nortriptyline, or cyclobenzaprine, may improve sleep but produce anticholinergic adverse effects and daytime drowsiness. Hypnotic agents, such as many benzodiazepines, are less useful overall because they generally do not prevent the frequent awakenings through the night in these patients. The combination of a tricyclic antidepressant at bedtime with a serotonin uptake inhibitor, such as fluoxetine, during the day may also be useful.

Nonsteroidal anti-inflammatory drugs (NSAIDs) and corticosteroids are typically not effective against FMS pain, although NSAIDs may be used if tendinitis or arthritis coexists with this disorder. Narcotics should be used only with extreme caution to control pain, preferably under the guidance of a pain clinic.

## TENDER POINTS OF FIBROMYALGIA

The patient with fibromyalgia syndrome may complain of specific areas of tenderness, which are indicated in the illustrations below.

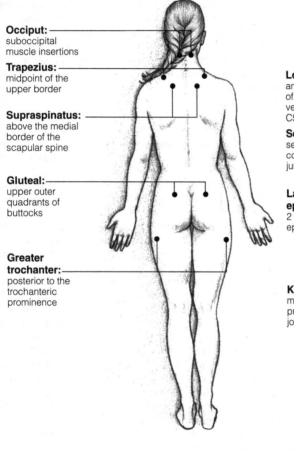

**Occiput:**
suboccipital
muscle insertions

**Trapezius:**
midpoint of the
upper border

**Supraspinatus:**
above the medial
border of the
scapular spine

**Gluteal:**
upper outer
quadrants of
buttocks

**Greater
trochanter:**
posterior to the
trochanteric
prominence

**Low cervical:**
anterior aspects
of the intertrans-
verse spaces at
C5 to C7

**Second rib:**
second
costochondral
junctions

**Lateral
epicondyle:**
2 cm distal to the
epicondyles

**Knee:**
medial fat pad
proximal to the
joint line

**Special considerations**
● Reassure the patient that FMS is common and, although chronic, can be treated.
● Explain to the patient that she may experience increased muscle pain when starting a new exercise program. If this occurs, suggest that she decrease the duration or intensity of the exercise. Encourage the patient not to stop exercising altogether, unless otherwise indicated, because even a limited amount of exercise each day may be beneficial.

# FOLIC ACID DEFICIENCY ANEMIA

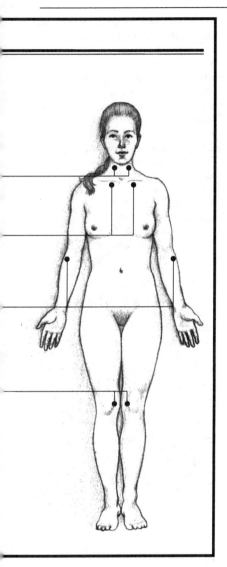

A common, slowly progressive megaloblastic anemia, folic acid deficiency anemia is most prevalent in infants, adolescents, pregnant and lactating females, alcoholics, elderly people, and people with malignant or intestinal diseases.

## Causes

Folic acid deficiency anemia results from a decreased level or lack of folate, a vitamin that is essential for red blood cell production and maturation. Causes include:

- *alcohol abuse* (may suppress metabolic effects of folate)
- *poor diet* (common in alcoholics, elderly people who live alone, and infants, especially those with infections or diarrhea)
- *impaired absorption* (due to intestinal dysfunction from such disorders as celiac disease, tropical sprue, and regional jejunitis and from bowel resection)
- *bacteria* competing for available folic acid
- *excessive cooking,* which can destroy a high percentage of folic acids in foods
- *limited storage capacity* in infants
- *prolonged drug therapy* (with anticonvulsants and estrogens)
- *increased folic acid requirement* during pregnancy, during rapid growth in infancy (common because of increased survival rate of preterm infants), during childhood and adolescence (because of general use of folate-poor cow's milk), and in patients with neoplastic diseases and some skin diseases (chronic exfoliative dermatitis).

- Advise the patient whose drug regimen includes a tricyclic antidepressant to take the dose 1 to 2 hours before bedtime, which may improve its benefits for sleep and reduce morning drowsiness.

## Signs and symptoms

Folic acid deficiency anemia gradually produces clinical features that are characteristic of other megaloblastic anemias without the neurologic manifestations. They include progressive fatigue, dyspnea, palpitations, weakness, glossitis, nausea, anorexia, headache, fainting, irritability, forgetfulness, pallor, and slight jaundice.

Folic acid deficiency anemia does not cause neurologic impairment unless it's associated with vitamin $B_{12}$ deficiency, as in pernicious anemia.

## Diagnosis

The Schilling test and a therapeutic trial of vitamin $B_{12}$ injections distinguish between folic acid deficiency anemia and pernicious anemia. Significant findings include macrocytosis, a decreased reticulocyte count, low platelet count, and a serum folate level less than 4 mg/ml.

## Treatment

Folic acid supplements and the elimination of contributing causes are the primary treatments. Supplements may be given orally (usually 1 to 5 mg/day) or parenterally (to patients who are severely ill, have malabsorption, or are unable to take oral medication).

➤ CLINICAL TIP The clinical features of anemia usually disappear within 1 to 2 weeks after administration of folate.

Many patients also respond favorably to a well-balanced diet.

If the patient has combined vitamin $B_{12}$ and folate deficiencies, folic acid replenishment alone may aggravate neurologic dysfunction.

## Special considerations

• Teach the patient to meet daily folic acid requirements by including a food from each food group in every meal.

• If the patient has a severe deficiency, explain that diet only reinforces folic acid supplementation and isn't therapeutic by itself.

• Urge compliance with the prescribed course of therapy. Advise the patient not to stop taking the supplements when he begins to feel better.

• If the patient has glossitis, emphasize the importance of good oral hygiene. Suggest regular use of mild or diluted mouthwash and a soft toothbrush.

• Monitor fluid and electrolyte balance, particularly in the patient who has severe diarrhea and is receiving parenteral fluid replacement therapy.

• Because anemia causes severe fatigue, schedule regular rest periods until the patient is able to resume normal activity.

• To prevent folic acid deficiency anemia, emphasize the importance of a well-balanced diet high in folic acid. Identify alcoholics with poor dietary habits, and try to arrange for appropriate counseling.

• Tell mothers who aren't breast-feeding to use commercially prepared formulas.

# FOLLICULITIS, FURUNCLES, AND CARBUNCLES

A bacterial infection of the hair follicle, folliculitis causes the formation of a pustule. The infection can be superficial (follicular impetigo or Bockhart's impetigo) or deep (sycosis barbae).

Furuncles, commonly known as boils, are another form of deep folliculitis. Carbuncles are a group of interconnected furuncles. The prognosis depends on the severity of the infection and the patient's physical condition and ability to resist infection.

## Causes

The most common cause of folliculitis, furuncles, or carbuncles is coagulase-positive *Staphylococcus aureus*. Predisposing factors include an infected wound, poor hygiene, debilitation, tight clothes, friction, and immunosuppressive therapy.

## Signs and symptoms

Folliculitis, furuncles, and carbuncles have different signs and symptoms.

● Folliculitis pustules usually appear on the scalp, arms, and legs in children and on the trunk, buttocks, and legs in adults.

● Furuncles are hard, painful nodules that commonly develop on the neck, face, axillae, and buttocks. For several days, these nodules enlarge and then rupture, discharging pus and necrotic material. After the nodules rupture, pain subsides, but erythema and edema may persist for days or weeks.

● Carbuncles are extremely painful, deep abscesses that drain through multiple openings onto the skin surface, usually around several hair follicles. Fever and malaise may accompany these lesions, which are now rather rare.

## Diagnosis

The obvious skin lesion confirms folliculitis, furuncles, or carbuncles. Wound culture usually shows *S. aureus*. In carbuncles, patient history reveals preexistent furuncles. A complete blood count may show an elevated white blood cell count (leukocytosis).

## Treatment

Appropriate treatment includes the following:

● Folliculitis is treated by cleaning the infected area thoroughly with antibacterial soap and water; applying warm, wet compresses to promote vasodilation and drainage from the lesions; applying topical antibiotics, such as mupirocin ointment or clindamycin or erythromycin solution; and, in extensive infection, administering systemic antibiotics (a cephalosporin or dicloxacillin).

● Furuncles may require incision and drainage of ripe lesions after application of warm, wet compresses and systemic antibiotics after drainage.

● Carbuncles require systemic antibiotic therapy as well as incision and drainage.

## Special considerations

● Care for folliculitis, furuncles, and carbuncles is basically supportive and emphasizes teaching the patient scrupulous personal and family hygiene measures. Taking the necessary precautions to prevent spreading infection is also an important part of care.

● Caution the patient never to squeeze a boil because this may cause it to rupture into the surrounding area.

● To avoid spreading bacteria to family members, urge the patient not to share towels and washcloths. Tell him that these items should be washed in hot water before being reused. The patient should change clothes and bedsheets daily, and they also should be washed in hot water. Encourage the patient to change dressings frequently and to discard them promptly in paper bags.

● Advise the patient with recurrent furuncles to have a physical examination because an underlying disease, such as diabetes, may be present.

❯ CLINICAL TIP Instruct men to use disposable razors to help decrease the spread of infection.

# FRAGILE X SYNDROME

Fragile X syndrome, characterized by learning disabilities and developmental delay, is believed to be the most prevalent inherited form of mental retardation. The fragile X gene is located on the X chromosome. Children and adults with unexplained mental retardation should be considered for fragile X testing. Affected individuals may also exhibit autistic-like behaviors, such as poor eye contact, speech abnormalities, and difficulty adapting to change. They may also be hyperactive.

➤ CLINICAL TIP Individuals with symptoms of autism should be considered for fragile X testing because 7% or more of these individuals test positive for this disorder.

## Causes

Fragile X syndrome is transmitted through X-linked dominant (or semi-dominant) inheritance; that is, the abnormal gene is located on the X (sex) chromosome. Females have two X chromosomes, whereas males have one X chromosome and one Y chromosome. A female carrier of fragile X has the gene on one of her X chromosomes; the other X chromosome is normal. There is a 50% chance of a carrier passing the abnormal gene to each offspring. Some carriers exhibit no signs of the disorder because of the protective effects of the normal X chromosome; others may be mentally retarded or have learning disabilities and show other signs of fragile X syndrome.

Most male offspring who inherit the abnormal gene on their single X chromosome from their mothers show characteristics of fragile X syndrome; a few males who inherit the gene exhibit no signs of the syndrome and are known as "nonpenetrant, normal transmitting males." These males will pass the abnormal gene to all their daughters but to none of their sons because the disorder can't be transmitted from male to male.

Fragile X syndrome occurs in about 1 in 1,500 males and 1 in 2,500 females. It has been reported in almost all races and ethnic populations.

## Signs and symptoms

Young children may have relatively few identifiable physical characteristics; behavioral or learning difficulties may be the initial presenting features.

Many adult patients display a prominent jaw and forehead and a head circumference that exceeds the 90th percentile. A long, narrow face with long or large ears that may be posteriorly rotated can be a helpful finding at all ages. Connective tissue abnormalities, including hyperextension of the fingers, a floppy mitral valve (in 80% of adults), and mild to severe pectus excavatum (funnel chest), have also been reported. Unusually large testes, found in most affected males after puberty, are an important identifying factor of the disorder.

The average IQ of a person with fragile X syndrome is comparable to that of a person with Down syndrome, but the behavioral characteristics are quite different. Hyperactivity, speech difficulties, language delay, and autistic-like behaviors may be attributed to other disorders, such as attention deficit hyperactivity disorder, and thus delay the diagnosis.

In carrier females, clinical signs may be milder and occur less frequently. The connective tissue manifestations may be as significant as in males. Many older female carriers exhibit the long face described for affected males.

## Diagnosis

Individuals with clinical signs of fragile X syndrome or relatives of an affected individual should undergo chromosomal analysis as well as deoxyribonucleic acid (DNA) analysis to determine whether they carry the fragile X gene. DNA analysis can differentiate affected males and nonpenetrant, normal transmitting males from normal males. It can also differentiate carrier females from noncarrier females. Prenatal diagnosis may also be available for most families.

Once a carrier has been identified in a family, other family members should be notified because they may also be carriers with an increased risk of having children with this disorder.

## Treatment

There is no cure for fragile X syndrome. Treatment is aimed at controlling individual symptoms. Surgery may be needed to repair a defective mitral valve.

## Special considerations

• Individuals who have been identified as carriers may experience guilt and grief; provide support to help the carrier and family members accept the diagnosis. (See *Educational needs in fragile X syndrome.*)

• Parents of an affected child may need help dealing with their grief over unmet expectations for the child; refer them for appropriate counseling if necessary.

• Refer the family (and possibly the extended family) to a genetic counselor to discuss the diagnosis, testing, and risk of recurrence in future offspring.

• Referral to a fragile X support group may be helpful.

---

✔ TEACHING CHECKLIST

## EDUCATIONAL NEEDS IN FRAGILE X SYNDROME

• Speech and language therapy
• Tightly structured classroom
• Visual clues to supplement verbal instructions
• Positive reinforcement of good behaviors
• Occupational, prevocational, or vocational training
• Physical therapy to assist with fine and gross motor delays
• Alternative teaching styles that decrease the child's anxiety and stimulate long-term memory, such as inclusion and indirect teaching

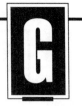

# GALLBLADDER AND BILE DUCT CANCERS

Cancer of the gallbladder is rare, constituting fewer than 1% of all cancer cases. It's usually found coincidentally in patients with cholecystitis; 1 in 400 cholecystectomies reveals cancer.

This disease is most prevalent in women over age 60. It's rapidly progressive and usually fatal; patients seldom live 1 year after diagnosis. The poor prognosis is due to late diagnosis; gallbladder cancer usually isn't diagnosed until after cholecystectomy, when it's typically in an advanced, metastatic stage.

Extrahepatic bile duct cancer is the cause of about 3% of all cancer deaths in the United States. It occurs in both men and women between ages 60 and 70 (incidence is slightly higher in men). The usual site is at the bifurcation in the common duct.

Cancer at the distal end of the common duct is often confused with pancreatic cancer. Characteristically, metastasis occurs in local lymph nodes and in the liver, lungs, and peritoneum.

## Causes

Many consider gallbladder cancer a complication of gallstones. This inference rests on circumstantial evidence from postmortem examinations: 60% to 90% of all gallbladder cancer patients also have gallstones. Postmortem data from patients with gallstones show gallbladder cancer in only 0.5%.

Adenocarcinoma accounts for 85% to 95% of all cases of gallbladder cancer; squamous cell carcinoma accounts for 5% to 15%. Mixed-tissue types are rare.

Lymph node metastasis is present in 25% to 70% of patients at diagnosis. Direct extension to the liver is common (46% to 89% of patients); direct extension to both the cystic and the common bile ducts as well as the stomach, colon, duodenum, and jejunum produces obstructions. Metastasis also occurs through the portal or hepatic veins to the peritoneum, ovaries, and lower lung lobes.

The cause of extrahepatic bile duct cancer isn't known, but statistics reveal an unexplained increased incidence of this cancer in patients with ulcerative colitis. This association may be due to a common cause — perhaps an immune mechanism or chronic use of certain drugs by the colitis patient.

## Signs and symptoms

Clinically, gallbladder cancer is almost indistinguishable from cholecystitis. The signs and symptoms of both disorders include pain in the epigastrium or right upper quadrant, weight loss, anorexia, nausea, vomiting, and jaundice. Chronic, progressively severe pain in an afebrile patient suggests cancer. With simple gallstones, the pain is sporadic.

Another telling clue to cancer is a palpable gallbladder (in the right upper quadrant) with obstructive jaundice. Some patients may also have hepatosplenomegaly.

### Signs of bile duct cancer

Progressive, profound jaundice is commonly the first sign of obstruction due to extrahepatic bile duct cancer. The jaundice is usually accompanied by chronic pain in the epigastrium or right upper quadrant, radiating to the back. Other common symptoms, if associated with active cholecystitis, include pruritus, skin excoriations, anorexia, weight loss, chills, and fever.

### Diagnosis

No test or procedure is in itself diagnostic of gallbladder cancer. However, the following laboratory tests support this diagnosis when they suggest hepatic dysfunction and extrahepatic biliary obstruction:

● *baseline studies* (complete blood count, routine urinalysis, electrolyte studies, enzymes)

● *liver function tests* (typically reveal elevated serum bilirubin, urine bile and bilirubin, and urobilinogen levels in more than 50% of patients as well as consistently elevated serum alkaline phosphatase levels)

● *occult blood in stools* (linked to the associated anemia)

● *cholecystography* (may show stones or calcification)

● *cholangiography* (may locate the site of common duct obstruction)

● *magnetic resonance imaging* (detects tumors).

The following tests help compile data that confirm extrahepatic bile duct cancer:

● *liver function tests* (indicate biliary obstruction: elevated levels of bilirubin [5 to 30 mg/dl], alkaline phosphatase, and blood cholesterol as well as prolonged prothrombin time)

● *endoscopic retrograde pancreatography* (identifies the tumor site and allows access for obtaining a biopsy specimen).

### Treatment

Surgical treatment of gallbladder cancer is essentially palliative and includes various procedures, such as cholecystectomy, common bile duct exploration, T-tube drainage, and wedge excision of hepatic tissue.

If the cancer invades gallbladder musculature, the survival rate is less than 5%, even with massive resection. Although some cases of long-term survival (4 to 5 years) have been reported, few patients survive longer than 6 months after surgery for gallbladder cancer.

Surgery is normally indicated to relieve the obstruction and jaundice that result from extrahepatic bile duct cancer. The type of procedure used to relieve obstruction depends on the site of the cancer. Such procedures may include cholecystoduodenostomy and T-tube drainage of the common duct.

➤ CLINICAL TIP   Other palliative measures for both kinds of cancer include radiation therapy, radiation implants (mostly used for local and incisional recurrences), and chemotherapy (with combinations of fluorouracil, doxorubicin, and lomustine). All these treatment measures have limited effects.

### Special considerations

After biliary resection:

● Monitor vital signs.

● Use strict aseptic technique when caring for the incision and the surrounding area.

● Place the patient in low Fowler's position.

● Prevent respiratory problems by encouraging deep breathing and coughing. The high incision makes the patient want to take shallow breaths; taking analgesics and splinting his abdomen with a pillow or an abdominal binder may make breathing easier.

• Monitor bowel sounds and bowel movements. Observe the patient's tolerance of his diet.

• Provide pain-control measures.

• Check intake and output carefully. Watch for electrolyte imbalance; monitor I.V. solutions to avoid overloading the cardiovascular system.

• Monitor the nasogastric tube, which will be in place for 24 to 72 hours postoperatively to relieve distention, and the T tube. Record the amount and color of drainage each shift. Secure the T tube to minimize tension on it and prevent its being pulled out.

• Help the patient and his family cope with their initial fears and reactions to the diagnosis by offering information and support.

• Before discharge, teach the patient how to manage the biliary catheter.

• Advise the patient of the adverse effects of both chemotherapy and radiation therapy, and monitor him for these effects.

# GASTRIC CANCER

Common throughout the world, gastric cancer affects all races. However, unexplained geographic and cultural differences in incidence occur; for example, mortality is high in Japan, Iceland, Chile, and Austria. In the United States, incidence has decreased 50% during the past 25 years, and the death rate from gastric cancer is one-third that of 30 years ago.

The decrease in gastric cancer incidence in the United States has been attributed, without proof, to the balanced American diet and to refrigeration, which reduces the number of nitrate-producing bacteria in food.

Incidence is highest in men over age 40. The prognosis depends on the stage of the disease at the time of diagnosis; overall, the 5-year survival rate is about 15%.

## Causes

The cause of gastric cancer is unknown. This cancer is often associated with gastritis with gastric atrophy, which is now thought to be a result of gastric cancer rather than a precursor state. Predisposing factors include environmental influences, such as smoking and high alcohol intake.

Genetic factors have also been implicated because this disease occurs more frequently among people with type A blood than among those with type O; similarly, it is more common in people with a family history of such cancer.

Dietary factors also seem related, including types of food preparation, physical properties of some foods, and certain methods of food preservation (especially smoking, pickling, and salting).

### Classification

According to gross appearance, gastric cancer can be classified as polypoid, ulcerating, ulcerating and infiltrating, or diffuse. The parts of the stomach affected by gastric cancer, listed in order of decreasing frequency, are the pylorus and antrum (50%), the lesser curvature (25%), the cardia (10%), the body of the stomach (10%), and the greater curvature (2% to 3%).

### Metastasis

Gastric cancer metastasizes rapidly to the regional lymph nodes, omentum, liver, and lungs by the following routes: walls of the stomach, duodenum, and esophagus; lymphatic system; adjacent organs; bloodstream; and peritoneal cavity.

## Signs and symptoms

Early clues to gastric cancer are chronic dyspepsia and epigastric discomfort, followed in later stages by weight loss, anorexia, a feeling of fullness after eating, anemia, and fatigue. If the cancer is in the cardia, the first symptom may be dysphagia and, later, vomiting (typically coffee-ground vomitus). Affected patients may also have blood in their stools.

The course of gastric cancer may be insidious or fulminating. The patient typically treats himself with antacids until the symptoms of advanced stages appear.

## Diagnosis

Diagnosis depends primarily on reinvestigations of persistent or recurring GI changes and complaints. To rule out other conditions that produce similar symptoms, a diagnostic evaluation must include the testing of blood, stools, and stomach fluid specimens.

Gastric cancer often requires the following studies for diagnosis:

• *Barium X-rays of the GI tract, with fluoroscopy* show changes (a tumor or filling defect in the outline of the stomach, loss of flexibility and distensibility, and abnormal gastric mucosa with or without ulceration).

• *Gastroscopy with fiber-optic endoscopy* helps rule out other diffuse gastric mucosal abnormalities by allowing direct visualization and gastroscopic biopsy to evaluate gastric mucosal lesions.

• *Photography with fiber-optic endoscopy* provides a permanent record of gastric lesions that can later be used to determine the progress of the disease and the effect of treatment.

The following studies may rule out metastasis to specific organs: computed tomographic scans, chest X-rays, liver and bone scans, and a liver biopsy. (See *Staging gastric cancer,* page 342.)

## Treatment

Surgery is often the treatment of choice. Excision of the lesion with appropriate margins is possible in more than one-third of patients. Even in patients whose disease isn't considered surgically curable, resection offers palliation and improves potential benefits from chemotherapy and radiation therapy.

### Types of surgery

The nature and extent of the lesion determine what kind of surgery is most appropriate. Common surgical procedures include subtotal gastrectomy and total gastrectomy.

When cancer involves the pylorus and antrum, gastrectomy removes the lower stomach and duodenum (gastrojejunostomy or Billroth II). If metastasis has occurred, the omentum and spleen may also have to be removed.

If gastric cancer has spread to the liver, peritoneum, or lymph glands, palliative surgery may include gastrostomy, jejunostomy, or a total or subtotal gastrectomy. Such surgery may temporarily relieve vomiting, nausea, pain, and dysphagia while allowing enteral nutrition to continue.

### Other treatments

Chemotherapy for GI cancers may help to control symptoms and prolong survival. Adenocarcinoma of the stomach has responded to several agents, including fluorouracil, carmustine, doxorubicin, cisplatin, methotrexate, and mitomycin.

Antiemetics can control nausea, which increases as the cancer advances. In the more advanced stages, sedatives and tranquilizers may be necessary to control overwhelming anxiety. Narcotics are often necessary to relieve severe and unremitting pain.

# STAGING GASTRIC CANCER

Both the prognosis and the treatment of gastric cancer depend on its type and stage. Using the TNM (tumor, node, metastasis) system, the American Joint Committee on Cancer describes the following stages of gastric cancer.

### Primary tumor

**TX** — primary tumor can't be assessed

**T0** — no evidence of primary tumor

**Tis** — carcinoma in situ: intraepithelial tumor doesn't penetrate the lamina propria

**T1** — tumor penetrates the lamina propria or submucosa

**T2** — tumor penetrates the muscularis propria or subserosa

**T3** — tumor penetrates the serosa (visceral peritoneum) without invading adjacent structures

**T4** — tumor invades adjacent structures

### Regional lymph nodes

**NX** — regional lymph nodes can't be assessed

**N0** — no evidence of regional lymph node metastasis

**N1** — involvement of perigastric lymph nodes within 3 cm of the edge of the primary tumor

**N2** — involvement of the perigastric lymph nodes more than 3 cm from the edge of the primary tumor or in lymph nodes along the left gastric, common hepatic splenic, or celiac arteries

### Distant metastasis

**MX** — distant metastasis can't be assessed

**M0** — no evidence of distant metastasis

**M1** — distant metastasis

### Staging categories

Gastric cancer stages progress from mild to severe as follows:

**Stage 0** — Tis, N0, M0

**Stage 1A** — T1, N0, M0

**Stage 1B** — T1, N1, M0; T2, N0, M0

**Stage II** — T1, N2, M0; T3, N0, M0

**Stage IIIA** — T2, N2, M0; T3, N1, M0; T4, N0, M0

**Stage IIIB** — T3, N2, M0; T4, N1, M0

**Stage IV** — T4, N2, M0; any T, any N, M1

---

Radiation therapy has been particularly useful when combined with chemotherapy in patients who have unresectable or partially resectable disease. It should be given on an empty stomach and shouldn't be used preoperatively because it may damage viscera and impede healing.

Treatment with antispasmodics and antacids may help relieve GI distress.

### Special considerations

• Before surgery, prepare the patient for its effects and for postsurgical procedures, such as insertion of a nasogastric (NG) tube for drainage and I.V. lines.

• Reassure the patient who is having a subtotal gastrectomy that he may eventually be able to eat normally.

• Prepare the patient who is having a total gastrectomy for slow recovery and only partial return to a normal diet.

• Emphasize the importance of changing position every 2 hours and of deep breathing.

• After any type of gastrectomy, pulmonary complications may result and oxygen may be needed. Regularly assist the patient with turning, coughing, and deep breathing. Turning the patient hourly and administering narcotic analgesics may prevent pulmonary problems. Incentive spirometry may also be needed for complete lung expansion. Proper positioning is important as well: semi-Fowler's position facilitates breathing and drainage.

● After gastrectomy, little (if any) drainage comes from the NG tube because no secretions form after stomach removal. Without a stomach for storage, many patients experience dumping syndrome. Intrinsic factor is absent from gastric secretions, leading to malabsorption of vitamin $B_{12}$.

● To prevent vitamin $B_{12}$ deficiency, the patient must take a replacement vitamin for the rest of his life as well as an iron supplement.

● During radiation therapy, encourage the patient to eat high-calorie, well-balanced meals. Offer fluids such as ginger ale to minimize such adverse effects as nausea and vomiting.

● Patients who experience poor digestion and absorption after gastrectomy need a special diet: frequent feedings of small amounts of clear liquids, increasing to small, frequent feedings of bland food.

● After total gastrectomy, patients must eat small meals for the rest of their lives.

➤ CLINICAL TIP Some patients need pancreatin and sodium bicarbonate after meals to prevent or control steatorrhea and dyspepsia.

● Wound dehiscence and delayed healing, stemming from decreased protein, anemia, and avitaminosis, may occur. Preoperative vitamin and protein replacement can prevent such complications.

● Observe the wound regularly for redness, swelling, failure to heal, and warmth. Parenteral administration of vitamin C may improve wound healing.

● Vitamin deficiency may result from obstruction, diarrhea, or an inadequate diet. Ascorbic acid, thiamine, riboflavin, nicotinic acid, and vitamin K supplements may be beneficial.

● Aside from meeting caloric needs, nutrition must provide adequate protein, fluid, and potassium intake to facilitate glycogen and protein synthesis.

● Anabolic agents may induce nitrogen retention. Steroids, antidepressants, wine, and brandy may boost the appetite.

When all treatments have failed:

● Concentrate on keeping the patient comfortable and free of pain, and provide as much psychological support as possible.

● If the patient is going home, discuss continuing care needs with the caregiver or refer the patient to an appropriate home health care agency.

# GASTRITIS

An inflammation of the gastric mucosa, gastritis may be acute or chronic. *Acute gastritis* produces mucosal reddening, edema, hemorrhage, and erosion. *Chronic gastritis* is common among elderly people and those with pernicious anemia. It's often present as chronic atrophic gastritis, in which all stomach mucosal layers are inflamed, with reduced numbers of chief and parietal cells.

## Causes

Acute and chronic gastritis vary in causative factors.

### Acute gastritis

Acute gastritis has a number of causes, including:

● chronic ingestion of irritating foods, spicy foods, or alcohol

● drugs, such as aspirin and other non-steroidal anti-inflammatory agents (in large doses), cytotoxic agents, caffeine, corticosteroids, antimetabolites, phenylbutazone, and indomethacin

• ingestion of poisons, especially DDT, ammonia, mercury, carbon tetrachloride, and corrosive substances
• endotoxins released from infecting bacteria, such as staphylococci, *Escherichia coli,* and salmonella.

Acute gastritis also may develop as a complication in acute illnesses, particularly major traumatic injuries, burns, infectious processes, major surgical procedures, and hepatic, renal, or respiratory failure.

### Chronic gastritis

Chronic gastritis may be associated with peptic ulcer disease, which causes chronic reflux of pancreatic secretions, bile, and bile acids from the duodenum into the stomach.

Recurring exposure to irritating substances, such as drugs, alcohol, cigarette smoke, and environmental agents, also may lead to chronic gastritis. Chronic gastritis may occur in patients with a history of pernicious anemia, underlying kidney disease, or diabetes mellitus.

Bacterial infection with *Helicobacter pylori* is a common cause of nonerosive chronic gastritis.

### Signs and symptoms

After exposure to the offending substance, the patient with acute gastritis typically reports a rapid onset of symptoms, such as epigastric discomfort, indigestion, cramping, anorexia, nausea, vomiting, and hematemesis. The symptoms last from a few hours to a few days. A patient with chronic gastritis may complain of similar symptoms or mild epigastric pain.

Erosive gastritis is usually asymptomatic. If symptoms are present, they include nausea, vomiting, anorexia, and epigastric pain. The patient with erosive gastritis probably will develop upper GI bleeding with coffee-ground emesis or melena.

### Diagnosis

The following tests are usually included to diagnose gastritis:
• *Fecal occult blood test* can detect occult blood in vomitus and stools if the patient has gastric bleeding.
• *Hemoglobin level and hematocrit* are low if significant bleeding has occurred.
• *Upper GI endoscopy* with biopsy confirms the diagnosis when performed within 24 hours of bleeding. An upper GI series may also be performed to exclude serious lesions.

➤ CLINICAL TIP  Upper endoscopy is contraindicated after ingestion of a corrosive agent.

### Treatment

*H. pylori* infection with gastritis may be eradicated with a number of triple-drug regimens. Eliminating the cause of gastritis is the first step to treating it.

Histamine$_2$-receptor antagonists, such as cimetidine and ranitidine, may block gastric secretions. Antacids may also be used as buffers.

For critically ill patients, antacids administered every 4 hours when the pH of the stomach is less than 4.0, with or without histamine-receptor antagonists, may reduce the frequency of gastritis attacks. Some patients also require analgesics. Until healing occurs, oxygen needs, blood volume, and fluid and electrolyte balance must be monitored.

When gastritis causes massive bleeding, treatment includes blood replacement, nasogastric lavage, angiography with vasopressin infused in normal saline solution and, sometimes, surgery.

Vagotomy and pyloroplasty have achieved limited success when conservative treatments have failed. Rarely, partial or total gastrectomy may be required.

Simply avoiding aspirin and spicy foods may relieve chronic gastritis. If symptoms develop or persist, antacids may be taken. If pernicious anemia is the cause, vitamin $B_{12}$ may be administered parenterally.

**Special considerations**

• For vomiting, give antiemetics and I.V. fluids. Monitor fluid intake and output and electrolyte levels.

• Monitor the patient for recurrent symptoms as food is reintroduced; provide a bland diet.

• Offer smaller, more frequent meals to reduce irritating gastric secretions. Eliminate foods that cause gastric upset.

• Administer antacids and other prescribed medications.

• If pain or nausea interferes with the patient's appetite, give analgesics or antiemetics 1 hour before meals.

• Tell the patient to avoid alcohol, caffeine, and irritating foods, such as spicy or highly seasoned foods.

• If the patient smokes, refer him to a smoking-cessation program.

• Urge the patient to seek immediate attention for recurring symptoms, such as hematemesis, nausea, and vomiting.

• Urge the patient to take prophylactic medications as prescribed.

• To reduce gastric irritation, advise the patient to take steroids with milk, food, or antacids.

• Instruct the patient to take antacids between meals and at bedtime and to avoid aspirin-containing compounds.

# GASTROENTERITIS

Also called intestinal flu, traveler's diarrhea, viral enteritis, and food poisoning, gastroenteritis is a self-limiting disorder characterized by diarrhea, nausea, vomiting, and abdominal cramping. It occurs in all age-groups and is a major cause of morbidity and mortality in underdeveloped nations.

In the United States, gastroenteritis ranks second to the common cold as a cause of lost work time and fifth as the cause of death among young children. It also can be life-threatening in elderly and debilitated people.

**Causes**

Gastroenteritis has many possible causes, including the following:

• bacteria (responsible for acute food poisoning): *Staphylococcus aureus, Salmonella, Shigella, Clostridium botulinum, Escherichia coli, Clostridium perfringens*

• amoebae: especially *Entamoeba histolytica*

• parasites: *Ascaris, Enterobius, Trichinella spiralis*

• viruses (may be responsible for traveler's diarrhea): adenovirus, echovirus, or coxsackievirus

• ingestion of toxins: plants or toadstools (mushrooms)

• drug reactions: antibiotics

• enzyme deficiencies

• food allergens.

The bowel reacts to any of these enterotoxins with hypermotility, producing severe diarrhea and secondary depletion of intracellular fluid.

**Signs and symptoms**

Clinical manifestations vary, depending on the pathologic organism and the level of GI tract involved. Gastroenteritis in adults is usually a self-limiting, nonfatal disease that produces diarrhea, abdominal discomfort (ranging from cramping to pain), nausea, and vomiting. Other possible symptoms include fever, malaise, and borborygmi.

In children and elderly and debilitated people, gastroenteritis produces the same symptoms, but the inability of these patients to tolerate electrolyte and fluid losses leads to a higher mortality.

## Diagnosis

Patient history can aid diagnosis of gastroenteritis. A stool culture should be obtained. Blood cultures are indicated in febrile patients.

## Treatment

Usually supportive, treatment consists of nutritional support and increased fluid intake.

An episode of acute gastroenteritis is self-limiting. When an episode is severe and produces symptoms for more than 3 or 4 days and the patient is a young child or an elderly or debilitated person, hospitalization may be necessary. Treatment may include fluid and electrolyte replacement, antibiotic therapy, and antiemetics.

## Special considerations

● Administer medications; correlate dosages, routes, and times appropriately with the patient's meals and activities; for example, give antiemetics 30 to 60 minutes before meals.

● If the patient is unable to tolerate food, replace lost fluids and electrolytes with clear liquids and sports-type drinks. Vary his diet to make it more enjoyable, and allow some choice of foods. Instruct the patient to avoid milk and milk products, which may exacerbate the condition.

● Record strict intake and output. Watch for signs of dehydration, such as dry skin and mucous membranes, fever, and sunken eyes.

● Wash your hands thoroughly after giving care to avoid spread of infection.

● Instruct the patient to perform warm sitz baths three times a day to relieve anal irritation.

> **CLINICAL TIP** If food poisoning is probable, contact public health authorities to interview patients and food handlers, and take samples of the suspected contaminated food.

● Educate regarding good hygiene to prevent recurrence. Instruct patients to thoroughly cook foods, especially pork; to refrigerate perishable foods, such as milk, mayonnaise, potato salad, and cream-filled pastry; and to always wash their hands with warm water and soap before handling food, especially after using the bathroom.

● Teach patients to clean utensils thoroughly, to avoid drinking water or eating raw fruit or vegetables when visiting a foreign country, and to eliminate flies and roaches in their home.

# GASTROESOPHAGEAL REFLUX

The backflow or reflux of gastric and duodenal contents into the esophagus and past the lower esophageal sphincter (LES), without associated belching or vomiting, is called gastroesophageal reflux. Reflux may or may not cause symptoms or pathologic changes. Persistent reflux may cause reflux esophagitis (inflammation of the esophageal mucosa). The prognosis varies with the underlying cause.

## Causes

The function of the LES — a high-pressure area in the lower esophagus, just above the stomach — is to prevent gastric contents from backing up into the esophagus. Normally, the LES creates pressure, closing the lower end of the esophagus, but relaxes after each swallow to allow food into the stomach.

Reflux occurs when LES pressure is deficient or when pressure within the stomach exceeds LES pressure.

The amount of time the reflux is in contact with the esophagus as well as the potency of the reflux relate to esophageal damage. Gastroesophageal reflux can also be related to delayed gastric emptying resulting from partial gastric outlet obstruction or gastroparesis. It may also be attributed to an abnormal esophageal clearance. In this instance, acid is not cleared and neutralized by esophageal peristalsis and salivary bicarbonates, as it is normally.

> **CLINICAL TIP** Gastroesophageal reflux may also be related to atypical symptoms, such as chronic cough, sore throat, asthma, and laryngitis, and atypical chest pain.

Predisposing factors include:
- pyloric surgery (alteration or removal of the pylorus), which allows reflux of bile or pancreatic juice
- long-term nasogastric (NG) intubation (more than 5 days)
- any agent that lowers LES pressure, such as food, alcohol, cigarettes, anticholinergics (atropine, belladonna, and propantheline), and other drugs (morphine, diazepam, and meperidine)
- hiatal hernia (especially in children)
- any condition or position that increases intra-abdominal pressure.

### Signs and symptoms

Gastroesophageal reflux doesn't always cause symptoms. The most common feature of this disorder is heartburn, which may become more severe 30 to 60 minutes after meals and on reclining and with vigorous exercise, bending, or lying down and may be relieved by antacids or sitting upright.

The pain of esophageal spasm resulting from reflux esophagitis tends to be chronic and may mimic that of angina pectoris, radiating to the neck, jaws, and arms. Other symptoms include odynophagia, which may be followed by a dull substernal ache from severe, long-term reflux; dysphagia from esophageal spasm, stricture, or esophagitis; bleeding (bright red or dark brown);

and Barrett's metaplasia. Many patients have a lesser degree of dyspeptic symptoms with or without heartburn.

Rarely, nocturnal regurgitation wakens the patient with coughing, choking, and a mouthful of saliva. Reflux may be associated with hiatal hernia. Direct hiatal hernia becomes clinically significant *only* when reflux is confirmed.

Pulmonary symptoms result from reflux of gastric contents into the throat and subsequent aspiration. They include chronic pulmonary disease or nocturnal wheezing, bronchitis, asthma, morning hoarseness, and cough.

In children, other signs consist of failure to thrive and forceful vomiting from esophageal irritation. Such vomiting sometimes causes aspiration pneumonia.

### Diagnosis

After a careful history and physical examination, tests to confirm gastroesophageal reflux include barium swallow fluoroscopy, esophageal pH probe, and esophagoscopy. In children, barium esophagography under fluoroscopic control can show reflux. Recurrent reflux after age 6 weeks is abnormal.

An acid perfusion (Bernstein) test can show that reflux is the cause of symptoms. Finally, endoscopy and a biopsy allow visualization and confirmation of pathologic changes in the mucosa.

### Treatment

Effective management relieves symptoms by reducing intra-abdominal pressure and reflux through gravity, neutralizing gastric contents, strengthening the LES with drug therapy and, in severe cases, performing surgery.

#### Positional therapy

To reduce intra-abdominal pressure and reflux, the patient should sleep in a reverse Trendelenburg position (with the

> **TEACHING CHECKLIST**
>
> # COPING WITH REFLUX
>
> ● Teach the patient what causes reflux, how to avoid reflux with an antireflux regimen (medication, diet, and positional therapy), and what symptoms to watch for and report.
> ● Instruct the patient to avoid any circumstance that increases intra-abdominal pressure (such as bending, coughing, vigorous exercise, tight clothing, constipation, and obesity) or any substance that reduces sphincter control (such as cigarettes, alcohol, fatty foods, and certain drugs).
> ● Advise the patient to sit upright, particularly after meals, and to eat small, frequent meals. Tell him to avoid highly seasoned food, acidic juices, alcoholic drinks, bedtime snacks, and foods high in fat or carbohydrates, which reduce lower esophageal sphincter pressure. The patient should avoid lying down for at least 2 hours after eating a meal.
> ● Tell the patient to take antacids as ordered (usually 1 hour and 3 hours after meals and at bedtime).

head of the bed elevated) and should avoid lying down after meals and late-night snacks. In uncomplicated cases, positional therapy is especially useful in infants and children.

### Antacids

Antacids given 1 hour and 3 hours after meals and at bedtime are effective for intermittent reflux. Hourly administration is necessary for intensive therapy. A nondiarrheal, nonmagnesium antacid (aluminum carbonate, aluminum hydroxide) may be preferred, depending on the patient's bowel status.

### Drug therapy

Bethanechol, a drug that helps to increase LES pressure, stimulates smooth-muscle contraction and decreases esophageal acidity after meals (proven with pH probe). Metoclopramide and cimetidine have also been used with beneficial results.

If possible, NG intubation should not be continued for more than 5 days because the tube interferes with sphincter integrity and itself allows reflux, especially when the patient lies flat.

### Surgery

Surgical intervention may be necessary to control severe and refractory symptoms, such as pulmonary aspiration, hemorrhage, obstruction, severe pain, perforation, incompetent LES, and associated hiatal hernia.

Surgical procedures that create an artificial closure at the gastroesophageal junction include the Belsey Mark IV operation (which invaginates the esophagus into the stomach) and the Hill or Nissen operation (which creates a gastric wraparound with or without fixation). Also, vagotomy or pyloroplasty may be combined with an antireflux regimen to modify gastric contents.

### Special considerations

● Teach the patient correct preparation for diagnostic testing. For example, he should not eat for 6 to 8 hours before having a barium X-ray or endoscopy.
● After surgery using a thoracic approach, carefully watch and record chest tube drainage and respiratory status. If needed, give chest physiotherapy and oxygen. Place the patient with an NG tube in semi-Fowler's position to help prevent reflux. Offer reassurance and emotional support.
● Teach the patient how to avoid and treat reflux. (See *Coping with reflux.*)

# GLAUCOMA

Glaucoma is a group of disorders characterized by intraocular pressure (IOP) high enough to damage the optic nerve. If untreated, it leads to gradual peripheral vision loss and, ultimately, blindness.

Glaucoma occurs in several forms: chronic open-angle (primary), acute angle-closure, low tension (normal IOP that is too high for a particular person), congenital (inherited as an autosomal recessive trait), and secondary to other causes.

Glaucoma is the second most common cause of blindness in the United States. About 2.5 million Americans are afflicted with the disease, but only 1 million know that they have it. Its incidence is highest among blacks, and it is the single most common cause of blindness in that group. The visual prognosis is good with early treatment.

## Causes

The cause of glaucoma varies according to the type of disorder:

• *Chronic open-angle glaucoma* results from overproduction of aqueous humor or from obstructed outflow of aqueous humor through the trabecular meshwork or the canal of Schlemm. This form of glaucoma frequently runs in families and affects 90% of all patients with glaucoma.

• *Acute angle-closure (narrow-angle) glaucoma* results from obstructed outflow of aqueous humor due to anatomically narrow angles between the anterior iris and the posterior corneal surface, shallow anterior chambers, a thickened iris that causes angle closure on pupil dilation, or a bulging iris that presses on the trabeculae, closing the angle. Adhesions in the angle, referred to as peripheral anterior synechiae, may be the cause.

• *Secondary glaucoma* can result from uveitis, trauma, or drugs (such as steroids). Neovascularization in the angle can result from vein occlusion or diabetes.

## Signs and symptoms

Clinical features vary with the form of glaucoma.

### Chronic open-angle glaucoma

Usually bilateral, chronic open-angle glaucoma has an insidious onset and a slowly progressive course. Symptoms appear late in the disease and include mild aching in the eyes, loss of peripheral vision, seeing halos around lights, and reduced visual acuity (especially at night) that's uncorrectable with glasses.

### Acute angle-closure glaucoma

An ophthalmic emergency, acute angle-closure glaucoma typically has a rapid onset. Symptoms include unilateral inflammation and pain, pressure over the eye, moderate pupil dilation that's nonreactive to light, a cloudy cornea, blurring and decreased visual acuity, photophobia, and seeing halos around lights.

Because increased IOP may induce nausea and vomiting, glaucoma may be misinterpreted as GI distress. Unless treated promptly, this acute form of glaucoma produces blindness in 3 to 5 days.

## Diagnosis

Loss of peripheral visual field, cupping of the optical disk, and increased IOP are the triad of signs that indicate glaucoma. Relevant diagnostic tests include the following:

• *Tonometry* (using an applanation, Schiøtz, or air-puff tonometer) measures IOP and provides a baseline for reference.

Normal IOP ranges between 8 and 21 mm Hg, but some patients who fall in the normal range develop signs and symptoms of glaucoma. On the other hand, some patients who have abnormally high pressure have no clinical effects.

Fingertip tension is another way to measure IOP. On gentle palpation of closed eyelids, one eye feels harder than the other in acute angle-closure glaucoma.

• *Slit-lamp examination* provides a look at the anterior structures of the eye, including the cornea, iris, and lens.

• *Gonioscopy*, by determining the angle of the anterior chamber of the eye, allows differentiation between chronic open-angle glaucoma and acute angle-closure glaucoma. The angle is normal in chronic open-angle glaucoma. In older patients, partial closure of the angle may also occur, so two forms of glaucoma may coexist.

• *Ophthalmoscopy* provides a look at the fundus, where cupping of the optic disk is visible in chronic open-angle glaucoma. This change appears later in chronic angle-closure glaucoma if the disease isn't brought under control. A pale disk appears in acute angle-closure glaucoma.

• *Perimetry or visual field tests* help evaluate the extent of chronic open-angle deterioration by determining peripheral vision loss.

• *Fundus photography* can monitor the disk for any changes.

## Treatment

Drug therapy is the treatment of choice for chronic open-angle glaucoma. If this fails, argon laser trabeculoplasty or trabeculectomy is performed. Acute angle-closure glaucoma is treated with drugs, laser iridotomy, or surgical peripheral iridectomy.

### Drug therapy for open-angle glaucoma

For chronic open-angle glaucoma, treatment initially decreases aqueous humor production through beta blockers, such as timolol (contraindicated for asthmatic patients or those with bradycardia) and betaxolol (a beta$_1$-receptor antagonist); alpha agonists, such as brimonidine (Alphagan), to lower IOP; and topical carbonic anhydrase inhibitors, such as dorzolamide (Trusopt).

Drug treatment also includes miotic eyedrops such as pilocarpine to facilitate the outflow of aqueous humor. Patients who are unresponsive to drug therapy may be candidates for iridectomy, a surgical filtering procedure that creates an opening for aqueous outflow.

> **CLINICAL TIP** The end stage of glaucoma may require a tube shunt (Moltino) or valve (Baerveldt) to keep IOP down.

### Argon laser trabeculoplasty

In argon laser trabeculoplasty, an argon laser beam is focused on the trabecular meshwork of an open angle. This produces a thermal burn that changes the surface of the meshwork and increases the outflow of aqueous humor.

### Trabeculectomy

In trabeculectomy, a flap of sclera is dissected free to expose the trabecular meshwork. This discrete tissue block is then removed and a peripheral iridectomy is performed. This procedure produces an opening for aqueous outflow under the conjunctiva, creating a filtering bleb.

### Treatment for angle-closure glaucoma

Acute angle-closure glaucoma is an ocular emergency that requires immediate treatment to lower the high IOP. If the pressure doesn't decrease with drug therapy, laser iridotomy or surgical peripheral iridectomy must be performed promptly to save the patient's vision.

Iridectomy relieves pressure by excising part of the iris to reestablish aqueous humor outflow. A prophylactic iridectomy is performed a few days later on the other eye to prevent an acute episode of glaucoma in that eye.

Preoperative drug therapy lowers IOP with I.V. mannitol and steroid drops to quell the inflammation. Acetazolamide is used as well as pilocarpine (which constricts the pupil, forcing the iris away from the trabeculae and allowing fluid to escape) and I.V. mannitol (20%) or oral glycerin (50%) to force fluid from the eye by making the blood hypertonic. Timolol (Timoptic) is used to decrease IOP. Severe pain may necessitate narcotic analgesics.

### Special considerations

• Stress the importance of meticulous compliance with prescribed drug therapy to prevent disk changes, loss of vision, and an increase in IOP.

• Give the patient with acute angle-closure glaucoma medications and prepare him physically and psychologically for laser iridotomy or surgical peripheral iridectomy.

• Postoperative care after laser peripheral iridectomy includes cycloplegic eyedrops (apraclonidine [Iopidine]) to relax the ciliary muscle and decrease inflammation, thus preventing adhesions. Cycloplegics must only be used in the affected eye. The use of these drops in the normal eye may precipitate an attack of acute angle-closure glaucoma in this eye, threatening the patient's residual vision.

• Encourage ambulation immediately after surgery.

• After surgical filtering, postoperative care includes cycloplegic dilation and topical antibiotic steroids to quell the inflammatory response to surgery.

• Stress the importance of glaucoma screening for early detection and prevention. All people over age 35, especially those with a family history of glaucoma, should have an annual tonometric examination.

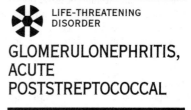

**LIFE-THREATENING DISORDER**

# GLOMERULONEPHRITIS, ACUTE POSTSTREPTOCOCCAL

Also called acute glomerulonephritis, acute poststreptococcal glomerulonephritis (APSGN) is a relatively common bilateral inflammation of the glomeruli. It follows a streptococcal infection of the respiratory tract or, less often, a skin infection, such as impetigo.

APSGN is most common in boys ages 6 to 10 but can occur at any age. Up to 95% of children and up to 70% of adults with APSGN recover fully; the remainder of patients may progress to chronic renal failure within months.

### Causes

APSGN results from the entrapment and collection of antigen-antibody complexes (produced as an immunologic mechanism in response to streptococci) in the glomerular capillary membranes, inducing inflammatory damage and impeding glomerular function.

Sometimes the immune complement further damages the glomerular membrane. The damaged and inflamed glomerulus loses the ability to be selectively permeable and allows red blood cells (RBCs) and proteins to filter through as the glomerular filtration rate (GFR) falls. Uremic poisoning may result.

## Signs and symptoms

APSGN begins within 1 to 3 weeks after untreated pharyngitis. Symptoms are mild to moderate edema, oliguria (< 400 ml/24 hours), proteinuria, azotemia, hematuria, and fatigue.

Mild to severe hypertension may result from either sodium or water retention (due to decreased GFR) and inappropriate renin release. Heart failure from hypervolemia leads to pulmonary edema.

## Diagnosis

A detailed patient history, assessment of clinical symptoms, and laboratory tests are needed to diagnose this disease. The following tests support the diagnosis:

● *Urinalysis* typically reveals proteinuria and hematuria. RBCs, white blood cells, and mixed cell casts are common findings in urinary sediment.

● *Blood tests* show elevated serum creatinine levels, low creatinine clearance, and impaired glomerular filtration.

● *Elevated antistreptolysin-0 titers* (in 80% of patients), *elevated streptozyme and anti-Dnase B titers, and low serum complement levels* verify recent streptococcal infection.

● *Throat culture* may also show group A beta-hemolytic streptococci.

● *Renal ultrasonography* may show a normal or slightly enlarged kidney.

● *Renal biopsy* may confirm the diagnosis in a patient with APSGN or may be used to assess renal tissue status.

## Treatment

The goals of treatment are relief of symptoms and prevention of complications. Vigorous supportive care includes bed rest, fluid and dietary sodium restrictions, and correction of electrolyte imbalances (possibly with dialysis, although this is seldom necessary).

Therapy may include diuretics, such as metolazone and furosemide, to reduce extracellular fluid overload and an antihypertensive such as hydralazine. The use of antibiotics to prevent secondary infection or transmission to others is controversial.

## Special considerations

● APSGN usually resolves within 2 weeks, so patient care is primarily supportive.

● Check vital signs and electrolyte values. Monitor intake and output and daily weight. Assess renal function daily through serum creatinine and blood urea nitrogen levels and urine creatinine clearance. Watch for signs of acute renal failure (oliguria, azotemia, and acidosis).

● Consult the dietitian to provide a diet high in calories and low in protein, sodium, potassium, and fluids.

● Protect the debilitated patient against secondary infection by providing good nutrition, using good hygienic technique, and preventing contact with infected people.

● Bed rest is necessary during the acute phase. Encourage the patient to gradually resume normal activities as symptoms subside.

● Provide emotional support for the patient and family. If the patient is on dialysis, explain the procedure fully.

● Advise the patient with a history of chronic upper respiratory tract infections to immediately report signs of infection (fever, sore throat).

● Tell the patient that follow-up examinations are necessary to detect chronic renal failure. Stress the need for regular blood pressure, urinary protein, and renal function assessments during the convalescent months to detect recurrence. After APSGN, gross hematuria may recur during nonspecific viral infections; abnormal urinary findings may persist for years.

CLINICAL TIP Encourage pregnant women with a history of APSGN to have frequent medical evaluations because pregnancy further stresses the kidneys and increases the risk of chronic renal failure.

# GLOMERULONEPHRITIS, CHRONIC

A slowly progressive disease, chronic glomerulonephritis is characterized by inflammation of the glomeruli, which results in sclerosis, scarring and, eventually, renal failure.

This condition usually remains subclinical until the progressive phase begins, marked by proteinuria, cylindruria (presence of granular tube casts), and hematuria. By the time it produces symptoms, chronic glomerulonephritis is usually irreversible.

## Causes

Common causes of chronic glomerulonephritis include primary renal disorders, such as membranoproliferative glomerulonephritis, membranous glomerulopathy, focal glomerulosclerosis, rapidly progressive glomerulonephritis and, less often, poststreptococcal glomerulonephritis.

Systemic disorders that may cause chronic glomerulonephritis include lupus erythematosus, Goodpasture's syndrome, and diabetes mellitus.

## Signs and symptoms

Chronic glomerulonephritis usually develops insidiously and asymptomatically, often over many years. It may suddenly become progressive at any time, producing nephrotic syndrome, hypertension, proteinuria, and hematuria.

### Late stages

In late stages, progressive chronic glomerulonephritis may accelerate to uremic symptoms, such as azotemia, nausea, vomiting, pruritus, dyspnea, malaise, and fatigability. Mild to severe edema and anemia may accompany these symptoms.

Severe hypertension may cause cardiac hypertrophy, leading to heart failure, and may accelerate the development of advanced renal failure, eventually necessitating dialysis or kidney transplantation.

## Diagnosis

Patient history and physical assessment seldom suggest glomerulonephritis. Suspicion develops from:

- *urinalysis,* which reveals proteinuria, hematuria, cylindruria, and red blood cell casts
- *rising blood urea nitrogen and serum creatinine levels*, which indicate advanced renal insufficiency
- *X-ray or ultrasonography,* which shows smaller kidneys
- *kidney biopsy,* which identifies underlying disease and provides data needed to guide therapy.

## Treatment

Effective treatment, essentially nonspecific and symptomatic, aims to control hypertension with antihypertensives and a sodium-restricted diet, to correct fluid and electrolyte imbalances through restrictions and replacement, to reduce edema with diuretics such as furosemide, and to prevent heart failure.

Treatment may also include antibiotics (for symptomatic urinary tract infections), dialysis, and transplantation.

## Special considerations

- Patient care is primarily supportive, focusing on continual observation and sound patient teaching.

• Accurately monitor vital signs, intake and output, and daily weight to evaluate fluid retention. Observe for signs of fluid, electrolyte, and acid-base imbalances.

• Ask the dietitian to plan low-sodium, high-calorie meals with adequate protein.

• Administer medications and provide good skin care (because of pruritus and edema) and oral hygiene. Instruct the patient to continue taking prescribed antihypertensives as scheduled, even if he's feeling better, and to report any adverse effects.

CLINICAL TIP   Advise the patient to take diuretics in the morning so he won't have to disrupt his sleep to void, and teach him how to assess ankle edema.

• Warn the patient to report signs of infection, particularly urinary tract infection, and to avoid contact with people who have infections. Urge follow-up examinations to assess renal function.

# GLYCOGEN STORAGE DISEASE

Consisting of at least eight distinct errors of metabolism — all inherited — glycogen storage disease alters the synthesis or degradation of glycogen, the form in which glucose is stored in the body.

Normally, muscle and liver cells store glycogen. Muscle glycogen is used in muscle contraction; liver glycogen can be converted into free glucose, which can then diffuse out of the liver cells to increase blood glucose levels.

Glycogen storage disease manifests as a dysfunction of the liver, heart, or musculoskeletal system. Symptoms vary from mild and easily controlled hypo-

glycemia to severe organ involvement that may lead to cardiac and respiratory failure.

## Causes

Almost all glycogen storage disease (types I through V and type VII) is transmitted as autosomal recessive traits. (See *Types of glycogen storage disease.*) The mode of transmission of type VI is unknown; type VIII may be an X-linked trait.

The most common type of glycogen storage disease is type I, glucose-6-phosphatase deficiency, or von Gierke's disease, which results from a deficiency of the liver enzyme glucose-6-phosphatase. It occurs in about 1 in 200,000 births, but the incidence may be higher in some populations. This enzyme converts glucose-6-phosphate into free glucose and is necessary for the release of stored glycogen and glucose into the bloodstream to relieve hypoglycemia.

Infants may die of acidosis before age 2; if they survive past this age, with proper treatment, they may grow normally and live to adulthood with only minimal hepatomegaly. Brief periods of fasting may produce irritability due to hypoglycemia and acidosis. Perspiration is excessive, and older children show heat intolerance. Easy bruising may be common. In older, untreated children, growth may be slow and sexual development may be incomplete. Hepatic adenomas are frequently seen by adolescence and may be premalignant lesions.

## Signs and symptoms

Primary clinical features of liver glycogen storage disease (types I, III, IV, VI, and VIII) are hepatomegaly and rapid onset of hypoglycemia and acidosis when food is withheld. Symptoms of muscle glycogen storage disease (types II, V, and VII) include poor muscle tone;

## TYPES OF GLYCOGEN STORAGE DISEASE

| TYPE | DEFICIENCY | INHERITANCE PATTERN |
|------|-----------|---------------------|
| I (von Gierke's) | Glucose-6-phosphatase | Autosomal recessive |
| II (Pompe's) | Alpha 1,4-glucosidase (acid maltase) | Probably autosomal recessive in most patients; late onset may be autosomal dominant |
| III (Cori's) | Debranching enzyme (amylo-1,6-glucosidase) | Autosomal recessive |
| IV (Andersen's) | Branching enzyme (amylo-1,4-1,6-transglucosidase) | Autosomal recessive |
| V (McArdle's) | Muscle phosphorylase | Autosomal recessive |
| VI (Hers') | Possible hepatic phosphorylase | Probably autosomal recessive |
| VII | Muscle phosphofructokinase | Probably autosomal recessive (rare) |
| VIII | Hepatic phosphorylase kinase | X-linked and autosomal recessive forms |

type II may result in death from heart failure.

In addition, type I may produce the following symptoms:

• *infants:* acidosis, hyperlipidemia, GI bleeding, coma

• *children:* low resistance to infection and, without proper treatment, short stature

• *adolescents:* gouty arthritis and nephropathy; chronic tophaceous gout; bleeding (especially epistaxis); small superficial vessels visible in skin, due to impaired platelet function; and fat deposits in cheeks, buttocks, and subcutaneous tissues.

Other symptoms include poor muscle tone; enlarged kidneys; xanthomas over extensor surfaces of the arms and legs; steatorrhea; multiple, bilateral, yellow lesions in fundi; and osteoporosis, probably secondary to a negative calcium balance. Proper treatment of glycogen storage disease should prevent all these effects.

### Diagnosis

Liver biopsies are the key tests in diagnosing type I glycogen storage disease.

• *Liver biopsy* confirms the diagnosis by showing normal glycogen synthetase and phosphorylase enzyme activities but reduced or absent glucose-6-phosphatase activity. Glycogen structure is normal, but levels are elevated.

• *Laboratory studies of plasma* demonstrate low glucose levels but high levels of free fatty acids, triglycerides, cholesterol, and uric acid. Serum analysis reveals high pyruvic acid and lactic acid levels. Diagnosis can be made prenatally for types II, III, and IV.

• *Injection of glucagon or epinephrine* increases pyruvic and lactic acid levels but doesn't increase blood glucose levels. The *glucose tolerance test* curve typically shows depletional hypoglycemia and reduced insulin output. An intrauterine diagnosis is possible.

## Treatment

For type I, the aims of treatment are to maintain glucose homeostasis and prevent secondary consequences of hypoglycemia through frequent feedings and a constant nocturnal nasogastric (NG) drip with an enteral nutrition formula or dextrose. Treatment includes a low-fat diet with normal amounts of protein and calories; carbohydrates should contain glucose or glucose polymers only.

Therapy for type III includes frequent feedings and a high-protein diet. Type IV requires a high-protein, high-calorie diet; bed rest; diuretics; sodium restriction; and paracentesis, if necessary, to relieve ascites.

Types V and VII require no treatment except avoidance of strenuous exercise. No treatment is necessary for types VI and VIII, and no effective treatment exists for type II.

## Special considerations

When managing type I disease:

> **CLINICAL TIP** Advise the patient or parents to include carbohydrate foods that contain mainly starch in the patient's diet and to sweeten foods with glucose only.

• Before discharge, teach the patient or a family member how to pass an NG tube, use a pump with alarm capacity, monitor blood glucose levels with glucose reagent strips, and recognize symptoms of hypoglycemia.

• Watch for signs of infection (fever, chills, myalgia) and hepatic encephalopathy (mental confusion, stupor, as-

terixis, coma) due to increased blood ammonia levels.

When managing other types:

• *Type II:* Explain test procedures, such as electromyography and EEG, thoroughly.

• *Type III:* Instruct the patient to eat a high-protein diet (eggs, nuts, fish, meat, poultry, and cheese).

• *Type IV:* Watch for signs of hepatic failure (nausea, vomiting, irregular bowel function, clay-colored stools, right upper quadrant pain, jaundice, dehydration, electrolyte imbalance, edema, and changes in mental status progressing to coma).

When caring for patients with type II, III, or IV glycogen storage disease, offer the parents reassurance and emotional support. Recommend and arrange for genetic counseling, if appropriate.

• *Types V through VIII*: Care for these patients is minimal. Explain the disorder to the patient and his family, and help them accept the limitations imposed by his particular type of glycogen storage disease.

# GOITER

Nontoxic or simple goiter — thyroid gland enlargement not caused by inflammation or a neoplasm — is commonly classified as endemic or sporadic.

*Endemic goiter* usually results from inadequate dietary intake of iodine associated with such factors as iodine-depleted soil and malnutrition. *Sporadic goiter* follows ingestion of certain drugs or foods.

Endemic goiter affects females more than males, especially during adolescence and pregnancy, when the demand on the body for thyroid hormone increases. Sporadic goiter affects no particular population segment. With appropriate treatment, the prognosis is good for either type.

## Causes

Simple goiter occurs when the thyroid gland can't produce and secrete enough thyroid hormone to meet metabolic requirements. As a result, the thyroid gland enlarges to compensate for inadequate hormone synthesis. Such compensation usually overcomes mild to moderate hormonal impairment.

Because thyroid-stimulating hormone (TSH) levels are generally within normal limits in patients with simple goiter, the disease probably results from impaired intrathyroidal hormone synthesis or depletion of glandular iodine, which increases the thyroid gland's sensitivity to TSH. Thyroid growth-stimulating immunoglobulins can also cause gland enlargement. However, increased levels of TSH may be transient and therefore missed.

### Endemic goiter

Endemic goiter usually results from inadequate dietary intake of iodine, which leads to inadequate production and secretion of thyroid hormone. The use of iodized salt prevents this deficiency.

### Sporadic goiter

Sporadic goiter commonly results from the ingestion of large amounts of goitrogenic foods or the use of goitrogenic drugs.

Goitrogenic foods contain agents that decrease thyroxine ($T_4$) production. Such foods include rutabagas, cabbage, soybeans, peanuts, peaches, peas, strawberries, spinach, and radishes.

Goitrogenic drugs include propylthiouracil, methimazole, iodides, and lithium. In a pregnant woman, such substances may cross the placenta and affect the fetus.

### Both types

Inherited defects may be responsible for insufficient $T_4$ synthesis or impaired iodine metabolism. Because families tend to congregate in a single geographic area, this familial factor may contribute to the incidence of both endemic and sporadic goiter.

## Signs and symptoms

Thyroid enlargement may range from a mildly enlarged gland to a massive, multinodular goiter. Because simple goiter doesn't alter the patient's metabolic state, clinical features arise solely from enlargement of the thyroid gland.

The patient may complain of respiratory distress and dysphagia from compression of the trachea and esophagus and from swelling and distention of the neck.

In addition, large goiters may obstruct venous return, produce venous engorgement and, in rare cases, induce development of collateral venous circulation in the chest. Such obstruction may cause dizziness or syncope when the patient raises his arms above his head.

## Diagnosis

An accurate diagnosis of simple goiter requires a thorough patient history and physical examination to rule out disorders with similar clinical effects, such as Graves' disease, Hashimoto's thyroiditis, and thyroid carcinoma. A detailed patient history also may reveal goitrogenic medications or foods or endemic influence.

The results of diagnostic laboratory tests include the following:
- *TSH:* high or normal
- *Serum $T_4$ concentrations:* low normal or normal
- *Iodine 131 uptake:* normal or increased (50% of the dose at 24 hours).

TEACHING CHECKLIST

## ✔ PATIENT INSTRUCTIONS IN GOITER

- To maintain constant hormone levels, instruct the patient to take prescribed thyroid hormone preparations at the same time each day.
- Instruct the patient and family members to identify and immediately report signs and symptoms of thyrotoxicosis. Such signs include increased pulse rate, palpitations, diarrhea, sweating, tremors, agitation, and shortness of breath.
- Instruct the patient with endemic goiter to use iodized salt to supply the daily 150 to 300 mcg of iodine necessary to prevent goiter.

### Treatment

The goal of treatment is to reduce thyroid hyperplasia. The following measures are used:

- Exogenous thyroid hormone replacement with levothyroxine is the treatment of choice; it decreases TSH secretion and allows the gland to rest. (See *Patient instructions in goiter*.)
- Small doses of iodine (Lugol's or potassium iodide solution) commonly relieve goiter caused by iodine deficiency. Sporadic goiter requires avoidance of known goitrogenic drugs and foods.
- A large goiter that is unresponsive to treatment may require subtotal thyroidectomy.

### Special considerations

- Measure the patient's neck circumference to check for progressive thyroid gland enlargement. Also check for the development of hard nodules in the gland, which may indicate carcinoma.
- Monitor the patient taking goitrogenic drugs for signs of sporadic goiter.
- Teach the patient about iodized salt, medications, and the symptoms of thyrotoxicosis.

# GONORRHEA

A common sexually transmitted disease, gonorrhea is an infection of the genitourinary tract (especially the urethra and cervix) and, occasionally, the rectum, pharynx, and eyes. Untreated gonorrhea can spread through the blood to the joints, tendons, meninges, and endocardium; in females, it can also lead to chronic pelvic inflammatory disease (PID) and sterility.

After adequate treatment, the prognosis in both males and females is excellent, although reinfection is common. Gonorrhea is especially prevalent among young people and people with multiple partners, particularly those between ages 19 and 25.

### Causes

Transmission of *Neisseria gonorrhoeae,* the organism that causes gonorrhea, almost exclusively follows sexual contact with an infected person. Children born of infected mothers can contract gonococcal ophthalmia neonatorum during passage through the birth canal. Children and adults with gonorrhea can contract gonococcal conjunctivitis by touching their eyes with contaminated hands.

### Signs and symptoms

Although many infected males are asymptomatic, after a 3- to 6-day incubation period, some develop symptoms of urethritis, including dysuria and purulent urethral discharge, with redness and swelling at the site of infection.

Most infected females remain asymptomatic but may develop inflammation and a greenish yellow discharge from the cervix — the most common gonorrheal symptoms in females.

Other clinical features vary according to the site involved:

• *urethra:* dysuria, urinary frequency and incontinence, purulent discharge, itching, red and edematous meatus

• *vulva:* occasional itching, burning, and pain due to exudate from an adjacent infected area. Vulval symptoms are more severe before puberty and after menopause.

• *vagina* (most common site in children over age 1): engorgement, redness, swelling, and profuse purulent discharge

• *pelvis:* severe pelvic and lower abdominal pain, muscle rigidity, tenderness, and abdominal distention. As the infection spreads, nausea, vomiting, fever, and tachycardia may develop in patients with salpingitis or PID.

• *liver:* right upper quadrant pain in patients with perihepatitis.

Other possible symptoms include pharyngitis, tonsillitis, rectal burning and itching, and bloody mucopurulent discharge.

### *Gonococcal septicemia*

Gonococcal septicemia is more common in females than in males. Its characteristic signs include tender papillary skin lesions on the hands and feet; these lesions may be pustular, hemorrhagic, or necrotic.

Gonococcal septicemia may also produce migratory polyarthralgia and polyarthritis and tenosynovitis of the wrists, fingers, knees, and ankles. Untreated septic arthritis leads to progressive joint destruction.

### *Eye involvement*

Signs of gonococcal ophthalmia neonatorum include lid edema, bilateral conjunctival infection, and abundant purulent discharge 2 to 3 days after birth. Adult conjunctivitis, most common in men, causes unilateral conjunctival redness and swelling. Untreated gonococcal conjunctivitis can progress to corneal ulceration and blindness.

### Diagnosis

A culture from the site of infection (urethra, cervix, rectum, or pharynx), grown on a Thayer-Martin or Transgrow medium, usually establishes the diagnosis by isolating the organism. A Gram stain showing gram-negative diplococci supports the diagnosis and may be sufficient to confirm gonorrhea in males.

Confirmation of gonococcal arthritis requires identification of gram-negative diplococci on smears made from joint fluid and skin lesions. Complement fixation and immunofluorescent assays of serum reveal antibody titers four times the normal rate. Culture of conjunctival scrapings confirms gonococcal conjunctivitis.

### Treatment

For adults and adolescents, the recommended treatment for uncomplicated gonorrhea caused by susceptible non-penicillinase-producing *N. gonorrhoeae* is a single 125-mg dose of ceftriaxone I.M.; for presumptive treatment of concurrent *Chlamydia trachomatis* infection, the treatment is 100 mg of doxycycline by mouth (P.O.) twice daily for 7 days.

A single dose of ceftriaxone and erythromycin for 7 days is recommended for pregnant patients and those allergic to penicillin.

The recommended initial regimen for disseminated gonococcal infection in adults and adolescents is 1 g of ceftriaxone I.M. or I.V. every 24 hours or, for patients allergic to beta-lactam antibiotics, 2 g of spectinomycin I.M. every 12 hours.

All regimens should be continued for 24 to 48 hours after improvement begins; then therapy may be switched to one of the following regimens to complete 1 full week of antimicrobial therapy: 400 mg of cefixime P.O. twice daily or 500 mg of ciprofloxacin P.O. twice daily. Ciprofloxacin is contraindicated in children, adolescents, and pregnant or lactating women.

Gonorrhea may also be treated with a single 1-g dose of azithromycin (Zithromax), per Centers for Disease Control and Prevention guidelines.

Treatment of gonococcal conjunctivitis requires a single 1-g dose of ceftriaxone I.M. and lavage of the infected eye with normal saline solution once.

Routine instillation of 1% silver nitrate or erythromycin drops into neo-nates' eyes has greatly reduced the incidence of gonococcal ophthalmia neonatorum.

### Special considerations
- Before treatment, establish whether the patient has any drug sensitivities, and watch closely for adverse effects during therapy.
- Warn the patient that until cultures prove negative, he's still infectious and can transmit gonococcal infection.
- Practice standard precautions.
- In the patient with gonococcal arthritis, apply moist heat to ease pain in affected joints.
- Urge the patient to inform sexual contacts of his infection so that they can seek treatment, even if cultures are negative. Advise them to avoid sexual intercourse until treatment is complete.

➤ CLINICAL TIP  Report all cases of gonorrhea to local public health authorities for follow-up on sexual contacts. Examine and test all people exposed to gonorrhea as well as newborn infants of infected mothers.
- Routinely instill two drops of 1% silver nitrate or erythromycin in the eyes of all neonates immediately after birth. Check newborn infants of infected mothers for signs of infection. Take specimens for culture from the infant's eyes, pharynx, and rectum.
- To prevent gonorrhea, tell patients to avoid anyone even *suspected* of being infected, to use condoms during intercourse, to wash their genitalia with soap and water before and after intercourse, and to avoid sharing washcloths or douche equipment.
- Report all cases of gonorrhea in children to child abuse authorities.

# GOUT

Gouty arthritis, or gout, is a metabolic disease marked by urate deposits in the joints, which cause painfully arthritic joints. It can strike any joint but favors those in the feet and legs. *Primary gout* usually occurs in men older than age 30 and in postmenopausal women. *Secondary gout* occurs in older people.

Gout follows an intermittent course and often leaves patients free of symptoms for years between attacks. Gout can lead to chronic disability or incapacitation and, rarely, severe hypertension and progressive renal disease. The prognosis is good with treatment.

### Causes
Although the exact cause of primary gout remains unknown, it seems linked to a genetic defect in purine metabolism, which causes overproduction of uric acid (hyperuricemia), retention of uric acid, or both.

In secondary gout, which develops during the course of another disease (such as obesity, diabetes mellitus, hypertension, sickle cell anemia, and renal disease), hyperuricemia results from the breakdown of nucleic acid.

Secondary gout can also follow drug therapy, especially the use of hydrochlorothiazide or pyrazinamide, which interferes with urate excretion. An increased concentration of uric acid leads to urate deposits, called tophi, in joints or tissues, causing local necrosis or fibrosis.

### Pseudogout

Another condition — pseudogout — results when calcium pyrophosphate crystals collect in the periarticular joint structures. (See *Pseudogout.*)

### Signs and symptoms

Gout develops in four stages: asymptomatic, acute, intercritical, and chronic.

### Asymptomatic stage

In asymptomatic gout, serum urate levels rise but produce no symptoms.

### Acute stage

As the disease progresses, it may cause hypertension or nephrolithiasis, with severe back pain. The first acute attack strikes suddenly and peaks quickly. Although it generally involves only one or a few joints, this initial attack is extremely painful. Affected joints appear hot, tender, inflamed, dusky red, or cyanotic.

The metatarsophalangeal joint of the great toe usually becomes inflamed first (podagra), followed by the instep, ankle, heel, knee, or wrist joints. Sometimes a low-grade fever is present. Mild acute attacks often subside quickly but recur at irregular intervals. Severe attacks may persist for days or weeks.

### Intercritical stage

Symptom-free intervals between gout attacks are called intercritical periods. Most patients have a second attack within 6 months to 2 years, but in some, the sec-

## PSEUDOGOUT

Also called calcium pyrophosphate disease, pseudogout results when calcium pyrophosphate crystals collect in periarticular joint structures. Without treatment, it leads to permanent joint damage in about one-half of the patients it affects, most of whom are elderly.

**Signs and symptoms**

Like gout, pseudogout causes abrupt joint pain and swelling, most commonly in the knee, wrist, ankle, and other peripheral joints. These recurrent, self-limiting attacks may be triggered by stress, trauma, surgery, severe dieting, thiazide therapy, and alcohol abuse. Associated symptoms are similar to those of rheumatoid arthritis.

**Diagnosis and treatment**

In pseudogout, the diagnosis depends on joint aspirations and a synovial biopsy to detect calcium pyrophosphate crystals. X-rays reveal calcific densities in the fibrocartilage and linear markings along bone ends. Blood tests may detect an underlying endocrine or metabolic disorder.

Effective treatment of pseudogout includes joint aspiration to relieve fluid pressure; instillation of steroids; administration of analgesics, phenylbutazone, salicylates, or other nonsteroidal anti-inflammatory drugs; and, if appropriate, treatment of the underlying endocrine or metabolic disorder.

ond attack is delayed for 5 to 10 years. Delayed attacks are more common in those who are untreated and last longer and are more severe than initial attacks.

Such attacks are also polyarticular, invariably affecting joints in the feet and legs, and sometimes accompanied by fever. A migratory attack sequentially strikes various joints and the Achilles tendon and is associated with either sub-deltoid or olecranon bursitis.

### Chronic stage

Eventually, chronic polyarticular gout sets in. This final, unremitting stage of the disease (chronic or tophaceous gout) is marked by persistent painful pol-yarthritis with large, subcutaneous tophi in cartilage, synovial membranes, tendons, and soft tissue.

Tophi form in the fingers, hands, knees, feet, ulnar sides of the forearms, helix of the ear, Achilles tendons and, rarely, internal organs, such as the kidneys and myocardium.

The skin over the tophus may ulcerate and release a chalky, white exudate or pus. Chronic inflammation and tophaceous deposits precipitate secondary joint degeneration, with eventual erosions, deformity, and disability. Kidney involvement with associated tubular damage leads to chronic renal dysfunction. Hypertension and albuminuria occur in some patients; urolithiasis is common.

### Diagnosis

The presence of monosodium urate monohydrate crystals in synovial fluid taken from an inflamed joint or a tophus establishes the diagnosis. Aspiration of synovial fluid (arthrocentesis) or tophaceous material reveals needlelike intracellular crystals of sodium urate.

Although hyperuricemia isn't specifically diagnostic of gout, the serum uric acid level is above normal. The urine uric acid level is usually higher in secondary gout than in primary gout.

Initially, X-ray examinations are normal. However, in chronic gout, X-rays show damage of the articular cartilage and subchondral bone. Outward displacement of the overhanging margin from the bone contour characterizes gout.

### Treatment

Correct management seeks to terminate an acute attack, reduce hyperuricemia, and prevent recurrence, complications, and the formation of renal calculi.

### Acute gout

Treatment for the patient with acute gout consists of bed rest, local application of heat or cold, and immobilization and protection of the inflamed, painful joints.

Analgesics, such as acetaminophen, relieve the pain associated with mild attacks, but acute inflammation requires concomitant treatment with colchicine (by mouth or I.V.) every hour for 8 hours until the pain subsides or until nausea, vomiting, cramping, or diarrhea develops.

Phenylbutazone or indomethacin in therapeutic doses may be used instead but is less specific. Resistant inflammation may require corticosteroids or corticotropin (I.V. drip or I.M.) or joint aspiration and an intra-articular corticosteroid injection.

### Chronic gout

Treatment of chronic gout consists of the following measures:.

• A continuing maintenance dosage of allopurinol is often given to suppress uric acid formation or control uric acid levels, preventing further attacks. This powerful drug should be used cautiously in patients with renal failure.

• Colchicine prevents recurrent acute attacks until uric acid returns to its normal level, but it doesn't affect the uric acid level. Uricosuric agents (probenecid and sulfinpyrazone) promote uric acid excretion and inhibit its accumulation, but their value is limited in patients with renal impairment. These drugs should not be given to patients with renal calculi.

• Other therapeutic measures include a few dietary restrictions, primarily the avoidance of alcohol and purine-rich foods. Obese patients should try to lose weight because obesity puts additional stress on painful joints.

• In some cases, surgery may be necessary to improve joint function or correct deformities. Tophi must be excised and drained if they become infected or ulcerated. They can also be excised to prevent ulceration, improve the patient's appearance, or make it easier for him to wear shoes or gloves.

### Special considerations

• Encourage bed rest, but use a bed cradle to keep bedcovers off extremely sensitive, inflamed joints.

• Give pain medication as needed, especially during acute attacks. Apply hot or cold packs to inflamed joints. Administer anti-inflammatory medication and other drugs, and watch for adverse effects. Be alert for GI disturbances with colchicine.

• Urge the patient to drink plenty of fluids (up to 2 L/day) to prevent formation of renal calculi.

• When forcing fluids, record intake and output accurately. Be sure to monitor serum uric acid levels regularly. Alkalinize urine with sodium bicarbonate or another agent, as needed.

> **CLINICAL TIP**  Watch for acute gout attacks 24 to 96 hours after surgery. Even minor surgery can precipitate an attack. Before and after surgery, administer colchicine to help prevent gout attacks as needed.

• Make sure the patient understands the importance of having serum uric acid levels checked periodically. Tell him to avoid high-purine foods, such as anchovies, liver, sardines, kidneys, sweetbreads, lentils, and alcoholic beverages (especially beer and wine), all of which raise the urate level.

• Explain the principles of a gradual weight reduction diet to obese patients. Such a diet features foods that contain moderate amounts of protein and little fat.

• Advise the patient who is receiving allopurinol, probenecid, and other drugs to report adverse effects, such as drowsiness, dizziness, nausea, vomiting, urinary frequency, and dermatitis, immediately.

• Warn the patient taking probenecid or sulfinpyrazone to avoid aspirin and other salicylates. Their combined effect causes urate retention.

• Inform the patient that long-term colchicine therapy is essential during the first 3 to 6 months of treatment with uricosuric drugs or allopurinol.

# GRAFT REJECTION SYNDROMES

As the clinical practice of solid organ transplantation evolves in sophistication and frequency, the focus on the mechanisms and subsequent treatment of graft rejection grows. Tissues commonly transplanted include the kidney, liver, heart, lung, and cornea. Bone marrow transplantation is unique, in that the host's immune system is markedly suppressed and an immune-mediated response can occur when cells in the transplanted bone marrow react against host antigens (called graft vs. host disease). The incidence of graft rejection has declined significantly with the improvement in compatibility screening techniques and immunosuppressive regimens.

### Causes

The donated organ, called an allograft if the donor and recipient are unrelated, is transplanted into the recipient, called the host. Rejection can occur when the host's immune responses are directed against the graft. The rapidity and reversibility of rejection depend on the various mechanisms involved, such as peritransplant ischemia and mechanical trauma, preformed antibody interactions with graft antigens, alloantigen-reactive T cells, and abnormal tissue remodeling.

Graft rejection syndromes can be divided into three subtypes, based on timing of onset and mechanisms involved.

### Hyperacute rejection
Hyperacute rejection occurs within minutes to hours after graft transplantation. This type of rejection has become rare, affecting less than 1% of transplant recipients due to improved pretransplant screenings. Hyperacute rejection occurs when circulating host antibodies recognize and bind to graft antigens (such as ABO blood group proteins or major histocompatibility complex proteins). Binding of these antibodies leads to initiation of the complement cascade, recruitment of neutrophils, platelet activation, damage to graft endothelial cells, and stimulation of coagulation reactions, which in turn lead to rapid thrombosis, loss of vascular integrity, tissue infarction, and loss of graft function.

### Acute rejection
Fifty percent of transplant patients experience acute rejection (with only 10% progressing to graft loss), which may occur several hours to days (even weeks) after transplantation. The incidence of acute rejection has decreased significantly with the successful use of immunosuppressants, such as cyclosporine and azathioprine. The incidence of graft loss has been reduced by newer antirejection therapies. Acute rejection occurs when alloantigen-reactive T cells from the host infiltrate the graft and are activated by contact with foreign, graft-related proteins presented to them by antigen-presenting cells. These T cells may lead to graft tissue damage either by direct killing of graft cells (cytolytic T cells) or by production of proinflammatory cytokines, such as tumor necrosis factor, interleukin-1, and interferon. These cytokines are vasoactive and perpetuate inflammatory cell recruitment and infiltration. As a result, graft inflammation progresses, leading to tissue distortion, vascular insufficiency, and cell destruction — all of which can eventually compromise graft function.

### Chronic rejection
Chronic rejection occurs in 50% of transplant patients within 10 years after transplantation. This form of rejection is characterized by the development of blood vessel luminal occlusion from progressive thickening of the intimal layers of medium and large arterial walls. Chronic rejection represents a pathologic tissue-remodeling response that develops at a variable rate after graft endothelial cells are traumatized by mechanical, ischemic, and immunologic injury during and after transplantation. These damaged vascular endothelial cells produce cytokines and tissue growth factors that initiate vascular repair, causing underlying smooth-muscle cells to begin proliferating. Large amounts of intimal matrix are produced, leading to increasingly occlusive vessel wall thickening. Slowly progressive reduction in blood flow results in regional tissue ischemia, cell death, and tissue fibrosis.

### Signs and symptoms
The signs and symptoms of graft rejection vary markedly, depending on the type of rejection, underlying illnesses, and type of organ transplanted. The most common evidence of rejection is rapid or gradual progression of organ dys-

function, such as oliguria and rising serum blood urea nitrogen and creatinine levels in the kidney; elevated transaminase levels, decreased albumin levels, and hypocoagulability in the liver; and hypotension, heart failure, and edema in the heart. Differentiation of the subtype of rejection is usually based on the timing.

## Diagnosis

Confirmation of a graft rejection can be made with a biopsy of the transplanted tissue. Graft tissue undergoing hyperacute rejection is characterized by large numbers of polymorphonuclear leukocytes within the graft blood vessels, widespread microthrombi, platelet accumulation, and interstitial hemorrhage. There is little or no interstitial inflammation. Acutely rejected tissue displays focal regions of perivascular infiltration of leukocytes, which become more widespread as the process progresses. Eventually, tissue distortion, cellular necrosis, and debris are seen. In chronic rejection, graft vessels display markedly thickened walls that may be occluded, and diffuse interstitial fibrosis is prominent. Leukocyte infiltration is usually mild or absent.

## Treatment

Management of transplant patients involves postoperative care after transplantation, close monitoring of the function of the grafted organ, immunosuppressive therapy for prevention and control of acute rejection, and surveillance with prophylactic measures against opportunistic infections. The primary method for managing hyperacute rejection is prevention. Avoidance of high-risk donor-recipient combinations and thorough pretransplant screening for cross-reactive antibodies are important. When a hyperacute rejection reaction is initiated, no pharmacologic

agents can halt it. Management becomes supportive until another donor organ can be found.

In acute rejection, immunosuppressants, usually given in combination regimens, can be effective. Commonly used agents include corticosteroids, cyclosporine, tacrolimus, and azathioprine. Newer antirejection therapies such as muromonab-CD3, an immunosuppressive monoclonal antibody directed at the CD3 molecule on T cells, are promising.

There is no accepted therapeutic strategy for treating chronic rejection. Preventive strategies to minimize peritransplant ischemia and reperfusion injury are under investigation and include such measures as the use of pulsatile graft perfusion devices during transport and peritransplant graft treatments to minimize release of mediators in response to vascular trauma.

> **CLINICAL TIP** Because graft rejection can be compounded by coexisting opportunistic infections, prophylaxis and early antibiotic or antiviral interventions are often indicated.

## Special considerations

● Pretransplant screening can indicate areas in which counseling and intervention may be useful to the patient and his family before transplantation.

● Graft rejection can be associated with a significant psychological as well as physical impact. The patient and his family may need extensive social support.

● Teach the patient how to recognize signs and symptoms of organ dysfunction. Instruct him to report fever, chills, or symptoms of infection immediately.

● Stress the importance of complying with immunosuppressive treatment. Explain to the patient that this compliance may be long term, if not lifelong.

# GRANULOCYTOPENIA AND LYMPHOCYTOPENIA

In *granulocytopenia*, a marked reduction in the number of circulating granulocytes occurs. Although this implies that all the granulocytes (neutrophils, basophils, and eosinophils) are reduced, granulocytopenia usually refers only to decreased neutrophils.

This disorder, which can occur at any age, is associated with infections and ulcerative lesions of the throat, GI tract, other mucous membranes, and skin. Its severest form is known as agranulocytosis.

*Lymphocytopenia (lymphopenia),* a rare disorder, is a deficiency of circulating lymphocytes (leukocytes produced mainly in lymph nodes).

In both granulocytopenia and lymphocytopenia, the total white blood cell (WBC) count may reach dangerously low levels (< 500/μl), leaving the body unprotected against infection. The prognosis in both disorders depends on the underlying cause and whether it can be treated. Untreated, severe granulocytopenia can be fatal in 3 to 6 days.

## Causes

Granulocytopenia and lymphocytopenia have several causes.

### Granulocytopenia

Granulocytopenia may result from decreased production of granulocytes in bone marrow, increased peripheral destruction of granulocytes, or greater utilization of granulocytes.

Decreased production of granulocytes in bone marrow generally stems from radiation or drug therapy; it's a common adverse effect of antimetabolites and alkylating agents and may occur in the patient who is hypersensitive to phenothiazines, sulfonamides (and some sulfonamide derivatives, such as chlorothiazide), antibiotics, or antiarrhythmic drugs.

Drug-induced granulocytopenia usually develops slowly and typically correlates with the dosage and duration of therapy. Production of granulocytes also decreases in such conditions as aplastic anemia and bone marrow cancers and in some hereditary disorders, such as infantile genetic agranulocytosis.

The growing loss of peripheral granulocytes is due to increased splenic sequestration, diseases that destroy peripheral blood cells (viral and bacterial infections), and drugs that act as haptens (carrying antigens that attack blood cells and causing acute idiosyncratic or non-dose-related drug reactions).

Infections such as infectious mononucleosis may result in granulocytopenia because of increased utilization of granulocytes.

### Lymphocytopenia

Similarly, lymphocytopenia may result from the decreased production, increased destruction, or loss of lymphocytes. Decreased production of lymphocytes may occur secondary to a genetic or thymic abnormality or to immunodeficiency disorders, such as ataxia-telangiectasia and thymic dysplasia. Increased destruction of lymphocytes may occur secondary to radiation therapy or chemotherapy (with alkylating agents).

Loss of lymphocytes may follow postsurgical thoracic duct drainage, intestinal lymphangiectasia, and impaired intestinal lymphatic drainage (as in Whipple's disease). Lymphocyte depletion can also result from elevated plasma corticoid levels (due to stress, corticotropin or steroid treatment, and heart failure).

Other associated disorders include Hodgkin's disease, leukemia, aplastic anemia, sarcoidosis, myasthenia gravis, lupus erythematosus, protein-calorie malnutrition, renal failure, terminal cancer, tuberculosis and, in infants, severe combined immunodeficiency disease (SCID).

### Signs and symptoms

Patients with granulocytopenia typically experience slowly progressive fatigue and weakness, followed by the sudden onset of signs of overwhelming infection (fever, chills, tachycardia, anxiety, headache, and extreme prostration); ulcers in the mouth or colon; pharyngeal ulceration, possibly with associated necrosis; pneumonia; and septicemia, possibly leading to septic shock and death.

If granulocytopenia is caused by an idiosyncratic drug reaction, signs of infection develop abruptly, without slowly progressive fatigue and weakness.

Patients with lymphocytopenia may exhibit enlarged lymph nodes, spleen, and tonsils and signs of an associated disease.

### Diagnosis

Granulocytopenia is diagnosed by a thorough patient history to check for precipitating factors. Physical examination for clinical effects of underlying disorders is also essential. The following test results confirm the diagnosis:

• A *complete blood count (CBC)* reveals a marked reduction in neutrophils ($< 500/\mu l$ leads to severe bacterial infections) and a WBC count lower than $2,000/\mu l$ with few observable granulocytes.

• *Examination of bone marrow* generally shows a scarcity of granulocytic precursor cells beyond the most immature forms, but this finding may vary, depending on the cause.

• A *lymphocyte count* less than $1,500/\mu l$ in adults or less than $3,000/\mu l$ in children indicates lymphocytopenia. Identifying the cause by evaluation of the patient's clinical status, bone marrow and lymph node biopsies, and other appropriate diagnostic tests helps establish the diagnosis.

### Treatment

Effective management of granulocytopenia must identify and eliminate the cause and control infection until the bone marrow can generate more leukocytes. This often means that drug or radiation therapy must be stopped and antibiotic treatment begun immediately, even while awaiting test results. Treatment may also include antifungal preparations.

Administration of a colony-stimulating factor, such as filgrastim or sargramostim, is another treatment used to stimulate bone marrow production of neutrophils. Spontaneous restoration of leukocyte production in bone marrow generally occurs within 1 to 3 weeks.

Treatment of lymphocytopenia includes eliminating the cause and managing any underlying disorders. For infants with SCID, therapy may include bone marrow transplantation.

### Special considerations

• Monitor vital signs frequently. Obtain cultures from blood, throat, urine, and sputum. Give antibiotics as scheduled.

• Explain the necessity for protective isolation (preferably with laminar air flow) to the patient and his family.

• Teach proper hand-washing technique and how to correctly use gowns and masks. Prevent patient contact with staff members or visitors with respiratory tract infections.

• Maintain adequate nutrition and hydration because malnutrition aggravates immunosuppression. Make sure the patient with mouth ulcers receives a high-calorie liquid diet; for example, high-protein milk shakes. Offer a straw to make drinking less painful.

• Provide warm saline water gargles and rinses, analgesics, and anesthetic lozenges because good oral hygiene promotes patient comfort and facilitates the healing process.

• Ensure adequate rest, which is essential to the mobilization of the body's defenses against infection. Provide good skin and perineal care.

• Monitor CBC and differential, blood culture results, serum electrolyte levels, intake and output, and daily weight.

➤ CLINICAL TIP  To help detect granulocytopenia and lymphocytopenia in the early, most treatable stages, monitor the WBC count of any patient receiving radiation therapy or chemotherapy. After the patient has developed bone marrow depression, he must zealously avoid exposure to infection.

• Advise the patient with known or suspected sensitivity to a drug that may lead to granulocytopenia or lymphocytopenia to alert medical personnel to this sensitivity in the future.

# GUILLAIN-BARRÉ SYNDROME

Also known as infectious polyneuritis, Landry-Guillain-Barré syndrome, and acute idiopathic polyneuritis, Guillain-Barré syndrome is an acute, rapidly progressive, and potentially fatal form of polyneuritis that causes muscle weakness and mild distal sensory loss.

This syndrome can occur at any age but is most common between ages 30 and 50; it affects both sexes equally. Recovery is spontaneous and complete in about 95% of patients, although mild motor or reflex deficits in the feet and legs may persist. The prognosis is best when symptoms clear between 15 and 20 days after onset.

## Causes
The precise cause of Guillain-Barré syndrome is unknown, but it may be a cell-mediated immune response with an attack on peripheral nerves in response to a virus. The major pathologic effect is segmental demyelination of the peripheral nerves.

Because this syndrome causes inflammation and degenerative changes in both the posterior (sensory) and the anterior (motor) nerve roots, signs of sensory and motor losses occur simultaneously.

### *Precipitating factors*
About 50% of patients with Guillain-Barré syndrome have a recent history of minor febrile illness, usually an upper respiratory tract infection or, less often, gastroenteritis. When infection precedes the onset of Guillain-Barré syndrome, signs of infection subside before neurologic features appear.

Other possible precipitating factors include surgery, rabies or swine influenza vaccination, viral illness, Hodgkin's or some other malignant disease, and systemic lupus erythematosus.

## Signs and symptoms
Muscle weakness, the major neurologic sign, usually appears in the legs first (ascending type) and then extends to the arms and facial nerves within 24 to 72 hours. Sometimes muscle weakness develops in the arms first (descending type) or in the arms and legs simultaneously. In milder forms of the disease, muscle weakness may affect only the cranial nerves or not occur.

Paresthesia, another common neurologic sign, sometimes precedes muscle weakness but vanishes quickly. Some patients with the disorder never develop this symptom.

Other clinical features include facial diplegia (possibly with ophthalmoplegia [ocular paralysis]), dysphagia or dysarthria and, less often, weakness of the muscles supplied by cranial nerve XI (spinal accessory nerve).

Muscle weakness develops so quickly that muscle atrophy doesn't occur, but hypotonia and areflexia do. Stiffness and pain in the form of a severe "charley horse" often occur.

### Three-phase course

The clinical course of Guillain-Barré syndrome is divided into three phases:
• The *initial phase* begins when the first definitive symptom develops; it ends 1 to 3 weeks later, when no further deterioration is noted.
• The *plateau phase* lasts from several days to 2 weeks.
• The *recovery phase* is believed to coincide with remyelination and axonal process regrowth. This phase extends over 4 to 6 months; patients with severe disease may take up to 2 years to recover, and recovery may not be complete.

### Complications

Significant complications of Guillain-Barré syndrome include mechanical ventilatory failure, aspiration pneumonia, sepsis, joint contractures, and deep vein thrombosis. Unexplained autonomic nervous system involvement may cause sinus tachycardia or bradycardia, hypertension, postural hypotension, and loss of bladder and bowel sphincter control.

### Diagnosis

A history of preceding febrile illness (usually a respiratory tract infection) and typical clinical features suggest Guillain-Barré syndrome.

Several days after onset of signs and symptoms, the cerebrospinal fluid (CSF) protein level begins to rise, peaking in 4 to 6 weeks, probably as a result of widespread inflammatory disease of the nerve roots. The CSF white blood cell count remains normal, but in severe disease, CSF pressure may rise above normal.

Probably because of predisposing infection, the complete blood count shows leukocytosis with the presence of immature forms early in the illness, but blood study results soon return to normal. Electromyography may show repeated firing of the same motor unit, instead of widespread sectional stimulation.

Nerve conduction velocities are slowed soon after paralysis develops. The diagnosis must rule out similar diseases, such as acute poliomyelitis.

### Treatment

Primarily supportive, treatment consists of endotracheal intubation or tracheotomy if the patient has difficulty clearing secretions.

A trial dose of prednisone may be given if the course of the disease is relentlessly progressive. If prednisone produces no noticeable improvement after 7 days, the drug is discontinued. Plasmapheresis is useful during the initial phase but offers no benefit if begun 2 weeks after onset.

### Special considerations

• Watch for ascending sensory loss, which precedes motor loss. Also, monitor vital signs and level of consciousness.
• Assess and treat respiratory dysfunction. If respiratory muscles are weak, take serial vital capacity recordings. Use a respirometer with a mouthpiece or a face mask for bedside testing.

- Obtain arterial blood gas measurements. Because neuromuscular disease results in primary hypoventilation with hypoxemia and hypercapnia, watch for a partial pressure of oxygen ($Pa_{O_2}$) below 70 mm Hg, which signals respiratory failure. Be alert for signs of a rising partial pressure of carbon dioxide (confusion, tachypnea).

- Auscultate for breath sounds, turn and reposition the patient regularly, and encourage coughing and deep breathing.

- Begin respiratory support at the first sign of dyspnea (in adults, a vital capacity < 800 ml; in children, < 12 ml/kg of body weight) or a decreasing $Pa_{O_2}$.

- If respiratory failure becomes imminent, establish an emergency airway with an endotracheal tube.

- Give meticulous skin care to prevent skin breakdown and contractures.

- Establish a strict turning schedule; inspect the skin (especially the sacrum, heels, and ankles) for breakdown, and reposition the patient every 2 hours.

- After each position change, stimulate circulation by carefully massaging pressure points. Also, use foam, gel, or alternating-pressure pads at points of contact.

- Perform passive range-of-motion exercises within the patient's pain limits, perhaps using a Hubbard tank. Remember that the proximal muscle groups of the thighs, shoulders, and trunk will be the most tender and cause the most pain on passive movement and turning.

- When the patient's condition stabilizes, change to gentle stretching and active assistance exercises.

- Assess the patient for signs of dysphagia (coughing, choking, "wet"-sounding voice, increased presence of rhonchi after feeding, drooling, delayed swallowing, regurgitation of food, and weakness in cranial nerves V, VII, IX, X, XI, or XII).

- Take measures to minimize aspiration: elevate the head of the bed, position the patient upright and leaning forward when eating, feed semisolid food, and check the mouth for food pockets.

- Encourage the patient to eat slowly and remain upright for 15 to 20 minutes after eating.

- A speech pathologist and modified video fluoroscopy can assist in identifying the best feeding strategies.

- If aspiration cannot be minimized by diet and position modification, nasogastric feeding is recommended.

- As the patient regains strength and can tolerate a vertical position, be alert for postural hypotension. Monitor blood pressure and pulse rate during tilting periods, and if necessary, apply toe-to-groin elastic bandages or an abdominal binder to prevent postural hypotension.

- Inspect the patient's legs regularly for signs of thrombophlebitis (localized pain, tenderness, erythema, edema, positive Homans' sign), a common complication of Guillain-Barré syndrome.

- To prevent thrombophlebitis, apply antiembolism stockings and give prophylactic anticoagulants as needed.

- If the patient has facial paralysis, give eye and mouth care every 4 hours.

- Protect the corneas with isotonic eyedrops and conical eye shields.

- Encourage adequate fluid intake (2,000 ml/day), unless contraindicated.

- Watch for urine retention. Measure and record intake and output every 8 hours, and offer the bedpan every 3 to 4 hours.

- If urine retention develops, begin intermittent catheterization as needed. Because the abdominal muscles are weak, the patient may need manual pressure on the bladder (Credé's method) before he can urinate.

- To prevent and relieve constipation, offer prune juice and a high-bulk diet. If necessary, give daily or alternate-day suppositories (glycerin or bisacodyl) or Fleet enemas.

• Before discharge, prepare a home care plan. Teach the patient how to transfer from bed to wheelchair and from wheelchair to toilet or tub and how to walk short distances with a walker or cane.

• Teach the family how to help the patient eat, compensating for facial weakness, and how to help him avoid skin breakdown. Stress the need for a regular bowel and bladder routine.

• Refer the patient for physical therapy, occupational therapy, and speech therapy, as needed.

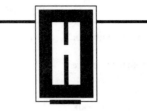

# HAEMOPHILUS INFLUENZAE INFECTION

*Haemophilus influenzae* is a common cause of epiglottitis, laryngotracheobronchitis, pneumonia, bronchiolitis, otitis media, and meningitis. Less commonly, it causes bacterial endocarditis, conjunctivitis, facial cellulitis, septic arthritis, and osteomyelitis.

*H. influenzae* pneumonia is an increasingly common nosocomial infection. It infects about one-half of all children before age 1 and virtually all children by age 3, although a new vaccine given at ages 2, 4, and 6 months has reduced this number.

## Cause

A small, gram-negative, pleomorphic aerobic bacillus, *H. influenzae* causes diseases in many organ systems but most frequently attacks the respiratory system. In exudates, this organism predominantly resembles a coccobacillus.

## Signs and symptoms

*H. influenzae* provokes a characteristic tissue response—acute suppurative inflammation.

When *H. influenzae* infects the larynx, trachea, and bronchial tree, it leads to mucosal edema and thick exudate; when it invades the lungs, it leads to bronchopneumonia.

In the pharynx, *H. influenzae* usually produces no remarkable changes, except when it causes epiglottitis, which generally affects both the laryngeal and the pharyngeal surfaces.

The pharyngeal mucosa may be reddened, rarely with soft yellow exudate. More commonly, it appears normal or shows only slight diffuse redness, even while severe pain makes swallowing difficult or impossible. These infections typically cause high fever and generalized malaise.

## Diagnosis

Isolation of the organism, usually with a blood culture, confirms *H. influenzae* infection. Other laboratory findings include:
- polymorphonuclear leukocytosis (15,000 to 30,000/µl)
- leukopenia (2,000 to 3,000/µl) in young children with severe infection
- *H. influenzae* bacteremia, found frequently in patients with meningitis.

## Treatment

*H. influenzae* infections usually respond to a 2-week course of ampicillin, but 30% of strains are resistant. Ceftriaxone, cefotaxime, or chloramphenicol is used concurrently until sensitivities are identified. Rifampin should be given before discharge to assure treatment success.

## Special considerations

- Maintain adequate respiratory function through proper positioning, humidification in children, and suctioning, as needed.
- Monitor the rate and type of respirations.
- Watch for signs of cyanosis and dyspnea, which necessitate intubation or a tracheotomy.
- For home treatment, suggest that the patient use a room humidifier or breathe moist air from a shower or bath, as necessary.
- Check the patient's history for drug allergies before giving antibiotics.

> **CLINICAL TIP** Monitor the complete blood count for signs of bone marrow depression when therapy includes chloramphenicol.

- Monitor intake (including I.V. infusions) and output. Watch for signs of dehydration, such as decreased skin turgor, parched lips, concentrated urine, decreased urine output, and increased pulse rate.
- Take preventive measures, such as giving the *H. influenzae* vaccine to children ages 2 (or younger) to 6, maintaining respiratory isolation, using proper hand-washing technique, properly disposing of respiratory secretions, placing soiled tissues in a plastic bag, and decontaminating all equipment.

---

 LIFE-THREATENING DISORDER

# HANTAVIRUS PULMONARY SYNDROME

---

Mainly occurring in the southwestern United States, *Hantavirus* pulmonary syndrome was first reported in May 1993. The syndrome, which rapidly progresses from flulike symptoms to respiratory failure and, possibly, death, is known for its high mortality.

The *Hantavirus* strain that causes disease in Asia and Europe — mainly hemorrhagic fever and kidney disease — is distinctly different from the one described in North America.

## Causes

A member of the Bunyaviridae family, the genus *Hantavirus* (first isolated in 1977) is responsible for hantavirus pulmonary syndrome. Disease transmission is associated with exposure to infected rodents, the primary reservoir for this virus.

Data suggest that the deer mouse is the main source, but piñon mice, brush mice, and western chipmunks in proximity to humans in rural areas are also sources.

Infected rodents manifest no apparent illness but shed the virus in feces, urine, and saliva. Human infection may occur from inhalation, ingestion (of contaminated food or water, for example), contact with rodent excrement, or rodent bites. Transmission from person to person or by mosquitos, fleas, or other arthropods has not been reported.

*Hantavirus* infections have been documented in people whose activities are associated with rodent contact, such as farming, hiking, or camping in rodent-infested areas, and occupying rodent-infested dwellings.

## Signs and symptoms

Noncardiogenic pulmonary edema distinguishes the syndrome. Common chief complaints include myalgia, fever, headache, nausea, vomiting, and cough. Respiratory distress typically follows the onset of a cough. Fever, hypoxia and, in some patients, serious hypotension typify the hospital course.

# SCREENING FOR *HANTAVIRUS* PULMONARY SYNDROME

The Centers for Disease Control and Prevention (CDC) has developed a screening procedure to track cases of hantavirus pulmonary syndrome. The screening criteria identify potential and actual cases.

## Potential cases

For a diagnosis of possible hantavirus pulmonary syndrome, a patient must have one of the following:

• a febrile illness (temperature equal to or above 101° F [38.3° C]) occurring in a previously healthy person and characterized by unexplained adult respiratory distress syndrome

• bilateral interstitial pulmonary infiltrates that develop within 1 week of hospitalization with respiratory compromise that requires supplemental oxygen

• an unexplained respiratory illness resulting in death and autopsy findings demonstrating noncardiogenic pulmonary edema without an identifiable specific cause of death.

## Exclusions

Of the patients who meet the criteria for having potential hantavirus pulmonary syndrome, the CDC excludes those who have any of the following:

• a predisposing underlying medical condition, for example, severe underlying pulmonary disease, solid tumors or hematologic cancers, congenital or acquired immunodeficiency disorders, and medical conditions such as rheumatoid arthritis and organ transplantation that require immunosuppressive therapy, such as steroids and cytotoxic chemotherapy

• an acute illness that provides a likely explanation for the respiratory illness (for example, a recent major trauma, burn, or surgery; recent seizures; or a history of aspiration, bacterial sepsis, another respiratory disorder such as respiratory syncytial virus in young children, influenza, and legionella pneumonia).

## Confirmed cases

Cases of confirmed hantavirus pulmonary syndrome must include the following:

• at least one serum sample or tissue specimen available for laboratory testing for evidence of hantavirus infection

• in a patient with a compatible clinical illness, serologic evidence (presence of hantavirus-specific immunoglobulin M [IgM] or rising titers of IgG), polymerase chain reaction for hantavirus ribonucleic acid, or positive immunohistochemistry for the hantavirus antigen.

---

Other signs and symptoms include a rising respiratory rate ($\geq$ 28 breaths per minute) and an increased heart rate ($\geq$ 120 beats per minute).

## Diagnosis

Despite efforts to identify clinical and laboratory features that distinguish hantavirus pulmonary syndrome from other infections with similar features, diagnosis is based on clinical suspicion along with a process of elimination developed by the Centers for Disease Control and Prevention (CDC) with the Council of State and Territorial Epidemiologists. (See *Screening for* Hantavirus *pulmonary syndrome.*)

*Note:* The CDC and state health departments can perform definitive testing for hantavirus exposure and antibody formation.

Laboratory tests usually reveal an elevated white blood cell count with a predominance of neutrophils, myeloid precursors, and atypical lymphocytes; elevated hematocrit; decreased platelet count; prolonged partial thromboplastin time; and a normal fibrinogen level.

Usually, laboratory findings demonstrate only minimal abnormalities in renal function, with serum creatinine levels no higher than 2.5 mg/dl.

Chest X-rays eventually show bilateral diffuse infiltrates in almost all patients (findings consistent with adult respiratory distress syndrome).

**Treatment**

Primarily supportive, treatment consists of maintaining adequate oxygenation, monitoring vital signs, and intervening to stabilize the patient's heart rate and blood pressure.

Drug therapy includes administering vasopressors, such as dopamine or epinephrine, for hypotension. Fluid volume replacement may also be ordered (with precautions not to overhydrate the patient).

Intravenous ribavirin early in the illness has shown benefit.

**Special considerations**

• Assess the patient's respiratory status and arterial blood gas values often.

• Monitor the patient's serum electrolyte levels, and correct imbalances as appropriate.

• Maintain a patent airway by suctioning. Ensure adequate humidification, and check ventilator settings frequently.

• In patients with hypoxemia, assess neurologic status frequently along with heart rate and blood pressure.

• Administer drug therapy, and monitor the patient's response.

• Provide I.V. fluid therapy based on the results of hemodynamic monitoring.

• Provide emotional support for the patient and his family.

> CLINICAL TIP Report cases of *Hantavirus* pulmonary syndrome to the state health department.

• Provide prevention guidelines. (Until more is known about *Hantavirus* pul-

monary syndrome, preventive measures focus on rodent control.)

# HEADACHE

The most common patient complaint, headache usually occurs as a symptom of an underlying disorder. Ninety percent of all headaches are vascular, muscle contraction, or a combination; 10% are due to underlying intracranial, systemic, or psychological disorders.

Migraine headaches, probably the most intensively studied, are throbbing, vascular headaches that usually begin to appear in childhood or adolescence and recur throughout adulthood. Affecting up to 10% of Americans, they're more common in females and have a strong familial incidence.

**Causes**

Most chronic headaches result from tension — muscle contraction — that may be caused by emotional stress, fatigue, menstruation, or environmental stimuli (such as noise, crowds, and bright lights).

Other possible causes include glaucoma; inflammation of the eyes or mucosa of the nasal or paranasal sinuses; diseases of the scalp, teeth, extracranial arteries, or external or middle ear; and muscle spasms of the face, neck, or shoulders.

In addition, headaches may be caused by vasodilators (such as nitrates, alcohol, and histamines), systemic disease, hypoxia, hypertension, head trauma and tumor, intracranial bleeding, abscess, and aneurysm.

*Migraine headache*

The cause of migraine headache is unknown, but these headaches are associated with constriction and dilation of intracranial and extracranial arteries. Certain biochemical abnormalities are thought to occur during a migraine attack. They include local leakage of a vasodilator polypeptide called neurokinin through the dilated arteries and a decrease in the plasma level of serotonin.

Several foods associated with migraine headache include aged or processed cheese and meats, alcoholic beverages (particularly red wine), food additives (such as monosodium glutamate), chocolate- and caffeine-containing foods, and nuts. Changes in the weather pattern, menstrual cycle fluctuations, sleep pattern changes, and too much or too little exercise can also trigger a migraine headache. In addition, one of the more common causes of a recurring headache is the rebound effect that occurs when the original treatment used to get rid of the headache triggers the next episode (as with narcotics).

### Headache pain

Pain may emanate from the pain-sensitive structures of the skin, scalp, muscles, arteries, and veins; cranial nerves V, VII, IX, and X; and cervical nerves 1, 2, and 3. Intracranial mechanisms of headache include traction or displacement of arteries, venous sinuses, or venous tributaries and inflammation or direct pressure on the cranial nerves with afferent pain fibers.

### Signs and symptoms

Migraine headaches and muscle contraction headaches have different signs and symptoms.

### Migraine headache

Initially, a migraine headache usually produces unilateral, pulsating pain that later becomes more generalized. The headache is often preceded by a scintillating scotoma, hemianopia, unilateral paresthesia, or speech disorders. The patient may experience irritability, anorex-

ia, nausea, vomiting, and photophobia. (See *Clinical features of headaches.*)

### Muscle contraction headache

This type of headache produces a dull, persistent ache; tender spots on the head and neck; and a feeling of tightness around the head, with a characteristic "hatband" distribution. The pain is often severe and unrelenting.

If caused by intracranial bleeding, the muscle contraction headache may result in neurologic deficits, such as paresthesia and muscle weakness; narcotics fail to relieve the pain in these cases. If the headache is caused by a tumor, pain is most severe when the patient awakens.

### Diagnosis

An accurate diagnosis requires a history of recurrent headaches and physical examination of the head and neck. Such examination includes percussion, auscultation for bruits, inspection for signs of infection, and palpation for defects, crepitus, and tender spots (especially after trauma).

A firm diagnosis also requires a complete neurologic examination, assessment for other systemic diseases (such as hypertension), and a psychosocial evaluation (when such factors are suspected).

Most patients may be diagnosed by a thorough history and physical examination. Magnetic resonance imaging, computed tomography, lumbar puncture, and serology may be beneficial. Neurologic deficits and an aneurysm must be ruled out if the headache is explosive and "the worst" in their lives.

### Treatment

Depending on the type of headache, treatment interventions range from relaxation techniques, massage, and biofeedback to pharmacologic agents. Tricyclic antidepressants, beta blockers, and anticonvulsants may be pre-

# CLINICAL FEATURES OF HEADACHE

The International Headache Society classifies migraines as occurring with or without an aura. The differentiating characteristics of each type are listed below.

## Migraines without an aura

Previously called common migraines or hemicrania simplex, migraine headaches without an aura are diagnosed when the patient has five attacks that include the following symptoms:
• untreated or unsuccessfully treated headache lasting 4 to 72 hours
• two of the following: pain that is unilateral, pulsating, moderate or severe in intensity, or aggravated by activity
• nausea, vomiting, photophobia, or phonophobia.

## Migraines with an aura

Previously called classic, classical, ophthalmic, hemiplegic, or aphasic migraines, migraine headaches with an aura are diagnosed when the patient has at least two attacks with three of the following characteristics:
• one or more reversible aura symptoms (indicates focal cerebral cortical or brain stem dysfunction)
• one or more aura symptoms that develop over more than 4 minutes, or two or more symptoms that occur in succession
• an aura symptom that lasts less than 60 minutes (per symptom)
• headache begins before, occurs with, or follows an aura with a free interval of less than 60 minutes.

Migraines with an aura also must have one of the following to be classified as a typical aura:
• homonymous visual disturbance
• unilateral paresthesia or numbness, or both
• unilateral weakness
• aphasia or other speech difficulty.
Migraines also have one of the following characteristics:
• history and physical and neurologic examinations are negative for a disorder
• examinations suggest a disorder that is ruled out by appropriate investigation
• a disorder is present but migraines don't occur for the first time in relation to the disorder.

## Tension-type headaches

In contrast to migraines, episodic tension-type headaches are diagnosed when the headache occurs on fewer than 180 days per year or the patient has fewer than 15 headaches a month and the following characteristics are present:
• headache lasts from 30 minutes to 7 days
• pain is pressing or tightening in quality, mild to moderate, bilateral, and not aggravated by activity
• photophobia or phonophobia sometimes occurs but usually not nausea or vomiting.

---

scribed for headache prevention; nonsteroidal anti-inflammatory drugs (NSAIDs), combination NSAIDs with caffeine, and ergotamines may be used for abortive measures. Narcotic agents are generally avoided or may be limited to twice weekly.

Abortive therapy using the synthetic form of serotonin (sumatriptan [Imitrex]) is now available in an oral form and as a nasal spray and can easily be carried for immediate use.

Other measures include identification and elimination of causative factors, stressors, or stimuli that might trigger an attack, such as in the migraine-type headache. Diet history and examination of lifestyle patterns may help identify causative agents.

## Special considerations

• Headaches seldom require hospitalization unless they are caused by a serious disorder. If that's the case, direct your care to the primary problem.

• Obtain a complete patient history: duration and location of the headache, time of day it usually begins, nature of the pain, the headache's concurrence with other symptoms such as blurred vision, and precipitating factors, such as tension, menstruation, loud noises, menopause, alcohol use, use of medications such as oral contraceptives, and prolonged fasting.

➤ CLINICAL TIP Have the patient keep a journal describing the events surrounding the headache. This can be used as a guide for the patient to avoid precipitating factors.

• Advise the patient to lie down in a dark, quiet room during an attack and to place ice packs on his forehead or a cold cloth over his eyes.

• Instruct the patient to take the prescribed medication at the onset of migraine symptoms, to prevent dehydration by drinking plenty of fluids after nausea and vomiting subside, and to use other headache-relief measures.

• Bear in mind that the patient with a migraine headache usually needs to be hospitalized only if nausea and vomiting are severe enough to induce dehydration and, possibly, shock.

# HEARING LOSS

Loss of hearing results from a mechanical or nervous impediment to the transmission of sound waves. Hearing loss is classified into three major forms:

• *Conductive loss* is the interrupted passage of sound from the external ear to the junction of the stapes and oval window.

• *Sensorineural loss* is impaired cochlear or acoustic (eighth cranial) nerve dysfunction, causing failure of transmission of sound impulses within the inner ear or brain.

• *Mixed loss* is a combination of conductive and sensorineural hearing loss.

Hearing loss may be partial or complete and is calculated from the American Medical Association formula: Hearing is 1.5% impaired for every decibel (dB) that the pure tone average exceeds 25 dB.

## Causes

Hearing loss may be congenital, or it may be caused by drugs, illness, loud noise, or aging.

### Congenital hearing loss

Hearing loss may be transmitted as a dominant, autosomal dominant, autosomal recessive, or sex-linked recessive trait. In neonates, it may also result from trauma, toxicity, or infection during pregnancy or delivery.

Predisposing factors include a family history of hearing loss or known hereditary disorders (such as otosclerosis), maternal exposure to rubella or syphilis during pregnancy, use of ototoxic drugs during pregnancy, prolonged fetal anoxia during delivery, and congenital abnormalities of the ears, nose, or throat.

Premature or low-birth-weight infants are most likely to have structural or functional hearing impairments; those with serum bilirubin levels greater than 20 mg/dl also risk hearing impairment from the toxic effect of high serum bilirubin levels on the brain.

In addition, trauma during delivery may cause intracranial hemorrhage and damage the cochlea or acoustic nerve.

### Sudden deafness

Sudden hearing loss may occur in a person with no prior hearing impairment. This condition is considered a medical emergency because prompt treatment may restore full hearing. Its causes and predisposing factors may include:

• acute infections, especially mumps (the most common cause of unilateral sensorineural hearing loss in children) and other bacterial and viral infections, such as rubella, rubeola, influenza, herpes zoster, and infectious mononucleosis, and mycoplasmal infections

• metabolic disorders, such as diabetes mellitus, hypothyroidism, and hyperlipoproteinemia

• vascular disorders, such as hypertension and arteriosclerosis

• head trauma or brain tumors

• ototoxic drugs, such as tobramycin, streptomycin, quinine, gentamicin, furosemide, and ethacrynic acid

• neurologic disorders, such as multiple sclerosis and neurosyphilis

• blood dyscrasias, such as leukemia and hypercoagulation.

### Noise-induced hearing loss

Hearing loss caused by loud noise may be transient or permanent and may follow prolonged exposure to loud noise (85 to 90 dB) or brief exposure to extremely loud noise (> 90 dB). Such hearing loss is common in workers subjected to constant industrial noise and in military personnel, hunters, and rock musicians.

### Presbycusis

An otologic effect of aging, presbycusis results from a loss of hair cells in the organ of Corti. This disorder causes sensorineural hearing loss, usually of high-frequency tones.

### Signs and symptoms

The four types of hearing loss have different signs and symptoms:

• Although congenital hearing loss may produce no obvious signs of hearing impairment at birth, a deficient response to auditory stimuli generally becomes apparent within 2 to 3 days of birth. As the child grows older, hearing loss impairs speech development.

• Sudden deafness may be conductive, sensorineural, or mixed, depending on its cause. Associated clinical features depend on the underlying cause.

• Noise-induced hearing loss causes sensorineural damage, the extent of which depends on the duration and intensity of the noise. Initially, the patient loses perception of certain frequencies (around 4,000 Hz) but with continued exposure eventually loses perception of all frequencies.

• Presbycusis usually produces tinnitus and the inability to understand the spoken word.

### Diagnosis

Patient, family, and occupational histories and a complete audiologic examination usually provide ample evidence of hearing loss and suggest possible causes or predisposing factors. The Weber and Rinne tests and other specialized audiologic tests differentiate between conductive and sensorineural hearing loss.

### Treatment

Measures for treating each type of hearing loss vary.

### Congenital hearing loss

After identifying the underlying cause, therapy for congenital hearing loss refractory to surgery consists of developing the patient's ability to communicate through sign language, speech reading, or other effective means.

Measures to prevent congenital hearing loss include aggressively immunizing children against rubella to reduce the risk of maternal exposure during pregnancy; educating pregnant women about the dangers of exposure to drugs, chemicals, or infection; and careful monitoring of the fetus during labor and delivery to prevent fetal anoxia.

### Sudden deafness

Treatment of sudden deafness requires prompt identification of the underlying cause. Prevention requires educating patients and health care professionals about the many causes of sudden deafness and the ways to recognize and treat them.

### Noise-induced hearing loss

Overnight rest usually restores normal hearing in those who have been exposed to noise levels greater than 90 dB for several hours but not in those who have been exposed to such noise repeatedly. As hearing deteriorates, treatment must include speech and hearing rehabilitation because hearing aids are seldom helpful.

Prevention of noise-induced hearing loss requires public recognition of the dangers of noise exposure and insistence on the use, as mandated by law, of protective devices such as earplugs during occupational exposure to noise.

### Presbycusis

Patients with presbycusis usually require a hearing aid.

### Special considerations

• When speaking to a patient with hearing loss who can read lips, stand directly in front of him with the light on your face and speak slowly and distinctly. Approach the patient within his visual range, and elicit his attention by raising your arm or waving; touching him may be unnecessarily startling.

• Don't smile, chew gum, or cover your mouth when talking. It makes lip reading more difficult.

• Make other staff members and hospital personnel aware of the patient's handicap and his established method of communication.

• Carefully explain all diagnostic tests and hospital procedures in a way the patient understands.

➤ CLINICAL TIP   Write out important statements or information for the patient. He may be embarrassed to tell you he did not hear everything you said.

• Make sure the patient with a hearing loss is in an area where he can observe unit activities and people approaching because such a patient depends totally on visual clues.

• When addressing an older patient, speak slowly and distinctly in a low tone; avoid shouting.

• Don't show annoyance by careless facial expressions.

• Provide emotional support and encouragement to the patient who is learning to use a hearing aid. Teach him how the aid works and how to maintain it.

• Assist the patient in setting realistic goals for recreational and leisure activities.

• Refer children with suspected hearing loss to an audiologist or otolaryngologist for further evaluation.

• To help prevent hearing loss, watch for signs of hearing impairment in patients receiving ototoxic drugs. Emphasize the danger of excessive exposure to noise; stress the danger of exposure to drugs, chemicals, and infection (especially rubella) to pregnant women; and encourage the use of protective devices in a noisy environment.

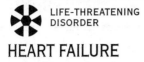

# HEART FAILURE

A syndrome characterized by myocardial dysfunction, heart failure leads to impaired pump performance (reduced cardiac output) or to frank heart failure and abnormal circulatory congestion. Congestion of systemic venous circulation may result in peripheral edema or hepatomegaly; congestion of pulmonary circulation may cause pulmonary edema, an acute, life-threatening emergency.

Pump failure usually occurs in a damaged left ventricle (left-sided heart failure) but may occur in the right ventricle (right-sided heart failure) either as a primary disorder or secondary to left-sided heart failure. Sometimes left- and right-sided heart failure develop simultaneously.

Although heart failure may be acute (as a direct result of myocardial infarction), it's generally a chronic disorder associated with retention of sodium and water by the kidneys. Advances in diagnostic and therapeutic techniques have greatly improved the outlook for patients with heart failure, but the prognosis still depends on the underlying cause and its response to treatment.

## Causes

Heart failure may result from a primary abnormality of the heart muscle (such as an infarction), inadequate myocardial perfusion due to coronary artery disease, or cardiomyopathy. Other causes include:

• mechanical disturbances in ventricular filling during diastole when there is too little blood for the ventricle to pump, as in mitral stenosis secondary to rheumatic heart disease or constrictive pericarditis and atrial fibrillation

• systolic hemodynamic disturbances, such as excessive cardiac workload due to volume overloading or pressure overload, that limit the heart's pumping ability.

These disturbances can result from mitral or aortic insufficiency, which causes volume overloading, and aortic stenosis or systemic hypertension, which results in increased resistance to ventricular emptying.

Reduced cardiac output triggers three compensatory mechanisms: ventricular dilation, hypertrophy, and increased sympathetic activity. These mechanisms improve cardiac output at the expense of increased ventricular work.

### Cardiac dilation

In cardiac dilation, an increase in end-diastolic ventricular volume (preload) causes increased stroke work and stroke volume during contraction, stretching cardiac muscle fibers beyond optimum limits and producing pulmonary congestion and pulmonary hypertension, which lead in turn to right-sided heart failure.

### Ventricular hypertrophy

In ventricular hypertrophy, an increase in muscle mass or the diameter of the left ventricle allows the heart to pump against increased resistance (impedance) to the outflow of blood.

An increase in ventricular diastolic pressure necessary to fill the enlarged ventricle may compromise diastolic coronary blood flow, limiting the oxygen supply to the ventricle and causing ischemia and impaired myocardial contractility.

### Increased sympathetic activity

As a response to decreased cardiac output and blood pressure, increased sympathetic activity occurs by enhancing

## PULMONARY EDEMA: HOW TO INTERVENE

Obtain the patient history, assist with diagnostic tests, and assess respiratory, mental, and cardiovascular status.

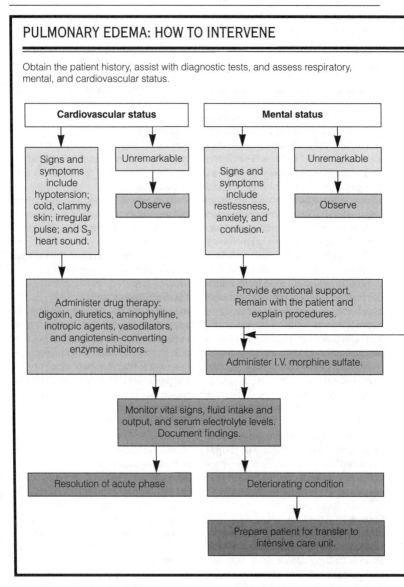

peripheral vascular resistance, contractility, heart rate, and venous return.

Signs of increased sympathetic activity, such as cool extremities and clamminess, may indicate impending heart failure. Increased sympathetic activity

also restricts blood flow to the kidneys, which respond by reducing the glomerular filtration rate and increasing tubular reabsorption of sodium and water, in turn expanding the circulating blood volume. This renal mechanism, if

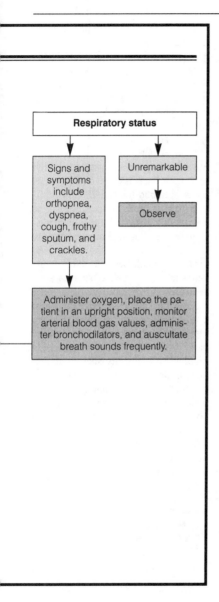

**Respiratory status**

→ Signs and symptoms include orthopnea, dyspnea, cough, frothy sputum, and crackles.

→ Unremarkable

→ Observe

→ Administer oxygen, place the patient in an upright position, monitor arterial blood gas values, administer bronchodilators, and auscultate breath sounds frequently.

comply with the prescribed treatment regimen.

### Signs and symptoms
Left-sided heart failure primarily produces pulmonary signs and symptoms; right-sided heart failure primarily produces systemic signs and symptoms. However, heart failure often affects both sides of the heart.

#### *Left-sided heart failure*
Clinical signs of left-sided heart failure include dyspnea, orthopnea, crackles, possibly wheezing, hypoxia, respiratory acidosis, cough, cyanosis or pallor, palpitations, arrhythmias, elevated blood pressure, and pulsus alternans.

#### *Right-sided heart failure*
Clinical signs of right-sided heart failure include dependent peripheral edema, hepatomegaly, splenomegaly, jugular vein distention, ascites, slow weight gain, arrhythmias, hepatojugular reflex, abdominal distention, nausea, vomiting, anorexia, weakness, fatigue, dizziness, and syncope.

#### *Complications*
These typically include pulmonary edema, venostasis with a predisposition to thromboembolism (associated primarily with prolonged bed rest), cerebral insufficiency, and renal insufficiency with severe electrolyte imbalance. (See *Pulmonary edema: How to intervene.*)

### Diagnosis
The following tests are used to diagnose heart failure:
● *Electrocardiography* reflects heart strain, enlargement, and ischemia. It may also reveal atrial enlargement, tachycardia, and extrasystole.
● *Chest X-ray* shows increased pulmonary vascular markings, interstitial

unchecked, can aggravate congestion and produce overt edema.

Chronic heart failure may worsen as a result of respiratory tract infections, pulmonary embolism, stress, increased sodium or water intake, and failure to

edema, pleural effusion, and cardiomegaly.

• *Pulmonary artery monitoring* typically demonstrates elevated pulmonary artery and pulmonary artery wedge pressures, elevated left ventricular end-diastolic pressure in left-sided heart failure, and elevated right atrial pressure or central venous pressure in right-sided heart failure.

• *Echocardiography* demonstrates left ventricular dysfunction with a reduced ejection fraction.

## Treatment

The aim of therapy is to improve pump function by reversing the compensatory mechanisms that are producing the symptoms. Heart failure can be controlled quickly by treatment consisting of:

• diuresis to reduce total blood volume and circulatory congestion

• prolonged bed rest

• digoxin to strengthen myocardial contractility

• vasodilators and angiotensin-converting enzyme inhibitors to increase cardiac output by reducing the impedance to ventricular outflow (afterload)

• antiembolism stockings to prevent venostasis and thromboembolus.

## Special considerations

During the acute phase:

• Place the patient in high Fowler's position, and give him supplemental oxygen to help him breathe more easily.

• Weigh the patient daily, and check for peripheral edema. Carefully monitor his I.V. intake and urine output, vital signs, and mental status. Auscultate the heart for abnormal sounds ($S_3$ gallop) and the lungs for crackles or rhonchi.

• Frequently monitor levels of blood urea nitrogen and serum creatinine, potassium, sodium, chloride, and magnesium.

• The patient should have continuous cardiac monitoring during acute and advanced stages to identify and treat arrhythmias promptly.

• To prevent deep vein thrombosis due to vascular congestion, assist the patient with range-of-motion exercises. Enforce bed rest and apply antiembolism stockings. Check regularly for calf pain and tenderness.

• Allow adequate rest periods.

Before discharge:

• Advise the patient to avoid foods high in sodium, such as canned or commercially prepared foods and dairy products, to curb fluid overload.

• Explain to the patient that the potassium he loses through diuretic therapy must be replaced by taking a prescribed potassium supplement and eating potassium-rich foods, such as bananas, apricots, and orange juice.

• Stress the need for regular checkups.

• Emphasize the importance of taking digoxin exactly as prescribed. Tell the patient to watch for and immediately report signs of toxicity, such as anorexia, vomiting, and yellow vision.

• Tell the patient to promptly report any pulse irregularities. He should also report dizziness, blurred vision, shortness of breath, persistent dry cough, palpitations, increased fatigue, paroxysmal nocturnal dyspnea, swollen ankles, decreased urine output, and rapid weight gain (5 to 21 lb [2.25 to 9.5 kg] in a week).

 LIFE-THREATENING DISORDER

# HEAT SYNDROME

Resulting from environmental or internal conditions that increase heat production or impair heat dissipation, heat syndrome falls into three categories: heat cramps, heat exhaustion, and heatstroke. (See *Managing heat syndrome.*)

# MANAGING HEAT SYNDROME

| TYPE AND PREDISPOSING FACTORS | SIGNS AND SYMPTOMS | MANAGEMENT |
|---|---|---|
| **HEAT CRAMPS** | | |
| • Commonly affect young adults<br>• Strenuous activity without training or acclimatization<br>• Normal to high temperature or high humidity | • Muscle twitching and spasms, weakness, severe muscle cramps<br>• Nausea<br>• Normal temperature or slight fever<br>• Normal central nervous system findings<br>• Diaphoresis | • Hospitalization is usually unnecessary.<br>• To replace fluid and electrolytes, give a balanced electrolyte drink.<br>• Loosen patient's clothing, and have him lie down in a cool place. Massage his muscles. If muscle cramps are severe, start an I.V. infusion with normal saline solution. |
| **HEAT EXHAUSTION** | | |
| • Commonly affects young people<br>• Physical activity without acclimatization<br>• Decreased heat dissipation<br>• High temperature and humidity | • Muscle cramps (infrequent)<br>• Nausea and vomiting<br>• Decreased blood pressure<br>• Thready, rapid pulse<br>• Cool, pallid skin<br>• Headache, mental confusion, syncope, giddiness<br>• Oliguria, thirst<br>• No fever<br>• Sweating | • Hospitalization is usually unnecessary but patient may need emergency evaluation.<br>• Immediately give a balanced electrolyte drink.<br>• Loosen patient's clothing, and put him in a shock position in a cool place. Massage his muscles. If cramps are severe, start an I.V. infusion.<br>• If needed, give oxygen. |
| **HEATSTROKE** | | |
| • Exertional heatstroke commonly affects young, healthy people who are involved in strenuous activity.<br>• Classic heatstroke commonly affects elderly, inactive people who have cardiovascular disease or who take drugs that influence temperature regulation. | • Hypertension followed by hypotension<br>• Atrial or ventricular tachycardia<br>• Hot, dry, red skin, which later turns gray; no diaphoresis<br>• Confusion, progressing to seizures and loss of consciousness<br>• Temperature higher than 104° F (40° C) | • Initiate ABCs (airway, breathing, and circulation) of life support.<br>• To lower patient's body temperature, cool rapidly with ice packs on arterial pressure points and hypothermia blankets.<br>• To replace fluids and electrolytes, start an I.V. infusion.<br>• Hospitalization is needed. |

*(continued)*

| MANAGING HEAT SYNDROME *(continued)* | | |
| --- | --- | --- |
| **TYPE AND PREDISPOSING FACTORS** | **SIGNS AND SYMPTOMS** | **MANAGEMENT** |
| **HEATSTROKE** *(continued)* | | |
| • High temperature and humidity without any wind | • Dilated pupils<br>• Slow, deep respirations; then Cheyne-Stokes respirations | • Insert nasogastric tube to prevent aspiration.<br>• Give a benzodiazepine to control seizures, I.V. chlorpromazine to reduce shivering, or mannitol to maintain urine output.<br>• Monitor temperature, intake, output, and cardiac status. Give dobutamine to correct cardiogenic shock. (Vasoconstrictors are contraindicated.) |

## Causes

Normally, humans adjust to excessive temperatures by complex cardiovascular and neurologic changes that are coordinated by the hypothalamus. Heat loss offsets heat production to regulate the body temperature. This is done by evaporation (sweating) or vasodilation, which cools the body's surface by radiation, conduction, and convection.

Heat production increases with exercise, infection, and use of drugs such as amphetamines.

Heat loss decreases with high temperatures or humidity, lack of acclimatization, excess clothing, obesity, dehydration, cardiovascular disease, sweat gland dysfunction, and use of drugs such as phenothiazines and anticholinergics.

When heat loss mechanisms fail to offset heat production, the body retains heat and heat syndrome may develop.

## Special considerations

• Heat illnesses are easily preventable, so it is important to educate the public about the various factors that cause them. This information is especially vital for athletes, laborers, and soldiers in field training.

CLINICAL TIP  Advise your patients to avoid heat syndrome by taking the following precautions in hot weather: rest frequently, avoid hot places, drink adequate fluids, and wear loose-fitting, lightweight clothing.

• Advise patients who are obese, elderly, or taking drugs that impair heat regulation to avoid overheating.

• Tell patients who have had heat cramps or heat exhaustion to increase their salt and water intake. They should also refrain from exercising until symptoms resolve, then resume exercises gradually with plenty of electrolyte-containing fluids and precautions to prevent overheating.

• Warn patients with heatstroke that residual hypersensitivity to high temperatures may persist for several months.

• Parents should be aware that young children and infants are at risk for overheating in hot weather.

# HEMOPHILIA

A hereditary bleeding disorder, hemophilia results from the deficiency of specific clotting factors. *Hemophilia A* (classic hemophilia), which affects more than 80% of all hemophiliacs, results from a deficiency of factor VIII; *hemophilia B* (Christmas disease), which affects 15% of hemophiliacs, results from a deficiency of factor IX.

The severity and prognosis of bleeding disorders vary with the degree of deficiency and the site of bleeding. The overall prognosis is best in mild hemophilia, which doesn't cause spontaneous bleeding and joint deformities.

Advances in treatment have greatly improved the prognosis, and many hemophiliacs live normal life spans. Surgical procedures can be done safely at special treatment centers for hemophiliacs under the guidance of a hematologist.

## Causes
Hemophilia A and hemophilia B are inherited as X-linked recessive traits. This means that female carriers have a 50% chance of transmitting the gene to each daughter, who would then be a carrier, and a 50% chance of transmitting the gene to each son, who would be born with hemophilia.

### Incidence
Hemophilia is the most common X-linked genetic disease, occurring in about 1.25 in 10,000 live male births. Hemophilia A is five times more common than hemophilia B. Hemophilia causes abnormal bleeding because of a specific clotting factor malfunction. After a person with hemophilia forms a platelet plug at a bleeding site, clotting factor deficiency impairs the capacity to form a stable fibrin clot.

## Signs and symptoms
Hemophilia produces abnormal bleeding, which may be mild, moderate, or severe, depending on the degree of factor deficiency.

### Mild hemophilia
The mild form of hemophilia frequently goes undiagnosed until adulthood because the patient with a mild deficiency doesn't bleed spontaneously or after minor trauma but has prolonged bleeding if challenged by major trauma or surgery. Postoperative bleeding continues as a slow ooze or ceases and starts again up to 8 days after surgery.

### Moderate and severe hemophilia
Moderate hemophilia causes symptoms similar to those of severe hemophilia but produces only occasional spontaneous bleeding episodes.

Severe hemophilia causes spontaneous bleeding. The first sign of severe hemophilia usually is excessive bleeding after circumcision. Later, spontaneous bleeding or severe bleeding after minor trauma may produce large subcutaneous and deep intramuscular hematomas.

Bleeding into joints and muscles causes pain, swelling, extreme tenderness and, possibly, permanent deformity. Bleeding near peripheral nerves may cause peripheral neuropathies, pain, paresthesia, and muscle atrophy.

If bleeding impairs blood flow through a major vessel, it can cause ischemia and gangrene. Pharyngeal, lingual, intracardial, intracerebral, and intracranial bleeding may lead to shock and death.

## Diagnosis
A history of prolonged bleeding after trauma or surgery (including dental ex-

tractions) or of episodes of spontaneous bleeding into muscles or joints usually indicates some defect in the hemostatic mechanism.

Specific coagulation factor assays can diagnose the type and severity of hemophilia. A positive family history can also help diagnose hemophilia, but 20% of all cases have no family history.

Characteristic findings in hemophilia A include:

- factor VIII assay 0% to 30% of normal
- prolonged activated partial thromboplastin time (APTT)
- normal platelet count and function, bleeding time, and prothrombin time.

Characteristics of hemophilia B include:

- deficient factor IX-C
- baseline coagulation results similar to those in hemophilia A, with normal factor VIII.

In hemophilia A or hemophilia B, the degree of factor deficiency determines severity:

- mild hemophilia — factor levels 5% to 40% of normal
- moderate hemophilia — factor levels 1% to 5% of normal
- severe hemophilia — factor levels < 1% of normal.

## Treatment

Hemophilia is not curable, but treatment can prevent crippling deformities and prolong life expectancy. Correct treatment quickly stops bleeding by increasing plasma levels of deficient clotting factors to help prevent disabling deformities that result from repeated bleeding into muscles and joints. Treatment varies according to the type of hemophilia.

- In hemophilia A, cryoprecipitated antihemophilic factor (AHF), lyophilized AHF, or both, given in doses large enough to raise clotting factor levels

above 25% of normal can permit normal hemostasis. Before surgery, AHF is administered to raise clotting factors to hemostatic levels. Levels are then kept within a normal range until the wound has completely healed.

- In hemophilia B, administration of factor IX concentrate during bleeding episodes increases factor IX levels.

A person with hemophilia who undergoes surgery needs careful management by a hematologist with expertise in hemophilia care. The patient requires replacement of the deficient factor before and after surgery. Such replacement may be necessary even for minor surgery such as a dental extraction.

In addition, aminocaproic acid is frequently used for oral bleeding to inhibit the active fibrinolytic system present in the oral mucosa. Preventive treatment teaches the patient how to avoid trauma, manage minor bleeding, and recognize bleeding that requires immediate medical intervention. (See *Managing hemophilia.*)

## Special considerations

During bleeding episodes:

- Give deficient clotting factor or plasma, as needed. The body uses up AHF in 48 to 72 hours, so repeat infusions, as needed, until bleeding stops.
- Apply cold compresses or ice bags, and raise the injured part.
- To prevent recurrence of bleeding, restrict activity for 48 hours after bleeding is under control.
- Control pain with an analgesic, such as acetaminophen, propoxyphene, codeine, or meperidine, as needed. Avoid I.M. injections because of possible hematoma formation at the injection site. Aspirin and aspirin-containing medications are contraindicated because they decrease platelet adherence and may increase the bleeding.

TEACHING CHECKLIST

# MANAGING HEMOPHILIA

Teach parents how to care for their child with hemophilia as follows.

## Risk for injury and bleeding

• Instruct parents to notify the doctor immediately after even a minor injury, but especially after an injury to the head, neck, or abdomen. Such injuries may require special blood factor replacement. Also, they should check with the doctor before allowing dental extractions or any other surgery.

• Stress the importance of regular, careful toothbrushing to prevent the need for dental surgery. The child should use a soft toothbrush.

• Teach parents to be alert for signs of severe internal bleeding, such as severe pain or swelling in a joint or muscle, stiffness, decreased joint movement, severe abdominal pain, severe headache, blood in the urine, and black, tarry stools.

## Risk for other disorders

• Because the child receives blood components, he's at risk for hepatitis. Early signs — headache, fever, decreased appetite, nausea, vomiting, abdominal tenderness, and pain over the liver — may appear 3 weeks to 6 months after treatment with blood components.

• Discuss the increased risk for human immunodeficiency virus (HIV) infection if the child received a blood product before routine screening of blood products for HIV began. Tell his parents to ask the doctor about periodic testing for HIV.

## Precautions and treatment

• Urge parents to make sure their child wears a medical identification bracelet at all times.

• *Warn parents never to give their child aspirin.* It can increase the ten-

dency to bleed. Advise them to give acetaminophen instead.

• Instruct parents to protect their child from injury but to avoid unnecessary restrictions that impair his development. For example, they can sew padded patches into the knees and elbows of a toddler's clothing to protect these joints during falls. They must forbid an older child to play contact sports such as football but can encourage swimming or playing golf.

• Teach parents to apply cold compresses or ice bags to an injured area and to elevate it or apply light pressure to a bleeding site. To prevent recurrence of bleeding, advise parents to restrict their child's activity for 48 hours after his bleeding is under control.

• If parents have been trained to give blood factor components at home to avoid hospitalization, make sure they know how to perform venipuncture and infusion techniques and don't delay treatment during bleeding episodes.

• Instruct parents to keep blood factor concentrate and infusion equipment on hand, even on vacation.

• Emphasize the importance of having the child keep routine appointments at the local hemophilia center.

## Importance of genetic screening

• Daughters should have genetic screening and testing to determine whether they are hemophilia carriers. Affected males should have counseling as well. If they mate with a noncarrier, 50% of their daughters will be carriers. If they mate with a carrier, each male or female child has a 25% chance of being affected.

• For more information, refer parents to the National Hemophilia Foundation.

If the patient has bled into a joint:
- Immediately elevate the joint.
- To restore joint mobility, begin range-of-motion exercises at least 48 hours after the bleeding is controlled. Tell the patient to avoid weight bearing until the bleeding stops and swelling subsides.

After bleeding episodes and surgery:
- Watch closely for signs of further bleeding, such as increased pain and swelling, fever, and shock.
- Closely monitor APTT.
- Teach parents special precautions to prevent bleeding episodes, signs of internal bleeding, and how to administer emergency first aid.
- Refer new patients to a hemophilia treatment center for evaluation. The center will devise a treatment plan for the patient's primary doctor and serve as a resource for everyone involved in the patient's care.
- People who have been exposed to the human immunodeficiency virus (HIV) through contaminated blood products need special support.

➤ CLINICAL TIP    Referral to a local or national acquired immunodeficiency syndrome support group may be helpful for patients who test positive for HIV.
- Refer the patient and family for genetic counseling to understand how the disease is inherited, and discuss prenatal testing.

# HEMORRHOIDS

Hemorrhoidal varices are part of the normal anatomy. Dilation and enlargement of the superior plexus of the superior hemorrhoidal veins located above the dentate line produce internal hemorrhoids. Enlargement of the plexus of the inferior hemorrhoidal veins located below the dentate line produces external hemorrhoids. External hemorrhoids may protrude from the rectum. Hemorrhoids occur in both sexes. Incidence is generally highest between ages 20 and 50.

## Causes
Hemorrhoids result from activities that increase intravenous pressure, resulting in distention and engorgement. Predisposing factors include prolonged sitting, straining at defecation, constipation, low-fiber diet, pregnancy, and obesity.

Other factors include hepatic disease, such as cirrhosis, amebic abscesses, or hepatitis; alcoholism; and anorectal infections.

## Signs and symptoms
Hemorrhoids are classified as *first-degree, second-degree, third-degree,* or *fourth degree,* depending on their severity. First-degree hemorrhoids are confined to the anal canal. Second-degree hemorrhoids occur when the hemorrhoids prolapse during straining but reduce spontaneously. Third-degree hemorrhoids are prolapsed hemorrhoids that require manual reduction after each bowel movement. Fourth-degree hemorrhoids are irreducible and chronically remain prolapsed. Signs and symptoms vary accordingly.
- Although first-degree hemorrhoids may produce no symptoms, they characteristically cause painless, intermittent bleeding during defecation. Bright red blood appears in stools or on toilet paper because of injury to the fragile mucosa covering the hemorrhoid. First-degree hemorrhoids may itch from poor anal hygiene.
- When second-degree hemorrhoids prolapse, they are usually painless and spontaneously return to the anal canal after defecation.

• Third-degree hemorrhoids cause constant discomfort and prolapse in response to any increase in intra-abdominal pressure. They must be manually reduced. Thrombosis of external hemorrhoids produces sudden rectal pain and a large, firm, subcutaneous lump that the patient can feel.

Hemorrhoids seldom cause severe bleeding leading to anemia.

➤ CLINICAL TIP Discomfort and pain usually does not occur with internal hemorrhoids. Thrombosed external hemorrhoids result in patients who strain while defecating, lift heavy objects, or have frequent bowel movements, such as those with inflammatory bowel disease.

### Diagnosis

Physical examination confirms external hemorrhoids. Anoscopy provides for visual examination of internal hemorrhoids.

### Treatment

Treatment depends on the type and severity of the hemorrhoids.

#### Nonsurgical treatments

Treatment includes measures to control pain, combat swelling and congestion, and regulate bowel habits. Patients can relieve constipation by consuming a high-fiber diet and increasing fluid intake by drinking eight to ten 8-oz glasses of water per day or by using bulking agents such as psyllium (Metamucil).

Venous congestion can be prevented by avoiding prolonged sitting on the toilet; local swelling and pain can be decreased with local anesthetic agents (lotions, creams, or suppositories) or astringents. Hydrocortisone (Anusol) suppositories may be used for edematous, prolapsed hemorrhoids in combination with warm sitz baths.

Hemorrhoids may be treated with injection sclerotherapy and rubber band ligation.

➤ CLINICAL TIP There is no evidence that topical cleaners or lotions (pads, foams, ointments) cause symptomatic hemorrhoids to shrink; they provide relief by soothing the area.

#### Hemorrhoidectomy

Hemorrhoidectomy is performed for patients with severe bleeding due to third- or fourth-degree hemorrhoids and those with thrombosed fourth-degree hemorrhoids. This procedure is contraindicated in patients with blood dyscrasias (acute leukemia, aplastic anemia, or hemophilia) or gastric cancer and during the first trimester of pregnancy.

### Special considerations

• To prepare the patient for outpatient hemorrhoidectomy, instruct him to administer an enema the night before and morning of surgery.

• Postoperatively, check for signs of prolonged rectal bleeding, administer adequate analgesics, and provide sitz baths.

• Before discharge, tell the patient that he can resume his regular diet.

• Instruct the patient to take a bulking agent, such as psyllium, about 1 hour after the evening meal to help ensure a daily bowel movement. Advise him to maintain regular bowel habits and avoid straining.

• Instruct the patient to avoid vigorous wiping and harsh soaps.

# HEMOTHORAX

In hemothorax, blood from damaged intercostal, pleural, mediastinal and, infrequently, lung parenchymal vessels enters the pleural cavity. Depending on the amount of bleeding and the underlying cause, hemothorax may be associated with varying degrees of lung collapse and mediastinal shift. Pneumothorax — air in the pleural cavity — often accompanies hemothorax.

## Causes

Hemothorax usually results from blunt or penetrating chest trauma; in fact, about 25% of patients with such trauma have hemothorax. Less often, it results from thoracic surgery, pulmonary infarction, neoplasm, dissecting thoracic aneurysm, or anticoagulant therapy.

## Signs and symptoms

The patient with hemothorax may experience chest pain, tachypnea, and mild to severe dyspnea, depending on the amount of blood in the pleural cavity and associated pathology. If respiratory failure results, the patient may appear anxious, restless, possibly stuporous, and cyanotic; marked blood loss produces hypotension and shock.

The affected side of the chest expands and stiffens and the unaffected side rises and falls with the patient's gasping respirations.

## Diagnosis

The following clinical test results, along with a history of trauma, strongly suggest hemothorax:

• *Percussion* reveals dullness and, on auscultation, decreased to absent breath sounds over the affected side.

• *Thoracentesis* yields blood or serosanguineous fluid.

• *Chest X-rays* show pleural fluid with or without mediastinal shift.

• *Arterial blood gas (ABG) analysis* may document respiratory failure.

• *Hemoglobin level* may be decreased, depending on blood loss.

## Treatment

Effective treatment stabilizes the patient's condition, stops the bleeding, evacuates blood from the pleural space, and reexpands the underlying lung. Mild hemothorax usually clears rapidly in 10 to 14 days, requiring only observation for further bleeding.

In severe hemothorax, thoracentesis serves not only as a diagnostic tool, but also as a method of removing fluid from the pleural cavity.

After the diagnosis is confirmed, a chest tube is inserted into the sixth intercostal space at the posterior axillary line. Suction may be used; a large-bore tube is used to prevent clot blockage. If the chest tube doesn't improve the patient's condition, he may need a thoracotomy to evacuate blood and clots and to control bleeding.

## Special considerations

• Give oxygen by face mask or nasal cannula.

• Give I.V. fluids and blood transfusions (monitored by a central venous pressure line), as needed, to treat shock. Monitor ABG levels often.

• Explain all procedures to the patient to allay his fears. Assist with thoracentesis. Warn the patient not to cough during this procedure.

• Observe chest tube drainage carefully, and record the volume drained at least every hour. Keep the chest tube open and free of clots. If the tube is warm and full of blood and the bloody fluid level in the water-seal bottle is rising rapidly, the patient may need immediate surgery.

• Watch the patient closely for pallor and gasping respirations. Monitor his vital signs diligently. Falling blood pressure and rising pulse and respiratory rates may indicate shock or massive bleeding.

# HEPATIC ENCEPHALOPATHY

Also known as hepatic coma, hepatic encephalopathy is a neurologic syndrome that results from the liver's failure to detoxify noxious agents that arise from the GI tract. Most common in patients with cirrhosis, this syndrome is caused primarily by ammonia intoxication of the brain. It may be acute and self-limiting or chronic and progressive.

Treatment requires correction of the precipitating cause and reduction of blood ammonia levels. In advanced stages, the prognosis is extremely poor, despite vigorous treatment.

## Causes

Hepatic encephalopathy develops as a result of rising blood ammonia levels. Several factors cause these levels to rise.

### Improper shunting of blood

Normally, the ammonia produced by protein breakdown in the bowel is metabolized to urea in the liver. When portal blood shunts past the liver, ammonia directly enters the systemic circulation and is carried to the brain.

Such shunting may result from the collateral venous circulation that develops in portal hypertension or from surgically created portal-systemic shunts. Cirrhosis further compounds this problem because impaired hepatocellular function prevents conversion of ammonia that reaches the liver.

### Other factors

Other factors that predispose to rising ammonia levels include excessive protein intake, sepsis, excessive accumulation of nitrogenous body wastes (from constipation or GI hemorrhage), and

bacterial action on protein and urea to form ammonia.

Certain other factors heighten the brain's sensitivity to ammonia intoxication: fluid and electrolyte imbalances (especially metabolic alkalosis), hypoxia, azotemia, impaired glucose metabolism, infection, and administration of sedatives, narcotics, and general anesthetics.

## Signs and symptoms

Clinical manifestations of hepatic encephalopathy vary, depending on the severity of neurologic involvement, and develop in four stages. Encephalopathy is usually graded by behavioral changes, the presence of asterixis, and EEG findings, with behavioral changes being the most apparent indicator.

• *Grade or stage I (prodromal stage):* mood fluctuation, sleep-wake reversal, forgetfulness; often overlooked because early symptoms, such as slight personality changes (disorientation, forgetfulness, slurred speech) and a slight tremor, are subtle

• *Grade or stage II (impending stage):* disorientation, confusion; may be incontinent; tremor progressing to asterixis, the hallmark of hepatic encephalopathy. Asterixis is characterized by quick, irregular extensions and flexions of the wrists and fingers when the wrists are held out straight and the hands flexed upward. Lethargy, aberrant behavior, and apraxia also occur.

• *Grade or stage III (stuporous stage):* hyperventilation; patient is stuporous but noisy and abusive when aroused.

• *Grade or stage IV (comatose stage):* hyperactive reflexes, a positive Babinski's sign, fetor hepaticus (musty, sweet breath odor), and coma.

## Diagnosis

Clinical features, a positive history of liver disease, and elevated serum ammonia levels in venous and arterial samples confirm hepatic encephalopathy. Other supportive test results include an EEG that slows as the disease progresses, an elevated bilirubin level, and prolonged prothrombin time.

## Treatment

Effective treatment stops the progression of encephalopathy by reducing blood ammonia levels. Such treatment eliminates ammonia-producing substances from the GI tract by:

● administration of lactulose to reduce the blood ammonia levels and use of sorbitol-induced catharsis to produce osmotic diarrhea

● reduction of dietary protein intake

● continuous aspiration of blood from the stomach

● administration of neomycin to suppress bacterial flora (preventing them from converting amino acids into ammonia).

### Lactulose

Lactulose traps ammonia in the bowel and promotes its excretion. It is effective because bacterial enzymes change lactulose to lactic acid, thereby rendering the colon too acidic for bacterial growth. At the same time, the resulting increase in free hydrogen ions prevents diffusion of ammonia through the mucosa; lactulose promotes conversion of systemically absorbable ammonia to ammonium, which is poorly absorbed and can be excreted.

The usual dosage of lactulose syrup is 30 to 45 ml by mouth (P.O.) three or four times daily. For acute hepatic coma, 300 ml diluted with 700 ml of water may be administered by retention enema. Lactulose therapy requires careful monitoring of fluid and electrolyte balance.

### Neomycin

Neomycin is usually given in a dose of 3 to 4 g daily P.O. or by retention enema. Although neomycin is nonabsorbable at the recommended dosage, an amount that exceeds 4 g daily may produce irreversible hearing loss and nephrotoxicity after prolonged use.

### Other treatments

Treatment may also include potassium supplements (80 to 120 mEq/day P.O. or I.V.) to correct alkalosis (from increased ammonia levels), especially if the patient is taking diuretics.

## Special considerations

● Frequently assess and record the patient's level of consciousness. Continually orient him to place and time.

● Keep a daily record of the patient's handwriting to monitor the progression of neurologic involvement.

● Monitor intake, output, and fluid and electrolyte balance. Check daily weight and measure abdominal girth. Immediately report signs of anemia (decreased hemoglobin), infection, alkalosis (increased serum bicarbonate levels), and GI bleeding (melena, hematemesis).

● Give prescribed drugs and watch for adverse effects.

● Consult with the dietitian to provide the specified low-protein diet, with carbohydrates supplying most of the calories. Provide good mouth care.

● Promote rest, comfort, and a quiet atmosphere. Discourage strenuous exercise.

● Use restraints if necessary, but avoid sedatives.

➤ CLINICAL TIP   Protect the comatose patient's eyes from corneal injury by using artificial tears or eye patches.

● Provide emotional support for the family of the patient with end-stage liver disease.

# HEPATITIS, NONVIRAL

Classified as toxic or drug-induced (idiosyncratic) hepatitis, nonviral hepatitis is an inflammation of the liver. Most patients recover from this illness, although a few develop fulminating hepatitis or cirrhosis.

## Causes

Nonviral hepatitis results from various causes.

- Alcohol overuse — follows heavy alcohol consumption
- Direct hepatotoxicity — hepatocellular damage and necrosis usually caused by toxins. It is dose-dependent and occurs primarily in connection with acetaminophen overdose.
- Idiosyncratic hepatotoxicity — follows a sensitization period of several weeks; caused by a host hypersensitivity to medications (isoniazid, methyldopa, mercaptopurine, lovastatin, pravastatin, dipyridamole, and halothane)
- Cholestatic reactions — caused by lack of bile excretion; possibly direct hepatotoxicity from oral contraceptives or anabolic steroids; hypersensitivity to phenothiazine derivatives such as chlorpromazine, antibiotics, thyroid medications, antidiabetic drugs, and cytotoxic drugs
- Metabolic and autoimmune disorders — acute exacerbations of subclinical liver disease, such as autoimmune hepatitis and Wilson's disease
- Infectious agents — systemic viruses, such as cytomegalovirus, mononucleosis or Epstein-Barr virus, measles virus, varicella zoster, adenovirus, herpes simplex virus, coxsackievirus, and human immunodeficiency virus; spirochetes such as those that cause syphilis and leptospirosis.

## Signs and symptoms

Clinical features of toxic and drug-induced hepatitis vary with the severity of the liver damage and the causative agent. In most patients, symptoms resemble those of viral hepatitis: anorexia, nausea, vomiting, jaundice, dark urine, hepatomegaly, possibly abdominal pain (with acute onset and massive necrosis), clay-colored stools, and pruritus with the cholestatic form of hepatitis.

⬤ CLINICAL TIP  Carbon tetrachloride poisoning also produces headache, dizziness, drowsiness, and vasomotor collapse; halothane-related hepatitis produces fever, moderate leukocytosis, and eosinophilia; chlorpromazine produces a rash, abrupt fever, arthralgias, lymphadenopathy, and epigastric or right upper quadrant pain.

## Diagnosis

Diagnostic findings include elevations in serum aspartate aminotransferase, alanine aminotransferase, both total and direct bilirubin (with cholestasis), and alkaline phosphatase levels; white blood cell (WBC) count; and eosinophil count (possible in the drug-induced type).

A liver biopsy may help identify the underlying pathology, especially infiltration with WBCs and eosinophils. Liver function tests have limited value in distinguishing between nonviral and viral hepatitis.

## Treatment

Effective treatment must remove the causative agent by lavage, catharsis, or hyperventilation, depending on the route of exposure. Acetylcysteine may serve as an antidote for toxic hepatitis caused by acetaminophen poisoning but doesn't prevent drug-induced hepatitis caused by other substances.

Corticosteroids may be prescribed for patients with drug-induced hepatitis.

**Special considerations**
To prevent this disease, teach the patient the proper use of drugs and the proper handling of cleaning agents and solvents.

# HEPATITIS, VIRAL

A fairly common systemic disease, viral hepatitis is marked by hepatocellular destruction, necrosis, and autolysis, leading to anorexia, jaundice, and hepatomegaly. In most patients, hepatic cells eventually regenerate with little or no residual damage. Old age and serious underlying disorders make complications more likely. The prognosis is poor if edema and end-stage liver disease develop.

There are five types of hepatitis:
• *Type A* (infectious or short-incubation hepatitis) is rising among homosexuals and in people with immunosuppression related to human immunodeficiency virus (HIV) infection. It's usually self-limiting and without a chronic form. About 40% of cases in the United States result from hepatitis A virus.
• *Type B* (serum or long-incubation hepatitis) also is increasing among HIV-positive individuals.

➤ CLINICAL TIP Hepatitis B is now considered a sexually transmitted disease because of its high incidence and rate of transmission by this route.

Routine screening of donor blood for the hepatitis B surface antigen (HBsAg) has decreased the incidence of post-transfusion cases, but transmission by needles shared by drug abusers remains a major problem. Acute signs and symptoms usually begin insidiously and last for 1 to 4 weeks. Urticaria or arthralgia that is experienced before any signs of jaundice is highly suggestive of hepati-

tis B infection. A chronic, potentially infectious state develops in about 10% of infected adults and in 70% to 90% of infected infants. This chronic state is associated with progressive liver disease in some individuals. Fulminant hepatitis can ensue, and there is an increased risk of primary hepatocellular carcinoma.
• *Type C* accounts for about 20% of all viral hepatitis cases and is primarily transmitted through blood and body fluids or obtained during tattooing.
• *Type D* (delta hepatitis) is responsible for about 50% of all cases of fulminant hepatitis, which has a high mortality. Developing in 1% of patients, fulminant hepatitis causes unremitting liver failure with encephalopathy. It progresses to coma and commonly leads to death within 2 weeks.

In the United States, type D hepatitis is confined to people who are frequently exposed to blood and blood products, such as I.V. drug users and hemophiliacs. It is transmitted parenterally and, less commonly, sexually.
• *Type E* (formerly grouped with type C under the name non-A, non-B hepatitis) occurs primarily in people who have recently returned from an endemic area (such as India, Africa, Asia, or Central America); it's more common in young adults and more severe in pregnant women.

**Causes**
The five major forms of viral hepatitis result from infection with the causative viruses: A, B, C, D, or E.

*Type A hepatitis*
Hepatitis A is highly contagious and usually transmitted by the fecal-oral route. It may also be transmitted parenterally.

> ◗ CLINICAL TIP I.V. drug abusers
> and recipients of multiple blood
product transfusions are at increased
risk for hepatitis A.

Hepatitis A usually results from ingestion of contaminated food, milk, or water. Outbreaks of this type are often traced to ingestion of seafood from polluted water.

### Type B hepatitis

Once thought to be transmitted only by the direct exchange of contaminated blood, hepatitis B is now also known to be transmitted by contact with human secretions and stool passed by health care workers, recipients of plasma-derived products, and hemodialysis patients. As a result, nurses, doctors, laboratory technicians, and dentists are frequently exposed to type B hepatitis, often as a result of wearing defective gloves.

Transmission also occurs during intimate sexual contact and through perinatal transmission.

### Type C hepatitis

Although hepatitis C viruses have been isolated, only a small percentage of patients have tested positive for them, perhaps reflecting the test's poor specificity. Usually, this type of hepatitis is transmitted through transfused blood from asymptomatic donors and receiving tattoos.

> ◗ CLINICAL TIP Most patients with
> hepatitis C are asymptomatic. Hepatitis C virus is associated with a high rate of chronic liver disease (chronic hepatitis, cirrhosis, and an increased risk of hepatocellular carcinoma), which develops in 50% to 80% of those infected. People who have chronic hepatitis C are considered infectious.

### Type D hepatitis

Hepatitis D is found only in patients with an acute or a chronic episode of hepatitis B and requires the presence of HBsAg. The type D virus depends on the double-shelled type B virus to replicate. For this reason, a type D infection can't outlast a type B infection.

Hepatitis D is rare in the United States, except in I.V. drug abusers.

### Type E hepatitis

Hepatitis E is transmitted enterically (oral-fecal and waterborne routes), much like type A. Because this virus is inconsistently shed in feces, detection is difficult.

## Signs and symptoms

Assessment findings are similar for the different types of hepatitis. Typically, signs and symptoms progress in three stages — prodromal (preicteric), clinical (icteric), and recovery (posticteric).

### Prodromal stage

In this stage, the patient typically complains of easy fatigue, anorexia (possibly with mild weight loss), generalized malaise, depression, headache, weakness, arthralgia, myalgia, photophobia, and nausea with vomiting. He also may describe changes in his senses of taste and smell.

Assessment of vital signs may reveal a temperature of 100° to 102° F (37.8° to 38.9° C). As the prodromal stage draws to a close, usually 1 to 5 days before the onset of the clinical jaundice stage, inspection of urine and stool specimens may reveal dark-colored urine and clay-colored stools.

### Clinical stage

If the patient has progressed to the clinical jaundice stage, he may report pruritus, abdominal pain or tenderness, and indigestion. Early in this stage, he may complain of anorexia; later, his appetite may return. Inspection of the sclerae, mucous membranes, and skin may reveal jaundice, which can last for 1 to 2 weeks.

Jaundice indicates that the damaged liver is unable to remove bilirubin from the blood, but it doesn't indicate the severity of the disease. Occasionally, hepatitis occurs without jaundice.

During the clinical jaundice stage, inspection of the skin may detect rashes, erythematous patches, and urticaria, especially if the patient has hepatitis B or C. Palpation may disclose abdominal tenderness in the right upper quadrant, an enlarged and tender liver and, in some cases, splenomegaly and cervical adenopathy.

### Recovery stage

During the recovery stage, most of the patient's symptoms decrease or subside. On palpation, a decrease in liver enlargement may be noted. The recovery phase commonly lasts from 2 to 12 weeks, although sometimes this phase lasts longer in patients with hepatitis B, C, or E.

### Diagnosis

In suspected viral hepatitis, a hepatitis profile is routinely performed. This study identifies antibodies specific to the causative virus, establishing the type of hepatitis as follows:

• *Type A:* Detection of an antibody to hepatitis A confirms the diagnosis.

• *Type B*: The presence of HBsAg and hepatitis B antibodies confirms the diagnosis.

• *Type C:* The diagnosis depends on serologic testing for the specific antibody 1 or more months after the onset of acute hepatitis. Until then, the diagnosis is established primarily by obtaining negative test results for hepatitis A, B, and D.

• *Type D:* The detection of intrahepatic delta antigens or immunoglobulin M

(IgM) antidelta antigens in acute disease (or IgM and IgG in chronic disease) establishes the diagnosis.

• *Type E:* Detection of hepatitis E antigens supports the diagnosis; the diagnosis may also be determined by ruling out hepatitis C.

Additional findings from liver function studies support the diagnosis:

• *Serum aspartate aminotransferase* and *serum alanine aminotransferase levels* are increased in the prodromal stage of acute viral hepatitis.

• *Serum alkaline phosphatase levels* are slightly increased.

• *Serum bilirubin levels* are elevated. Levels may continue to be high late in the disease, especially in severe cases.

• *Prothrombin time (PT)* is prolonged (> 3 seconds longer than normal indicates severe liver damage).

• *White blood cell counts* commonly reveal transient neutropenia and lymphopenia followed by lymphocytosis.

• *Liver biopsy* is performed if chronic hepatitis is suspected. (It's performed for acute hepatitis only if the diagnosis is questionable.)

### Treatment

No specific drug therapy has been developed for hepatitis, with the exception of hepatitis C, which has been treated somewhat successfully with interferon alfa-2b. Instead, the patient is advised to rest in the early stages of the illness and to combat anorexia by eating small, high-protein meals.

> CLINICAL TIP The largest meal should be eaten in the morning because nausea tends to intensify as the day progresses.

Protein intake should be reduced if signs of precoma — lethargy, confusion, and mental changes — develop.

In acute viral hepatitis, hospitalization usually is required only for patients with severe symptoms (severe nausea, vomiting, change in mental status, and PT > 3 seconds above normal) or complications. Parenteral nutrition may be required if the patient experiences persistent vomiting and is unable to maintain oral intake.

Antiemetics (diphenhydramine or prochlorperazine) may be given 30 minutes before meals to relieve nausea and prevent vomiting; phenothiazines have a cholestatic effect and should be avoided. For severe pruritus, the resin cholestyramine may be given.

**Special considerations**
- Before the patient is discharged, discuss restrictions and how to prevent a recurrence of hepatitis. (See *Preventing a recurrence of hepatitis.*)
- Enteric precautions are used when caring for patients with type A or E hepatitis. Practice standard precautions for all patients.
- Stress the importance of thorough hand washing.
- Inform visitors about isolation precautions.
- Provide rest periods throughout the day. Schedule treatments and tests so the patient can rest between bouts of activity.
- Because inactivity may make the patient anxious, include diversional activities as part of his care. Gradually add activities as the patient begins to recover.
- Encourage the patient to eat. Provide small, frequent meals. Minimize medications.
- Force fluids (at least 4,000 ml/day). Encourage the anorectic patient to drink fruit juices. Also offer chipped ice and effervescent soft drinks to maintain hydration without inducing vomiting.
- Administer supplemental vitamins and commercial feedings. If symptoms are severe and the patient can't tolerate oral intake, provide parenteral nutrition and hydration.
- Monitor the patient's weight daily, and record intake and output. Observe stools for color, consistency, and amount, and record the frequency of bowel movements.
- Watch for signs of fluid shift, such as weight gain and orthostasis.
- Watch for signs of hepatic coma, dehydration, pneumonia, vascular problems, and pressure ulcers.
- In fulminant hepatitis, maintain electrolyte balance and a patent airway, prevent infections, and control bleeding. Correct hypoglycemia and any other complications while awaiting liver regeneration and repair.

---

TEACHING CHECKLIST

## PREVENTING A RECURRENCE OF HEPATITIS

- Before discharge, emphasize the importance of having regular medical checkups for at least 1 year. The patient will have an increased risk of developing hepatocellular carcinoma.
- Warn the patient against using any alcohol or nonprescription drugs for 1 year.
- Teach the patient to recognize the signs of recurrence.
- Encourage appropriate vaccinations.
- Discuss the use of medications.
- Teach the patient how to protect himself against other viruses.
- Stress the need for personal safety.

# HERNIATED DISK

Also called a ruptured or slipped disk or a herniated nucleus pulposus, a herniated disk occurs when all or part of the nucleus pulposus — the soft, gelatinous, central portion of an intervertebral disk — is forced through the disk's weakened or torn outer ring (anulus fibrosus).

When this happens, the extruded disk may impinge on spinal nerve roots as they exit from the spinal canal or on the spinal cord itself, resulting in back pain and other signs of nerve root irritation. Herniated disks usually occur in adults (mostly men) under age 45.

## Causes

Herniated disks may result from severe trauma or strain or may be related to intervertebral joint degeneration. In older patients, whose disks have begun to degenerate, minor trauma may cause herniation. About 90% of herniated disks occur in the lumbar and lumbosacral regions, 8% occur in the cervical area, and 1% to 2% occur in the thoracic area.

Patients with a congenitally small lumbar spinal canal or with osteophyte formation along the vertebrae may be more susceptible to nerve root compression with a herniated disk and more likely to have neurologic symptoms.

## Signs and symptoms

The overriding symptom of lumbar herniated disk is severe low back pain that radiates to the buttocks, legs, and feet, usually unilaterally. When herniation follows trauma, the pain may begin suddenly, subside in a few days, and then recur at shorter intervals and with progressive intensity.

Sciatic pain follows, beginning as a dull pain in the buttocks. Valsalva's maneuver, coughing, sneezing, and bending intensify the pain, which is often accompanied by muscle spasms. A herniated disk may also cause sensory and motor loss in the area innervated by the compressed spinal nerve root and, in later stages, weakness and atrophy of leg muscles.

## Diagnosis

Obtaining a careful patient history is vital because the mechanisms that intensify disk pain are diagnostically significant. The following test results support the diagnosis:

● The *straight-leg-raising test* and its variants are perhaps the best tests for diagnosing a herniated disk. For this test, the patient lies in a supine position while the examiner places one hand on the patient's ilium, to stabilize the pelvis, and the other hand under the ankle and then slowly raises the patient's leg. The test is positive only if the patient complains of posterior leg (sciatic) pain, not back pain.

● In *LeSegue's test,* the patient lies flat while the thigh and knee are flexed to a 90-degree angle. Resistance and pain as well as loss of ankle or knee-jerk reflex indicate spinal root compression.

● *X-rays of the spine* are essential to rule out other abnormalities but may not diagnose a herniated disk because a marked disk prolapse can be present despite a normal X-ray.

● *Peripheral vascular status check,* including posterior tibial and dorsalis pedis pulses and the skin temperature of extremities, helps rule out ischemic disease, another cause of leg pain or numbness.

● Aside from the physical examination and X-rays, *myelography, computed tomography,* and *magnetic resonance imaging* provide the most specific diagnostic information, showing spinal canal compression by herniated disk material.

## Treatment

Treatment measures are initially conservative and consist of several weeks of bed rest (possibly with pelvic traction), heat applications, an exercise program, and medication. If neurologic impairment progresses rapidly, surgery may be necessary.

### Drug therapy

Aspirin reduces inflammation and edema at the site of injury; rarely, corticosteroids such as dexamethasone may be prescribed for the same purpose. Muscle relaxants, especially diazepam or methocarbamol, also may be beneficial.

### Surgery

A herniated disk that fails to respond to conservative treatment may necessitate surgery. The most common procedure, laminectomy, involves excision of a portion of the lamina and removal of the protruding disk.

If laminectomy doesn't alleviate pain and disability, a spinal fusion may be necessary to overcome segmental instability. Laminectomy and spinal fusion are sometimes performed concurrently to stabilize the spine.

### Other treatments

Chemonucleolysis—injection of the enzyme chymopapain into the herniated disk to dissolve the nucleus pulposus—is a possible alternative to laminectomy. Microdiskectomy can also be used to remove fragments of the nucleus pulposus.

## Special considerations

• Herniated disk requires supportive care, careful patient teaching, and strong emotional support to help the patient cope with the discomfort and frustration of chronic low back pain.
• If the patient requires myelography, reinforce the need for this test and tell the patient to expect some pain. Assure him that he'll receive a sedative before the test, if needed, to keep him as calm and comfortable as possible.
• Before myelography, question the patient carefully about allergies to iodides, iodine-containing substances, or seafood because such allergies may indicate sensitivity to the test's radiopaque dye.
• After myelography, urge the patient to remain in bed with his head elevated (especially if metrizamide was used) and to drink plenty of fluids. Monitor intake and output. Watch for seizures and an allergic reaction.
• During conservative treatment, watch for any deterioration in neurologic status (especially during the first 24 hours after admission), which may indicate an urgent need for surgery.
• Apply antiembolism stockings, as prescribed, and encourage the patient to move his legs, as allowed. Provide high-topped sneakers to prevent footdrop. Work closely with the physical therapy department to ensure a consistent regimen of leg- and back-strengthening exercises.
• Remind the patient to cough, deep-breathe, and use an incentive spirometer to prevent pulmonary complications.
• Assess for bowel function. Use a fracture bedpan for the patient on complete bed rest.
• After laminectomy, microdiskectomy, or spinal fusion, enforce bed rest. If a blood drainage system (Hemovac) is in use, check the tubing frequently for kinks and a secure vacuum. Empty the Hemovac at the end of each shift, and record the amount and color of drainage.
• Report colorless moisture on dressings (possibly cerebrospinal fluid leakage) or excessive drainage immediately. Observe the neurovascular status of the legs (color, motion, temperature, sensation).
• Monitor vital signs, and check for bowel sounds and abdominal distention.

Use the logrolling technique to turn the patient.

> **CLINICAL TIP** Administer analgesics, especially 30 minutes before initial attempts at sitting or walking. Help the patient during his first attempt to walk. Provide a straight-backed chair for limited sitting.

• Teach the patient who has undergone spinal fusion how to wear a brace. Assist with straight-leg-raising and toe-pointing exercises as necessary.

• Before discharge, teach proper body mechanics — bending at the knees and hips (never at the waist), standing straight, and carrying objects close to the body.

• Advise the patient to lie down when tired and to sleep on his side (never on his abdomen) on an extra-firm mattress or a bed board. Urge him to maintain proper weight to prevent lordosis caused by obesity.

• Before chemonucleolysis, ask the patient about allergies to meat tenderizers (chymopapain is a similar substance). Such an allergy contraindicates the use of this enzyme, which can produce severe anaphylaxis in a sensitive patient. Enforce bed rest. Administer analgesics and apply heat, as needed. Assist with special exercises, and tell the patient to continue these exercises after discharge.

• Tell the patient who must receive a muscle relaxant of possible adverse effects, especially drowsiness. Warn him to avoid activities that require alertness until he has built up a tolerance to the drug's sedative effects.

# HERPES SIMPLEX

A recurrent viral infection, herpes simplex is caused by *Herpesvirus hominis* (HVH), a widespread infectious agent. Herpes Type 1, which is transmitted by oral and respiratory secretions, affects the skin and mucous membranes and commonly produces cold sores and fever blisters.

Herpes Type 2 primarily affects the genital area and is transmitted by sexual contact. Cross-infection may result from orogenital sex.

## Causes

About 85% of all HVH infections are subclinical. The others produce localized lesions and systemic reactions. After the first infection, a patient is a carrier susceptible to recurrent infections, which may be provoked by fever, menses, stress, heat, and cold. In recurrent infections, the patient usually has no constitutional signs and symptoms.

### Incidence

Primary HVH is the leading cause of gingivostomatitis in children ages 1 to 3. It causes the most common nonepidemic encephalitis and is the second most common viral infection in pregnant women. It can pass to the fetus transplacentally and, in early pregnancy, may cause spontaneous abortion or premature birth.

Herpes is equally common in males and females. It occurs worldwide and is most prevalent among children in lower socioeconomic groups who live in crowded environments. Saliva, stool, urine, skin lesions, and purulent eye exudate are potential sources of infection.

## Signs and symptoms

Primary infection in childhood may be generalized or localized.

In neonates, HVH symptoms usually appear 1 to 2 weeks after birth. They range from localized skin lesions to a disseminated infection of such organs as the liver, lungs, and brain. Common complications include seizures, mental retardation, blindness, chorioretinitis, deafness, microcephaly, diabetes insipidus, and spasticity. Neonates with disseminated disease have a high mortality.

### Generalized infection

After an incubation period of from 2 to 12 days, onset of generalized infection begins with fever, pharyngitis, erythema, and edema. After brief prodromal tingling and itching, typical primary lesions erupt as vesicles on an erythematous base, eventually rupturing and leaving a painful ulcer, followed by a yellowish crust. Healing begins 7 to 10 days after onset and is complete in 3 weeks.

Vesicles may form on any part of the oral mucosa, especially the tongue, gingiva, and cheeks. In generalized infection, vesicles occur with submaxillary lymphadenopathy, increased salivation, halitosis, anorexia, and a temperature as high as 105° F (40.6° C). Herpetic stomatitis may lead to severe dehydration in children.

A generalized infection usually runs its course in 4 to 10 days. In this form, virus reactivation causes cold sores — single or grouped vesicles in and around the mouth.

### Localized infection

Genital herpes usually affects adolescents and young adults. Typically painful, the initial attack produces fluid-filled vesicles that ulcerate and heal in 1 to 3 weeks. Fever, regional lymphadenopathy, and dysuria may also occur.

Usually, herpetic keratoconjunctivitis is unilateral and causes only local symptoms: conjunctivitis, regional adenopathy, blepharitis, and vesicles on the lid. Other ocular symptoms may be excessive lacrimation, edema, chemosis, photophobia, and purulent exudate.

### Other signs and symptoms

Both types of HVH can cause acute sporadic encephalitis with an altered level of consciousness, personality changes, and seizures. Other effects include smell and taste hallucinations and neurologic abnormalities such as aphasia.

Herpetic whitlow, an HVH finger infection, commonly affects health care workers. First the finger tingles and then it becomes red, swollen, and painful. Vesicles with a red halo erupt and may ulcerate or coalesce. Other effects may include satellite vesicles, fever, chills, malaise, and a red streak up the arm.

## Diagnosis

Typical lesions may suggest HVH infection. Confirmation requires isolation of the virus from local lesions and a histologic biopsy. A rise in antibodies and moderate leukocytosis may support the diagnosis.

## Treatment

Symptomatic and supportive therapy is essential. Generalized primary infection usually requires an analgesic-antipyretic to reduce fever and relieve pain. Anesthetic mouthwashes such as viscous lidocaine may reduce the pain of gingivostomatitis, enabling the patient to eat and preventing dehydration. Drying agents such as calamine lotion make labial lesions less painful.

Refer patients with eye infections to an ophthalmologist. Topical corticosteroids are contraindicated in active infection, but idoxuridine, trifluridine, and vidarabine are effective.

A 5% acyclovir ointment may bring relief to patients with genital herpes or to immunosuppressed patients with HVH skin infections. Intravenous acyclovir helps treat more severe infections. (See *Treating and preventing herpes simplex,* page 404.)

## TREATING AND PREVENTING HERPES SIMPLEX

• Teach the patient with genital herpes to use warm compresses or take sitz baths several times a day. Tell him to use a drying agent such as povidone-iodine solution, to increase his fluid intake, and to avoid all sexual contact during the active stage.
• Recommend that pregnant women with *Herpesvirus hominus* infection have weekly viral cultures of the cervix and external genitalia starting at 32 weeks' gestation.
• Instruct patients with herpetic whitlow not to share towels or utensils with uninfected people. Educate staff members and other susceptible people about the risk of contracting the disease.
• Tell patients with cold sores not to kiss infants or people with eczema. (Those with genital herpes pose no risk to infants if their hygiene is meticulous.)

### Special considerations
• Abstain from direct patient care if you have herpetic whitlow.
• Patients with central nervous system infection alone need no isolation.
• Teach patients how to care for themselves during an outbreak of HVH and how to avoid infecting others.

# HERPES ZOSTER

Also called shingles, herpes zoster is an acute unilateral and segmental inflammation of the dorsal root ganglia caused by infection with the herpesvirus varicella-zoster, which also causes chickenpox. This infection usually occurs in adults. It produces localized vesicular skin lesions confined to a dermatome and severe neuralgic pain in peripheral areas innervated by the nerves arising in the inflamed root ganglia.

The prognosis is good unless the infection spreads to the brain. Eventually, most patients recover completely, except for possible scarring and, in corneal damage, visual impairment. Occasionally, neuralgia may persist for months or years.

Herpes zoster is found primarily in adults, especially those older than age 50. It seldom recurs.

## Causes
Herpes zoster results from reactivation of varicella virus that has lain dormant in the cerebral ganglia (extramedullary ganglia of the cranial nerves) or the ganglia of posterior nerve roots since a previous episode of chickenpox.

Exactly how or why this reactivation occurs isn't clear. Some believe that the virus multiplies as it is reactivated and that it is neutralized by antibodies remaining from the initial infection. But if effective antibodies aren't present, the virus continues to multiply in the ganglia, destroy the host neuron, and spread down the sensory nerves to the skin.

## Signs and symptoms
Herpes zoster usually runs a typical course with classic signs and symptoms. Serious complications sometimes occur.

### Onset of disease
Herpes zoster begins with fever and malaise. Within 2 to 4 days, severe deep pain, pruritus, and paresthesia or hyperesthesia develop, usually on the trunk and occasionally on the arms and legs in a dermatomal distribution. Pain may

be continuous or intermittent and usually lasts from 1 to 4 weeks.

### Skin lesions

Up to 2 weeks after the first symptoms, small, red, nodular skin lesions erupt on the painful areas. These lesions commonly spread unilaterally around the thorax or vertically over the arms or legs. Sometimes nodules don't appear, but when they do, they quickly become vesicles filled with clear fluid or pus.

About 10 days after they appear, the vesicles dry and form scabs. (See *Skin lesions in herpes zoster.*) When they rupture, such lesions often become infected and, in severe cases, may lead to the enlargement of regional lymph nodes; they may even become gangrenous. Intense pain may occur before the rash appears and after the scabs form.

### Cranial nerve involvement

Occasionally, herpes zoster involves the cranial nerves, especially the trigeminal and geniculate ganglia or the oculomotor nerve. Geniculate zoster may cause vesicle formation in the external auditory canal, ipsilateral facial palsy, hearing loss, dizziness, and loss of taste.

Trigeminal ganglion involvement causes eye pain and, possibly, corneal and scleral damage and impaired vision. Rarely, oculomotor involvement causes conjunctivitis, extraocular weakness, ptosis, and paralytic mydriasis.

### Rare complications

In rare cases, herpes zoster leads to generalized central nervous system infection, muscle atrophy, motor paralysis (usually transient), acute transverse myelitis, and ascending myelitis. More often, generalized infection causes acute retention of urine and unilateral paralysis of the diaphragm. In postherpetic neuralgia, a complication most com-

## SKIN LESIONS IN HERPES ZOSTER

Characteristic skin lesions in herpes zoster are fluid-filled vesicles that dry and form scabs after about 10 days.

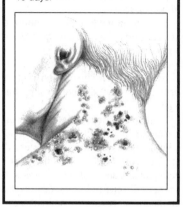

mon in elderly patients, intractable neuralgic pain may persist for years. Scars may be permanent.

## Diagnosis

A positive diagnosis of herpes zoster usually isn't possible until the characteristic skin lesions develop. Before then, the pain may mimic that of appendicitis, pleurisy, or other conditions. Diagnostic test results include the following:

• *Examination of vesicular fluid and infected tissue* shows eosinophilic intranuclear inclusions and varicella virus.

• *Lumbar puncture* shows increased cerebrospinal fluid pressure; examination of cerebrospinal fluid shows increased protein levels and, possibly, pleocytosis.

• *Staining antibodies from vesicular fluid and identification under fluorescent light* differentiate herpes zoster from localized herpes simplex.

## Treatment

No specific treatment exists. The primary goal of supportive treatment is to relieve itching and neuralgic pain with calamine lotion or another antipruritic; aspirin, possibly with codeine or another analgesic; and, occasionally, collodion or tincture of benzoin applied to unbroken lesions.

If bacteria have infected ruptured vesicles, treatment usually includes an appropriate systemic antibiotic.

Trigeminal zoster with corneal involvement calls for instillation of idoxuridine ointment or another antiviral agent.

To help a patient cope with the intractable pain of postherpetic neuralgia, administer a systemic corticosteroid, such as cortisone or, possibly, corticotropin, to reduce inflammation as well as tranquilizers, sedatives, or tricyclic antidepressants with phenothiazines.

Acyclovir seems to stop progression of the rash and prevent visceral complications. In immunocompromised patients — both children and adults — acyclovir therapy may be administered I.V. The drug appears to prevent disseminated, life-threatening disease in some patients.

➤ CLINICAL TIP  Acyclovir and famciclovir shorten the duration of pain and symptoms in normal adults.

## Special considerations

● Keep the patient comfortable, maintain meticulous hygiene, and prevent infection. During the acute phase, encourage him to get adequate rest and give supportive care to promote proper healing of lesions.

● Apply calamine lotion liberally to the lesions. If lesions are severe and widespread, apply a wet dressing.

● Instruct the patient to avoid scratching the lesions.

● If vesicles rupture, apply a cold compress.

● To decrease the pain of oral lesions, tell the patient to use a soft toothbrush, eat a soft diet, and use saline mouthwash.

● To minimize neuralgic pain, never withhold or delay administration of analgesics. Give them exactly on schedule because the pain of herpes zoster can be severe. In postherpetic neuralgia, avoid narcotic analgesics because of the danger of addiction.

● Repeatedly reassure the patient that herpetic pain will eventually subside. Provide the patient with diversionary activity to take his mind off the pain and pruritus.

# HIATAL HERNIA

Hiatus or hiatal hernia is a defect in the diaphragm that permits a portion of the stomach to pass through the diaphragmatic opening into the chest. Three types of hiatal hernia can occur: *sliding hernia, paraesophageal ("rolling") hernia,* and *mixed hernia,* which includes features of both. (See *Two types of hiatal hernia.*)

In a sliding hernia, both the stomach and the gastroesophageal junction slip up into the chest, so that the gastroesophageal junction is above the diaphragmatic hiatus. In paraesophageal hernia, a part of the greater curvature of the stomach rolls through the diaphragmatic defect. Treatment can prevent such complications as strangulation of the herniated intrathoracic portion of the stomach.

## Causes

Usually, hiatal hernia results from muscle weakening that's common with aging and may be secondary to esophageal cancer, kyphoscoliosis, trauma, and certain surgical procedures. It may also result from certain diaphragmatic malformations that may cause congenital weakness.

In hiatal hernia, the muscular collar around the esophageal and diaphragmatic junction loosens, permitting the lower portion of the esophagus and the stomach to rise into the chest when intra-abdominal pressure increases (possibly causing gastroesophageal reflux). Such increased intra-abdominal pressure may result from ascites, pregnancy, obesity, constrictive clothing, bending, straining, coughing, Valsalva's maneuver, or extreme physical exertion.

*Incidence*
A sliding hernia is 3 to 10 times more common than paraesophageal and mixed hernias combined. The incidence of hiatal hernia is higher in women than in men (especially the paraesophageal type) and increases with age.

*Signs and symptoms*
Typically, a paraesophageal hernia produces no symptoms; it is usually an incidental finding on barium swallow. Because this type of hernia leaves the closing mechanism of the cardiac sphincter unchanged, it seldom causes acid reflux and reflux esophagitis.

Symptoms result from displacement or stretching of the stomach and may include a feeling of fullness in the chest or pain that resembles angina pectoris. Even if it produces no symptoms, this type of hernia needs surgical treatment because of the high risk of strangulation.

A sliding hernia without an incompetent sphincter produces no reflux or symptoms and, consequently, doesn't require treatment. When a sliding hernia does cause symptoms, they're typical of

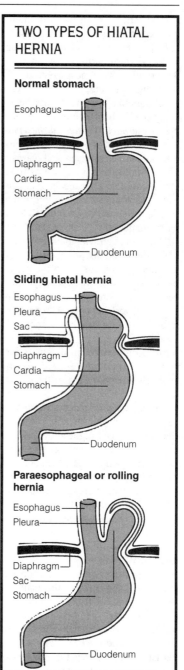

## TWO TYPES OF HIATAL HERNIA

**Normal stomach**

Esophagus
Diaphragm
Cardia
Stomach
Duodenum

**Sliding hiatal hernia**

Esophagus
Pleura
Sac
Diaphragm
Cardia
Stomach
Duodenum

**Paraesophageal or rolling hernia**

Esophagus
Pleura
Diaphragm
Sac
Stomach
Duodenum

gastric reflux (resulting from the incompetent lower esophageal sphincter [LES]) and may include the following:

• *Pyrosis* (heartburn) occurs from 1 to 4 hours after eating and is aggravated by reclining, belching, and increased intra-abdominal pressure. It may be accompanied by regurgitation or vomiting.

• *Retrosternal or substernal chest pain* results from reflux of gastric contents, distention of the stomach, and spasm or altered motor activity. Chest pain occurs most often after meals or at bedtime and is aggravated by reclining, belching, and increased intra-abdominal pressure.

Other common symptoms reflect possible complications.

• *Dysphagia* occurs when the hernia produces esophagitis, esophageal ulceration, or stricture, especially with ingestion of very hot or cold foods, alcoholic beverages, or a large amount of food.

• *Bleeding* may be mild or massive, frank or occult; the source may be esophagitis or erosions of the gastric pouch.

• *Severe pain and shock* result from incarceration, in which a large portion of the stomach is caught above the diaphragm. (This usually occurs with paraesophageal hernia.) Incarceration may lead to the perforation of a gastric ulcer as well as strangulation and gangrene of the herniated portion of the stomach. This requires immediate surgery.

## Diagnosis

Hiatal hernia is diagnosed based on typical clinical features and the results of the following laboratory studies and procedures:

• *Chest X-ray* occasionally shows an air shadow behind the heart with a large hernia and infiltrates in the lower lobes if the patient has aspirated.

• In a *barium study,* the hernia may appear as an outpouching that contains barium at the lower end of the esophagus. (Small hernias are difficult to recognize.) This study also shows diaphragmatic abnormalities.

• *Endoscopy and biopsy* differentiate between hiatal hernia, varices, and other small gastroesophageal lesions; identify the mucosal junction and the edge of the diaphragm indenting the esophagus; and can rule out malignant tumors that otherwise might be difficult to detect.

• *Esophageal motility studies* assess the presence of esophageal motor abnormalities before surgical repair of the hernia.

• *pH studies* assess for reflux of gastric contents.

• *Acid perfusion (Bernstein) test* indicates that heartburn results from esophageal reflux when perfusion of hydrogen chloride through the nasogastric (NG) tube provokes this symptom.

The following laboratory tests may indicate GI bleeding as a complication of hiatal hernia:

• *Complete blood count* may show hypochromic microcytic anemia when bleeding from esophageal ulceration occurs.

• *Stool guaiac test* may be positive.

• *Analysis of gastric contents* may reveal blood.

## Treatment

The primary goals of treatment are to relieve symptoms by minimizing or correcting the incompetent cardia and to manage and prevent complications. Medical therapy is used initially because symptoms usually respond to it and hiatal hernia may recur after surgery.

### *Medical therapy*

Medical therapy attempts to modify or reduce reflux by changing the quantity or quality of refluxed gastric contents, strengthening the LES muscle pharmacologically, or decreasing the amount of reflux through gravity.

Specific measures include restricting any activity that increases intra-abdominal pressure (coughing, straining, bending), giving antiemetics and cough suppressants, avoiding constrictive clothing, modifying diet, giving stool softeners or laxatives to prevent straining during defecation, and discouraging smoking because it stimulates gastric acid production.

Modifying the diet means eating small, frequent, bland meals at least 2 hours before lying down (no bedtime snacks); eating slowly; and avoiding spicy foods, fruit juices, alcoholic beverages, and coffee. Antacids also modify the fluid refluxed into the esophagus and are probably the best treatment for intermittent reflux.

To reduce the amount of reflux, the overweight patient should lose weight to decrease intra-abdominal pressure. Elevating the head of the bed about 6″ (15 cm) reduces gastric reflux by gravity.

Drug therapy to strengthen cardiac sphincter tone may include a cholinergic agent such as bethanecol. Metoclopramide has also been used to stimulate smooth-muscle contraction, increase LES tone, and decrease reflux after eating.

### Surgery

Failure to control symptoms medically or the onset of such complications as stricture, bleeding, pulmonary aspiration, strangulation, or incarceration necessitates an antireflux surgical repair.

Surgery creates an artificial closing mechanism at the gastroesophageal junction to strengthen the LES's barrier function. A transabdominal fundoplication is performed by wrapping the fundus of the stomach around the lower esophagus to prevent reflux of stomach contents. An abdominal or a thoracic approach may be used. Laparoscopic surgery to repair the hernia is now commonplace.

### Special considerations

● To enhance compliance with treatment, instruct the patient about the causes of this disorder. Explain proposed treatments, diagnostic tests, and significant symptoms.

● Prepare the patient for diagnostic tests as needed. After endoscopy, watch for signs of perforation (falling blood pressure, rapid pulse, shock, and sudden pain).

● Before surgery, reinforce patient teaching about the procedure and any preoperative and postoperative considerations.

● Postoperatively, monitor intake and output, including NG tube drainage.

> CLINICAL TIP Never manipulate an NG tube in a patient with a hiatal hernia surgical repair.

● If a thoracic approach was used, the patient will have chest tubes in place. Carefully observe chest tube drainage and respiratory status, and perform pulmonary physiotherapy.

● Monitor NG tube patency and security to prevent distention of the stomach during the healing period. Distention can cause a breakdown of the repair.

● Instruct the patient that a barium swallow will be performed on the 6th to 7th postoperative day to look for the unobstructed passage of barium into the stomach before starting solid foods.

● Inform the patient that slight dysphagia may be experienced in the first few weeks after surgery. This will gradually disappear.

● Instruct the patient to eat small, frequent meals.

● Counsel the patient that increased flatus and mild gastric distention may occur due to trapping of air in the stomach from air swallowing. Air swallowing should be consciously avoided.

• Instruct the patient to take all medications in liquid or crushed form for at least 6 months to avoid a drug-induced esophageal injury.

# HODGKIN'S DISEASE

A neoplastic disease, Hodgkin's disease is characterized by painless, progressive enlargement of lymph nodes, spleen, and other lymphoid tissue resulting from proliferation of lymphocytes, histiocytes, eosinophils, and Reed-Sternberg giant cells. The latter cells are its special histologic feature.

Untreated, Hodgkin's disease follows a variable but relentlessly progressive and ultimately fatal course. Advances in therapy have made Hodgkin's disease potentially curable, even in advanced stages, and appropriate treatment yields a 5-year survival rate of about 90%.

## Causes

The cause of Hodgkin's disease is unknown. This disease is most common in young adults and occurs more often in men than in women. It occurs in all races but is slightly more common in whites. Incidence peaks in two age-groups: ages 15 to 38 and after age 50, except in Japan, where it occurs exclusively among people over age 50.

## Signs and symptoms

Symptoms vary, depending on the stage of the disease.

### Early signs

The first sign of Hodgkin's disease is usually a painless swelling of one of the cervical lymph nodes (but sometimes the axillary, mediastinal, or inguinal lymph nodes), occasionally in a patient who has a history of recent upper respiratory tract infection.

In older patients, the first symptoms may be nonspecific: persistent fever, night sweats, fatigue, weight loss, and malaise. Rarely, if the mediastinum is initially involved, Hodgkin's disease may produce respiratory symptoms.

Another early and characteristic indication of Hodgkin's disease is pruritus, which, although mild at first, becomes acute as the disease progresses. Other symptoms depend on the degree and location of systemic involvement.

Lymph nodes may enlarge rapidly, producing pain and obstruction, or slowly and painlessly for months or years. It's not unusual to see the lymph nodes "wax and wane," but they usually don't return to normal.

### Late signs

Sooner or later, most patients develop systemic manifestations, including enlargement of retroperitoneal nodes and nodular infiltrations of the spleen, liver, and bones. At this late stage, other symptoms include edema of the face and neck, progressive anemia, possibly jaundice, nerve pain, and increased susceptibility to infection.

## Diagnosis

Diagnostic measures for confirming Hodgkin's disease include a thorough medical history and a complete physical examination, followed by a lymph node biopsy checking for abnormal histiocyte proliferation of Reed-Sternberg cells and nodular fibrosis and necrosis.

Other appropriate diagnostic tests include bone marrow, liver, mediastinal, lymph node, and spleen biopsies; routine chest X-ray; abdominal computed tomographic scan; lung scan; bone scan; and lymphangiography to detect lymph node or organ involvement. Laparoscopy and a lymph node biopsy are performed to complete staging.

Hematologic tests show mild to severe normocytic anemia, normochromic anemia (in 50% of patients), and an elevated, normal, or reduced white blood cell count and differential showing any combination of neutrophilia, lymphocytopenia, monocytosis, and eosinophilia. An elevated serum alkaline phosphatase level indicates liver or bone involvement.

The same diagnostic tests are also used for staging. A staging laparotomy is necessary for patients under age 55 and those without obvious stage III or stage IV disease, lymphocyte predominance subtype histology, or medical contraindications. Diagnosis must rule out other disorders that enlarge the lymph nodes. (See *Staging Hodgkin's disease,* page 412.)

### Treatment

Appropriate therapy (chemotherapy, radiation therapy, or both, depending on the stage of the disease) is based on a careful physical examination with accurate histologic interpretation and proper clinical staging. Correct and timely treatment allows longer survival and even induces an apparent cure in many patients.

#### Chemotherapy and radiation therapy

Radiation therapy is used alone for stage I and stage II and in combination with chemotherapy for stage III. Chemotherapy is used for stage IV, sometimes inducing a complete remission. The well-known MOPP protocol (mechlorethamine, vincristine [Oncovin], procarbazine, and prednisone) was the first to provide significant cures in patients with generalized Hodgkin's disease.

Another useful combination is ABVD (doxorubicin [Adriamycin], bleomycin,

vinblastine, and dacarbazine). Treatment with these drugs may require concomitant antiemetics, sedatives, or antidiarrheals to combat GI adverse effects.

#### Other treatments

New treatments include high-dose chemotherapeutic agents with autologous bone marrow transplantation or autologous peripheral blood stem cell transfusions. Biotherapy alone hasn't proved effective.

### Special considerations

Because many patients with Hodgkin's disease receive radiation therapy or chemotherapy as outpatients, tell the patient to observe the following precautions:

● Watch for and promptly report adverse effects of radiation therapy and chemotherapy (particularly anorexia, nausea, vomiting, diarrhea, fever, and bleeding).

● Minimize adverse effects of radiation therapy by maintaining good nutrition (aided by eating small, frequent meals of favorite foods), drinking plenty of fluids, pacing activities to counteract therapy-induced fatigue, and keeping the skin in radiated areas dry.

➤ CLINICAL TIP Control pain and bleeding of stomatitis by using a soft toothbrush, cotton swab, or anesthetic mouthwash such as viscous lidocaine; by applying petroleum jelly to the patient's lips; and by avoiding astringent mouthwashes.

● If a female patient is of childbearing age, advise her to delay pregnancy until prolonged remission because radiation therapy and chemotherapy can cause genetic mutations and spontaneous abortions.

● Because the patient with Hodgkin's disease has usually been healthy until this point, he's likely to be especially distressed. Provide emotional support

## STAGING HODGKIN'S DISEASE

Treatment of Hodgkin's disease depends on the stage it has reached — that is, the number, location, and degree of involved lymph nodes. The Ann Arbor Classification System, adopted in 1971, divides Hodgkin's disease into four stages, which are then subdivided into categories.

Category A includes patients with undefined signs and symptoms, and category B includes patients who experience such defined signs as recent unexplained weight loss, fever, and night sweats.

### Stage I
Hodgkin's disease appears in a single lymph node region (I) or a single extralymphatic organ (IE).

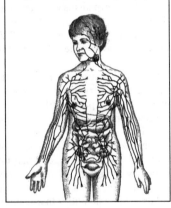

### Stage II
The disease appears in two or more nodes on the same side of the diaphragm (II) and in an extralymphatic organ (IIE).

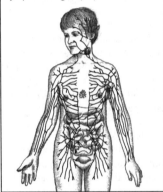

### Stage III
Hodgkin's disease spreads to both sides of the diaphragm (III) and perhaps to an extralymphatic organ (IIIE), the spleen (IIIS), or both (IIIES).

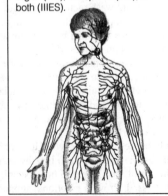

### Stage IV
The disease disseminates, involving one or more extralymphatic organs or tissues, with or without associated lymph node involvement.

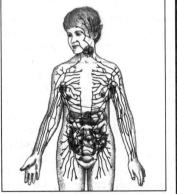

and offer appropriate reassurance. Ease the patient's anxiety by sharing your optimism about his prognosis.

● Make sure the patient and his family know that the local chapter of the American Cancer Society is available for information, financial assistance, and supportive counseling.

# HUNTINGTON'S DISEASE

Also called Huntington's chorea, hereditary chorea, chronic progressive chorea, and adult chorea, Huntington's disease is a hereditary disease in which degeneration in the cerebral cortex and basal ganglia causes chronic progressive chorea (involuntary and irregular movements) and cognitive deterioration, ending in dementia.

Huntington's disease usually strikes people between ages 25 and 55 (the average age is 35); however, 2% of cases occur in children, and 5%, as late as age 60. Death usually results 10 to 15 years after onset from suicide, heart failure, or pneumonia.

## Causes

Huntington's disease is transmitted as an autosomal dominant trait, and either sex can transmit and inherit it. Each child of a parent with this disease has a 50% chance of inheriting it; the child who inherits it can pass it on to his own children.

Because of hereditary transmission, Huntington's disease is prevalent in areas where affected families have lived for several generations. Genetic testing is now offered to those with a known family history of the disease.

## Signs and symptoms

The onset of this disease is insidious. The patient eventually becomes totally dependent — emotionally and physically — through loss of musculoskeletal control.

> CLINICAL TIP   Although Huntington's disease is associated with some types of psychiatric illness, it has a clinically different presentation and cause.

### Neurologic manifestations

Gradually, the patient develops progressively severe choreic movements. Such movements are rapid, often violent, and purposeless. Initially, they are unilateral and more prominent in the face and arms than in the legs, progressing from mild fidgeting to grimacing, tongue smacking, dysarthria (indistinct speech), athetoid movements (especially of the hands) related to emotional state, and torticollis.

Bradykinesia (slow movements) is often accompanied by rigidity. Muscle strength is generally maintained. The combination of chorea, bradykinesia, and normal muscle strength results in impairment of both voluntary and involuntary movement.

Another neurologic manifestation is dysphagia, which is seen in a large percentage of patients in the advanced stages. Dysarthria generally presents early in the disease process and may be complicated by perseveration (persistent repetition of a reply), oral apraxia (difficulty coordinating movement of the mouth), and aprosody (inability to accurately reproduce or interpret the tone of language).

### Cognitive manifestations

Dementia is an early indication of the disease and is subcortical in nature. Unlike patients with Alzheimer's disease, Huntington patients have no significant impairment of immediate memory. When problems with recent memory occur, they may be due to retrieval rather than encoding problems. Comprehension of information is preserved. Because the disease primarily affects the frontal lobes, deficits of executive function (planning, organizing, regulating, and programming) are common. Impulse control is also impaired, whereas insight into loss of cognitive function is retained.

### Psychiatric manifestations
Psychiatric symptoms may precede movement alteration by several years. Depression is the earliest symptom. Other common personality changes include irritability, lability, impulsiveness, and aggressive behavior. Depression may also have a manic component. Psychosis and obsessive-compulsive behavior are not common.

### Diagnosis
Huntington's disease can be detected by positron emission tomography and deoxyribonucleic acid analysis. The diagnosis is based on a characteristic clinical history: progressive chorea and dementia, onset of the disorder early in middle age (ages 35 to 40), and confirmation of a genetic link.

A computed tomography scan and magnetic resonance imaging demonstrate brain atrophy. Molecular genetics may detect the gene for Huntington's disease in people at risk while they're still asymptomatic.

### Treatment
Because Huntington's disease has no known cure, treatment is supportive, protective, and aimed at relieving symptoms. Tranquilizers as well as chlorpromazine, haloperidol, and imipramine help control choreic movements, but they can't stop mental deterioration. They also alleviate discomfort and depression, making the patient easier to manage. However, tranquilizers increase patient rigidity.

To control choreic movements without rigidity, choline may be prescribed. Institutionalization is often necessary because of mental deterioration.

### Special considerations
• Provide physical support by attending to the patient's basic needs, such as hygiene, skin care, bowel and bladder care, and nutrition. Increase this support as mental and physical deterioration make him increasingly immobile.
• Assist in designing a behavioral plan that deals with the disruptive and aggressive behavior and impulse control problems. Reinforce positive behaviors, and maintain consistency with all caregiving.
• Offer emotional support to the patient and his family. Teach them about the disease, and listen to their concerns and special problems. Keep in mind the patient's dysarthria, and allow him extra time to express himself, thereby decreasing frustration. Teach the family to participate in the patient's care.
• Stay alert for possible suicide attempts. Control the patient's environment to protect him from suicide or other self-inflicted injury. Pad the side rails of the bed but avoid restraints, which may cause the patient to injure himself with violent, uncontrolled movements.
• If the patient has difficulty walking, provide a walker to help him maintain his balance.
• If the patient has dysphagia, minimize the potential for aspiration, infection, malnutrition, and pneumonitis.
• Make sure affected families receive genetic counseling. All affected family members should realize that each of their offspring has a 50% chance of inheriting this disease.

- Refer people at risk who desire genetic testing to specialized centers where psychosocial support is available.
- Refer the patient and his family to appropriate community organizations.
- For more information about this degenerative disease, refer the patient and his family to the Huntington's Disease Association.

# HYDROCEPHALUS

An excessive accumulation of cerebrospinal fluid (CSF) within the ventricular spaces of the brain, hydrocephalus occurs most often in neonates. It can also occur in adults as a result of injury or disease. In infants, hydrocephalus enlarges the head, and in both infants and adults, the resulting compression can damage brain tissue.

With early detection and surgical intervention, the prognosis improves but remains guarded. Even after surgery, such complications as developmental delay, impaired motor function, and vision loss can persist. Without surgery, the prognosis is poor: Mortality may result from increased intracranial pressure (ICP) in people of all ages; infants may also die prematurely of infection and malnutrition.

## Causes

Hydrocephalus may result from an obstruction in CSF flow (noncommunicating hydrocephalus) or from faulty absorption of CSF (communicating hydrocephalus).

### Noncommunicating hydrocephalus

In this type of hydrocephalus, the obstruction occurs most frequently between the third and fourth ventricles, at the aqueduct of Sylvius, but it can also occur at the outlets of the fourth ventricle (foramina of Luschka and Magendie) or, rarely, at the foramen of Monro.

This obstruction may result from faulty fetal development, infection (syphilis, granulomatous diseases, meningitis), a tumor, a cerebral aneurysm, or a blood clot (after intracranial hemorrhage).

### Communicating hydrocephalus

In this type of hydrocephalus, faulty absorption of CSF may result from surgery to repair a myelomeningocele, adhesions between meninges at the base of the brain, or meningeal hemorrhage. Rarely, a tumor in the choroid plexus causes overproduction of CSF, producing hydrocephalus.

## Signs and symptoms

In infants, the unmistakable sign of hydrocephalus is enlargement of the head clearly disproportionate to the infant's growth. Other characteristic changes include distended scalp veins; thin, shiny, fragile-looking scalp skin; and underdeveloped neck muscles. (See *Characteristics of hydrocephalus*, page 416.)

In severe hydrocephalus, the roof of the orbit is depressed, the eyes are displaced downward, and the sclerae are prominent. A high-pitched, shrill cry as well as abnormal muscle tone in the legs, irritability, anorexia, and projectile vomiting often occur.

In adults and older children, indicators of hydrocephalus include a decreased level of consciousness (LOC), ataxia, incontinence, and impaired intellect.

In infants, the fontanels may not feel full due to the infant's inability to increase the head circumference when the brain is under pressure. Because the sutures aren't fused, the skull widens to accommodate the pressure.

## CHARACTERISTICS OF HYDROCEPHALUS

In infants, changes characteristic of hydrocephalus include marked enlargement of the head; distended scalp veins; thin, shiny, and fragile-looking scalp skin; and underdeveloped neck muscles.

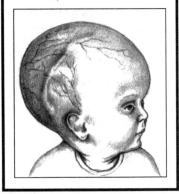

### Diagnosis

In infants, abnormally large head size for the patient's age strongly suggests hydrocephalus. Skull X-rays show thinning of the skull with separation of sutures and widening of the fontanels.

Other diagnostic tests, including angiography, computed tomography, and magnetic resonance imaging, can differentiate between hydrocephalus and intracranial lesions and can also demonstrate the Arnold-Chiari deformity, which may occur in an infant with hydrocephalus.

### Treatment

Surgical correction is the only treatment for hydrocephalus. Usually, such surgery consists of insertion of a ventriculoperitoneal shunt, which transports excess fluid from the lateral ventricle into the peritoneal cavity.

A less common procedure is insertion of a ventriculoatrial shunt, which drains fluid from the brain's lateral ventricle into the right atrium of the heart, where the fluid makes its way into the venous circulation.

Complications of surgery include shunt infection, septicemia (after ventriculoatrial shunt), adhesions and paralytic ileus, migration, peritonitis, and intestinal perforation (with peritoneal shunt).

### Special considerations

On initial assessment:
- Obtain a complete history from the patient or the family. Note the patient's general behavior, especially irritability, apathy, and decreased LOC.
- Perform a neurologic assessment. Examine the eyes: pupils should be equal and reactive to light. In adults and older children, evaluate movements and motor strength in the extremities. (Watch especially for ataxia.)
- Irritability, restlessness, and change in cognitive function are all indicators of increased ICP in both adults and children. A change in eating, sleeping, and pitch of cry are strong indicators of increased ICP in infants.

Before surgery to insert a shunt:
- Encourage maternal-infant bonding when possible. When caring for the infant yourself, hold him on your lap for feeding, stroke and cuddle him, and speak soothingly.
- Check the fontanels for tension or fullness, and measure and record head circumference.

➤ CLINICAL TIP  To appropriately assess fontanels, lay the infant down and then elevate him to a sitting position. Truly tense fontanels will be present in the sitting position. Remember that if the infant is crying, fontanel pressure will increase. This would not be indicative of hydrocephalus.

On the patient's chart, draw a picture showing where to measure the head so that other staff members measure it in the same place, or mark the forehead with ink.

• To prevent postfeeding aspiration and hypostatic pneumonia, place the infant on his side and reposition him every 2 hours, or prop him up in an infant seat.

• To prevent skin breakdown, make sure his earlobe is flat, and place a sheepskin or rubber foam under his head.

• When turning the infant, move his head, neck, and shoulders with his body to reduce strain on his neck.

• Feed the infant slowly. To lessen the strain from the weight of the infant's head on your arm while holding him during feeding, place his head, neck, and shoulders on a pillow.

After surgery:

• Place the infant on the side opposite the operative site, with his head level with his body.

• Check temperature, pulse rate, blood pressure, and LOC. Also check the fontanels daily for fullness. Watch for irritability, which may be an early sign of increased ICP and shunt malfunction.

• Watch for signs of infection, especially meningitis: fever, stiff neck, irritability, or tense fontanels. Also watch for redness, swelling, and other signs of local infection over the shunt tract. Check the dressing often for drainage.

• Listen for bowel sounds after ventriculoperitoneal shunt.

• Check the infant's growth and development periodically, and help the parents set goals consistent with ability and potential.

• Help the parents focus on their child's strengths, not his weaknesses. Discuss special education programs, and emphasize the infant's need for sensory stimulation appropriate for his age.

• Teach the parents to watch for signs of shunt malfunction, infection, and paralytic ileus. Tell them that shunt insertion requires periodic surgery to lengthen the shunt as the child grows older, to correct malfunctioning, or to treat infection.

# HYDRONEPHROSIS

An abnormal dilation of the renal pelvis and the calyces of one or both kidneys, hydronephrosis is caused by an obstruction of urine flow in the genitourinary tract. Although partial obstruction and hydronephrosis may not produce symptoms initially, the pressure built up behind the area of obstruction eventually results in symptomatic renal dysfunction.

## Causes
Almost any type of obstructive uropathy can result in hydronephrosis. The most common causes are benign prostatic hyperplasia, urethral strictures, and calculi; less common causes include strictures or stenosis of the ureter or bladder outlet, congenital abnormalities, abdominal tumors, blood clots, neurogenic bladder, and tumors of the ureter and bladder.

### Sites of obstruction
If obstruction is in the urethra or bladder, hydronephrosis is usually bilateral; if obstruction is in a ureter, it's usually unilateral. Obstructions distal to the bladder cause the bladder to dilate and act as a buffer zone, delaying hydronephrosis. Total obstruction of urine flow with dilation of the collecting system ultimately causes complete cortical atrophy and cessation of glomerular filtration.

## Signs and symptoms

Clinical features of hydronephrosis vary with the cause of the obstruction. In some patients, hydronephrosis produces no symptoms or only mild pain and slightly decreased urine flow; in others, it may produce severe, colicky renal pain or dull flank pain that may radiate to the groin and gross urinary abnormalities, such as hematuria, pyuria, dysuria, alternating oliguria and polyuria, and complete anuria.

Other symptoms of hydronephrosis include nausea, vomiting, abdominal fullness, pain on urination, dribbling, and hesitancy. Unilateral obstruction may cause pain on only one side, usually in the flank area.

### *Complications*

The most common complication of an obstructed kidney is infection (pyelonephritis) due to stasis that exacerbates renal damage and may create a life-threatening crisis. Paralytic ileus frequently accompanies acute obstructive uropathy.

## Diagnosis

Although the patient's clinical features may suggest hydronephrosis, excretory urography, retrograde pyelography, renal ultrasonography, and renal function studies are necessary to confirm it.

## Treatment

The goals of treatment are to preserve renal function and prevent infection through surgical removal of the obstruction, such as dilation for stricture of the urethra and prostatectomy for benign prostatic hyperplasia.

If renal function has already been affected, therapy may include a diet low in protein, sodium, and potassium. This diet is designed to stop the progression of renal failure before surgery.

Inoperable obstructions may require decompression and drainage of the kidney, using a nephrostomy tube placed temporarily or permanently in the renal pelvis. Concurrent infection requires appropriate antibiotic therapy.

## Special considerations

● Explain hydronephrosis as well as the purpose of excretory urography and other diagnostic procedures. Find out whether the patient is allergic to the dye used in excretory urography.

● Administer medication for pain as needed.

● Postoperatively, closely monitor intake and output, vital signs, and fluid and electrolyte status. Watch for a rising pulse rate and cold, clammy skin, which indicate possible impending hemorrhage and shock. Monitor renal function studies daily.

● If a nephrostomy tube has been inserted, check it frequently for bleeding and patency. Irrigate the tube, but don't clamp it.

● If the patient is to be discharged with a nephrostomy tube in place, teach him how to care for it properly.

➤ CLINICAL TIP   To prevent progression of hydronephrosis to irreversible renal disease, urge older men (especially those with family histories of benign prostatic hyperplasia or prostatitis) to have routine medical checkups. Teach them to recognize and report symptoms of hydronephrosis (colicky pain, hematuria) or urinary tract infection.

# HYPERALDOSTERONISM

In hyperaldosteronism, hypersecretion of the mineralocorticoid aldosterone by the adrenal cortex causes excessive reabsorption of sodium and water and excessive renal excretion of potassium.

## Causes

Hyperaldosteronism may be primary or secondary. Most cases of primary hyperaldosteronism are due to benign aldosterone-producing adrenal adenomas. The remainder are due to bilateral adrenal hyperplasia. Rarely, adrenal carcinoma can cause primary hyperaldosteronism. The incidence is three times higher in women than in men and is highest between ages 30 and 50.

In primary hyperaldosteronism, chronic aldosterone excess is independent of the renin-angiotensin system and in fact suppresses plasma renin activity. This aldosterone excess enhances sodium reabsorption by the kidneys, which leads to mild hypernatremia and, simultaneously, hypokalemia and increased extracellular fluid volume. Expansion of intravascular fluid volume also occurs and results in volume-dependent hypertension and increased cardiac output.

Excessive ingestion of English black licorice or licorice-like substances can produce a syndrome similar to primary hyperaldosteronism due to the mineralocorticoid action of glycyrrhizic acid.

Secondary hyperaldosteronism results from an extra-adrenal abnormality that stimulates the adrenal gland to increase production of aldosterone. For example, conditions that reduce renal blood flow (renal artery stenosis) and extracellular fluid volume or produce a sodium deficit activate the renin-angiotensin system and, subsequently, increase aldosterone secretion. Thus, secondary hyperaldosteronism may result from conditions that induce hypertension through increased renin production (such as Wilms' tumor), ingestion of oral contraceptives, and pregnancy.

Secondary hyperaldosteronism may also result from disorders unrelated to hypertension. Such disorders may or may not cause edema. For example, nephrotic syndrome, hepatic cirrhosis with ascites, and heart failure commonly induce edema; Bartter's syndrome and salt-losing nephritis don't.

## Signs and symptoms

Most clinical effects of hyperaldosteronism result from hypokalemia, which increases neuromuscular irritability and produces muscle weakness, fatigue, headaches, paresthesia, and intermittent, flaccid paralysis.

Hypokalemia interferes with normal insulin secretion and can worsen glucose control in diabetic patients with hyperaldosteronism. Hypertension and its accompanying complications are also common. Another characteristic finding is loss of renal concentrating ability, resulting in polyuria and polydipsia. Azotemia indicates chronic potassium depletion nephropathy.

➤ CLINICAL TIP Consider primary hyperaldosteronism in those hypertensive patients with spontaneous hypokalemia or significant hypokalemia on modest diuretic dosing.

## Diagnosis

Persistently low serum potassium levels in a nonedematous patient who isn't taking diuretics, doesn't have obvious GI losses (from vomiting or diarrhea), and has a normal sodium intake suggest hyperaldosteronism.

If hypokalemia develops in a hypertensive patient shortly after starting treatment with potassium-wasting diuretics (such as thiazides), and if it persists after the diuretic has been discontinued and potassium replacement therapy has been instituted, evaluation for hyperaldosteronism is necessary.

A low plasma renin level that fails to increase appropriately during volume depletion (upright posture, sodium depletion) and a high plasma aldosterone level during volume expansion by salt loading confirm primary hyperaldosteronism in a hypertensive patient without edema.

The serum bicarbonate level is often elevated, with ensuing alkalosis due to hydrogen and potassium ion loss in the distal renal tubules.

Other tests show markedly increased urine aldosterone levels and increased plasma aldosterone levels. In secondary hyperaldosteronism, plasma renin levels are increased.

A suppression test is useful to differentiate between primary and secondary hyperaldosteronism. During this test, the patient receives desoxycorticosterone I.M. for 3 days while plasma aldosterone levels and urine metabolites are continuously measured. These levels decrease in secondary hyperaldosteronism but remain the same in primary hyperaldosteronism. Simultaneously, renin levels are low in primary hyperaldosteronism and high in secondary hyperaldosteronism.

Other findings include electrocardiogram signs of hypokalemia (ST-segment depression and flattened U waves), chest X-ray showing left ventricular hypertrophy from chronic hypertension, and localization of the tumor by adrenal angiography, computed tomography, or magnetic resonance imaging.

### Treatment

The treatment for aldosterone-producing adenoma is unilateral adrenalectomy. Potassium-sparing diuretics (spironolactone and amiloride) are used to control hyperaldosteronism in patients with bilateral hyperplasia or those with unilateral adenoma who are unable to undergo surgery.

Treatment of secondary hyperaldosteronism must include correction of the underlying cause.

### Special considerations

• Monitor and record urine output, blood pressure, weight, and serum potassium levels.

• Watch for hypokalemia-induced cardiac arrhythmias, paresthesia, and weakness. Give potassium replacement as ordered.

• Ask the dietitian to provide a low-sodium, high-potassium diet.

• After adrenalectomy, watch for weakness, hyponatremia, rising serum potassium levels, and signs of adrenal hypofunction, especially hypotension.

• If the patient is taking spironolactone or amiloride, advise him to watch for signs of hyperkalemia. Tell him that impotence and gynecomastia may follow long-term use of spironolactone.

• Tell the patient who must take steroid hormone replacement to wear a medical identification bracelet.

# HYPERHIDROSIS

The excessive secretion of sweat from the eccrine glands, hyperhydrosis usually occurs in the axillae (typically after puberty) and on the palms and soles (often starting during infancy or childhood).

### Causes

Possible causes of hyperhidrosis include the following:

• Genetic factors may contribute to the development of hyperhidrosis and, in susceptible individuals, emotional stress appears to be the most common cause. Increased central nervous system (CNS) impulses may provoke excessive release of acetylcholine, producing a heightened sweat response.

• Exercise and a hot climate can cause profuse sweating in these patients.

• Certain drugs, such as antipyretics, emetics, meperidine, and anticholinesterase, can increase sweating.

• In addition, hyperhidrosis may occur as a clinical manifestation of an underlying disorder. Infections and chronic diseases, such as tuberculosis, malaria, and lymphoma, may cause excessive nighttime sweating. Diabetic patients often demonstrate hyperhidrosis during a hypoglycemic crisis.

• Other predisposing conditions include pheochromocytomas; cardiovascular disorders, such as shock and heart failure; CNS disturbances (most often lesions of the hypothalamus); withdrawal from drugs or alcohol; menopause; and Graves' disease.

### Signs and symptoms
Axillary hyperhidrosis frequently produces such extreme sweating that patients often ruin their clothes in 1 day and develop contact dermatitis from clothing dyes; similarly, hyperhidrosis of the soles can easily damage a pair of shoes.

Profuse sweating from both the soles and the palms hinders the patient's ability to work and interact socially. Patients with this condition often report increased emotional strain.

### Diagnosis
Clinical observations and the patient history confirm hyperhidrosis.

### Treatment
The treatment of choice is the application of 20% aluminum chloride in absolute ethanol. (Most antiperspirants contain a 5% solution.) Formaldehyde may also be used but may lead to allergic contact sensitization.

Glutaraldehyde produces less contact sensitivity than formaldehyde but stains the skin; it is used more often on the feet than on the hands as a soak or applied directly several times a week and then weekly as needed. Therapy sometimes includes anticholinergics, except in patients with glaucoma or benign prostatic hyperplasia.

Severe hyperhidrosis unresponsive to conservative therapy may require local axillary removal of sweat glands or, as a last resort, a cervicothoracic or lumbar sympathectomy.

➤ CLINICAL TIP   Another form of effective treatment involves iontophoresis of water into involved areas of skin by a device that may be purchased by the patient.

### Special considerations
• Provide support and reassurance because hyperhidrosis may be socially embarrassing.

• Tell the patient to apply aluminum chloride in absolute ethanol nightly to dry axillae, soles, or palms. The area should be covered with plastic wrap for 6 to 8 hours, preferably overnight, and then washed with soap and water. Repeat this procedure for several nights until profuse daytime sweating subsides. Frequency of treatments can then be reduced.

• Advise the patient with hyperhidrosis of the soles to wear leather sandals and white or colorfast cotton socks.

# HYPERLIPOPROTEINEMIA

About one in five persons with elevated plasma lipid and lipoprotein levels has hyperlipoproteinemia, an inherited disorder marked by increased plasma concentrations of one or more lipoproteins. Hyperlipoproteinemia may also occur secondary to other conditions, such as diabetes, pancreatitis, hypothyroidism, and renal disease.

This disorder affects lipid transport in serum and produces varied clinical changes, from relatively mild symptoms that can be corrected by dietary management to potentially fatal pancreatitis.

Hyperlipoproteinemia occurs as five distinct metabolic disorders. Types I and III are transmitted as autosomal recessive traits; types II, IV, and V are transmitted as autosomal dominant traits.

## Causes

Each type of hyperlipoproteinemia has distinct causes and incidence. (See *Types of hyperlipoproteinemia.*)

## Signs and symptoms

Clinical features of hyperlipoproteinemia vary according to the type of disorder:

● *Type I:* recurrent attacks of severe abdominal pain similar to pancreatitis, usually preceded by fat intake; abdominal spasm, rigidity, or rebound tenderness; hepatosplenomegaly with liver or spleen tenderness; papular or eruptive xanthomas (pinkish yellow cutaneous deposits of fat) over pressure points and extensor surfaces; lipemia retinalis (reddish white retinal vessels); malaise; anorexia; and fever

● *Type II:* tendinous xanthomas (firm masses) on the Achilles tendons and tendons of the hands and feet, tuberous xanthomas, xanthelasma, juvenile corneal arcus (opaque ring surrounding the corneal periphery), accelerated atherosclerosis and premature coronary artery disease (CAD), and recurrent polyarthritis and tenosynovitis

● *Type III:* peripheral vascular disease manifested by claudication or tuboeruptive xanthomas (soft, inflamed, pedunculated lesions) over the elbows and knees; palmar xanthomas on the hands, particularly fingertips; premature atherosclerosis

● *Type IV:* predisposition to atherosclerosis and early CAD, exacerbated by excessive calorie intake, obesity, diabetes, and hypertension

● *Type V:* abdominal pain (most common), pancreatitis, peripheral neuropathy, eruptive xanthomas on extensor surfaces of the arms and legs, lipemia retinalis, and hepatosplenomegaly.

## Diagnosis

Diagnostic findings vary among the five types of hyperlipoproteinemia.

## Treatment

The first goal is to identify and treat any underlying problem such as diabetes. If no underlying problem exists, the primary treatment for types II, III, and IV is dietary management, especially restriction of cholesterol intake. Drug therapy (cholestyramine, clofibrate, or niacin) may also be used to lower the plasma triglyceride or cholesterol level when diet alone is ineffective.

### Type I

In type I hyperlipoproteinemia, treatment requires long-term weight reduction, with fat intake restricted to less than 20 g/day. A 20- to 40-g/day medium-chain triglyceride diet may be ordered to supplement caloric intake. The patient should also avoid alcoholic beverages to decrease plasma triglycerides. The prognosis is good with treatment; without treatment, death can result from pancreatitis.

### Type II

For type II, dietary management to restore normal lipid levels and decrease the risk of atherosclerosis includes restriction of cholesterol intake to less than 300 mg/day for adults and less than 150 mg/day for children; triglyceride levels must be restricted to less than 100 mg/day

# TYPES OF HYPERLIPOPROTEINEMIA

| TYPE | CAUSES AND INCIDENCE | DIAGNOSTIC FINDINGS |
|---|---|---|
| **I**<br>(Frederickson's hyperlipoprotein-emia, fat-induced hyperlipemia, idiopathic familial) | • Deficient or abnormal lipoprotein lipase, resulting in decreased or absent postheparin lipolytic activity<br>• Relatively rare<br>• Present at birth | • Chylomicrons (very-low-density lipoprotein [VLDL], low-density lipoprotein [LDL], and high-density lipoprotein) in plasma 14 hours or more after last meal<br>• Highly elevated serum chylomicron and triglyceride levels; slightly elevated serum cholesterol level<br>• Lower serum lipoprotein lipase level<br>• Leukocytosis |
| **II**<br>(Familial hyperbetalipoproteinemia, essential familial hypercholesterolemia) | • Deficient cell surface receptor that regulates LDL degradation and cholesterol synthesis, resulting in increased levels of plasma LDL over joints and pressure points<br>• Onset between ages 10 and 30 | • Increased plasma concentrations of LDL<br>• Increased serum LDL and cholesterol levels<br>• Increased LDL levels in amniotic fluid |
| **III**<br>(Familial broad-beta disease, xanthoma tuberosum) | • Unknown underlying defect results in deficient conversion of triglyceride-rich VLDL to LDL.<br>• Uncommon; usually occurs after age 20 but can occur earlier in men | • Abnormal serum beta-lipoprotein level<br>• Elevated cholesterol and triglyceride levels<br>• Slightly elevated glucose tolerance<br>• Hyperuricemia |
| **IV**<br>(Endogenous hypertriglyceridemia, hyperbetalipoproteinemia) | • Usually occurs secondary to obesity, alcoholism, diabetes, or emotional disorders<br>• Relatively common, especially in middle-aged men | • Elevated VLDL levels<br>• Abnormal levels of triglycerides in plasma; variable increase in serum<br>• Normal or slightly elevated serum cholesterol level<br>• Mildly abnormal glucose tolerance<br>• Family history<br>• Early coronary artery disease |
| **V**<br>(Mixed hyper-triglyceridemia, mixed hyperlipidemia) | • Defective triglyceride clearance causes pancreatitis; usually secondary to another disorder, such as obesity or nephrosis<br>• Uncommon; onset usually occurs late in adolescence or early in adulthood. | • Chylomicrons in plasma<br>• Elevated plasma VLDL levels<br>• Elevated serum cholesterol and triglyceride levels |

for children and adults. The diet should also be high in polyunsaturated fats.

In familial hypercholesterolemia, nicotinic acid with a bile acid usually normalizes low-density lipoprotein levels. For severely affected children, portacaval shunt is a last resort to reduce plasma cholesterol levels.

The prognosis remains poor regardless of treatment; in homozygotes, myocardial infarction usually causes death before age 30.

### Type III

For type III, dietary management includes restriction of cholesterol intake to less than 300 mg/day; carbohydrates must also be restricted, and polyunsaturated fats are increased. Clofibrate and niacin help lower blood lipid levels. Weight reduction is helpful. With strict adherence to the prescribed diet, the prognosis is good.

### Type IV

For type IV, weight reduction may normalize blood lipid levels without additional treatment. Long-term dietary management includes restricted cholesterol intake, increased polyunsaturated fats, and avoidance of alcoholic beverages. Clofibrate and niacin may lower plasma lipid levels.

The prognosis remains uncertain because of predisposition to premature CAD.

### Type V

The most effective treatment for type V is weight reduction and long-term maintenance of a low-fat diet. Alcoholic beverages must be avoided. Niacin, clofibrate, gemfibrozil, and a 20- to 40-g/day medium-chain triglyceride diet may prove helpful.

The prognosis is uncertain because of the risk of pancreatitis. Increased fat intake may cause recurrent bouts of illness, possibly leading to pseudocyst formation, hemorrhage, and death.

### Special considerations

● Care for patients with hyperlipoproteinemia emphasizes careful monitoring for adverse reactions to drugs and teaching the importance of long-term dietary management.

● Administer cholestyramine before meals or before bedtime. This drug must not be given with other medications. Watch for adverse reactions, such as nausea, vomiting, constipation, steatorrhea, rashes, and hyperchloremic acidosis. Also watch for malabsorption of other medications and fat-soluble vitamins.

● Give clofibrate as prescribed. Watch for adverse reactions, such as cholelithiasis, cardiac arrhythmias, intermittent claudication, thromboembolism, nausea, weight gain (from fluid retention), and myositis.

➤ CLINICAL TIP *Don't* administer niacin to patients with active peptic ulcers or liver disease. Use with caution in patients with diabetes. In other patients, watch for adverse reactions, such as flushing, pruritus, hyperpigmentation, and exacerbation of inactive peptic ulcers.

● Urge the patient to adhere to his diet (usually 1,000 to 1,500 calories/day), to avoid excess sugar and alcoholic beverages, to minimize intake of saturated fats (higher in meats, coconut oil), and to increase intake of polyunsaturated fats (vegetable oils).

● Instruct the patient, for the 2 weeks preceding serum cholesterol and serum triglyceride tests, to maintain a steady weight and to adhere strictly to the prescribed diet. He should also fast for 12 hours before the test.

● Instruct women with elevated serum lipid levels to avoid oral contraceptives or drugs that contain estrogen.

# HYPERPARATHYROIDISM

Characterized by overactivity of one or more of the four parathyroid glands, hyperparathyroidism results from excessive secretion of parathyroid hormone (PTH). Such hypersecretion of PTH promotes bone resorption and leads to hypercalcemia and hypophosphatemia. (See *Bone resorption in primary hyperparathyroidism.*)

Increased renal and GI absorption of calcium occurs.

Primary hyperparathyroidism is now commonly diagnosed by elevated calcium levels found on laboratory profiles in asymptomatic patients. It affects women two to three times more frequently than men.

### Causes

Hyperparathyroidism may be primary or secondary:

• In primary hyperparathyroidism, one or more of the parathyroid glands enlarges, increasing PTH secretion and elevating serum calcium levels. The most common cause is a single adenoma. Primary hyperparathyroidism is also a component of multiple endocrine neoplasia, in which all four glands are usually involved.

• In secondary hyperparathyroidism, excessive compensatory production of PTH stems from a hypocalcemia-producing abnormality outside the parathyroid gland, such as rickets, vitamin D deficiency, chronic renal failure, and osteomalacia due to phenytoin (Dilantin).

### Signs and symptoms

The clinical effects of primary hyperparathyroidism result from hypercalcemia and are typically present in several body systems.

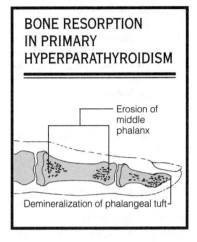

**BONE RESORPTION IN PRIMARY HYPERPARATHYROIDISM**

Erosion of middle phalanx

Demineralization of phalangeal tuft

• *Renal:* nephrocalcinosis due to elevated levels of calcium and, possibly, recurring nephrolithiasis, which may lead to renal insufficiency. Renal manifestations, including polyuria, are the most common effects of hyperparathyroidism.

• *Skeletal and articular:* chronic low back pain and easy fracturing due to bone degeneration; bone tenderness; chondrocalcinosis; osteopenia and osteoporosis, especially on the vertebrae; erosions of the juxta-articular surface; subchondrial fractures; traumatic synovitis; and pseudogout

• *GI:* pancreatitis, causing constant, severe epigastric pain that radiates to the back; peptic ulcers, causing abdominal pain, anorexia, nausea, and vomiting

• *Neuromuscular:* muscle weakness and atrophy, particularly in the legs

• *Central nervous system:* psychomotor and personality disturbances, depression, overt psychosis, stupor and, possibly, coma

• *Other:* skin necrosis, cataracts, calcium microthrombi to lungs and pancreas, polyuria, anemia, and subcutaneous calcification.

Similarly, in secondary hyperparathyroidism, decreased serum calcium levels may produce the same features of calcium imbalance with skeletal deformities of the long bones (rickets, for example) as well as symptoms of the underlying disease.

### Diagnosis

Findings differ in primary and secondary disease.

#### Primary disease

In primary disease, a high concentration of serum PTH on radioimmunoassay with accompanying hypercalcemia confirms the diagnosis. In addition, X-rays show diffuse demineralization of bones, bone cysts, outer cortical bone absorption, and subperiosteal erosion of the phalanges and distal clavicles.

Microscopic examination of the bone with such tests as X-ray spectrophotometry typically demonstrates increased bone turnover. Laboratory tests reveal elevated urine and serum calcium, chloride, and alkaline phosphatase levels and decreased serum phosphorus levels.

Hyperparathyroidism may also raise uric acid and creatinine levels and increase basal acid secretion and serum immunoreactive gastrin. Increased serum amylase levels may indicate acute pancreatitis.

#### Secondary disease

Laboratory findings in secondary hyperparathyroidism show normal or slightly decreased serum calcium levels and variable serum phosphorus levels, especially when hyperparathyroidism is due to rickets, osteomalacia, or kidney disease. The patient history may reveal familial kidney disease, seizure disorders, or drug ingestion.

Other laboratory values and physical examination findings identify the cause of secondary hyperparathyroidism.

### Treatment

Effective treatment varies, depending on the cause of the disease.

#### Primary disease

Treatment for primary hyperparathyroidism may include surgery to remove the adenoma or, depending on the extent of hyperplasia, all but half of one gland (the remaining part of the gland is necessary to maintain normal PTH levels). Such surgery may relieve bone pain within 3 days. However, renal damage may be irreversible.

CLINICAL TIP  Patients with primary hyperparathyroidism should be considered for surgery when:

• calcium levels are greater than or equal to 1 mg/dl above normal
• osteoporosis or hypercalcemia is present
• recurrent peptic ulcer disease is present
• nephrolithiasis is present
• impaired kidney function is noted
• patient is young or consistent follow-up is unavailable.

Preoperatively — or if surgery isn't feasible or necessary — other treatments can decrease calcium levels. They include forcing fluids, limiting dietary intake of calcium, and promoting sodium and calcium excretion through forced diuresis using normal saline solution (up to 6 L in life-threatening circumstances), furosemide, or ethacrynic acid.

Other treatments include administering oral sodium or potassium phosphate, subcutaneous calcitonin, I.V. mithramycin, or I.V. biphosphonates. In primary hyperparathyroidism, surgery is the only definitive therapy. There are no effective long-term medical therapies for hyperparathyroidism.

Therapy for potential postoperative magnesium and phosphate deficiencies includes I.V. administration of magnesium and phosphate or sodium phosphate solution given by mouth or retention enema. In addition, during the first 4 to 5 days after surgery, when serum calcium falls to low normal levels, supplemental calcium may be necessary; vitamin D or calcitriol may also be used to raise the serum calcium level.

### Secondary disease

Treatment of secondary hyperparathyroidism must correct the underlying cause of parathyroid hyperplasia. It consists of vitamin D therapy or, in the patient with kidney disease, administration of an oral calcium preparation for hyperphosphatemia.

In the patient with renal failure, dialysis is necessary to lower phosphorus levels and may have to continue for the remainder of the patient's life.

In the patient with chronic secondary hyperparathyroidism, the enlarged glands may not revert to normal size and function even after calcium levels have been controlled.

## Special considerations

• Care emphasizes prevention of complications from the underlying disease and its treatment.

• Obtain pretreatment baseline serum potassium, calcium, phosphate, and magnesium levels because these values may change abruptly during treatment.

• During hydration to reduce the serum calcium level, record intake and output accurately. Strain the urine to check for calculi. Provide at least 3 L of fluid a day, including cranberry or prune juice to increase urine acidity and help prevent calculus formation.

• Obtain blood samples and urine specimens to measure sodium, potassium, and magnesium levels, especially for the patient taking furosemide.

• Auscultate for breath sounds often. Listen for signs of pulmonary edema in the patient receiving large amounts of saline solution I.V., especially if he has lung or heart disease.

• Monitor the patient receiving digitalis glycosides carefully because elevated calcium levels can rapidly produce toxic effects.

• Because the patient is predisposed to pathologic fractures, take safety precautions to minimize the risk of injury. Assist him with walking, keep the bed at its lowest position, and raise the side rails. Lift the immobilized patient carefully to minimize bone stress.

• Schedule care to allow the patient with muscle weakness as much rest as possible.

• Watch for signs of peptic ulcer, and administer antacids as appropriate.

After parathyroidectomy:

• Check frequently for respiratory distress, and keep a tracheotomy tray at bedside. Watch for postoperative complications, such as laryngeal nerve damage and, rarely, hemorrhage. Monitor intake and output carefully.

• Check for swelling at the operative site. Place the patient in semi-Fowler's position, and support his head and neck with sandbags to decrease edema, which may cause pressure on the trachea.

• Watch for signs of mild tetany, such as complaints of tingling in the hands and around the mouth. These symptoms should subside quickly but may be prodromal signs of tetany, so keep calcium gluconate I.V. available for emergency administration. Watch for increased neuromuscular irritability and other signs of severe tetany.

• Ambulate the patient as soon as possible postoperatively, even though he may find this uncomfortable, because pressure on bones speeds up bone recalcification.

• Check laboratory results for low serum calcium and magnesium levels.

• Monitor the patient's mental status, and watch for listlessness. In the patient with persistent hypercalcemia, check for muscle weakness and psychiatric symptoms.

• Before discharge, advise the patient of the possible adverse effects of drug therapy. Emphasize the need for periodic follow-up through laboratory blood tests. If hyperparathyroidism wasn't corrected surgically, warn the patient to avoid calcium-containing antacids and thiazide diuretics.

# HYPERSPLENISM

A syndrome marked by exaggerated splenic activity and, possibly, splenomegaly (enlargement of the spleen), hypersplenism results in peripheral blood cell deficiency as the spleen traps and destroys peripheral blood cells.

## Causes

Hypersplenism may be idiopathic (primary) or secondary to an extrasplenic disorder, such as chronic malaria, polycythemia vera, and rheumatoid arthritis. In hypersplenism, the spleen's normal filtering and phagocytic functions accelerate indiscriminately, automatically removing antibody-coated, aging, and abnormal cells, even though some cells may be functionally normal.

The spleen may also temporarily sequester normal platelets and red blood cells (RBCs), withholding them from circulation. In this manner, the enlarged spleen may trap as much as 90% of the body's platelets and up to 45% of its RBC mass.

## Signs and symptoms

Most patients with hypersplenism develop anemia, leukopenia, or thrombocytopenia, often with splenomegaly. They may contract frequent bacterial infections, bruise easily, hemorrhage spontaneously from the mucous membranes and GI or genitourinary tract, and suffer ulcerations of the mouth, legs, and feet. They commonly develop fever, weakness, and palpitations.

Patients with secondary hypersplenism may have other clinical abnormalities, depending on the underlying disease.

## Diagnosis

Splenomegaly and evidence of abnormal splenic destruction or sequestration of RBCs or platelets are necessary to diagnose hypersplenism.

• The most definitive test measures the accumulation of erythrocytes in the spleen and liver after I.V. infusion of chromium-labeled RBCs or platelets. A high spleen-to-liver ratio of radioactivity indicates splenic destruction or sequestration.

• Complete blood count shows a decreased hemoglobin level (as low as 4 g/dl), white blood cell count (< 4,000/µl), platelet count (< 125,000/µl), and reticulocyte count.

• Splenic biopsy, scan, and angiography may be useful; a biopsy is hazardous, however, and should be avoided if possible.

## Treatment

Splenectomy is indicated only in transfusion-dependent patients who are refractory to medical therapy. Splenectomy seldom cures the patient but does correct the effects of cytopenia.

Postoperative complications include infection and thromboembolic disease. Occasionally, splenectomy may result in accelerated blood cell destruction in the bone marrow and liver. Secondary hypersplenism necessitates treatment of the underlying disease.

**Special considerations**
• If splenectomy is scheduled, administer preoperative transfusions of blood or blood products (fresh frozen plasma, platelets) to replace deficient blood elements. Symptoms or complications of any underlying disorder should be treated also.
• Postoperatively, monitor vital signs, observing for signs of shock.
• Check for excessive drainage or apparent bleeding.
• Watch for infection, thromboembolism, and abdominal distention.

CLINICAL TIP To decrease chances of infection in the splenectomy patient, pneumococcal vaccine (Pneumovax) should be administered before discharge. In addition, patient teaching should include signs of infection to report, how to prevent acquiring community infections, and ways to optimize health (such as nutrition and exercise).
• Keep the nasogastric tube patent; listen for bowel sounds.
• Instruct the patient to perform deep-breathing exercises, and encourage early ambulation to prevent respiratory complications and venous stasis.

# HYPERTENSION

An intermittent or a sustained elevation in diastolic or systolic blood pressure, hypertension occurs as two major types: essential (idiopathic) hypertension, the most common, and secondary hypertension, which results from kidney disease or another identifiable cause. Malignant hypertension is a severe, fulmi-

nant form of hypertension common to both types.

Hypertension is a major cause of cerebrovascular accident (CVA), heart disease, and renal failure. The prognosis is good if this disorder is detected early and if treatment begins before complications develop. Severely elevated blood pressure (hypertensive crisis) may be fatal.

**Causes**
Hypertension affects 15% to 20% of adults in the United States. If untreated, it carries a high mortality.

*Risk factors*
Family history, race (most common in blacks), stress, obesity, a high intake of saturated fats or sodium, use of tobacco, sedentary lifestyle, and aging are risk factors for essential hypertension.

CLINICAL TIP Systolic hypertension poses a risk that is equal to or greater than diastolic elevations. It is commonly seen in elderly people and presents a risk for CVA or myocardial infarction (MI).

Secondary hypertension may result from renovascular disease; pheochromocytoma; primary hyperaldosteronism; Cushing's syndrome; thyroid, pituitary, or parathyroid dysfunction; coarctation of the aorta; pregnancy; neurologic disorders; and use of oral contraceptives or other drugs, such as cocaine, epoetin alfa, and cyclosporine.

*Blood pressure regulators*
Cardiac output and peripheral vascular resistance determine blood pressure. Increased blood volume, cardiac rate, and stroke volume as well as arteriolar vasoconstriction can raise blood pressure. The link to sustained hypertension is unclear. Hypertension may also result from the failure of the following intrinsic regulatory mechanisms:

• Renal hypoperfusion causes the release of renin, which is converted by angiotensinogen, a liver enzyme, to angiotensin I. Angiotensin I is converted to angiotensin II, a powerful vasoconstrictor. The resulting vasoconstriction increases afterload.

Angiotensin II stimulates adrenal secretion of aldosterone, which increases sodium reabsorption. Hypertonic-stimulated release of antidiuretic hormone from the pituitary gland follows, increasing water reabsorption, plasma volume, cardiac output, and blood pressure.

• Autoregulation changes the diameter of an artery to maintain perfusion despite fluctuations in systemic blood pressure. The intrinsic mechanisms responsible include stress relaxation (vessels gradually dilate when blood pressure rises to reduce peripheral resistance) and capillary fluid shift (plasma moves between vessels and extravascular spaces to maintain intravascular volume).

• When the blood pressure drops, baroreceptors in the aortic arch and carotid sinuses decrease their inhibition of the medulla's vasomotor center, which increases sympathetic stimulation of the heart by norepinephrine. This in turn increases cardiac output by strengthening the contractile force, increasing the heart rate, and augmenting peripheral resistance by vasoconstriction.

Stress can also stimulate the sympathetic nervous system to increase cardiac output and peripheral vascular resistance.

## Signs and symptoms

Hypertension usually doesn't produce clinical effects until vascular changes in the heart, brain, or kidneys occur. Highly elevated blood pressure damages the intima of small vessels, resulting in fibrin accumulation in the vessels, development of local edema and, possibly, intravascular clotting.

Symptoms produced by this process depend on the location of the damaged vessels:
• *brain:* CVA
• *retina:* blindness
• *heart:* MI
• *kidneys:* proteinuria, edema and, eventually, renal failure.

Hypertension increases the heart's workload, causing left ventricular hypertrophy and, later, left ventricular failure, left- and right-sided heart failure, and pulmonary edema.

## Diagnosis

Serial blood pressure measurements that are greater than 140/90 mm Hg in people under age 50 or greater than 150/95 mm Hg in those over age 50 confirm hypertension. Auscultation may reveal bruits over the abdominal aorta and the carotid, renal, and femoral arteries; ophthalmoscopy reveals arteriovenous nicking and, in hypertensive encephalopathy, papilledema.

The patient history and the following additional tests may show predisposing factors and help identify an underlying cause such as kidney disease:
• *Urinalysis:* The presence of protein, red blood cells, and white blood cells may indicate glomerulonephritis.
• *Excretory urography:* Renal atrophy indicates chronic kidney disease; one kidney that is more than ⅝" (1.5 cm) shorter than the other suggests unilateral kidney disease.
• *Serum potassium:* Levels less than 3.5 mEq/L may indicate adrenal dysfunction (primary hyperaldosteronism).
• *Blood urea nitrogen (BUN) and serum creatinine levels:* A BUN level that is normal or elevated to more than 20 mg/dl and a serum creatinine level that is normal or elevated to more than 1.5 mg/dl suggest kidney disease.

Other tests help detect cardiovascular damage and other complications:
• *Electrocardiography* may show left ventricular hypertrophy or ischemia.
• *Chest X-ray* may show cardiomegaly.
• *Echocardiography* may show left ventricular hypertrophy.
• *Oral captopril challenge* tests for renovascular hypertension. This functional diagnostic test depends on the abrupt inhibition of circulating angiotensin II by angiotensin-converting enzyme (ACE) inhibitors, removing the major support for perfusion through a stenotic kidney. The acutely ischemic kidney immediately releases more renin and undergoes a marked decrease in glomerular filtration rate and renal blood flow.
• *Renal arteriography* may show renal artery stenosis.

### Treatment
Secondary hypertension treatment focuses on correcting the underlying cause and controlling hypertensive effects.

The National Institutes of Health recommend the following stepped-care approach for treating primary hypertension:
• *Step 1:* Help the patient initiate necessary lifestyle modifications, including weight reduction, moderation of alcohol intake, regular physical exercise, reduction of sodium intake, and smoking cessation.
• *Step 2:* If the patient fails to achieve the desired blood pressure or make significant progress, continue lifestyle modifications and begin drug therapy. Preferred drugs include diuretics and beta blockers. These drugs have proved effective in reducing cardiovascular morbidity and mortality.

If diuretics or beta-adrenergic blockers are ineffective or unacceptable, the doctor may prescribe ACE inhibitors,

calcium antagonists, alpha$_1$-receptor antagonists, or alpha- and beta-adrenergic antagoists. These drugs, although effective in reducing blood pressure, have yet to prove effective in reducing morbidity and mortality.
• *Step 3:* If the patient fails to achieve the desired blood pressure or make significant progress, increase the drug dosage, substitute a drug in the same class, or add a drug from a different class.
• *Step 4:* If the patient fails to achieve the desired blood pressure or make significant progress, add a second or third agent or a diuretic (if one isn't already prescribed). Second or third agents may include direct-acting vasodilators, alpha$_1$-receptor antagonists, and peripherally acting adrenergic neuron antagonists.

> **CLINICAL TIP** The treatment for renal artery stenosis includes the use of ACE inhibitors and renal artery stents.

#### Hypertensive emergencies
Examples of hypertensive emergencies include hypertensive encephalopathy, intracranial hemorrhage, acute left-sided heart failure with pulmonary edema, and dissecting aortic aneurysm. Hypertensive emergencies are also associated with eclampsia and severe pregnancy-related hypertension, unstable angina, and acute MI.

Typically, hypertensive emergencies require parenteral administration of a vasodilator or an adrenergic inhibitor or oral administration of a selected drug, such as nifedipine, captopril, clonidine, or labetalol, to rapidly reduce blood pressure.

Hypertension without accompanying symptoms or target organ disease seldom requires emergency drug therapy.

## Special considerations

- To encourage adherence to antihypertensive therapy, suggest that the patient establish a daily routine for taking his medication. Warn that uncontrolled hypertension may cause stroke and heart attack.

- Tell the patient to report adverse reactions to drugs.

- Advise the patient to avoid high-sodium antacids and over-the-counter cold and sinus medications, which contain harmful vasoconstrictors.

- Encourage a change in the patient's dietary habits. Help the obese patient plan a weight-reduction diet; tell him to avoid high-sodium foods (pickles, potato chips, canned soups, cold cuts) and table salt.

- Help the patient examine and modify his lifestyle, for example, by reducing stress and exercising regularly.

If a patient is hospitalized with hypertension:

- Find out if he was taking his prescribed medication. If he wasn't, ask why. If the patient can't afford the medication, refer him to an appropriate social service agency.

- Tell the patient and his family to keep a record of drugs used in the past, noting especially which ones were or were not effective. Suggest recording this information on a card so that the patient can show it to his doctor.

- Tell the patient who has a renal artery stent to expect an increase in urine output the first few days after the procedure.

When routine blood pressure screening reveals elevated pressure:

- Make sure the cuff size is appropriate for the patient's upper arm circumference.

- Measure the pressure in both arms in lying, sitting, and standing positions.

- Ask the patient if he smoked, drank a beverage containing caffeine, or was emotionally upset before the measurement.

- Advise the patient to return for blood pressure testing at frequent and regular intervals.

To help identify hypertension and prevent untreated hypertension:

- Participate in public education programs dealing with hypertension and ways to reduce risk factors.

- Encourage public participation in blood pressure screening programs. Routinely screen all patients, especially those at risk (blacks and people with family histories of hypertension, CVA, or heart attack).

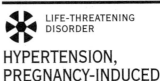

LIFE-THREATENING DISORDER

# HYPERTENSION, PREGNANCY-INDUCED

Toxemia of pregnancy, or pregnancy-induced hypertension (PIH), usually develops late in the second trimester or in the third trimester. *Preeclampsia,* the nonconvulsive form of toxemia, develops in about 7% of pregnancies. It may be mild or severe, and the incidence is significantly higher in low socioeconomic groups.

*Eclampsia* is the convulsive form of toxemia. About 5% of women with preeclampsia develop eclampsia; of these, about 15% die of toxemia itself or its complications. Fetal mortality is high because of the increased incidence of premature delivery.

## Causes

The cause of PIH is unknown, but it appears to be related to inadequate prenatal care (especially poor nutrition), parity (more prevalent in primigravidas), multiple pregnancies, preexisting diabetes mellitus, and hypertension.

Age is also a factor. Adolescents and primaparas over age 35 are at higher risk for preeclampsia. Other theories postulate a long list of potential toxic sources, such as autolysis of placental infarcts, autointoxication, uremia, maternal sensitization to total proteins, and pyelonephritis.

**Signs and symptoms**
- Mild preeclampsia generally produces the following signs: hypertension, proteinuria, generalized edema, and a sudden weight gain of more than 3 lb (1.36 kg) a week during the second trimester or more than 1 lb (0.45 kg) a week during the third trimester.
- Severe preeclampsia is marked by increased hypertension and proteinuria, which eventually lead to the development of oliguria. Hemolysis, elevated liver enzyme levels, and a low platelet count (the HELLP syndrome) is often severe.

❯ CLINICAL TIP A daughter whose mother had toxemia is at high risk for developing HELLP syndrome with new pregnancy.

Other symptoms that indicate worsening preeclampsia include blurred vision due to retinal arteriolar spasms, epigastric pain or heartburn, irritability, emotional tension, and severe frontal headache.
- In eclampsia, all the clinical manifestations of preeclampsia are magnified and associated with seizures and possibly coma, premature labor, stillbirth, renal failure, and liver damage.

**Diagnosis**
The following findings suggest mild preeclampsia:
- *elevated blood pressure readings:* 140 mm Hg systolic or a rise of 30 mm Hg

or more above the patient's normal systolic pressure measured on two occasions, 6 hours apart; 90 mm Hg diastolic or a rise of 15 mm Hg or more above the patient's normal diastolic pressure measured on two occasions, 6 hours apart
- *proteinuria:* > 500 mg/24 hours.

The following findings suggest severe preeclampsia:
- *much higher blood pressure readings:* 160/110 mm Hg or higher on two occasions, 6 hours apart, while on bed rest
- *increased proteinuria:* ≥ 5 g/24 hours
- *oliguria:* urine output ≤ 400 ml/24 hours
- *deep tendon reflexes:* possibly hyperactive as central nervous system (CNS) irritability increases.

Typical clinical features — especially seizures — with typical findings for severe preeclampsia strongly suggest eclampsia. An ophthalmoscopic examination may reveal vascular spasm, papilledema, retinal edema or detachment, and arteriovenous nicking or hemorrhage.

Real-time ultrasonography and stress and nonstress tests evaluate fetal well-being. In the stress test, oxytocin stimulates contractions; fetal heart tones are then monitored electronically.

In the nonstress test, fetal heart tones are monitored electronically during periods of fetal activity without oxytocin stimulation. Electronic monitoring reveals stable or increased fetal heart tones during periods of fetal activity.

**Treatment**
Adequate nutrition, good prenatal care, and control of preexisting hypertension with hydralazine (Apresoline) during pregnancy decrease the incidence and severity of preeclampsia. Early recognition and prompt treatment of preeclampsia can prevent progression to eclampsia.

Therapy for preeclampsia is designed to halt the disorder's progress—specifically, the early effects of eclampsia, such as seizures, residual hypertension, and renal shutdown—and to ensure fetal survival. Some doctors advocate the prompt induction of labor, especially if the patient is near term; others follow a more conservative approach.

***Conservative measures***
Therapy may include sedatives such as phenobarbital along with complete bed rest to relieve anxiety, reduce hypertension, and evaluate response to therapy. If renal function remains adequate, a high-protein, low-sodium, low-carbohydrate diet with increased fluid intake is recommended.

If blood pressure fails to respond to bed rest and sedation and persistently rises above 160/100 mm Hg or if CNS irritability increases, magnesium sulfate may produce general sedation, promote diuresis, reduce blood pressure, and prevent seizures.

***Cesarean section***
If these measures fail to improve the patient's condition or if fetal life is endangered (as determined by stress or nonstress tests), cesarean section or oxytocin induction may be required to terminate the pregnancy.

***Treatment for seizures***
Emergency treatment of eclamptic seizures consists of immediate administration of I.V. diazepam, followed by magnesium sulfate (I.V. drip), oxygen administration, and electronic fetal monitoring. After the patient's condition stabilizes, a cesarean section may be performed.

**Special considerations**
• Monitor regularly for changes in blood pressure, pulse and respiratory rates, fetal heart tones, vision, level of consciousness, and deep tendon reflexes and for headache unrelieved by medication. Assess these signs before administering medications. Absence of patellar reflexes may indicate magnesium sulfate toxicity.
• Assess fluid balance by measuring intake and output and by checking daily weight.
• Observe for signs of fetal distress by closely monitoring the results of stress and nonstress tests.
• Instruct the patient to lie in a left lateral position to increase venous return, cardiac output, and renal blood flow.
• Keep emergency resuscitative equipment and drugs (including diazepam and magnesium sulfate) available in case of seizures and cardiac or respiratory arrest. Also keep calcium gluconate at the bedside because it counteracts the toxic effects of magnesium sulfate.
• To protect the patient from injury, maintain seizure precautions. Don't leave an unstable patient unattended.
• Give emergency treatment to the patient having seizures. Provide a quiet, darkened room until the patient's condition stabilizes, and enforce absolute bed rest. Carefully monitor administration of magnesium sulfate; give oxygen. Don't administer anything by mouth. Insert an indwelling urinary catheter for accurate measurement of intake and output.
• Provide emotional support for the patient and family.

**CLINICAL TIP** If the patient's condition necessitates premature delivery, point out that infants of mothers with toxemia are usually small for gestational age but sometimes fare better than other premature babies of the same weight, possibly because they've developed adaptive responses to stress in utero.

# HYPOGLYCEMIA

An abnormally low glucose level in the bloodstream, hypoglycemia occurs when glucose burns up too rapidly, when the glucose release rate falls behind tissue demands, or when excessive insulin enters the bloodstream.

Hypoglycemia is classified as reactive or fasting. *Reactive hypoglycemia* results from the reaction to the disposition of meals or the administration of excessive insulin. *Fasting hypoglycemia* causes discomfort during long periods of abstinence from food, for example, in the early morning hours before breakfast.

Although hypoglycemia is a specific endocrine imbalance, its symptoms are often vague and depend on how quickly the patient's glucose levels drop. If not corrected, severe hypoglycemia may result in coma, irreversible brain damage, and death.

## Causes
The two forms of hypoglycemia have different causes and occur in different types of patients.

### Reactive hypoglycemia
Several forms of reactive hypoglycemia occur. In a diabetic patient, it may result from administration of too much insulin or—less commonly—too much oral antidiabetic medication. In a mildly diabetic patient (or one in the early stages of diabetes mellitus), reactive hypoglycemia may result from delayed and excessive insulin production after carbohydrate ingestion.

Similarly, a nondiabetic patient may suffer reactive hypoglycemia from a sharp increase in insulin output after a meal. Sometimes called *postprandial hypoglycemia,* this type of reactive hypoglycemia usually disappears when the patient eats something sweet.

In some patients, reactive hypoglycemia may have no known cause (idiopathic reactive) or may result from total parenteral nutrition due to gastric dumping syndrome or from impaired glucose tolerance.

### Fasting hypoglycemia
This type of hypoglycemia usually results from an excess of insulin or insulin-like substance or from a decrease in counterregulatory hormones. It can be *exogenous,* resulting from such external factors as alcohol or drug ingestion, or *endogenous,* resulting from organic problems.

Endogenous hypoglycemia may result from tumors or liver disease. Insulinomas, small islet cell tumors in the pancreas, secrete excessive amounts of insulin, which inhibits hepatic glucose production. They are generally benign (in 90% of patients).

Extrapancreatic tumors, although uncommon, can also cause hypoglycemia by increasing glucose utilization and inhibiting glucose output. Such tumors occur primarily in the mesenchyma, liver, adrenal cortex, GI system, and lymphatic system. They may be benign or malignant.

Among nonendocrine causes of fasting hypoglycemia are severe liver diseases, including hepatitis, cancer, cirrhosis, and liver congestion associated with heart failure. All these conditions reduce the uptake and release of glycogen from the liver.

Some endocrine causes include destruction of pancreatic islet cells; adrenocortical insufficiency, which contributes to hypoglycemia by reducing the production of cortisol and cortisone needed for gluconeogenesis; and pituitary insufficiency, which reduces corticotropin and growth hormone levels.

### Causes in infants and children

Hypoglycemia is at least as common in neonates and children as it is in adults. Usually, infants develop hypoglycemia because of an increased number of cells per unit of body weight and because of increased demands on stored liver glycogen to support respirations, thermoregulation, and muscle activity.

In full-term neonates, hypoglycemia may occur 24 to 72 hours after birth and is usually transient. In infants who are premature or small for gestational age, onset of hypoglycemia is much more rapid — it can occur as soon as 6 hours after birth — due to their small, immature livers, which produce much less glycogen. A rare cause of hypoglycemia in infants is nesidioblastosis, a benign condition of the insulin-producing islet cells. The treatment is surgical.

Maternal disorders that can produce hypoglycemia in infants within 24 hours after birth include diabetes mellitus, pregnancy-induced hypertension, erythroblastosis, and glycogen storage disease.

### Signs and symptoms

Reactive hypoglycemia causes fatigue, malaise, nervousness, irritability, trembling, tension, headache, hunger, cold sweats, and rapid heart rate. The same clinical effects usually characterize fasting hypoglycemia.

In addition, fasting hypoglycemia may cause central nervous system (CNS) disturbances, for example, blurred or double vision, confusion, motor weakness, hemiplegia, seizures, and coma.

In infants and children, signs and symptoms of hypoglycemia are vague. A neonate's refusal to feed may be the primary clue to underlying hypoglycemia. Associated CNS effects include tremors, twitching, weak or high-pitched cry, sweating, limpness, seizures, and coma.

### Diagnosis

Reagent or glucose reagent strips provide quick screening methods for determining blood glucose level. A color change that corresponds to less than 45 mg/dl indicates the need for a venous blood sample.

Laboratory testing confirms the diagnosis by showing decreased blood glucose values. The following values indicate hypoglycemia:
- *full-term infants:* < 30 mg/dl before a feeding; < 40 mg/dl after a feeding
- *preterm infants:* < 20 mg/dl before a feeding; < 30 mg/dl after a feeding
- *children and adults:* < 40 mg/ dl before a meal; < 50 mg/dl after a meal.

In addition, a 5-hour glucose tolerance test may be administered to provoke reactive hypoglycemia. After a 12-hour fast, laboratory testing to detect plasma insulin and plasma glucose levels may identify fasting hypoglycemia.

### Treatment

Reactive hypoglycemia and fasting hypoglycemia require different treatments.

### Reactive hypoglycemia

Effective treatment of reactive hypoglycemia requires dietary modification to help delay glucose absorption and gastric emptying. Usually, this includes small, frequent meals; ingestion of complex carbohydrates, fiber, and fat; and avoidance of simple sugars, alcohol, and fruit drinks.

The patient may also receive anticholinergic drugs to slow gastric emptying and intestinal motility and to inhibit vagal stimulation of insulin release.

## Fasting hypoglycemia

In fasting hypoglycemia, surgery and drug therapy are usually required. In patients with insulinoma, removal of the tumor is the treatment of choice. Drug therapy may include nondiuretic thiazides such as diazoxide to inhibit insulin secretion, streptozocin, and hormones, such as glucocorticoids and long-acting glycogen.

## In neonates

Therapy for neonates who have hypoglycemia or who are at risk of developing it includes preventive measures. A hypertonic solution of dextrose 10%, calculated at 5 to 10 ml/kg of body weight administered I.V. over 10 minutes and followed by 4 to 8 mg/kg/minute for maintenance, should correct a severe hypoglycemic state in neonates.

To reduce the chance of hypoglycemia in high-risk infants, they should receive feedings — either breast milk or a solution of dextrose 5% or 10% in water — as soon after birth as possible.

### Special considerations

● Watch for signs of hypoglycemia (such as poor feeding) in high-risk infants.

● Monitor infusion of hypertonic glucose in the neonate to avoid hyperglycemia, circulatory overload, and cellular dehydration. Terminate glucose solutions gradually to prevent hypoglycemia caused by hyperinsulinemia.

● Monitor the effects of drug therapy, and watch for the development of adverse effects.

● Teach the patient which foods to include in his diet (complex carbohydrates, fiber, fat) and which foods to avoid (simple sugars, alcohol). Refer the patient and his family for dietary counseling as appropriate.

# HYPOPARATHYROIDISM

A deficiency of parathyroid hormone (PTH), hypoparathyroidism is caused by disease, injury, or congenital malfunction of the parathyroid glands. Because the parathyroid glands primarily regulate calcium balance, hypoparathyroidism causes hypocalcemia, producing neuromuscular symptoms ranging from paresthesia to tetany.

The clinical effects of hypoparathyroidism are usually correctable with replacement therapy. Some complications of long-term hypocalcemia, such as cataracts and basal ganglion calcifications, are irreversible.

### Causes

Hypoparathyroidism may be acute or chronic and is classified as idiopathic or acquired:

● Idiopathic hypoparathyroidism may result from an autoimmune genetic disorder or the congenital absence of the parathyroid glands.

● Acquired hypoparathyroidism often results from accidental removal of or injury to the parathyroid glands during thyroidectomy or other neck surgery or, rarely, from massive thyroid irradiation. It may also result from ischemic infarction of the parathyroid glands during surgery or from hemochromatosis, sarcoidosis, amyloidosis, tuberculosis, neoplasms, or trauma.

● Acquired, reversible hypoparathyroidism may result from hypomagnesemia-induced impairment of hormone synthesis and release, from suppression of normal gland function due to hypercalcemia, or from delayed maturation of parathyroid function.

PTH isn't regulated by the pituitary or hypothalamus. It normally maintains blood calcium levels by increasing bone resorption and GI absorption of calcium. It also maintains an inverse relationship between serum calcium and phosphate levels by inhibiting phosphate reabsorption in the renal tubules. Abnormal PTH production disrupts this balance. Incidence of the idiopathic and reversible forms is highest in children; incidence of the irreversible acquired form is highest in older patients who have undergone surgery for hyperthyroidism or other head and neck conditions.

## Signs and symptoms
Although mild hypoparathyroidism may be asymptomatic, it usually produces hypocalcemia and high serum phosphate levels that affect the central nervous system (CNS) as well as other body systems.

### Chronic hypoparathyroidism
In the chronic form, the disease typically causes neuromuscular irritability, increased deep tendon reflexes, Chvostek's sign (hyperirritability of the facial nerve, producing a characteristic spasm when it's tapped), dysphagia, organic brain syndrome, psychosis, mental deficiency in children, and tetany.

Chronic tetany may cause difficulty in walking and a tendency to fall. It can lead to laryngospasm, stridor and, eventually, cyanosis and seizures.

### Acute hypoparathyroidism
More severe than chronic tetany, acute (overt) tetany begins with a tingling in the fingertips, around the mouth and, occasionally, in the feet. This tingling spreads and becomes more severe, producing muscle tension and spasms and consequent adduction of the thumbs, wrists, and elbows. Pain varies with the degree of muscle tension but seldom affects the face, legs, and feet.

Like chronic tetany, acute tetany may cause laryngospasm, stridor, cyanosis, and seizures. These CNS abnormalities tend to be exaggerated during hyperventilation, pregnancy, infection, withdrawal of thyroid hormone, and administration of diuretics and before menstruation.

Other clinical effects include abdominal pain; dry, lusterless hair; spontaneous hair loss; brittle fingernails that develop ridges or fall out; dry, scaly skin; cataracts; and weakened tooth enamel, which causes teeth to stain, crack, and decay easily.

Hypocalcemia may induce cardiac arrhythmias and eventually lead to heart failure.

## Diagnosis
The following test results confirm the diagnosis of hypoparathyroidism:
• *radioimmunoassay for PTH:* decreased PTH concentration
• *serum calcium:* decreased level
• *serum phosphorus:* increased level
• *electrocardiography (ECG):* prolonged QT and ST intervals due to hypocalcemia.

The following test helps provoke clinical evidence of hypoparathyroidism: Inflating a blood pressure cuff on the upper arm to between diastolic and systolic blood pressure and maintaining this inflation for 3 minutes elicits Trousseau's sign (carpal spasm).

## Treatment
Because calcium absorption from the small intestine requires the presence of vitamin D, treatment includes vitamin D and calcium supplements. Such therapy is usually lifelong, except for the reversible form of the disease.

If the patient is unable to tolerate vitamin D because of hepatic or renal problems, calcitriol may be used.

Acute, life-threatening tetany requires immediate I.V. administration of 10% calcium gluconate to raise serum calcium levels. The patient who's awake and

> ✓ **TEACHING CHECKLIST**
>
> ## DISCHARGE INSTRUCTIONS IN HYPOPARATHYROIDISM
>
> ● Advise the patient to follow a high-calcium, low-phosphorus diet, and tell him which foods are permitted.
> ● For the patient on drug therapy, emphasize the importance of checking serum calcium levels at least three times a year. Instruct him to watch for signs of hypercalcemia and to keep medications away from light and heat.
> ● Instruct the patient with scaly skin to use creams to soften his skin.
> ● Tell the patient to keep his nails trimmed to prevent them from splitting.

able to cooperate can help raise serum calcium levels by breathing into a paper bag and then inhaling his own carbon dioxide; this produces hypoventilation and mild respiratory acidosis.

Sedatives and anticonvulsants may control spasms until calcium levels rise. Chronic tetany requires maintenance therapy with oral calcium and vitamin D supplements.

**Special considerations**

● While awaiting the diagnosis of hypoparathyroidism in a patient with a history of tetany, maintain a patent I.V. line and keep I.V. calcium available. Because the patient is vulnerable to seizures, maintain seizure precautions.

● Keep a tracheotomy tray and endotracheal tube at bedside because laryngospasm may result from hypocalcemia.

● For the patient with tetany, administer 10% calcium gluconate slow I.V. (1 mg/minute) and maintain a patent airway. Such a patient may also require intubation, and sedation with I.V. diazepam.

● Monitor vital signs often after administration of I.V. diazepam to make certain blood pressure and heart rate return to normal.

● When caring for the patient with chronic hypoparathyroidism, particularly a child, stay alert for minor muscle twitching (especially in the hands) and for signs of laryngospasm (respiratory stridor or dysphagia) because these effects may signal onset of tetany.

● Because the patient with chronic disease has prolonged QT intervals on an ECG, watch for heart block and signs of decreasing cardiac output.

● Closely monitor the patient receiving both digitalis glycosides and calcium because calcium potentiates the effect of digitalis glycosides. Stay alert for signs of digitalis toxicity (arrhythmias, nausea, fatigue, visual changes).

● Do careful patient teaching. (See *Discharge instructions in hypoparathyroidism.*)

# HYPOPITUITARISM

Hypopituitarism, also known as panhypopituitarism, is a complex syndrome marked by metabolic dysfunction, sexual immaturity, and growth retardation (when it occurs in childhood), resulting from a deficiency of the hormones secreted by the anterior pituitary gland. Panhypopituitarism refers to a generalized condition caused by partial or total failure of all six of this gland's vital hormones—corticotropin, thyroid-stimulating hormone (TSH), luteinizing hormone (LH), follicle-stimulating hormone (FSH), human growth hormone (HGH), and prolactin. Partial hypopituitarism and complete hypopituitarism occur in adults and children; in children, these diseases may cause dwarfism and delayed puberty. The prognosis may be good with adequate replacement therapy and correction of the underlying causes.

## Causes

The most common cause of primary hypopituitarism is a tumor. Other causes include congenital defects (hypoplasia or aplasia of the pituitary gland); pituitary infarction (most often from postpartum hemorrhage); partial or total hypophysectomy by surgery, irradiation, or chemical agents; and, rarely, granulomatous disease (tuberculosis, for example). Occasionally, hypopituitarism may have no identifiable cause, or it may be related to autoimmune destruction of the gland. Secondary hypopituitarism stems from a deficiency of releasing hormones produced by the hypothalamus—either idiopathic or possibly resulting from infection, trauma, or a tumor.

Primary hypopituitarism usually develops in a predictable pattern of hormonal failures. It generally starts with hypogonadism from gonadotropin failure (decreased FSH and LH levels). In adults, it causes cessation of menses in women and impotence in men. GH deficiency follows; in children, this causes short stature, delayed growth, and delayed puberty. Subsequent failure of thyrotropin (decreased TSH levels) causes hypothyroidism; finally, adrenocortical failure (decreased corticotropin levels) results in adrenal insufficiency. When hypopituitarism follows surgical ablation or trauma, the pattern of hormonal events may not necessarily follow this sequence.

Sometimes damage to the hypothalamus or neurohypophysis from one of the above leads to diabetes insipidus.

## Signs and symptoms

Clinical features of hypopituitarism develop slowly and vary with the severity of the disorder and the number of deficient hormones. Signs and symptoms of hypopituitarism in adults may include gonadal failure (secondary amenorrhea, impotence, infertility, decreased libido), diabetes insipidus, hypothyroidism (fatigue, lethargy, sensitivity to cold, menstrual disturbances), and adrenocortical insufficiency (hypoglycemia, anorexia, nausea, abdominal pain, orthostatic hypotension).

Postpartum necrosis of the pituitary (Sheehan's syndrome) characteristically causes failure of lactation, menstruation, and growth of pubic and axillary hair as well as symptoms of thyroid and adrenocortical failure.

In children, hypopituitarism causes retarded growth and delayed puberty. Dwarfism usually isn't apparent at birth, but early signs begin to appear during the first few months of life; by age 6 months, growth retardation is obvious. Although these children generally enjoy good health, pituitary dwarfism may cause chubbiness due to fat deposits in the lower trunk, delayed secondary tooth eruption and, possibly, hypoglycemia. Growth continues at less than one-half the normal rate—sometimes into the patient's 20s or 30s—to an average height of 4′ (122 cm) with normal proportions.

When hypopituitarism strikes before puberty, it prevents development of secondary sex characteristics (including facial and body hair). In males, it produces undersized testes, penis, and prostate gland; absent or minimal libido; and inability to initiate and maintain an erection. In females, it usually causes immature development of the breasts, sparse or absent pubic and axillary hair, and primary amenorrhea.

Panhypopituitarism may induce a host of mental and physiologic abnormalities, including lethargy, psychosis, orthostatic hypotension, bradycardia, anemia, and anorexia. Clinical manifestations of hormonal deficiencies resulting from pituitary destruction don't become apparent until 75% of the gland is destroyed. Total loss of all hormones released by the anterior pituitary is fatal unless treated.

Neurologic signs associated with hypopituitarism and produced by pituitary tumors include headache, bilateral temporal hemianopia, loss of visual acuity and, possibly, blindness. Acute hypopituitarism resulting from surgery or infection is often associated with fever, hypotension, vomiting, and hypoglycemia — all characteristic of adrenal insufficiency.

## Diagnosis

In suspected hypopituitarism, evaluation must confirm hormonal deficiency due to impairment or destruction of the anterior pituitary gland and rule out disease of the target organs (adrenals, gonads, and thyroid) or the hypothalamus. Low serum levels of thyroxine ($T_4$), for example, indicate diminished thyroid gland function, but further tests are necessary to identify the source of this dysfunction as the thyroid, pituitary, or hypothalamus.

Radioimmunoassay showing decreased plasma levels of some or all pituitary hormones, accompanied by end-organ hypofunction, suggests pituitary failure and eliminates target gland disease. Failure of thyrotropin-releasing hormone administration to increase TSH or prolactin concentrations rules out hypothalamic dysfunction as the cause of hormonal deficiency.

Provocative tests are helpful in pinpointing the source of low cortisol levels. Oral metyrapone blocks cortisol synthesis, which should stimulate pituitary secretion of corticotropin and the adrenal precursors of cortisol, measured in urine as hydroxycorticosteroids. Insulin-induced hypoglycemia also stimulates corticotropin secretion. Persistently low levels of corticotropin indicate pituitary or hypothalamic failure. These tests require careful medical supervision because they may precipitate an adrenal crisis.

Diagnosis of hypopituitarism requires measurement of GH levels in the blood after administration of regular insulin (inducing hypoglycemia) or levodopa. These drugs should provoke increased secretion of GH. Persistently low GH levels, despite provocative testing, confirm GH deficiency. Computed tomography scan, magnetic resonance imaging, or cerebral angiography confirms the presence of intrasellar or extrasellar tumors.

## Treatment

Replacement of hormones secreted by the target glands is the most effective treatment for hypopituitarism. Hormone replacement therapy includes cortisol, $T_4$, and androgen or cyclic estrogen. Prolactin need not be replaced. The patient of reproductive age may benefit from cyclic administration of FSH and human chorionic gonadotropin to induce ovulation.

➤ CLINICAL TIP In hypopituitarism, the TSH levels become an unreliable marker for thyroid hormone replacement. Therefore, follow free $T_4$ levels in this patient.

Somatrem, identical to GH but the product of recombinant deoxyribonucleic acid technology, has replaced growth hormones derived from human sources. It's effective for treating dwarfism and stimulates growth increases as great as 6″ (15 cm) in the 1st year of treatment. The growth rate tapers off in subsequent years. After pubertal changes have occurred, the effects of somatrem therapy are limited. Occasionally, a child becomes unresponsive to somatrem therapy, even with larger doses, perhaps because antibodies have formed against it. In such refractory patients, small doses of androgen may again stimulate growth, but extreme caution is necessary to prevent premature closure of the epiphyses. Children with hypopituitarism may also need replacement of adrenal and thyroid hormones and, as they approach puberty, sex hormones.

### Special considerations

● Caring for patients with hypopituitarism requires an understanding of hormonal effects and skilled physical and psychological support.

● Monitor the results of all laboratory tests for hormonal deficiencies, and know what they mean. Until hormone replacement therapy is complete, check for signs of thyroid deficiency (increasing lethargy), adrenal deficiency (weakness, orthostatic hypotension, hypoglycemia, fatigue, and weight loss), and gonadotropin deficiency (decreased libido, lethargy, and apathy).

● Watch for anorexia in the patient with panhypopituitarism. Help plan a menu that contains his favorite foods — ideally, high-calorie foods. Monitor for weight loss or gain.

● Record temperature, blood pressure, and heart rate every 4 to 8 hours. Check eyelids, nail beds, and skin for pallor, which indicates anemia.

● Prevent infection by giving meticulous skin care. Because the patient's skin is probably dry, use oil or lotion instead of soap. If body temperature is low, provide additional clothing and covers, as needed, to keep the patient warm.

● Darken the room if the patient has a tumor that is causing headaches and visual disturbances. Help with any activity that requires good vision, such as reading the menu. The patient with bilateral hemianopia has impaired peripheral vision, so be sure to stand where he can see you and advise the family to do the same.

● During insulin testing, monitor closely for signs of hypoglycemia (initially, slow cerebration, tachycardia, diaphoresis, and nervousness, progressing to seizures). Keep dextrose 50% in water available for I.V. administration to correct hypoglycemia rapidly.

● To prevent orthostatic hypotension, be sure to keep the patient supine during levodopa testing.

● Instruct the patient to wear a medical identification bracelet. Teach him and family members how to administer steroids parenterally in case of an emergency.

● Refer the family of a child with dwarfism to appropriate community resources for psychological counseling because the emotional stress caused by this disorder increases as the child becomes more aware of his condition.

# HYPOTHYROIDISM IN ADULTS

Hypothyroidism, a state of low serum thyroid hormone, results from hypothalamic, pituitary, or thyroid insufficiency. The disorder can progress to life-threatening myxedema coma. Hypothyroidism is more prevalent in women than in men; in the United States, incidence is rising significantly in people ages 40 to 50.

## Causes

Hypothyroidism results from inadequate production of thyroid hormone, usually because of dysfunction of the thyroid gland due to surgery (thyroidectomy), radiation therapy (particularly with $^{131}$I), inflammation, chronic autoimmune thyroiditis (Hashimoto's disease) or, rarely, conditions such as amyloidosis and sarcoidosis. It may also result from pituitary failure to produce thyroid-stimulating hormone (TSH), hypothalamic failure to produce thyrotropin-releasing hormone, inborn errors of thyroid hormone synthesis, inability to synthesize thyroid hormone because of iodine deficiency (usually dietary), or the use of antithyroid medications such as propylthiouracil.

In patients with hypothyroidism, infection, exposure to cold, and sedatives may precipitate myxedema coma.

### Signs and symptoms

Typically, the early clinical features of hypothyroidism are vague: fatigue, forgetfulness, sensitivity to cold, unexplained weight gain, and constipation. As the disorder progresses, characteristic myxedematous signs and symptoms appear: decreasing mental stability; dry, flaky, inelastic skin; puffy face, hands, and feet; hoarseness; periorbital edema; upper eyelid droop; dry, sparse hair; and thick, brittle nails.

Cardiovascular involvement leads to decreased cardiac output, slow pulse rate, signs of poor peripheral circulation and, occasionally, an enlarged heart. Other common effects include anorexia, abdominal distention, menorrhagia, decreased libido, infertility, ataxia, and nystagmus. Reflexes show delayed relaxation time (especially in the Achilles tendon).

Progression to myxedema coma is usually gradual, but when stress aggravates severe or prolonged hypothy-

roidism, coma may develop abruptly. Clinical effects include progressive stupor, hypoventilation, hypoglycemia, hyponatremia, hypotension, and hypothermia.

### Diagnosis

Radioimmunoassay confirms hypothyroidism with low triiodothyronine ($T_3$) and thyroxine ($T_4$) levels.

Supportive laboratory findings include:

- increased TSH level when hypothyroidism is due to thyroid insufficiency; decreased TSH level when hypothyroidism is due to hypothalamic or pituitary insufficiency
- elevated levels of serum cholesterol, alkaline phosphatase, and triglycerides
- normocytic, normochromic anemia.

In myxedema coma, laboratory tests may also show low serum sodium levels as well as decreased pH and increased partial pressure of carbon dioxide, indicating respiratory acidosis.

### Treatment

Therapy for hypothyroidism consists of gradual thyroid hormone replacement with levothyroxine ($T_4$) and, occasionally, liothyronine ($T_3$).

CLINICAL TIP The TSH level is the most reliable marker to follow in primary hypothyroidism. It should be kept within the normal range.

During myxedema coma, effective treatment supports vital functions while restoring euthyroidism. To support blood pressure and pulse rate, treatment includes I.V. administration of levothyroxine and hydrocortisone to correct possible pituitary or adrenal insufficiency. Hypoventilation requires oxygenation and respiratory support.

Other supportive measures include fluid replacement and antibiotics for infection.

**Special considerations**

To manage the hypothyroid patient:

• Provide a high-bulk, low-calorie diet, and encourage activity to combat constipation and promote weight loss. Administer cathartics and stool softeners as needed.

• After thyroid replacement therapy begins, watch for symptoms of hyperthyroidism, such as restlessness, sweating, and excessive weight loss.

• Tell the patient to report signs of aggravated cardiovascular disease, such as chest pain and tachycardia.

• To prevent myxedema coma, tell the patient to continue his course of thyroid medication even if his symptoms subside.

• Warn the patient to report infection immediately and to make sure any doctor who prescribes drugs for him knows about the underlying hypothyroidism.

Treatment of myxedema coma requires supportive care:

• Check frequently for signs of decreasing cardiac output (such as falling urine output).

• Monitor temperature until stable. Provide extra blankets and clothing and a warm room to compensate for hypothermia. Rapid rewarming may cause vasodilation and vascular collapse.

• Record intake and output and daily weight. As treatment begins, urine output should increase and body weight should decrease.

• Turn the edematous bedridden patient every 2 hours, and provide skin care, particularly around bony prominences, at least once a shift.

• Avoid sedation when possible or reduce the dose because hypothyroidism delays metabolism of many drugs.

• Maintain a patent I.V. line. Monitor serum electrolyte levels carefully when administering I.V. fluids.

• Monitor vital signs carefully when administering levothyroxine because rapid correction of hypothyroidism can cause adverse cardiac effects. Report chest pain or tachycardia immediately. Watch for hypertension and heart failure in the elderly patient.

• Check arterial blood gas values for indications of hypoxia and respiratory acidosis to determine whether the patient needs ventilatory assistance.

• Because myxedema coma may have been precipitated by an infection, check possible sources of infection, such as blood or urine, and obtain sputum cultures.

# HYPOTHYROIDISM IN CHILDREN

Deficiency of thyroid hormone secretion during fetal development and early in infancy results in infantile cretinism (congenital hypothyroidism). Untreated hypothyroidism is characterized in infants by respiratory difficulties, persistent jaundice, and hoarse crying and in older children by stunted growth (dwarfism), bone and muscle dystrophy, and mental deficiency.

Cretinism is three times more common in girls than in boys. Early diagnosis and treatment allow the best prognosis; infants treated before age 3 months usually grow and develop normally. Athyroid children who remain untreated beyond age 3 months and children with acquired hypothyroidism who remain untreated beyond age 2 suffer irreversible mental retardation; their skeletal abnormalities are reversible with treatment.

**Causes**

In infants, cretinism usually results from defective embryonic development that causes congenital absence or underdevelopment of the thyroid gland. The next most common cause can be traced to an inherited enzymatic defect in the synthesis of thyroxine ($T_4$) caused by an autosomal recessive gene. Less frequently, antithyroid drugs taken during pregnancy produce cretinism in infants. In children older than age 2, cretinism usually results from chronic autoimmune thyroiditis.

## Signs and symptoms

The weight and length of an infant with infantile cretinism appear normal at birth, but characteristic signs of hypothyroidism develop by the time he's 3 to 6 months old. In a breast-fed infant onset of most symptoms may be delayed until weaning because breast milk contains small amounts of thyroid hormone.

Typically, an infant with cretinism sleeps excessively, seldom cries (except for occasional hoarse crying), and is inactive. Because of this, his parents may describe him as a "good baby—no trouble at all." Such behavior actually results from lowered metabolism and progressive mental impairment. The infant with cretinism also exhibits abnormal deep tendon reflexes, hypotonic abdominal muscles, a protruding abdomen, and slow, awkward movements. He has feeding difficulties, develops constipation and, because his immature liver can't conjugate bilirubin, becomes jaundiced.

His large, protruding tongue obstructs respiration, making breathing loud and noisy and forcing him to open his mouth to breathe. He may have dyspnea on exertion; anemia; abnormal facial features — such as a short forehead; puffy, wide-set eyes (periorbital edema); wrinkled eyelids; and a broad, short, upturned nose — and a dull expression, resulting from mental retardation. His skin is cold and mottled because of poor circulation, and his hair is dry, brittle, and dull. Teeth erupt late and tend to decay

early, body temperature is below normal, and pulse rate is slow.

In the child who acquires hypothyroidism after age 2, appropriate treatment can prevent mental retardation. However, growth retardation becomes apparent in short stature (due to delayed epiphyseal maturation, particularly in the legs), obesity, and a head that appears abnormally large because the arms and legs are stunted. An older child may show delayed or accelerated sexual development.

## Diagnosis

A high serum level of thyroid-stimulating hormone (TSH) associated with low triiodothyronine and $T_4$ levels points to cretinism. Because early detection and treatment can minimize the effects of cretinism, many states require measurement of infant thyroid hormone levels at birth.

Thyroid scan and [131]I uptake tests show decreased uptake levels and confirm the absence of thyroid tissue in athyroid children. Increased gonadotropin levels are compatible with sexual precocity in older children and may coexist with hypothyroidism. An electrocardiogram shows bradycardia and flat or inverted T waves in untreated infants. Hip, knee, and thigh X-rays reveal the absence of the femoral or tibial epiphyseal line and delayed skeletal development that is markedly inappropriate for the child's chronological age. A low $T_4$ level associated with a normal TSH level suggests hypothyroidism secondary to hypothalamic or pituitary disease, a rare condition.

## Treatment

Early detection is mandatory to prevent irreversible mental retardation and permit normal physical development.

Treatment of infants younger than age 1 consists of replacement therapy with oral levothyroxine, beginning with moderate doses. Dosage gradually increases to levels sufficient for lifelong maintenance. (Rapid increase in dosage may precipitate thyrotoxicity.) Doses are proportionately higher in children than in adults because children metabolize thyroid hormone more quickly. Therapy in older children includes levothyroxine.

### Special considerations

Prevention, early detection, comprehensive parent teaching, and psychological support are essential. Know the early signs. Be especially wary if parents emphasize how good and how quiet their new baby is.

• During early management of infantile cretinism, monitor blood pressure and pulse rate; report hypertension and tachycardia immediately. But remember — normal infant heart rate is about 120 beats/minute. If the infant's tongue is unusually large, position him on his side and observe him frequently to prevent airway obstruction. Check rectal temperature every 2 to 4 hours. Keep the infant warm and his skin moist.

• Inform the parents that the child will require lifelong treatment with thyroid supplements. Teach them to recognize the signs of overdose: rapid pulse rate, irritability, insomnia, fever, sweating, and weight loss. Stress the need to comply with the treatment regimen to prevent further mental impairment.

• Provide support to help the parents deal with a child who may be mentally retarded. Help them adopt a positive but realistic attitude and focus on their child's strengths rather than his weaknesses. Encourage them to provide stimulating activities to help the child reach his maximum potential. Refer them to appropriate community resources for support.

# HYPOVOLEMIC SHOCK

In hypovolemic shock, reduced intravascular blood volume causes circulatory dysfunction and inadequate tissue perfusion. Without sufficient blood or fluid replacement, hypovolemic shock syndrome may lead to irreversible cerebral and renal damage, cardiac arrest and, ultimately, death. (See *What happens in hypovolemic shock.*) Hypovolemic shock requires early recognition of signs and symptoms and prompt, aggressive treatment to improve the prognosis.

### Causes

Hypovolemic shock usually results from acute blood loss—about one-fifth of the total volume. Such massive blood loss may result from GI bleeding, internal hemorrhage (hemothorax, hemoperitoneum), or external hemorrhage (accidental or surgical trauma) or from any condition that reduces circulating intravascular plasma volume or other body fluids, such as in severe burns. Other underlying causes of hypovolemic shock include intestinal obstruction, peritonitis, acute pancreatitis, ascites and dehydration from excessive perspiration, severe diarrhea or protracted vomiting, diabetes insipidus, diuresis, and inadequate fluid intake.

### Signs and symptoms

Hypovolemic shock produces a syndrome of hypotension with narrowing pulse pressure; decreased sensorium; tachycardia; rapid, shallow respirations; reduced urine output (< 25 ml/hour); and cold, pale, clammy skin. Metabolic acidosis with an accumulation of lactic acid develops as a result of tissue anoxia as cellular metabolism shifts from aerobic to anaerobic pathways.

# WHAT HAPPENS IN HYPOVOLEMIC SHOCK

In hypovolemic shock, vascular fluid volume loss causes extreme tissue hypoperfusion. Internal fluid losses can result from hemorrhage or third-space fluid shifting. External fluid loss can result from severe bleeding or from severe diarrhea, diuresis, or vomiting. Inadequate vascular volume leads to decreased venous return and cardiac output. The resulting drop in arterial blood pressure activates the body's compensatory mechanisms in an attempt to increase vascular volume. If compensation is unsuccessful, decompensation and death may occur.

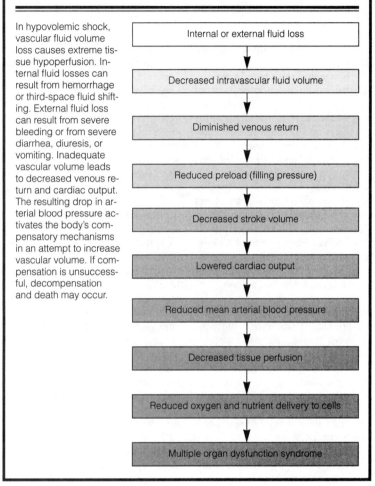

Internal or external fluid loss

Decreased intravascular fluid volume

Diminished venous return

Reduced preload (filling pressure)

Decreased stroke volume

Lowered cardiac output

Reduced mean arterial blood pressure

Decreased tissue perfusion

Reduced oxygen and nutrient delivery to cells

Multiple organ dysfunction syndrome

Disseminated intravascular coagulation (DIC) is a possible complication of hypovolemic shock.

## Diagnosis
No single symptom or diagnostic test establishes the diagnosis or severity of shock. Characteristic laboratory findings include:

● elevated potassium, serum lactate, and blood urea nitrogen levels
● increased urine specific gravity (> 1.020) and urine osmolality
● decreased blood pH and partial pressure of arterial oxygen and increased partial pressure of arterial carbon dioxide.

In addition, gastroscopy, aspiration of gastric contents through a nasogastric tube, and X-rays identify internal bleeding sites; coagulation studies may detect coagulopathy from DIC.

## Treatment

Emergency treatment measures must include prompt and adequate blood and fluid replacement to restore intravascular volume and raise blood pressure. Normal saline solution or lactated Ringer's solution and then possibly plasma proteins (albumin) or other plasma expanders may produce adequate volume expansion until whole blood can be matched. A rapid solution infusion system can provide these crystalloids or colloids at high flow rates. Application of a pneumatic antishock garment may be helpful. Treatment may also include oxygen administration, identification of bleeding site, control of bleeding by direct measures (such as application of pressure and elevation of an extremity) and, possibly, surgery.

## Special considerations

Management of hypovolemic shock necessitates prompt, aggressive supportive measures and careful assessment and monitoring of vital signs. Follow these priorities:

• Check for a patent airway and adequate circulation. If blood pressure and heart rate are absent, start cardiopulmonary resuscitation.

• Record blood pressure, pulse rate, peripheral pulses, respiratory rate, and other vital signs every 15 minutes and monitor the electrocardiogram continuously. A systolic blood pressure lower than 80 mm Hg usually results in inadequate coronary artery blood flow, cardiac ischemia, arrhythmias, and further complications of low cardiac output. When blood pressure drops below 80 mm Hg, increase the oxygen flow rate and notify the doctor immediately. A progressive drop in blood pressure accompanied by a thready pulse generally signals inadequate cardiac output from reduced intravascular volume. Notify the doctor, and increase the infusion rate.

• Start I.V. lines with normal saline or lactated Ringer's solution, using a large-bore catheter (14G), which allows easier administration of later blood transfusions.

➤ CLINICAL TIP  Don't start I.V. lines in the legs of a patient in shock who has suffered abdominal trauma because infused fluid may escape through the ruptured vessel into the abdomen.

• An indwelling urinary catheter may be inserted to measure hourly urine output. If output is less than 30 ml/hour in adults, increase the fluid infusion rate, but watch for signs of fluid overload, such as an increase in pulmonary artery wedge pressure (PAWP). Notify the doctor if urine output does not improve. An osmotic diuretic such as mannitol may be ordered to increase renal blood flow and urine output. Determine how much fluid to give by checking blood pressure, urine output, central venous pressure (CVP), or PAWP.

➤ CLINICAL TIP  To increase accuracy, CVP should be measured at the level of the right atrium, using the same reference point on the chest each time.

• Draw an arterial blood sample to measure arterial blood gas (ABG) values. Administer oxygen by face mask or airway to ensure adequate oxygenation of tissues. Adjust the oxygen flow rate to a higher or lower level, as ABG measurements indicate.

• Draw venous blood for complete blood count and electrolyte, type and crossmatch, and coagulation studies.

• During therapy, assess skin color and temperature and note any changes. Cold, clammy skin may be a sign of continuing peripheral vascular constriction, indicating progressive shock.

➤ CLINICAL TIP   Watch for signs of impending coagulopathy (petechiae, bruising, bleeding or oozing from the gums or venipuncture sites).

• Explain all procedures and their purpose. Throughout these emergency measures, provide emotional support to the patient and his family.

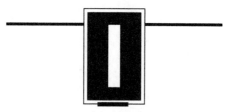

# IDIOPATHIC THROMBOCYTOPENIC PURPURA

Idiopathic thrombocytopenic purpura (ITP), thrombocytopenia that results from immunologic platelet destruction, may be acute (postviral thrombocytopenia) or chronic (Werlhof's disease, purpura hemorrhagica, essential thrombocytopenia, autoimmune thrombocytopenia). Acute ITP usually affects children between ages 2 and 6; chronic ITP mainly affects adults under age 50, especially women between ages 20 and 40.

The prognosis for acute ITP is excellent; nearly four out of five patients recover without treatment. The prognosis for chronic ITP is good; remissions lasting weeks or years are common, especially among women.

## Causes
ITP may be an autoimmune disorder because antibodies that reduce the life span of platelets have been found in nearly all patients. The spleen probably helps to remove platelets modified by the antibody. Acute ITP usually follows a viral infection, such as rubella and chickenpox, and can follow immunization with a live virus vaccine. Chronic ITP seldom follows infection and is often linked to immunologic disorders, such as systemic lupus erythematosus. It's also linked to drug reactions.

## Signs and symptoms
Clinical features of ITP common to all forms of thrombocytopenia include petechiae, ecchymoses, and mucosal bleeding from the mouth, nose, or GI tract. Generally, hemorrhage is a rare physical finding. Purpuric lesions may occur in vital organs, such as the lungs, kidneys, or brain, and may prove fatal.

In acute ITP, which commonly occurs in children, onset is usually sudden and without warning, causing easy bruising, epistaxis, and bleeding gums. Onset of chronic ITP is insidious.

## Diagnosis
Platelet count less than 20,000/µl and prolonged bleeding time suggest ITP. Platelet size and morphologic appearance may be abnormal; anemia may be present if bleeding has occurred.

As in thrombocytopenia, bone marrow studies show an abundance of megakaryocytes and a shortened circulating platelet survival time (hours or days). Occasionally, platelet antibodies may be found in vitro, but this diagnosis is usually inferred from platelet survival data and the absence of an underlying disease.

## Treatment
Acute ITP may be allowed to run its course without intervention or may be treated with glucocorticoids or immune globulin. For chronic ITP, corticosteroids

may be the initial treatment of choice. Patients who fail to respond within 1 to 4 months or who need high steroid dosage are candidates for splenectomy, which has an 85% success rate. Alternative treatments include immunosuppression, high-dose I.V. gamma globulin, and immunoabsorption apheresis using staphylococcal protein-A columns.

> **CLINICAL TIP** Before splenectomy, the patient may require blood, blood components, and vitamin K to correct anemia and coagulation defects. After splenectomy, he may need blood and component replacement and platelet concentrate. Normally, platelets increase spontaneously after splenectomy.

### Special considerations
- Patient care for ITP is essentially the same as for other types of thrombocytopenia, with emphasis on teaching the patient to observe for petechiae, ecchymoses, and other signs of recurrence.
- Monitor patients receiving immunosuppressive therapy for signs of bone marrow depression, infection, mucositis, GI ulcers, and severe diarrhea or vomiting.
- Tell the patient to avoid aspirin and ibuprofen.

# IMPETIGO

A contagious, superficial skin infection, impetigo (also known as impetigo contagiosa) occurs in nonbullous and bullous forms. This vesiculopustular eruptive disorder spreads most easily among infants, young children, and elderly people.

Predisposing factors such as poor hygiene, anemia, malnutrition, and a warm climate favor outbreaks of this infection, most of which occur during the late summer and early fall. Impetigo can complicate chickenpox, eczema, and other skin conditions marked by open lesions.

### Causes
Coagulase-positive *Staphylococcus aureus* and, less commonly, group A beta-hemolytic streptococci usually produce nonbullous impetigo; *S. aureus* (especially of phage type 71) generally causes bullous impetigo.

### Signs and symptoms
*Common nonbullous impetigo* typically begins with a small red macule that turns into a vesicle, becoming pustular with a honey-colored crust within hours. When the vesicle breaks, a thick yellow crust forms from the exudate. Autoinoculation may cause satellite lesions. Other features include pruritus, burning, and regional lymphadenopathy.

A rare but serious complication of streptococcal impetigo is glomerulonephritis.

In *bullous impetigo*, a thin-walled vesicle opens and a thin, clear crust forms on the subsequent eruption. It commonly appears on exposed areas.

### Diagnosis
Characteristic lesions suggest impetigo (see *Recognizing impetigo vesicles,* page 452.) Microscopic visualization of the causative organism in a Gram stain of vesicle fluid usually confirms *S. aureus* infection and justifies antibiotic therapy.

Culture and sensitivity testing of fluid or denuded skin may indicate the most appropriate antibiotic, but therapy shouldn't be delayed for laboratory results, which can take 3 days.

### Treatment
Generally, treatment consists of systemic antibiotics (usually a pencillinase-resistant penicillin, cephalosporin, or erythromycin) for 10 days. A topical

## RECOGNIZING IMPETIGO VESICLES

In impetigo, when the vesicles break, crust forms from the exudate. This infection is especially contagious among young children.

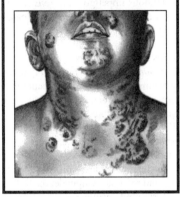

antibiotic such as mupirocin ointment may be used for minor infections.

Therapy also includes removal of the exudate by washing the lesions two or three times a day with soap and water or, for stubborn crusts, using warm soaks or compresses of normal saline or a diluted soap solution.

### Special considerations
• Urge the patient not to scratch because this spreads impetigo. Advise parents to cut the child's fingernails.
• Give medications as necessary; remember to check for penicillin allergy. Stress the need to continue prescribed medications for 7 to 10 days, even after the lesions have healed.
• Teach the patient or family how to care for impetiginous lesions. To prevent further spread of this highly contagious infection, encourage frequent bathing using a bactericidal soap.

• Tell the patient not to share towels, washcloths, or bed linens with family members. Emphasize the importance of following proper hand-washing technique.

➤ CLINICAL TIP  Check family members for impetigo. If this infection is present in a schoolchild, notify the school.

# INCLUSION CONJUNCTIVITIS

Inclusion conjunctivitis is an acute ocular inflammation resulting from infection by *Chlamydia trachomatis*. Although inclusion conjunctivitis occasionally becomes chronic, the prognosis is generally good with treatment. If untreated, it may run a course of 3 to 9 months.

### Causes
*C. trachomatis* is an obligate intracellular organism. It usually infects the urethra in males and the cervix in females and is transmitted during sexual activity.

Because contaminated cervical secretions infect the eyes of the neonate during birth, inclusion conjunctivitis is an important cause of ophthalmia neonatorum. Rarely, inclusion conjunctivitis results from autoinfection, by hand-to-eye transfer of the organism from the genitourinary tract.

### Signs and symptoms
Inclusion conjunctivitis develops 5 to 10 days after contamination (it takes longer to develop than gonococcal ophthalmia). In a neonate, the lower eyelids redden and a thick, purulent discharge develops. In children and adults, follicles appear inside the lower eyelids; such follicles don't form in infants because the lymphoid tissue isn't yet well developed. Children and adults also de-

velop preauricular lymphadenopathy and, as complications, otitis media and, occasionally, interstitial pneumonia.

Inclusion conjunctivitis may persist for weeks or months, possibly with superficial corneal involvement. In neonates, pseudomembranes may form, which can lead to conjunctival scarring.

## Diagnosis

Clinical features and a history of sexual contact with an infected person suggest inclusion conjunctivitis. Examination of Giemsa-stained conjunctival scraping reveals cytoplasmic inclusion bodies in conjunctival epithelial cells, many polymorphonuclear leukocytes, and a negative culture for bacteria.

## Treatment

Treatment consists of eyedrops of 1% tetracycline in oil, erythromycin ophthalmic ointment, or sulfonamide eyedrops five or six times daily for 2 weeks for infants and oral tetracycline or erythromycin for 3 weeks for adults. In severe disease, adults may require concomitant systemic sulfonamide therapy. The patient's sexual partner should also be examined and treated.

Prophylactic tetracycline or erythromycin ointment is applied once 1 hour after delivery.

> CLINICAL TIP   The Credé prophylaxis does not protect against inclusion conjunctivitis.

## Special considerations

● Keep the patient's eyes as clean as possible, using aseptic technique. Clean the eyes from the inner to the outer canthus. Apply warm soaks as needed. Record the amount and color of drainage.
● Remind the patient not to rub his eyes, which can irritate them.
● If the patient's eyes are sensitive to light, keep the room dark or suggest that he wear dark glasses.

● To prevent further spread of inclusion conjunctivitis, wash your hands thoroughly before and after administering eye medications.
● Suggest a pelvic examination for the mother of an infected neonate or for any adult with inclusion conjunctivitis.
● Obtain a history of recent sexual contacts, so the contacts can be examined for inclusion conjunctivitis.

# INFERTILITY, FEMALE

Infertility affects about 10% to 15% of all couples in the United States. About 40% to 50% of all infertility is attributed to the female. (See also "Male Infertility," page 456.) After extensive investigation and treatment, about 50% of these infertile couples achieve pregnancy. Of the 50% who don't, 10% have no pathologic basis for infertility; the prognosis in this group becomes extremely poor if pregnancy isn't achieved after 3 years.

## Causes

The causes of female infertility may be functional, anatomic, or psychological.

### Functional causes

Complex hormonal interactions determine the normal function of the female reproductive tract and require an intact hypothalamic-pituitary-ovarian axis, a system that stimulates and regulates the production of hormones necessary for normal sexual development and function.

Any defect or malfunction of this system axis can cause infertility due to insufficient gonadotropin secretions (both luteinizing hormone [LH] and follicle-stimulating hormone). The ovary controls and is controlled by the hypothalamus through a system of negative and positive feedback mediated by estrogen production. Insufficient gonadotropin levels may result from infections, tumors, or neurologic disease of the hypothalamus or pituitary gland. Hypothyroidism also impairs fertility.

### Anatomic causes

The anatomic causes of female infertility include the following:

● Ovarian factors related to anovulation and oligo-ovulation (infrequent ovulation) are a major cause of infertility. Presumptive signs of ovulation include regular menses, cyclic changes reflected in basal body temperature readings, postovulatory progesterone levels, and endometrial changes due to the presence of progesterone. The absence of presumptive signs suggests anovulation.

Ovarian failure, in which no ova are produced by the ovaries, may result from ovarian dysgenesis or premature menopause. Amenorrhea is often associated with ovarian failure. Oligo-ovulation may be due to a mild hormonal imbalance in gonadotropin production and regulation and may be caused by polycystic disease of the ovary or abnormalities in the adrenal or thyroid gland that adversely affect hypothalamic-pituitary functioning.

● *Uterine abnormalities* may include a congenitally absent uterus, bicornuate or double uterus, leiomyomas, or Asherman's syndrome, in which the anterior and posterior uterine walls adhere because of scar tissue formation.

● *Tubal and peritoneal factors* are due to faulty tubal transport mechanisms and unfavorable environmental influences that affect the sperm, ova, or recently fertilized ovum. Tubal loss or impairment may occur secondary to ectopic pregnancy.

Frequently, tubal and peritoneal factors result from anatomic abnormalities: bilateral occlusion of the tubes due to salpingitis (resulting from gonorrhea,

tuberculosis, or puerperal sepsis), peritubal adhesions (resulting from endometriosis, pelvic inflammatory disease [PID], use of an intrauterine device for contraception, diverticulosis, or childhood rupture of the appendix), and uterotubal obstruction due to tubal spasm.

● *Cervical factors* may include a malfunctioning cervix that produces deficient or excessively viscous mucus and is impervious to sperm, preventing entry into the uterus. The cervix may also be stenotic or dilated.

**>** CLINICAL TIP  Make sure the patient is not pregnant if the cervix is dilated.

In cervical infection, viscous mucus may contain spermicidal macrophages. The existence of cervical antibodies that immobilize sperm has been proven.

### Psychological problems

Such problems probably account for relatively few cases of infertility. Occasionally, ovulation may stop because of stress, which results in failure of the body to release LH. Marital discord may affect the frequency of intercourse. More often, psychological problems result from, rather than cause, infertility.

### Signs and symptoms

The inability to achieve pregnancy after having regular intercourse without contraception for at least 1 year suggests infertility.

### Diagnosis

The diagnosis requires a complete physical examination and health history, including specific questions on the patient's reproductive and sexual function, past diseases, mental state, previous surgery, types of contraception used in the past, and family history. Irregular, painless menses may indicate anovulation. A history of PID may suggest fallopian tube blockage.

### Tests that assess ovulation

- *Basal body temperature graph* shows a sustained elevation in body temperature after ovulation until just before onset of menses, indicating the approximate time of ovulation. Oral temperatures are taken every morning before rising.
- *Endometrial biopsy,* done on or about day 5 after the basal body temperature rises, provides histologic evidence that ovulation has occurred.
- *Progesterone blood levels,* measured when they should be highest, can show a luteal phase deficiency. Over-the-counter ovulation predictor kits are less expensive and quite accurate.

The following procedures assess structural integrity of the fallopian tubes, ovaries, and uterus:

- *Hysterosalpingography* provides radiologic evidence of tubal obstruction and abnormalities of the uterine cavity by injecting radiopaque contrast fluid through the cervix.
- *Endoscopy* confirms the results of hysterosalpingography and visualizes the endometrial cavity by hysteroscopy or explores the posterior surface of the uterus, fallopian tubes, and ovaries by culdoscopy. Laparoscopy allows visualization of the abdominal and pelvic areas.

### Male-female interaction studies

- *Postcoital test (Sims-Huhner test)* examines the cervical mucus for motile sperm cells after intercourse that takes place at midcycle (as close to ovulation as possible).
- *Immunologic or antibody testing* detects spermicidal antibodies in the sera of the female. Further research is being conducted in this area.

### Treatment

Effective treatment depends on identifying the underlying abnormality.

### Functional infertility

In hyperactivity or hypoactivity of the adrenal or thyroid gland, hormone therapy is necessary; a progesterone deficiency requires progesterone replacement. Anovulation necessitates treatment with clomiphene, human menopausal gonadotropins, or human chorionic gonadotropin; ovulation usually occurs several days after such treatment.

If mucus production decreases (an adverse effect of clomiphene), small doses of estrogen to improve the quality of cervical mucus may be given concomitantly.

### Anatomic infertility

Surgical restoration may correct certain anatomic causes of infertility, such as fallopian tube obstruction. Surgery may also be necessary to remove tumors located in or near the hypothalamus or pituitary gland. Endometriosis requires drug therapy (danazol or medroxyprogesterone, or noncyclic administration of oral contraceptives), surgical removal of areas of endometriosis, or both.

Other options, often controversial and involving emotional and financial cost, include surrogate mothering, frozen embryos, in vitro fertilization, and artificial insemination.

### Special considerations

- Management includes providing the infertile couple with emotional support and information about diagnostic and treatment techniques.
- Explain the procedures thoroughly.
- Encourage the patient and her partner to talk about their feelings, and listen to what they have to say with a nonjudgmental attitude.
- If the patient requires surgery, tell her what to expect postoperatively; this depends on which procedure is to be performed.

# INFERTILITY, MALE

Male infertility may be suspected whenever a couple fails to achieve pregnancy after about 1 year of regular unprotected intercourse. About 40% to 50% of infertility problems in the United States are totally or partially attributed to the male. (See also "Female Infertility," page 453.)

## Causes
Some of the factors that cause male infertility include:
• *varicocele,* a mass of dilated and tortuous varicose veins in the spermatic cord
• *semen disorders,* such as volume or motility disturbances or inadequate sperm density
• *proliferation of abnormal or immature sperm,* with variations in the size and shape of the head
• *systemic disease,* such as diabetes mellitus, neoplasms, liver and kidney diseases, and viral disturbances, especially mumps orchitis
• *genital infection,* such as gonorrhea, tuberculosis, and herpes
• *disorders of the testes,* such as cryptorchidism, Sertoli-cell–only syndrome, varicocele, and ductal obstruction (caused by absence or ligation of the vas deferens or infection)
• *genetic defects,* such as Klinefelter's syndrome (chromosomal pattern XXY, eunuchoidal habitus, gynecomastia, small testes) or Reifenstein's syndrome (chromosomal pattern 46XY, reduced testosterone, azoospermia, eunuchoidism, gynecomastia, hypospadias)
• *immune disorders,* such as autoimmune infertility and allergic orchitis
• *endocrine imbalance* (rare) that disrupts pituitary gonadotropins, inhibiting spermatogenesis, testosterone production, or both; such imbalances occur in Kallmann's syndrome, panhypopituitarism, hypothyroidism, and congenital adrenal hyperplasia
• *chemicals* and *drugs* that can inhibit gonadotropins or interfere with spermatogenesis, such as arsenic, methotrexate, medroxyprogesterone acetate, nitrofurantoin, monoamine oxidase inhibitors, and some antihypertensives
• *sexual problems,* such as erectile dysfunction, ejaculatory incompetence, and low libido.

Other factors include age, occupation, trauma to the testes, and tight-fitting clothing that constricts the scrotum and affects sperm production.

## Signs and symptoms
The obvious indication of male infertility is failure to impregnate a fertile woman. Clinical features may include:
• atrophied testes
• empty scrotum
• scrotal edema
• varicocele or anteversion of the epididymis
• inflamed seminal vesicles
• beading or abnormal nodes on the spermatic cord and vas deferens
• penile nodes, warts, or plaques or hypospadias
• prostatic enlargement, nodules, swelling, or tenderness.

In addition, male infertility is often apt to induce troublesome negative emotions in a couple, such as anger, hurt, disgust, guilt, and loss of self-esteem.

## Diagnosis
A detailed patient history may reveal abnormal sexual development, delayed puberty, infertility in previous relationships, and a medical history of prolonged fever, mumps, impaired nutritional status, previous surgery, or trauma to the genitalia.

After a thorough patient history and physical examination, the most conclusive test for male infertility is semen analysis. Other laboratory tests include gonadotropin assay to determine the integrity of the pituitary gonadal axis, serum testosterone levels to determine organ response to luteinizing hormone (LH), urine 17-ketosteroid levels to measure testicular function, and a testicular biopsy to help clarify unexplained oligospermia and azoospermia. Vasography and seminal vesiculography may be necessary.

### Treatment

When anatomic dysfunctions or infections cause infertility, treatment consists of correcting the underlying problem. A varicocele requires surgical repair or removal.

For patients with sexual dysfunctions, treatment includes education, counseling or therapy (on sexual techniques, coital frequency, and reproductive physiology), and proper nutrition with vitamin supplements.

Decreased follicle-stimulating hormone levels may respond to vitamin B therapy; decreased LH levels may respond to chorionic gonadotropin therapy. A normal or elevated LH level requires low dosages of testosterone. Decreased testosterone levels, decreased semen motility, and volume disturbances may respond to chorionic gonadotropin.

Patients with oligospermia who have a normal history and physical examination, normal hormonal assay results, and no signs of systemic disease require emotional support and counseling, adequate nutrition, multivitamins, and selective therapeutic agents, such as clomiphene, chorionic gonadotropin, and low dosages of testosterone. Obvious alternatives to such treatment are adoption and artificial insemination.

---

**TEACHING CHECKLIST**

## PREVENTING MALE INFERTILITY

Help prevent male infertility by encouraging patients to:

● have regular physical examinations
● protect their testicles during athletic activities
● receive early treatment for sexually transmitted diseases
● ask about surgical correction of anatomic defects.

---

### Special considerations

● Help prevent male infertility through patient education. (See *Preventing male infertility.*)
● Educate the couple, as necessary, regarding reproductive and sexual functions and about factors that may interfere with fertility, such as the use of lubricants and douches.
● Urge men with oligospermia to avoid habits that may interfere with normal spermatogenesis by elevating scrotal temperature, such as wearing tight underwear and athletic supporters, taking hot tub baths, and habitually riding a bicycle. Explain that cool scrotal temperatures are essential for adequate spermatogenesis.
● When possible, advise infertile couples to join group programs to share their feelings and concerns with other couples who have the same problem.

# INFLUENZA

Also called the grippe or the flu, influenza is an acute, highly contagious infection of the respiratory tract that results from three types of *Myxovirus in-*

*fluenzae.* It occurs sporadically or in epidemics (usually during the colder months). Epidemics tend to peak within 2 to 3 weeks after initial cases and subside within 1 month.

Although influenza affects all age-groups, its incidence is highest in schoolchildren. Its severity is greatest in the very young, elderly people, and those with chronic diseases. In these groups, influenza may even lead to death. The catastrophic pandemic of 1918 was responsible for an estimated 20 million deaths. The most recent pandemics — in 1957, 1968, and 1977 — began in mainland China.

## Causes
Transmission of influenza occurs through inhalation of a respiratory droplet from an infected person or by indirect contact, such as the use of a contaminated drinking glass. The virus then invades the epithelium of the respiratory tract, causing inflammation and desquamation.

One of the remarkable features of the influenza virus is its capacity for antigenic variation. Such variation leads to infection by strains of the virus to which little or no immunologic resistance is present in the population at risk. Antigenic variation is characterized as *antigenic drift* (minor changes that occur yearly or every few years) and *antigenic shift* (major changes that lead to pandemics). Influenza viruses are classified into three groups:

- Type A, the most prevalent, strikes every year, with new serotypes causing epidemics every 3 years.
- Type B also strikes annually but only causes epidemics every 4 to 6 years.
- Type C is endemic and causes only sporadic cases.

## Signs and symptoms
After an incubation period of 24 to 48 hours, flu symptoms begin to appear: the sudden onset of chills, a temperature of 101° to 104° F (38.3° to 40° C), headache, malaise, myalgia (particularly in the back and limbs), a nonproductive cough and, occasionally, laryngitis, hoarseness, conjunctivitis, rhinitis, and rhinorrhea.

These symptoms usually subside in 3 to 5 days, but cough and weakness may persist. Fever is usually higher in children than in adults. Also, cervical adenopathy and croup are likely to be associated with influenza in children. In some patients (especially elderly ones), lack of energy and easy fatigability may persist for several weeks.

### Complications
Fever that persists longer than 3 to 5 days signals the onset of complications. The most common complication is pneumonia, which can be primary influenza viral pneumonia or secondary to bacterial infection. Influenza may also cause myositis, exacerbation of chronic obstructive pulmonary disease, Reye's syndrome and, rarely, myocarditis, pericarditis, transverse myelitis, and encephalitis.

## Diagnosis
At the beginning of an influenza epidemic, early cases are usually mistaken for other respiratory disorders. Because signs and symptoms are not pathognomonic, isolation of *M. influenzae* through the inoculation of chicken embryos (with nasal secretions from infected patients) is essential at the first sign of an epidemic. In addition, nose and throat cultures and increased serum antibody titers help confirm this diagnosis.

After these measures confirm an influenza epidemic, diagnosis requires only observation of clinical signs and symptoms. Uncomplicated cases show a decreased white blood cell count with an increase in lymphocytes.

## Treatment

Uncomplicated influenza is treated with bed rest, adequate fluid intake, aspirin or acetaminophen (in children) to relieve fever and muscle pain, and guaifenesin or another expectorant to relieve nonproductive coughing. Prophylactic antibiotics are not recommended because they have no effect on the influenza virus.

Amantadine (an antiviral agent) has proved to be effective in reducing the duration of signs and symptoms in influenza A infection. In influenza complicated by pneumonia, supportive care (fluid and electrolyte supplements, oxygen, assisted ventilation) and treatment of bacterial superinfection with appropriate antibiotics are necessary. No specific therapy exists for cardiac, central nervous system, or other complications.

## Special considerations

● Advise the patient to use mouthwashes and increase his fluid intake. Warm baths or heating pads may relieve myalgia. Give him nonnarcotic analgesics and antipyretics as needed.
● Screen visitors to protect the patient from bacterial infection and the visitor from influenza. Use respiratory precautions.
● Teach the patient proper disposal of tissues and proper hand-washing technique to prevent the virus from spreading.
● Watch for signs and symptoms of developing pneumonia, such as crackles, another temperature rise, and coughing accompanied by purulent or bloody sputum. Assist the patient in a gradual return to his normal activities.
● Educate patients about influenza immunizations. For high-risk patients and health care personnel, suggest annual inoculations at the start of the flu season (late autumn). Remember, that such vaccines are made from chicken embryos and must not be given to people who are hypersensitive to eggs, feathers, or chickens. The vaccine administered is based on the previous year's virus and is usually about 75% effective.
● All people receiving the vaccine should be made aware of possible adverse effects (discomfort at the vaccination site, fever, malaise and, rarely, Guillain-Barré syndrome). Although the vaccine has not been proven harmful to the fetus, it's not recommended for pregnant women, except those who are highly susceptible to influenza, such as those with chronic diseases.

◀ CLINICAL TIP   For people who are hypersensitive to eggs, amantadine is an effective alternative to the vaccine.

# INGUINAL HERNIA

A hernia occurs when part or all of a viscus protrudes from a normal location in the body. Most hernias are protrusions of part of the abdominal viscus through the abdominal wall. Although many kinds of abdominal hernias are possible, inguinal hernias are most common.

In an inguinal hernia, the large or small intestine, omentum, or bladder protrudes into the inguinal canal. Hernias can be reducible (if the hernia can be manipulated back into place with relative ease by the contents being pushed back into the abdominal cavity), incarcerated (if the hernia can't be reduced because adhesions have formed in the hernial sac), or strangulated (part of the herniated intestine becomes twisted or edematous, seriously interfering with normal blood flow and peristalsis and possibly leading to intestinal obstruction and necrosis).

## Causes

In males, during the 7th month of gestation, the testes normally descend into the scrotum, preceded by the peritoneal sac. If the sac closes improperly, it leaves an opening through which the intestine can slip. In either sex, a hernia can result from weak abdominal muscles (caused by congenital malformation, trauma, or aging) or increased intra-abdominal pressure (due to heavy lifting, pregnancy, obesity, or straining). An inguinal hernia may be indirect or direct.

### Indirect inguinal hernia

The more common form, an indirect inguinal hernia results from weakness in the fascial margin of the internal inguinal ring. An indirect inguinal hernia enters the inguinal canal through the internal inguinal ring and emerges through the external inguinal ring. The indirect inguinal hernia extends down the inguinal canal, often into the scrotum or labia. An indirect inguinal hernia may develop at any age, is three times more common in males, and is especially prevalent in infants under age 1.

### Direct inguinal hernia

A direct inguinal hernia results from a weakness in the fascial floor of the inguinal canal. Portions of the bowel or omentum protrude through the floor of the inguinal canal to emerge through the external ring extending above the inguinal ligament. Instead of entering the canal through the internal ring, the hernia passes through the posterior inguinal wall, protrudes directly through the fascia transversalis of the canal (in an area known as Hesselbach's triangle), and comes out at the external ring.

## Signs and symptoms

Inguinal hernia usually causes a lump over the herniated area when the patient stands or strains. The lump disappears when the patient is supine. Tension on the herniated contents may cause a sharp, steady pain in the groin, which fades when the hernia is reduced.

**CLINICAL TIP** The patient complains of a dull ache or bulge in the groin area. Initial herniation may be noted as a short period of burning sensation when straining.

Strangulation produces severe pain and may lead to partial or complete bowel obstruction and even intestinal necrosis. Partial bowel obstruction may cause anorexia, vomiting, pain and tenderness in the groin, an irreducible mass, and diminished bowel sounds. Complete obstruction may cause shock, high fever, absent bowel sounds, and bloody stools. In an infant, an inguinal hernia often coexists with an undescended testis or a hydrocele.

## Diagnosis

In a patient with a large hernia, physical examination reveals an obvious swelling or lump in the inguinal area. In the patient with a small hernia, the affected area may simply appear full. Palpation of the inguinal area while the patient is performing Valsalva's maneuver confirms the diagnosis.

To detect a hernia in a male patient, the patient is asked to stand with his ipsilateral leg slightly flexed and his weight resting on the other leg. The examiner inserts an index finger into the lower part of the scrotum and invaginates the scrotal skin so the finger advances through the external inguinal ring to the internal ring (about $1\frac{1}{2}''$ to $2''$ [4 to 5 cm] through the inguinal canal). The patient is then told to cough. If the examiner feels pressure against the fingertip, an indirect hernia exists; if pressure is felt against the side of the finger, a direct hernia exists.

A patient history of sharp or "catching" pain when lifting or straining may help confirm the diagnosis. A suspected bowel obstruction requires X-rays and a white blood cell count (which may be elevated).

## Treatment

If the hernia is reducible, the pain may be temporarily relieved by pushing the hernia back into place. A truss may keep the abdominal contents from protruding into the hernial sac, although it won't cure the hernia. This device is especially beneficial for an elderly or a debilitated patient for whom surgery is potentially hazardous.

### Herniorrhaphy

Herniorrhaphy, the treatment of choice, returns the contents of the hernial sac to the abdominal cavity and closes the opening. It's commonly performed under local anesthestic as an outpatient procedure. Another effective surgical procedure is hernioplasty, which reinforces the weakened area with steel mesh, fascia, or wire. Complications can include urine retention, wound infection, hydrocele formation, and scrotal edema.

### Bowel resection

A strangulated or necrotic hernia necessitates bowel resection. Rarely, an extensive resection may require temporary colostomy. In either case, resection lengthens postoperative recovery and requires antibiotics, parenteral fluids, and electrolyte replacements.

## Special considerations

- Apply a truss only after hernia reduction. For best results, apply it in the morning, while the patient is in bed.
- Watch for signs of incarceration and strangulation.

CLINICAL TIP Don't try to reduce an incarcerated hernia because this may induce perforation of the bowel. If severe intestinal obstruction arises because of hernial strangulation, a nasogastric tube may be inserted promptly to empty the stomach and relieve pressure on the hernial sac.

- Before surgery, closely monitor vital signs. Administer I.V. fluids and analgesics for pain as needed. Control fever with acetaminophen or tepid sponge baths as necessary. Place the patient in Trendelenburg's position to reduce pressure on the hernia site.
- Give special reassurance and support to a child scheduled for hernia repair. Encourage him to ask questions, and answer them as simply as possible. Offer appropriate diversions to distract him from the impending surgery.
- After surgery, evaluate the patient's ability to void. Check the incision and dressing at least three times a day for drainage, inflammation, and swelling. Check for normal bowel sounds and watch for fever.
- Observe carefully for postoperative scrotal swelling. To reduce such swelling, support the scrotum with a rolled towel and apply an ice bag.
- Encourage fluid intake to maintain hydration and prevent constipation. Teach deep-breathing exercises, and show the patient how to splint the incision before coughing.
- Before discharge, warn the patient against lifting or straining. In addition, tell him to watch for signs of infection at the incision site and to keep the incision clean and covered until the sutures are removed.

# INSECT BITES AND STINGS

Among the most common traumatic complaints are insect bites and stings, the more serious of which include those of ticks, brown recluse spiders, black widow spiders, scorpions, bees, wasps, and yellow jackets. For information on each type, see *Comparing insect bites and stings,* pages 462 to 467.

*(Text continues on page 466.)*

# COMPARING INSECT BITES AND STINGS

| GENERAL INFORMATION | CLINICAL FEATURES |
| --- | --- |

### TICK

| | |
| --- | --- |
| • Common in woods and fields throughout the United States<br>• Attaches to host in any of its life stages (larva, nymph, adult); fastens to host with its teeth, then secretes a cementike material to reinforce attachment<br>• Flat, brown, speckled body about ¼" (6.25 mm) long; has eight legs<br>• Also transmits Rocky Mountain spotted fever and Lyme disease | • Itching may be sole symptom; or after several days, host may develop tick paralysis (acute flaccid paralysis, starting as paresthesia and pain in legs and resulting in respiratory failure from bulbar paralysis). |

### BROWN RECLUSE (VIOLIN) SPIDER

| | |
| --- | --- |
| • Common to south-central United States; usually found in dark areas (outdoor privy, barn, woodshed)<br>• Dark brown violin on its back; three pairs of eyes; female more dangerous than male<br>• Most bites occur between April and October. | • Venom is coagulotoxic. Reaction begins 2 to 8 hours after bite.<br>• Localized vasoconstriction causes ischemic necrosis at bite site. Small, reddened puncture wound forms a bleb and becomes ischemic. In 3 to 4 days, center becomes dark and hard. Within 2 to 3 weeks, an ulcer forms.<br>• Minimal initial pain increases over time.<br>• Other symptoms include fever, chills, malaise, weakness, nausea, vomiting, edema, seizures, joint pain, petechiae, cyanosis, and phlebitis.<br>• Rarely, thrombocytopenia and hemolytic anemia develop, leading to death within first 24 to 48 hours (usually in a child or a patient with a previous history of cardiac disease). Prompt and appropriate treatment results in recovery |

### BLACK WIDOW SPIDER

| | |
| --- | --- |
| • Common throughout the United States, particularly in warmer climates; usually found in dark areas (outdoor privy, barn, woodshed) | • Venom is neurotoxic. Age, size, and sensitivity of patient determine the severity and progression of symptoms.<br>• Pinprick sensation, followed by dull, numbing pain (may go unnoticed)<br>• Edema and tiny, red bite marks |

| TREATMENT | SPECIAL CONSIDERATIONS |
|---|---|
| • Removal of tick<br>• Local antipruritics for itching papule<br>• Mechanical ventilation for respiratory failure | • To remove a tick, cover it with a tissue or gauze pad soaked in mineral, salad, or machine oil or alcohol. This blocks the tick's breathing pores and causes it to withdraw from the skin. If the tick doesn't disengage after the pad has been in place for ½ hour, carefully remove it with tweezers, taking care to remove all parts.<br>• To reduce the risk of being bitten, teach the patient to keep away from wooded areas, to wear protective clothes, and to carefully examine his body for ticks after being outdoors.<br>• Teach patients how to safely remove ticks. |
| • No known specific treatment<br>• Combination therapy with corticosteroids, antibiotics, antihistamines, tranquilizers, I.V. fluids, and tetanus prophylaxis<br>• Lesion excision in first 10 to 12 hours relieves pain. A split-thickness skin graft closes the wound. Without grafting, healing may take 6 to 8 weeks.<br>• A large chronic ulcer may require skin grafting. | • Clean the lesion with a 1:20 Burow's aluminum acetate solution, and apply antibiotic ointment as ordered.<br>• Take a complete patient history, including allergies and other preexisting medical problems.<br>• Reassure the patient with a disfiguring ulcer that skin grafting can improve his appearance.<br>• To prevent brown recluse bites, tell patients to spray or wear gloves and heavy clothes when working around woodpiles or sheds, to inspect outdoor working clothes for spiders before use, and to discourage children from playing near infested areas. |
| • Neutralization of venom using antivenin I.V., preceded by desensitization when skin or eye tests show sensitivity to horse serum<br>• Calcium gluconate I.V. to control muscle spasms | • Take a complete patient history, including allergies and other preexisting medical problems.<br>• Have epinephrine and emergency resuscitation equipment on hand in case of anaphylactic reaction to antivenin. |

*(continued)*

## COMPARING INSECT BITES AND STINGS *(continued)*

| GENERAL INFORMATION | CLINICAL FEATURES |
|---|---|

### BLACK WIDOW SPIDER *(continued)*

| | |
|---|---|
| • Female is coal black with red or orange hourglass on ventral side; female larger than male (male doesn't bite)<br>• Mortality less than 1% (increased risk among the elderly, infants, and those with allergies) | • Rigidity of stomach muscles and severe abdominal pain (10 to 40 minutes after bite)<br>• Muscle spasms in extremities<br>• Ascending paralysis, causing difficulty swallowing and labored, grunting respirations<br>• Other symptoms include extreme restlessness, vertigo, sweating, chills, pallor, seizures (especially in children), hyperactive reflexes, hypertension, tachycardia, thready pulse, circulatory collapse, nausea, vomiting, headache, ptosis, eyelid edema, urticaria, pruritus, and fever. |

### SCORPION

| | |
|---|---|
| • Common throughout the United States (30 different species); two deadly species in southwestern states<br>• Curled tail with stinger on end; eight legs; 3″ (7.5 cm) long<br>• Most stings occur during warmer months.<br>• Mortality less than 1% (increased risk among the elderly and children) | *Local reaction:*<br>• Local swelling and tenderness, sharp burning sensation, skin discoloration, paresthesia, lymphangitis with regional gland swelling<br>*Systemic reaction (neurotoxic):*<br>• Immediate sharp pain; hyperesthesia; drowsiness; itching of nose, throat, and mouth; impaired speech (due to sluggish tongue); generalized muscle spasms, including jaw muscle spasms, laryngospasms, incontinence, seizures, nausea, vomiting, and drooling<br>• Symptoms last from 24 to 78 hours; bite site recovers last.<br>• Anaphylaxis is rare.<br>• Death may follow cardiovascular or respiratory failure.<br>• The prognosis is poor if symptoms progress rapidly in first few hours. |

| TREATMENT | SPECIAL CONSIDERATIONS |
|---|---|
| • Muscle relaxants such as diazepam for severe muscle spasms<br>• Frequent vital signs checks during the first 12 hours<br>• Epinephrine or antihistamines<br>• Oxygen by nasal cannula or mask<br>• Tetanus immunization<br>• Antibiotics to prevent infection | • Keep the patient quiet and warm and the affected part immobile.<br>• Clean the bite site with an antiseptic; apply ice to relieve pain and swelling and to slow circulation.<br>• Check vital signs frequently during the first 12 hours after the bite. Report any changes to the doctor. Symptoms usually subside in 3 to 4 hours.<br>• When giving analgesics, monitor respiratory status.<br>• To prevent black widow spider bites, tell the patient to spray areas of infestation with creosote at least every 2 months, to wear gloves and heavy clothing when working around woodpiles or sheds, to inspect outdoor working clothes for spiders before putting them on, and to discourage children from playing near infested areas. |
| • Antivenin (made from cat serum), if available. (Contact Antivenin Lab, Arizona State University, Tempe, Arizona.)<br>• Calcium gluconate I.V for muscle spasm<br>• Phenobarbital I.M. for seizures<br>• Emetine S.C. to relieve pain (Opiates such as morphine and codeine are contraindicated because they enhance the venom's effects.) | • Take a complete patient history, including allergies and other preexisting medical conditions.<br>• Immobilize the patient, and apply a tourniquet proximal to the sting.<br>• Pack the area extending beyond the tourniquet in ice. After 5 minutes of ice pack, remove the tourniquet.<br>• Monitor vital signs. Watch closely for signs of respiratory distress. (Keep emergency resuscitation equipment available.) |

*(continued)*

## COMPARING INSECT BITES AND STINGS *(continued)*

| GENERAL INFORMATION | CLINICAL FEATURES |
|---|---|
| **BEE, WASP, AND YELLOW JACKET** | |
| • When a honeybee (rounded abdomen) or a bumblebee (over 1″ [2.5 cm] long; furry, rounded abdomen) stings, its stinger remains in the victim; the bee flies away and dies.<br>• A wasp or yellow jacket (slender body with elongated abdomen) retains its stingers and can sting repeatedly. | *Local reaction:*<br>• Painful wound (protruding stinger from bees), edema, urticaria, pruritus<br>*Systemic reaction (anaphylaxis):*<br>• Symptoms of hypersensitivity usually appear within 20 minutes and may include weakness, chest tightness, dizziness, nausea, vomiting, abdominal cramps, and throat constriction. The shorter the interval between the sting and systemic symptoms, the worse the prognosis. Without prompt treatment, symptoms may progress to cyanosis, coma, and death. |

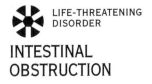

LIFE-THREATENING
DISORDER

# INTESTINAL OBSTRUCTION

An intestinal obstruction is a partial or complete blockage of the lumen in the small or large bowel. A small-bowel obstruction is far more common (90% of patients) and usually more serious. A complete obstruction in any part of the bowel, if untreated, can cause death within hours from shock and vascular collapse. Intestinal obstructions are most likely to occur from adhesions caused by previous abdominal surgery, external hernias, volvulus, Crohn's disease, radiation enteritis, intestinal wall hematomas (after trauma or anticoagulant therapy), and neoplasms.

## Causes

Adhesions and strangulated hernias usually cause small-bowel obstructions; carcinomas usually cause large-bowel obstructions. A mechanical intestinal obstruction results from foreign bodies (fruit pits, gallstones, worms) or compression of the bowel wall due to stenosis, intussusception, volvulus of the sigmoid or cecum, tumors, or atresia.

A nonmechanical obstruction results from physiologic disturbances, such as paralytic ileus (see *Paralytic ileus,* page 469), electrolyte imbalances, toxicity (uremia, generalized infection), neurogenic abnormalities (spinal cord lesions), and thrombosis or embolism of mesenteric vessels.

The three forms of intestinal obstruction are:
• *simple:* blockage prevents intestinal contents from passing with no other complications

| TREATMENT | SPECIAL CONSIDERATIONS |
|---|---|
| • Atropine to counteract parasympathetic effects of venom if needed<br>• Antihistamines and corticosteroids (in urticaria)<br>• Tetanus prophylaxis<br>• In anaphylaxis, oxygen by nasal cannula or mask and epinephrine 1:1,000 S.C. or I.M.<br>• In bronchospasm, albuterol and corticosteroids<br>• In hypotension, epinephrine and isoproterenol | • If the stinger is in place, scrape it off. Don't pull it; this action releases more toxin.<br>• Clean the site and apply ice.<br>• Watch the patient carefully for signs of anaphylaxis. Keep emergency resuscitation equipment available.<br>• Tell a patient who is allergic to bee stings to wear a medical identification bracelet or carry a card and to carry an anaphylaxis kit. Teach him how to use the kit, and refer him to an allergist for hyposensitization.<br>• To prevent bee stings, tell the patient to avoid wearing bright colors and going barefoot, to avoid flowers and fruit that attract bees, and to use insect repellent. |

• *strangulated:* blood supply to part or all of the obstructed section is cut off in addition to blockage of the lumen

• *close-looped:* both ends of a bowel section are occluded, isolating it from the rest of the intestine.

In all three forms, the physiologic effects are similar: When intestinal obstruction occurs, fluid, air, and gas collect near the site. Peristalsis increases temporarily as the bowel tries to force its contents through the obstruction, injuring intestinal mucosa and causing distention at and above the site of the obstruction. This distention blocks the flow of venous blood and halts normal absorptive processes. As a result, the bowel begins to secrete water, sodium, and potassium into the fluid pooled in the lumen. This results in distention and enormous amounts of fluid in the gut.

An obstruction in the upper intestine results in metabolic alkalosis from dehydration and loss of gastric hydrochloric acid; a lower obstruction causes slow-er dehydration and loss of intestinal alkaline fluids, resulting in metabolic acidosis. Ultimately, an intestinal obstruction may lead to ischemia, necrosis, and death.

### Signs and symptoms
Clinical features depend on the location and extent of the obstruction.

#### Partial small-bowel obstruction
Colicky pain, nausea, vomiting, constipation, and abdominal distention characterize small-bowel obstruction. Signs and symptoms of dehydration are present.

Auscultation reveals bowel sounds, borborygmi, and rushes; occasionally, they are loud enough to be heard without a stethoscope. Palpation elicits abdominal tenderness with moderate distention; rebound tenderness occurs when the obstruction has caused strangulation with ischemia. In late stages, signs of hypovolemic shock result from progressive dehydration and plasma loss.

### Complete small-bowel obstruction

In a complete small-intestinal (small-bowel) obstruction, vigorous peristaltic waves propel bowel contents toward the mouth instead of the rectum. Spasms may occur every 3 to 5 minutes and last about 1 minute each, with persistent epigastric or periumbilical pain. Small amounts of mucus and blood may be passed. The higher the obstruction, the earlier and more severe the vomiting. Vomitus initially contains gastric juice, then bile, and finally fecal contents of the ileum. Constipation develops in complete obstruction. There is minimal or no fever. Abdominal distention is pronounced. Mild tenderness is present. Peristaltic rushes and high-pitched tinkles occur during paroxysms of pain. Visible peristalsis may be noted.

### Partial large-bowel obstruction

Symptoms of large-bowel obstruction develop more slowly because the colon can absorb fluid from its contents and distend well beyond its normal size. Constipation may be the only clinical effect for days. Colicky abdominal pain may appear suddenly, producing spasms that last less than 1 minute each and recur every few minutes. Continuous hypogastric pain and nausea may develop, but vomiting is initially absent.

Large-bowel obstruction can cause dramatic abdominal distention: Loops of large bowel may become visible on the abdomen.

### Complete large-bowel obstruction

Eventually, a complete large-bowel obstruction may cause fecal vomiting, continuous pain, or localized peritonitis.

Patients with a partial obstruction may display any of the above symptoms in a milder form. Leakage of liquid stools around the obstruction is common in partial obstruction.

## Diagnosis

Progressive, colicky abdominal pain and distention, with or without nausea and vomiting, suggest bowel obstruction. Plain abdominal radiography confirms the diagnosis.

> **CLINICAL TIP** Small-bowel obstruction must be distinguished from adynamic ileus. Pancreatitis, acute gastroenteritis, appendicitis, and acute mesenteric ischemia must be ruled out.

Abdominal films show the presence and location of intestinal gas or fluid. In small-bowel obstructions, a typical "stepladder" pattern emerges, with alternating fluid and gas levels apparent in 3 to 4 hours. In large-bowel obstructions, a barium enema reveals a distended, air-filled colon or a closed loop of sigmoid with extreme distention (in sigmoid volvulus).

Laboratory results that support this diagnosis include:

- decreased sodium, chloride, and potassium levels (due to vomiting)
- slightly elevated white blood cell count (with necrosis, peritonitis, or strangulation)
- increased serum amylase level (possibly from irritation of the pancreas by a bowel loop).

## Treatment

Initial therapy consists of correcting fluid and electrolyte imbalances, decompressing the bowel to relieve vomiting and distention, and treating shock and peritonitis. A strangulated obstruction usually necessitates blood replacement as well as I.V. fluid administration. Nasogastric tube suction is necessary to relieve vomiting and abdominal distention.

Close monitoring of the patient's condition determines the duration of treatment; if the patient fails to improve or

# PARALYTIC ILEUS

Paralytic (adynamic) ileus is a physiologic form of intestinal obstruction that may develop in the small bowel after abdominal surgery. It causes decreased or absent intestinal motility that usually disappears spontaneously after 2 to 3 days.

## Causes
This condition can develop as a response to trauma, toxemia, or peritonitis or as a result of electrolyte deficiencies (especially hypokalemia) and the use of certain drugs, such as pain medications, ganglionic blocking agents, and anticholinergics. It can also result from vascular causes, such as thrombosis and embolism.

## Signs and symptoms
Clinical effects of paralytic ileus include severe, continuous abdominal discomfort with nausea and vomiting. Abdominal distention is also present. Bowel sounds are diminished or absent. The patient may be severely constipated or may pass flatus and small, liquid stools.

## Treatment
Paralytic ileus that lasts longer than 48 hours necessitates intubation for decompression and nasogastric suctioning. Isotonic fluids should be administered to restore intravascular volume and correct electrolyte disorders.

When paralytic ileus results from surgical manipulation of the bowel, treatment may also include administration of prokinetic agents, such as metoclopramide, erythromycin, and cisapride.

## Special considerations
When caring for patients with paralytic ileus, warn those receiving cholinergic agents to expect certain paradoxical adverse effects, such as intestinal cramps and diarrhea. Check frequently for returning bowel sounds.

---

if his condition deteriorates, surgery is necessary. Surgery is performed on all patients with large-bowel obstruction.

Total parenteral nutrition may be appropriate if the patient suffers a protein deficit from chronic obstruction, postoperative or paralytic ileus, or infection.

Drug therapy includes analgesics and sedatives. Antibiotics are given for peritonitis due to bowel strangulation or infarction. Broad-spectrum antibiotics should be given to provide anaerobic and gram-negative coverage.

## Special considerations
• Effective management of intestinal obstruction, a life-threatening condition that often causes overwhelming pain and distress, requires skillful supportive care and keen observation.
• Monitor vital signs frequently. A drop in blood pressure may indicate reduced circulating blood volume due to blood loss from a strangulated hernia. Remember, as much as 10 L of fluid can collect in the small bowel, drastically reducing plasma volume. Observe the patient closely for signs of shock (pallor, rapid pulse, and hypotension).
• Assess for signs of metabolic alkalosis (changes in sensorium; slow, shallow respirations; hypertonic muscles; tetany) or acidosis (shortness of breath on exertion; disorientation; and, later, deep and rapid breathing, weakness, and malaise).
• Watch for signs and symptoms of secondary infection, such as fever and chills.
• Monitor urine output carefully to assess renal function, circulating blood volume, and possible urine retention caused by bladder compression by the distended intestine. If you suspect blad-

der compression, catheterize the patient for residual urine. Also, measure abdominal girth frequently to detect progressive distention.

• Provide fastidious mouth and nose care if the patient has vomited or undergone decompression by intubation. Observe for signs of dehydration (thick, swollen tongue; dry, cracked lips; dry oral mucous membranes).

• Record the amount and color of drainage from the decompression tube. Irrigate the tube with normal saline solution to maintain patency. If a weighted tube has been inserted, check periodically to make sure it's advancing. Assist the patient to turn from side to side (or ambulate) to facilitate passage of the tube.

• Maintain the patient in semi-Fowler's position as much as possible to promote pulmonary ventilation and ease respiratory distress from abdominal distention. Auscultate for bowel sounds, and observe for signs of returning peristalsis (passage of flatus and mucus through the rectum).

• Explain all diagnostic and therapeutic procedures to the patient, and answer any questions he may have. Inform the patient that these procedures are necessary to relieve the obstruction and reduce pain.

• Prepare the patient and his family for the possibility of surgery, and provide emotional support and positive reinforcement afterward. Arrange for an enterostomal therapist to visit the patient who has had an ostomy.

# INTUSSUSCEPTION

In intussusception, a portion of the bowel telescopes (invaginates) into an adjacent distal portion. Intussusception may be fatal, especially if treatment is delayed for a strangulated intestine.

## Causes

Intussusception is most common in infants and occurs three times more often in males than in females. It typically occurs between ages 3 months and 3 years, with a peak incidence between ages 6 and 9 months.

Studies suggest that intussusception may be linked to viral infections because seasonal peaks are noted — in the late spring and early summer, coinciding with the peak incidence of enteritis, and in the midwinter, coinciding with the peak incidence of respiratory tract infections.

The cause of most cases of intussusception in infants is unknown. In older children, polyps, alterations in intestinal motility, hemangioma, lymphosarcoma, lymphoid hyperplasia, or Meckel's diverticulum may trigger the process. In adults, intussusception usually results from benign or malignant tumors (65% of patients). It may also result from polyps, Meckel's diverticulum, gastroenterostomy with herniation, or an appendiceal stump.

When a bowel segment (the intussusceptum) invaginates, peristalsis propels it along the bowel, pulling more bowel along with it; the receiving segment is the intussuscipiens. This invagination produces edema, hemorrhage from venous engorgement, incarceration, and obstruction. If treatment is delayed for longer than 24 hours, strangulation of the intestine usually occurs, with gangrene, shock, and perforation.

## Signs and symptoms

In an infant or a child, intussusception produces four cardinal clinical effects:

• intermittent attacks of severe colicky abdominal pain, which cause the child to scream, draw up his legs to his abdomen, turn pale and diaphoretic and, possibly, display grunting respirations. Between bouts of colic, the infant is often sleepy or lethargic.

• initially, vomiting of stomach contents; later, vomiting of bile-stained or fecal material

• "currant jelly" stools, which contain a mixture of blood and mucus

• tender, distended abdomen, with a palpable, sausage-shaped right upper quadrant mass; often, the viscera are absent from the right lower quadrant.

In adults, intussusception produces nonspecific, chronic, and intermittent symptoms, including colicky abdominal pain and tenderness, vomiting, diarrhea (occasionally constipation), bloody stools, and weight loss. Abdominal pain usually localizes in the right lower quadrant, radiates to the back, and increases with eating. Adults with severe intussusception may develop strangulation with excruciating pain, abdominal distention, and tachycardia.

## Diagnosis

The following test results confirm intussusception:

• *Barium enema* confirms colonic intussusception when it shows the characteristic coiled-spring sign; it also delineates the extent of intussusception.

• *Upright abdominal X-rays* may show a soft-tissue mass and signs of complete or partial obstruction with dilated loops of bowel.

• *White blood cell count* up to 15,000/µl indicates obstruction; > 15,000/µl, strangulation; > 20,000/µl, bowel infarction should be considered.

## Treatment

In children, therapy may include hydrostatic reduction or surgery. Surgery is indicated for children with recurrent intussusception, for those who show signs of shock or peritonitis, and for those in whom symptoms have been present longer than 24 hours. In adults, surgery is always the treatment of choice.

### Hydrostatic reduction

During hydrostatic reduction, the radiologist drips a barium solution into the rectum from a height of not more than 3′ (0.9 m); fluoroscopy traces the progress of the barium. If the procedure is successful, there is free flow of contrast into the ileum and the mass disappears. Inability to show this suggests incomplete reduction and necessitates surgical exploration.

### Surgery

During surgery, manual reduction is attempted first. After compressing the bowel above the intussusception, the surgeon attempts to milk the intussusception back through the bowel. If manual reduction fails or if the bowel is gangrenous or strangulated, the surgeon performs a resection of the affected bowel segment. An incidental appendectomy is also performed.

## Special considerations

• Monitor vital signs before and after surgery. A change in temperature may indicate sepsis; infants may become hypothermic at the onset of infection. Tachycardia and hypotension may be signs of peritonitis.

• Monitor fluid intake and output. Watch for signs of dehydration and bleeding. Administer I.V. fluids, blood, or blood products, as necessary.

• Nasogastric (NG) intubation is performed to decompress the intestine and minimize vomiting. Monitor NG drainage, and replace lost volume as required.

• Monitor the patient who has undergone hydrostatic reduction for passage of stools and barium, a sign that the reduction was successful. Keep in mind that a few patients will have a recurrence of intussusception, usually within the first 36 to 48 hours after the reduction.

- Postoperatively, administer broad-spectrum antibiotics and provide meticulous wound care. Monitor the incision for inflammation, drainage, and suture separation (dehiscence).
- Encourage the patient to deep-breathe and cough productively, to use incentive spirometry, and to assume the semi-Fowler position when doing so. Teach the patient to splint the incision when he coughs.
- Oral fluids may be given postoperatively when bowel sounds and peristalsis resume. The patient's diet can be advanced as tolerated.
- Monitor for abdominal distention after the patient resumes a normal diet.
- Offer reassurance and emotional support to the child and his parents. This condition is considered a pediatric emergency, and parents are often unprepared for their child's hospitalization and possible surgery; they may feel guilty for not seeking medical attention sooner.
- To minimize the stress of hospitalization, encourage the parents to participate in their child's care as much as possible.

# IRON DEFICIENCY ANEMIA

In iron deficiency anemia, an inadequate supply of iron for optimal formation of red blood cells (RBCs) results in smaller (microcytic) cells with less color on staining. Body stores of iron, including plasma iron, decrease, as does transferrin, which binds with and transports iron. Insufficient body stores of iron lead to a depleted RBC mass and, in turn, a decreased hemoglobin (Hb) concentration (hypochromia) and decreased oxygen-carrying capacity of the blood. A common disease worldwide, iron deficiency anemia affects 10% to 30% of the adult population of the United States.

## Causes

Iron deficiency anemia may result from:
- inadequate dietary intake of iron (< 2 mg/day), as in prolonged, unsupplemented (not eating solid foods after age 6 months) breast- or bottle-feeding of infants and during periods of stress, such as rapid growth in children and adolescents
- iron malabsorption, as in chronic diarrhea, partial or total gastrectomy, and malabsorption syndromes such as celiac disease
- blood loss secondary to drug-induced GI bleeding (from anticoagulants, aspirin, steroids) or due to heavy menses, hemorrhage from trauma, GI ulcers, cancer, or bleeding varices
- pregnancy, which diverts maternal iron to the fetus for erythropoiesis
- intravascular hemolysis-induced hemoglobinuria or paroxysmal nocturnal hemoglobinuria
- mechanical erythrocyte trauma caused by a prosthetic heart valve or vena cava filters.

Iron deficiency anemia occurs most commonly in premenopausal women, infants (particularly premature and low-birth-weight infants), children, and adolescents (especially girls).

## Signs and symptoms

Because of the gradual progression of iron deficiency anemia, many patients are initially asymptomatic. They tend not to seek medical treatment until anemia is severe.

At advanced stages, decreased Hb and the consequent decrease in the blood's oxygen-carrying capacity cause the patient to develop dyspnea on exertion, fatigue, listlessness, pallor, inability to concentrate, irritability, headache, and a susceptibility to infection. Decreased oxygen perfusion causes the heart to compensate with increased cardiac output and tachycardia.

In chronic iron deficiency anemia, nails become spoon-shaped and brittle, the corners of the mouth crack, the tongue turns smooth, and the patient complains of dysphagia or may develop pica. Associated neuromuscular effects include vasomotor disturbances, numbness and tingling of the extremities, and neuralgic pain.

## Diagnosis

Blood studies (serum iron, total iron-binding capacity, ferritin levels) and stores in bone marrow may confirm iron deficiency anemia. However, the results of these tests can be misleading because of complicating factors, such as infection, pneumonia, blood transfusion, and iron supplements. Characteristic blood study results include:

- low Hb levels (males, < 12 g/dl; females, < 10 g/dl)
- low hematocrit (males, < 47 ml/dl; females, < 42 ml/dl)
- low serum iron levels, with high iron-binding capacity
- low serum ferritin levels
- low RBC count, with microcytic and hypochromic cells (in early stages, RBC count may be normal, except in infants and children)
- decreased mean corpuscular Hb in severe anemia.

Bone marrow studies reveal depleted or absent iron stores (done by staining) and normoblastic hyperplasia.

The diagnosis must rule out other forms of anemia, such as those that result from thalassemia minor, cancer, and chronic inflammatory, liver, and kidney disease.

## Prevention

Public health professionals can play a vital role in the prevention of iron deficiency anemia by:

- teaching the basics of a nutritionally balanced diet — red meats, green vegetables, eggs, whole wheat, iron-fortified bread, cereals, and milk. (No food in itself contains enough iron to *treat* iron deficiency anemia; an average-sized person with anemia would have to eat at least 10 lb [4.5 kg] of steak daily to receive therapeutic amounts of iron.)
- emphasizing the need for high-risk individuals — such as premature infants, children under age 2, and pregnant women — to receive prophylactic oral iron, as ordered by a doctor. (Children under age 2 should also receive supplemental cereals and formulas high in iron.)
- assessing a family's dietary habits for iron intake and noting the influence of childhood eating patterns, cultural food preferences, and family income on adequate nutrition.
- encouraging families with deficient iron intake to eat meat, fish, or poultry; whole or enriched grain; and foods high in ascorbic acid.
- carefully assessing a patient's drug history because certain drugs, such as pancreatic enzymes and vitamin E, may interfere with iron metabolism and absorption and because aspirin, steroids, and other drugs may cause GI bleeding. (Teach patients who must take gastric irritants to take these medications with meals or milk.)

## Treatment

The first priority of treatment is to determine the underlying cause of anemia. When this is determined, iron replacement therapy can begin. The treatment of choice is an oral preparation of iron or a combination of iron and ascorbic acid (which enhances iron absorption). In some cases, iron may have to be administered parenterally, for instance, if the patient is noncompliant to the oral preparation, if he needs more iron than he can take orally, if malab-

CLINICAL TIP

## INJECTING IRON SOLUTIONS

For deep I.M. injections of iron solutions, use the Z-track technique to avoid subcutaneous irritation and discoloration from leaking medication:

Choose a 19G to 20G 2″ to 3″ needle. After drawing up the solution, change to a fresh needle to avoid tracking the solution through to subcutaneous tissue. Draw 0.5 cc of air into the syringe as an "air-lock."

Displace the skin and fat at the injection site (in the upper outer quadrant of the buttocks or the ventrogluteal site only) firmly to one side. Clean the area.

Insert the needle. Aspirate to check for entry into a blood vessel. Inject the solution slowly, followed by the 0.5 cc of air in the syringe. Pull the needle straight out.

Keeping the tissues displaced with your finger, wait 10 seconds. Then release the tissues.

Apply direct pressure to the site but don't massage it. Caution the patient against vigorous exercise for 15 to 30 minutes.

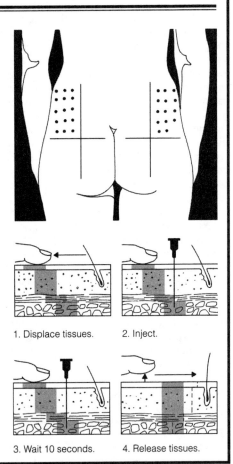

1. Displace tissues.

2. Inject.

3. Wait 10 seconds.

4. Release tissues.

sorption prevents adequate iron absorption, or if a maximum rate of Hb regeneration is desired. (See *Injecting iron solutions*.)

Because a total-dose I.V. infusion of supplemental iron is painless and requires fewer injections, it's usually preferred over I.M. administration. Pregnant patients and elderly patients with severe anemia, for example, should receive a total-dose infusion of iron dextran in normal saline solution over 8 hours. To minimize the risk of an allergic reaction to iron, an I.V. test dose of 0.5 ml should be given first.

### Special considerations
• Review guidelines for managing anemia with the patient and his family. (See *Supportive management in anemia*.)

## SUPPORTIVE MANAGEMENT IN ANEMIA

Follow these guidelines to help manage the patient with anemia.

### Nutritional needs
• If the patient is fatigued, urge him to eat small, frequent meals throughout the day.
• If the patient has oral lesions, suggest soft, cool, bland foods.
• If the patient has dyspepsia, eliminate spicy foods and include milk and dairy products in his diet.
• If the patient is anorexic and irritable, encourage his family to bring his favorite foods from home (unless his diet is restricted) and to keep him company during meals, if possible.

### Activities
• If during physical activity the patient's pulse accelerates rapidly and he develops hypotension with hyperpnea, diaphoresis, light-headedness, palpitations, shortness of breath, or weakness, the activity is too strenuous.
• Tell the patient to pace his activities and allow for frequent rest periods.

### Infection precautions
• Instruct the patient to avoid crowds and other sources of infection. Encourage him to practice good hand-washing technique. Stress the importance of receiving necessary immunizations and prompt medical treatment for any sign of infection.

### Diagnostic tests
• Explain erythropoiesis, the function of blood, and the purpose of diagnostic and therapeutic procedures.

### Complications
• Instruct the patient on signs of bleeding that may exacerbate anemia. Sources may include stool, ecchymotic areas, gingival bleeding, and hematuria.
• If the patient is confined to strict bed rest, teach the family and patient how to perform range-of-motion exercises. Stress the importance of frequent turning, coughing, and deep breathing.
• Warn the patient to move about and change positions slowly to minimize dizziness induced by cerebral hypoxia.

---

• Monitor the patient's compliance with the prescribed iron supplement therapy. Advise the patient not to stop therapy, even if he feels better, because replacement of iron stores takes time.
• Advise the patient that milk or an antacid interferes with absorption but that vitamin C can increase absorption. Instruct the patient to drink liquid supplemental iron through a straw to prevent staining his teeth.
• Tell the patient to report adverse reactions, such as nausea, vomiting, diarrhea, constipation, fever, and severe stomach pain, which may require a dosage adjustment.

• If the patient receives iron I.V., monitor the infusion rate carefully, and observe for an allergic reaction. Stop the infusion and begin supportive treatment immediately if the patient shows signs of an adverse reaction. Also, watch for dizziness and headache and for thrombophlebitis around the I.V. site.
• Use the Z-track injection method when administering iron I.M. to prevent skin discoloration, scarring, and irritating iron deposits in the skin.
• Because an iron deficiency may recur, advise regular checkups.

# IRRITABLE BOWEL SYNDROME

Also referred to as spastic colon or spastic colitis, irritable bowel syndrome is marked by chronic symptoms of abdominal pain, alternating constipation and diarrhea, and abdominal distention. This disorder is extremely common; 20% of patients, however, never seek medical attention.

## Causes

This functional disorder is generally associated with psychological stress; however, it may result from physical factors, such as diverticular disease, ingestion of irritants (coffee, raw fruits or vegetables), lactose intolerance, abuse of laxatives, food poisoning, and colon cancer.

## Signs and symptoms

Irritable bowel syndrome characteristically produces intermittent, crampy lower abdominal pain. The pain is usually relieved by defecation or passage of flatus. It typically occurs during the day. Pain intensifies with stress or 1 to 2 hours after meals. The patient may experience constipation alternating with diarrhea, with one being the dominant problem. Mucus is usually passed through the rectum. Abdominal distention and bloating are common.

## Diagnosis

A history and physical examination should be performed. A careful patient history is required to determine contributing psychological factors, such as a recent stressful life change. The diagnosis must also rule out other disorders, such as amebiasis, diverticulitis, colon cancer, and lactose intolerance. Appropriate diagnostic procedures include sigmoidoscopy, colonoscopy, barium enema, rectal biopsy, and stool examination for blood, parasites, and bacteria.

## Treatment

Therapy aims to relieve symptoms and includes counseling to help the patient understand the relation between stress and his illness. Strict dietary restrictions aren't beneficial, but food irritants should be investigated and the patient instructed to avoid them. Rest and heat applied to the abdomen are helpful, as is judicious use of sedatives (phenobarbital) and antispasmodics (propantheline, diphenoxylate with atropine sulfate). However, with chronic use, the patient may become dependent on these drugs. If the cause of irritable bowel syndrome is chronic laxative abuse, bowel training may help correct the condition.

## Special considerations

➤ CLINICAL TIP Because the patient with irritable bowel syndrome isn't hospitalized, focus your care on patient teaching.

• Instruct the patient to avoid irritating foods, and encourage development of regular bowel habits.

• Help the patient deal with stress, and warn against dependence on sedatives or antispasmodics.

• Encourage regular checkups because irritable bowel syndrome is associated with a higher-than-normal incidence of diverticulitis and colon cancer. For patients over age 40, emphasize the need for a yearly flexible sigmoidoscopy and rectal examination.

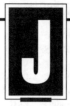

# JAW DISLOCATION
OR FRACTURE

Jaw dislocation is a displacement of the temporomandibular joint. Jaw fracture is a break in one or both of the two maxillae (upper jawbones) or the mandible (lower jawbone). Treatment can usually restore jaw alignment and function.

### Causes
Simple fractures or dislocations are usually caused by a manual blow along the jawline; more serious compound fractures often result from car accidents and penetration injuries.

### Signs and symptoms
Malocclusion is the most obvious sign of dislocation or fracture. Other signs include mandibular pain, swelling, ecchymosis, loss of function, and asymmetry. In addition, mandibular fractures that damage the alveolar nerve produce paresthesia or anesthesia of the chin and lower lip. Maxillary fractures produce infraorbital paresthesia and often accompany fractures of the nasal and orbital complex.

### Diagnosis
Abnormal maxillary or mandibular mobility during physical examination and a history of trauma suggest fracture or dislocation. X-rays can confirm diagnosis but a computed tomography scan is usually necessary for accurate diagnosis and ultimate repair.

### Treatment
As in all traumatic injuries, check first for a patent airway, adequate ventilation, and pulses; then control hemorrhage and check for other injuries. As necessary, maintain a patent airway with an oropharyngeal airway, nasotracheal intubation, or a tracheotomy. Relieve pain with analgesics as needed.

After the patient stabilizes, surgical reduction and fixation by wiring restores mandibular and maxillary alignment. Maxillary fractures may also require reconstruction and repair of soft-tissue injuries.

Teeth and bones are never removed during surgery unless unavoidable. If the patient has lost teeth from trauma, the surgeon will decide whether they can be reimplanted. If they can, he will reimplant them within 6 hours, while they're still viable. Viability is increased if the tooth is placed in milk. Dislocations are usually manually reduced under anesthesia.

### Special considerations
After reconstructive surgery:
• Position the patient on his side, with his head slightly elevated. A nasogastric tube is usually in place, with low suction to remove gastric contents and prevent nausea, vomiting, and aspiration of vomitus.
• As necessary, suction the nasopharynx through the nose, or by pulling the

cheek away from the teeth and inserting a small suction catheter through any natural gap between teeth.

• If the patient isn't intubated, provide nourishment through a straw. If he has a natural gap between his teeth, insert the straw there — if not, one or two teeth may have to be extracted. However, extraction is avoided when possible.

• Start the diet with clear liquids; after the patient can tolerate fluids, offer milk shakes, broth, juices, pureed foods, and nutritional supplements.

• If the patient is unable to tolerate oral fluids, I.V. therapy can maintain hydration postoperatively.

• Administer antiemetics, as needed, to minimize nausea and prevent aspiration of vomitus (a very real danger in a patient whose jaw is wired). Keep a pair of wire cutters at the bedside to snip the wires should the patient vomit. A dental water-pulsator may be used for mouth care while the wires are intact.

• Because the patient will have difficulty talking while his jaw is wired, provide a Magic Slate or pencil and paper, and suggest appropriate diversions.

# JUVENILE RHEUMATOID ARTHRITIS

Affecting children under age 16, juvenile rheumatoid arthritis (JRA), also known as juvenile chronic arthritis, is an immune-mediated inflammatory disorder of the connective tissues characterized by joint swelling and pain or tenderness. It may also involve organs, such as the skin, heart, lungs, liver, spleen, and eyes, producing extra-articular signs and symptoms.

JRA has three major types: systemic (Still's disease or acute febrile type), polyarticular, and pauciarticular.

Depending on the type, this disease can occur as early as age 6 weeks — although rarely before 6 months — with peaks of onset between ages 1 and 3, and 8 and 12. Considered the major chronic rheumatic disorder of childhood, JRA affects an estimated 150,000 to 250,000 children in the United States: the overall incidence is twice as high in girls, with variation among the types.

## Causes

The cause of JRA remains puzzling. Research continues to test several theories, such as those linking JRA to genetic factors or to an abnormal immune response. Viral or bacterial (particularly streptococcal) infection, trauma, and emotional stress may be precipitating factors, but their relationship to JRA remains unclear.

## Signs and symptoms

Signs and symptoms vary with the type of JRA.

### Systemic JRA

Affecting boys and girls almost equally, systemic JRA accounts for approximately 20% to 30% of cases. The affected children may have mild, transient arthritis or frank polyarthritis associated with fever and rash.

CLINICAL TIP   Joint involvement may not be evident at first, but the child's behavior may clearly suggest joint pain. Such a child may want to constantly sit in a flexed position, may not walk much, or may refuse to walk at all. Young children with JRA are noticeably irritable and listless.

Fever in systemic JRA occurs suddenly and spikes to 103° F (39.4° C) or higher once or twice daily, usually in the late afternoon, then rapidly returns to normal or subnormal. (This "sawtooth" or intermittent spiking fever pattern helps differentiate JRA from other inflammatory disorders.) When fever spikes, an evanescent rheumatoid rash often appears, consisting of small, pale or salmon pink macules, most commonly on the trunk and proximal extremities and occasionally on the face, palms, and soles.

Massaging or applying heat intensifies this rash, which is usually most conspicuous where the skin has been rubbed or subjected to pressure, such as that from underclothing.

Other signs and symptoms of systemic JRA may include hepatosplenomegaly, lymphadenopathy, pleuritis, pericarditis, myocarditis, and nonspecific abdominal pain.

### Polyarticular JRA

This form of the disorder affects girls four to nine times more often than boys and may be seronegative or seropositive for rheumatoid factor (RF). It involves five or more joints and usually develops insidiously. Most commonly involved joints are the wrists, elbows, knees, ankles, and small joints of the hands and feet.

Polyarticular JRA can also affect larger joints, including the temporomandibular joints and those of the cervical spine, hips, and shoulders. These joints become swollen, tender, and stiff.

Usually, the arthritis is symmetrical; it may be remittent or indolent. The patient may run a low-grade fever with daily peaks. Listlessness and weight loss can occur, possibly with lymphadenopathy and hepatosplenomegaly. Other signs of polyarticular JRA include subcutaneous nodules on the elbows or heels and noticeable developmental retardation.

Seropositive polyarticular JRA, the more severe type, usually occurs late in childhood and can cause destructive arthritis that mimics adult RA.

### Pauciarticular JRA

Involving few joints (usually no more than four), pauciarticular JRA most often affects the knees and other large joints. It accounts for 45% of cases. Three major subtypes exist:

• *Pauciarticular JRA with chronic iridocyclitis* most commonly strikes girls under age 6 and involves the knees, elbows, ankles, or iris. Inflammation of the iris and ciliary body is often asymptomatic but may produce pain, redness, blurred vision, and photophobia. Young girls who test positive for antinuclear antibody (ANA) are at highest risk for eye complications.

• *Pauciarticular JRA with sacroiliitis* usually strikes boys (9:1) over age 8, who tend to be HLA-B27–positive. This subtype is characterized by lower extremity arthritis that produces hip, sacroiliac, heel, and foot pain and Achilles tendinitis. These patients may later develop the sacroiliac and lumbar arthritis characteristic of ankylosing spondylitis. Some also experience acute iritis, but not as frequently as those with the first subtype.

• The third subtype includes patients with joint involvement who test negative for ANA and HLA-B27 and who don't develop iritis. Characterized by asymmetrical involvement of large or small joints, this subtype can strike at any age during childhood. These patients have a better prognosis than those with the first or second subtype, although some may progress to polyarticular disease.

Common to all types of JRA is joint stiffness in the morning or after periods of inactivity. Growth disturbances may also occur, resulting in overgrowth or undergrowth adjacent to inflamed joints.

### Diagnosis

Persistent joint pain and the rash and fever clearly point to JRA. Laboratory

tests are useful for ruling out other inflammatory or even malignant diseases that can mimic JRA and for monitoring disease activity and response to therapy.
• *Complete blood count* shows decreased hemoglobin levels, neutrophilia, and thrombocytosis.
• *Erythrocyte sedimentation rate, complement (C)-reactive protein, haptoglobin, immunoglobulins,* and *C3 levels* may be elevated.
• *ANA test* may be positive in patients who have pauciarticular JRA with chronic iridocyclitis.
• *RF* is present in 15% of JRA cases, as compared with 85% of RA cases.
• Positive *HLA-B27* test may forecast later development of ankylosing spondylitis.
• Early *X-ray* changes include soft-tissue swelling, effusion, and periostitis in affected joints. Later, osteoporosis and accelerated bone growth may appear, followed by subchondral erosions, joint space narrowing, bone destruction, and fusion.

## Treatment
Successful management of JRA usually involves administration of anti-inflammatory drugs, physical therapy, carefully planned nutrition and exercise, and regular eye examinations. Both the child and his parents must be involved in therapy.

Aspirin is the initial drug of choice, with the dosage based on the child's weight. However, other nonsteroidal anti-inflammatory drugs (NSAIDs) may also be used. If these prove ineffective, methotrexate has been shown to be a useful second-line agent. In addition, gold salts, hydroxychloroquine, penicillamine, and sulfasalazine may be considered. Responses to the agents may differ among the various subtypes of JRA. Because of adverse effects, systemic steroids are generally reserved for treatment of systemic complications that

are resistant to NSAIDs, such as pericarditis and iritis. However, intra-articular steroids can be very effective in managing pauci- and polyarticular JRA.

> **CLINICAL TIP** Joint rest (by splinting) used for up to three days after joint injections with corticosteroids may improve anti-inflammatory response.

Corticosteroids and mydriatic drugs are commonly used for iridocyclitis. Low-dose cytotoxic drug therapy is currently being investigated.

Physical therapy promotes regular exercise to maintain joint mobility and muscle strength, thereby preventing contractures, deformity, and disability. Good posture, gait training, and joint protection are also beneficial. Splints help reduce pain, prevent contractures, and maintain correct joint alignment.

Generally, the prognosis for JRA is good, although disabilities can occur. Surgery is usually limited to soft-tissue releases to improve joint mobility. Joint replacement is delayed until the child has matured physically and can handle vigorous rehabilitation.

## Special considerations
• Encourage the child to be as independent as possible and to develop a positive attitude toward school, social development, and vocational planning.
• Schedule regular slit-lamp examinations to help ensure early diagnosis and treatment of iridocyclitis.
• Children with pauciarticular JRA with chronic iridocyclitis should be checked every 3 months during periods of active disease and every 6 months during remissions.

> **CLINICAL TIP** Stress the need for regular eye exams even in the absence of joint symptoms. Iridocyclitis may be asymptomatic and, if undiagnosed and untreated, can lead to loss of vision.

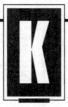

# KAPOSI'S SARCOMA

Initially, this cancer of the lymphatic cell wall was described as a rare blood vessel sarcoma, occurring mostly in elderly Italian and Jewish men. In recent years, the incidence of Kaposi's sarcoma has risen dramatically along with the incidence of acquired immunodeficiency syndrome (AIDS). Currently, it's the most common AIDS-related cancer.

Kaposi's sarcoma causes structural and functional damage. When associated with AIDS, it progresses aggressively, involving the lymph nodes, the viscera and, possibly, GI structures.

## Causes

The exact cause of Kaposi's sarcoma is unknown, but the disease may be related to immunosuppression. Genetic or hereditary predisposition is also suspected.

## Signs and symptoms

The initial sign of Kaposi's sarcoma is one or more obvious lesions in various shapes, sizes, and colors (ranging from red-brown to dark purple) that appear most commonly on the skin, buccal mucosa, hard and soft palates, lips, gums, tongue, tonsils, conjunctivae, and sclerae.

In advanced disease, the lesions may join, becoming one large plaque. Untreated lesions may appear as large, ulcerative masses.

Other signs and symptoms include:
- a health history of AIDS
- pain (if the sarcoma advances beyond the early stages or if a lesion breaks down or impinges on nerves or organs)
- edema from lymphatic obstruction
- dyspnea (in cases of pulmonary involvement), wheezing, hypoventilation, and respiratory distress from bronchial blockage.

The most common extracutaneous sites are the lungs and GI tract (esophagus, oropharynx, and epiglottis).

Signs and symptoms of disease progression and metastasis include severe pulmonary involvement and GI involvement leading to digestive problems.

## Diagnosis

The diagnosis is made following a tissue biopsy that identifies the lesion's type and stage. Then, a computed tomography scan may be performed to detect and evaluate possible metastasis. (See *Laubenstein's stages of Kaposi's sarcoma,* page 482.)

## Treatment

In Kaposi's sarcoma, treatment isn't indicated for all patients. Indications include cosmetically offensive, painful, or obstructive lesions of rapidly progressing disease.

Radiation therapy, chemotherapy, and biotherapy with biological response modifiers are treatment options. Radi-

## LAUBENSTEIN'S STAGES OF KAPOSI'S SARCOMA

The following staging system was proposed by L.J. Laubenstein for use in evaluating and treating patients who have acquired immunodeficiency syndrome and Kaposi's sarcoma:

*Stage I*—locally indolent cutaneous lesions
*Stage II*—locally aggressive cutaneous lesions
*Stage III*—mucocutaneous and lymph node involvement
*Stage IV*—visceral involvement.

Within each stage, a patient may have different symptoms classified as a stage subtype—A or B—as follows:
• Subtype A—no systemic signs or symptoms
• Subtype B—one or more systemic signs and symptoms, including 10% weight loss, fever of unknown origin that exceeds 100° F (37.8° C) for more than 2 weeks, chills, lethargy, night sweats, anorexia, and diarrhea.

ation therapy alleviates symptoms, including pain from obstructing lesions in the oral cavity or extremities and edema caused by lymphatic blockage. It may also be used for cosmetic improvement.

Chemotherapy includes combinations of doxorubicin, vinblastine, vincristine, and etoposide (VP-16).

Biotherapy with interferon alfa-2b may be administered for AIDS-related Kaposi's sarcoma. The treatment reduces the number of skin lesions but is ineffective in advanced disease.

**Special considerations**
• The patient who's coping poorly may need a referral for psychological counseling. Family members may also need help in coping with the patient's disease and with any associated demands that the disorder places upon them.
• As appropriate, allow the patient to participate in self-care decisions whenever possible, and encourage him to participate in self-care measures as much as he can.
• Inspect the patient's skin every shift. Look for new lesions and skin breakdown. If the patient has painful lesions, help him into a more comfortable position.
• Follow universal precautions when caring for the patient.
• Administer pain medications. Suggest distractions, and help the patient with relaxation techniques.
• To help the patient adjust to changes in his appearance, urge him to share his feelings, and provide encouragement.
• Monitor the patient's weight daily.
• Supply the patient with high-calorie, high-protein meals. If he can't tolerate regular meals, provide him with frequent smaller meals. Consult with the dietitian, and plan meals around the patient's treatment.
• If the patient can't take food by mouth, administer I.V. fluids. Also provide antiemetics and sedatives.
• Be alert for adverse effects of radiation therapy or chemotherapy—such as anorexia, nausea, vomiting, and diarrhea—and take steps to prevent or alleviate them.
• Reinforce the explanation of treatments. Make sure the patient understands which adverse reactions to expect and how to manage them. For example, during radiation therapy, instruct the patient to keep irradiated skin dry to avoid possible breakdown and subsequent infection.
• Explain all prescribed medications, including any possible adverse effects and drug interactions.

- Explain infection-prevention techniques and, if necessary, demonstrate basic hygiene measures to prevent infection. Advise the patient not to share his toothbrush, razor, or other items that may be contaminated with blood. These measures are especially important if the patient also has AIDS.

- Help the patient plan daily periods of alternating activity and rest to help him cope with fatigue. Teach energy-conservation techniques. Encourage him to set priorities, accept the help of others, and delegate nonessential tasks.

- Explain the proper use of assistive devices, when appropriate, to ease ambulation and promote independence.

- Stress the need for ongoing treatment and care.

- As appropriate, refer the patient to support groups offered by the social services department.

- If the patient's prognosis is poor (less than 6 months to live), suggest immediate hospice care.

- Explain the benefits of initiating and executing advance directives and a durable power of attorney.

# KERATITIS

Inflammation of the cornea (keratitis) may be acute or chronic, superficial or deep. Superficial keratitis is fairly common and may develop at any age. The prognosis is good with treatment. Untreated, recurrent keratitis may lead to blindness.

## Causes
Keratitis may result from exposure (such as in Bell's palsy where the eyelids don't close). It may also result from infection by herpes simplex virus, type 1 (known as dendritic keratitis because of a char-acteristic branched lesion of the cornea resembling the veins of a leaf). Less commonly, it stems from bacterial and fungal infections and, rarely, from congenital syphilis.

## Signs and symptoms
Unilateral keratitis may produce mild irritation, tearing, and photophobia. If the infection is in the center of the cornea, it may produce blurred vision. Left untreated, corneal opacities can occur. When keratitis results from exposure, it usually affects the lower portion of the cornea.

## Diagnosis
A slit-lamp examination reveals the depth of the keratitis. If keratitis is due to herpes simplex virus, staining the eye with a fluorescein strip produces one or more small branchlike (dendritic) lesions; touching the cornea with cotton reveals reduced corneal sensation. Vision testing may show slightly decreased acuity. The patient history may reveal a recent infection of the upper respiratory tract accompanied by cold sores.

## Treatment
In acute keratitis due to herpes simplex virus, treatment consists of trifluridine eyedrops or vidarabine ointment. A broad-spectrum antibiotic may prevent secondary bacterial infection.

Chronic dendritic keratitis may respond more quickly to vidarabine. Long-term topical therapy may be necessary. (Corticosteroid therapy is contraindicated in dendritic keratitis or any other viral or fungal disease of the cornea.) Treatment for fungal keratitis consists of natamycin.

Keratitis due to exposure requires application of moisturizing ointment to the exposed cornea and of a plastic bubble eye shield or eye patch. Treatment for severe corneal scarring may include keratoplasty (cornea transplantation).

## Special considerations
● Look for keratitis in patients predisposed to cold sores. Explain that stress, trauma, fever, colds, and overexposure to the sun may trigger flare-ups.

▶ CLINICAL TIP Protect the exposed corneas of unconscious patients by cleaning the eyes daily, applying moisturizing ointment, or covering the eyes with an eye shield.

# KIDNEY CANCER

Kidney cancer is also known as nephrocarcinoma, renal cell carcinoma, hypernephroma, and Grawitz's tumor. It usually occurs in older adults, with about 85% of tumors originating in the kidneys and others resulting from metastasis from other primary sites. Renal pelvic tumors and Wilms' tumor occur primarily in children.

Kidney tumors, which usually are large, firm, nodular, encapsulated, unilateral, and solitary, can be separated histologically into clear cell, granular, and spindle cell types. The prognosis, which sometimes seems better for the clear cell type, probably depends on the cancer stage. (See *Staging kidney cancer.*) The 5-year survival rate for kidney cancer is about 50%; the 10-year survival rate is lower.

## Causes
The causes of kidney cancer aren't known. However, the incidence of this cancer is rising, possibly as a result of exposure to environmental carcinogens as well as increased longevity. Even so, kidney cancer accounts for only about 2% of all adult cancers. It's twice as common in men as in women and usually strikes after age 40.

## Signs and symptoms
Kidney cancer produces a classic clinical triad — hematuria, pain, and a palpable mass — but any one of these features may be the first sign of cancer. Microscopic or gross hematuria (which may be intermittent) suggests that the cancer has spread to the renal pelvis.

Constant abdominal or flank pain may be dull or, if the cancer causes bleeding or blood clots, acute and colicky. The mass is generally smooth, firm, and nontender. All three signs of kidney cancer coexist in only about 10% of patients.

Other symptoms include fever (perhaps from hemorrhage or necrosis); hypertension (from compression of the renal artery with renal parenchymal ischemia); rapidly progressing hypercalcemia (possibly from ectopic parathyroid hormone production by the tumor); and urine retention. Weight loss, edema in the legs, nausea, and vomiting are signs of advanced kidney cancer.

▶ CLINICAL TIP Patients may also present with bone pain or fracture from a metastatic lesion.

## Diagnosis
Studies to identify kidney cancer usually include computed tomography scans, excretory urography and retrograde pyelography, ultrasound, cystoscopy (to rule out associated bladder cancer), and nephrotomography or renal angiography to distinguish a kidney cyst from a tumor.

Related tests include liver function studies showing increased levels of alkaline phosphatase, bilirubin, alanine aminotransferase, and aspartate aminotransferase, as well as prolonged prothrombin time. Such results may point to liver metastasis, but if metastasis hasn't occurred, these abnormalities reverse after the tumor has been resected.

# STAGING KIDNEY CANCER

Using the TNM (tumor, node, metastasis) system, the American Joint Committee on Cancer has established the following stages for kidney cancer.

### Primary tumor
*TX*—primary tumor can't be assessed

*T0*—no evidence of primary tumor

*T1*—tumor 2.5 cm or less in greatest dimension and limited to the kidney

*T2*—tumor greater than 2.5 cm in greatest dimension and limited to the kidney

*T3*—tumor extends into major veins or invades adrenal gland or perinephric tissues, but not beyond Gerota's fascia

*T3a*—tumor extends into adrenal gland or perinephric tissues, but not beyond Gerota's fascia

*T3b*—tumor grossly extends into renal veins or vena cava

*T4*—tumor extends beyond Gerota's fascia

### Regional lymph nodes
*NX*—regional lymph nodes can't be assessed

*N0*—no evidence of regional lymph node metastasis

*N1*—metastasis in a single lymph node, 2 cm or less in greatest dimension

*N2*—metastasis in a single lymph node between 2 and 5 cm in greatest dimension, or metastasis to several lymph nodes, none more than 5 cm in greatest dimension

*N3*—metastasis in a lymph node, more than 5 cm in greatest dimension

### Distant metastasis
*MX*—distant metastasis can't be assessed

*M0*—no known distant metastasis

*M1*—distant metastasis

### Staging categories
Kidney cancer progresses from mild to severe as follows:

*Stage I*—T1, N0, M0

*Stage II*—T2, N0, M0

*Stage III*—TI, N1, M0; T2, N1, M0; T3a, N0, M0; T3a, N1, M0; T3b, N0, M0; T3b, N1, M0

*Stage IV*—any N, M0; any T, N2, M0; any T, N3, M0; any T, any N, M1

---

Routine laboratory findings of hematuria, anemia (unrelated to blood loss), polycythemia, hypercalcemia, and increased erythrocyte sedimentation rate call for more testing to rule out kidney cancer. A bone scan should also be performed to rule out skeletal metastasis.

### Treatment
Radical nephrectomy, with or without regional lymph node dissection, offers the only chance of cure. Because the disease is radiation-resistant, radiation is used only if the cancer spreads to the perinephric region or the lymph nodes, or if the primary tumor or metastatic sites can't be fully excised. In such cases, high radiation doses are used.

Chemotherapy has been only erratically effective against kidney cancer. Chlorambucil, fluorouracil, cyclophosphamide, vinblastine, lomustine, vincristine, cisplatin, tamoxifen, teniposide, interferons, and hormones, such as medroxyprogesterone and testosterone, have been used, usually with poor results. Biotherapy (lymphokine-activated killer cells with recombinant-interleukin-2) shows promise but causes adverse reactions. Interferon is somewhat effective in advanced disease.

## Special considerations

- Meticulous postoperative care, supportive treatment during other therapy, and psychological support can hasten recovery and minimize complications.
- Before surgery, assure the patient that his body will adapt to the loss of a kidney.
- Teach the patient about such expected postoperative procedures as diaphragmatic breathing, coughing properly, splinting his incision, and others.
- After surgery, encourage diaphragmatic breathing and coughing.
- Assist the patient with leg exercises, and turn him every 2 hours.
- Check dressings often for excessive bleeding. Watch for signs of internal bleeding, such as restlessness, sweating, and increased pulse rate.
- Place the patient on the operative side to allow the pressure of adjacent organs to fill the dead space at the operative site, improving dependent drainage. If possible, help the patient walk within 24 hours after surgery.
- Maintain adequate fluid intake, and monitor intake and output. Monitor laboratory results for anemia, polycythemia, or abnormal blood values that may point to bone or liver involvement or that may result from radiation or chemotherapy.
- Treat adverse effects of medication.
- Stress the need to comply with the prescribed outpatient treatment regimen.

# KYPHOSIS

Also known as roundback, kyphosis is an anteroposterior curving of the spine that causes a bowing of the back, commonly at the thoracic, but sometimes at the thoracolumbar or sacral, level.

Normally, the spine displays some convexity, but excessive thoracic kyphosis is pathologic. Kyphosis occurs in children and adults.

## Causes

Congenital kyphosis is rare but usually severe, with resultant cosmetic deformity and reduced pulmonary function.

### *Adolescent kyphosis*

Also called Scheuermann's disease, juvenile kyphosis, and vertebral epiphysitis, adolescent kyphosis is the most common form of this disorder. It may result from growth retardation or a vascular disturbance in the vertebral epiphysis (usually at the thoracic level) during periods of rapid growth, or from congenital deficiency in the thickness of the vertebral plates.

Other causes include infection, inflammation, aseptic necrosis, and disk degeneration. The subsequent stress of weight bearing on the compromised vertebrae may result in the thoracic hump often seen in adolescents with kyphosis. Symptomatic adolescent kyphosis is more prevalent in girls than in boys and occurs most often between ages 12 and 16.

### *Adult kyphosis*

Also known as adult roundback, adult kyphosis may result from aging and associated degeneration of intervertebral disks, atrophy, and osteoporotic collapse of the vertebrae; from endocrine disorders such as hyperparathyroidism, and Cushing's disease; and from prolonged steroid therapy.

Adult kyphosis may also result from conditions such as arthritis, Paget's disease, polio, compression fracture of the thoracic vertebrae, metastatic tumor, plasma cell myeloma, or tuberculosis.

In both children and adults, kyphosis may also result from poor posture.

Disk lesions called Schmorl's nodes may develop in anteroposterior curving of the spine and are localized protrusions of nuclear material through the cartilage plates and into the spongy bone of the vertebral bodies. If the anterior portions of the cartilage are destroyed, bridges of new bone may transverse the intervertebral space, causing ankylosis.

## Signs and symptoms

Clinical features vary with the type of kyphosis.

### Adolescent features

Development of adolescent kyphosis is usually insidious, often occurring after a history of excessive sports activity, and may be asymptomatic except for the obvious curving of the back (sometimes more than 90 degrees). In some adolescents, kyphosis may produce mild pain at the apex of the curve (about 50% of patients), fatigue, tenderness or stiffness in the involved area or along the entire spine, and prominent vertebral spinous processes at the lower dorsal and upper lumbar levels, with compensatory increased lumbar lordosis, and hamstring tightness.

In rare case, kyphosis may induce neurologic damage: spastic paraparesis secondary to spinal cord compression or herniated nucleus pulposus. In both adolescent and adult forms of kyphosis that aren't due to poor posture alone, the spine won't straighten out when the patient assumes a recumbent position.

### Adult features

Adult kyphosis produces a characteristic roundback appearance, possibly associated with pain, weakness of the back, and generalized fatigue. Unlike the adolescent form, adult kyphosis rarely produces local tenderness, except in senile osteoporosis with recent compression fracture.

## Diagnosis

Physical examination reveals curvature of the thoracic spine in varying degrees of severity. X-rays may show vertebral wedging, Schmorl's nodes, irregular end plates and, possibly, mild scoliosis of 10 to 20 degrees.

Adolescent kyphosis must be distinguished from tuberculosis and other inflammatory or neoplastic diseases that cause vertebral collapse; the severe pain, bone destruction, or systemic symptoms associated with these diseases help to rule out a diagnosis of kyphosis. Other sites of bone disease, primary sites of cancer, and infection must also be evaluated, possibly by a vertebral biopsy.

## Treatment

For kyphosis caused by poor posture alone, treatment may consist of therapeutic exercises, bed rest on a firm mattress (with or without traction), and a brace to straighten the kyphotic curve until spinal growth is complete.

Corrective exercises include pelvic tilts to decrease lumbar lordosis, hamstring stretches to overcome muscle contractures, and thoracic hyperextensions to flatten the kyphotic curve. These exercises may be performed in or out of the brace.

Lateral X-rays taken every 4 months evaluate correction. Gradual weaning from the brace can begin after maximum correction of the kyphotic curve, vertebral wedging has decreased, and the spine has reached full skeletal maturity. Loss of correction indicates that weaning from the brace has been too rapid, and time out of the brace is decreased accordingly.

Treatment for both adolescent and adult kyphosis also includes appropriate measures for the underlying cause

# MANAGING KYPHOSIS

- Explain how to perform therapeutic exercises and emphasize good posture.
- Tell the patient to use bed rest when pain is severe.
- Remind the patient to use a firm mattress or bed board to offer good support.
- Explain how to use the brace and encourage compliance with the prescribed use of the brace.
- Teach the patient good skin care to prevent skin breakdown from brace usage.
- Caution the patient that only an orthotist should adjust the brace.

and, possibly, spinal arthrodesis for relief of symptoms. Although rarely necessary, surgery may be recommended when kyphosis causes neurologic damage, a spinal curve greater than 60 degrees, or intractable and disabling back pain in a patient with full skeletal maturity. Preoperative measures may include halo-femoral traction.

Corrective surgery includes a posterior spinal fusion with spinal instrumentation, iliac bone grafting, and plaster immobilization. Anterior spinal fusion followed by immobilization in plaster may be necessary when kyphosis produces a spinal curve greater than 70 degrees.

**Special considerations**
- Effective management of kyphosis requires first-rate supportive care for patients in traction or a brace, skillful patient teaching, and sensitive emotional support. For more patient-teaching information, see *Managing kyphosis*.

- If corrective surgery is needed, explain all preoperative tests thoroughly, as well as the need for postoperative traction or casting if applicable.
- After surgery, check the patient's neurovascular status every 2 to 4 hours for the first 48 hours, and watch for any changes.
- Turn the patient often by logrolling him.
- Offer pain medication every 3 or 4 hours for the first 48 hours.
- Institute blood product replacement as needed.
- Accurately measure fluid intake and output, including urine specific gravity.
- Insert a nasogastric tube and an indwelling urinary catheter as needed; a rectal tube may also be necessary if paralytic ileus causes abdominal distention.
- Provide meticulous skin care. Check the skin at the cast edges several times a day; use heel and elbow protectors to prevent skin breakdown.
- Change dressings as necessary.
- Assist during the removal of sutures and application of a new cast (usually about 10 days after surgery).
- Encourage gradual ambulation (often with the use of a tilt-table in the physical therapy department).
- At discharge, provide detailed, written cast care instructions. Tell the patient to immediately report pain, burning, skin breakdown, loss of feeling, tingling, numbness, or cast odor.
- Advise the patient to drink plenty of liquids to avoid constipation and to report any illness (especially abdominal pain or vomiting) immediately.
- Arrange for home visits by a home care nurse.

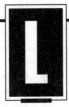

# LABYRINTHITIS

An inflammation of the labyrinth of the inner ear, labyrinthitis frequently incapacitates the patient by producing severe vertigo that lasts for 3 to 5 days; symptoms gradually subside over a 3- to 6-week period. This disorder is rare, although viral labyrinthitis is often associated with upper respiratory tract infections.

## Causes

Labyrinthitis is usually caused by viral infection. It may be a primary infection; the result of trauma; or a complication of influenza, otitis media, or meningitis. In chronic otitis media, cholesteatoma formation erodes the bone of the labyrinth, allowing bacteria to enter from the middle ear. Toxic drug ingestion is another possible cause of labyrinthitis.

## Signs and symptoms

Because the inner ear controls both hearing and balance, this infection typically produces severe vertigo (with any movement of the head) and sensorineural hearing loss. Vertigo begins gradually but peaks within 48 hours, causing loss of balance and falling in the direction of the affected ear.

Other associated signs and symptoms include spontaneous nystagmus, with jerking movements of the eyes toward the unaffected ear; nausea, vomiting, and giddiness; with cholesteatoma, signs of middle ear disease; and, with severe bacterial infection, purulent drainage. To minimize symptoms such as giddiness and nystagmus, the patient may assume a characteristic posture — lying on the side of the unaffected ear and looking in the direction of the affected ear.

## Diagnosis

A typical clinical picture and history of upper respiratory tract infection suggest labyrinthitis. Typical diagnostic measures include culture and sensitivity testing to identify the infecting organism, if purulent drainage is present, and audiometric testing.

When an infectious etiology can't be found, additional testing must be done to rule out a brain lesion or Ménière's disease.

## Treatment

Symptomatic treatment includes bed rest, with the head immobilized between pillows; oral meclizine to control vertigo; and massive doses of antibiotics to combat diffuse purulent labyrinthitis. Oral fluids can prevent dehydration from vomiting; for severe nausea and vomiting, I.V. fluids may be necessary.

When conservative management fails, treatment necessitates surgical excision of the cholesteatoma and drainage of the infected areas of the middle and inner ear. Prevention is possible by early and vigorous treatment of predisposing conditions, such as otitis media and any local or systemic infection.

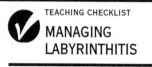

TEACHING CHECKLIST

## MANAGING LABYRINTHITIS

- Tell the patient to avoid sudden position changes.
- Help the patient assess how much his disability will affect his daily life.
- Work with the patient to identify hazards in the home (such as throw rugs and dark stairways).
- Discuss the patient's anxieties and concerns about vertigo attacks and decreased hearing.
- Stress the importance of maintaining or resuming normal diversions or social activities when balance disturbance is absent.

### Special considerations
- Keep the side rails up to prevent falls.
- If vomiting is severe, administer antiemetics. Record intake and output, and give I.V. fluids as necessary.
- Tell the patient that recovery may take as long as 6 weeks. During this time, he should limit activities that vertigo may make hazardous.
- If recovery doesn't occur within 4 to 6 weeks, a computed tomography scan should be performed to rule out an intracranial lesion.
- Review teaching points with the patient. (See *Managing labyrinthitis*.)

# LARYNGEAL CANCER

The most common form of laryngeal cancer is squamous cell carcinoma (95%); rare forms include adenocarcinoma, sarcoma, and others. Such cancer may be intrinsic or extrinsic.

An *intrinsic* tumor is on the true vocal cord and tends not to spread because underlying connective tissues lack lymph nodes. An *extrinsic* tumor is on some other part of the larynx and tends to spread early. Laryngeal cancer is nine times more common in males than in females; most victims are between ages 50 and 65.

### Causes
In laryngeal cancer, major predisposing factors include smoking and alcoholism; minor factors include chronic inhalation of noxious fumes and familial tendency.

Laryngeal cancer is classified according to its location:
- supraglottis (false vocal cords)
- glottis (true vocal cords)
- subglottis (downward extension from the vocal cords [rare]).

### Signs and symptoms
In intrinsic laryngeal cancer, the dominant and earliest symptom is hoarseness that persists longer than 3 weeks; in extrinsic cancer, it's a lump in the throat or pain or burning in the throat when drinking citrus juice or hot liquid. Later clinical effects of metastasis include dysphagia, dyspnea, cough, enlarged cervical lymph nodes, and pain radiating to the ear.

### Diagnosis
Any hoarseness that lasts longer than 2 weeks requires visualization of the larynx by laryngoscopy.

A firm diagnosis also requires xeroradiography, a biopsy, laryngeal tomography, computed tomography scan, or laryngography to define the borders of the lesion, and a chest X-ray to detect metastasis. (See *Staging laryngeal cancer.*)

# STAGING LARYNGEAL CANCER

The TNM (tumor, node, metastasis) classification system developed by the American Joint Committee on Cancer describes laryngeal cancer stages and guides treatment. The T stages cover supraglottic, glottic, and subglottic tumors.

## Primary tumor
*TX*—primary tumor unassessible
*T0*—no evidence of primary tumor
*Tis*—carcinoma in situ

## Supraglottic tumor stages
*T1*—tumor confined to one subsite in supraglottis; vocal cords retain motion
*T2*—tumor extends to other sites in supraglottis or to glottis; vocal cords retain motion
*T3*—tumor confined to larynx, but vocal cords lose motion; or tumor extends to the postcricoid area, the pyriform sinus, or the preepiglottic space, and vocal cords lose motion; or both
*T4*—tumor extends through thyroid cartilage or extends to tissues beyond the larynx (such as the oropharynx or soft tissues of the neck), or both

## Glottic tumor stages
*T1*—tumor confined to vocal cords, which retain normal motion; may involve anterior or posterior commissures
*T2*—tumor extends to supraglottis, subglottis, or both; vocal cords may lose motion
*T3*—tumor confined to larynx, but vocal cords lose motion
*T4*—tumor extends through thyroid cartilage, to tissues beyond the larynx (such as the oropharynx or soft tissues of the neck), or both

## Subglottic tumor stages
*T1*—tumor confined to subglottis
*T2*—tumor extends to vocal cords; vocal cords may lose motion
*T3*—tumor confined to larynx with vocal cord fixation
*T4*—tumor extends through cricoid or thyroid cartilage, to tissues beyond the larynx, or both

## Regional lymph nodes
*NX*—regional lymph nodes can't be assessed
*N0*—no evidence of regional lymph node metastasis
*N1*—metastasis in a single ipsilateral lymph node 3 cm or less in greatest dimension
*N2*—metastasis in one or more ipsilateral lymph nodes, or in bilateral or contralateral nodes, larger than 3 cm but less than 6 cm in greatest dimension
*N3*—metastasis in a node larger than 6 cm in greatest dimension

## Distant metastasis
*MX*—distant metastasis unassessible
*M0*—no evidence of distant metastasis
*MI*—distant metastasis

## Staging categories
Laryngeal cancer progresses from mild to severe as follows:
*Stage 0*—Tis, N0, M0
*Stage I*—T1, N0, M0
*Stage II*—T2, N0, M0
*Stage III*—T3, N0, M0; T1, N1, M0; T2, N1, M0; T3, N1, M0
*Stage IV*—T4, N0 or N1, M0; any T, N2 or N3, M0; any T, any N, M1

## Treatment
Early lesions are treated with surgery or radiation; advanced lesions with surgery, radiation, and chemotherapy. The chemotherapeutic agents may include methotrexate, cisplatin, bleomycin, fluorouracil, and vincristine.

The treatment goal is to eliminate the cancer and preserve speech. If speech preservation isn't possible, speech rehabilitation may include esophageal speech or prosthetic devices; surgical techniques to construct a new voice box are still experimental. Surgical procedures vary with tumor size and can include cordectomy, partial or total laryngectomy, supraglottic laryngectomy, or total laryngectomy with laryngoplasty.

### Special considerations

● Psychological support and good preoperative and postoperative care can minimize complications and speed recovery.

Before partial or total laryngectomy:

● Instruct the patient to maintain good oral hygiene. If appropriate, instruct a male patient to shave off his beard.

● Encourage the patient to express his concerns before surgery. Help him choose a temporary nonspeaking method of communication (such as writing).

● If appropriate, arrange for a laryngectomee to visit him. Explain postoperative procedures (suctioning, nasogastric [NG] tube feeding, care of laryngectomy tube) and their results (breathing through the neck, speech alteration). Also prepare him for other functional losses: He won't be able to smell, blow his nose, whistle, gargle, sip, or suck on a straw.

After partial laryngectomy:

● Give I.V. fluids and, usually, tube feedings for the first 2 days postoperatively; then resume oral fluids. Keep the tracheostomy tube (inserted during surgery) in place until edema subsides.

● Keep the patient from using his voice until he has medical permission (usually 2 to 3 days postoperatively). Then caution him to whisper until healing is complete.

After total laryngectomy:

● As soon as the patient returns to his bed, place him on his side and elevate his head 30 to 45 degrees. When you move him, remember to support his neck.

● The patient will probably have a laryngectomy tube in place until his stoma heals (about 7 to 10 days). This tube is shorter and thicker than a tracheostomy tube but requires the same care.

● Watch for crusting and secretions around the stoma, which can cause skin breakdown. To prevent crust formation, provide adequate room humidification. Remove crusting with petroleum jelly, antimicrobial ointment, and moist gauze.

● Teach stoma care.

● Watch for fistula formation (redness, swelling, secretions on suture line). A fistula may form between the reconstructed hypopharynx and the skin. This eventually heals spontaneously but may take weeks or months.

● Watch for carotid artery rupture (bleeding), which usually occurs in patients who have had preoperative radiation, particularly those with a fistula that constantly bathes the carotid artery with oral secretions. If carotid rupture occurs, apply pressure to the site; call for help immediately and take the patient to the operating room for carotid ligation.

● Watch for tracheostomy stenosis (constant shortness of breath), which occurs weeks to months after laryngectomy; treatment includes fitting the patient with successively larger tracheostomy tubes until he can tolerate insertion of a large one.

● If the patient has a fistula, feed him through an NG tube; otherwise, food will leak through the fistula and delay healing.

● Monitor vital signs (be especially alert for fever, which indicates infection).

● Record fluid intake and output, and watch for dehydration.

● Provide frequent mouth care.

> **CLINICAL TIP** Suction gently unless otherwise instructed. Don't

attempt deep suctioning, which could penetrate the suture line. Suction through both the tube and the patient's nose because the patient can no longer blow air through his nose; suction his mouth gently.

• After insertion of a drainage catheter (usually connected to a blood drainage system or a GI drainage system), don't stop suction until drainage is minimal. After catheter removal, check dressings for drainage.

• Give analgesics as necessary.

• If the patient has an NG feeding tube, check tube placement and elevate the patient's head to prevent aspiration.

• Reassure the patient that speech rehabilitation may help him speak again. Encourage him to contact the International Association of Laryngectomees and other sources of support.

---

> **TEACHING CHECKLIST**
>
> ## MANAGING REFLUX LARYNGITIS
>
> ─────────────
>
> To prevent gastric reflux, which can lead to laryngitis, give the patient the following instructions:
>
> • Elevate the head of the bed (by elevating the mattress). Sleeping on additional pillows won't be sufficient.
> • Avoid alcohol and coffee. Explain other dietary recommendations as needed.
> • Avoid eating for 3 to 4 hours before going to bed.
> • Take antacids and $H_2$-receptor antagonists as prescribed.

# LARYNGITIS

A common disorder, laryngitis is acute or chronic inflammation of the vocal cords. Acute laryngitis may occur as an isolated infection or as part of a generalized bacterial or viral upper respiratory tract infection. Repeated attacks of acute laryngitis cause inflammatory changes associated with chronic laryngitis.

## Causes

Acute laryngitis usually results from infection (primarily viral) or excessive use of the voice, an occupational hazard in certain vocations (for example, teaching, public speaking, singing). It may also result from leisure-time activities (such as cheering at a sports event), inhalation of smoke or fumes, or aspiration of caustic chemicals. Causes of chronic laryngitis include chronic upper respiratory tract disorders (sinusitis, bronchitis, nasal polyps, allergy), mouth breathing, smoking, constant exposure to dust or other irritants, and alcohol abuse. Reflux laryngitis is caused by regurgitation of gastric acid into the hypopharynx. (See *Managing reflux laryngitis*.)

## Signs and symptoms

Acute laryngitis typically begins with hoarseness, ranging from mild to complete loss of voice. Associated clinical features include pain (especially when swallowing or speaking), dry cough, fever, laryngeal edema, and malaise. In chronic laryngitis, persistent hoarseness is usually the only symptom. In reflux laryngitis, hoarseness and dysphagia are present but heartburn isn't.

## Diagnosis

Indirect laryngoscopy confirms the diagnosis by revealing red, inflamed and, occasionally, hemorrhagic vocal cords, with rounded rather than sharp edges and exudate. Bilateral swelling may be present. In severe cases or if toxicity is a concern, a culture of the exudate is obtained.

### Treatment

Primary treatment consists of resting the voice. For viral infection, symptomatic care includes analgesics and throat lozenges for pain relief. Bacterial infection requires antibiotic therapy. Severe, acute laryngitis may necessitate hospitalization. When laryngeal edema results in airway obstruction, tracheotomy may be necessary. In chronic laryngitis, effective treatment must eliminate the underlying cause. In reflux laryngitis, postural and dietary changes along with antacids and $H_2$-receptor antagonists combine for effective treatment.

### Special considerations

• Explain to the patient why he shouldn't talk, and place a sign over the bed to remind others of this restriction. Provide a Magic Slate or a pad and pencil for communication. Mark the intercom panel so other facility personnel are aware that the patient can't answer.
• Minimize the need to talk by trying to anticipate the patient's needs.
• Suggest that the patient maintain adequate humidification by using a vaporizer or humidifier during the winter, by avoiding air conditioning during the summer (because it dehumidifies), by using medicated throat lozenges, and by not smoking. Urge him to complete the prescribed antibiotics.
• Obtain a detailed patient history to help determine the cause of chronic laryngitis. Encourage modification of predisposing habits.

# LEGIONNAIRES' DISEASE

An acute bronchopneumonia, Legionnaires' disease is produced by a fastidious, gram-negative bacillus. It derives its name and notoriety from the peculiar, highly publicized disease that struck 182 people (29 of whom died) at an American Legion convention in Philadelphia in July 1976.

This disease may occur epidemically or sporadically, usually in late summer or early fall. Its severity ranges from a mild illness, with or without pneumonitis, to multilobar pneumonia, with a mortality as high as 15%. A milder, self-limiting form (Pontiac syndrome) subsides within a few days but leaves the patient fatigued for several weeks; this form mimics Legionnaires' disease but produces few or no respiratory symptoms, no pneumonia, and no fatalities.

### Causes

The causative agent of Legionnaires' disease, *Legionella pneumophila,* is an aerobic, gram-negative bacillus that's probably transmitted by an airborne route. In past epidemics, it has spread through cooling towers or evaporation condensers in air-conditioning systems. However, *Legionella* bacilli also flourish in soil and excavation sites. The disease doesn't spread from person to person.

Legionnaires' disease occurs more often in men than in women and is most likely to affect:
• middle-aged to elderly people
• immunocompromised people (particularly those receiving corticosteroids, for example, after a transplant), or those

with lymphoma or other disorders associated with delayed hypersensitivity
• patients with a chronic underlying disease, such as diabetes, chronic renal failure, or chronic obstructive pulmonary disease
• alcoholics
• cigarette smokers (three to four times more likely to develop Legionnaires' disease than nonsmokers).

### Signs and symptoms

The multisystem clinical features of Legionnaires' disease follow a predictable sequence, although onset of the disease may be gradual or sudden.

After a 2- to 10-day incubation period, nonspecific, prodromal signs and symptoms appear, including diarrhea, anorexia, malaise, diffuse myalgias and generalized weakness, headache, recurrent chills, and an unremitting fever, which develops within 12 to 48 hours with a temperature as high as 105° F (40.5° C). A cough then develops that initially is nonproductive but eventually may produce grayish, nonpurulent and, occasionally, blood-streaked sputum.

Other characteristic features include nausea, vomiting, disorientation, mental sluggishness, confusion, mild temporary amnesia, pleuritic chest pain, tachypnea, dyspnea, fine crackles and, in 50% of patients, bradycardia. Patients who develop pneumonia may also experience hypoxia. Other complications include hypotension, delirium, heart failure, arrhythmias, acute respiratory failure, renal failure, and shock (usually fatal).

### Diagnosis

The patient history focuses on possible sources of infection and predisposing conditions. In addition, a chest X-ray shows patchy, localized infiltration, which progresses to multilobar consolidation (usually involving the lower lobes), pleural effusion and, in fulminant disease, opacification of the entire lung.

Auscultation reveals fine crackles, progressing to coarse crackles as the disease advances.

Abnormal test findings include leukocytosis, an increased erythrocyte sedimentation rate, an increase in liver enzyme levels (alanine aminotransferase, aspartate aminotransferase, alkaline phosphatase), hyponatremia, decreased partial pressure of arterial oxygen and, initially, decreased partial pressure of arterial carbon dioxide. Bronchial washings and blood, pleural fluid, and sputum tests rule out other infections.

Definitive tests include direct immunofluorescence of respiratory tract secretions and tissue, a culture of *L. pneumophila,* and indirect fluorescent antibody testing of serum comparing acute samples with convalescent samples drawn at least 3 weeks later. A urine specimen for *L. pneumophila* antigen may also be performed. A convalescent serum showing a fourfold or greater rise in antibody titer for *Legionella* confirms this diagnosis.

### Treatment

Antibiotic treatment begins as soon as Legionnaires' disease is suspected and diagnostic material is collected; it shouldn't await laboratory confirmation. Erythromycin is the drug of choice, but if it's not effective alone, rifampin can be added to the regimen. If erythromycin is contraindicated, rifampin or rifampin with tetracycline may be used.

Supportive therapy includes administration of antipyretics, fluid replacement, circulatory support with pressor drugs if necessary, and oxygen administration by mask, cannula, or mechanical ventilation.

## Special considerations

• Closely monitor the patient's respiratory status. Evaluate chest wall expansion, depth and pattern of respirations, cough, and chest pain.

> CLINICAL TIP Watch for restlessness, which may indicate that the patient is hypoxemic and requires suctioning, repositioning, or more aggressive oxygen therapy.

• Continually monitor the patient's vital signs, pulse oximetry or arterial blood gas values, level of consciousness, and dryness and color of the lips and mucous membranes. Watch for signs of shock (decreased blood pressure, thready pulse, diaphoresis, clammy skin).

• Keep the patient comfortable; avoid chills and exposure to drafts. Provide mouth care frequently. If necessary, apply soothing cream to the nostrils.

• Replace fluid and electrolytes as needed. The patient with renal failure may require dialysis.

• Provide mechanical ventilation and other respiratory therapy as needed. Teach the patient how to cough effectively, and encourage deep-breathing exercises. Stress the need to continue these measures until recovery is complete.

• Give antibiotics as necessary, and observe carefully for adverse effects.

---

# LEUKEMIA, ACUTE

---

Acute leukemia is a malignant proliferation of white blood cell precursors (blasts) in bone marrow or lymph tissue and their accumulation in peripheral blood, bone marrow, and body tissues.

The most common forms are acute lymphoblastic (lymphocytic) leukemia (ALL), characterized by the abnormal growth of lymphocyte precursors (lymphoblasts); acute myeloblastic (myelogenous) leukemia (AML), in which myeloid precursors (myeloblasts) rapidly accumulate; and acute monoblastic (monocytic) leukemia, or Schilling's type, characterized by a marked increase in monocyte precursors (monoblasts). Other variants include acute myelomonocytic leukemia and acute erythroleukemia.

Untreated, acute leukemia is invariably fatal, usually because of complications that result from leukemic cell infiltration of bone marrow or vital organs. With treatment, the prognosis varies.

In ALL, treatment induces remissions in 90% of children (average survival time: 5 years) and in 65% of adults (average survival time: 1 to 2 years). Children ages 2 to 8 have the best survival rate with intensive therapy.

In AML, the average survival time is only 1 year after diagnosis, even with aggressive treatment. In acute monoblastic leukemia, treatment induces remissions lasting 2 to 10 months in 50% of children; adults survive only about 1 year after diagnosis, even with treatment.

## Causes

Research on predisposing factors isn't conclusive but points to some combination of viruses (viral remnants have been found in leukemic cells), genetic and immunologic factors, and exposure to radiation and certain chemicals.

Pathogenesis isn't clearly understood, but immature, nonfunctioning white blood cells (WBCs) appear to accumulate first in the tissue where they originate (lymphocytes in lymph tissue, granulocytes in bone marrow). These immature WBCs then spill into the bloodstream and from there infiltrate

## WHAT HAPPENS IN LEUKEMIA

This illustration shows how white blood cells (agranulocytes and granulocytes) proliferate in the bloodstream in leukemia, overwhelming red blood cells (RBCs) and platelets.

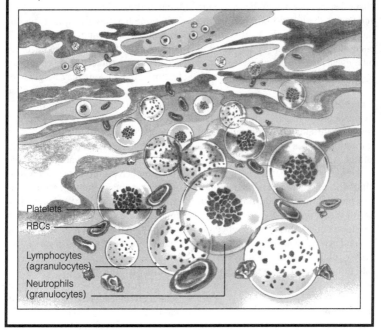

Platelets
RBCs
Lymphocytes (agranulocytes)
Neutrophils (granulocytes)

other tissues, eventually causing organ malfunction because of encroachment or hemorrhage. (See *What happens in leukemia.*)

### *Incidence*

Acute leukemia is more common in males than in females, in whites (especially people of Jewish descent), in children between ages 2 and 5 (80% of all leukemias in this age-group are ALL), and in people who live in urban and industrialized areas. Acute leukemia ranks 20th in causes of cancer-related deaths among people of all age-groups. Among children, however, it's the most common form of cancer. In the United States, an estimated 11,000 people develop acute leukemia annually.

### Signs and symptoms

Signs of acute leukemia are the sudden onset of high fever accompanied by thrombocytopenia and abnormal bleeding, such as nosebleeds, gingival bleeding, purpura, ecchymoses, petechiae, easy bruising after minor trauma, and prolonged menses. Nonspecific symptoms, such as low-grade fever, weakness, and lassitude, may persist for days or months before visible symptoms appear.

Other insidious signs include pallor, chills, and recurrent infections. In addition, ALL, AML, and acute monoblastic leukemia may cause dyspnea, anemia, fatigue, malaise, tachycardia, palpitations, systolic ejection murmur, and abdominal or bone pain. When leukemic cells cross the blood-brain barrier and thereby escape the effects of systemic chemotherapy, the patient may develop meningeal leukemia (confusion, lethargy, headache).

## Diagnosis

Typical clinical findings and bone marrow aspirate showing a proliferation of immature WBCs confirm acute leukemia. An aspirate that's dry or free of leukemic cells in a patient with typical clinical findings requires a bone marrow biopsy, usually of the posterior superior iliac spine.

Blood counts show thrombocytopenia and neutropenia. A differential leukocyte count determines cell type. Lumbar puncture detects meningeal involvement.

## Treatment

Systemic chemotherapy aims to eradicate leukemic cells and induce remission. Chemotherapy varies according to the type of leukemia:

• meningeal leukemia — intrathecal instillation of methotrexate or cytarabine with cranial radiation

• ALL — vincristine, prednisone, high-dose cytarabine, L-asparaginase, AMSA, and daunorubicin. Because there's a 40% risk of meningeal leukemia in ALL, intrathecal methotrexate or cytarabine is given. Radiation therapy is given for testicular infiltration.

• AML—a combination of I.V. daunorubicin and cytarabine or, if these drugs fail to induce remission, a combination of cyclophosphamide, vincristine, prednisone, or methotrexate; high-dose cytarabine alone or along with other drugs; amsacrine; etoposide; and 5-azacytidine and mitoxantrone

• acute monoblastic leukemia — cytarabine and thioguanine with daunorubicin or doxorubicin.

A bone marrow transplant may be possible. Treatment also may include antibiotic, antifungal, and antiviral drugs and granulocyte injections to control infection. Transfusions may be given of platelets (to prevent bleeding) and red blood cells (to prevent anemia).

## Special considerations

• For the leukemia patient, emphasize comfort, minimize the adverse effects of chemotherapy, promote preservation of veins, manage complications, and provide teaching and psychological support. Because so many of these patients are children, be especially sensitive to their emotional needs and those of their families.

Before treatment:

• Explain the course of the disease, treatments, and adverse effects of medications.

• Teach the patient and his family how to recognize infection (fever, chills, cough, sore throat) and abnormal bleeding (bruising, petechiae) and how to stop such bleeding (applying pressure and ice to the area).

• Promote good nutrition. Explain that chemotherapy may cause weight loss and anorexia, so encourage the patient to eat and drink high-calorie, high-protein foods and beverages. However, chemotherapy and adjunctive prednisone may cause weight gain, so dietary counseling and teaching are helpful.

• Help establish an appropriate rehabilitation for the patient during remission.

For supportive care:

• Watch for signs of meningeal leukemia (confusion, lethargy, head-ache). If these occur, know how to manage care after intrathecal chemotherapy. After such instillation, place the patient in Trendelenburg's position for 30 minutes. Force fluids and keep the patient supine for 4 to 6 hours.

• Check the lumbar puncture site often for bleeding.

• If the patient receives cranial radiation, teach him about potential adverse effects, and do what you can to minimize them.

• Prevent hyperuricemia, a possible result of rapid chemotherapy-induced leukemic cell lysis. Force fluids to about 2 qt (2 L) daily, and give acetazolamide, sodium bicarbonate tablets, and allopurinol. Check urine pH often — it should be above 7.5. Watch for a rash or another hypersensitivity reaction to allopurinol.

• Watch for early signs of cardiotoxicity, such as arrhythmias, and signs of heart failure if the patient receives daunorubicin or doxorubicin.

• Control infection by placing the patient in a private room and imposing reverse isolation, if necessary. (The benefits of reverse isolation are controversial.) Coordinate patient care so the leukemic patient doesn't come in contact with staff who also care for patients with infections or infectious diseases. Avoid using indwelling urinary catheters and giving I.M. injections because they provide an avenue for infection. Screen staff and visitors for contagious diseases, and watch for any signs of infection.

• Provide thorough skin care by keeping the patient's skin and perianal area clean, applying mild lotions or creams to keep skin from drying and cracking, and thoroughly cleaning skin before all invasive skin procedures. Use strict aseptic technique and a metal scalp vein needle (metal butterfly needle) when starting I.V. lines. If the patient receives total parenteral nutrition, provide scrupulous subclavian catheter care.

• Monitor the patient's temperature every 4 hours.

➤ CLINICAL TIP  A patient with a temperature over 101° F (38.3° C) and a decreased WBC count should receive prompt antibiotic therapy.

• Watch for bleeding; if it occurs, apply ice compresses and pressure, and elevate the extremity. Avoid giving I.M. injections, aspirin, and aspirin-containing drugs. Also avoid taking rectal temperatures, giving rectal suppositories, and doing digital examinations.

• Prevent constipation by providing adequate hydration, a high-residue diet, stool softeners, and mild laxatives, and by encouraging walking.

• Control mouth ulceration by checking often for obvious ulcers and gum swelling and by providing frequent mouth care and saline rinses.

• Tell the patient to use a soft toothbrush and to avoid hot, spicy foods and overuse of commercial mouthwashes. Also check the rectal area daily for induration, swelling, erythema, skin discoloration, or drainage.

• Minimize stress by providing a calm, quiet atmosphere that is conducive to rest and relaxation. For children particularly, be flexible with patient care and visiting hours to promote maximum interaction with family and friends and to allow time for schoolwork and play.

• For those patients who are refractory to chemotherapy and in the terminal phase of the disease, supportive nursing care aims to provide comfort; management of pain, fever, and bleeding; and patient and family support. Provide the opportunity for religious counseling. Discuss the option of home or hospice care.

# LEUKEMIA, CHRONIC GRANULOCYTIC

Chronic granulocytic leukemia (CGL) is also known as chronic myelogenous (or myelocytic) leukemia. The disease is characterized by the abnormal overgrowth of granulocytic precursors (myeloblasts, promyelocytes, metamyelocytes, and myelocytes) in bone marrow, peripheral blood, and body tissues.

CGL is most common in young and middle-aged adults and is slightly more common in men than in women; it's rare in children. In the United States, approximately 3,000 to 4,000 cases of CGL develop annually, accounting for roughly 20% of all leukemias.

The clinical course of CGL proceeds in two distinct phases: the *insidious chronic phase,* with anemia and bleeding abnormalities and, eventually, the *acute phase (blastic crisis),* in which myeloblasts, the most primitive granulocytic precursors, proliferate rapidly. This disease is invariably fatal. Average survival time is 3 to 4 years after onset of the chronic phase and 3 to 6 months after onset of the acute phase.

## Causes

Almost 90% of patients with CGL have the Philadelphia (Ph[1]) chromosome, an abnormality discovered in 1960 in which the long arm of chromosome 22 is translocated, usually to chromosome 9. Radiation and carcinogenic chemicals may induce this chromosome abnormality. Myeloproliferative diseases also seem to increase the incidence of CGL, and some clinicians suspect that an unidentified virus causes this disease.

## Signs and symptoms

Typically, CGL induces the following clinical effects:

● anemia (fatigue, weakness, decreased exercise tolerance, pallor, dyspnea, tachycardia, and headache)

● thrombocytopenia, with resulting bleeding and clotting disorders (retinal hemorrhage, ecchymoses, hematuria, melena, bleeding gums, nosebleeds, and easy bruising)

● hepatosplenomegaly, with abdominal discomfort and pain in splenic infarction from leukemic cell infiltration.

Other symptoms include sternal and rib tenderness from leukemic infiltrations of the periosteum; low-grade fever; weight loss; anorexia; renal calculi or gouty arthritis from increased uric acid excretion; occasionally, prolonged infection and ankle edema; and, rarely, priapism and vascular insufficiency.

## Diagnosis

In patients with typical clinical changes, chromosomal analysis of peripheral blood or bone marrow showing Ph[1] and low leukocyte alkaline phosphatase levels confirms CGL. Other relevant laboratory results include:

● White blood cell abnormalities: leukocytosis (leukocyte count ranging from 50,000/μl to as high as 250,000/μl), occasional leukopenia (leukocyte count < 5,000/μl), neutropenia (neutrophil count < 1,500/μl) despite a high leukocyte count, and increased circulating myeloblasts

● hemoglobin: often below 10 g/dl

● hematocrit; low (<30%)

● platelet count: thrombocytosis (>1 million/μl) common

● serum uric acid level: possibly >8 mg/dl

● bone marrow aspirate or biopsy: hypercellular, characteristically shows bone marrow infiltration by significantly increased number of myeloid elements (a biopsy is done only if aspirate is dry); in the acute phase, myeloblasts predominate

• computed tomography scan: may identify the organs affected by leukemia.

## Treatment

Aggressive chemotherapy has so far failed to produce remission in CGL. Consequently, the goal of treatment in the chronic phase is to control leukocytosis and thrombocytosis. The most commonly used oral agents are busulfan and hydroxyurea. Aspirin is commonly given to prevent stroke if the patient's platelet count is over 1 million/µl.

Ancillary CGL treatments include:
• local splenic radiation or splenectomy to increase platelet count and decrease adverse effects related to splenomegaly
• leukapheresis (selective leukocyte removal) to reduce leukocyte count
• allopurinol to prevent secondary hyperuricemia or colchicine to relieve gout due to elevated serum uric acid levels
• prompt treatment of infections that may result from chemotherapy-induced bone marrow suppression.

During the acute phase of CGL, lymphoblastic or myeloblastic leukemia may develop. Treatment is similar to that for acute lymphoblastic leukemia. Remission, if achieved, is commonly short lived. Bone marrow transplant may produce long asymptomatic periods in the early phase of illness but has been less successful in the accelerated phase. Despite vigorous treatment, CGL usually progresses after onset of the acute phase.

For more information on treatment during the acute phase, see "Acute Leukemia," pages 496 to 499.

## Special considerations

• In patients with CGL, meticulous supportive care, psychological support, and careful patient teaching help make the

---

TEACHING CHECKLIST

## MANAGING CHRONIC GRANULOCYTIC LEUKEMIA

Because the patient with CGL often receives outpatient chemotherapy throughout the chronic phase, sound patient teaching is essential.

• Explain the adverse effects of chemotherapy and the related signs and symptoms.
• Describe the signs of infection and caution the patient to report them promptly.
• Explain the signs of thrombocytopenia and what preventative measures the patient can take (such as avoiding aspirin).
• Teach the patient what to do if he starts to bleed (such as external pressure).
• Emphasize the need for adequate rest and a high-calorie, high-protein diet.

---

most of remissions and minimize complications.
• Reinforce the explanation of the disease and its treatment to the patient and his family.

Throughout the chronic phase of CGL when the patient is hospitalized:
• If the patient has persistent anemia, schedule laboratory tests and physical care with frequent rest periods in between, and assist the patient with walking if necessary.
• Regularly check the patient's skin and mucous membranes for pallor, petechiae, and bruising.
• For more patient-teaching information, see *Managing chronic granulocytic leukemia.*

- To minimize bleeding, suggest a soft-bristled toothbrush, an electric razor, and other safety precautions.
- To minimize the abdominal discomfort of splenomegaly, provide small, frequent meals.
- For the same reason, prevent constipation with a stool softener or laxative as needed. Ask the dietary department to provide a high-bulk diet, and maintain adequate fluid intake.
- To prevent atelectasis, stress the need for coughing and deep-breathing exercises.

# LEUKEMIA, CHRONIC LYMPHOCYTIC

A generalized, progressive disease that's common in elderly people, chronic lymphocytic leukemia is marked by an uncontrollable spread of abnormal, small lymphocytes in lymphoid tissue, blood, and bone marrow. The prognosis is poor if anemia, thrombocytopenia, neutropenia, bulky lymphadenopathy, and severe lymphocytosis are present.

Nearly all patients with chronic lymphocytic leukemia are men over age 50. According to the American Cancer Society, chronic lymphocytic leukemia accounts for almost one-third of new leukemia cases annually.

## Causes

Although the cause of chronic lymphocytic leukemia is unknown, researchers suspect hereditary factors (higher incidence has been recorded within families), still-undefined chromosome abnormalities, and certain immunologic defects (such as ataxia-telangiectasia or acquired agammaglobulinemia). The disease doesn't seem to be associated with radiation exposure.

## Signs and symptoms

Chronic lymphocytic leukemia is the most benign and the most slowly progressive form of leukemia. Clinical signs derive from the infiltration of leukemic cells in bone marrow, lymphoid tissue, and organ systems.

### Early stages

In early stages, patients usually complain of fatigue, malaise, fever, and nodal enlargement. They're particularly susceptible to infection.

### Advanced stages

In advanced stages, patients may experience severe fatigue and weight loss, with liver or spleen enlargement, bone tenderness, and edema from lymph node obstruction. Pulmonary infiltrates may appear when lung parenchyma is involved. Skin infiltrations, manifested by macular to nodular eruptions, occur in about half the cases of chronic lymphocytic leukemia.

As the disease progresses, bone marrow involvement may lead to anemia, pallor, weakness, dyspnea, tachycardia, palpitations, bleeding, and infection. Opportunistic fungal, viral, and bacterial infections commonly occur in late stages.

## Diagnosis

Typically, chronic lymphocytic leukemia is an incidental finding during a routine blood test that reveals numerous abnormal lymphocytes. In early stages, the white blood cell (WBC) count is mildly but persistently elevated. Granulocytopenia is the rule, but the WBC count climbs as the disease progresses.

Blood studies also show a hemoglobin count below 11 g, hypogammaglobulinemia, and depressed serum globulin levels. Other common findings include neutropenia ($< 1,500/\mu l$), lymphocytosis ($> 10,000/\mu l$), and thrombocytopenia ($< 150,000/\mu l$). Bone marrow aspiration and biopsy show lymphocytic invasion.

### Treatment
Systemic chemotherapy includes alkylating agents, usually chlorambucil or cyclophosphamide, and sometimes steroids (prednisone) when autoimmune hemolytic anemia or thrombocytopenia occurs.

When chronic lymphocytic leukemia causes obstruction or organ impairment or enlargement, local radiation treatment can be used to reduce organ size. Allopurinol can be given to prevent hyperuricemia, a relatively uncommon finding.

### Special considerations
• Focus patient care on relieving symptoms and preventing infection. Clean the patient's skin daily with mild soap and water. Frequent soaks may be ordered. Watch for signs of infection: temperature over 100° F (37.8° C), chills, redness, or swelling of any body part.
• Watch for signs of thrombocytopenia (easy bruising, nosebleeds, bleeding gums, and black, tarry stools) and anemia (pale skin, weakness, fatigue, dizziness, and palpitations).
• Advise the patient to avoid aspirin and products containing aspirin. Explain that many medications contain aspirin. Teach him how to recognize aspirin variants on medication labels.
• Explain chemotherapy and its possible adverse effects.

> **CLINICAL TIP** If the patient will be discharged, tell him to avoid coming in contact with obviously ill people, especially children with common contagious childhood diseases.

• Urge the patient to eat high-protein foods and drink high-calorie beverages.
• Stress the importance of follow-up care, frequent blood tests, and taking all medications exactly as prescribed.

• Teach the patient the signs of recurrence (swollen lymph nodes in the neck, axilla, and groin; increased abdominal size or discomfort), and tell him to notify his doctor immediately if he detects any of these signs.
• Provide emotional support and be a good listener. Most patients with chronic lymphocytic leukemia are elderly and many are frightened. Try to keep their spirits up by concentrating on little things, such as improving their personal appearance, providing a pleasant environment, and asking questions about their families. If possible, provide opportunities for their favorite activities.

---

**LIFE-THREATENING DISORDER**

# LIVER ABSCESS

A liver abscess occurs when bacteria or protozoa destroy hepatic tissue, producing a cavity, which fills with infectious organisms, liquefied liver cells, and leukocytes. Necrotic tissue then walls off the cavity from the rest of the liver.

Liver abscess occurs equally in men and women, usually in those over age 50. Death occurs in 15% of affected patients despite treatment.

### Causes
Underlying causes of liver abscess include benign or malignant biliary obstruction along with cholangitis, extrahepatic abdominal sepsis, and trauma or surgery to the right upper quadrant. Liver abscesses also occur from intra-arterial chemoembolizations or cryosurgery in the liver, which causes necrosis of tumor cells and potential infection.

The method by which bacteria reach the liver reflects the underlying causes. Biliary tract disease is the most common cause of liver abscess. Liver abscess after intra-abdominal sepsis (such as with diverticulitis) is most likely to be caused by hematogenous spread through the portal bloodstream. Hematogenous spread by hepatic arterial flow may occur in infectious endocarditis. Abscesses arising from hematogenous transmission are usually caused by a single organism; those arising from biliary obstruction are usually caused by a mixed flora. Patients with metastatic cancer to the liver, diabetes mellitus, and alcoholism are more likely to develop a liver abscess. The organisms that predominate in liver abscess are gram-negative aerobic bacilli, enterococci, streptococci, and anaerobes. Amebic liver abscesses are caused by *Entamoeba histolytica*.

### Signs and symptoms
The clinical manifestations of a liver abscess depend on the degree of involvement. Some patients are acutely ill; in others, the abscess is recognized only at autopsy, after death from another illness.

The onset of symptoms of a pyogenic abscess is usually sudden; in an amebic abscess, the onset is more insidious. Common signs include abdominal pain, weight loss, fever, chills, diaphoresis, nausea, vomiting, and anemia. Signs of right pleural effusion, such as dyspnea and pleural pain, develop if the abscess extends through the diaphragm. Liver damage may cause jaundice.

### Diagnosis
Ultrasonography and computed tomography (CT) scan with contrast medium can accurately define intrahepatic lesions and allow assessment of intra-abdominal pathology. Percutaneous needle aspiration of the abscess can also be performed with diagnostic tests to identify the causative organism. Contrast-aided magnetic resonance imaging may also become an accurate method for diagnosing hepatic abscesses.

Abnormal laboratory values include elevated levels of serum aspartate aminotransferase, alanine aminotransferase, alkaline phosphatase, and bilirubin; an increased white blood cell count: and decreased serum albumin levels. In pyogenic abscess, a blood culture can identify the bacterial agent; in amebic abscess, a stool culture and serologic and hemagglutination tests can isolate *E. histolytica.*

### Treatment
Antibiotic therapy along with drainage is the preferred treatment for most hepatic abscesses. Percutaneous drainage either with ultrasound or CT guidance is usually sufficient to evacuate pus. Surgery may be performed to drain pus in unstable patients with continued sepsis (despite attempted nonsurgical treatment) and for patients with persistent fevers (lasting longer than 2 weeks) after percutaneous drainage and appropriate antibiotic therapy.

Before the causative organism is identified, antibiotics should be started to treat aerobic gram-negative bacilli, streptococci, and anaerobic bacilli including *Bacteroides* species. A common combination is ampicillin, an aminoglycoside with either metronidazole or clindamycin. Third-generation cephalosporins can be substituted for the aminoglycosides in patients at risk for renal toxicity. When the causative organisms are identified, the antibiotic regimen should be modified to match the patient's sensitivities. I.V. antibiotics should be administered for 14 days and then replaced with oral preparations to complete a 6-week course.

## Special considerations
• Provide supportive care, monitor vital signs (especially temperature), and maintain fluid and nutritional intake.
• Administer anti-infectives and antibiotics as necessary, and watch for possible adverse effects. Stress the importance of compliance with therapy.
• Explain diagnostic and surgical procedures.
• Watch carefully for complications of abdominal surgery, such as hemorrhage or infection.

➤ CLINICAL TIP  Prepare the patient for I.V. antibiotic administration as an outpatient with home care support.

# LIVER CANCER

A rare form of cancer, liver cancer (primary and metastatic hepatic carcinoma) has a high mortality It's responsible for roughly 2% of all cancers in the United States and for 10% to 50% in Africa and parts of Asia. Liver cancer is most prevalent in men (particularly over age 60); incidence increases with age. It's rapidly fatal, usually within 6 months, from GI hemorrhage, progressive cachexia, hepatic failure, or metastasis.

Most primary liver tumors (90%) originate in the parenchymal cells and are hepatomas (hepatocellular carcinoma, primary lower-cell carcinoma). Some primary tumors originate in the intrahepatic bile ducts and are known as cholangiomas (cholangiocarcinoma, cholangiocellular carcinoma). Rarer tumors include a mixed-cell type, Kupffer cell sarcoma and hepatoblastomas (which occur almost exclusively in children and are usually resectable and curable).

The liver is one of the most common sites of metastasis from other primary cancers, particularly those of the colon, rectum, stomach, pancreas, esophagus, lung, or breast or melanoma. In the United States, metastatic liver carcinoma occurs over 20 times more often than primary carcinoma and, after cirrhosis, is the leading cause of liver-related death. At times, liver metastasis may appear as a solitary lesion, the first sign of recurrence after a remission.

## Causes
The immediate cause of liver cancer is unknown, but it may be a congenital disease in children. Adult liver cancer may result from environmental exposure to carcinogens, such as the chemical compound aflatoxin (a mold that grows on rice and peanuts), thorium dioxide (a contrast medium formerly used in liver radiography), *Senecio* alkaloids and, possibly, androgens and oral estrogens.

### Risk factors
Roughly 30% to 70% of patients with hepatomas also have cirrhosis. (Hepatomas are 40 times more likely to develop in a cirrhotic liver than in a normal one.) Whether cirrhosis is a premalignant state, or alcohol and malnutrition predispose the liver to develop hepatomas, is still unclear. Another risk factor is exposure to the hepatitis B virus, although this risk will probably decrease with the availability of the hepatitis B vaccine.

## Signs and symptoms
Clinical effects of liver cancer include:
• a mass in the right upper quadrant
• tender, nodular liver on palpation
• severe pain in the epigastrium or the right upper quadrant
• bruit, hum, or rubbing sound if the tumor involves a large part of the liver.

- weight loss, weakness, anorexia, fever
- occasional jaundice or ascites
- occasional evidence of metastasis through the venous system to the lungs, from lymphatics to the regional lymph nodes, or by direct invasion of the portal veins
- dependent edema.

## Diagnosis

The confirming test for liver cancer is a needle or open biopsy of the liver. Liver cancer is difficult to diagnose in the presence of cirrhosis, but several tests can help identify it:

- *Liver function studies* (aspartate aminotransferase, alanine aminotransferase, alkaline phosphatase, lactate dehydrogenase, and bilirubin) show abnormal liver function.
- *Alpha-fetoprotein level* increases above 500 µg/ml.
- *Chest X-ray* may rule out metastasis.
- *Liver scan* may show filling defects.
- *Arteriography* may define large tumors.
- *Electrolyte studies* may indicate an increased retention of sodium (resulting in functional renal failure) and hypoglycemia, leukocytosis, hypercalcemia, or hypocholesterolemia.

## Treatment

Because liver cancer is often in an advanced stage at diagnosis, few hepatic tumors are resectable. A resectable tumor must be a single tumor in one lobe, without cirrhosis, jaundice, or ascites. Resection is done by lobectomy or partial hepatectomy.

Radiation therapy for unresectable tumors is usually palliative. However, because of the liver's low tolerance for radiation, this therapy hasn't increased survival.

Another method of treatment is chemotherapy with I.V. fluorouracil, methotrexate, streptozocin, lomustine, or doxorubicin or with regional infusion of fluorouracil or floxuridine (catheters are placed directly into the hepatic artery or left brachial artery for continuous infusion for 7 to 21 days, or permanent implantable pumps are used on an outpatient basis for long-term infusion).

Appropriate treatment for liver metastasis may include resection by lobectomy or chemotherapy with mitomycin or fludarabine. (The results are similar to those in hepatoma.) Liver transplantation is now an alternative for some patients.

## Special considerations

- Patient care should emphasize comprehensive supportive measures and emotional support.
- Control edema and ascites. Monitor the patient's diet throughout. Most patients need a special diet that restricts sodium, fluids (no alcohol allowed), and protein.
- Weigh the patient daily, and note intake and output accurately. Watch for signs of ascites—peripheral edema, orthopnea, or dyspnea on exertion. If ascites is present, measure and record abdominal girth daily.
- To increase venous return and prevent edema, elevate the patient's legs whenever possible.
- Monitor respiratory function. Note any increase in respiratory rate or shortness of breath. Bilateral pleural effusion (noted on chest X-ray) is common, as is metastasis to the lungs. Watch carefully for signs of hypoxemia from intrapulmonary arteriovenous shunting.
- Relieve fever. Administer sponge baths and aspirin suppositories if there are no signs of GI bleeding. Avoid acetaminophen because the diseased liver can't metabolize it. High fever indicates infection and requires antibiotics.

• Provide meticulous skin care. Turn the patient frequently and keep his skin clean to prevent pressure ulcers. Apply lotion to prevent chafing, and administer an antipruritic such as diphenhydramine for severe itching.

• Watch for encephalopathy. Many patients develop end-stage symptoms of ammonia intoxication, including confusion, restlessness, irritability, agitation, delirium, asterixis, lethargy and, finally, coma.

• Monitor the patient's serum ammonia level, vital signs, and neurologic status.

> **CLINICAL TIP** Be prepared to control ammonia accumulation with sorbitol (to induce osmotic diarrhea), neomycin (to reduce bacterial flora in the GI tract), lactulose (to control bacterial elaboration of ammonia), and sodium polystyrene sulfonate (to lower the potassium level).

• If a transhepatic catheter is used to relieve obstructive jaundice, irrigate it frequently with the prescribed solution (normal saline or, sometimes, 5,000 units of heparin in 500 ml of dextrose 5% in water).

• Monitor vital signs frequently for any indication of bleeding or infection.

• After surgery, give standard postoperative care. Watch for intraperitoneal bleeding and sepsis, which may precipitate a coma. Monitor for renal failure by checking urine output, blood urea nitrogen, and creatinine levels hourly.

---

**LIFE-THREATENING DISORDER**

# LUNG ABSCESS

---

A lung abscess is a lung infection accompanied by pus accumulation and tissue destruction. The abscess may be putrid (due to anaerobic bacteria) or nonputrid (due to anaerobes or aerobes), and often has a well-defined border. The availability of effective antibiotics has made lung abscesses much less common than they were in the past.

## Causes

A lung abscess is a manifestation of necrotizing pneumonia, often the result of aspiration of oropharyngeal contents. Poor oral hygiene with dental or gingival (gum) disease is strongly associated with a putrid lung abscess. Septic pulmonary emboli commonly produce cavitary lesions. Infected cystic lung lesions and cavitating bronchial carcinoma must be distinguished from lung abscesses.

## Signs and symptoms

The clinical effects of lung abscess include a cough that may produce bloody, purulent, or foul-smelling sputum; pleuritic chest pain; dyspnea; excessive sweating; chills; fever; headache; malaise; diaphoresis; and weight loss.

Complications include rupture into the pleural space, which results in empyema and, rarely, massive hemorrhage. A chronic lung abscess may cause localized bronchiectasis. Failure of an abscess to improve with antibiotic treatment suggests a possible underlying neoplasm or other causes of obstruction.

## Diagnosis

The following tests are used to diagnose a lung abscess:

• *Auscultation of the chest* may reveal crackles and decreased breath sounds.

• *Chest X-ray* shows a localized infiltrate with one or more clear spaces, usually containing air-fluid levels.

• *Percutaneous aspiration of an abscess* or *bronchoscopy* may be used to obtain cultures to identify the causative organism. Bronchoscopy is only used if abscess resolution is eventful and the patient's condition permits it,

• *Blood cultures, Gram stain,* and *culture of sputum* are also used to detect the causative organism.

• *White blood cell count* commonly exceeds 10,000/µl.

### Treatment

Antibiotic therapy often lasts for months until radiographic resolution or definite stability occurs. Symptoms usually disappear in a few weeks. Postural drainage may facilitate discharge of necrotic material into upper airways, where expectoration is possible; oxygen therapy may relieve hypoxemia. A poor response to therapy requires resection of the lesion or removal of the diseased section of the lung. All patients need rigorous follow-up and serial chest X-rays.

### Special considerations

• Provide chest physiotherapy (including coughing and deep breathing).

• Increase fluid intake to loosen secretions, and provide a quiet, restful atmosphere.

➤ CLINICAL TIP   To prevent a lung abscess in the unconscious patient and the patient with seizures, first prevent aspiration of secretions. Do this by suctioning the patient and by positioning him to promote drainage of secretions.

# LUNG CANCER

Lung cancer usually develops within the wall or epithelium of the bronchial tree. Its most common types are epidermoid (squamous cell) carcinoma, small cell (oat cell) carcinoma, adeno-carcinoma, and large cell (anaplastic) carcinoma.

Although the prognosis is usually poor, it varies with the extent of spread at the time of diagnosis and the growth rate of the specific cell type. Only about 13% of patients with lung cancer survive 5 years after diagnosis. Lung cancer is the most common cause of cancer death in men and is fast becoming the most common cause in women, even though it's largely preventable.

### Causes

Most experts agree that lung cancer is attributable to inhalation of carcinogenic pollutants by a susceptible host. Who is most susceptible? Any smoker over age 40, especially if he began to smoke before age 15, has smoked a whole pack or more per day for 20 years, or works with or near asbestos.

Pollutants in tobacco smoke cause progressive lung cell degeneration. Lung cancer is 10 times more common in smokers than in nonsmokers; indeed, 80% of lung cancer patients are or were smokers.

Cancer risk is determined by the number of cigarettes smoked daily, the depth of inhalation, how early in life smoking began, and the nicotine content of cigarettes. Two other factors also increase susceptibility: exposure to carcinogenic industrial and air pollutants (asbestos, uranium, arsenic, nickel, iron oxides, chromium, radioactive dust, and coal dust), and familial susceptibility.

### Signs and symptoms

Because early-stage lung cancer usually produces no symptoms, this disease is often in an advanced state at diagnosis. The following late-stage symptoms often lead to a diagnosis:

• with epidermoid and small cell carcinomas: smoker's cough, hoarseness, wheezing, dyspnea, hemoptysis, and chest pain

- with adenocarcinoma and large cell carcinoma: fever, weakness, weight loss, anorexia, and shoulder pain.

In addition to their obvious interference with respiratory function, lung tumors may also alter the production of hormones that regulate body function or homeostasis. Clinical conditions that result from such changes are known as hormonal paraneoplastic syndromes:

- *Gynecomastia* may result from large cell carcinoma.
- *Hypertrophic pulmonary osteoarthropathy* (bone and joint pain from cartilage erosion due to abnormal production of growth hormone) may result from large cell carcinoma and adenocarcinoma.
- *Cushing's* and *carcinoid syndromes* may result from small cell carcinoma. *Hypercalcemia* may result from epidermoid tumors.

Metastatic symptoms vary greatly, depending on the effect of tumors on intrathoracic and distant structures:

- *bronchial obstruction:* hemoptysis, atelectasis, pneumonitis, dyspnea
- *recurrent nerve invasion:* hoarseness, vocal cord paralysis
- *chest wall invasion:* piercing chest pain; increasing dyspnea; severe shoulder pain, radiating down the arm
- *local lymphatic spread:* cough, hemoptysis, stridor, pleural effusion
- *phrenic nerve involvement:* dyspnea; shoulder pain; unilateral paralyzed diaphragm, with paradoxical motion
- *esophageal compression:* dysphagia
- *vena caval obstruction:* venous distention and edema of the face, neck, chest, and back
- *pericardial involvement:* pericardial effusion, tamponade, arrhythmias
- *cervical thoracic sympathetic nerve involvement:* miosis, ptosis, exophthalmos, reduced sweating.

Distant metastasis may involve any part of the body, most commonly the central nervous system, liver, and bone.

### Diagnosis

Typical clinical findings may strongly suggest lung cancer, but a firm diagnosis requires further evidence, including the following:

- *Chest X-ray* usually shows an advanced lesion, but it can detect a lesion up to 2 years before symptoms appear. It also indicates tumor size and location.
- *Sputum cytology,* which is 75% reliable, requires a specimen coughed up from the lungs and tracheobronchial tree, *not* postnasal secretions or saliva.
- *Computed tomography (CT) scan* of the chest may help to delineate the tumor's size and its relationship to surrounding structures.
- *Bronchoscopy* can locate the tumor site. Bronchoscopic washings provide material for cytologic and histologic examination. The flexible fiber-optic bronchoscope increases the test's effectiveness.
- A *needle biopsy* of the lungs uses biplane fluoroscopic visual control to detect peripherally located tumors. This allows a firm diagnosis in 80% of patients.
- *Tissue biopsy* of accessible metastatic sites includes supraclavicular and mediastinal node and pleural biopsies.
- *Thoracentesis* allows chemical and cytologic examination of pleural fluid.

Additional studies include preoperative mediastinoscopy or mediastinotomy to rule out involvement of mediastinal lymph nodes (which would preclude curative pulmonary resection).

Other tests to detect metastasis include a bone scan, bone marrow biopsy (recommended in small cell carcinoma), and a CT scan of the brain or abdomen.

# STAGING LUNG CANCER

Using the TNM (tumor, node, metastasis) classification system, the American Joint Committee on Cancer stages lung cancer as follows.

### Primary tumor

*TX*—primary tumor can't be assessed, or malignant tumor cells detected in sputum or bronchial washings but undetected by X-ray or bronchoscopy

*T0*—no evidence of primary tumor

*Tis*—carcinoma in situ

*T1*—tumor 3 cm or less in greatest dimension, surrounded by normal lung or visceral pleura; no bronchoscopic evidence of cancer closer to the center of the body than the lobar bronchus

*T2*—tumor larger than 3 cm; or one that involves the main bronchus and is 2 cm or more from the carina; or one that invades the visceral pleura; or one that's accompanied by atelectasis or obstructive pneumonitis that extends to the hilar region but doesn't involve the entire lung

*T3*—tumor of any size that extends into neighboring structures, such as the chest wall, diaphragm, or mediastinal pleura; or a tumor in the main bronchus that doesn't involve but is less than 2 cm from the carina; or a tumor that's accompanied by atelectasis or obstructive pneumonitis of the entire lung

*T4*—tumor of any size that invades the mediastinum, heart, great vessels, trachea, esophagus, vertebral body, or carina; or a tumor with malignant pleural effusion

### Regional lymph nodes

*NX*—regional lymph nodes can't be assessed

*N0*—no detectable metastasis to lymph nodes

*N1*—metastasis to the ipsilateral peribronchial or hilar lymph nodes or both

*N2*—metastasis to the ipsilateral mediastinal or subcarinal lymph nodes or both

*N3*—metastasis to the contralateral mediastinal or hilar lymph nodes, the ipsilateral or contralateral scalene lymph nodes, or the supraclavicular lymph nodes

### Distant metastasis

*MX*—distant metastasis can't be assessed

*M0*—no evidence of distant metastasis

*M1*—distant metastasis

### Staging categories

Lung cancer progresses from mild to severe as follows:

*Occult carcinoma*—TX, N0, M0

*Stage 0*—Tis, N0, M0

*Stage I*—T1, N0, M0; T2, N0, M0

*Stage II*—T1, N1, M0; T2, N1, M0

*Stage IIIA*—T1, N2, M0; T2, N2, M0; T3, N0, M0; T3, N1, M0; T3, N2, M0

*Stage IIIB*—any T, N3, M0; T4, any N, M0

*Stage IV*—any T, any N, M1

---

After histologic confirmation, staging determines the extent of the disease and helps in planning treatment and predicting the prognosis. (See *Staging lung cancer.*)

## Treatment

Various combinations of surgery, radiation, and chemotherapy may improve the prognosis and prolong survival. Nevertheless, because treatment usually begins at an advanced stage, it's largely palliative.

### Surgery

Unless the tumor is nonresectable, or other conditions rule out surgery, excision is the primary treatment for stage

I, stage II, or selected stage III squamous cell carcinoma, adenocarcinoma, and large cell carcinoma. Surgery may include partial removal of a lung (wedge resection, segmental resection, lobectomy, radical lobectomy) or total removal (pneumonectomy, radical pneumonectomy).

### Radiation

Preoperative radiation therapy may reduce tumor bulk to allow for surgical resection. Preradiation chemotherapy helps improve response rates. Radiation therapy is ordinarily recommended for stage I and stage II lesions, if surgery is contraindicated, and for stage III lesions when the disease is confined to the involved hemithorax and the ipsilateral supraclavicular lymph nodes.

Generally, radiation therapy is delayed until 1 month after surgery, to allow the wound to heal, and is then directed to the part of the chest most likely to develop metastasis. High-dose radiation therapy or radiation implants may also be used.

### Chemotherapy

Another treatment is chemotherapy including combinations of fluorouracil, vincristine, mitomycin, cisplatin, and vindesine, which produce a response rate of about 40% but have a minimal effect on overall survival. Promising combinations for treating small cell carcinomas include cyclophosphamide with doxorubicin and vincristine; cyclophosphamide with doxorubicin, vincristine, and etoposide; and etoposide with cisplatin, cyclophosphamide, and doxorubicin.

### Laser therapy

Still largely experimental, laser therapy involves direction of laser energy through a bronchoscope to destroy local tumors.

### Special considerations

Comprehensive supportive care and patient teaching can minimize complications and speed recovery from surgery, radiation, and chemotherapy.

Before surgery:
• Supplement and reinforce information about the disease and the surgical procedure.
• Explain expected postoperative procedures, such as the insertion of an indwelling urinary catheter, use of an endotracheal or chest tube (or both), dressing changes, and I.V. therapy.
• Teach the patient how to perform coughing, deep diaphragmatic breathing, and range-of-motion (ROM) exercises.
• Inform the patient that he may take nothing by mouth after midnight the night before surgery, that he'll shower with a soaplike antibacterial agent the night or morning before surgery, and that he'll be given preoperative medications, such as a sedative and an anticholinergic, to dry secretions.

After thoracic surgery:
• Maintain a patent airway, and monitor chest tubes to reestablish normal intrathoracic pressure and prevent postoperative and pulmonary complications.
• Check vital signs every 15 minutes during the first hour after surgery, every 30 minutes during the next 4 hours, and then every 2 hours. Watch for abnormal respiration and other changes.
• Suction the patient often, and encourage him to begin deep breathing and coughing as soon as possible. Check secretions often. Initially, sputum will be thick and dark with blood, but it should become thinner and grayish yellow within a day.
• Monitor and record closed chest drainage. Keep chest tubes patent and draining effectively.

> **CLINICAL TIP** Position the patient on the surgical side to promote drainage and lung reexpansion.

● Watch for and report foul-smelling discharge and excessive drainage on dressing. Usually, the dressing is removed after 24 hours, unless the wound appears infected.
● Monitor intake and output. Maintain adequate hydration.
● Watch for and treat infection, shock, hemorrhage, atelectasis, dyspnea, mediastinal shift, and pulmonary embolus.
● To prevent pulmonary embolus, apply antiembolism stockings and encourage ROM exercises.

If the patient is receiving chemotherapy and radiation:
● Explain possible adverse effects of radiation and chemotherapy. Watch for, treat, and (when possible) try to prevent them.
● Ask the dietary department to provide soft, nonirritating foods that are high in protein, and encourage the patient to eat high-calorie between-meal snacks.
● Give antiemetics and antidiarrheals as needed.
● Schedule patient care activities in a way that helps the patient conserve his energy.
● During radiation therapy, administer skin care to minimize skin breakdown. If the patient receives radiation therapy in an outpatient setting, warn him to avoid tight clothing, exposure to the sun, and harsh ointments on his chest. Teach him exercises to help prevent shoulder stiffness.

Teach high-risk patients ways to reduce their chances of developing lung cancer:
● Refer smokers who want to quit to local branches of the American Cancer Society, Smokenders, or other smoking cessation programs or suggest group therapy, individual counseling, or hypnosis.

● Encourage patients with recurring or chronic respiratory infections and those with chronic lung disease who detect any change in the character of a cough to see their doctor promptly for evaluation.

# LUPUS ERYTHEMATOSUS

A chronic inflammatory disorder of the connective tissues, lupus erythematosus appears in two forms: *discoid lupus erythematosus,* which affects only the skin, and *systemic lupus erythematosus (SLE),* which affects multiple organ systems (as well as the skin) and can be fatal. Like rheumatoid arthritis, SLE is characterized by recurring remissions and exacerbations, which are especially common during the spring and summer.

The annual incidence of SLE averages 27.5 cases per 1 million whites and 75.4 cases per 1 million blacks. SLE strikes women 8 times as often as men, increasing to 15 times as often during childbearing years. It occurs worldwide but is most prevalent among Asians and blacks. The prognosis improves with early detection and treatment but remains poor for patients who develop cardiovascular, renal, or neurologic complications or severe bacterial infections.

## Causes
The exact cause of SLE remains a mystery, but available evidence points to interrelated immunologic, environmental, hormonal, and genetic factors.

### Immune dysregulation
Immune dysregulation, in the form of autoimmunity, is thought to be the prime causative mechanism. In autoimmunity, the body produces antibodies against

components of its own cells, such as the antinuclear antibody (ANA). The formed antigen-antibody complexes can activate the body's immunity and damage tissues. One significant feature in patients with SLE is their ability to produce antibodies against many different tissue components, such as red blood cells, neutrophils, platelets, lymphocytes, or almost any organ or tissue in the body.

### Predisposing factors
Physical or mental stress, streptococcal or viral infections, exposure to sunlight or ultraviolet light, immunization, pregnancy, and abnormal estrogen metabolism may all affect the development of this disease in a genetically susceptible individual.

SLE also may be triggered or aggravated by treatment with certain drugs, for example, procainamide, hydralazine, anticonvulsants and, less frequently, penicillins, sulfa drugs, and oral contraceptives.

### Signs and symptoms
The onset of SLE may be acute or insidious and produces no characteristic clinical pattern. However, symptoms commonly include fever, weight loss, malaise, fatigue, rashes, and polyarthralgia. SLE may involve any organ system.

### Joint and skin effects
In 90% of patients, joint involvement is similar to that in rheumatoid arthritis (although the arthritis of lupus is usually nonerosive). Skin lesions are most commonly an erythematous rash in areas exposed to light. The classic butterfly rash over the nose and cheeks occurs in fewer than 50% of the patients. A scaly papular rash (which mimics psoriasis) may also develop, especially in sun-exposed areas. Ultraviolet rays often provoke or aggravate skin eruptions. (See *Discoid lupus erythematosus,* page 514.) Vasculitis can develop (especially in the digits), possibly leading to infarctive lesions, necrotic leg ulcers, or digital gangrene. Raynaud's phenomenon appears in about 20% of patients. Patchy alopecia and painless ulcers of the mucous membranes are common.

### Cardiopulmonary effects
About 50% of SLE patients develop signs of pulmonary abnormalities, such as pleurisy, pleural effusions, pneumonitis, pulmonary hypertension and, rarely, pulmonary hemorrhage. Cardiac involvement may include pericarditis, myocarditis, endocarditis, and early coronary atherosclerosis.

### Renal effects
Onset of glomerulonephritis may be evidenced by microscopic hematuria, pyuria, and urine sediment with cellular casts. Renal disease may progress to kidney failure, particularly when untreated. Urinary tract infections may result from heightened susceptibility to infection.

### Neurologic effects
Seizure disorders and mental dysfunction may indicate neurologic damage. Central nervous system (CNS) involvement may produce emotional instability, psychosis, and organic brain syndrome. Headaches, irritability, and depression are common. (See *Signs of systemic lupus erythematosus,* page 515.)

### Systemic effects
Constitutional symptoms of SLE include aching, malaise, fatigue, low-grade or spiking fever, chills, anorexia, and weight loss. Lymph node enlargement (diffuse or local, and nontender), abdominal pain, nausea, vomiting, di-

---

# DISCOID LUPUS ERYTHEMATOSUS

Discoid lupus erythematosus (DLE) is a form of lupus erythematosus marked by chronic skin eruptions that, if untreated, can lead to scarring and permanent disfigurement. About 1 out of 20 patients with DLE later develops systemic lupus erythematosus (SLE).

### Causes
The exact cause of DLE is unknown, but some evidence suggests an autoimmune defect. An estimated 60% of patients with DLE are women in their late twenties or older. This disease is rare in children.

### Clinical features
DLE lesions are raised, red, scaling plaques, with follicular plugging and central atrophy. The raised edges and sunken centers give them a coinlike appearance. Although these lesions can appear anywhere on the body, they usually erupt on the face, scalp, ears, neck, and arms or on any part of the body that's exposed to sunlight.

Such lesions can resolve completely or may cause hypopigmentation or hyperpigmentation, atrophy, and scarring. Facial plaques sometimes assume the butterfly pattern characteristic of SLE. Hair tends to become brittle or may fall out in patches; alopecia can be permanent.

### Diagnosis
As a rule, the patient history and the appearance of the rash itself are diagnostic. A lupus erythematosus cell test is positive in fewer than 10% of patients. A skin biopsy of lesions reveals immunoglobulins or complement components. SLE must be ruled out.

### Treatment
Patients with DLE should avoid prolonged exposure to the sun, fluorescent lighting, or reflected sunlight. They should wear protective clothing, use sunscreening agents, avoid engaging in outdoor activities during periods of most intense sunlight (between 10 a.m. and 2 p.m.), and report any changes in the lesions. Drug treatment consists of topical, intralesional, or systemic medication, as in SLE.

---

arrhea, and constipation may occur. Women may experience irregular menstrual periods or amenorrhea during the active phase of SLE.

Because SLE usually strikes women of childbearing age, questions related to pregnancy often arise. Available evidence indicates that a woman with SLE can have a safe, successful pregnancy if she has no serious renal or neurologic impairment.

### Diagnosis
Diagnostic tests for patients with SLE include a complete blood count with differential, which may show anemia and a decreased white blood cell count; platelet count, which may be decreased; erythrocyte sedimentation rate, which is often elevated; and serum electrophoresis, which may show hypergammaglobulinemia.

Specific tests for SLE include the following:

• *ANA, anti-double-stranded deoxyribonucleic acid (dsDNA), and lupus erythematosus cell tests* are positive in active SLE; because the anti-dsDNA test is rarely positive in other conditions, it's the most specific test for SLE. However, if the patient is in remission, anti-dsDNA results may be reduced or ab-

## SIGNS OF SYSTEMIC LUPUS ERYTHEMATOSUS

Diagnosing systemic lupus erythematosus (SLE) is difficult because SLE often mimics other diseases, symptoms may be vague, and symptoms vary greatly from patient to patient.

For these reasons, the American Rheumatism Association has issued a list of criteria for classifying SLE, to be used primarily for consistency in epidemiologic surveys. Usually, four or more of these signs are present at some time during the course of the disease:
- malar or discoid rash
- photosensitivity
- oral or nasopharyngeal ulcerations
- nonerosive arthritis (of two or more peripheral joints)
- pleuritis or pericarditis
- profuse proteinuria (exceeding 0.5 g/day) or excessive cellular casts in the urine
- seizures or psychoses
- hemolytic anemia, leukopenia, lymphopenia, or thrombocytopenia
- anti-dsDNA or antiSmith antibody test or positive findings of antiphospholipid antibodies (elevated IgG or IgM anticardiolipin antibodies, positive test for lupus anticoagulant, or false-positive serologic tests for syphilis)
- abnormal titer of antinuclear antibody.

sent (because anti-dsDNA correlates with disease activity, especially renal involvement, and helps monitor the patient's response to therapy). Other autoantibodies commonly found include anti-SM (also highly specific for SLE), anti-SSA, anti-SSB, and anti-RNP.

- *Urine studies* may show red blood cells and white blood cells, urine casts and sediment, and significant protein loss (more than 0.5 g/24 hours).
- *Blood studies* reveal decreased serum complement (C3 and C4) levels, which indicate active disease.
- *Chest X-ray* may show pleurisy or lupus pneumonitis.
- *Electrocardiography* may show a conduction defect with cardiac involvement or pericarditis.
- Kidney biopsy determines the stage of the disease and the extent of renal involvement.

Some patients show a positive lupus *anticoagulant test* and a positive *anticardiolipin test.* Such patients are prone to antiphospholipid syndrome (thrombosis, abortion, and thrombocytopenia).

### Treatment

Patients with mild disease require little or no medication. Nonsteroidal antiinflammatory compounds, including aspirin, control arthritis symptoms in many patients. Skin lesions need topical treatment. Corticosteroid creams, such as hydrocortisone or triamcinolone, are recommended for acute lesions.

Refractory skin lesions are treated with intralesional corticosteroids or antimalarials such as hydroxychloroquine. Because hydroxychloroquine can cause retinal damage, such treatment requires ophthalmologic examination every 6 months.

#### Corticosteroids

The treatment of choice, corticosteroids are used for systemic symptoms of SLE, for acute generalized exacerbations, or for serious disease related to vital organ systems, such as pleuritis, pericarditis, lupus nephritis, vasculitis, and CNS involvement. Initial doses equivalent to 60 mg or more of prednisone often bring noticeable improvement within 48 hours.

As soon as symptoms are under control, steroid dosage is tapered down slowly. (Rising serum complement levels and decreasing anti-dsDNA titers indicate that the patient is responding to the treatment.) Diffuse proliferative glomerulonephritis, a major complication of SLE, requires treatment with large doses of steroids and cytotoxic therapy (such as cyclophosphamide). If renal failure occurs, dialysis or a kidney transplant may be necessary. Antihypertensive drugs and dietary changes may also be warranted in renal disease. SLE patients on long-term steroids are at a particular risk for osteonecrosis of the hips.

**Special considerations**
• Careful assessment, supportive measures, emotional support, and patient teaching are all important parts of caring for patients with SLE.
• Watch for constitutional symptoms: joint pain or stiffness, weakness, fever, fatigue, and chills. Observe for dyspnea, chest pain, and any edema of the extremities.
• Note the size, type, and location of skin lesions.
• Check urine for hematuria, scalp for hair loss, and skin and mucous membranes for petechiae, bleeding, ulceration, pallor, and bruising.
• Provide a balanced diet. Foods high in protein, vitamins, and iron help maintain optimum nutrition and prevent anemia. However, renal involvement may mandate a low-sodium, low-protein diet.
• Urge the patient to get plenty of rest. Schedule diagnostic tests and procedures to allow adequate rest.
• Explain all tests and procedures. Tell the patient that several blood samples are needed initially, then periodically, to monitor his progress.

• Apply heat packs to relieve joint pain and stiffness.
• Encourage regular exercise to maintain full range of motion (ROM) and prevent contractures. Teach ROM exercises, as well as body alignment and postural techniques. Arrange for physical therapy and occupational counseling as appropriate.
• Explain the expected benefit of prescribed medications, and watch for adverse effects, especially when the patient is taking high doses of corticosteroids.
• Advise the patient receiving cyclophosphamide to maintain adequate hydration. If prescribed, give mesna to prevent hemorrhagic cystitis and ondansetron to prevent nausea and vomiting.
• Monitor vital signs, intake and output, weight, and laboratory reports. Check pulse rates and observe for orthopnea. Check stools and GI secretions for blood.
• Observe for hypertension, weight gain, and other signs of renal involvement.
• Assess for signs of neurologic damage: personality change, paranoid or psychotic behavior, ptosis, or diplopia. Take seizure precautions. If Raynaud's phenomenon is present, warm and protect the patient's hands and feet.
• Offer cosmetic tips, such as suggesting the use of hypoallergenic makeup, and refer the patient to a hairdresser who specializes in scalp disorders.
• Advise the patient to purchase medications in quantity, if possible. Warn against "miracle" drugs for the relief of arthritis symptoms.
• Refer the patient to the Lupus Foundation of America and the Arthritis Foundation as necessary.
• For more patient-teaching information, see *Managing lupus*.

## MANAGING LUPUS

- Remember to schedule regular checkups and keep your appointments. Routine blood tests and frequent blood pressure screening can detect a flare-up of lupus in the early stages.
- Report unexplained symptoms such as weight loss, fever, extreme fatigue, or persistent fluid retention.
- Eat a balanced diet and participate in a low-impact exercise program to maintain your energy level and control your weight.
- Take a calcium supplement and a multivitamin with vitamin D to reduce your risk for osteoporosis if you're taking prednisone. Check with your doctor for dosage information.
- Avoid intense sun exposure because it can trigger symptoms. Wear a wide-brimmed hat and long-sleeved clothing outdoors, and stay indoors during the brightest hours of the day. Always apply sunblock and repeat the application to attain the best protection.
- Report any fever or other sign of infection to your doctor because antibiotic intervention may be needed.

- Consult your doctor before dental or genitourinary procedures because you may need to take antibiotics first to prevent infection.
- Check with your doctor to see if he recommends yearly flu and pneumonia shots for you.
- Practice effective birth control if you have active lupus (particularly with kidney involvement) or if you're taking cytotoxic medications. Very active lupus and drug therapy pose significant risks for both mother and child. Some patients with lupus can have successful pregnancies, but planning and discussion with your doctor is essential.
- Follow your medication regimen for the best long-term lupus management.
- Check with your doctor or pharmacist regarding special information about your medications (such as taking medications before, after, or with meals) to derive the most benefit from the medications and avoid adverse effects.

# LYME DISEASE

A multisystemic disorder, Lyme disease is caused by the spirochete, *Borrelia burgdorferi,* which is carried by the minute tick *Ixodes dammini* or another tick in the Ixodidae family. It often begins in the summer with the classic skin lesion called erythema chronicum migrans (ECM). Weeks or months later, cardiac or neurologic abnormalities sometimes develop, possibly followed by arthritis.

Initially, Lyme disease was identified in a group of children in Lyme, Connecticut. Now Lyme disease is known to occur primarily in three parts of the United States:

- in the northeast, from Massachusetts to Maryland
- in the midwest, in Wisconsin and Minnesota
- in the west, in California and Oregon.

Although Lyme disease is endemic to these areas, cases have been reported in 43 states and 20 other countries, including Germany, Switzerland, France, and Australia.

## Causes

Lyme disease occurs when a tick injects spirochete-laden saliva into the bloodstream or deposits fecal matter on the skin. After incubating for 3 to 32 days, the spirochetes migrate out to the skin, causing ECM. Then they disseminate to other skin sites or organs by the bloodstream or lymph system.

The spirochetes' life cycle isn't completely clear: They may survive for years in the joints or they may trigger an inflammatory response in the host and then die.

## Signs and symptoms

Typically, Lyme disease has three stages.

### Stage 1

ECM heralds stage 1 with a red macule or papule, often at the site of a tick bite. This lesion often feels hot and itchy and may grow to more than 20″ (50 cm) in diameter. Within a few days, more lesions may erupt along with a malar rash, conjunctivitis, or diffuse urticaria. In 3 to 4 weeks, lesions are replaced by small red blotches, which persist for several more weeks.

Malaise and fatigue are constant, but other findings are intermittent: headache, fever, chills, achiness, and regional lymphadenopathy. Less common effects are meningeal irritation, mild encephalopathy, migrating musculoskeletal pain, and hepatitis. A persistent sore throat and dry cough may appear several days before ECM.

### Stage 2

Weeks to months later, the second stage begins with neurologic abnormalities — fluctuating meningoencephalitis with peripheral and cranial neuropathy — that usually resolve after days or months. Facial palsy is especially noticeable. Cardiac abnormalities, such as a brief, fluctuating atrioventricular heart block, may also develop.

### Stage 3

Characterized by arthritis, stage 3 begins weeks or years later. Migrating musculoskeletal pain leads to frank arthritis with marked swelling, especially in the large joints. Recurrent attacks may precede chronic arthritis with severe cartilage and bone erosion.

## Diagnosis

Because isolation of *B. burgdorferi* is unusual in humans and because indirect immunofluorescent antibody tests are marginally sensitive, diagnosis often rests on the characteristic ECM lesion and related clinical findings, especially in endemic areas. Mild anemia and an elevated erythrocyte sedimentation rate, leukocyte count, serum immunoglobulin M level, and aspartate aminotransferase level support the diagnosis.

## Treatment

A 10- to 20-day course of oral tetracycline is the treatment of choice for adults. Penicillin and erythromycin are alternates. Oral penicillin is usually prescribed for children. When given in the early stages, these drugs can minimize later complications. When given during the late stages, high-dose penicillin I.V. may be a successful treatment. There is now a vaccine (Lymerix) available to prevent Lyme disease. For maximal effectiveness, it's given as a series of three injections.

➤ CLINICAL TIP  Neurologic abnormalities are best treated with I.V. ceftriaxone or I.V. penicillin.

## Special considerations

• Take a detailed patient history, asking about travel to endemic areas and exposure to ticks.

● Check for drug allergies, and administer antibiotics carefully.

● For a patient with arthritis, help with range-of-motion and strengthening exercises, but avoid overexertion.

● Assess the patient's neurologic function and level of consciousness frequently. Watch for signs of increased intracranial pressure and cranial nerve involvement, such as ptosis, strabismus, and diplopia.

● Check for cardiac abnormalities, such as arrhythmias and heart block.

# LYMPHOMAS, MALIGNANT

Also known as non-Hodgkin's lymphomas and lymphosarcomas, malignant lymphomas are a heterogeneous group of malignant diseases originating in lymph glands and other lymphoid tissue. Nodular lymphomas have a better prognosis than the diffuse form of the disease, but in both, the prognosis is worse than in Hodgkin's disease.

## Causes

The cause of malignant lymphomas is unknown, although some theories suggest a viral source. Up to 35,000 new cases appear annually in the United States. Malignant lymphomas are two to three times more common in males than in females and occur in all age-groups.

Although rare in children, these lymphomas occur one to three times more often and cause twice as many deaths as Hodgkin's disease in children under age 15. Incidence rises with age (median age is 50). Malignant lymphomas seem linked to certain races and ethnic groups, with increased incidence in whites and people of Jewish ancestry.

## Signs and symptoms

Usually, the first indication of malignant lymphoma is swelling of the lymph glands, enlarged tonsils and adenoids, and painless, rubbery nodes in the cervical or supraclavicular areas. In children, these nodes are usually in the cervical region, and the disease causes dyspnea and coughing.

As the lymphoma progresses, the patient develops symptoms specific to the area involved and systemic complaints of fatigue, malaise, weight loss, fever, and night sweats.

## Diagnosis

A positive diagnosis requires histologic evaluation of biopsied lymph nodes of tonsils, bone marrow, liver, bowel, or skin; or of tissue removed during exploratory laparotomy. A biopsy differentiates malignant lymphoma from Hodgkin's disease. (See *Classifying malignant lymphomas,* page 520.)

Other tests include bone and chest X-rays, lymphangiography, a liver and spleen scan, computed tomography scan of the abdomen, and excretory urography. Laboratory tests include a complete blood count (which may show anemia), uric acid level (elevated or normal), serum calcium level (elevated if bone lesions are present), serum protein level (normal), and liver function studies.

## Treatment

Radiation therapy is used mainly in the early localized stage of the disease. Total nodal irradiation is often effective for both nodular and diffuse histologies.

Chemotherapy is most effective with multiple combinations of antineoplastic agents. For example, cyclophosphamide, doxorubicin, vincristine (Oncovin), and prednisone (CHOP) can induce a complete remission in 70% to 80% of patients with a nodular histology and in

# CLASSIFYING MALIGNANT LYMPHOMAS

Staging and classifying systems for malignant lymphomas include the National Cancer Institute's (NCI) system, the Rappaport Histologic Classification, and the Lukes-Collins Classification.

*Note:* The NCI also cites a "miscellaneous" category, which includes these lymphomas: composite, mycosis fungoides, histiocytic, extramedullary plasmacytoma, and unclassifiable

| NCI | RAPPAPORT | LUKES-COLLINS |
|-----|-----------|---------------|
| **LOW GRADE** | | |
| • Small lymphocytic<br>• Follicular, predominantly small cleaved cell<br>• Follicular mixed, small and large cell | • Diffuse well-differentiated lymphocytic<br>• Nodular poorly differentiated lymphocytic<br>• Nodular mixed lymphoma | • Small lymphocytic and plasmacytoid lymphocytic<br>• Small cleaved follicular center cell, follicular only, or follicular and diffuse<br>• Small cleaved follicular center cell, follicular; large cleaved follicular center cell, follicular |
| **INTERMEDIATE GRADE** | | |
| • Follicular, predominantly large cell<br>• Diffuse, small cleaved cell<br>• Diffuse mixed, small and large cell<br>• Diffuse large cell, cleaved or noncleaved | • Nodular histiocytic lymphoma<br>• Diffuse poorly differentiated lymphoma<br>• Diffuse mixed lymphocytic-histiocytic<br>• Diffuse histiocytic lymphoma | • Large cleaved or noncleaved follicular center cell, or both, follicular<br>• Small cleaved follicular center cell, diffuse<br>• Small cleaved, large cleaved, or large noncleaved follicular center cell, diffuse<br>• Large cleaved or noncleaved follicular center cell, diffuse |
| **HIGH GRADE** | | |
| • Diffuse large cell immunoblastic<br>• Large cell, lymphoblastic<br>• Small noncleaved cell | • Diffuse histiocytic lymphoma<br>• Lymphoblastic, convoluted or nonconvoluted<br>• Undifferentiated, Burkitt's and non-Burkitt's diffuse undifferentiated lymphoma | • Immunoblastic sarcoma, T-cell or B-cell type<br>• Convoluted T cell<br>• Small noncleaved follicular center cell |

20% to 55% of patients with a diffuse histology. Other combinations — such as methotrexate, bleomycin, doxorubicin, cyclophosphamide, vincristine, and prednisone (M-BACOP) — induce prolonged remission and sometimes cure the diffuse form.

### Special considerations

• Observe the patient who's receiving radiation or chemotherapy for anorexia, nausea, vomiting, or diarrhea. Plan small, frequent meals scheduled around treatment.

• If the patient can't tolerate oral feedings, administer I.V. fluids and, as necessary, give antiemetics and sedatives.

• Instruct the patient to keep irradiated skin dry.

• Provide emotional support by informing the patient and family about the prognosis and diagnosis and by listening to their concerns. If needed, refer the patient and family to the local chapter of the American Cancer Society for information and counseling.

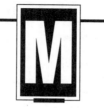

# MACULAR DEGENERATION

Macular degeneration, which is atrophy or degeneration of the macular disk, accounts for about 12% of all cases of blindness in the United States and for about 17% of new cases of blindness. It's one of the causes of severe irreversible loss of central vision in people over age 50.

Two types of age-related macular degeneration occur. The dry, or *atrophic,* form is characterized by atrophic pigment epithelial changes and is most often associated with a slow, progressive distortion of straight lines or edges and central visual loss. The wet, or *exudative,* form causes rapid onset of visual impairment. It's characterized by subretinal neovascularization that causes leakage, hemorrhage, and fibrovascular scar formation, which produce significant loss of central vision.

## Causes

Age-related macular degeneration results from the formation of drusen (clumps of epithelium) or subretinal neovascular membrane in the macular region. No predisposing conditions have been identified. However, it may be hereditary.

Underlying pathologic changes occur primarily at the level of the retinal pigment epithelium, Bruch's membrane, and choriocapillaris in the macular region. Drusen (bumps), which are common in elderly people, appear as yellow deposits beneath the pigment epithelium and may be prominent in the macula.

## Signs and symptoms

The patient notices a change in central vision; for example, he may notice a blank spot in the center of the page when reading.

## Diagnosis

The following tests are used to diagnose macular degeneration:
- *indirect ophthalmoscopy:* may reveal gross macular changes.
- *Amsler's grid:* reveals central visual field distortion
- *I.V. fluorescein angiography:* may show leaking vessels as fluorescein dye flows into the tissues from the subretinal neovascular net.

## Treatment

Laser photocoagulation reduces the incidence of severe visual loss in patients with subretinal neovascularization.

## Special considerations

- Inform patients who have bilateral central vision loss of the low-vision rehabilitation services that are available to them.
- Special devices, such as low-vision optical aids, are available to improve the quality of life in patients with good peripheral vision.

# MALIGNANT MELANOMA

A neoplasm that arises from melanocytes, malignant melanoma is relatively rare and accounts for only 1% to 2% of all types of cancer. The three types of melanomas are *superficial spreading melanoma, nodular malignant melanoma,* and *lentigo maligna melanoma.*

Melanoma is slightly more common in women than in men and is rare in children. Peak incidence occurs between the ages of 50 and 70, although the incidence in younger age-groups is increasing.

Melanoma spreads through the lymphatic and vascular systems and metastasizes to the regional lymph nodes, skin, liver, lungs, and central nervous system (CNS). Its course is unpredictable, however, and recurrence and metastasis may occur more than 5 years after resection of the primary lesion.

The prognosis varies with tumor thickness. Generally, superficial lesions are curable, while deeper lesions tend to metastasize. The Breslow Level Method measures tumor depth from the granular level of the epidermis to the deepest melanoma cell. Melanoma lesions less than 0.76 mm deep have an excellent prognosis, while deeper lesions (more than 0.76 mm) are at risk for metastasis. The prognosis is better for a tumor on an extremity (which is drained by one lymphatic network) than for one on the head, neck, or trunk (drained by several networks).

## Causes

Several factors may influence the development of melanoma:
● *Excessive exposure to sunlight.* Melanoma is most common in sunny, warm areas and often develops on parts of the body that are exposed to the sun.
● *Skin type.* Most persons who develop melanoma have blond or red hair, fair skin, and blue eyes; are prone to sunburn; and are of Celtic or Scandinavian ancestry. Melanoma is rare among blacks; when it does develop, it usually arises in lightly pigmented areas (the palms, plantar surface of the feet, or mucous membranes).
● *Hormonal factors.* Pregnancy may increase risk and exacerbate growth.
● *Family history.* Melanoma occurs slightly more often within families.
● *Past history of melanoma.* A person who has had one melanoma is at greater risk of developing a second.

## Signs and symptoms

Common sites for melanoma are on the head and neck in men, on the legs in women, and on the backs of people exposed to excessive sunlight. Up to 70% arise from a preexisting nevus. They rarely appear in the conjunctiva, choroid, pharynx, mouth, vagina, or anus.

Suspect melanoma when any skin lesion or nevus enlarges, changes color, becomes inflamed or sore, itches, ulcerates, bleeds, undergoes textural changes, or shows signs of surrounding pigment regression (halo nevus or vitiligo).

Each type of melanoma has special characteristics:
● *Superficial spreading melanoma,* the most common form, usually develops between the ages of 40 and 50. This lesion arises on an area of chronic irritation. In women, it's most common between the knees and ankles; in blacks and Asians, on the toe webs and soles (lightly pigmented areas subject to trauma).

Characteristically, this melanoma has a red, white, and blue color over a brown or black background and an irregular,

## STAGING MALIGNANT MELANOMA

Several systems exist for staging malignant melanoma, including the TNM (tumor, node, metastasis) system, developed by the American Joint Committee on Cancer, and Clark's system, which classifies tumor progression according to skin layer penetration.

### Primary tumor

*TX*—primary tumor can't be assessed

*T0*—no evidence of primary tumor

*Tis*—melanoma in situ (atypical melanotic hyperplasia, severe melanotic dysplasia), not an invasive lesion (Clark's level 1)

*T1*—tumor 0.75 mm thick or less that invades the papillary dermis (Clark's level II)

*T2*—tumor between 0.75 and 1.5 mm thick, or tumor invades the interface between the papillary and reticular dermis (Clark's level III), or both

*T3*—tumor between 1.5 and 4 mm thick, or tumor invades the reticular dermis (Clark's level IV), or both

*T3a*—tumor between 1.5 and 3 mm thick

*T3b*—tumor between 3 and 4 mm thick

*T4*—tumor more than 4 mm thick, or tumor invades subcutaneous tissue

(Clark's level V), or tumor has one or more satellites within 2 cm of the primary tumor

*T4a*—tumor more than 4 mm thick, or tumor invades subcutaneous tissue, or both

*T4b*—one or more satellites exist within 2 cm of the primary tumor

### Regional lymph nodes

*NX*—regional lymph nodes can't be assessed

*N0*—no evidence of regional lymph node involvement

*N0*—metastasis 3 cm or less in greatest dimension in any regional lymph node

*N1*—metastasis greater than 3 cm in greatest dimension in any regional lymph node, or in-transit metastasis, or both

notched margin. Its surface is irregular, with small elevated tumor nodules that may ulcerate and bleed. Horizontal growth may continue for many years; when vertical growth begins, the prognosis worsens.

• *Nodular malignant melanoma* usually develops between the ages of 40 and 50, grows vertically, invades the dermis, and metastasizes early. This lesion is usually a polypoidal nodule, with uniformly dark discoloration (it may be grayish), and looks like a blackberry. Occasionally, this melanoma is flesh-colored, with flecks of pigment around its base (possibly inflamed).

• *Lentigo maligna melanoma* is relatively rare. It arises from a lentigo maligna on an exposed skin surface and usually occurs between the ages of 60 and 70.

This lesion looks like a large (1″ to 2″ [3- to 6-cm]), flat freckle of tan, brown, black, whitish, or slate color, and has irregularly scattered black nodules on the surface. It develops slowly, usually over many years, and eventually may ulcerate. This melanoma commonly develops under the fingernails, on the face, and on the back of the hands.

### Diagnosis

A skin biopsy with histologic examination can distinguish malignant melanoma from a benign nevus, seborrheic keratosis, and pigmented basal cell epithelioma; it can also determine tumor

**Distant metastasis**

*MX*— distant metastasis can't be assessed

*M0*— no evidence of distant metastasis

*M1*— distant metastasis

*M1a*— metastasis in skin, subcutaneous tissue, or lymph nodes beyond the regional nodes.

*M1b*— visceral metastasis

**Staging categories**

Malignant melanoma progresses from mild to severe as follows:

*Stage I*— T1, N0, M0; T2, N0, M0

*Stage II*— T3, N0, M0

*Stage III*— T4, N0, M0; any T, N1, M0; any T, N2, M0

*Stage IV*— any T, any N, M1

**Clark's levels**

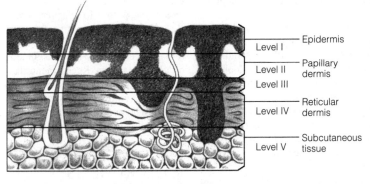

Level I — Epidermis

Level II — Papillary dermis

Level III

Level IV — Reticular dermis

Level V — Subcutaneous tissue

thickness. Physical examination, paying particular attention to lymph nodes, can point to metastatic involvement. (See *Staging malignant melanoma.*)

Baseline laboratory studies include a complete blood count with differential, erythrocyte sedimentation rate, platelet count, liver function studies, and urinalysis. Depending on the depth of tumor invasion and metastasis, baseline diagnostic studies may also include a chest X-ray and computed tomography (CT) scan of the chest and abdomen. Signs of bone metastasis may call for a bone scan; CNS metastasis, a CT scan of the brain.

**Treatment**

A patient with malignant melanoma requires surgical resection to remove the tumor. The extent of resection depends on the size and location of the primary lesion. Closure of a wide resection may require a skin graft. Surgical treatment may also include regional lymphadenectomy.

Deep primary lesions may merit adjuvant chemotherapy and biotherapy to eliminate or reduce the number of tumor cells. Radiation therapy is usually reserved for metastatic disease; it doesn't prolong survival but may reduce tumor size and relieve pain.

Regardless of the treatment method, melanomas require close, long-term follow-up to detect metastasis and recurrences.

➤ CLINICAL TIP   About 13% of recurrences develop more than 5 years after the primary surgery.

**Special considerations**
• Management of the melanoma patient requires careful physical, psychological, and social assessment. Preoperative teaching, meticulous postoperative care, and psychological support can make the patient more comfortable, speed recovery, and prevent complications.
• After diagnosis, review the explanation of treatment options. Tell the patient what to expect before and after surgery, what the wound will look like, and what type of dressing he'll have.
• Warn the patient that the donor site for a skin graft may be as painful as the tumor excision site, if not more so. Honestly answer any questions he may have about surgery, chemotherapy, and radiation.
• After surgery, be careful to prevent infection. Check dressings often for excessive drainage, foul odor, redness, or swelling.
• If surgery included lymphadenectomy, minimize lymphedema by applying an antiembolism stocking and instructing the patient to keep the extremity elevated.
• During chemotherapy, know which adverse reactions to expect and take measures to minimize them. For instance, give an antiemetic to reduce nausea and vomiting.
    When preparing for discharge:
• Emphasize the need for close follow-up to detect recurrences early. Explain that recurrences and metastasis, if they occur, are often delayed, so follow-up must continue for years.
• Tell the patient how to recognize signs of recurrence.

• Provide psychological support. Encourage the patient to verbalize his fears.
    In advanced metastatic disease:
• Control and prevent pain with consistent, regularly scheduled administration of analgesics. *Don't* wait to relieve pain until after it occurs.
• Make referrals for home care, social services, and spiritual and financial assistance as needed.
• If the patient is dying, identify the needs of patient, family, and friends, and provide appropriate support and care.

➤ CLINICAL TIP   To help prevent malignant melanoma, stress the detrimental effects of overexposure to solar radiation, especially to fair-skinned, blue-eyed patients. Recommend that they use a sunblock or sunscreen. In all physical examinations, especially in fair-skinned people, look for unusual nevi or other skin lesions.

# MALLORY-WEISS SYNDROME

Mild to massive and usually painless bleeding due to a tear in the mucosa or submucosa of the cardia or lower esophagus characterizes Mallory-Weiss syndrome. Such a tear, usually singular and longitudinal, results from prolonged or forceful vomiting. Sixty percent of these tears involve the cardia; 15%, the terminal esophagus; and 25%, the region across the esophagogastric junction. Mallory-Weiss syndrome is most common in men over age 40, especially alcoholics.

**Causes**
The direct cause of a tear in Mallory-Weiss syndrome is forceful or prolonged vomiting, probably when the upper

esophageal sphincter fails to relax during vomiting. This lack of sphincter coordination is more common after excessive intake of alcohol. Other factors and conditions that may also increase intra-abdominal pressure and predispose to esophageal tearing include coughing, straining during bowel movements, trauma, seizures, childbirth, hiatal hernia, esophagitis, gastritis, and atrophic gastric mucosa.

> **CLINICAL TIP** Patients with portal hypertension are at a higher risk for continuous or recurrent bleeding. Monitoring for signs of hemorrhage is advised.

### Signs and symptoms

Typically, Mallory-Weiss syndrome begins with vomiting of blood or passing large amounts of blood rectally a few hours to several days after normal vomiting. This bleeding, which may be accompanied by epigastric or back pain, may range from mild to massive but is generally more profuse than in esophageal rupture.

In Mallory-Weiss syndrome, the blood vessels are only partially severed, preventing retraction and closure of the lumen. Massive bleeding — most likely when the tear is on the gastric side, near the cardia — may quickly lead to fatal shock.

### Diagnosis

Identifying esophageal tears by fiberoptic endoscopy confirms Mallory-Weiss syndrome. These lesions, which usually occur near the gastroesophageal junction, appear as erythematous longitudinal cracks in the mucosa when recently produced and as raised, white streaks surrounded by erythema in older tears. Other helpful diagnostic measures include the following:

• *Angiography* (selective celiac arteriography) can determine the bleeding site but not the cause; this is used when endoscopy isn't available.

• *Gastrotomy* may be performed at the time of surgery.

• *Hematocrit* helps quantify blood loss.

### Treatment

Appropriate treatment varies with the severity of bleeding. Usually, GI bleeding stops spontaneously, requiring supportive measures and careful observation but no definitive treatment. However, if bleeding continues, treatment may include:

• angiographic infusion of a vasoconstrictor (vasopressin) into the superior mesenteric artery or direct infusion into a vessel that leads to the bleeding artery

• transcatheter embolization or thrombus formation with an autologous blood clot or other hemostatic material (insertion of artificial material, such as a shredded absorbable gelatin sponge or, less often, the patient's own clotted blood through a catheter into the bleeding vessel to aid thrombus formation)

• surgery to suture each laceration (for massive recurrent or uncontrollable bleeding).

### Special considerations

• Evaluate respiratory status, monitor arterial blood gas measurements, and administer oxygen as necessary.

• Assess the amount of blood loss, and record related symptoms, such as hematemesis and melena (including color, amount, consistency, and frequency).

• Monitor hematologic status (hemoglobin, hematocrit, red blood cells). Draw blood for coagulation studies (prothrombin time, partial thromboplastin time, and platelet count) and typing and crossmatching.

• Try to keep three units of matched whole blood on hand at all times. Until blood is available, insert a large-bore

(14G to 18G) I.V. line, and start a temporary infusion of normal saline solution.

• Monitor the patient's vital signs, central venous pressure, urine output, and overall clinical status.

• Explain diagnostic procedures carefully.

• Keep the patient warm.

• Obtain a history of recent medications taken, dietary habits, and use of alcohol.

• Avoid giving the patient medications that may cause nausea or vomiting. Administer antiemetics, as necessary, to prevent postoperative retching and vomiting.

• Reassure the patient that bleeding will subside.

• Advise the patient to avoid alcohol, aspirin, and other irritating substances.

# MASTITIS AND BREAST ENGORGEMENT

Mastitis (parenchymatous inflammation of the mammary glands) and breast engorgement (congestion) are disorders that may affect lactating females. Mastitis occurs postpartum in about 1%, mainly in primiparas who are breast-feeding. It occurs occasionally in nonlactating females and rarely in males. All breast-feeding mothers develop some degree of engorgement, but it's especially likely to be severe in primiparas. The prognosis for both disorders is good.

## Causes

Mastitis develops when a pathogen that typically originates in the nursing infant's nose or pharynx invades breast tissue through a fissured or cracked nipple and disrupts normal lactation. The most common pathogen of this type is *Staphylococcus aureus;* less frequently, it's *Staphylococcus epidermidis* or beta-hemolytic streptococci. Rarely, mastitis may result from disseminated tuberculosis or the mumps virus. Predisposing factors include a fissure or abrasion on the nipple; blocked milk ducts; and an incomplete let-down reflex, usually due to emotional trauma. Blocked milk ducts can result from a tight bra or prolonged intervals between breast-feedings.

Causes of breast engorgement include venous and lymphatic stasis and alveolar milk accumulation.

## Signs and symptoms

Mastitis may develop anytime during lactation but usually begins 3 to 4 weeks postpartum with fever (101° F [38.3° C] or higher in acute mastitis), malaise, and flulike symptoms. The breasts (or, occasionally, one breast) become tender, hard, swollen, and warm. Unless mastitis is treated adequately, it may progress to breast abscess.

Breast engorgement generally starts with onset of lactation (day 2 to day 5 postpartum). The breasts undergo changes similar to those in mastitis, and body temperature may be elevated. Engorgement may be mild, causing only slight discomfort, or severe, causing considerable pain. A severely engorged breast can interfere with the infant's capacity to feed because of his inability to position his mouth properly on the swollen, rigid breast.

## Diagnosis

In a lactating female with breast discomfort or other signs of inflammation, cultures of expressed milk confirm generalized mastitis; cultures of breast skin surface confirm localized mastitis. Such cultures also determine the appropriate antibiotic treatment. Obvious swelling of lactating breasts confirms engorgement.

## Treatment

Antibiotic therapy, the primary treatment for mastitis, generally consists of penicillin G to combat staphylococcus; erythromycin or kanamycin is used for penicillin-resistant strains. Although symptoms usually subside 2 to 3 days after treatment begins, antibiotic therapy should continue for 10 days. Other appropriate measures include analgesics for pain and, rarely, when antibiotics fail to control the infection and mastitis progresses to breast abscess, incision and drainage of the abscess.

The goal of treatment of breast engorgement is to relieve discomfort and control swelling, and may include analgesics to alleviate pain, and ice packs and an uplift support bra to minimize edema. Rarely, oxytocin nasal spray may be necessary to release milk from the alveoli into the ducts. To facilitate breast-feeding, the mother may manually express excess milk before a feeding so the infant can grasp the nipple properly.

## Special considerations

If the patient has mastitis:
• Isolate the patient and her infant to prevent the spread of infection to other nursing mothers. Explain mastitis to the patient and why isolation is necessary.
• Obtain a complete patient history, including a drug history, especially allergy to penicillin.
• Assess and record the cause and amount of discomfort. Give analgesics, as needed.
• Reassure the mother that breast-feeding during mastitis won't harm her infant because he's the source of the in-

fection. Tell her to offer the infant the affected breast first to promote complete emptying of the breast and prevent clogged ducts. However, if an open abscess develops, tell her to stop breast-feeding with this breast and use a breast pump until the abscess heals. She should continue to breast-feed on the unaffected side.

➤ CLINICAL TIP   Suggest applying a warm, wet towel to the affected breast or taking a warm shower to help her relax and improve her ability to breast-feed.
• To prevent mastitis and relieve its symptoms, teach the patient good health care, breast care, and breast-feeding habits. Advise her to always wash her hands before touching her breasts.
• Instruct the patient to combat fever by getting plenty of rest, drinking sufficient fluids, and following prescribed antibiotic therapy.

If the patient has breast engorgement:
• Assess and record the level of discomfort. Give analgesics, and apply ice packs as needed.
• Teach the patient how to express excess breast milk manually. She should do this just before nursing to enable the infant to get the swollen areola into his mouth. Caution against excessive expression of milk between feedings because this stimulates milk production and prolongs engorgement.
• Explain that because breast engorgement is caused by the physiologic processes of lactation, breast-feeding is the best remedy. Suggest breast-feeding every 2 to 3 hours and at least once during the night.
• Ensure that the mother wears a well-fitted nursing bra that isn't too tight.

# MÉNIÈRE'S DISEASE

Also known as endolymphatic hydrops, Ménière's disease is a labyrinthine dysfunction that produces severe vertigo, sensorineural hearing loss, and tinnitus. It usually affects adults, men slightly more often than women, between the ages of 30 and 60. After multiple attacks over several years, this disorder leads to residual tinnitus and hearing loss.

## Causes

Ménière's disease may result from overproduction or decreased absorption of endolymph, which causes endolymphatic hydrops or endolymphatic hypertension, with consequent degeneration of the vestibular and cochlear hair cells.

This condition may stem from autonomic nervous system dysfunction that produces a temporary constriction of blood vessels supplying the inner ear. In some women, premenstrual edema may precipitate attacks of Ménière's disease.

## Signs and symptoms

Ménière's disease produces three characteristic effects: severe vertigo, tinnitus, and sensorineural hearing loss. Fullness or blocked feeling in the ear is also quite common. Violent paroxysmal attacks last from 10 minutes to several hours. During an acute attack, other symptoms include severe nausea, vomiting, sweating, giddiness, and nystagmus. Also, vertigo may cause loss of balance and falling to the affected side.

To lessen these symptoms, the patient may assume a characteristic posture — lying on the unaffected ear and looking in the direction of the affected ear. Initially, the patient may be asymptomatic between attacks, except for residual tinnitus that worsens during an attack.

> ➤ CLINICAL TIP Such attacks may occur several times a year, or remissions may last as long as several years. These attacks become less frequent as hearing loss progresses (usually unilateral); they may cease when hearing loss is total.

## Diagnosis

The presence of all three typical symptoms suggests Ménière's disease. Audiometric studies indicate a sensorineural hearing loss and loss of discrimination and recruitment. Electronystagmography, electrocochleography, a computed tomography scan, magnetic resonance imaging, and X-rays of the internal meatus may be necessary for differential diagnosis.

## Treatment

In Ménière's disease, treatment with atropine may stop an attack in 20 to 30 minutes. Epinephrine or diphenhydramine may be necessary in a severe attack; dimenhydrinate, meclizine, diphenhydramine, or diazepam may be effective in a milder attack.

Long-term management includes use of a diuretic or vasodilator and restricted sodium intake (<2 g/day). Prophylactic antihistamines or mild sedatives (phenobarbital, diazepam) may also be helpful. If Ménière's disease persists after 2 years of treatment, produces incapacitating vertigo, or resists medical management, surgery may be necessary. Destruction of the affected labyrinth permanently relieves symptoms but at the expense of irreversible hearing loss. Systemic streptomycin is reserved for patients in whom the disease is bilateral and no other treatment can be considered.

## Special considerations

If the patient is in the facility during an attack of Ménière's disease:

• Advise him against reading and exposure to glaring lights to reduce dizziness.

• Keep the side rails of the patient's bed up to prevent falls. Tell him not to get out of bed or walk without assistance.

• Instruct the patient to avoid sudden position changes and any tasks that vertigo makes hazardous because an attack can begin quite rapidly.

Before surgery:

• If the patient is vomiting, record fluid intake and output and characteristics of vomitus. Administer antiemetics as necessary, and give small amounts of fluid frequently.

After surgery:

• Record intake and output carefully.

• Tell the patient to expect dizziness and nausea for 1 or 2 days after surgery.

• Give prophylactic antibiotics and antiemetics as required.

• For more patient-teaching information, see *Managing Ménière's disease.*

---

**LIFE-THREATENING DISORDER**

# MENINGITIS

---

In meningitis, the brain and the spinal cord meninges become inflamed, usually as a result of bacterial infection. Such inflammation may involve all three meningeal membranes — the dura mater, arachnoid, and pia mater.

The prognosis is good and complications are rare, especially if the disease is recognized early and the infecting organism responds to antibiotics. However, mortality in untreated meningitis is 70% to 100%. The prognosis is poorer for infants and elderly people.

---

**TEACHING CHECKLIST**

## MANAGING MÉNIÈRE'S DISEASE

• Follow a low-sodium diet.
• Avoid tobacco, alcohol, and caffeine as directed.
• Stress management can reduce frequency and severity of some vertiginous attacks.
• Maintain your diversional and social activities.
• Try not to let the fear of vertigo stop you from participating in daily activities when vertigo is absent.

---

## Causes

Meningitis is almost always a complication of another bacterial infection — bacteremia (especially from pneumonia, empyema, osteomyelitis, and endocarditis), sinusitis, otitis media, encephalitis, myelitis, or brain abscess — usually caused by *Neisseria meningitidis, Haemophilus influenzae, Streptococcus pneumoniae,* and *Escherichia coli.*

Meningitis may also follow skull fracture, a penetrating head wound, lumbar puncture, or ventricular shunting procedures. Aseptic meningitis may result from a virus or other organism. Sometimes no causative organism can be found.

Meningitis often begins as an inflammation of the pia-arachnoid, which may progress to congestion of adjacent tissues and destroy some nerve cells.

## Signs and symptoms

Typical signs include the following features.

### Cardinal signs

The cardinal signs of meningitis are those of infection (fever, chills, malaise) and of increased intracranial pressure (headache, vomiting and, rarely, papilledema).

### Meningeal irritation

Signs of meningeal irritation include nuchal rigidity, positive Brudzinski's and Kernig's signs, exaggerated and symmetrical deep tendon reflexes, and opisthotonos (a spasm in which the back and extremities arch backward so that the body rests on the head and heels).

### Other manifestations

Other features of meningitis are sinus arrhythmias; irritability; photophobia, diplopia, and other visual problems; and delirium, deep stupor, and coma. An infant may show signs of infection but often is simply fretful and refuses to eat. Such an infant may vomit a great deal, leading to dehydration; this prevents a bulging fontanel and thus masks this important sign of increased intracranial pressure (ICP).

As the illness progresses, twitching, seizures (in 30% of infants), or coma may develop. Most older children have the same symptoms as adults. In subacute meningitis, onset may be insidious.

### Diagnosis

A lumbar puncture showing typical findings in cerebrospinal fluid (CSF) and positive Brudzinski's and Kernig's signs usually establish this diagnosis. (See *Two telltale signs of meningitis.*) The lumbar puncture usually indicates elevated CSF pressure from obstructed CSF outflow at the arachnoid villi. The fluid may appear cloudy or milky white, depending on the number of white blood cells present. CSF protein levels tend to be high; glucose levels may be low.

(In subacute meningitis, CSF findings may vary.) CSF culture and sensitivity tests usually identify the infecting organism, unless it's a virus.

Other useful tests include the following:

• *Cultures* of blood, urine, and nose and throat secretions; a *chest X-ray; electrocardiography;* and a *physical examination,* with special attention to skin, ears, and sinuses, can uncover the primary infection site.

• *Blood tests* commonly reveal leukocytosis and serum electrolyte abnormalities.

• *Computed tomography scan* can rule out cerebral hematoma, hemorrhage, or tumor.

### Treatment

In meningitis, treatment includes appropriate antibiotic therapy and vigorous supportive care.

### Antibiotics

Usually, I.V. antibiotics are given for at least 2 weeks and are followed by oral antibiotics. Such antibiotics include penicillin G, ampicillin, or nafcillin. However, if the patient is allergic to penicillin, anti-infective therapy includes tetracycline, chloramphenicol, or kanamycin.

Other drugs include a digitalis glycoside, such as digoxin, to control arrhythmias, mannitol to decrease cerebral edema, an anticonvulsant (usually given I.V.) or a sedative to reduce restlessness, and aspirin or acetaminophen to relieve headache and fever.

### Supportive care

Supportive measures include bed rest, fever reduction, and measures to prevent dehydration. Isolation is necessary if nasal cultures are positive. Of course, treatment includes appropriate therapy

# TWO TELLTALE SIGNS OF MENINGITIS

### Brudzinski's sign
To test for *Brudzinski's sign,* place the patient in a dorsal recumbent position; then put your hands behind his neck and bend it forward. Pain and resistance may indicate meningeal inflammation, neck injury, or arthritis. However, if the patient also flexes the hips and knees in response to this manipulation, chances are he has meningitis.

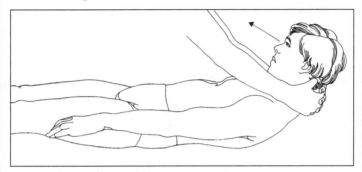

### Kernig's sign
To test for *Kernig's sign,* place the patient in a supine position. Flex his leg at the hip and knee, then straighten the knee. Pain or resistance points to meningitis.

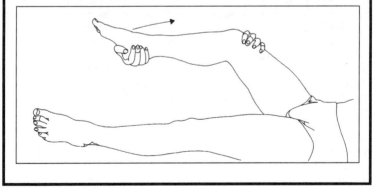

for any coexisting conditions, such as endocarditis or pneumonia.

To prevent meningitis, prophylactic antibiotics are sometimes used after ventricular shunting procedures, skull fracture, or penetrating head wounds, but this use is controversial.

### Special considerations
● Assess neurologic function often. Observe the patient's level of consciousness, and check for signs of increased ICP (plucking at the bedcovers, vomiting, seizures, a change in motor function and vital signs). Also watch for

> CLINICAL TIP

## OMINOUS SIGNS IN MENINGITIS

Be especially alert for deterioration in the patient's condition as evidenced by:

- temperature increase up to 102° F (38.9° C)
- reduced level of consciousness
- onset of seizures
- altered respirations.

signs of cranial nerve involvement (ptosis, strabismus, diplopia).

- Watch for deterioration in the patient's condition, which may signal an impending crisis. (See *Ominous signs in meningitis.*)
- Monitor fluid balance. Maintain adequate fluid intake to avoid dehydration, but avoid fluid overload because of the danger of cerebral edema. Measure central venous pressure and intake and output accurately.
- Watch for adverse reactions to I.V. antibiotics and other drugs. To avoid infiltration and phlebitis, check the I.V. site often, and change the site according to facility policy.
- Position the patient carefully to prevent joint stiffness and neck pain. Turn him often, according to a planned positioning schedule. Assist with range-of-motion exercises.
- Maintain adequate nutrition and elimination. It may be necessary to provide small, frequent meals or supplement these meals with nasogastric tube or parenteral feedings.
- To prevent constipation and minimize the risk of increased ICP resulting from straining during defecation, give the patient a mild laxative or stool softener.

- Ensure the patient's comfort. Provide mouth care regularly. Maintain a quiet environment. Darkening the room may decrease photophobia.
- Relieve headache with a nonnarcotic analgesic, such as aspirin or acetaminophen, as needed. (Narcotics interfere with accurate neurologic assessment.)
- Provide reassurance and support. The patient may be frightened by his illness and frequent lumbar punctures. If he's delirious or confused, attempt to reorient him often.
- Reassure the family that the delirium and behavior changes caused by meningitis usually disappear.
- If a severe neurologic deficit appears permanent, refer the patient to a rehabilitation program as soon as the acute phase of this illness has passed.
- To help prevent meningitis, teach patients with chronic sinusitis or other chronic infections the importance of proper medical treatment.
- Follow strict aseptic technique when treating patients with head wounds or skull fractures.

# MENINGOCOCCAL INFECTIONS

Two major meningococcal infections (meningitis and meningococcemia) are caused by the gram-negative bacteria *Neisseria meningitidis,* which also causes primary pneumonia, purulent conjunctivitis, endocarditis, sinusitis, and genital infection.

Meningococcemia occurs as simple bacteremia, fulminant meningococcemia and, rarely, chronic meningococcemia. It often accompanies meningitis. (For more information on meningitis, see "Meningitis," pages 531 to

534.) Meningococcal infections may occur sporadically or in epidemics; virulent infections may be fatal within a matter of hours.

## Causes

Meningococcal infections occur most often among children (ages 6 months to 1 year) and men, usually military recruits, because of overcrowding.

*N. meningitidis* has seven serogroups (A, B, C, D, X, Y, Z); group A causes most epidemics. These bacteria are often present in upper respiratory flora. Transmission takes place through inhalation of an infected droplet from a carrier (an estimated 2% to 38% of the population). The bacteria then localize in the nasopharynx.

Following an incubation period of approximately 3 or 4 days, the bacteria spread through the bloodstream to the joints, skin, adrenal glands, lungs, and central nervous system. The tissue damage that results (possibly due to the effects of bacterial endotoxins) produces symptoms and, in fulminant meningococcemia and meningococcal bacteremia, progresses to hemorrhage, thrombosis, and necrosis.

## Signs and symptoms

Clinical features of meningococcal infection vary. Symptoms of *meningococcal bacteremia* include a sudden, spiking fever; headache; sore throat; cough; chills; myalgia (in the back and legs); arthralgia; tachycardia; tachypnea; mild hypotension; and a petechial, nodular, or maculopapular rash.

In 10% to 20% of patients, this progresses to *fulminant meningococcemia,* with extreme prostration, enlargement of skin lesions, disseminated intravascular coagulation (DIC), and shock. Unless it is treated promptly, fulminant meningococcemia results in death from respiratory or heart failure in 6 to 24 hours.

Characteristics of *chronic meningococcemia* include intermittent fever, maculopapular rash, joint pain, and enlarged spleen.

## Diagnosis

Isolation of *N. meningitidis* through a positive blood culture, cerebrospinal fluid (CSF) culture, or lesion scraping confirms the diagnosis except in nasopharyngeal infections, because *N. meningitidis* exists as part of the normal nasopharyngeal flora.

Tests that support the diagnosis include counterimmunoelectrophoresis of the CSF or blood, a low white blood cell count and, in patients with skin or adrenal hemorrhages, decreased platelet and clotting levels. Diagnostic evaluation must rule out Rocky Mountain spotted fever and vascular purpuras.

## Treatment

As soon as meningococcal infection is suspected, treatment begins with large doses of aqueous penicillin G, ampicillin, or a cephalosporin, such as cefoxitin and moxalactam; or, for the patient who's allergic to penicillin, chloramphenicol I.V. Therapy may also include mannitol for cerebral edema, heparin I.V. for DIC, dopamine for shock, and digoxin and a diuretic if heart failure develops.

Supportive measures include fluid and electrolyte maintenance, proper ventilation (patent airway and oxygen if necessary), insertion of an arterial or central venous pressure (CVP) line to monitor cardiovascular status, and bed rest.

Chemoprophylaxis with rifampin or minocycline is useful for facility workers who come in close contact with the patient; minocycline can also temporarily eradicate the infection in carriers.

**Special considerations**

• The dosages of I.V. antibiotics should be adjusted as necessary to maintain blood and CSF drug levels.

• Enforce bed rest in early stages. Provide a dark, quiet, restful environment.

• Maintain adequate ventilation with oxygen or a ventilator if necessary. Suction and turn the patient frequently.

• Keep accurate intake and output records to maintain proper fluid and electrolyte levels. Monitor blood pressure, pulse, arterial blood gas levels, and CVP.

• Watch for complications, such as DIC, arthritis, endocarditis, and pneumonia.

• If the patient is receiving chloramphenicol, monitor his complete blood count.

• Check the patient's drug history for allergies before giving antibiotics.

**CLINICAL TIP** To prevent the spread of meningococcal infection:

• Impose respiratory isolation until the patient has received antibiotic therapy for 24 hours.

• Label all meningococcal specimens. Deliver them to the laboratory quickly because meningococci are very sensitive to changes in humidity and temperature.

• Report all meningococcal infections to public health department officials.

---

**LIFE-THREATENING DISORDER**

# METABOLIC ACIDOSIS

---

A physiologic state of excess acid accumulation and deficient base bicarbonate, metabolic acidosis is produced by an underlying pathologic disorder. Symptoms result from the body's attempts to correct the acidotic condition through compensatory mechanisms in the lungs, kidneys, and cells.

Metabolic acidosis is more prevalent among children, who are vulnerable to acid-base imbalance because their metabolic rates are faster and their ratios of water to total-body weight are lower. Severe or untreated metabolic acidosis can be fatal.

**Causes**

Metabolic acidosis usually results from excessive burning of fats in the absence of usable carbohydrates. This can be caused by diabetic ketoacidosis, chronic alcoholism, malnutrition, or a low-carbohydrate, high-fat diet — all of which produce more keto acids than the metabolic process can handle.

Other causes include:

• *anaerobic carbohydrate metabolism:* a decrease in tissue oxygenation or perfusion, as occurs with pump failure after myocardial infarction, or when pulmonary or hepatic disease, shock, or anemia forces a shift from aerobic to anaerobic metabolism, causing a corresponding rise in the lactic acid level

• *renal insufficiency and failure (renal acidosis):* underexcretion of metabolized acids or the inability to conserve base

• *diarrhea and intestinal malabsorption:* loss of sodium bicarbonate from the intestines, causing the bicarbonate buffer system to shift to the acidic side. For example, ureteroenterostomy and Crohn's disease can also induce metabolic acidosis.

Less frequently, metabolic acidosis results from salicylate intoxication (overuse of aspirin), exogenous poisoning, or Addison's disease with an increased excretion of sodium and chloride and the retention of potassium ions (due to a deficiency of glucocorticoids and mineralocorticoids).

## Signs and symptoms

In mild acidosis, symptoms of the underlying disease may obscure any direct clinical evidence. Metabolic acidosis typically begins with headache and lethargy, progressing to drowsiness, central nervous system depression, Kussmaul's respirations (as the lungs attempt to compensate by "blowing off" carbon dioxide), stupor and, if the condition is severe and goes untreated, coma and death.

Associated GI distress usually produces anorexia, nausea, vomiting, and diarrhea and may lead to dehydration. Underlying diabetes mellitus may cause fruity breath from catabolism of fats and excretion of accumulated acetone through the lungs.

## Diagnosis

Arterial pH below 7.35 confirms metabolic acidosis. In severe acidotic states, pH may fall to 7.10 and partial pressure of arterial carbon dioxide may be normal or less than 34 mm Hg as compensatory mechanisms take hold. The bicarbonate level may be less than 22 mEq/L. Supportive findings include:

• *urine pH:* < 4.5 in the absence of renal disease

• *serum potassium levels:* > 5.5 mEq/L from chemical buffering

• *glucose:* > 150 mg/dl in diabetes

• *serum ketone bodies:* elevated in diabetes mellitus

• *plasma lactic acid:* elevated in lactic acidosis

• *anion gap:* > 14 mEq/L, indicating metabolic acidosis.

These values result from increased acid production or renal insufficiency. (See *Defining the anion gap.*)

## DEFINING THE ANION GAP

The anion gap is the difference between concentrations of serum cations and anions — determined by measuring one cation (sodium) and two anions (chloride and bicarbonate). The normal concentration of sodium is 140 mEq/L; of chloride, 102 mEq/L; and of bicarbonate, 26 mEq/L Thus, the anion gap between *measured* cations (actually sodium alone) and *measured* anions is about 12 mEq/L (140 minus 128).

Concentrations of potassium, calcium, and magnesium (*unmeasured* cations), or proteins, and phosphate, sulfate, and organic acids (*unmeasured* anions) aren't needed to measure the anion gap. Added together, the concentration of unmeasured cations would be about 11 mEq/L; of unmeasured anions, about 23 mEq/L. Thus, the normal anion gap between unmeasured cations and anions is about 12 mEq/L (23 minus 11) — give or take 2 mEq/L for normal variation.

An anion gap over 14 mEq/L indicates *metabolic acidosis.* It may result from the accumulation of excess organic acids or from retention of hydrogen ions, which chemically bond with bicarbonate and decrease bicarbonate levels.

## Treatment

In metabolic acidosis, treatment consists of administration of sodium bicarbonate I.V. for severe cases, evaluation and correction of electrolyte imbalances and, ultimately, correction of the underlying cause. For example, in diabetic ketoacidosis, a low-dose continuous I.V. infusion of insulin is recommended.

**Special considerations**

• Keep sodium bicarbonate ampules handy for emergency administration. Frequently monitor vital signs, laboratory results, and level of consciousness because changes can occur rapidly.

• In diabetic acidosis, watch for secondary changes due to hypovolemia, such as decreasing blood pressure.

• Record intake and output accurately to monitor renal function.

• Watch for signs of excessive serum potassium—weakness, flaccid paralysis, and arrhythmias, possibly leading to cardiac arrest. After treatment, check for overcorrection to hypokalemia.

> **CLINICAL TIP** Because metabolic acidosis commonly causes vomiting, position the patient to prevent aspiration.

• Prepare for possible seizures with seizure precautions.

• Provide good oral hygiene. Use sodium bicarbonate washes to neutralize mouth acids, and lubricate the patient's lips with lemon and glycerine swabs.

• To prevent metabolic acidosis, carefully observe patients receiving I.V. therapy or who have intestinal tubes in place, as well as those suffering from shock, hyperthyroidism, hepatic disease, circulatory failure, or dehydration.

• Teach the patient with diabetes how to routinely test urine for sugar and acetone, and encourage strict adherence to insulin or oral antidiabetic therapy.

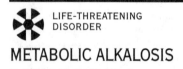

LIFE-THREATENING
DISORDER

# METABOLIC ALKALOSIS

A clinical state marked by decreased amounts of acid or increased amounts of base bicarbonate, metabolic alkalosis causes metabolic, respiratory, and renal responses, producing characteristic symptoms—most notably, hypoventilation. This condition always occurs secondary to an underlying cause. With early diagnosis and prompt treatment, the prognosis is good; however, untreated metabolic alkalosis may lead to coma and death.

**Causes**

Metabolic alkalosis results from loss of acid, retention of base, or renal mechanisms associated with decreased serum levels of potassium and chloride.

*Loss of acid*

Causes of critical acid loss include vomiting, nasogastric tube drainage or lavage without adequate electrolyte replacement, fistulas, and the use of steroids and certain diuretics (furosemide, thiazides, and ethacrynic acid).

Hyperadrenocorticism is another cause of severe acid loss. Cushing's disease, primary hyperaldosteronism, and Bartter's syndrome, for example, all lead to retention of sodium and chloride and urinary loss of potassium and hydrogen.

*Retention of base*

Excessive retention of base can result from excessive intake of bicarbonate of soda or other antacids (usually for treatment of gastritis or peptic ulcer), excessive intake of absorbable alkali (as in milk-alkali syndrome), administration of excessive amounts of I.V. fluids with high concentrations of bicarbonate or lactate, or respiratory insufficiency—all of which cause chronic hypercapnia from high levels of plasma bicarbonate.

**Signs and symptoms**

Clinical features of metabolic alkalosis result from the body's attempt to correct the acid-base imbalance, primarily through hypoventilation. Other manifestations include irritability, picking at bedclothes (carphology), twitching, confusion, nausea, vomiting, and diarrhea (which aggravates alkalosis).

Cardiovascular abnormalities — such as atrial tachycardia — and respiratory disturbances — such as cyanosis and apnea — also occur. In the alkalotic patient, diminished peripheral blood flow during repeated blood pressure checks may provoke carpopedal spasm in the hand — a possible sign of impending tetany (Trousseau's sign). Uncorrected metabolic alkalosis may progress to seizures and coma.

### Diagnosis
A blood pH greater than 7.45 and a bicarbonate level above 29 mEq/L confirm the diagnosis. A partial pressure of carbon dioxide greater than 45 mm Hg indicates attempts at respiratory compensation. Serum electrolyte levels show a potassium level of 3.5 mEq/L and a chloride level of 98 mEq/L. Other characteristic findings include:
• *urine pH* of about 7 (usually)
• *urinalysis* revealing alkalinity after the renal compensatory mechanism begins to excrete bicarbonate
• *electrocardiography* that may show a low T wave merging with a P wave and atrial tachycardia.

### Treatment
The goal of treatment is to correct the underlying cause of metabolic alkalosis. Therapy for severe alkalosis may include cautious administration of ammonium chloride I.V. to release hydrogen chloride and restore the concentration of extracellular fluid and chloride levels.

Potassium chloride and normal saline solution (except in the presence of heart failure) are usually sufficient to replace losses from gastric drainage. Electrolyte replacement with potassium chloride and discontinuing diuretics correct

metabolic alkalosis resulting from potent diuretic therapy.

### Special considerations
• When administering ammonium chloride 0.9%, limit the infusion rate to 1¼ hours; faster administration may cause hemolysis of red blood cells. Avoid overdosage because it may cause overcorrection to metabolic acidosis. Don't give ammonium chloride to a patient with signs of hepatic or renal disease.

➤ CLINICAL TIP Dilute potassium when giving I.V. containing potassium salts. Monitor the infusion rate to prevent damage to blood vessels; watch for signs of phlebitis.
• Watch closely for signs of muscle weakness, tetany, or decreased activity.
• Monitor vital signs frequently, and record intake and output to evaluate respiratory, fluid, and electrolyte status. Remember, respiratory rate usually decreases in an effort to compensate for alkalosis. Hypotension and tachycardia may indicate electrolyte imbalance, especially hypokalemia.
• To prevent metabolic alkalosis, warn patients against overusing alkaline agents. Irrigate nasogastric tubes with isotonic saline solution instead of plain water to prevent loss of gastric electrolytes. Monitor I.V. fluid concentrations of bicarbonate or lactate.
• Teach patients with ulcers to recognize signs of milk-alkali syndrome: a distaste for milk, anorexia, weakness, and lethargy.

# METHICILLIN-RESISTANT *STAPHYLOCOCCUS AUREUS*

Methicillin-resistant *Staphylococcus aureus* (MRSA) is a mutation of very common bacterium spread easily by direct person-to-person contact. Once limited to large teaching hospitals and tertiary care centers, MRSA is now endemic in nursing homes, long-term – care facilities, and even community hospitals. Patients most at risk for MRSA include immunosuppressed patients, burn patients, intubated patients, and those with central venous catheters, surgical wounds, or dermatitis.

Others at risk include those with prosthetic devices, heart valves, and postoperative wound infections. Other risk factors include prolonged hospital stays, extended therapy with multiple or broad-spectrum antibiotics, and close proximity to those colonized or infected with MRSA. Also at risk are patients with acute endocarditis, bacteremia, cervicitis, meningitis, pericarditis, and pneumonia.

## Causes

MRSA enters health care facilities through an infected or colonized patient or a colonized health care worker. Although MRSA has been recovered from environmental surfaces, it's transmitted mainly by health care workers' hands. Many colonized individuals become silent carriers. The most frequent site of colonization is the anterior nares (40% of adults and most children become transient nasal carriers). Other sites include the groin, axilla, and the gut, though these sites aren't as common. Typically, MRSA colonization is diagnosed by isolating bacteria from nasal secretions.

In individuals where the natural defense system breaks down, such as after an invasive procedure, trauma or chemotherapy, the normally benign bacteria can invade tissue, proliferate, and cause infection. Today up to 90% of *S. aureus* isolates or strains are penicillin-resistant, and about 27% of all *S. au-*

*reus* isolates are resistant to methicillin, a penicillin derivative. These strains may also resist cephalosporins, aminoglycosides, erythromycin, tetracycline, and clindamycin.

MRSA has become prevalent with the overuse of antibiotics. Over the years, overuse has given once-susceptible bacteria the chance to develop defenses against antibiotics. This new capability allows resistant strains to flourish when antibiotics knock out their more sensitive cousins.

## Diagnosis

MRSA can be cultured from the suspected site with the appropriate culture method. For example, MRSA in a wound infection can be swabbed for culture. Blood, urine, and sputum cultures will reveal sources of MRSA.

## Treatment

To eradicate MRSA colonization in the nares, the doctor may order topical mupirocin applied inside the nostrils. Other protocols involve combining a topical agent and an oral antibiotic. Most facilities keep patients in isolation until surveillance cultures are negative.

To attack MRSA infection, vancomycin is the drug of choice. A serious adverse effect (mostly caused by histamine release) is itching, which can progress to anaphylaxis. Some doctors also add rifampin, but whether rifampin acts synergistically or antagonistically when given with vancomycin is controversial.

## Special considerations

• Personnel in contact with the patients should wash hands before and after patient care.

**➤ CLINICAL TIP** Good hand washing is the most effective way to prevent MRSA from spreading.

• Use an antiseptic soap such as chlorhexidine because bacteria have been cultured from worker's hands after they've washed with milder soap. One study showed that without proper hand washing, MRSA could survive on health care workers' hands for up to 3 hours.

• Contact isolation precautions should be used when in contact with the patient. A private room should be used, as well as dedicated equipment and disinfection of the environment.

• Change gloves when contaminated or when moving from a "dirty" area of the body to a clean one.

• Instruct family and friends to wear protective clothing when they visit the patient and show them how to dispose of it.

• Provide teaching and emotional support to the patient and family members.

• Consider grouping infected patients together and having the same nursing staff care for them.

• Equipment used on the patient should not be laid on the bed or bed stand and should be wiped with appropriate disinfectant before leaving the room.

• Ensure judicious and careful use of antibiotics. Encourage doctors to limit antibiotic use.

• Instruct the patient to take antibiotics for the full prescription period, even if he begins to feel better.

# MONONUCLEOSIS

Infectious mononucleosis is an acute infectious disease caused by the Epstein-Barr virus (EBV), a member of the herpes group. It primarily affects young adults and children, although in children it's usually so mild that it's often overlooked.

Characteristically, infectious mononucleosis produces fever, sore throat, and cervical lymphadenopathy (the hallmarks of the disease), as well as hepatic dysfunction, increased lymphocytes and monocytes, and development and persistence of heterophil antibodies. The prognosis is excellent, and major complications are uncommon.

## Causes

Apparently, the reservoir of EBV is limited to humans. Infectious mononucleosis probably spreads by the oropharyngeal route because about 80% of patients carry EBV in their throats during the acute infection and for an indefinite period afterward.

It can also be transmitted by blood transfusion and has been reported after cardiac surgery as the "post-pump perfusion" syndrome. Infectious mononucleosis is probably contagious from before symptoms develop until the fever subsides and oropharyngeal lesions disappear.

Infectious mononucleosis is fairly common in the United States, Canada, and Europe, and both sexes are affected equally. Incidence varies seasonally among college students (most common in the early spring and early fall) but not among the general population.

## Signs and symptoms

The symptoms of mononucleosis mimic those of many other infectious diseases, including hepatitis, rubella, and toxoplasmosis. Typically, after an incubation period of about 10 days in children and from 30 to 50 days in adults, infectious mononucleosis produces prodromal symptoms, such as headache, malaise, and fatigue.

After 3 to 5 days, patients typically develop a triad of symptoms: sore throat, cervical lymphadenopathy, and temperature fluctuations, with an evening peak of 101° to 102° F (38.3° to 38.9° C) Splenomegaly, hepatomegaly, stomatitis, exudative tonsillitis, or pharyngitis may also develop.

Sometimes, early in the illness, a maculopapular rash that resembles rubella develops; also, jaundice occurs in about 5% of patients. Major complications are rare but may include splenic rupture, aseptic meningitis, encephalitis, hemolytic anemia, and Guillain-Barré syndrome. Symptoms usually subside from 6 to 10 days after onset of the disease but may persist for weeks.

### Diagnosis
Physical examination demonstrating the clinical triad suggests infectious mononucleosis. The following abnormal laboratory results confirm it:
● *White blood cell (WBC) count* increases 10,000 to 20,000/µl during the second and third weeks of illness. Lymphocytes and monocytes account for 50% to 70% of the total WBC count; 10% of the lymphocytes are atypical.
● *Heterophil antibodies* (agglutinins for sheep red blood cells) in serum drawn during the acute illness and at 3- to 4-week intervals rise to four times normal.
● *Indirect immunofluorescence* shows antibodies to EBV and cellular antigens. Such testing is usually more definitive than heterophil antibodies.
● *Liver function studies* are abnormal.

### Treatment
Infectious mononucleosis resists prevention and antimicrobial treatment. Thus, therapy is essentially supportive: relief of symptoms, bed rest during the acute febrile period, and aspirin or another salicylate for headache and sore throat.

If severe throat inflammation causes airway obstruction, steroids can be used to relieve swelling and avoid tracheotomy. Splenic rupture, marked by sudden abdominal pain, requires splenectomy. About 20% of patients with infectious mononucleosis will also have streptococcal pharyngotonsillitis; these patients should receive antibiotic therapy for at least 10 days.

### Special considerations
Because uncomplicated infectious mononucleosis doesn't require hospitalization, patient teaching is essential. Convalescence may take several weeks, usually until the patient's WBC count returns to normal.
● During the acute illness, stress the need for bed rest. If the patient is a student, tell him he may continue less demanding school assignments and see his friends but should avoid long, difficult projects until after recovery.
● To minimize throat discomfort, encourage the patient to drink milk shakes, fruit juices, and broths, and also to eat cool, bland foods.

> CLINICAL TIP Advise the patient to use saline gargles and aspirin as needed.

# MULTIPLE ENDOCRINE NEOPLASIA

Multiple endocrine neoplasia (MEN), including Werner's syndrome and Sipple's syndrome, is a hereditary disorder in which two or more endocrine glands develop hyperplasia, adenoma, or carcinoma, concurrently or consecutively.

Two of the types that occur are well documented: MEN I (Werner's syndrome), the most common form, involves hyperplasia and adenomatosis of the parathyroid glands, islet cells of the pancreas, pituitary and, rarely, thyroid and adrenal glands; MEN II (Sipple's syndrome) involves medullary carcinoma of the thyroid, with hyperplasia and adenomatosis of the adrenal medulla (pheochromocytoma) and parathyroid glands.

## Causes

MEN usually results from autosomal dominant inheritance, affects both males and females, and may occur at any time from adolescence to old age.

## Signs and symptoms

Clinical effects of MEN may develop in various combinations and orders, depending on the glands involved.

### MEN I

The most common symptom of MEN I is peptic ulceration, associated with the Zollinger-Ellison syndrome (marked by increased gastrin production from non-beta islet cell tumors of the pancreas). Hypoglycemia may result from pancreatic beta islet cell tumors, with increased insulin production.

When MEN I affects the parathyroid glands, it produces signs of hyperparathyroidism, including hypercalcemia (because the parathyroids are primarily responsible for the regulation of calcium and phosphorus levels). When MEN causes a pituitary tumor, it usually triggers pituitary hyperfunction but can also result in hypofunction. MEN I rarely produces renal or skeletal complications.

### MEN II

Characteristic features of MEN II with medullary carcinoma of the thyroid include enlarged thyroid mass, with resultant increased calcitonin. With tumors of the adrenal medulla (pheochromocytomas), symptoms include headache, tachyarrhythmias, and hypertension; with adenomatosis or hyperplasia of the parathyroid glands,

symptoms result from renal calculi and hypercalcemia. Cushing's syndrome may occur from ectopic corticotropin.

## Diagnosis

Investigating symptoms of pituitary tumor, hypoglycemia, hypercalcemia, or GI hemorrhage may lead to a diagnosis of MEN.

Diagnostic tests must be used to carefully evaluate each affected endocrine gland. For example, radioimmunoassay showing increased levels of gastrin in patients with peptic ulceration and Zollinger-Ellison syndrome suggests the need for follow-up studies for MEN I because 50% of patients with Zollinger-Ellison syndrome have MEN. After confirmation of MEN, family members must also be assessed for this inherited syndrome.

## Treatment

Treatment must eradicate the tumors. Subsequent therapy controls residual symptoms.

### MEN I

In patients with MEN I, peptic ulceration is usually the most urgent clinical feature, so primary treatment emphasizes control of bleeding or resection of necrotic tissue. In hypoglycemia caused by insulinoma, oral administration of diazoxide or glucose can keep blood glucose levels within acceptable limits. Subtotal (partial) pancreatectomy is required to remove the tumor.

Because all parathyroid glands have the potential for neoplastic enlargement, subtotal parathyroidectomy may also be required. Transsphenoidal surgery may be required for pituitary lesions.

### MEN II

In MEN II, treatment of an adrenal medullary tumor includes antihypertensives and resection of the tumor.

## Special considerations

• If MEN involves the pancreas, monitor blood glucose levels frequently. If it affects the adrenal glands, monitor blood pressure closely, especially during drug therapy.

• Manage peptic ulcers, hypoglycemia, and other complications as needed.

• If a pituitary tumor is suspected, watch for signs of pituitary trophic hormone dysfunction, which may affect any of the endocrine glands.

• Be aware that pituitary apoplexy (sudden severe headache, altered level of consciousness, visual disturbances) may occur.

# MULTIPLE MYELOMA

Multiple myeloma is also known as malignant plasmacytoma, plasma cell myeloma, and myelomatosis. It's a disseminated neoplasm of marrow plasma cells that infiltrates bone to produce osteolytic lesions throughout the skeleton (flat bones, vertebrae, skull, pelvis, ribs); in late stages, it infiltrates the body organs (liver, spleen, lymph nodes, lungs, adrenal glands, kidneys, skin, and GI tract). Multiple myeloma strikes about 9,600 people yearly — mostly men over age 40.

The prognosis is usually poor because the disease is commonly diagnosed after it has already infiltrated the vertebrae, pelvis, skull, ribs, clavicles, and sternum. By then, skeletal destruction is widespread and, without treatment, leads to vertebral collapse; about 52% of patients die within 3 months of diagnosis and 90% within 2 years. Early diagnosis and treatment prolong the lives of many patients by 3 to 5 years. Death usually follows complications, such as infection, renal failure, hematologic disorders, fractures, hypercalcemia, hyperuricemia, or dehydration.

## Signs and symptoms

The earliest symptom of multiple myeloma is often back pain. This disease should be considered in diagnosis or treatment of elderly patients with new onset of low back pain. Arthritic symptoms may also occur: achiness, joint swelling, and tenderness, possibly from vertebral compression. Other effects include fever, malaise, slight evidence of peripheral neuropathy (such as peripheral paresthesia), pathologic fractures, and easy bruising.

As multiple myeloma progresses, symptoms of vertebral compression may become acute, accompanied by anemia, weight loss, thoracic deformities (ballooning), and loss of body height — 5″ (13 cm) or more — due to vertebral collapse.

Renal complications such as pyelonephritis (caused by tubular damage from large amounts of Bence Jones protein, hypercalcemia, and hyperuricemia) may occur. (See *Bence Jones protein.*) Severe, recurrent infection such as pneumonia may follow damage to nerves associated with respiratory function.

## Diagnosis

After a physical examination and a careful medical history, the following diagnostic tests and nonspecific laboratory abnormalities confirm the presence of multiple myeloma:

• *Complete blood count* shows moderate or severe anemia. The differential may show 40% to 50% lymphocytes but seldom more than 3% plasma cells. An elevated erythrocyte sedimentation rate results from increased clumping of red blood cells (rouleaux formation) caused by increased concentration of serum immunoprotein.

- *Urine studies* may show Bence Jones protein and hypercalciuria. Absence of Bence Jones protein doesn't rule out multiple myeloma; however, its presence almost invariably confirms the disease.
- *Bone marrow aspiration* detects myelomatous cells (an abnormal number of immature plasma cells).
- *Serum electrophoresis* shows an elevated globulin spike that's electrophoretically and immunologically abnormal.

> **CLINICAL TIP**  Urine protein electrophoresis may detect cases that are missed by serum electrophoresis.

- *X-rays* during early stages may show only diffuse osteoporosis. Eventually, they show multiple, sharply circumscribed osteolytic (punched-out) lesions, particularly on the skull, pelvis, and spine — the characteristic lesions of multiple myeloma.
- *Excretory urography* can assess renal involvement. To avoid precipitation of Bence Jones protein, iothalamate or diatrizoate is used instead of the usual contrast medium. Also, although oral fluid restriction is usually the standard procedure before excretory urography, patients with multiple myeloma receive large quantities of fluid, generally orally but sometimes I.V. before this test is done.

### Treatment

Long-term treatment of multiple myeloma consists mainly of chemotherapy to suppress plasma cell growth and control pain. Some combinations include cyclophosphamide, doxorubicin, and prednisone; and carmustine, doxorubicin, and prednisone. Also, adjuvant local radiation reduces acute lesions, such as collapsed vertebrae, and relieves localized pain.

Other treatment usually includes a melphalan-prednisone combination in

## BENCE JONES PROTEIN

The hallmark of multiple myeloma, this protein (a light chain of gamma globulin) was named for Henry Bence Jones, an English doctor who in 1848 noticed that patients with a curious bone disease excreted a unique protein — unique in that it coagulated at 113° to 131° F (45° to 55° C), then redissolved when heated to boiling.

It remained for Otto Kahler, an Austrian, to demonstrate in 1889 that Bence Jones protein was related to myeloma. Bence Jones protein isn't found in the urine of *all* multiple myeloma patients, but it's almost never found in patients without this disease.

high intermittent doses or low continuous daily doses, and analgesics for pain. For spinal cord compression, the patient may require a laminectomy; for renal complications, dialysis.

Because the patient may have bone demineralization and may lose large amounts of calcium into blood and urine, he's a prime candidate for renal calculi, nephrocalcinosis and, eventually, renal failure due to hypercalcemia. Hypercalcemia is managed with hydration, diuretics, corticosteroids, oral phosphate, and I.V. mithramycin to decrease serum calcium levels.

### Special considerations

- Push fluids; encourage the patient to drink 3,000 to 4,000 ml of fluids daily, particularly before excretory urography. Monitor his fluid intake and output. (Daily output should be at least 1,500 ml.)
- Encourage the patient to walk. (Immobilization increases bone demineralization and vulnerability to pneumo-

nia.) Give analgesics, as needed, to lessen pain.

● Never allow the patient to walk unaccompanied; be sure that he uses a walker or other supportive aid to prevent falls. Since the patient is particularly vulnerable to pathologic fractures, he may be fearful. Give reassurance, and allow him to move at his own pace.

● Prevent complications by watching for fever or malaise, which may signal the onset of infection, and for signs of other problems, such as severe anemia and fractures.

● If the patient is bedridden, change his position every 2 hours. Give passive range-of-motion and deep-breathing exercises. When he can tolerate them, promote active exercises.

● If the patient is taking melphalan (a phenylalanine derivative of nitrogen mustard that depresses bone marrow), make sure that his blood count (platelet and white blood cell) is taken before each treatment.

● If the patient is taking prednisone, watch closely for infection because this drug often masks it.

● Whenever possible, get the patient out of bed within 24 hours after laminectomy. Check for hemorrhage, motor or sensory deficits, and loss of bowel or bladder function. Position the patient as necessary, maintain alignment, and logroll when turning.

● Provide emotional support for the patient and his family. Help relieve their anxiety by clearly explaining diagnostic tests (including painful procedures, such as bone marrow aspiration and biopsy), treatments, and the prognosis. If needed, refer them to an appropriate community resource for additional support.

# MULTIPLE SCLEROSIS

Multiple sclerosis (MS) is caused by demyelination of the white matter of the brain and spinal cord and damage to nerve fibers and their targets. In MS, sporadic patches of axon demyelination and nerve fiber loss occur throughout the central nervous system, inducing widely disseminated and varied neurologic dysfunction. Characterized by exacerbations and remissions, MS is a major cause of chronic disability in young adults.

▶ CLINICAL TIP New evidence of nerve fiber loss may provide an explanation for the invisible neurologic deficits experienced by many patients with MS. The axons decide the presence or absence of function. Loss of myelin doesn't correlate with loss of function.

The prognosis varies. MS may progress rapidly, disabling the patient by early adulthood or causing death within months of onset. However, 70% of patients lead active, productive lives with prolonged remissions.

Terms to describe MS forms include:

● *elapsing-remitting* — clear relapses (or acute attacks or exacerbations) with full recovery or partial recovery and lasting disability. Between the attacks there is no worsening of the disease.

● *primary progressive* — steady progression or worsening of the disease from the onset with minor recovery or plateaus. This form is uncommon and may involve different brain and spinal cord damage than other forms.

● *secondary progressive* — begins as a pattern of clear-cut relapses and recovery, but becomes steadily progressive and worsens between acute attacks.

• *progressive relapsing* — steadily progressive from the onset, but also has clear acute attacks. This form is rare.

## Causes

The exact cause of MS is unknown, but current theories suggest a slow-acting or latent viral infection and an autoimmune response. Other theories suggest that environmental and genetic factors may also be linked to MS.

Emotional stress, overwork, fatigue, pregnancy, and acute respiratory infections may precede the onset of this illness.

MS usually begins between the ages of 20 and 40 (the average age of onset is 27). It affects three women for every two men and five whites for every black. Incidence is low in Japan; it's generally higher among urban populations and upper socioeconomic groups. A family history of MS and living in a cold, damp climate increase the risk.

## Signs and symptoms

Clinical findings in MS depend on the extent and site of myelin destruction, the extent of remyelination, and the adequacy of subsequent restored synaptic transmission.

Signs and symptoms in MS may be transient, or they may last for hours or weeks. They may wax and wane with no predictable pattern, vary from day to day, and be bizarre and difficult for the patient to describe.

In most patients, visual problems and sensory impairment, such as burning, pins and needles, and electrical sensations, are the first signs that something may be wrong.

Other characteristic changes include the following:

• *ocular disturbances* — optic neuritis, diplopia, ophthalmoplegia, blurred vision, and nystagmus

• *muscle dysfunction* — weakness, paralysis ranging from monoplegia to quadriplegia, spasticity, hyperreflexia, intention tremor, and gait ataxia

• *urinary disturbances* — incontinence, frequency, urgency, and frequent infections

• *bowel disturbances* — involuntary evacuation or constipation

• *fatigue* — often the most debilitating symptom.

Associated signs and symptoms include poorly articulated or scanning speech and dysphagia. Clinical effects may be so mild that the patient is unaware of them or so intense that they are debilitating.

## Diagnosis

Because early symptoms may be mild, years may elapse between onset of the first signs and the diagnosis. Diagnosis of this disorder requires evidence of two or more neurologic attacks. Periodic testing and close observation of the patient are necessary, perhaps for years, depending on the course of the disease.

The following tests may be performed:

• *Magnetic resonance imaging* may detect MS lesions.

• *EEG* is abnormal in one-third of patients.

• *Lumbar puncture* shows an elevated gamma globulin fraction of immunoglobulin G but normal total cerebrospinal fluid (CSF) protein levels. An elevated CSF gamma globulin level is significant only when serum gamma globulin levels are normal; it reflects hyperactivity of the immune system due to chronic demyelination. In addition, the WBC level in CSF may be elevated.

• *Electrophoresis* can detect oligoclonal bands of immunoglobulin in CSF. Present in most patients, they can be found even when the percentage of gamma globulin in CSF is normal.

A differential diagnosis must rule out spinal cord compression, foramen magnum tumor (which may mimic the exacerbations and remissions of MS), multiple small strokes, syphilis or another infection, thyroid disease, and chronic fatigue syndrome.

## Treatment
The aim of treatment is threefold: to treat the acute exacerbation, the disease process, and the related signs and symptoms.

### *Acute exacerbation*
I.V. methylprednisone followed by oral prednisone has been shown to be effective for speeding recovery for acute attacks. Other drugs, such as azathioprine (Imuran) or methotrexate and cytoxin, may be used.

### *Treating the disease*
Three drugs (Betaseron, Avonex, and glatiramen [Copaxone]) may reduce the frequency and severity of relapses and slow central nervous system damage. Betaseron and Avonex (both interferon-$B_1$) and Copaxone (a combination of four amino acids) are currently available for relapsing-remitting MS.

### *Treating signs and symptoms*
● *Spasticity* occurs as a result of opposing muscle groups relaxing and contracting at the same time. Stretching and range-of-motion exercises, coupled with correct positioning, are helpful in relaxing muscles and maintaining function.

➤ CLINICAL TIP When working with a spastic extremity, never try to force it open. Gently rotate the extremity toward the direction it's being pulled and then gradually rotate it outward. Repeat, and go a little further with each

attempt. Applying pressure to the contracted area can help with relaxation. Avoid touching the palm of the hand or sole of the foot. Minimize spasticity by holding the heel of the foot and by folding the hand open from the outer edges.

Drug therapy for spasticity includes Baclofen (Lioresal) and tizanidine (Zanaflex). For severe spasticity, Botox injections, intrathecal injections, nerve blocks, and surgery may be necessary.

● *Fatigue* in MS is characterized by an overwhelming feeling of exhaustion that can occur at any time of the day without warning. The cause is unknown. Changes in environmental conditions, such as heat and humidity, can aggravate fatigue. Frequent rest periods, aerobic exercise, and cooling techniques (air conditioning, breezes, water sprays) can minimize fatigue. The drugs Symmetrel, Cylert, and Ritalin have proven beneficial as have antidepressants to manage fatigue.

● *Bladder problems* may arise from failure to store urine, failure to empty the bladder or, more commonly, a combination of both. Treatment ranges from simple strategies such as drinking cranberry juice to the placement of an indwelling urinary catheter and suprapubic tubes. Intermittent self-catheterization and postvoiding catheterization programs are very beneficial. In addition, anticholinergic medications may be helpful.

● *Bowel problems,* such as constipation and involuntary evacuation of stool, can be managed by increasing fiber. Bulking agents such as Metamucil assist in relief and prevention of bowel problems. Other bowel-training strategies, such as daily suppositories and rectal stimulation, may be necessary.

● *Sensory symptoms,* such as pain, numbness, burning, and tingling sensations, can be well managed by low-dose tricyclic antidepressants, phenytoin, or carbamazepine.

• *Cognitive dysfunction* is experienced by 50% of patients with MS. Cognitive problems tend to be minor in nature with retrieval of information being the most frequently experienced symptom. For more severe issues, a neuropsychological consultation could be beneficial.

• *Motor dysfunction,* such as problems with balance, strength, and muscle coordination, may present in MS. Adaptive devices and physical therapy intervention help to maintain mobility.

• *Other symptoms* such as tremors may be treated with beta blockers, sedatives, or diuretics. Dysarthria requires a speech therapy consultation. Vertigo may be managed with antihistamines, vision therapy, or exercises. Vision changes may require vision therapy or adaptive lenses.

**Special considerations**

• Emphasize the need to avoid stress, infections, and fatigue and to maintain independence by developing new ways of performing daily activities.

• Be sure to tell the patient to avoid exposure to bacterial and viral infections.

• Stress the importance of eating a nutritious, well-balanced diet that contains sufficient fiber to prevent constipation.

• Encourage adequate fluid intake and regular urination.

• Watch for adverse reactions to drug therapy.

• Copaxone reactions occur immediately after injection. The patient may experience transient flushing, chest pain, palpitations, and dyspnea, which last only a few seconds. Usually no additional treatment is needed.

• Patients receiving Betaseron or Avonex require routine laboratory monitoring (complete blood count with differential), blood urea nitrogen, creatinine, alanine aminotransferase, and urinalysis.

❯ CLINICAL TIP Nonsteroidal antiinflammatory drugs (NSAIDs) administered with bedtime injections of Betaseron have been helpful in minimizing adverse effects (flulike symptoms, site reactions, suicidal ideation). Subcutaneous site rotation is necessary. Betaseron injections are given every other day, and the medication must be refrigerated. Avonex reactions are similar to Betaseron, with I.M. injections once per week. Copaxone is administered in daily subcutaneous injections.

• Promote emotional stability. Help the patient establish a daily routine to maintain optimal functioning.

• Inform the patient that exacerbations are unpredictable, necessitating physical and emotional adjustments in his lifestyle.

• For more information, refer the patient to the National Multiple Sclerosis Society.

# MUMPS

Also known as infectious or epidemic parotitis, mumps is an acute viral disease caused by a paramyxovirus. It's most prevalent in children older than age 5 but younger than age 9. Infants under age 1 seldom get this disease because of passive immunity from maternal antibodies. Peak incidence occurs during late winter and early spring. The prognosis for complete recovery is good, although mumps sometimes causes complications.

**Causes**

The mumps paramyxovirus is found in the saliva of an infected person and is transmitted by droplets or by direct con-

## SITE OF PAROTID INFLAMMATION IN MUMPS

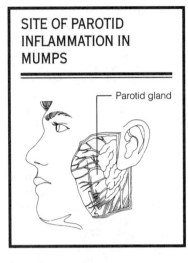

Parotid gland

tact. The virus is present in the saliva 6 days before to 9 days after onset of parotid gland swelling; the 48-hour period immediately preceding onset of swelling is probably the time of highest communicability.

The incubation period ranges from 14 to 25 days (the average is 18 days). One attack of mumps (even if unilateral) almost always confers lifelong immunity.

### Signs and symptoms

The clinical features of mumps vary widely. An estimated 30% of susceptible people have subclinical illness.

Mumps usually begins with prodromal symptoms that last for 24 hours and include myalgia, anorexia, malaise, headache, and low-grade fever, followed by an earache that's aggravated by chewing, parotid gland tenderness and swelling, a temperature of 101° to 104° F (38.3° to 40° C), and pain when chewing or when drinking sour or acidic liquids.

Simultaneously with the swelling of the parotid gland or several days later, one or more of the other salivary glands may become swollen. (See *Site of parotid inflammation in mumps*.)

### Complications

Epididymo-orchitis and mumps meningitis are complications of mumps. Epididymo-orchitis, which occurs in approximately 25% of postpubertal males who contract mumps, produces abrupt onset of testicular swelling and tenderness, scrotal erythema, lower abdominal pain, nausea, vomiting, fever, and chills.

Swelling and tenderness may last for several weeks; epididymitis may precede or accompany orchitis. In 50% of men with mumps-induced orchitis, the testicles show some atrophy, but sterility is extremely rare.

Mumps meningitis complicates mumps in 10% of patients and affects males three to five times more often than females. Symptoms include fever, meningeal irritation (nuchal rigidity, headache, and irritability), vomiting, drowsiness, and a lymphocyte count in cerebrospinal fluid ranging from 500 to 2,000/μl.

Recovery is usually complete. Less common effects are pancreatitis, deafness, arthritis, myocarditis, encephalitis, pericarditis, oophoritis, and nephritis.

### Diagnosis

In mumps, a diagnosis is usually made after the characteristic signs and symptoms develop, especially parotid gland enlargement with a history of exposure to mumps. Serologic antibody testing can verify the diagnosis when parotid or other salivary gland enlargement is absent. If comparison between a blood sample obtained during the acute phase of illness and another sample obtained 3 weeks later shows a fourfold rise in antibody titer, the patient most likely had mumps.

## Treatment

Effective treatment includes analgesics for pain, antipyretics for fever, and adequate fluid intake to prevent dehydration from fever and anorexia. If the patient can't swallow, I.V. fluid replacement may be necessary.

### Special considerations

• Stress the need for bed rest during the febrile period.

• Give analgesics, and apply warm or cool compresses to the neck to relieve pain.

• Give antipyretics and tepid sponge baths for fever.

• To prevent dehydration, encourage the patient to drink fluids; to minimize pain and anorexia, advise him to avoid spicy, irritating foods and those that require a lot of chewing.

• During the acute phase, observe the patient closely for signs of central nervous system involvement, such as an altered level of consciousness and nuchal rigidity.

➤ CLINICAL TIP Respiratory isolation is advocated for mumps. Precautions should be taken by all personnel in contact with the patient.

• Emphasize the importance of routine immunization with live attenuated mumps virus (paramyxovirus) at age 15 months and for susceptible patients (especially males) who are approaching or are past puberty.

• Remember, immunization within 24 hours of exposure may prevent or attenuate the actual disease. Immunity against mumps lasts at least 12 years.

• Report all cases of mumps to local public health authorities.

➤ CLINICAL TIP The patient should be excluded from school or the workplace for 9 days from the onset of mumps.

# MUSCULAR DYSTROPHY

Muscular dystrophy is actually a group of congenital disorders characterized by progressive symmetrical wasting of skeletal muscles without neural or sensory defects. Paradoxically, these wasted muscles tend to enlarge because of connective tissue and fat deposits, giving an erroneous impression of muscle strength.

Four main types of muscular dystrophy occur: *Duchenne's (pseudohypertrophic) muscular dystrophy,* which accounts for 50% of all cases; *Becker's (benign pseudohypertrophic) muscular dystrophy; facioscapulohumeral (Landouzy-Dejerine) dystrophy;* and *limb-girdle dystrophy.*

The prognosis varies. Duchenne's muscular dystrophy generally strikes during early childhood and usually results in death by age 20. Patients with Becker's muscular dystrophy live into their 40s. Facioscapulohumeral and limb-girdle dystrophies usually don't shorten life expectancy.

### Causes

Muscular dystrophy is caused by various genetic mechanisms. Duchenne's and Becker's muscular dystrophies are X-linked recessive disorders. They result from defects in the gene coding for the muscle protein dystrophin. The defect can be mapped genetically to the Xp21 locus.

Duchenne's and Becker's muscular dystrophies affect males almost exclusively. The incidence of Duchenne's muscular dystrophy in males is 13 to 33 per 100,000. Becker's muscular dystrophy occurs in about 1 to 3 males per 100,000.

Facioscapulohumeral dystrophy is an autosomal dominant disorder. Limb-girdle dystrophy may be inherited in several ways, but it's usually an autosomal recessive trait. These two types affect both sexes about equally.

## Signs and symptoms

Although the four types of muscular dystrophy cause progressive muscular deterioration, the degree of severity and the age of onset vary.

### Duchenne's muscular dystrophy

Duchenne's muscular dystrophy begins insidiously, between the age of 3 and 5. It affects leg and pelvic muscles initially but eventually spreads to the involuntary muscles. Muscle weakness produces a waddling gait, toe-walking, and lordosis.

Children with this disorder have difficulty climbing stairs, fall down often, can't run properly, and their scapulae flare out (or "wing") when they raise their arms. Calf muscles especially become enlarged and firm. Muscle deterioration progresses rapidly, and contractures develop. Usually, these children are confined to wheelchairs by ages 9 to 12.

Late in the disease, progressive weakening of cardiac muscle causes tachycardia, electrocardiogram abnormalities, and pulmonary complications. Death commonly results from sudden heart failure, respiratory failure, or infection.

### Becker's muscular dystrophy

Signs and symptoms of Becker's muscular dystrophy resemble those of Duchenne's muscular dystrophy, but they progress more slowly. Although symptoms start around age 5, the patient can still walk well beyond age 15 — sometimes into his 40s.

### Facioscapulohumeral dystrophy

This is a slowly progressive and relatively benign form of muscular dystrophy that commonly begins before age 10 but may develop during early adolescence. It weakens the muscles of the face, shoulders, and upper arms at first but eventually spreads to all voluntary muscles, producing a pendulous lower lip and absence of the nasolabial fold.

Early symptoms include inability to pucker the mouth or whistle, abnormal facial movements, and absence of facial movements when laughing or crying. Other signs consist of diffuse facial flattening that leads to a masklike expression, winging of the scapulae, inability to raise the arms above the head, and, in infants, inability to suckle.

### Limb-girdle dystrophy

This form follows a similarly slow course and often causes only slight disability. Usually, it begins between the ages of 6 and 10; less often, in early adulthood. Muscle weakness first appears in the upper arm and pelvic muscles. Other symptoms include winging of the scapulae, lordosis with abdominal protrusion, waddling gait, poor balance, and inability to raise the arms.

## Diagnosis

Typical clinical findings, family history, and test findings are used to diagnose the disease. If another family member has muscular dystrophy, its clinical characteristics can indicate the type of dystrophy the patient has and how he may be affected.

Electromyography typically demonstrates short, weak bursts of electrical activity in affected muscles. A muscle biopsy shows variations in the size of muscle fibers and, in later stages, fat and connective tissue deposits. In Duchenne's muscle dystrophy, a muscle biopsy reveals an absence of dystrophin.

Immunologic and molecular biological techniques now available in specialized medical centers facilitate accurate prenatal and postnatal diagnosis of Duchenne's and Becker's muscular dystrophies. These techniques also help to identify a person as a carrier.

In addition, these newer techniques are replacing muscle biopsy and serum creatine kinase tests as diagnostic procedures.

### Treatment

To date, scientists have found no treatment that can stop the progressive muscle impairment of muscular dystrophy. However, orthopedic appliances as well as exercise, physical therapy, and surgery to correct contractures can help preserve the patient's mobility and independence.

Family members who are carriers of muscular dystrophy should receive genetic counseling regarding the risk of transmitting this disease.

### Special considerations

• Comprehensive long-term care and follow-up, patient and family teaching, and psychological support can help the patient and family deal with this disorder.

• When respiratory involvement occurs in Duchenne's muscular dystrophy, encourage coughing, deep-breathing exercises, and diaphragmatic breathing. Teach parents how to recognize early signs of respiratory complications.

• Encourage and assist with active and passive range-of-motion exercises to preserve joint mobility and prevent muscle atrophy.

• Advise the patient to avoid long periods of bed rest and inactivity; if necessary, limit his TV viewing and other sedentary activities.

• Refer the patient for physical therapy. Splints, braces, surgery to correct contractures, trapeze bars, overhead slings, and a wheelchair can help preserve mobility. A footboard or high-topped sneakers and a foot cradle increase comfort and prevent footdrop.

• Because inactivity may cause constipation, encourage adequate fluid intake, increase dietary bulk, and obtain an order for a stool softener.

• Because such a patient is prone to obesity because of reduced physical activity, help him and his family plan a low-calorie, high-protein, high-fiber diet.

CLINICAL TIP    Always allow the patient plenty of time to perform even simple physical tasks because he's likely to be slow and awkward.

• Encourage communication among family members to help them deal with the emotional strain this disorder produces. Provide emotional support to help the patient cope with continual changes in body image.

• If necessary, refer adult patients for sexual counseling.

• Refer those who must acquire new job skills for vocational rehabilitation. (Contact the Department of Labor and Industry in your state for more information.)

• For information on social services and financial assistance, refer patients and their families to the Muscular Dystrophy Association.

• Refer family members for genetic counseling.

# MYASTHENIA GRAVIS

Myasthenia gravis produces sporadic but progressive weakness and abnormal fatigability of striated (skeletal) muscles, which are exacerbated by exercise and repeated movement but improved by anticholinesterase drugs. Usually,

---

this disorder affects muscles innervated by the cranial nerves (face, lips, tongue, neck, and throat), but it can affect any muscle group.

Myasthenia gravis follows an unpredictable course of periodic exacerbations and remissions. (See *Coping with lifelong myasthenia gravis.)* There is no known cure. Drug treatment has improved the prognosis and allows patients to lead relatively normal lives, except during exacerbations. When the disease involves the respiratory system, it may be life-threatening.

## Causes
Myasthenia gravis causes a failure in transmission of nerve impulses at the neuromuscular junction. Theoretically, such impairment may result from an autoimmune response, ineffective acetylcholine release, or inadequate muscle fiber response to acetylcholine.

Myasthenia gravis affects 1 in 25,000 people at any age, but incidence peaks between the ages of 20 and 40. It's three times more common in women than in men in this age-group, but after age 40, the incidence is similar.

About 20% of infants born to myasthenic mothers have transient (or occasionally persistent) myasthenia. This disease may coexist with immune and thyroid disorders; about 15% of myasthenic patients have thymomas. Remissions occur in about 25% of patients.

## Signs and symptoms
The dominant symptoms of myasthenia gravis are skeletal muscle weakness and fatigability. In the early stages, easy fatigability of certain muscles may appear with no other findings. Later, it may be severe enough to cause paralysis. Typically, myasthenic muscles are strongest in the morning but weaken throughout the day, especially after exercise. Short rest periods temporarily restore muscle function.

### Progressive muscle weakness
More and more muscles become weak, and eventually some muscles may lose function entirely. Resulting symptoms

depend on the muscle group affected; they become more intense during menses and after emotional stress, prolonged exposure to sunlight or cold, or infections.

Onset may be sudden or insidious. In many patients, weak eye closure, ptosis, and diplopia are the first signs that something is wrong.

Myasthenic patients usually have blank and expressionless faces and nasal vocal tones. They experience frequent nasal regurgitation of fluids and have difficulty chewing and swallowing. Because of this, they often worry about choking. Their eyelids droop, and they may have to tilt their heads back to see. Their neck muscles may become too weak to support their heads without bobbing.

In patients with weakened respiratory muscles, decreased tidal volume and vital capacity make breathing difficult and predispose them to pneumonia and other respiratory tract infections. Respiratory muscle weakness (myasthenic crisis) may be severe enough to require an emergency airway and mechanical ventilation.

### Diagnosis

Muscle fatigability that improves with rest strongly suggests a diagnosis of myasthenia gravis. Tests for this neurologic condition record the effect of exercise and subsequent rest on muscle weakness. Electromyography, with repeated neural stimulation, may help confirm this diagnosis.

The classic proof of myasthenia gravis is improved muscle function after an I.V. injection of edrophonium or neostigmine. In myasthenic patients, muscle function improves within 30 to 60 seconds and lasts up to 30 minutes. Long-standing ocular muscle dysfunction may fail to respond to such testing. This test can differentiate a myasthenic

crisis from a cholinergic crisis (caused by acetylcholine overactivity at the neuromuscular junction). The acetylcholine receptor antibody titer may be elevated in generalized myasthenia. Evaluation should rule out thyroid disease and thymoma. Rheumatoid arthritis, lupus erythematosus, and polymyositis are often associated with myasthenia gravis.

### Treatment

In myasthenia gravis, treatment is aimed at relieving symptoms. Anticholinesterase drugs, such as neostigmine and pyridostigmine, counteract fatigue and muscle weakness and allow about 80% of normal muscle function. However, these drugs become less effective as the disease worsens. Decreasing the immune response toward acetylcholine receptors at the neuromuscular junction is the goal of immunosuppressant therapy. Corticosteroids, azathioprine, cyclosporine, and cyclophosphamide are used in a progressive fashion (when the previous drug response is poor, the next one is used). To suppress the immune system during acute relapses, gamma globulin (IgG) may also be used. Plasmapheresis is used in severe exacerbations.

Patients with thymomas require a thymectomy, which may cause remission in some cases of adult-onset myasthenia. Acute exacerbations that cause severe respiratory distress necessitate emergency treatment. Tracheotomy, positive-pressure ventilation, and vigorous suctioning to remove secretions usually produce improvement in a few days.

Because anticholinesterase drugs aren't effective in myasthenic crisis, they're stopped until respiratory function improves. Myasthenic crisis requires immediate hospitalization and vigorous respiratory support.

## Special considerations

• Careful baseline assessment, early recognition and treatment of potential crises, supportive measures, and thorough patient teaching can minimize exacerbations and complications. Continuity of care is essential.

• Establish an accurate neurologic and respiratory baseline. Thereafter, monitor tidal volume and vital capacity regularly. The patient may need a ventilator and frequent suctioning to remove accumulating secretions.

• Be alert for signs of an impending crisis (increased muscle weakness, respiratory distress, difficulty in talking or chewing).

• Space administration of drugs evenly, and give them on time to prevent relapses. Be prepared to give atropine for anticholinesterase overdose or toxicity.

• Plan exercise, meals, patient care, and activities to make the most of energy peaks. For example, give medication 20 to 30 minutes before meals to facilitate chewing or swallowing. Allow the patient to participate in self-care.

• When swallowing is difficult, give soft, solid foods instead of liquids to lessen the risk of choking.

• After a severe exacerbation, try to increase social activity as soon as possible.

• Patient teaching is essential because myasthenia gravis is usually a lifelong condition.

➤ CLINICAL TIP  Teach the patient to avoid or closely monitor the effects of certain drugs. Curare-like drugs, local anesthetics, common cold products, tonic water and antiarrhythmics containing quinine, aminoglycoside antibiotics, tetracyclines, morphine sulphate, beta blockers, and calcium channel blockers may worsen muscle weakness by impairing the transmission of impulses across the neuromuscular junction.

# MYELITIS AND ACUTE TRANSVERSE MYELITIS

Myelitis, or inflammation of the spinal cord, can result from several diseases. Poliomyelitis affects the cord's gray matter and produces motor dysfunction; leukomyelitis affects only the white matter and produces sensory dysfunction. These types of myelitis can attack any level of the spinal cord, causing partial destruction or scattered lesions.

Acute transverse myelitis, which affects the entire thickness of the spinal cord, produces both motor and sensory dysfunctions. This form of myelitis, which has a rapid onset, is the most devastating.

The prognosis depends on the severity of cord damage and prevention of complications. If spinal cord necrosis occurs, the prognosis for complete recovery is poor. Even without necrosis, residual neurologic deficits usually persist after recovery. Patients who develop spastic reflexes early in the course of the illness are more likely to recover than those who don't.

## Causes

Acute transverse myelitis has a variety of causes. It often follows acute infectious diseases, such as measles or pneumonia (the inflammation occurs after the infection has subsided), and primary infections of the spinal cord itself, such as syphilis or acute disseminated encephalomyelitis.

Acute transverse myelitis can accompany demyelinating diseases, such as acute multiple sclerosis, and inflammatory and necrotizing disorders of the spinal cord, such as hematomyelia.

Certain toxic agents (carbon monoxide, lead, and arsenic) can cause a type of myelitis in which acute inflammation (followed by hemorrhage and possible necrosis) destroys the entire circumference (myelin, axis cylinders, and neurons) of the spinal cord.

Other forms of myelitis may result from poliovirus, herpes zoster, herpesvirus B, or rabies virus; disorders that cause meningeal inflammation, such as syphilis, abscesses and other suppurative conditions, and tuberculosis; smallpox or polio vaccination; parasitic and fungal infections; and chronic adhesive arachnoiditis.

### Signs and symptoms

In acute transverse myelitis, onset is rapid, with motor and sensory dysfunctions below the level of spinal cord damage appearing in 1 to 2 days.

Patients with acute transverse myelitis develop flaccid paralysis of the legs (sometimes beginning in just one leg) with loss of sensory and sphincter functions. Such sensory loss may follow pain in the legs or trunk. Reflexes disappear in the early stages but may reappear later. The extent of damage depends on which level of the spinal cord is affected; transverse myelitis rarely involves the arms. If spinal cord damage is severe, it may cause shock (hypotension and hypothermia).

### Diagnosis

Paraplegia of rapid onset usually points to acute transverse myelitis. In such patients, neurologic examination confirms paraplegia or neurologic deficit below the level of the spinal cord lesion and absent or, later, hyperactive reflexes. Cerebrospinal fluid may be normal or show increased lymphocyte or protein levels.

CLINICAL TIP  Diagnostic evaluation must rule out a spinal cord tumor and identify the cause of any underlying infection.

### Treatment

No effective treatment exists for acute transverse myelitis. However, this condition requires appropriate treatment of any underlying infection. Some patients with postinfectious or multiple sclerosis-induced myelitis have received steroid therapy, but its benefits aren't clear.

### Special considerations

• Frequently assess vital signs. Watch carefully for signs of spinal shock (hypotension and excessive sweating).

• Prevent contractures with range-of-motion exercises and proper alignment.

• Watch for signs of urinary tract infections from indwelling urinary catheters.

• Prevent skin infections and pressure ulcers with meticulous skin care. Check pressure points often and keep skin clean and dry; use a water bed or another pressure-relieving device.

• Initiate rehabilitation immediately. Assist the patient with physical therapy, bowel and bladder training, and any lifestyle changes that his condition requires.

---

**LIFE-THREATENING DISORDER**

# MYOCARDIAL INFARCTION

In myocardial infarction (MI), also known as heart attack, reduced blood flow through one of the coronary arteries results in myocardial ischemia and necrosis. In cardiovascular disease, the leading cause of death in the United States and western Europe, death usually results from the cardiac damage or complications of MI.

Mortality is high when treatment is delayed; almost half of all sudden deaths due to an MI occur before hospitalization, within 1 hour of the onset of symptoms. The prognosis improves if vigorous treatment begins immediately.

## Causes

Predisposing factors include:
- positive family history
- hypertension
- smoking
- elevated levels of serum triglycerides, total cholesterol, and low-density lipoproteins
- diabetes mellitus
- obesity or excessive intake of saturated fats, carbohydrates, or salt
- sedentary lifestyle
- aging
- stress or a Type A personality (aggressive, ambitious, competitive, addicted to work, chronically impatient)
- drug use, especially cocaine.

Men and postmenopausal women are more susceptible to MI than premenopausal women, although incidence is rising among females, especially those who smoke and take oral contraceptives.

The site of the MI depends on the vessels involved. Occlusion of the circumflex branch of the left coronary artery causes a lateral wall infarction; occlusion of the anterior descending branch of the left coronary artery, an anterior wall infarction.

True posterior or inferior wall infarctions generally result from occlusion of the right coronary artery or one of its branches. Right ventricular infarctions can also result from right coronary artery occlusion, can accompany inferior infarctions, and may cause right heart failure. In transmural MI, tissue damage extends through all myocardial layers; in subendocardial MI, only in the innermost and possibly the middle layers.

## Signs and symptoms

The cardinal symptoms of MI is persistent, crushing substernal pain that may radiate to the left arm, jaw, neck, or shoulder blades. Such pain is often described as heavy, squeezing, or crushing and may persist for 12 hours or more. However, in some MI patients — particularly older adults or diabetics — pain may not occur at all; in others, it may be mild and confused with indigestion.

In patients with coronary artery disease, angina of increasing frequency, severity, or duration (especially if not provoked by exertion, a heavy meal, or cold and wind) may signal impending infarction.

### Other features

Other clinical effects include a feeling of impending doom, fatigue, nausea, vomiting, and shortness of breath. Some patients may have no symptoms. The patient may experience catecholamine responses, such as coolness in extremities, perspiration, anxiety, and restlessness. Fever is unusual at the onset of an MI, but a low-grade fever may develop during the next few days. Blood pressure varies; hypotension or hypertension may be present.

### Complications

The most common post-MI complications include recurrent or persistent chest pain, arrhythmias, left ventricular failure (resulting in heart failure or acute pulmonary edema), and cardiogenic shock. Unusual but potentially lethal complications that may develop soon after infarction include thromboembolism; papillary muscle dysfunction or rupture, causing mitral insufficiency; rupture of the ventricular septum, causing ventricular septal defect; rupture of the myocardium; and ventricular aneurysm.

Up to several months after infarction, Dressler's syndrome may develop (pericarditis, pericardial friction rub, chest pain, fever, leukocytosis and, possibly, pleurisy or pneumonitis). (See *Complications of myocardial infarction,* pages 560 and 561.)

### Diagnosis

Persistent chest pain, ST-segment changes on the electrocardiogram (ECG), and elevated levels of total creatine kinase (CK) and the CK-MB isoenzyme over a 72-hour period usually confirm MI. Auscultation may reveal diminished heart sounds, gallops and, in papillary dysfunction, the apical systolic murmur of mitral insufficiency over the mitral valve area.

When clinical features are equivocal, assume that the patient has had an MI until tests rule it out. Diagnostic test results include the following:

● *serial 12-lead ECG:* ECG abnormalities may be absent or inconclusive during the first few hours following an MI. When present, characteristic abnormalities include serial ST-segment depression in subendocardial MI and ST-segment elevation in transmural MI.

● *serial serum enzyme levels:* CK levels are elevated specifically, CK-MB or troponin levels.

● *echocardiography:* may show ventricular wall motion abnormalities in patients with a transmural MI.

Scans using I.V. technetium 99 can identify acutely damaged muscle by picking up radioactive nucleotide, which appears as a "hot spot" on the film. They are useful in localizing a recent MI.

### Treatment

The goals of treatment are to relieve chest pain, to stabilize heart rhythm, to reduce cardiac workload, to revascularize the coronary artery, and to preserve myocardial tissue. Arrhythmias,

the predominant problem during the first 48 hours after the infarction, may require antiarrhythmics, possibly a pacemaker and, rarely, cardioversion.

To preserve myocardial tissue, thrombolytic therapy should be started I.V. within 3 hours after the onset of symptoms (unless contraindications exist). Thrombolytic therapy includes either streptokinase, alteplase, recombinant tissue plasminogen activator (t-PA), retivase, or urokinase.

Percutaneous transluminal coronary angioplasty (PTCA) may be another option. If PTCA is performed soon after the onset of symptoms, the thrombolytic agent may be administered directly into the coronary artery.

Other treatments consist of:

● aspirin (5 g) to inhibit platelet aggregation (should be initiated within 24 hours after onset of symptoms)

● lidocaine or other drugs, such as procainamide, quinidine, bretylium, or disopyramide, for ventricular arrhythmias

● atropine I.V. or a temporary pacemaker for heart block or bradycardia

● nitroglycerin (sublingual, topical, transdermal, or I.V.) or isosorbide dinitrate (sublingual, oral, or I.V.) to relieve pain by redistributing blood to ischemic areas of the myocardium, increasing cardiac output, and reducing myocardial workload

● diltiazem and verapamil (sublingual, oral, or I.V.), which may prevent reinfarction and ischemia in a non-Q-wave MI

● heparin I.V. (usually follows thrombolytic therapy)

● morphine I.V. for pain and sedation

● bed rest with bedside commode to decrease cardiac workload

● oxygen administration at a modest flow rate for 3 to 6 hours (a lower concentration is necessary if the patient has chronic obstructive pulmonary disease)

# COMPLICATIONS OF MYOCARDIAL INFARCTION

| COMPLICATION | DIAGNOSIS | TREATMENT |
|---|---|---|
| Arrhythmias | • Electrocardiography (ECG) shows premature ventricular contractions, ventricular tachycardia, or ventricular fibrillation; in inferior wall myocardial infarction (MI), bradycardia and junctional rhythms or atrioventricular block; in anterior wall MI, tachycardia or heart block. | • Antiarrhythmics, atropine, cardioversion, and pacemaker |
| Heart failure | • In left ventricular failure, chest X-rays show venous congestion, cardiomegaly, and Kerley's B lines.<br>• Catheterization shows increased pulmonary artery pressure (PAP) and central venous pressure. | • Diuretics, vasodilators, inotropic agents, and digitalis glycosides |
| Cardiogenic shock | • Catheterization shows decreased cardiac output and increased PAP and pulmonary artery wedge pressure (PAWP).<br>• Signs include hypotension, tachycardia, S3, S4, decreased level of consciousness, decreased urine output, neck vein distention, and cool, pale skin. | • I.V. fluids, vasodilators, diuretics, digitalis glycosides, intra-aortic balloon pump (IABP), and beta-adrenergic stimulants |
| Rupture of left ventricular papillary muscle | • Auscultation reveals apical holosystolic murmur. Inspection of jugular vein pulse or hemodynamic monitoring shows increased v waves.<br>• Dyspnea is prominent.<br>• Color-flow and Doppler echocardiogram show mitral insufficiency. Pulmonary artery catheterization shows increased PAP and PAWP. | • Nitroprusside<br>• IABP<br>• Surgical replacement of the mitral valve with possible concomitant myocardial revascularization (in patients with significant coronary artery disease) |
| Ventricular septal rupture | • In left-to-right shunt, auscultation reveals holosystolic murmur and thrill.<br>• Catheterization shows increased PAP and PAWP.<br>• Confirmation by increased oxygen saturation of right ventricle and pulmonary artery.<br>• Color-flow/Doppler echocardiography demonstrates left-to-right blood flow across the septum. | • Surgical correction, IABP, nitroglycerin, nitroprusside, low-dose inotropic agents, or pacemaker |

## COMPLICATIONS OF MYOCARDIAL INFARCTION *(continued)*

| COMPLICATION | DIAGNOSIS | TREATMENT |
|---|---|---|
| Pericarditis or Dressler's syndrome | • Auscultation reveals a friction rub.<br>• Chest pain is relieved by sitting up. | • Nonsteroidal anti-inflammatory drugs or corticosteroids |
| Ventricular aneurysm | • Chest X-ray may show cardiomegaly.<br>• ECG may show arrhythmias and persistent ST-segment elevation.<br>• Left ventriculography or echocardiography shows altered or paradoxical left ventricular motion. | • Cardioversion, defibrillation, antiarrhythmics, vasodilators, anticoagulants, digitalis glycosides, and diuretics. If conservative treatment fails, surgical resection is necessary. |
| Thromboembolism | • Severe dyspnea and chest pain or neurologic changes<br>• Nuclear scan shows ventilation-perfusion mismatch.<br>• Angiography shows arterial blockage. | • Oxygen and heparin |

• drugs to increase myocardial contractility or blood pressure

• beta-adrenergic blockers, such as propranolol or timolol, after acute MI to help prevent reinfarction

• pulmonary artery catheterization to detect left or right ventricular failure and to monitor the patient's response to treatment

• angiotensin-converting enzyme inhibitors to improve survival rate in a low ejection fraction (large anterior wall MI).

**Special considerations**

• Care for patients who have suffered an MI is directed toward detecting complications, preventing further myocardial damage, and promoting comfort, rest, and emotional well-being. Most MI patients receive treatment in the coronary care unit (CCU), where they're under constant observation for complications.

• On admission to the CCU, monitor and record the patient's ECG, blood pressure, temperature, and heart and breath sounds.

• Assess and record the severity and duration of pain; administer analgesics. Avoid I.M. injections; absorption from the muscle is unpredictable.

• Check the patient's blood pressure after giving nitroglycerin, especially the first dose.

• Frequently monitor the ECG to detect rate changes or arrhythmias. Place rhythm strips in the patient's chart periodically for evaluation.

• During episodes of chest pain, obtain ECG, blood pressure, and pulmonary artery catheter measurements for changes.

• Watch for signs and symptoms of fluid retention (crackles, cough, tachypnea, edema), which may indicate impending heart failure. Carefully monitor daily weight, intake and output, respirations, serum enzyme levels, and blood pressure.

• Auscultate for adventitious breath sounds periodically (patients on bed rest frequently have atelectatic crackles, which may disappear after coughing) and for $S_3$ or $S_4$ gallops.

• Organize patient care and activities to maximize periods of uninterrupted rest.

• Ask the dietary department to provide a clear liquid diet until nausea subsides. A low-cholesterol, low-sodium, caffeine-free diet may be ordered.

• Provide a stool softener to prevent straining during defecation, which causes vagal stimulation and may slow the heart rate. Allow use of a bedside commode, and provide as much privacy as possible.

• Assist with range-of-motion exercises. If the patient is completely immobilized by a severe MI, turn him often.

• Antiembolism stockings help prevent venostasis and thrombophlebitis.

• Provide emotional support, and help reduce stress and anxiety; administer tranquilizers as needed.

• Explain procedures and answer questions. Explaining the CCU environment and routine can ease anxiety. Involve the patient's family in his care as much as possible.

To prepare for discharge:

• Promote adherence measures by thoroughly explaining the prescribed medication regimen and other treatment measures.

• Warn about adverse reactions to drugs, and advise the patient to watch for and report signs of toxicity (anorexia, nausea, vomiting, and yellow vision, for example, if the patient is receiving digoxin).

• Review dietary restrictions with the patient. If he must follow a low-sodium or low-fat and low-cholesterol diet, provide a list of foods that he should avoid. Ask the dietitian to speak to the patient and his family.

• Counsel the patient to resume sexual activity progressively.

➤ CLINICAL TIP Advise the patient to report typical or atypical chest pain. Postinfarction syndrome may develop, producing chest pain that must be differentiated from recurrent MI, pulmonary infarct, or heart failure.

• If the patient has a Holter monitor in place, explain its purpose and use.

• Stress the need to stop smoking.

• Encourage participation in a cardiac rehabilitation program.

# MYOCARDITIS

Myocarditis is focal or diffuse inflammation of the cardiac muscle (myocardium). It may be acute or chronic and can occur at any age. Frequently, myocarditis fails to produce specific cardiovascular symptoms or electrocardiogram (ECG) abnormalities, and recovery is usually spontaneous, without residual defects. Occasionally, myocarditis is complicated by heart failure; rarely, it may lead to cardiomyopathy.

## Causes

Myocarditis may result from:

• *viral infections* (most common cause in the United States and western Europe): coxsackievirus A and B strains and, possibly, poliomyelitis, influenza, rubeola, rubella, and adenoviruses and echoviruses

• *bacterial infections:* diphtheria, tuberculosis, typhoid fever, tetanus, and staphylococcal, pneumococcal, and gonococcal infections

• *hypersensitive immune reactions:* acute rheumatic fever and postcardiotomy syndrome

• *radiation therapy:* large doses of radiation to the chest in treating lung or breast cancer

• *chemical poisons:* such as chronic alcoholism

• *parasitic infections:* especially South American trypanosomiasis (Chagas' disease) in infants and immunosuppressed adults; also, toxoplasmosis

• *helminthic infections:* such as trichinosis.

### Signs and symptoms

Myocarditis usually causes nonspecific symptoms — such as fatigue, dyspnea, palpitations, and fever — that reflect the accompanying systemic infection. Occasionally, it may produce mild, continuous pressure or soreness in the chest (unlike the recurring, stress-related pain of angina pectoris).

Although myocarditis is usually self-limiting, it may induce myofibril degeneration that results in right and left heart failure, with cardiomegaly, neck vein distention, dyspnea, persistent fever with resting or exertional tachycardia disproportionate to the degree of fever, and supraventricular and ventricular arrhythmias.

Sometimes myocarditis recurs or produces chronic valvulitis (when it results from rheumatic fever), cardiomyopathy, arrhythmias, and thromboembolism.

### Diagnosis

The patient history commonly reveals recent febrile upper respiratory tract infection, viral pharyngitis, or tonsillitis. A physical examination shows supraventricular and ventricular arrhythmias, $S_3$ and $S_4$ gallops, a faint $S_1$, possibly a murmur of mitral insufficiency (from papillary muscle dysfunction) and, if pericarditis is present, a pericardial friction rub.

Electrocardiography typically shows diffuse ST-segment and T-wave abnormalities (as in pericarditis), conduction defects (prolonged PR interval), and other supraventricular arrhythmias.

Stool and throat cultures may identify the causative bacteria. An endomyocardial biopsy is used to confirm the diagnosis, but a negative biopsy doesn't exclude the diagnosis. A repeat biopsy may be needed.

Laboratory tests can't unequivocally confirm myocarditis, but the following findings support this diagnosis:

• *Cardiac enzyme levels* (creatine kinase [CK], the CK-MB isoenzyme, aspartate aminotransferase, and lactate dehydrogenase) are elevated.

• *White blood cell count* and *erythrocyte sedimentation rate* are increased.

• *Antibody titers* (such as antistreptolysin O titer in rheumatic fever) are elevated.

### Treatment

In MI, treatment includes antibiotics for bacterial infection, modified bed rest to decrease the cardiac workload, and careful management of complications. Heart failure requires restriction of activity to minimize myocardial oxygen consumption, supplemental oxygen therapy, sodium restriction, diuretics to decrease fluid retention, and digitalis glycosides to increase myocardial contractility. However, digitalis glycosides must be administered cautiously because some patients with myocarditis show a paradoxical sensitivity to even small doses.

Arrhythmias necessitate prompt but cautious administration of antiarrhythmics, such as quinidine or procainamide, because these drugs depress myocardial contractility. Thromboembolism requires anticoagulation therapy. Treatment with corticosteroids or other immunosuppressants is controversial and therefore limited to combating life-threatening complications such as intractable heart failure.

### Special considerations
• Assess cardiovascular status frequently, watching for signs of heart failure, such as dyspnea, hypotension, and tachycardia. Check for changes in cardiac rhythm or conduction.
• Observe for signs of digitalis toxicity (anorexia, nausea, vomiting, blurred vision, cardiac arrhythmias) and for complicating factors that may potentiate toxicity, such as electrolyte imbalances or hypoxia.
• Stress the importance of bed rest. Assist with bathing as necessary; provide a bedside commode, which puts less stress on the heart than using a bedpan. Reassure the patient that activity limitations are temporary.
• Offer diversional activities that are physically undemanding.

➤ CLINICAL TIP During recovery, recommend that the patient resume normal activities slowly and avoid competitive sports.

# MYRINGITIS, INFECTIOUS

Acute infectious myringitis is characterized by inflammation, hemorrhage, and effusion of fluid into the tissue at the end of the external ear canal and the tympanic membrane. This self-limiting disorder (resolving spontaneously within 3 days to 2 weeks) often follows acute otitis media or upper respiratory tract infection and frequently occurs epidemically in children.

Chronic granular myringitis, a rare inflammation of the squamous layer of the tympanic membrane, causes gradual hearing loss. Without specific treatment, this condition can lead to stenosis of the ear canal, as granulation extends from the tympanic membrane to the external ear.

### Causes
Acute infectious myringitis usually follows viral infection but may also result from infection with bacteria (pneumococci, *Haemophilus influenzae,* beta-hemolytic streptococci, staphylococci) or any other organism that may cause acute otitis media. Myringitis is a rare sequela of atypical pneumonia caused by *Mycoplasma pneumoniae.* The cause of chronic granular myringitis is unknown.

### Signs and symptoms
Acute infectious myringitis begins with severe ear pain, commonly accompanied by tenderness over the mastoid process. Small, reddened, inflamed blebs form in the canal, on the tympanic membrane and, with bacterial invasion, in the middle ear.

Fever and hearing loss are rare unless fluid accumulates in the middle ear or a large bleb totally obstructs the external auditory meatus. Spontaneous rupture of these blebs may cause bloody discharge. Chronic granular myringitis produces pruritus, purulent discharge, and gradual hearing loss.

### Diagnosis
In acute infectious myringitis, the diagnosis is based on a physical examination showing characteristic blebs and on a typical patient history. Culture and sensitivity testing of exudate identifies secondary infection. In chronic granular myringitis, physical examination may

reveal granulation extending from the tympanic membrane to the external ear.

**Treatment**

Hospitalization usually isn't required for acute infectious myringitis. Treatment consists of measures to relieve pain. Analgesics, such as aspirin or acetaminophen, and application of heat to the external ear are usually sufficient, but severe pain may necessitate the use of codeine.

Systemic or topical antibiotics prevent or treat secondary infection. Incision of the blebs and evacuation of serum and blood may relieve pressure and help drain exudate, but these measures don't speed recovery.

Treatment of chronic granular myringitis consists of systemic antibiotics or local anti-inflammatory antibiotic combination eardrops, and surgical excision and cautery. If stenosis is present, surgical reconstruction is necessary.

**Special considerations**

• Stress the importance of completing prescribed antibiotic therapy.
• Teach the patient how to instill topical antibiotics (eardrops). When necessary, explain incision of the blebs.

➤ CLINICAL TIP To help prevent acute infectious myringitis, advise early treatment of acute otitis media.

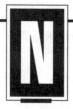

# NASAL PAPILLOMAS

A papilloma is a benign epithelial tissue overgrowth within the intranasal mucosa. Inverted papillomas grow into the underlying tissue, usually at the junction of the antrum and the ethmoidal sinus; they generally occur singly but sometimes are associated with squamous cell cancer.

Exophytic papillomas, which also tend to occur singly, arise from epithelial tissue, commonly on the surface of the nasal septum. Both types of papillomas are most prevalent in males. Recurrence is likely, even after surgical excision.

### Causes
A papilloma may arise as a benign precursor of a neoplasm or as a response to tissue injury or viral infection, but its cause is unknown.

### Signs and symptoms
Both inverted and exophytic papillomas typically produce symptoms related to unilateral nasal obstruction—stuffiness, postnasal drip, headache, shortness of breath, dyspnea and, rarely, severe respiratory distress, nasal drainage, and infection. Epistaxis is most likely to occur with exophytic papillomas.

### Diagnosis
On examination of the nasal mucosa, inverted papillomas usually appear large, bulky, highly vascular, and edematous; color varies from dark red to gray; consistency, from firm to friable. Exophytic papillomas are commonly raised, firm, and rubbery-pink to gray and securely attached by a broad or pedunculated base to the mucous membrane. Histologic examination of excised tissue confirms the diagnosis.

### Treatment
The most effective treatment is wide surgical excision or diathermy, with careful inspection of adjacent tissues and sinuses to rule out extension. The use of surgical lasers is another option. Aspirin or acetaminophen and decongestants may relieve symptoms.

### Special considerations
● If bleeding occurs, have the patient sit upright, and instruct him to expectorate blood into an emesis basin. Compress both sides of the patient's nose against the septum for 10 to 15 minutes and apply ice compresses to the nose.
● Check for airway obstruction. Place your hand under the patient's nostrils to assess air exchange, and watch for signs of mild shortness of breath.
● If surgery is scheduled, tell the patient what to expect postoperatively. Instruct him not to blow his nose. (The packing is usually removed 12 to 24 hours after surgery.)
● Postoperatively, monitor vital signs and respiratory status. Use pulse oximetry to monitor oxygen saturation levels.

• As needed, administer analgesics and facilitate breathing with a cool-mist vaporizer. Provide mouth care.

• Frequently change the mustache dressing or drip pad to ensure proper absorption of drainage. Record the type and amount of drainage.

**CLINICAL TIP** While the nasal packing is in place, expect scant, usually bright red, clotted drainage. Remember that the amount of drainage often increases for a few hours after the packing is removed.

• Because papillomas tend to recur, tell the patient to seek medical attention at the first sign of nasal discomfort, discharge, or congestion that doesn't subside with conservative treatment.

• Encourage regular follow-up visits to detect early signs of recurrence.

• For more postoperative patient-teaching information, see *Papillomas: Recovering after surgery.*

## NASAL POLYPS

Benign and edematous growths, nasal polyps are usually multiple, mobile, and bilateral. Nasal polyps may become large and numerous enough to cause nasal distention and enlargement of the bony framework, possibly occluding the airway. They're more common in adults than in children and tend to recur.

### Causes

Nasal polyps are usually produced by the continuous pressure resulting from a chronic allergy that causes prolonged mucous membrane edema in the nose and sinuses. Other predisposing factors include chronic sinusitis, chronic rhinitis, and recurrent nasal infections.

TEACHING CHECKLIST

## PAPILLOMAS: RECOVERING AFTER SURGERY

Review these points with your patient prior to discharge after nasal papilloma surgery.

• Nasal edema will persist for 10 to 14 days; minimal blood-tinged mucus drainage will be present for 10 to 14 days; discomfort can be expected for 7 to 10 days, but actual pain should be reported to the doctor.

• Elevate the head of the bed to facilitate breathing, reduce swelling, and promote adequate drainage.

• Don't blow your nose for 10 days.

• Sneeze with your mouth open to avoid increasing intranasal pressure and bleeding.

• Avoid lifting, straining, and exercise for at least 14 days or as instructed by the doctor.

• Avoid smoking and other noxious fumes that may irritate the nose.

### Signs and symptoms

Nasal obstruction is the primary indication of nasal polyps. Such obstruction causes anosmia, a sensation of fullness in the face, nasal discharge, headache, and shortness of breath. Associated clinical features are usually symptomatic of allergic rhinitis.

### Diagnosis

The following tests are used to diagnose nasal polyps:

• *X-rays of sinuses and nasal passages* reveal soft-tissue shadows over the affected areas.

• *Examination with a nasal speculum* shows a dry, red surface, with clear or gray growths. Large growths may resemble tumors.

TEACHING CHECKLIST

## NASAL POLYPS: RECOVERING AFTER SURGERY

Review these teaching points with your patient before discharge.

• Nasal edema will persist for 10 to 14 days; minimal blood-tinged mucus drainage will be present for 10 to 14 days; discomfort can be expected for 7 to 10 days, but actual pain should be reported to the doctor.
• Don't blow your nose for 10 days.
• Sneeze with your mouth open to avoid increasing intranasal pressure and bleeding.
• Increase humidification by using a bedside humidifier.
• Avoid lifting, straining, and exercise for at least 14 days or as instructed by the doctor.
• Avoid smoking and other noxious fumes that may irritate the nose.

Nasal polyps occurring in children require further testing to rule out cystic fibrosis and Peutz-Jeghers syndrome.

## Treatment

Generally, treatment consists of corticosteroids (either by direct injection into the polyps or by local spray) to temporarily reduce the polyp. Treatment of the underlying cause may include antihistamines to control allergy and antibiotic therapy if infection is present. Local application of an astringent shrinks hypertrophied tissue. However, medical management alone is rarely effective.

Consequently, the treatment of choice is polypectomy, which is usually performed under a local anesthetic. The use of surgical lasers is becoming more popular. Continued recurrence may require surgical opening of the ethmoid and maxillary sinuses and evacuation of diseased tissue.

## Special considerations

• Give antihistamines, as needed, to the patient with allergies.
• Prepare the patient for scheduled surgery by telling him what to expect postoperatively, for example, nasal packing for 1 to 2 days after surgery.

After surgery:

• Monitor for excessive bleeding or other drainage, and promote patient comfort.
• Elevate the head of the bed to facilitate breathing, reduce swelling, and promote adequate drainage.
• Change the mustache dressing or drip pad, as needed, and record the consistency, amount. and color of nasal drainage.
• Intermittently apply ice compresses over the nostrils to lessen swelling, prevent bleeding, and relieve pain.
• If nasal bleeding occurs — most likely after packing is removed — have the patient sit upright, monitor his vital signs, and advise him not to swallow blood.

CLINICAL TIP   Compress the outside of the patient's nose against the septum for 10 to 15 minutes. If bleeding persists, nasal packing may be necessary.
• For more postoperative patient-teaching information, see *Nasal polyps: Recovering after surgery.*

To prevent nasal polyps, instruct patients with allergies to avoid exposure to allergens and to take antihistamines at the first sign of an allergic reaction. Also, advise them to avoid overuse of nose drops and sprays.

✸ LIFE-THREATENING
DISORDER

# NEAR DROWNING

Near drowning refers to surviving — temporarily, at least — the physiologic effects of hypoxemia and acidosis that result from submersion in fluid. Hypoxemia and acidosis are the primary problems in victims of near drowning.

Near drowning occurs in three forms:
• "dry" — the victim doesn't aspirate fluid but suffers respiratory obstruction or asphyxia (10% to 15% of patients)
• "wet" — the victim aspirates fluid and suffers from asphyxia or secondary changes due to fluid aspiration (about 85% of patients)
• secondary — the victim suffers recurrence of respiratory distress (usually aspiration pneumonia or pulmonary edema) within minutes or 1 to 2 days after a near-drowning incident.

## Causes

In the United States, drowning claims nearly 8,000 lives annually. No statistics are available for near-drowning incidents. Near drowning results from an inability to swim or, in swimmers, from panic, a boating accident, a heart attack or a blow to the head while in the water, drinking heavily before swimming, or a suicide attempt.

### Results of aspiration

Regardless of the tonicity of the fluid aspirated, hypoxemia is the most serious consequence of near drowning, followed by metabolic acidosis. Other consequences depend on the kind of water aspirated.

After freshwater aspiration, changes in the character of lung surfactant result in exudation of protein-rich plasma into the alveoli. This, plus increased capillary permeability, leads to pulmonary edema and hypoxemia.

After saltwater aspiration, the hypertonicity of sea water exerts an osmotic force, which pulls fluid from pulmonary capillaries into the alveoli. The resulting intrapulmonary shunt causes hypoxemia. Also, the pulmonary capillary membrane may be injured and induce pulmonary edema. In both kinds of near drowning, pulmonary edema and hypoxemia occur secondary to aspiration.

## Signs and symptoms

Near-drowning victims can display a host of clinical problems: apnea, shallow or gasping respirations, substernal chest pain, asystole, tachycardia, bradycardia, restlessness, irritability, lethargy, fever, confusion, unconsciousness, vomiting, abdominal distention, and a cough that produces a pink, frothy fluid.

## Diagnosis

A history of near drowning along with characteristic features and auscultation of crackles and rhonchi are required for a diagnosis. Supportive tests include:
• *blood tests:* may show leukocytosis
• *arterial blood gas (ABG) analysis:* shows decreased oxygen content, a low bicarbonate level, and low pH
• *electrocardiography:* shows supraventricular tachycardia, occasional premature ventricular contractions, nonspecific ST segment, and T-wave abnormalities.

## Treatment

• Begin emergency treatment with cardiopulmonary resuscitation (CPR) and administration of 100% oxygen.
• Stabilize the patient's neck in case he has a cervical injury.

• When the patient arrives at the facility, assess for a patent airway. Establish one if necessary.

• Continue CPR, intubate the patient, and provide respiratory assistance such as mechanical ventilation with positive end-expiratory pressure if needed.

• Assess ABG and pulse oximetry values.

• If the patient's abdomen is distended, insert a nasogastric tube. (Intubate the patient first if he's unconscious.)

• Start I.V. lines; insert an indwelling urinary catheter.

• Give medications as necessary. Much controversy exists about the benefits of drug treatment of near-drowning victims. However, such treatment may include sodium bicarbonate for acidosis, corticosteroids for cerebral edema, antibiotics to prevent infections, and bronchodilators to ease bronchospasms.

**Special considerations**

• Observe for pulmonary complications and signs of delayed drowning (confusion, substernal pain, adventitious breath sounds). Suction often. Pulmonary artery catheters may be useful in assessing cardiopulmonary status.

▶ CLINICAL TIP  Remember, all near-drowning victims should be admitted for an observation period of 24 to 48 hours because of the possibility of delayed drowning.

• Monitor vital signs, intake and output, and peripheral pulses. Check for skin perfusion. Watch for signs of infection.

• To facilitate breathing, raise the head of the bed slightly.

• To prevent near drowning, advise swimmers to avoid drinking alcohol before swimming, to observe water safety measures, and to take a water safety course sponsored by the Red Cross, YMCA, or YWCA.

---

◆ LIFE-THREATENING DISORDER

# NECROTIZING ENTEROCOLITIS

Neonatal necrotizing enterocolitis (NEC) is a clinical condition characterized by an initial mucosal intestinal injury that may progress to transmural bowel necrosis. Although NEC occurs frequently, its cause is unknown. NEC is the leading surgical emergency in neonates in North America.

With early detection, the survival rate is 60% to 80%. Infectious complications associated with bowel necrosis include bacterial peritonitis, systemic sepsis, and intra-abdominal abscess formation.

**Causes**

NEC occurs most often in premature infants ($<34$ weeks' gestation) and those of low birth weight ($<5$ lb [2.3 kg]). NEC is occurring more frequently, possibly because of the higher incidence and survival of premature and low-birth-weight infants.

▶ CLINICAL TIP  More than 90% of NEC cases occur after initiation of feedings.

One in ten infants who develop NEC is full-term. Among premature and low-birth-weight infants in intensive care nurseries, incidence varies from 1% to 12%. NEC is associated with 2% of all infant deaths.

*Possible risk factors*

The exact cause of NEC is unknown. Suggested predisposing factors include birth asphyxia, postnatal hypotension, respiratory failure, hypothermia, sepsis, acidosis, and structural cardiac defects as well as pharmacologic associations, such as cocaine exposure and indomethacin treatment.

NEC may also be a response to significant prenatal stress, such as premature rupture of membranes, placenta previa, maternal sepsis, toxemia of pregnancy, or breech or cesarean birth.

### *Causative theory*
According to current theory, NEC develops when the infant suffers perinatal hypoxemia due to shunting of blood from the gut to more vital organs. Subsequent mucosal ischemia provides an ideal medium for bacterial growth. Hypertonic formula may increase bacterial activity because—unlike maternal breast milk—it doesn't provide protective immunity and because it contributes to the production of hydrogen gas. As the bowel swells and breaks down, gas-forming bacteria invade damaged areas, producing free air in the intestinal wall. This may result in fatal perforation and peritonitis.

### Signs and symptoms
Any infant who has suffered from perinatal hypoxemia has the potential for developing NEC. A distended (especially tense or rigid) abdomen, with gastric retention, is the earliest and most common sign of oncoming NEC, usually appearing from 1 to 10 days after birth.

Other clinical features are increasing residual gastric contents (which may contain bile), bilious vomitus, and occult or gross blood in stools. One-fourth of patients have bloody diarrhea. A red or shiny, taut abdomen may indicate peritonitis.

Nonspecific signs and symptoms include thermal instability, lethargy, metabolic acidosis, jaundice, and disseminated intravascular coagulation (DIC).

The major complication is perforation, which requires surgery.

Recurrence of NEC and mechanical and functional abnormalities of the intestine, especially stricture, are the usual cause of residual intestinal malfunction in any infant who survives acute NEC and may develop as late as 3 months postoperatively.

### Diagnosis
Successful treatment of NEC relies on early recognition based on the following diagnostic test results:

● *Anteroposterior and lateral abdominal X-rays* confirm the diagnosis by showing nonspecific intestinal dilation and, in later stages of NEC, pneumatosis cystoides intestinalis (gas or air in the intestinal wall). Portal vein gas and fixed or thickened small bowel loops are also important radiographic findings. Sequential screening films are taken every 6 to 8 hours during the early disease stages.
● *Platelet count* may fall below 50,000/μl.
● *Serum sodium levels* are decreased.
● *Arterial blood gas (ABG) levels* show metabolic acidosis (a result of sepsis).
● *Bilirubin levels* show infection-induced breakdown of red blood cells.
● *Blood and stool cultures* identify the infecting organism.
● *Guaiac test* detects occult blood in stools.

### Treatment
Up to 90% of infants with NEC can be managed without surgery. The first signs of NEC necessitate discontinuation of oral intake to rest the injured bowel. I.V. fluids, including total parenteral nutrition, maintain fluid and electrolyte balance and nutrition during this time; passage of a nasogastric (NG) tube allows bowel decompression.

Correction of hypoxemia, hypotension, acidosis, and any other reversible

> **CLINICAL TIP**
>
> # RECOGNIZING OMINOUS SIGNS IN NECROTIZING ENTEROCOLITIS
>
> When an infant suffers perinatal hypoxemia, be alert for the following signs of gastric distention and perforation:
>
> - apnea
> - cardiovascular shock
> - sudden drop in temperature
> - sudden listlessness and ragdoll limpness
>
> - bradycardia
> - increasing abdominal tenderness, edema, erythema, or involuntary abdominal rigidity.

medical problems is needed. Optimizing cardiac performance is necessary. Serial physical examinations, platelet counts, lactate levels, and ABG levels are the most useful indications of progressive sepsis.

### Antibiotic therapy

Drug therapy consists of parenteral administration of broad-spectrum antibiotics to suppress bacterial flora and prevent bowel perforation. (These drugs can also be administered through an NG tube if necessary.)

### Surgery

Surgery is indicated if the patient shows any of the following signs or symptoms: signs of perforation (free intraperitoneal air on X-ray) or symptoms of peritonitis, respiratory insufficiency (caused by severe abdominal distention), progressive and intractable acidosis, or DIC. Surgery removes all necrotic and acutely inflamed bowel and creates a temporary colostomy or ileostomy.

### Special considerations

- Be alert for signs of gastric distention and perforation. (See *Recognizing ominous signs in necrotizing enterocolitis.*)

- Take axillary temperatures to avoid perforating the bowel.
- Prevent cross-contamination by disposing of soiled diapers properly and washing hands after diaper changes.
- Prepare the parents for a potential deterioration in their infant's condition. Explain all treatments, including why feedings are withheld.
- After surgery, the infant needs mechanical ventilation. Gently suction secretions, and monitor respirations often.
- Replace fluids lost through NG tube and stoma drainage. Include drainage losses in output records. Weigh the infant daily. A daily weight gain of 0.35 to 0.7 oz (9.9 to 19.8 g) indicates a good response to therapy.
- An infant with a temporary colostomy or ileostomy should be referred to an enterostomal therapy nurse to assist the patient and family in meeting needs.
- Encourage the parents to participate in their infant's physical care after his condition is no longer critical.
- Because of the infant's small abdomen, the suture line is near the stoma. Maintaining a clean suture line may be problematic. Good skin care is essential because the immature infant's skin is fragile and vulnerable to excoriation

and the active enzymes in bowel secretions, which are corrosive.

● Improvise infant-sized colostomy bags from urine collection bags, medicine cups, or condoms. Karaya gum is helpful in making a seal.

● Watch for wound disruption, infection, dehiscence, and excoriation — potential dangers because of severe catabolism.

● Watch for intestinal malfunction from stricture or short-bowel syndrome. Such complications usually develop 1 month after the infant resumes normal feedings.

● Encourage parental visits.

● To help prevent NEC, encourage mothers to breast-feed because breast milk contains live macrophages that fight infection and has a low pH that inhibits the growth of many organisms. Also, colostrum — fluid secreted before the milk — contains high concentrations of immunoglobulin A, which directly protects the bowel from infection, and which the neonate lacks for several days postpartum.

● Instruct mothers that they may refrigerate their milk for 48 hours but shouldn't freeze or heat it because this destroys antibodies. Tell them to use plastic — not glass — containers because leukocytes adhere to glass.

● To maintain an adequate milk supply, breast-feeding mothers should pump milk while the baby can't take anything by mouth.

# NEPHROTIC SYNDROME

Nephrotic syndrome (NS) is characterized by marked proteinuria, hypoalbuminemia, hyperlipemia, and edema. Although NS isn't a disease itself, it results from a specific glomerular defect and indicates renal damage. The prognosis is highly variable, depending on the underlying cause. Some forms may progress to end-stage renal failure.

## Causes

About 75% of NS cases result from primary (idiopathic) glomerulonephritis. Classifications include the following:

● In *lipid nephrosis (nil lesions)* — the main cause of NS in children — the glomeruli appear normal by light microscopy. Some tubules may contain increased lipid deposits.

● *Membraneous glomerulonephritis* — the most common lesion in adult idiopathic NS — is characterized by uniform thickening of the glomerular basement membrane containing dense deposits. It can eventually progress to renal failure.

● *Focal glomerulosclerosis* can develop spontaneously at any age, follow kidney transplantation, or result from heroin abuse. Reported incidence of this condition is 10% in children with NS and up to 20% in adults. Lesions initially affect the deeper glomeruli, causing hyaline sclerosis, with later involvement of the superficial glomeruli. These lesions generally cause slowly progressive deterioration in renal function. Remissions occur occasionally.

● In *membranoproliferative glomerulonephritis*, slowly progressive lesions develop in the subendothelial region of the basement membrane. These lesions may follow infection, particularly streptococcal infection. This disease occurs primarily in children and young adults.

Other causes of NS include metabolic diseases such as diabetes mellitus; collagen-vascular disorders, such as systemic lupus erythematosus and polyarteritis nodosa; circulatory diseases, such as heart failure and sickle-cell anemia; nephrotoxins, such as mercury, gold, and nonsteroidal anti-inflamma-

## PATHOPHYSIOLOGY OF NEPHROTIC SYNDROME

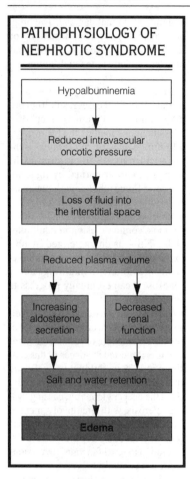

### Signs and symptoms

The dominant clinical feature of nephrotic syndrome is mild to severe dependent edema of the ankles or sacrum, or periorbital edema, especially in children. Such edema may lead to ascites, pleural effusion, and swollen external genitalia. (See *Pathophysiology of nephrotic syndrome.*)

Accompanying symptoms may include orthostatic hypotension, lethargy, anorexia, depression, and pallor. Major complications are malnutrition, infection, coagulation disorders, thromboembolic vascular occlusion, and accelerated atherosclerosis.

### Diagnosis

Consistent proteinuria in excess of 3.5 g/24 hours strongly suggests NS; examination of urine also reveals an increased number of hyaline, granular, and waxy, fatty casts, and oval fat bodies. Serum values that support the diagnosis are increased cholesterol, phospholipids, and triglycerides and decreased albumin levels. Histologic identification of the lesion requires a kidney biopsy.

### Treatment

Effective treatment of NS necessitates correction of the underlying cause if possible. Supportive treatment consists of protein replacement with a nutritional diet of 1.5 g protein/kg of body weight, with restricted sodium intake; diuretics for edema; and antibiotics for infection.

Some patients respond to an 8-week course of corticosteroid therapy (such as prednisone), followed by a maintenance dose. Others respond better to a combination course of prednisone and azathioprine or cyclophosphamide.

### Special considerations

● Frequently check urine protein. (Urine containing protein appears frothy.)

tory drugs (NSAIDs); allergic reactions; infections, such as tuberculosis or hepatitis B; preeclampsia toxemia; hereditary nephritis; multiple myeloma; and other neoplastic diseases. These diseases increase glomerular protein permeability, leading to the increased urinary excretion of protein, especially albumin, and subsequent hypoalbuminemia.

- Measure blood pressure while the patient is supine and also while he's standing; be alert for a drop in blood pressure that exceeds 20 mm Hg.

- After a kidney biopsy, watch for bleeding and shock.

- Monitor intake and output and check weight at the same time each morning — after the patient voids and before he eats — and while he's wearing the same kind of clothing

- Ask the dietitian to plan a high-protein, low-sodium diet.

- Provide good skin care because the patient with NS usually has edema.

> **CLINICAL TIP** To avoid thrombophlebitis, encourage activity and exercise, and provide antiembolism stockings as needed.

- Watch for and teach the patient and family how to recognize adverse reactions to drug therapy, such as bone marrow toxicity from cytotoxic immunosuppressives and cushingoid signs and symptoms (muscle weakness, mental changes, acne, moon face, hirsutism, girdle obesity, purple striae, amenorrhea) from long-term steroid therapy.

- Other steroidal complications include masked infections, increased susceptibility to infections, ulcers, GI bleeding, and steroid-induced diabetes; a steroid crisis may occur if the drug is discontinued abruptly.

- To prevent GI complications, administer steroids with food or milk. Omeprazole, misoprostol, or an antacid may be prescribed concurrently to prevent gastric ulcers.

- Explain that the adverse effects of steroids will subside when therapy stops.

- Offer the patient and family reassurance and support, especially during the acute phase, when edema is severe and the patient's body image changes.

# NEURAL TUBE DEFECTS

Neural tube defects (NTDs) are serious birth defects that involve the spine or brain; they result from failure of the neural tube to close at approximately 28 days after conception. The most common forms of NTD are spina bifida (50% of cases), anencephaly (40%), and encephalocele (10%).

Spina bifida occulta is the most common and least severe spinal cord defect. It's characterized by incomplete closure of one or more vertebrae without protrusion of the spinal cord or meninges.

However, in more severe forms of spina bifida, incomplete closure of one or more vertebrae causes protrusion of the spinal contents in an external sac or cystic lesion (spina bifida cystica). Spina bifida cystica has two classifications: myelomeningocele (meningomyelocele) and meningocele. In myelomeningocele, the external sac contains meninges, cerebrospinal fluid (CSF), and a portion of the spinal cord or nerve roots distal to the conus medullaris. When the spinal nerve roots end at the sac, motor and sensory functions below the sac are terminated. In meningocele, less severe than myelomeningocele, the sac contains only meninges and CSF. Meningocele may produce no neurologic symptoms.

In encephalocele, a saclike portion of the meninges and brain protrudes through a defective opening in the skull. Usually, it's in the occipital area, but it may also occur in the parietal, nasopharyngeal, or frontal area.

In anencephaly, the most severe form of NTD, the closure defect occurs at the cranial end of the neuroaxis and, as a result, part or all of the top of the skull is missing, severely damaging the brain.

Portions of the brain stem and spinal cord may also be missing. No diagnostic or therapeutic efforts are helpful; this condition is invariably fatal.

## Causes

NTDs may be isolated birth defects, may result from exposure to a teratogen, or may be part of a multiple malformation syndrome (for example, chromosomal abnormalities such as trisomy 18 or 13 syndrome). Isolated NTDs (those not due to a specific teratogen or associated with other malformations) are believed to be caused by a combination of genetic and environmental factors. Although most of the specific environmental triggers are unknown, recent research has identified a lack of folic acid in the mother's diet as one of the risk factors.

The incidence of NTDs varies greatly among countries and by region in the United States. For example, the incidence is significantly higher in the British Isles and low in southern China and Japan. In the United States, North and South Carolina have at least twice the incidence of NTDs as most other parts of the country. These birth defects are also more common in whites than in blacks.

## Signs and symptoms

Spina bifida occulta is often accompanied by a depression or dimple, tuft of hair, soft fatty deposits, port wine nevi, or a combination of these abnormalities on the skin over the spinal defect; however, such signs may be absent. Spina bifida occulta doesn't usually cause neurologic dysfunction but occasionally is associated with foot weakness or bowel and bladder disturbances. Such disturbances are especially likely during rapid growth phases, when the spinal cord's ascent within the vertebral column may be impaired by its abnormal adherence to other tissues.

In both myelomeningocele and meningocele, a saclike structure protrudes over the spine. Like spina bifida occulta, meningocele seldom causes neurologic deficit. But myelomeningocele, depending on the level of the defect, causes permanent neurologic dysfunction, such as flaccid or spastic paralysis and bowel and bladder incontinence. Associated disorders include trophic skin disturbances (ulcerations, cyanosis), clubfoot, knee contractures, hydrocephalus (in about 90% of patients), and possibly mental retardation, Arnold-Chiari syndrome (in which part of the brain protrudes into the spinal canal), and curvature of the spine.

Clinical effects of encephalocele vary with the degree of tissue involvement and location of the defect. However, surviving infants are usually severely mentally retarded with paralysis and hydrocephalus common.

## Diagnosis

Amniocentesis can detect elevated alpha-fetoprotein (AFP) levels in amniotic fluid, which indicates the presence of an open neural tube defect. Measuring acetylcholinesterase levels can confirm the diagnosis. (Biochemical testing will usually miss closed NTDs.) Because 5% to 7% of NTDs are associated with chromosomal abnormalities, a fetal karyotype should be done in addition to the biochemical tests.

Maternal serum AFP screening in combination with other serum markers, such as human chorionic gonadotropin (HCG), free betaHCG, or unconjugated estriol, may be offered to some patients who aren't scheduled for amniocentesis, such as those with a lower risk of NTDs and those who will be under age 34½ at the time of delivery. Although this screening test can't diagnose either an open NTD or a chromosomal abnormality, it can estimate a fetus's risk of such a defect. The majority of patients with abnormal maternal serum AFP levels won't have an affected child but they should be offered diagnostic testing by amniocentesis. If the amniocentesis results are normal, abnormal AFP levels may still indicate an increased risk for perinatal complications, such as premature rupture of the membranes, abruptio placentae, or fetal death. Ultrasound may be used when the fetus has an increased risk of an open NTD based on either the family history or abnormal serum screening results; however, this test alone can't identify all open NTDs or ventral wall defects.

If the NTD isn't diagnosed before birth, other tests are used to make the diagnosis. For example, spina bifida occulta is often overlooked, although it's occasionally palpable and spinal X-ray can show the bone defect. Myelography can differentiate it from other spinal abnormalities, especially spinal cord tumors.

Myelomeningocele and meningocele are obvious on examination; transillumination of the protruding sac can sometimes distinguish between them. (In meningocele, it typically transilluminates; in myelomeningocele, it doesn't.) In myelomeningocele, a pinprick examination of the legs and trunk shows the level of sensory and motor involvement; skull X-rays, cephalic measurements, and computed tomography (CT) scan demonstrate associated hydrocephalus. Other appropriate laboratory tests in patients with myelomeningocele include urinalysis, urine cultures, and tests for renal function starting in the neonatal period and continuing at regular intervals.

In encephalocele, X-rays show a basilar bony skull defect. CT scan and ultrasonography further define the defect.

## Treatment

Prompt neurosurgical repair and aggressive management may improve the condition of children with some NTDs, but serious and permanent handicaps are likely.

Spina bifida occulta usually requires no treatment. Treatment of meningocele consists of surgical closure of the protruding sac and continual assessment of growth and development. Treatment of myelomeningocele requires repair of the sac and supportive measures to promote independence and prevent further complications. Surgery doesn't reverse neurologic deficits. A shunt may be needed to relieve associated hydrocephalus.

Treatment of encephalocele includes surgery during infancy to place protruding tissues back in the skull, excise the sac, and correct associated craniofacial abnormalities.

## Special considerations

When an NTD has been diagnosed prenatally, refer the prospective parents to a genetic counselor, who can provide information and support the couple's decisions on how to manage the pregnancy.

● Recent research sponsored by the March of Dimes and others has indicated that the risk of an open NTD may be reduced 50% to 70% in pregnant women who take a daily multivitamin with folic acid.

➤ CLINICAL TIP Urge all women of childbearing age to take such a vitamin supplement until menopause or the end of childbearing potential. (See *Folic acid supplement recommendations,* page 578.)

● The parents of a child with an NTD will need assistance from doctors, nurses, surgeons, rehabilitation providers, and social workers. Help to coordinate such assistance as needed. Obviously,

# FOLIC ACID SUPPLEMENT RECOMMENDATIONS

The following recommendations for folic acid supplement dosages have been endorsed by the Centers for Disease Control and Prevention, the U.S. Public Health Service, the March of Dimes Birth Defects Foundation, and the Spina Bifida Association of America, among other groups.

### All women of childbearing age

All women who are capable of becoming pregnant should:
- consume 0.4 mg of folic acid daily to reduce their risk of having a child with spina bifida or another neural tube defect (NTD)
- continue to consume 0.4 mg of folic acid daily when pregnant until their health care provider prescribes other prenatal vitamins.

### Women at high risk

Women with a previous pregnancy affected by an NTD should:
- receive genetic counseling before their next pregnancy
- consume 0.4 mg of folic acid daily
- when actively trying to become pregnant (at least 1 month before conception), increase their dosage of folic acid to 4 mg daily (by taking a separate folic acid supplement, not by increasing their intake of multivitamins)
- continue to take 4 mg of folic acid daily through the first 3 months of pregnancy.

care is most complex when the neurologic deficit is severe. Immediate goals include psychological support to help parents accept the diagnosis and pre- and postoperative care. Long-term goals include patient and family teaching and measures to prevent contractures, pressure ulcers, urinary tract infections (UTIs), and other complications.

Before surgery:
- Prevent local infection by cleaning the defect gently with sterile saline solution or other solutions as ordered. Inspect the defect often for signs of infection, and cover it with sterile dressings moistened with sterile saline solution. Prevent skin breakdown by placing sheepskin or a foam pad under the infant. Keep skin clean, and apply lotion to knees, elbows, chin, and other pressure areas. Give antibiotics as ordered.
- Handle the infant carefully, and don't apply pressure to the defect. Usually, the infant can't wear a diaper or a shirt until after surgical correction because it will irritate the sac, so keep him warm in an infant Isolette. Hold and cuddle the infant; on your lap, position him on his abdomen; teach parents to do the same.
- Provide adequate time for parent-child bonding if possible.
- Measure head circumference daily, and watch for signs of hydrocephalus and meningeal irritation, such as fever or nuchal rigidity. Be sure to mark the spot so you get accurate readings.
- Contractures can be minimized by passive range-of-motion exercises and casting. To prevent hip dislocation, moderately abduct hips with a pad between the knees, or with sandbags and ankle rolls.
- Monitor intake and output. Watch for decreased skin turgor, dryness, or other signs of dehydration. Provide meticulous skin care to genitals and buttocks to prevent infection.
- Ensure adequate nutrition.

After surgery:
- Watch for hydrocephalus, which can be a complication following surgery. Measure the infant's head circumference as ordered.

• Monitor vital signs often. Watch for signs of shock, infection, and increased intracranial pressure (ICP), such as projectile vomiting. Frequently assess the infant's fontanels. Remember that before age 2, infants don't show typical signs of increased ICP because suture lines aren't fully closed. In infants, the most telling sign is bulging fontanels.

• Change the dressing regularly as ordered, and check and report any signs of drainage, wound rupture, and infection.

• Place the infant in the prone position to protect and assess the site.

• If leg casts have been applied to treat deformities, watch for signs that the child is outgrowing the cast. Regularly check distal pulses to ensure adequate circulation.

To help parents cope with their infant's physical problems and successfully meet long-term treatment goals:

• Teach them to recognize early signs of complications, such as hydrocephalus, pressure ulcers, and UTIs.

• Provide psychological support and encourage a positive attitude. Help parents work through their feelings of guilt, anger, and helplessness.

• Encourage parents to begin training their child in a bladder routine by age 3. Emphasize the need for increased fluid intake to prevent UTIs. Teach intermittent catheterization and conduit hygiene as ordered.

• To prevent constipation and bowel obstruction, stress the need for increased fluid intake, a high-bulk diet, exercise, and a stool softener, as ordered. If possible, teach parents to help empty their child's bowel by telling him to bear down, and giving a glycerin suppository as needed.

• Urge early recognition of developmental lags (a possible result of hydrocephalus). If present, stress the importance of follow-up IQ assessment to help plan realistic educational goals. The child may need to attend a school with special facilities. Also, stress the need for stimulation to ensure maximum mental development. Help parents plan activities appropriate to their child's age and abilities.

• Refer parents for genetic counseling, and suggest that amniocentesis be performed in future pregnancies. Also refer parents to the Spina Bifida Association of America.

# NEURITIS, PERIPHERAL

Also known as multiple neuritis, peripheral neuropathy, and polyneuritis, peripheral neuritis is the degeneration of peripheral nerves supplying mainly the distal muscles of the extremities. It results in muscle weakness with sensory loss and atrophy, and decreased or absent deep tendon reflexes. This syndrome is associated with a noninflammatory degeneration of the axon and myelin sheaths, chiefly affecting the distal muscles of the extremities.

Although peripheral neuritis can occur at any age, its incidence is highest in men between the ages of 30 and 50. Because onset is usually insidious, patients may compensate by overusing unaffected muscles; however, onset is rapid with severe infection and chronic alcohol intoxication. If the cause can be identified and eliminated, the prognosis is good.

## Causes

Causes of peripheral neuritis include:

• chronic intoxication (ethyl alcohol, arsenic, lead, carbon disulfide, benzene, phosphorus, and sulfonamides)

• infectious diseases (meningitis, diphtheria, syphilis, tuberculosis, pneumonia, mumps, and Guillain-Barré syndrome)

• metabolic and inflammatory disorders (gout, diabetes mellitus, rheumatoid arthritis, polyarteritis nodosa, systemic lupus erythematosus)

• nutritive diseases (beriberi and other vitamin deficiencies and cachectic states).

### Signs and symptoms

The clinical effects of peripheral neuritis develop slowly, and the disease usually affects the motor and sensory nerve fibers. Neuritis typically produces flaccid paralysis, wasting, loss of reflexes, pain of varying intensity, loss of ability to perceive vibratory sensations, and paresthesia, hyperesthesia, or anesthesia in the hands and feet.

Deep tendon reflexes are diminished or absent, and atrophied muscles are tender or hypersensitive to pressure or palpation. Footdrop may also be present. Cutaneous manifestations include glossy, red skin and decreased sweating.

➤ CLINICAL TIP Patients often have a history of clumsiness and may complain of frequent vague sensations.

### Diagnosis

The patient history and physical examination delineate the characteristic distribution of motor and sensory deficits. Electromyography may show a delayed action potential if this condition impairs motor nerve function.

### *Treatment*

Effective treatment of peripheral neuritis consists of supportive measures to relieve pain, adequate bed rest, and physical therapy as needed. Most important, the underlying cause must be identified and corrected. For instance, it's essential to identify and remove the toxic agent, correct nutritional and vitamin deficiencies (the patient needs a high-calorie diet rich in vitamins, especially B complex), or counsel the patient to avoid alcohol.

### Special considerations

• Relieve pain with correct positioning, analgesics, or possibly phenytoin, which has been used experimentally for neuritic pain, especially if associated with diabetic neuropathy.

• Instruct the patient to rest and refrain from using the affected extremity.

• To prevent pressure ulcers, apply a foot cradle. To prevent contractures, arrange for the patient to obtain splints, boards, braces, or other orthopedic appliances.

• After the pain subsides, passive range-of-motion exercises or massage may be beneficial. Electrotherapy is advocated for nerve and muscle stimulation.

# NEUROGENIC ARTHROPATHY

Most common in men over age 40, neurogenic arthropathy (Charcot's arthropathy) is a progressively degenerative disease of peripheral and axial joints, resulting from impaired sensory innervation. The loss of sensation in the joints causes progressive deterioration, resulting from unrecognized trauma (especially repeated minor episodes) or primary disease, which leads to laxity of supporting ligaments and eventual disintegration of the affected joints.

### Causes

In adults, the most common cause of neurogenic arthropathy is diabetes mellitus. Other causes include tabes dorsalis (especially among patients ages 40 to 60), syringomyelia (which progresses to neurogenic arthropathy in about 25% of patients), myelopathy of pernicious anemia, spinal cord trauma, paraplegia, hereditary sensory neuropathy, and Charcot-Marie-Tooth disease. Rarely, amyloidosis, peripheral nerve injury, myelomeningocele (in children), leprosy, or alcoholism causes neurogenic arthropathy.

Frequent intra-articular injections of corticosteroids have also been linked to neurogenic arthropathy. The analgesic effect of the corticosteroids may mask symptoms and allow continuous damaging stress to accelerate joint destruction.

### Signs and symptoms
Neurogenic arthropathy begins insidiously with swelling, warmth, increased mobility, and instability in a single joint or in many joints. It can progress to deformity. The first clue to vertebral neuroarthropathy, which progresses to gross spinal deformity, may be nothing more than a mild, persistent backache. Characteristically, pain is minimal despite obvious deformity.

The specific joint that's affected varies. Diabetes usually attacks the joints and bones of the feet; tabes dorsalis attacks the large weight-bearing joints, such as the knee, hip, ankle, or lumbar and dorsal vertebrae (Charcot spine); syringomyelia, the shoulder, elbow, or cervical intervertebral joint. Neurogenic arthropathy related to intra-articular injection of corticosteroids usually develops in the hip or knee joint.

### Diagnosis
A patient history of painless joint deformity and underlying primary disease suggests neurogenic arthropathy. The physical examination may reveal bone fragmentation in advanced disease. X-rays confirm the diagnosis and assess the severity of joint damage.

In the early stage of the disease, soft tissue swelling or effusion may be the only overt effect; in the advanced stage, articular fracture, subluxation, erosion of articular cartilage, periosteal new bone formation, and excessive growth of marginal loose bodies (osteophytosis) or resorption may be seen.

Other diagnostic measures include:
- *vertebral examination:* narrowing of disk spaces, deterioration of vertebrae, and osteophyte formation, leading to ankylosis and deforming kyphoscoliosis
- *synovial biopsy:* bony fragments and bits of calcified cartilage.

### Treatment
Effective management relieves associated pain with analgesics and immobilization, using crutches, splints, braces, and restriction of weight bearing.

In severe disease, surgery may include arthrodesis or, in severe diabetic neuropathy, amputation. However, surgery risks further damage through nonunion and infection.

### Special considerations
- Assess the pattern of pain and give analgesics as needed.
- Check sensory perception, range of motion, alignment, joint swelling, and the status of underlying disease.
- Teach the patient joint protection techniques; to avoid physically stressful actions that may cause pathologic fractures; and to take safety precautions, such as removing throw rugs and clutter that may cause falls.
- Advise the patient to report severe joint pain, swelling, or instability.

> CLINICAL TIP  Warm compresses may be applied to relieve local pain and tenderness.
- Teach the patient the proper technique for using crutches or other orthopedic devices. Stress the importance of prop-

er fitting and regular professional readjustment of such devices and the importance of good skin care. Warn that impaired sensation might allow damage from these aids without discomfort.
• Emphasize the need to continue regular treatment of the underlying disease.

# NEUROGENIC BLADDER

Also known as neuromuscular dysfunction of the lower urinary tract, neurologic bladder dysfunction, and neuropathic bladder, neurogenic bladder refers to all types of bladder dysfunction caused by an interruption of normal bladder innervation. Subsequent complications include incontinence, residual urine retention, urinary infection, stone formation, and renal failure. A neurogenic bladder can be spastic (hypertonic, reflex, or automatic), flaccid (hypotonic, atonic, nonreflex, or autonomous), or uncoordinated (dyssynergic).

## Causes

At one time, neurogenic bladder was thought to result primarily from spinal cord injury; now, it appears to stem from a host of underlying conditions:
• *cerebral disorders,* such as cerebrovascular accident, brain tumor (meningioma and glioma), Parkinson's disease, multiple sclerosis, dementia, and incontinence caused by aging
• *spinal cord disease or trauma,* such as spinal stenosis (causing cord compression) or arachnoiditis (causing adhesions between the membranes covering the cord), cervical spondylosis, myelopathies from hereditary or nutritional deficiencies and, rarely, tabes dorsalis

• *disorders of peripheral innervation,* including autonomic neuropathies resulting from endocrine disturbances such as diabetes mellitus (most common)
• *metabolic disturbances,* such as hypothyroidism, porphyria, or uremia (infrequent)
• *acute infectious diseases* such as Guillain-Barré syndrome
• *heavy metal toxicity*
• *chronic alcoholism*
• *collagen diseases* such as systemic lupus erythematosus
• *vascular diseases* such as atherosclerosis
• *distant effects of cancer* such as primary oat cell carcinoma of the lung
• *herpes zoster*
• *sacral agenesis.*

An upper motor neuron lesion (above S2 to S4) causes spastic neurogenic bladder, with spontaneous contractions of the detrusor muscles, elevated intravesical voiding pressure, bladder wall hypertrophy with trabeculation, and urinary sphincter spasms.

A lower motor neuron lesion (below S2 to S4) causes flaccid neurogenic bladder, with decreased intravesical pressure, increased bladder capacity and large residual urine retention, and poor detrusor contraction.

## Signs and symptoms

Neurogenic bladder produces a wide range of clinical signs, depending on the underlying cause and its effect on the structural integrity of the bladder. Usually, this disorder causes some degree of incontinence, changes in initiation or interruption of micturition, and an inability to empty the bladder completely. Other symptoms of neurogenic bladder include vesicoureteral reflux, deterioration or infection in the upper urinary tract, and hydroureteral nephrosis.

## Spastic neurogenic bladder

Depending on the site and extent of the spinal cord lesion, spastic neurogenic bladder may produce involuntary or frequent scanty urination without a feeling of bladder fullness and possibly spontaneous spasms of the arms and legs. Anal sphincter tone may be increased.

Tactile stimulation of the abdomen, thighs, or genitalia may precipitate voiding and spontaneous contractions of the arms and legs. With cord lesions in the upper thoracic (cervical) level, bladder distention can trigger hyperactive autonomic reflexes, resulting in severe hypertension, bradycardia, and headaches.

## Flaccid neurogenic bladder

Features of flaccid neurogenic bladder may be associated with overflow incontinence, diminished anal sphincter tone, and a greatly distended bladder (this is evident on percussion or palpation), but without the accompanying feeling of bladder fullness due to sensory impairment.

## Diagnosis

The patient's history may include a condition or disorder that can cause neurogenic bladder, incontinence, and disruptions of micturition patterns. The following tests will help evaluate the patient's bladder function:

• *Voiding cystourethrography* evaluates bladder neck function, vesicoureteral reflux, and continence.

• *Urodynamic studies* help evaluate how urine is stored in the bladder, how well the bladder empties, and the rate of movement of urine out of the bladder during voiding. These studies consist of four components:

– *Urine flow study (uroflow)* shows diminished or impaired urine flow.

– *Cystometry* evaluates bladder nerve supply, detrusor muscle tone, and intravesical pressures during bladder filling and contraction.

– *Urethral pressure profile* determines urethral function with respect to the length of the urethra and the outlet pressure resistance.

– *Sphincter electromyelography* correlates the neuromuscular function of the external sphincter with bladder muscle function during bladder filling and contraction. This evaluates how well the bladder and urinary sphincter muscles work together.

• *Retrograde urethrography* reveals the presence of strictures and diverticula. This test may not be performed on a routine basis.

## Treatment

The goals of treatment are to maintain the integrity of the upper urinary tract, control infection, and prevent urinary incontinence through evacuation of the bladder, drug therapy, surgery or, less commonly, neural blocks and electrical stimulation.

### Bladder evacuation

Techniques of bladder evacuation include Credé's method, Valsalva's maneuver, and intermittent self-catheterization.

Credé's method (application of manual pressure over the lower abdomen) and Valsalva's maneuver (performing forced exhalation against a closed glottis) promote complete emptying of the bladder. (For more patient-teaching information, see *Dealing with neurogenic bladder,* page 584.)

After appropriate instruction, most patients can perform Credé's method themselves; however, even when performed properly, this method isn't always successful and doesn't always eliminate the need for catheterization.

Intermittent self-catheterization — more effective than either Credé's

# DEALING WITH NEUROGENIC BLADDER

In your patient teaching for neurogenic bladder, cover the following topics:

• Explain all diagnostic tests clearly so the patient understands the procedure, the time involved, and the possible results. Assure him that the lengthy diagnostic process is necessary to identify the most effective treatment plan.
• Explain the treatment plan to the patient in detail.
• Encourage the patient to drink plenty of fluids to prevent calculus formation and infection form urinary stasis.
• Teach the patient bladder evacuation techniques, such as Credé's method, Valsalva's maneuver, and intermittent self-catheterization. Generally, a male can perform this procedure more easily, but a female can learn self-catheterization with the help of a mirror. Intermittent self-catheterization, in conjunction with a bladder-retraining program, is especially useful for patients with flaccid neurogenic bladder.
• Counsel the patient regarding sexual activities. Remember, the incontinent patient feels embarrassed and distressed. Provide emotional support.

## Drug therapy

In neurogenic bladder, drug therapy may include bethanechol and phenoxybenzamine to facilitate bladder emptying, and propantheline, methantheline, flavoxate, dicyclomine, and imipramine to facilitate urine storage.

## Surgery

When conservative treatment fails, surgery may correct the structural impairment through transurethral resection of the bladder neck, urethral dilatation, external sphincterotomy, or urinary diversion procedures. Implantation of an artificial urinary sphincter may be necessary if permanent incontinence follows surgery for neurogenic bladder.

## Special considerations

Care for patients with neurogenic bladder varies according to the underlying cause and the method of treatment.

• Use strict aseptic technique during insertion of an indwelling urinary catheter (a temporary measure to drain the incontinent patient's bladder). Don't interrupt the closed drainage system for any reason.
• Obtain urine specimens with a syringe and small-bore needle inserted through the aspirating port of the catheter itself (below the junction of the balloon instillation site). Irrigate in the same manner if necessary.
• Clean the catheter insertion site with soap and water at least twice a day.
• Don't allow the catheter to become encrusted.
• Use a sterile applicator to apply antibiotic ointment around the meatus after catheter care. Keep the drainage bag below the tubing, and don't raise the bag above the level of the bladder.
• Clamp the tubing, or empty the bag before transferring the patient to a wheelchair or stretcher to prevent accidental urine reflux.

method or Valsalva's maneuver — has proved to be a major advance in the treatment of neurogenic bladder because it allows complete emptying of the bladder without the risks that an indwelling urinary catheter poses.

**CLINICAL TIP** If urine output is considerable, empty the bag more frequently than once every 8 hours because bacteria can multiply in standing urine and migrate up the catheter and into the bladder.

• Watch for signs of infection (fever, cloudy or foul-smelling urine).

• Try to keep the patient as mobile as possible. Perform passive range-of-motion exercise if necessary.

• If urinary diversion procedure is to be performed, arrange for consultation with an enterostomal therapist, and coordinate the care.

• Before discharge, teach the patient and his family evacuation techniques as necessary (Credé's method, intermittent self-catheterization).

# NOSE, FRACTURED

The most common facial fracture, a fractured nose usually results from blunt injury and is often associated with other facial fractures. The severity of the fracture depends on the direction, force, and type of the blow.

A severe, comminuted fracture may cause extreme swelling or bleeding that may jeopardize the airway and require tracheotomy during early treatment. Inadequate or delayed treatment may cause permanent nasal displacement, septal deviation, and obstruction.

## Causes

In low-energy injuries, noncomminuted nasal bone fragments are caused by low-velocity trauma. Such injuries could occur in the following situations:

• injuries created during fistfights (hand or fist blows only, no blunt instruments)

• uncomplicated falls, such as tripping

• low-velocity motor vehicle collision.

In high-energy injuries, a higher amount of energy is absorbed by the nasal-facial skeleton, with comminution of bone fragments and associated injuries to the soft tissue and orbital-facial skeleton. These injuries would include:

• injuries sustained from a leveraged blow to the nose using an object such as a stick, pipe, or other blunt object

• falls from heights

• sport injuries with fast-moving projectiles, such as a ball or puck

• high-velocity motor vehicle collisions.

## Signs and symptoms

Immediately after the injury, a nosebleed may occur, and soft-tissue swelling may quickly obscure the break. After several hours, pain, periorbital ecchymoses, and nasal displacement and deformity are prominent. A possible complication is septal hematoma, which may lead to abscess formation, resulting in vascular septic necrosis and saddle nose deformity.

## Diagnosis

Palpation, X-rays, and clinical findings, such as a deviated septum, confirm a nasal fracture. The diagnosis also requires a full patient history, including the cause of the injury and the amount of nasal bleeding. Watch for clear fluid drainage, which may suggest a cerebrospinal fluid (CSF) leak and a basilar skull fracture. A computed tomography (CT) scan may be necessary.

## Treatment

Treatment restores normal facial appearance and reestablishes bilateral nasal passage after swelling subsides. Reduction of the fracture corrects alignment; immobilization (intranasal packing and an external splint shaped to the nose and taped) maintains it. Reduction is best accomplished in the operating

TEACHING CHECKLIST

## COPING WITH A NOSE FRACTURE

Review the following points with your patient prior to discharge.

• Tell the patient that he may be required to wear the external splint at night for an additional time.
• Remind the patient to be gentle with his nose and to keep his head elevated.
• Advise the patient to perform no strenuous lifting or activity for 4 additional weeks and no contact sports for at least 6 weeks (and only then after clearance by the doctor).
• Caution the patient not to wear glasses for 6 weeks because pressure from the glasses can permanently indent the nasal bridge.

• Because the patient will find breathing more difficult as the swelling increases, instruct him to breathe slowly through his mouth.
• To warm the inhaled air during cold weather, tell the patient to cover his mouth with a handkerchief or scarf.
• To prevent subcutaneous emphysema or intracranial air penetration (and potential meningitis), warn the patient not to blow his nose.
• After packing and splinting, apply ice in a plastic bag.
• Before discharge, tell the patient that ecchymoses should fade after about 2 weeks.
• For more patient-teaching information, see *Coping with a nose fracture.*

room under local anesthesia for adults and general anesthesia for children.

**CLINICAL TIP** Early or late repair is possible, but most doctors prefer to delay reduction for 5 to 10 days after the injury, especially if severe swelling is present.

CSF leakage calls for close observation, a CT scan of the basilar skull, and antibiotic therapy; septal hematoma requires incision and drainage to prevent necrosis.

**Special considerations**

• Start treatment immediately. While waiting for X-rays, apply ice packs to the nose to minimize swelling. Wrap the ice packs in a light towel to prevent ice from directly contacting the skin,
• To control anterior bleeding, gently apply local pressure. Posterior bleeding is rare and requires an internal tamponade applied in the emergency department.

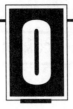

# OBSESSIVE-COMPULSIVE DISORDER

Obsessive thoughts and compulsive behaviors represent recurring efforts to control overwhelming anxiety, guilt, or unacceptable impulses that persistently enter the consciousness. The word *obsession* refers to a recurrent idea, thought, impulse, or image that is intrusive and inappropriate and causes marked anxiety or distress.

*A compulsion* is a ritualistic, repetitive, and involuntary defensive behavior. Performing a compulsive behavior reduces the patient's anxiety and increases the probability that the behavior will recur. Compulsions are often associated with obsessions.

Patients with obsessive-compulsive disorder are prone to abuse psychoactive substances, such as alcohol and anxiolytics, in an attempt to relieve their anxiety. In addition, other anxiety disorders and major depression often coexist with obsessive-compulsive disorder.

Obsessive-compulsive disorder is typically a chronic condition with remissions and flare-ups. Mild forms of the disorder are relatively common in the population at large.

## Causes

The cause of obsessive-compulsive disorder is unknown. Some studies suggest the possibility of brain lesions, but the most useful research and clinical studies base an explanation on psychological theories. In addition, major depression, organic brain syndrome, and schizophrenia may contribute to the onset of obsessive-compulsive disorder.

## Signs and symptoms

The psychiatric history of a patient with this disorder may reveal the presence of obsessive thoughts, words, or mental images that persistently and involuntarily invade the consciousness.

Some common obsessions include thoughts of violence (such as stabbing, shooting, maiming, or hitting), thoughts of contamination (images of dirt, germs, or feces), repetitive doubts and worries about a tragic event, and repeating or counting images, words, or objects in the environment. The patient recognizes that the obsessions are a product of his own mind and that they interfere with normal daily activities.

The patient's history also may reveal the presence of compulsions, irrational and recurring impulses to repeat a certain behavior. Common compulsions include repetitive touching, sometimes combined with counting; doing and undoing (for instance, opening and closing doors or rearranging things); washing (especially hands); and checking (to be sure no tragedy has occurred since the last time he checked). The patient's anxiety often is so strong that he will avoid the situation or the object that evokes the impulse.

## DIAGNOSING OBSESSIVE-COMPULSIVE DISORDER

The diagnosis of obsessive-compulsive disorder is made when the patient's signs and symptoms meet the established criteria in the *DSM-IV.*

**Obsessions or compulsions**
Obsessions are defined as all of the following.
• Recurrent and persistent thoughts, impulses, or images that are experienced, at some time during the disturbance, as intrusive and inappropriate and that cause marked anxiety or distress.
• The thoughts, impulses, or images are not simply excessive worries about real-life problems.
• The person attempts to ignore or suppress such thoughts or impulses or to neutralize them with some other thought or action.
• The person recognizes that the obsessions are the products of his mind and not externally imposed.
Compulsions are defined by all of the following.
• Repetitive behaviors or mental acts performed by the person, who feels driven to perform them in response to an obsession or according to rules that must be applied rigidly.
• The behavior or mental acts are aimed at preventing or reducing distress or preventing some dreaded event or situation. However, either the activity is not connected in a realistic way with what it is designed to neu-

tralize or prevent, or it is clearly excessive.
• The patient recognizes that his behavior is excessive or unreasonable (this may not be true for young children or for patients whose obsessions have evolved into overvalued ideas).

**Additional criteria**
• At some point, the person recognizes that the obsessions or compulsions are excessive or unreasonable.
• The obsessions or compulsions cause marked distress, are time consuming (take more than 1 hour a day), or significantly interfere with the person's normal routine, occupational functioning, or usual social activities or relationships.
• If another Axis I disorder is present, the content of the obsession is unrelated to it; for example, the ideas, thoughts, or images are not about food in the presence of an eating disorder, about drugs in the presence of a psychoactive substance abuse disorder, or about guilt in a major depressive disorder.
• The disturbance is not due to the direct physiologic effects of a substance or a general medical condition.

When the obsessive-compulsive phenomena are mental, observation may reveal no behavioral abnormalities. However, compulsive acts may be observed, although feelings of shame, nervousness, or embarrassment may prompt the patient to try limiting these acts to his own private time.

You'll need to evaluate the impact of obsessive-compulsive phenomena on the patient's normal routine. He'll typically report moderate to severe im-

pairment of social and occupational functioning.

### Diagnosis
For characteristic findings in patients with this condition, see *Diagnosing obsessive-compulsive disorder.*

### Treatment
Obsessive-compulsive disorder is tenacious, but with treatment, improvement occurs in 60% to 70% of patients. Current treatment usually involves a com-

# BEHAVIORAL THERAPIES

The following behavioral therapies are used to treat the patient with obsessive-compulsive disorder.

### Aversion therapy
Application of a painful stimulus creates an aversion to the obsession that leads to undesirable behavior (compulsion).

### Thought stopping
This technique breaks the habit of fear-inducing anticipatory thoughts. The patient learns to stop unwanted thoughts by saying the word "stop" and then focusing his attention on achieving calmness and muscle relaxation.

### Thought switching
To replace fear-inducing self-instructions with competent self-instructions, the patient learns to replace negative thoughts with positive ones until the positive thoughts become strong enough to overcome the anxiety-provoking ones.

### Flooding
This frequent, full-intensity exposure (through the use of imagery) to an object that triggers a symptom must be used with caution because it produces extreme discomfort.

### Implosion therapy
A form of desensitization, implosion therapy calls for repeated exposure to a highly feared object.

### Response prevention
Preventing compulsive behavior by distraction, persuasion, or redirection of activity, this form of behavioral therapy may require hospitalization or involvement of the family to be effective.

bination of medication and cognitive behavioral therapy. Other types of psychotherapy may also be helpful.

Effective medications include clomipramine, a tricyclic antidepressant; selective serotonin reuptake inhibitors, such as fluoxetine, paroxetine, sertraline, and fluvoxamine; and the benzodiazepine clonazepam.

Behavioral therapies—aversion therapy, thought stopping, thought switching, flooding, implosion therapy, and response prevention—have also been effective (see *Behavioral therapies.*)

## Special considerations
• Approach the patient unhurriedly.

➤ CLINICAL TIP Provide an accepting atmosphere; don't appear shocked, amused, or critical of the ritualistic behavior.

• Keep the patient's physical health in mind. For example, compulsive hand washing may cause skin breakdown, and rituals or preoccupations may cause inadequate food and fluid intake and exhaustion. Provide for basic needs, such as rest, nutrition, and grooming, if the patient becomes involved in ritualistic thoughts and behaviors to the point of self-neglect.

• Let the patient know you're aware of his behavior. For example, you might say, "I noticed you've made your bed three times today; that must be very tiring for you."

• Help the patient explore feelings associated with the behavior. For example, ask him, "What do you think about while you are performing your chores?"

• Make reasonable demands and set reasonable limits, explaining their purpose clearly. Avoid creating situations that increase frustration and provoke anger, which may interfere with treatment.

• Explore patterns leading to the behavior or recurring problems.

• Listen attentively, offering feedback.

• Engage the patient in activities to create positive accomplishments and raise his self-esteem and confidence.

• Encourage active diversional activities, such as whistling or humming a tune, to divert attention from the unwanted thoughts and to promote a pleasurable experience.

• Help the patient develop new ways to solve problems and more effective coping skills by setting limits on unacceptable behavior (for example, by limiting the number of times per day he may indulge in compulsive behavior). Gradually shorten the time allowed. Help him focus on other feelings or problems for the remainder of the time.

• Identify insight and improved behavior (reduced compulsive behavior and fewer obsessive thoughts). Evaluate behavioral changes by your own observations and the patient's reports.

• Identify disturbing topics of conversation that reflect underlying anxiety or terror.

• When interventions don't work, reevaluate them and recommend alternative strategies.

• Help the patient identify progress and set realistic expectations of himself and others.

• Explain how to channel emotional energy to relieve stress (for example, through sports and creative endeavors). In addition, teach the patient relaxation and breathing techniques to help reduce anxiety.

• Work with the patient and other treatment team members to establish behavioral goals and to help the patient tolerate anxiety in pursuing these goals.

# OSGOOD-SCHLATTER DISEASE

Also called osteochondrosis, Osgood-Schlatter disease is a painful, incomplete separation of the epiphysis of the tibial tubercle from the tibial shaft. Severe disease may cause permanent tubercle enlargement.

## Causes

Osgood-Schlatter disease probably results from trauma, before the complete fusion of the epiphysis to the main bone has occurred (between the ages of 10 and 15). Such trauma may be a single violent action or repeated knee flexion against tight quadriceps muscle. Other causes include locally deficient blood supply and genetic factors.

## Signs and symptoms

The patient complains of constant aching and pain and tenderness below the kneecap that worsens during any activity that causes forceful contraction of the patellar tendon on the tubercle, such as ascending or descending stairs. Such pain may be associated with some obvious soft-tissue swelling, localized heat, and local tenderness.

## Diagnosis

Physical examination supports the diagnosis: The examiner forces the tibia into internal rotation while slowly extending the patient's knee from 90 degrees of flexion; at about 30 degrees, such flexion produces pain that subsides immediately with external rotation of the tibia.

X-rays may be normal or show epiphyseal separation and soft-tissue swelling for up to 6 months after onset;

eventually, they may show bone fragmentation.

## Treatment

Treatment usually consists of immobilization of the leg for 6 to 8 weeks and supportive measures. Full extension immobilization of the leg through reinforced elastic knee support, plaster cast, or splint allows revascularization and reossification of the tubercle and minimizes the pull of the quadriceps.

Supportive measures include activity restrictions, aspirin and, possibly, cortisone injections into the joint to relieve tenderness. In very mild cases, simple restriction of predisposing activities (bicycling, running) may be adequate.

**▶ CLINICAL TIP** Rarely, conservative measures fail, and surgery may be necessary. Such surgery includes removal or fixation of the epiphysis or drilling holes through the tubercle to the main bone to form channels for rapid revascularization.

## Special considerations

● Monitor the patient's circulation, sensation, and pain, and watch for excessive bleeding after surgery.

● Assess daily for limitation of motion. Administer analgesics as needed.

● Make sure the knee support or splint isn't too tight. Keep the cast dry and clean, and "petal" it around the top and bottom margins to avoid skin irritation.

● Teach proper use of crutches.

● Tell the patient to protect the injured knee with padding and to avoid trauma and repeated flexion (running, contact sports).

● Monitor for muscle atrophy.

● Emphasize that restrictions are temporary

# OSTEOARTHRITIS

The most common form of arthritis, osteoarthritis is chronic, causing deterioration of the joint cartilage and formation of reactive new bone at the margins and subchondral areas of the joints. This degeneration results from a breakdown of chondrocytes, most often in the hips and knees.

## Causes

Osteoarthritis is widespread, occurring equally in both sexes. Incidence is after age 40; its earliest symptoms generally begin in middle age and may progress with advancing age.

The degree of disability depends on the site and severity of involvement; it can range from minor limitation of the fingers to severe disability in persons with hip or knee involvement. The rate of progression varies, and joints may remain stable for years in an early stage of deterioration.

Primary osteoarthritis, a normal part of aging, results from many things, including metabolic, genetic, chemical, and mechanical factors. Secondary osteoarthritis usually follows an identifiable predisposing event — most commonly trauma, congenital deformity, or obesity — and leads to degenerative changes.

## Signs and symptoms

The most common symptom of osteoarthritis is a deep, aching joint pain, particularly after exercise or weight bearing, usually relieved by rest. Other symptoms include:

● stiffness in the morning and after exercise (relieved by rest)

● aching during changes in weather

● "grating" of the joint during motion

# VIEWING OSTEOARTHRITIS

Involvement of the interphalangeal joints produces irreversible changes in the distal joints (Heberden's nodes) and the proximal joints (Bouchard's nodes). These nodes can be painless initially, with gradual progression to or sudden flare-ups of redness, swelling, tenderness, and impaired sensation and dexterity.

**Heberden's nodes**

**Bouchard's nodes**

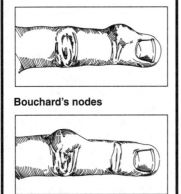

of systemic symptoms rules out an inflammatory joint disorder. X-rays of the affected joint help confirm diagnosis of osteoarthritis but may be normal in the early stages. X-rays may require many views and typically show:
- narrowing of joint space or margin
- cystlike bony deposits in joint space and margins
- sclerosis of the subchondral space
- joint deformity due to degeneration or articular damage
- bony growths at weight-bearing areas
- fusion of joints.

No laboratory test is specific for osteoarthritis.

## Treatment

The goal of treatment is to relieve pain, maintain or improve mobility, and minimize disability. Medications include aspirin (or other nonnarcotic analgesics), phenylbutazone, indomethacin, fenoprofen, ibuprofen, propoxyphene and, in some cases, intra-articular injections of corticosteroids. Such injections, given every 4 to 6 months, may delay the development of nodes in the hands.

Effective treatment also reduces stress by supporting or stabilizing the joint with crutches, braces, cane, walker, cervical collar, or traction. Other supportive measures include massage, moist heat, paraffin dips for hands, protective techniques for preventing undue stress on the joints, adequate rest (particularly after activity) and, occasionally, exercise when the knees are affected.

Surgical treatment, reserved for patients who have severe disability or uncontrollable pain, may include the following:
- *arthroplasty* (partial or total): replacement of deteriorated part of joint with prosthetic appliance
- *arthrodesis:* surgical fusion of bones; used primarily in spine (laminectomy)

- altered gait contractures
- limited movement.

These symptoms increase with poor posture, obesity, and occupational stress.

Osteoarthritis of the interphalangeal joints produces irreversible changes in the distal joints (Heberden's nodes) and proximal joints (Bouchard's nodes). These nodes may be painless at first but eventually become red, swollen, and tender, causing numbness and loss of dexterity. (See *Viewing osteoarthritis.*)

## Diagnosis

A thorough physical examination confirms typical symptoms, and the absence

• *osteoplasty:* scraping and lavage of deteriorated bone from joint

• *osteotomy:* change in alignment of bone to relieve stress by excision of wedge of bone or cutting of bone.

**Special considerations**

• Promote adequate rest, particularly after activity. Plan rest periods during the day, and provide for adequate sleep at night. Moderation is the key — teach the patient to "pace" daily activities.

• Assist with physical therapy, and encourage the patient to perform gentle, isometric range-of-motion (ROM) exercises.

• If the patient needs surgery, provide appropriate preoperative and postoperative care.

• Provide emotional support and reassurance to help the patient cope with limited mobility. Explain that osteoarthritis is *not* a systemic disease.

• Specific patient care depends on the affected joint:

– *Hand:* Apply hot soaks and paraffin dips to relieve pain, as necessary.

– *Spine (lumbar and sacral):* Recommend firm mattress (or bed board) to decrease morning pain.

– *Spine (cervical):* Check cervical collar for constriction; watch for redness with prolonged use.

– *Hip:* Use moist heat pads to relieve pain and administer antispasmodic drugs as necessary. Assist with ROM and strengthening exercises, always making sure the patient gets the proper rest afterward. Check crutches, cane, braces, and walker for proper fit, and teach the patient how to use them correctly. For example, the patient with unilateral joint involvement should use an orthopedic appliance (such as a cane or walker) on the normal side. Advise the use of cushions when sitting, as well as the use of an elevated toilet seat.

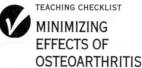

TEACHING CHECKLIST

## MINIMIZING EFFECTS OF OSTEOARTHRITIS

Review the following teaching points with your patient.

• Explain the need for adequate rest during the day, after exertion, and at night.

• Remind the patient to take medications as prescribed and to report adverse reactions immediately.

• Instruct the patient to avoid overexertion.

• Describe proper posture in standing, walking, stooping, and picking up objects.

• Recommend that the patient avoid weight-bearing activities.

• Encourage the patient to wear well-fitting shoes that are supportive. Remind him not to allow the heels to become too worn down.

• Recommend that he perform range-of-motion exercises gently.

• Discuss the importance of maintaining proper body weight.

• Tell the patient to avoid activities that require repeated impact on joints.

– *Knee:* Twice daily, assist with prescribed ROM exercises, exercises to maintain muscle tone, and progressive resistance exercises to increase muscle strength. Provide elastic supports or braces if needed.

• For more patient-teaching information, see *Minimizing effects of osteoarthritis.*

❯ CLINICAL TIP Tell the patient to install safety devices at home, such as guard rails in the bathroom. The patient's living area may need to be assessed for safety and prevention of injuries.

# OSTEOMYELITIS

A pyogenic bone infection, osteomyelitis may be chronic or acute. It commonly results from a combination of local trauma — usually quite trivial but resulting in hematoma formation — and an acute infection originating elsewhere in the body. Although osteomyelitis often remains localized, it can spread through the bone to the marrow, cortex, and periosteum.

Acute osteomyelitis is usually a blood-borne disease, which most often affects rapidly growing children. Chronic osteomyelitis (rare) is characterized by multiple draining sinus tracts and metastatic lesions.

Osteomyelitis occurs more often in children than in adults — and particularly in boys — usually as a complication of an acute localized infection. The most common sites in children are the lower end of the femur and the upper end of the tibia, humerus, and radius. In adults, the most common sites are the pelvis and vertebrae, generally the result of contamination associated with surgery or trauma.

The incidence of both chronic and acute osteomyelitis is declining, except in drug abusers. With prompt treatment, the prognosis for acute osteomyelitis is very good; for chronic osteomyelitis, which is more prevalent in adults, the prognosis is still poor.

## Causes

The most common pyogenic organism in osteomyelitis is *Staphylococcus aureus;* others include *Streptococcus pyogenes, Pneumococcus, Pseudomonas aeruginosa, Escherichia coli,* and *Proteus vulgaris.* Typically, these organisms find a culture site in a hematoma from recent trauma or in a weakened area, such as the site of local infection (for example, furunculosis), and spread directly to bone.

As the organisms grow and form pus within the bone, tension builds within the rigid medullary cavity, forcing pus through the haversian canals. This forms a subperiosteal abscess that deprives the bone of its blood supply and eventually may cause necrosis. In turn, necrosis stimulates the periosteum to create new bone (involucrum); the old bone (sequestrum) detaches and works its way out through an abscess or the sinuses. By the time sequestrum forms, osteomyelitis is chronic.

## Signs and symptoms

Onset of acute osteomyelitis is usually rapid, with sudden pain in the affected bone, and tenderness, heat, swelling, and restricted movement over it. Associated systemic symptoms may include tachycardia, sudden fever, nausea, and malaise.

Generally, the clinical features of both chronic and acute osteomyelitis are the same, except that chronic infection can persist intermittently for years, flaring up spontaneously after minor trauma. Sometimes, however, the only symptom of chronic infection is the persistent drainage of pus from an old pocket in a sinus tract.

## Diagnosis

Patient history, physical examination, and the following laboratory tests help to confirm osteomyelitis:
- *White blood cell count* shows leukocytosis.
- *Erythrocyte sedimentation rate* and *C-reactive protein (CRP)* are elevated; however CRP appears to be a better diagnostic tool.
- *Blood cultures* identify the causative organism.

X-rays may not show bone involvement until the disease has been active for some time, usually 2 to 3 weeks. Bone scans can detect early infection. Diagnosis must rule out poliomyelitis, rheumatic fever, myositis, and bone fractures.

> CLINICAL TIP Computed tomography scan and magnetic resonance imaging may be necessary to delineate the extent of infection.

### Treatment

Treatment varies for acute and chronic osteomyelitis.

#### *Acute osteomyelitis*

Acute osteomyelitis should be treated before a definitive diagnosis. Treatment includes:

• administration of large doses of I.V. antibiotics (usually a penicillinase-resistant penicillin, such as nafcillin or oxacillin, or a cephalosporin) after blood cultures are taken
• early surgical drainage to relieve pressure buildup and sequestrum formation
• immobilization of the affected bone by plaster cast, traction, or bed rest
• supportive measures, such as administration of analgesics and I.V. fluids.

If an abscess forms, treatment includes incision and drainage, followed by a culture of the drainage. Antibiotic therapy to control infection may include administration of systemic antibiotics; intracavitary instillation of antibiotics through closed-system continuous irrigation with low intermittent suction; limited irrigation with blood drainage system with suction (Hemovac); or local application of packed, wet, antibiotic-soaked dressings.

#### *Chronic osteomyelitis*

In chronic osteomyelitis, surgery is usually required to remove dead bone (sequestrectomy) and to promote drainage (saucerization). The prognosis is poor even after surgery. Patients are often in great pain and require prolonged hospitalization. Resistant chronic osteomyelitis in an arm or leg may necessitate amputation.

Some facilities also use hyperbaric oxygen to increase the activity of naturally occurring leukocytes.

Free tissue transfers and local muscle flaps are also used to fill in dead space and increase blood supply.

### Special considerations

The caregiver's major concerns are to control infection, protect the bone from injury, and offer meticulous supportive care.

• Use strict aseptic technique when changing dressings and irrigating wounds.
• If the patient is in skeletal traction for compound fractures, cover insertion points of pin tracks with small, dry dressings, and tell him not to touch the skin around the pins and wires.
• Administer I.V. fluids to maintain adequate hydration as necessary.
• Provide a diet high in protein and vitamin C.
• Assess vital signs and wound appearance daily, and monitor daily for new pain, which may indicate secondary infection.
• Carefully monitor suctioning equipment. Keep containers filled of solution being instilled. Monitor the amount of solution instilled and suctioned.
• Support the affected limb with firm pillows. Keep the limb level with the body; don't let it sag.
• Provide good skin care. Turn the patient gently every 2 hours and watch for signs of developing pressure ulcers.
• Provide good cast care. Support the cast with firm pillows and "petal" the edges with pieces of adhesive tape or moleskin to smooth rough edges.

• Check circulation and drainage: If a wet spot appears on the cast, circle it with a marking pen and note the time of appearance (on the cast). Be aware of how much drainage is expected. Check the circled spot at least every 4 hours. Watch for any enlargement.

• Protect the patient from mishaps, such as jerky movements and falls, which may threaten bone integrity.

• Be alert for sudden pain, crepitus, or deformity. Watch for any sudden malposition of the limb, which may indicate fracture.

• Provide emotional support and appropriate diversions.

• Before discharge, teach the patient how to protect and clean the wound and, most importantly, how to recognize signs of recurring infection (increased temperature, redness, localized heat, and swelling).

• Stress the need for follow-up examinations.

• Instruct the patient to seek prompt treatment for possible sources of recurrence—blisters, boils, styes, and impetigo.

# OSTEOPOROSIS

In osteoporosis, a metabolic bone disorder, the rate of bone resorption accelerates while the rate of bone formation slows down, causing a loss of bone mass. Bones affected by this disease lose calcium and phosphate salts and thus become porous, brittle, and abnormally vulnerable to fracture.

Osteoporosis may be primary or secondary to an underlying disease. Primary osteoporosis is often called senile or postmenopausal osteoporosis because it most commonly develops in elderly, postmenopausal women.

## Causes

The cause of primary osteoporosis is unknown; however, a mild but prolonged negative calcium balance, resulting from an inadequate dietary intake of calcium, may be an important contributing factor—as may declining gonadal adrenal function, faulty protein metabolism due to estrogen deficiency, and a sedentary lifestyle.

Causes of secondary osteoporosis include prolonged therapy with steroids or heparin, total immobilization or disuse of a bone (as with hemiplegia, for example), alcoholism, malnutrition, malabsorption, scurvy, lactose intolerance, hyperthyroidism, osteogenesis imperfecta, and Sudeck's atrophy (localized to hands and feet, with recurring attacks).

## Signs and symptoms

Osteoporosis is usually discovered when an elderly person bends to lift something, hears a snapping sound, then feels a sudden pain in the lower back. Vertebral collapse, producing a backache with pain that radiates around the trunk, is the most common presenting feature. Any movement or jarring aggravates the backache.

In another common pattern, osteoporosis can develop insidiously, with increasing deformity, kyphosis, loss of height, and a markedly aged appearance. As vertebral bodies weaken, spontaneous wedge fractures, pathologic fractures of the neck and femur, Colles' fractures after a minor fall, and hip fractures are all common.

Osteoporosis primarily affects the weight-bearing vertebrae. Only when the condition is advanced or severe, as in Cushing's syndrome or hyperthyroidism, do comparable changes occur in the skull, ribs, and long bones.

## Diagnosis

Differential diagnosis must exclude other causes of rarefying bone disease, especially those affecting the spine, such as metastatic carcinoma and advanced multiple myeloma. Initial evaluation attempts to identify the specific cause of osteoporosis through the patient history. Diagnostic tests include the following:

• *X-rays* show typical degeneration in the lower thoracic and lumbar vertebrae. The vertebral bodies may appear flattened and may look denser than normal. Loss of bone mineral becomes evident in later stages.

• *Dual* or *single photon absorptiometry* allows measurement of bone mass, which helps to assess the extremities, hips, and spine.

• *Serum calcium, phosphorus,* and *alkaline phosphatase* are all within normal limits, but *parathyroid hormone* may be elevated.

• *Bone biopsy* shows thin, porous, but otherwise normal-looking bone.

## Treatment

Effective treatment aims to prevent additional fractures and control pain. A physical therapy program, emphasizing gentle exercise and activity, is an important part of the treatment. Estrogen, to be started within 3 years after menopause, may be given to decrease the rate of bone resorption; sodium fluoride, to stimulate bone formation; and calcium and vitamin D, to support normal bone metabolism. However, drug therapy merely arrests osteoporosis and doesn't cure it.

Weakened vertebrae should be supported, usually with a back brace. Surgery can correct pathologic fractures of the femur by open reduction and internal fixation. Colles' fracture requires reduction with plaster immobilization for 4 to 10 weeks.

## Prevention

The incidence of senile osteoporosis may be reduced through adequate intake of dietary calcium and regular exercise. Hormonal and fluoride treatments may also offer some preventive benefit.

Secondary osteoporosis can be prevented through effective treatment of the underlying disease, as well as steroid therapy, early mobilization after surgery or trauma, decreased alcohol consumption, careful observation for signs of malabsorption, and prompt treatment of hyperthyroidism.

## Special considerations

• Focus on the patient's fragility, stressing careful positioning, ambulation, and prescribed exercises.

• Check the patient's skin daily for redness, warmth, and new sites of pain, which may indicate new fractures. Encourage activity; help the patient walk several times daily.

• Perform passive range-of-motion exercises, or encourage the patient to perform active exercises. Make sure she regularly attends scheduled physical therapy sessions.

• Institute safety precautions such as keeping side rails up. Move the patient gently and carefully at all times. Explain to the patient's family and ancillary facility personnel how easily an osteoporotic patient's bones can fracture.

• Provide a balanced diet, high in nutrients that support skeletal metabolism: vitamin D, calcium, and protein. Administer analgesics and heat to relieve pain.

• Make sure the patient and her family clearly understand the prescribed drug regimen. Tell them how to recognize significant adverse reactions and to report them immediately. Also tell the patient to report any new pain sites immediately, especially after trauma, no matter how slight.

• Advise the patient to sleep on a firm mattress and avoid excessive bed rest. Make sure she knows how to wear her back brace.

> **CLINICAL TIP** Thoroughly explain osteoporosis to the patient and her family. If they don't understand the nature of this disease, they may feel that they could have prevented the fractures if they had been more careful.

• Teach the patient good body mechanics — to stoop before lifting anything and to avoid twisting movements and prolonged bending.

• Instruct the female patient taking estrogen in the proper technique for self-examination of the breasts. Tell her to perform this examination at least once a month and to report any lumps immediately. Emphasize the need for regular gynecologic exams. Tell her to report abnormal bleeding promptly.

# OTITIS EXTERNA

Also known as external otitis and swimmer's ear, otitis externa is an inflammation of the skin of the external ear canal and auricle. It may be acute or chronic and it's most common in the summer. With treatment, acute otitis externa usually subsides within 7 days (although it may become chronic) and tends to recur.

## Causes
Otitis externa usually results from bacterial infection with an organism, such as *Pseudomonas, Proteus vulgaris,* streptococci, or *Staphylococcus aureus;* sometimes it stems from a fungus, such as *Aspergillus niger* or *Candida albicans* (fungal otitis externa is most common in the tropics). Occasionally, chronic otitis externa results from dermatologic conditions, such as seborrhea or psoriasis. Predisposing factors include:

• swimming in contaminated water; cerumen creates a culture medium for the waterborne organism

• cleaning the ear canal with a cotton swab, bobby pin, finger, or other foreign objects; this irritates the ear canal and possibly introduces the infecting microorganism

• exposure to dust, hair care products, or other irritants, which causes the patient to scratch his ear, excoriating the auricle and canal

• regular use of earphones, earplugs, or earmuffs, which trap moisture in the ear canal, creating a culture medium for infection

• chronic drainage from a perforated tympanic membrane.

## Signs and symptoms
Acute otitis externa characteristically produces moderate to severe pain that is exacerbated by manipulation of the auricle or tragus, clenching the teeth, opening the mouth, or chewing. Its other clinical effects may include fever, foul-smelling aural discharge, regional cellulitis, and partial hearing loss.

Fungal otitis externa may be asymptomatic, although *A. niger* produces a black or gray blotting paper–like growth in the ear canal. In chronic otitis externa, pruritus replaces pain, which may lead to scaling and skin thickening with a resultant narrowing of the lumen. An aural discharge may also occur. Asteatosis (lack of cerumen) is common.

## Diagnosis
Physical examination confirms otitis externa. In acute otitis externa, otoscopy reveals a swollen external ear canal (sometimes to the point of complete closure), periauricular lymphadenopathy (tender nodes in front of the tragus, be-

hind the ear, or in the upper neck) and, occasionally, regional cellulitis.

In fungal otitis externa, removal of growth shows thick red epithelium. Microscopic examination or culture and sensitivity tests can identify the causative organism and determine antibiotic treatment. Pain on palpation of the tragus or auricle distinguishes acute otitis externa from otitis media.

In chronic otitis externa, physical examination shows thick red epithelium in the ear canal. Severe chronic otitis externa may reflect underlying diabetes mellitus, hypothyroidism, or nephritis.

### Treatment
Treatment varies, depending on the type of otitis externa.

#### *Acute otitis externa*
To relieve the pain of acute otitis externa, treatment includes heat therapy to the periauricular region (heat lamp; hot, damp compresses; heating pad), aspirin or acetaminophen, and codeine. Instillation of antibiotic eardrops (with or without hydrocortisone) follows cleaning of the ear and removal of debris. If fever persists or regional cellulitis develops, a systemic antibiotic is necessary.

#### *Fungal otitis externa*
As with other forms of this disorder, fungal otitis externa necessitates careful cleaning of the ear. Application of a keratolytic or 2% salicylic acid in cream containing nystatin may help treat otitis externa resulting from candidal organisms.

Instillation of slightly acidic eardrops creates an unfavorable environment in the ear canal for most fungi as well as *Pseudomonas.*

#### *Chronic otitis externa*
Primary treatment consists of cleaning the ear and removing debris. Supplemental therapy includes instillation of antibiotic eardrops or application of antibiotic ointment or cream (neomycin, bacitracin, or polymyxin, possibly combined with hydrocortisone). Another ointment contains phenol, salicylic acid, precipitated sulfur, and petroleum jelly and produces exfoliative and antipruritic effects.

For mild chronic otitis externa, treatment may include instilling antibiotic eardrops once or twice weekly and wearing specially fitted earplugs while showering, shampooing, or swimming.

### Special considerations
If the patient has acute otitis externa:
- Monitor vital signs, particularly temperature. Watch for and record the type and amount of aural drainage.
- Remove debris and gently clean the ear canal with mild Burow's solution (aluminum acetate). Place a wisp of cotton soaked with solution into the ear, and apply a saturated compress directly to the auricle. Afterward, dry the ear gently but thoroughly. (In severe otitis externa, cleaning may be delayed until after initial treatment with antibiotic eardrops.)
- To instill eardrops in an adult, pull the pinna upward and backward to straighten the canal. For children, pull the pinna downward and backward. To ensure that the drops reach the epithelium, insert a wisp of cotton moistened with eardrops.
- If the patient has chronic otitis externa, clean the ear thoroughly. Use wet soaks intermittently on oozing or infected skin. If the patient has a chronic fungal infection, clean the ear canal well, then apply an exfoliative ointment.

To prevent otitis externa:

• Suggest using lamb's wool earplugs coated with petroleum jelly to keep water out of the ears when showering or shampooing.

• Tell the patient to wear earplugs or to keep his head above water when swimming and to instill two or three drops of 3% boric acid solution in 70% alcohol before and after swimming to toughen the skin of the external car canal.

• Warn against cleaning the ears with cotton swabs or other objects.

• Urge prompt treatment of otitis media to prevent perforation of the tympanic membrane.

• If the patient is diabetic, evaluate him for malignant otitis externa.

CLINICAL TIP  Hearing aid users who are prone to otitis externa should consider having the device vented to improve aeration of the external ear canal.

# OTITIS MEDIA

Inflammation of the middle ear, otitis media may be suppurative or secretory, acute or chronic. Acute otitis media is common in children; its incidence rises during the winter months, paralleling the seasonal rise in nonbacterial respiratory tract infections.

With prompt treatment, the prognosis for acute otitis media is excellent; however, prolonged accumulation of fluid within the middle ear cavity causes chronic otitis media, with possible perforation of the tympanic membrane. Chronic suppurative otitis media may lead to scarring, adhesions, and severe structural or functional ear damage; chronic secretory otitis media, with its persistent inflammation and pressure, may cause conductive hearing loss.

## Causes

Otitis media results from disruption of eustachian tube patency. (See *Site of otitis media.*)

### Suppurative otitis media

In the suppurative form, respiratory tract infection, allergic reaction, nasotracheal intubation, or positional changes allow nasopharyngeal flora to reflux through the eustachian tube and colonize the middle ear. Suppurative otitis media usually results from bacterial infection with pneumococci, *Haemophilus influenzae* (the most common cause in children under age 6), *Moraxella catarrhalis,* beta-hemolytic streptococci, staphylococci (most common cause in children age 6 or older), or gram-negative bacteria.

Predisposing factors include the normally wider, shorter, more horizontal eustachian tubes and increased lymphoid tissue in children as well as anatomic anomalies. Chronic suppurative otitis media results from inadequate treatment of acute otitis episodes or from infection by resistant strains of bacteria or, rarely, tuberculosis.

### Secretory otitis media

In this form of otitis media, obstruction of the eustachian tube causes a buildup of negative pressure in the middle ear that promotes transudation of sterile serous fluid from blood vessels in the membrane of the middle ear. Such effusion may be secondary to eustachian tube dysfunction from viral infection or allergy. It may also follow barotrauma (pressure injury caused by inability to equalize pressures between the environment and the middle ear), as can occur during rapid aircraft descent in a person with an upper respiratory tract infection or during rapid underwater ascent in scuba diving (barotitis media).

## SITE OF OTITIS MEDIA

The shaded areas of the middle ear in the illustration below denote sites of otitis media.

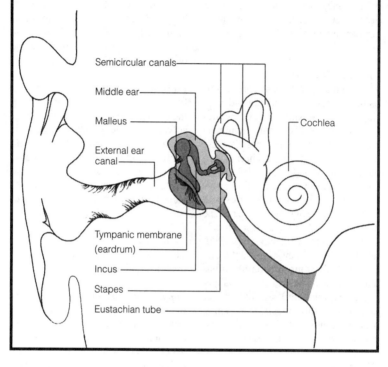

Chronic secretory otitis media follows persistent eustachian tube dysfunction from mechanical obstruction (adenoidal tissue overgrowth, tumors), edema (allergic rhinitis, chronic sinus infection), or inadequate treatment of acute suppurative otitis media.

### Signs and symptoms

Clinical features vary with the specific type of the disorder.

#### *Suppurative otitis media*

Symptoms of acute suppurative otitis media include severe, deep, throbbing pain (from pressure behind the tympanic membrane); signs of upper respiratory tract infection (sneezing, coughing); mild to very high fever; hearing loss (usually mild and conductive); dizziness; nausea; and vomiting.

Other possible effects include bulging of the tympanic membrane with concomitant erythema and purulent drainage in the ear canal from tympanic membrane rupture. However, many patients are asymptomatic.

#### *Secretory otitis media*

In acute secretory otitis media, a severe conductive hearing loss varies from 15 to 35 db, depending on the thickness and amount of fluid in the middle ear cavity — and, possibly, a sensation of fullness in the ear and popping, crackling, or clicking sounds on swallowing or with jaw movement. Accumulation of fluid may also cause the patient to hear an echo when he speaks and to experience a vague feeling of top-heaviness.

### Chronic otitis media

The cumulative effects of chronic otitis media include thickening and scarring of the tympanic membrane, decreased or absent tympanic membrane mobility, cholesteatoma (a cystlike mass in the middle ear) and, in chronic suppurative otitis media, a painless, purulent discharge. The extent of associated conductive hearing loss varies with the size and type of tympanic membrane perforation and ossicular destruction.

If the tympanic membrane has ruptured, the patient may state that the pain has suddenly stopped. Complications may include abscesses (brain, subperiosteal, and epidural), sigmoid sinus or jugular vein thrombosis, septicemia, meningitis, suppurative labyrinthitis, facial paralysis, and otitis externa.

### Diagnosis

Diagnostic tests also vary with the specific type of otitis media.

### Suppurative otitis media

In acute suppurative otitis media, otoscopy reveals obscured or distorted bony landmarks of the tympanic membrane. Pneumatoscopy can show decreased tympanic membrane mobility, but this procedure is painful with an obviously bulging, erythematous tympanic membrane. The pain pattern is diagnostically significant: In acute suppurative otitis media, for example, pulling the auricle *doesn't* exacerbate the pain.

### Secretory otitis media

In acute secretory otitis media, otoscopic examination reveals tympanic membrane retraction, which causes the bony landmarks to appear more prominent.

Examination also detects clear or amber fluid behind the tympanic membrane. If hemorrhage into the middle ear has occurred, as in barotrauma, the tympanic membrane appears blue-black.

### Chronic otitis media

In patients with chronic otitis media, the history discloses recurrent or unresolved otitis media. Otoscopy shows thickening and sometimes scarring, and decreased mobility of the tympanic membrane; pneumatoscopy, decreased or absent tympanic membrane movement. History of recent air travel or scuba diving suggests barotitis media.

### Treatment

The type of otitis media dictates the treatment guidelines.

### Suppurative otitis media

In acute suppurative otitis media, antibiotic therapy includes ampicillin or amoxicillin. In areas with a high incidence of beta-lactamase–producing *H. influenzae* and in patients who aren't responding to ampicillin or amoxicillin, amoxicillin/clavulanate potassium may be used.

For those who are allergic to penicillin derivatives, therapy may include cefaclor or cotrimoxazole. Severe, painful bulging of the tympanic membrane usually necessitates myringotomy. Broad-spectrum antibiotics can help prevent acute suppurative otitis media in high-risk patients. In patients with recurring otitis, antibiotics must be used with discretion to prevent development of resistant strains of bacteria.

➤ CLINICAL TIP   Most patients who are receiving antibiotic therapy for acute otitis media have significant improvement in 48 hours.

### Secretory otitis media

For patients with acute secretory otitis media, inflation of the eustachian tube by performing Valsalva's maneuver several times a day may be the only treatment required. Otherwise, nasopharyngeal decongestant therapy may be helpful. It should continue for at least 2 weeks and sometimes indefinitely, with periodic evaluation.

If decongestant therapy fails, myringotomy and aspiration of middle ear fluid are necessary, followed by insertion of a polyethylene tube into the tympanic membrane, for immediate and prolonged equalization of pressure. The tube falls out spontaneously after 9 to 12 months. Concomitant treatment of the underlying cause (such as elimination of allergens, or adenoidectomy for hypertrophied adenoids) may also be helpful in correcting this disorder.

### Chronic otitis media

Treatment of chronic otitis media includes broad-spectrum antibiotics, such as amoxicillin/clavulanate potassium or cefuroxime, for exacerbations of acute otitis media; elimination of eustachian tube obstruction; treatment of otitis externa; myringoplasty and tympanoplasty to reconstruct middle ear structures when thickening and scarring are present; and, possibly, mastoidectomy. Cholesteatoma requires excision.

### Special considerations

● Explain all diagnostic tests and procedures.
● After myringotomy, maintain drainage flow. Don't place cotton or plugs deep in the ear canal; however, sterile cotton may be placed loosely in the external ear to absorb drainage.

● To prevent infection, change the cotton whenever it gets damp, and wash hands before and after giving ear care. Watch for headache, fever, severe pain, or disorientation.
● After tympanoplasty, reinforce dressings, and observe for excessive bleeding from the ear canal. Administer analgesics as needed. Warn the patient against blowing his nose or getting the ear wet when bathing.
● Encourage the patient to complete the prescribed course of antibiotic treatment. If nasopharyngeal decongestants are ordered, teach correct instillation.

➤ CLINICAL TIP  Most children will have an effusion present at the completion of a 10- to 14-day course of antibiotic therapy. Effusion may last up to 12 weeks before spontaneous clearance can be expected.

● Suggest application of heat to the ear to relieve pain.
● Advise the patient with acute secretory otitis media to watch for and immediately report pain and fever — signs of secondary infection.

To prevent otitis media:
● Teach recognition of upper respiratory tract infections and encourage early treatment.
● Instruct parents not to feed their infant in a supine position or put him to bed with a bottle. This prevents reflux of nasopharyngeal flora.
● To promote eustachian tube patency, instruct the patient to perform Valsalva's maneuver several times daily.
● Identify and treat allergies.

# OTOSCLEROSIS

The most common cause of conductive deafness, otosclerosis is the slow formation of spongy bone in the otic cap-

## OTOSCLEROSIS: RECOVERING AFTER SURGERY

Review the following points with the patient prior to discharge.

- Instruct the patient to sneeze and cough with his mouth open for 2 weeks after surgery to prevent dislodgment of the graft or prosthesis.
- Inform the patient that he may hear a variety of noises, such as cracking or popping; reassure him that this is normal.
- Tell the patient that the ear packing or middle ear fluid decreases hearing in the affected ear and it can seem as if he's talking in a barrel.
- Reassure the patient that minor ear discomfort is expected and urge him to take the prescribed pain medication. Stress that excessive ear pain should be reported to the doctor.
- Occasionally a small amount of bleeding from the ear occurs; reassure the patient that this is normal. Excessive ear drainage should be reported to the doctor.
- Explain that some patients initially find the improvement in hearing after stapes surgery so great that it causes sensitivity or distress. This usually di-

minishes as the patient adapts to his improved hearing level.
- Before discharge, instruct the patient to avoid loud noises and sudden pressure changes (such as those that occur while diving or flying) until healing is complete (usually 6 months).
- Advise the patient not to blow his nose for at least 1 week to prevent contaminated air and bacteria from entering the eustachian tube.
- Stress the importance of protecting the ears against cold; avoiding any activities that provoke dizziness, such as straining, bending, or heavy lifting; and, if possible, avoiding contact with anyone who has an upper respiratory tract infection.
- Teach the patient and his family how to change the external ear dressing (eye pad or gauze pad) and care for the incision.
- Emphasize the need to complete the prescribed antibiotic regimen and to return for scheduled follow-up care.

sule, particularly at the oval window. It occurs in at least 10% of whites and is twice as prevalent in females as in males, usually between the ages of 15 and 30. There's a positive family history in 55% of patients. With surgery, the prognosis is good.

### Causes
Otosclerosis appears to result from a genetic factor transmitted as an autosomal dominant trait; many patients report family histories of hearing loss (excluding presbycusis). Pregnancy may trigger the onset of this condition.

### Signs and symptoms
Spongy bone in the otic capsule immobilizes the footplate of the normally mobile stapes, disrupting the conduction of vibrations from the tympanic membrane to the cochlea. This causes progressive unilateral hearing loss, which may advance to bilateral deafness. Other symptoms include tinnitus and paracusis of Willis (hearing conversation better in a noisy environment than in a quiet one).

### Diagnosis
Early diagnosis is based on a Rinne test that shows bone conduction lasting longer than air conduction (normally,

the reverse is true). As otosclerosis progresses, bone conduction also deteriorates.

• *Audiometric testing* reveals hearing loss ranging from 60 db, in early stages, to total loss.

• *Weber's test* detects sound lateralizing to the more affected ear.

• *Physical examination* reveals a normal tympanic membrane.

**Treatment**

Effective treatment consists of stapedectomy (removal of the stapes) and insertion of a prosthesis to restore partial or total hearing. This procedure is performed on only one ear at a time, beginning with the ear that has suffered greater damage. Alternative surgery includes stapedotomy (creation of a small hole in the stapes' footplate, through which a wire and piston are inserted).

Postoperatively, treatment includes hospitalization for 2 or 3 days and antibiotics to prevent infection. If surgery isn't possible, a hearing aid (air conduction aid with molded ear insert receiver) enables the patient to hear conversation in normal surroundings, although this therapy isn't as effective as stapedectomy.

**Special considerations**

• During the first 24 hours after surgery, keep the patient lying flat, with the affected ear facing upward (to maintain the position of the graft).

• Enforce bed rest with bathroom privileges for 48 hours. Because the patient may be dizzy, keep the side rails up and assist him with ambulation.

• Assess for pain and vertigo, which may be relieved with repositioning or prescribed medication.

• For more patient-teaching information, see *Otosclerosis: Recovering after surgery.*

# OVARIAN CANCER

After cancer of the lung, breast, and colon, primary ovarian cancer ranks as the most common cause of cancer deaths among American women. In women with previously treated breast cancer, metastatic ovarian cancer is more common than cancer at any other site.

The prognosis varies with the histologic type and stage of the disease but is generally poor because ovarian tumors produce few early signs and are usually advanced at diagnosis. Although about 40% of women with ovarian cancer survive for 5 years, the overall survival rate hasn't improved significantly.

Three main types of ovarian cancer exist:

• *Primary epithelial tumors* account for 90% of all ovarian cancers and include serous cystoadenocarcinoma, mucinous cystoadenocarcinoma, and endometrioid and mesonephric malignancies. Serous cystoadenocarcinoma is the most common type and accounts for 50% of all cases.

• *Germ cell tumors* include endodermal sinus malignancies, embryonal carcinoma (a rare ovarian cancer that appears in children), immature teratomas, and dysgerminoma.

• *Sex cord (stromal) tumors include granulosa cell tumors* (which produce estrogen and may have feminizing effects), granulosatheca cell tumors, and the rare arrhenoblastomas (which produce androgen and have virilizing effects).

**Causes**

Exactly what causes ovarian cancer isn't known, but its incidence is noticeably higher in women of upper socioeconomic levels between the ages of 20 and 54. However, it can occur during childhood. Other contributing factors include age at menopause; infertility; celibacy; high-fat diet; exposure to asbestos, talc, and industrial pollutants; nulliparity; familial tendency; and history of breast or uterine cancer.

Primary epithelial tumors arise in the müllerian epithelium; germ cell tumors, in the ovum itself; and sex cord tumors, in the ovarian stroma (the ovary's supporting framework).

Ovarian tumors spread rapidly intraperitoneally by local extension or surface seeding and, occasionally, through the lymphatics and the bloodstream. Generally, extraperitoneal spread is through the diaphragm into the chest cavity, which may cause pleural effusions. Other types of metastasis are rare.

### Signs and symptoms

Typically, symptoms vary with the size of the tumor. Occasionally, in the early stages, ovarian cancer causes vague abdominal discomfort, dyspepsia, and other mild GI disturbances. As it progresses, it causes urinary frequency, constipation, pelvic discomfort, abdominal distention, and weight loss.

Tumor rupture, torsion, or infection may cause pain, which, in young patients, may mimic appendicitis. Granulosa cell tumors have feminizing effects (such as bleeding between periods in premenopausal women); conversely, arrhenoblastomas have virilizing effects. Advanced ovarian cancer causes ascites, rarely postmenopausal bleeding and pain, and symptoms relating to metastatic sites (most often pleural effusions).

### Diagnosis

In ovarian cancer, diagnosis requires clinical evaluation, a complete patient history, surgical exploration, and histologic studies. Preoperative evaluation includes a complete physical examination, including pelvic examination with Pap smear (positive in only a small number of women with ovarian cancer) and the following special tests:

- abdominal ultrasonography, computed tomography scan, or X-ray (may delineate tumor size)
- complete blood count, blood chemistries, and electrocardiography
- excretory urography for information on renal function and possible urinary tract anomalies or obstruction
- chest X-ray for distant metastasis and pleural effusions
- barium enema (especially in patients with GI symptoms) to reveal obstruction and size of tumor
- lymphangiography to show lymph node involvement
- mammography to rule out primary breast cancer
- liver function studies or a liver scan in patients with ascites
- ascites fluid aspiration for identification of typical cells by cytology
- laboratory tumor marker studies, such as ovarian carcinoma antigen, carcinoembryonic antigen, and human chorionic gonadotropin.

Despite extensive testing, accurate diagnosis and staging are impossible without exploratory laparotomy, including lymph node evaluation and tumor resection. (See *Staging ovarian cancer.*)

### Treatment

Depending on the stage of the disease and the patient's age, treatment of ovarian cancer requires varying combinations of surgery, chemotherapy and, in some cases, radiation.

#### Conservative treatment

Occasionally, in girls or young women with a unilateral encapsulated tumor who wish to maintain fertility, the fol-

## STAGING OVARIAN CANCER

The International Federation of Gynecology and Obstetrics uses the staging system below for ovarian cancer.

**Stage I**—growth limited to the ovaries

**Stage IA**—growth limited to one ovary; no ascites; no tumor on the external surface; capsule intact

**Stage IB**—growth limited to both ovaries; no ascites; no tumor on the external surfaces; capsules intact

**Stage IC**—tumor either Stage IA or IB but on surface of one or both ovaries; or with capsule ruptured; or with ascites containing malignant cells or with positive peritoneal washings

**Stage II**—growth involving one or both ovaries with pelvic extension

**Stage IIA**—extension or metastasis, or both, to the uterus or tubes (or both)

**Stage IIB**—extension to pelvic tissues

**Stage IIIC**—tumor either Stage IIA or IIB, but with tumor on surface of one or both ovaries; or with capsule (or capsules) ruptured; or with ascites present containing malignant cells or with positive peritoneal washings

**Stage III**—tumor involving one or both ovaries with peritoneal implants outside the pelvis or positive retroperitoneal or inguinal nodes; superficial liver metastasis equals Stage III; tumor limited to the true pelvis but with confirmed extension to small bowel or omentum

**Stage IIIA**—tumor grossly limited to the true pelvis with negative nodes but with confirmed microscopic seeding of abdominal peritoneal surfaces

**Stage IIIB**—tumor of one or both ovaries with confirmed implants of abdominal peritoneal surfaces, none exceeding 2 cm in dimension; nodes are negative

**Stage IIIC**—abdominal implants greater than 2 cm or positive retroperitoneal or inguinal nodes or both

**Stage IV**—growth involving one or both ovaries with distant metastasis (such as pleural effusion and abnormal cells or parenchymal liver metastasis)

lowing conservative approach may be appropriate:

• resection of the involved ovary

• biopsies of the omentum and the uninvolved ovary

• peritoneal washings for cytologic examination of pelvic fluid

• careful follow-up, including periodic chest X-rays to rule out lung metastasis.

### Aggressive treatment

Ovarian cancer usually requires more aggressive treatment, including total abdominal hysterectomy and bilateral salpingo-oophorectomy with tumor resection, omentectomy, appendectomy, lymph node biopsies with lymphadenectomy, tissue biopsies, and peritoneal washings.

Complete tumor resection is impossible if the tumor has matted around other organs or if it involves organs that can't be resected. Bilateral salpingo-oophorectomy in a prepubertal girl necessitates hormone replacement therapy, beginning at puberty, to induce the development of secondary sex characteristics.

Chemotherapy extends survival time in most ovarian cancer patients. Unfortunately, it is largely palliative in advanced disease, but prolonged remissions are being achieved in some patients.

Chemotherapeutic drugs useful in ovarian cancer include melphalan, chlorambucil, thiotepa, methotrexate, cyclophosphamide, doxorubicin, vincristine, vinblastine, dactinomycin, bleomycin, paclitaxel, and cisplatin. These drugs are usually given in combination and they may be administered intraperitoneally.

Radiation therapy is generally not used for ovarian cancer because the resulting myelosuppression would limit the effectiveness of chemotherapy.

***Other treatments***
Radioisotopes have been used as adjuvant therapy, but they cause small-bowel obstructions and stenosis.

In addition, I.V. administration of biological response modifiers — interleukin-2, interferon, and monoclonal antibodies — is currently being investigated.

**Special considerations**
Because the treatment of ovarian cancer varies widely, so must the care of the patient.

Before surgery:
• Thoroughly explain all preoperative tests, the expected course of treatment, and surgical and postoperative procedures.
• In premenopausal women, explain that bilateral oophorectomy artificially induces early menopause, so they may experience hot flashes, headaches, palpitations, insomnia, depression, and excessive perspiration.

After surgery:
• Monitor vital signs frequently, and check I.V. fluids often. Monitor intake and output, while maintaining good catheter care. Check the dressing regularly for excessive drainage or bleeding, and watch for signs of infection.
• Provide abdominal support, and watch for abdominal distention. Encourage coughing and deep breathing. Reposition the patient often, and encourage her to walk shortly after surgery.
• Monitor and treat adverse effects of radiation and chemotherapy.

▶ CLINICAL TIP  If the patient is receiving immunotherapy, watch for flulike symptoms that may last 12 to 24 hours after drug administration. Give aspirin or acetaminophen for fever. Keep the patient well covered with blankets, and provide warm liquids to relieve chills. Administer an antiemetic as needed.
• Enlist the help of a social worker, chaplain, and other members of the health care team for additional supportive care.

# OVARIAN CYSTS

Usually ovarian cysts are nonneoplastic sacs on an ovary that contain fluid or semisolid material. Although these cysts are usually small and produce no symptoms, they require thorough investigation as possible sites of malignant change.

Common ovarian cysts include follicular cysts, lutein cysts (granulosa-lutein [corpus luteum] and theca-lutein cysts), and polycystic (or sclerocystic) ovarian disease. Ovarian cysts can develop anytime between puberty and menopause, including during pregnancy. Granulosa-lutein cysts occur infrequently, usually during early pregnancy. The prognosis for nonneoplastic ovarian cysts is excellent.

**Causes**
*Follicular cysts* are generally very small and arise from follicles that overdistend instead of going through the atretic stage of the menstrual cycle. When such cysts

persist into menopause, they secrete excessive amounts of estrogen in response to the hypersecretion of follicle-stimulating hormone and luteinizing hormone that normally occurs during menopause.

*Granulosa-lutein cysts,* which occur within the corpus luteum, are functional, nonneoplastic enlargements of the ovaries caused by excessive accumulation of blood during the hemorrhagic phase of the menstrual cycle.

*Theca-lutein cysts* are commonly bilateral and filled with clear, straw-colored fluid; they are often associated with hydatidiform mole, choriocarcinoma, or hormone therapy (with human chorionic gonadotropin [HCG] or clomiphene citrate).

*Polycystic ovarian disease* is part of the Stein-Leventhal syndrome and stems from endocrine abnormalities.

## Signs and symptoms

Small ovarian cysts (such as follicular cysts) usually don't produce symptoms unless torsion or rupture causes signs of an acute abdomen (abdominal tenderness, distention, and rigidity). Large or multiple cysts may induce mild pelvic discomfort, low back pain, dyspareunia, or abnormal uterine bleeding secondary to a disturbed ovulatory pattern. Ovarian cysts with torsion induce acute abdominal pain similar to that of appendicitis.

Granulosa-lutein cysts that appear early in pregnancy may grow as large as 2″ to 2½″ (5 to 6 cm) in diameter and produce unilateral pelvic discomfort and, if rupture occurs, massive intraperitoneal hemorrhage. In nonpregnant women, these cysts may cause delayed menses, followed by prolonged or irregular bleeding. Polycystic ovarian disease may also produce secondary amenorrhea, oligomenorrhea, or infertility.

## Diagnosis

Generally, characteristic clinical features suggest ovarian cysts. Visualization of the ovaries through ultrasound, laparoscopy, or surgery (often for another condition) confirms ovarian cysts.

Extremely elevated HCG titers strongly suggest theca-lutein cysts.

In polycystic ovarian disease, physical examination demonstrates bilaterally enlarged polycystic ovaries. Tests reveal slightly elevated urinary 17-ketosteroid levels and anovulation (shown by basal body temperature graphs and endometrial biopsy). Direct visualization must rule out paraovarian cysts of the broad ligament, salpingitis, endometriosis, and neoplastic cysts.

## Treatment

The type of cyst dictates the treatment method.

### Follicular cysts

This type of cyst generally doesn't require treatment because it tends to disappear spontaneously within 60 days. However, if it interferes with daily activities, administration of oral clomiphene citrate for 5 days or I.M. progesterone (also for 5 days) reestablishes the ovarian hormonal cycle and induces ovulation. Oral contraceptives may also accelerate involution of functional cysts (including both types of lutein cysts and follicular cysts).

### Granulosa-lutein and theca-lutein cysts

If granulosa-lutein cysts occur during pregnancy, treatment is symptomatic because they diminish during the third trimester and rarely require surgery. Theca-lutein cysts disappear spontaneously after elimination of the hydatidiform mole, destruction of choriocarcinoma, or discontinuation of HCG or clomiphene citrate therapy.

### Polycystic ovarian disease

Treatment of polycystic ovarian disease may include the administration of such drugs as clomiphene citrate to induce ovulation, medroxyprogesterone acetate for 10 days of every month for the patient who doesn't want to become pregnant, or low-dose oral contraceptives for the patient who needs reliable contraception.

Surgery, in the form of laparoscopy or exploratory laparotomy with possible ovarian cystectomy or oophorectomy, may become necessary if an ovarian cyst is found to be persistent or suspicious.

## Special considerations

● Carefully explain the nature of the particular cyst, the type of discomfort — if any — that the patient is likely to experience, and how long the condition is expected to last.

● Preoperatively, watch for signs of cyst rupture, such as increasing abdominal pain, distention, and rigidity. Monitor vital signs for fever, tachypnea, or hypotension, which may indicate peritonitis or intraperitoneal hemorrhage. Administer sedatives, as ordered, to ensure adequate rest before surgery.

● Postoperatively, encourage frequent movement in bed and early ambulation as ordered. Early ambulation effectively prevents pulmonary embolism.

● Provide emotional support. Offer appropriate reassurance if the patient fears cancer or infertility.

➤ CLINICAL TIP Before discharge, advise the patient to increase her activities at home gradually — preferably over 4 to 6 weeks. Tell her to abstain from intercourse and to use tampons and douches during this period.

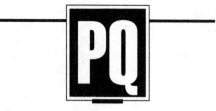

# PAGET'S DISEASE

Also known as osteitis deformans, Paget's disease is a slowly progressive metabolic bone disease characterized by an initial phase of excessive bone resorption (osteoclastic phase), followed by a reactive phase of excessive abnormal bone formation (osteoblastic phase). The new bone structure, which is chaotic, fragile, and weak, causes painful deformities of both external contour and internal structure.

Paget's disease usually localizes in one or several areas of the skeleton (most frequently the lower torso), but occasionally, skeletal deformity is widely distributed. It can be fatal, particularly when it is associated with heart failure (widespread disease creates a continuous need for high cardiac output), bone sarcoma, or giant cell tumors.

## Causes

Paget's disease occurs worldwide but is extremely rare in Asia, the Middle East, Africa, and Scandinavia. In the United States, it affects approximately 2.5 million people over age 40 (mostly men).

Although its exact cause is unknown, one theory holds that early viral infection (possibly with mumps virus) causes a dormant skeletal infection that erupts many years later as Paget's disease. In 5% of the patients, the involved bone will undergo malignant changes.

## Signs and symptoms

Clinical effects of Paget's disease vary.

### Pain

Early stages may be asymptomatic, but when pain does develop, it is usually severe and persistent and may coexist with impaired movement resulting from impingement of abnormal bone on the spinal cord or sensory nerve root. Such pain intensifies with weight bearing.

### Other features

The patient with skull involvement shows characteristic cranial enlargement over frontal and occipital areas (hat size may increase) and may complain of headaches. Other deformities include kyphosis (spinal curvature due to compression fractures of pagetic vertebrae), accompanied by a barrel-shaped chest and asymmetrical bowing of the tibia and femur, which often reduces height. Pagetic sites are warm and tender and are susceptible to pathologic fractures after minor trauma. Pagetic fractures heal slowly and often incompletely.

Bony impingement on the cranial nerves may cause blindness and hearing loss with tinnitus and vertigo. Other complications include hypertension, renal calculi, hypercalcemia, gout, heart failure, and a waddling gait (from softening of pelvic bones).

## Diagnosis

X-rays taken before overt symptoms develop show increased bone expansion and density. A bone scan, which is more sensitive than X-rays, clearly shows early pagetic lesions (radioisotope concentrates in areas of active disease). Bone biopsy reveals characteristic mosaic pattern. Other laboratory findings include:

• anemia
• elevated serum alkaline phosphatase levels (an index of osteoblastic activity and bone formation)
• elevated 24-hour urine levels for hydroxyproline (amino acid excreted by kidneys and an index of osteoclastic hyperactivity). Increasing use of routine chemistry screens — which include serum alkaline phosphatase — is making early diagnosis more common.

## Treatment

If the patient is asymptomatic, treatment isn't needed. The patient with symptoms requires drug therapy, which may include:

• *calcitonin* (a hormone, given subcutaneously or I.M.) and *etidronate* (oral) to retard bone resorption (which relieves bone lesions) and reduce serum alkaline phosphate and urinary hydroxyproline secretion. Although calcitonin requires long-term maintenance therapy, there is noticeable improvement after the first few weeks of treatment; etidronate produces improvement after 1 to 3 months.

• *mithramycin,* a cytotoxic antibiotic, to decrease calcium, urinary hydroxyproline, and serum alkaline phosphatase levels. This drug produces remission of symptoms within 2 weeks and biochemical improvement in 1 to 2 months. However, mithramycin may destroy platelets or compromise renal function.

Self-administration of calcitonin and etidronate helps patients with Paget's disease lead near-normal lives. Nevertheless, these patients may need surgery to reduce or prevent pathologic fractures, correct secondary deformities, and relieve neurologic impairment.

To decrease the risk of excessive bleeding due to hypervascular bone, drug therapy with calcitonin and etidronate or mithramycin must precede surgery. Joint replacement is difficult because bonding material (methyl methacrylate) doesn't set properly on pagetic bone.

Other treatments vary according to symptoms. Aspirin, indomethacin, or ibuprofen usually controls pain,

## Special considerations

• To evaluate the effectiveness of analgesics, assess level of pain daily. Watch for new areas of pain or restricted movements — which may indicate new fracture sites — and sensory or motor disturbances, such as difficulty in hearing, seeing, or walking.

• Monitor serum calcium and alkaline phosphatase levels.

• If the patient is confined to prolonged bed rest, prevent pressure ulcers by providing good skin care. Reposition the patient frequently, and use a flotation mattress. Provide high-topped sneakers to prevent footdrop.

• Monitor intake and output. Encourage adequate fluid intake to minimize renal calculi formation.

• Demonstrate how to inject calcitonin properly and rotate injection sites. Warn the patient that adverse effects may occur (nausea, vomiting, local inflammatory reaction at injection site, facial flushing, itching of hands, and fever). Reassure him that these effects are usually mild and infrequent.

• To help the patient adjust to the changes in lifestyle imposed by this disease, teach him how to pace activities and, if necessary, how to use assistive devices.

• Encourage the patient to follow a recommended exercise program — avoiding both immobilization and excessive activity. Suggest a firm mattress or a bed board to minimize spinal deformities.

• Warn against imprudent use of analgesics.

• To prevent falls at home, advise removal of throw rugs and other small obstacles.

• Emphasize the importance of regular checkups, including the eyes and ears.

> CLINICAL TIP   Tell the patient receiving etidronate to take this medication with fruit juice 2 hours before or after meals (milk or other high-calcium fluids impair absorption), to divide daily dosage to minimize adverse effects, and to watch for and report stomach cramps, diarrhea, fractures, and increasing or new bone pain.

• Tell the patient receiving mithramycin to watch for signs of infection, easy bruising, bleeding, and temperature elevation, and to report for regular follow-up laboratory tests.

• Help the patient and family make use of community support resources, such as a visiting nurse or home health agency. For more information, refer them to the Paget's Disease Foundation.

# PANCREATIC CANCER

A deadly GI cancer, pancreatic cancer progresses rapidly. Pancreatic tumors are almost always adenocarcinomas and most arise in the head of the pancreas. Rarer tumors are those of the body and tail of the pancreas and islet cell tumors. The two main tissue types are cylinder cell and large, fatty, granular cell.

## Causes

Pancreatic cancer occurs most commonly in men between the ages of 35 and 70. Geographically, the incidence is highest in Israel, the United States, Sweden, and Canada.

Evidence suggests that pancreatic cancer is linked to inhalation or absorption of the following carcinogens, which are then excreted by the pancreas:
• cigarettes
• foods high in fat and protein
• food additives
• industrial chemicals, such as beta-naphthalene, benzidine, and urea.

Possible predisposing factors are chronic pancreatitis, diabetes mellitus, and chronic alcohol abuse.

## Signs and symptoms

The most common features of pancreatic carcinoma are weight loss, abdominal or low back pain, jaundice, and diarrhea. (See *Types of pancreatic cancer,* page 614.) Other generalized effects include fever, skin lesions (usually on the legs), and emotional disturbances, such as depression, anxiety, and premonition of fatal illness.

## Diagnosis

Definitive diagnosis requires a laparotomy with a biopsy. Other tests used to detect pancreatic cancer include:
• *ultrasound* — can identify a mass but not its histology
• *computed tomography scan* — similar to ultrasound but shows greater detail
• *angiography* — shows vascular supply of tumor
• *endoscopic retrograde cholangiopancreatography* — allows visualization, instillation of contrast medium, and specimen biopsy
• *magnetic resonance imaging* — shows tumor size and location in great detail.

Laboratory tests supporting this diagnosis include serum bilirubin (increased), serum amylase and serum lipase (sometimes elevated), prothrom-

## TYPES OF PANCREATIC CANCER

| PATHOLOGY | CLINICAL FEATURES |
|---|---|
| **HEAD OF PANCREAS** | |
| • Often obstructs ampulla of Vater and common bile duct<br>• Directly metastasizes to duodenum<br>• Adhesions anchor tumor to spine, stomach, and intestines. | • Jaundice (predominant symptom) — slowly progressive, unremitting; may cause skin (especially of the face and genitals) to turn olive green or black<br>• Pruritus — often severe<br>• Weight loss — rapid and severe (as great as 30 lb [13.6 kg]); may lead to emaciation, weakness, and muscle atrophy<br>• Slowed digestion, gastric distention, nausea, diarrhea. and steatorrhea with clay-colored stools<br>• Liver and gallbladder enlargement from lymph node metastasis to biliary tract and duct wall results in compression and obstruction; gallbladder may be palpable (Courvoisier's sign).<br>• Dull, nondescript, continuous abdominal pain radiating to upper right quadrant; relieved by bending forward<br>• GI hemorrhage and biliary infection common |
| **BODY AND TAIL OF PANCREAS** | |
| • Large nodular masses become fixed to retropancreatic tissues and spine.<br>• Direct invasion of spleen, left kidney, suprarenal gland, diaphragm<br>• Involvement of celiac plexus results in thrombosis of splenic vein and spleen infarction. | *Body*<br>• Pain (predominant symptom) — usually epigastric, develops slowly and radiates to back; relieved by bending forward or sitting up; intensified by lying supine; most intense 3 to 4 hours after eating; when celiac plexus is involved, pain is more intense and lasts longer<br>• Venous thrombosis and thrombophlebitis — frequent; may precede other symptoms by months<br>• Splenomegaly (from infarction), hepatomegaly (occasionally), and jaundice (rarely)<br>*Tail*<br>Symptoms result from metastasis:<br>• Abdominal tumor (most common finding) produces a palpable abdominal mass; abdominal pain radiates to left hypochondrium and left chest.<br>• Anorexia leads to weight loss, emaciation, and weakness<br>• Splenomegaly and upper GI bleeding |

bin time (prolonged), and aspartate aminotransferase and alanine aminotransferase (elevations indicate necrosis of liver cells).

Additional pertinent studies are alkaline phosphatase (marked elevation occurs with biliary obstruction); plasma insulin immunoassay (shows measurable serum insulin in the presence of islet cell tumors); hemoglobin and hematocrit (may show mild anemia); fasting blood glucose (may indicate hypoglycemia or hyperglycemia); and stools (occult blood may signal ulceration in GI tract or ampulla of Vater).

## STAGING PANCREATIC CANCER

Using the TNM (tumor, node, metastasis) system, the American Joint Committee on Cancer has established the following stages for pancreatic cancer.

**Primary tumor**
*TX*— primary tumor can't be assessed
*T0*— no evidence of primary tumor
*T1*— tumor limited to the pancreas
*T1a* — tumor 2 cm or less in greatest dimension
*1Ib*— tumor more than 2 cm in greatest dimension
*T2*— tumor penetrates the duodenum, bile duct, or peripancreatic tissues
*T3*— tumor penetrates the stomach, spleen, colon, or adjacent large vessels

**Regional lymph nodes**
*NX*— regional lymph nodes can't be assessed

*N0*— no evidence of regional lymph node metastasis
*N1* — regional lymph node metastasis

**Distant metastasis**
*MX*— distant metastasis can't be assessed
*M0*— no known distant metastasis
*M1*— distant metastasis

**Staging categories**
Pancreatic cancer progresses from mild to severe as follows:
*Stage I*— T1, N0, M0; T2, N0, M0
*Stage II*— T3, N0, M0
*Stage III*— any T, N1, M0
*Stage IV*— any T, any N, M1

**Treatment**

In pancreatic cancer, treatment is rarely successful because this disease has usually metastasized widely at diagnosis. (See *Staging pancreatic cancer.*)

Therapy consists of surgery and, possibly, radiation and chemotherapy. Small advances have been made in the survival rate with surgery:

• Total pancreatectomy may increase survival time by resecting a localized tumor or by controlling postoperative gastric ulceration.

• Cholecystojejunostomy, choledochoduodenostomy, and choledochojejunostomy have partially replaced radical resection to bypass obstructing common bile duct. extensions, thus decreasing the incidence of jaundice and pruritus.

• Whipple's operation, or pancreatoduodenectomy, has a high mortality but can produce wide lymphatic clearance, except with tumors located near the portal vein, superior mesenteric vein and artery, and celiac axis. This rarely used procedure removes the head of the pancreas, the duodenum, and portions of the body and tail of the pancreas, stomach, jejunum, pancreatic duct, and distal portion of the bile duct.

• Gastrojejunostomy is performed if radical resection isn't indicated and duodenal obstruction is expected to develop later.

Although pancreatic carcinoma generally responds poorly to chemotherapy, recent studies using combinations of fluorouracil, streptozocin, ifosfamide, and doxorubicin show a trend toward longer survival time. Other medications used in pancreatic cancer include:

• antibiotics (oral, I.V., or I.M.)— to prevent infection and relieve symptoms

• anticholinergics (particularly propantheline)— to decrease GI tract spasm

and motility and reduce pain and secretions
- antacids (oral or by nasogastric [NG] tube) — to decrease secretion of pancreatic enzymes and suppress peptic activity, thereby reducing stress-induced damage to gastric mucosa
- diuretics — to mobilize extracellular fluid from ascites
- insulin — to provide adequate exogenous insulin supply after pancreatic resection
- narcotics — to relieve pain, but only after analgesics fail because morphine, meperidine, and codeine can lead to biliary tract spasm and increase common bile duct pressure
- pancreatic enzymes (average dose is 0.5 to 1 mg with meals — to assist in digestion of proteins, carbohydrates, and fats when pancreatic juices are insufficient because of surgery or obstruction.

Radiation therapy is usually ineffective except as an adjunct to chemotherapy or as a palliative measure.

**Special considerations**
Before surgery:
- Ensure that the patient is medically stable, particularly regarding nutrition (this may take 4 to 5 days). If the patient can't tolerate oral feedings, provide total parenteral nutrition and I.V. fat emulsions to correct deficiencies and maintain positive nitrogen balance.
- Give blood transfusions (to combat anemia), vitamin K (to overcome prothrombin deficiency), antibiotics (to prevent postoperative complications), and gastric lavage (to maintain gastric decompression), as necessary.
- Tell the patient about expected postoperative procedures and expected adverse effects of radiation and chemotherapy.

After surgery:
- Watch for and report complications, such as fistula, pancreatitis, fluid and electrolyte imbalance, infection, hemorrhage, skin breakdown, nutritional deficiency, hepatic failure, renal insufficiency, and diabetes.
- If the patient is receiving chemotherapy, treat adverse effects symptomatically.

Throughout this illness, provide meticulous supportive care as follows:
- Monitor fluid balance, abdominal girth, metabolic state, and weight daily. In weight loss, replace nutrients I.V., orally, or by NG tube; in weight gain (due to ascites), impose dietary restrictions, such as a low-sodium or fluid-retention diet as required. Maintain a 2,500 calorie diet.
- Serve small, frequent, nutritious meals by enlisting the dietitian's services. Administer an oral pancreatic enzyme at mealtimes, if needed. As necessary, give antacids to prevent stress ulcers.
- To prevent constipation, administer laxatives, stool softeners, and cathartics as required; modify diet; and increase fluid intake. To increase GI motility, position the patient properly at mealtime, and help him walk when he can.
- Administer pain medication, antibiotics, and antipyretics, as necessary. Note time, site (if injected), and response.
- Watch for signs of hypoglycemia or hyperglycemia; administer glucose or an antidiabetic agent as necessary. Monitor blood glucose and urine acetone levels.
- Provide meticulous skin care to avoid pruritus and necrosis.

> **CLINICAL TIP** Prevent excoriation in a pruritic patient by clipping his nails and having him wear cotton gloves.

- Watch for signs of upper GI bleeding; test stools and vomitus for occult blood, and keep a flow sheet of hemoglobin and hematocrit values.

- To control active bleeding, promote gastric vasoconstriction with prescribed medication. Replace any fluid loss.

- Ease discomfort from pyloric obstruction with an NG tube.

- To prevent thrombosis, apply antiembolism stockings and assist in range-of-motion exercises. If thrombosis occurs, elevate the patient's legs, and give an anticoagulant or aspirin, as required.

---

**LIFE-THREATENING DISORDER**

# PANCREATITIS

---

Pancreatitis, inflammation of the pancreas, occurs in acute and chronic forms. In pancreatitis, the enzymes normally excreted by the pancreas digest pancreatic tissue (autodigestion). Acute pancreatitis can range from mild self-limiting episodes of abdominal discomfort to severe systemic illness associated with fluid sequestration, metabolic disorder, hypotension, sepsis, and death. Life-threatening illness is associated with pancreatic hemorrhage or necrosis in about 10% of patients.

In 90% of patients with acute pancreatitis, the disease occurs as a mild, self-limiting illness and requires only simple supportive care. In the remaining 10% of patients, the disease can evolve into a severe form with significant complications, a lengthy duration, and a significant mortality rate.

## Causes

The most common causes of pancreatitis are biliary tract disease and alcoholism, but it can also result from pancreatic carcinoma, trauma, or certain drugs, such as glucocorticoids, sulfon-amides, chlorothiazide, and azathioprine.

This disease also may develop as a complication of peptic ulcer, mumps, or hypothermia. Rarer causes are stenosis or obstruction of the sphincter of Oddi, hypercalcemia, duodenal obstruction, hyperlipemia, ischemia from vasculitis or vascular disease, viral infections, mycoplasmal pneumonia, scorpion venom, and pregnancy. It may also be familial or idiopathic.

Pancreatitis may also develop in a patient after surgery. This occurrence has the highest morbidity and mortality. Whatever the cause, complications from acute pancreatitis are possible.

> **CLINICAL TIP** Determining the cause of pancreatitis is useful both for managing and predicting complications.

## Signs and symptoms

In many patients, the first and only symptom of mild pancreatitis is steady epigastric pain centered close to the umbilicus. The pain usually begins as a gradually increasing mid-epigastric pain reaching its maximum intensity several hours after the beginning of the illness. In pancreatitis resulting from alcohol ingestion, the pain commences 12 to 48 hours after an episode of binge drinking. Nausea and vomiting generally accompany the abdominal pain. However, a severe attack causes extreme pain, persistent vomiting, abdominal rigidity, diminished bowel activity (suggesting peritonitis), right or left pleural effusion, or left hemidiaphragm elevation.

Severe pancreatitis may produce extreme malaise and restlessness, mottled skin, tachycardia, and diaphoresis. Hypotension, hypovolemia, hypoperfusion, sepsis, and shock may ensue. Pulmonary complications and secondary pancreatic infections, such as pancreatic abscess

# CHRONIC PANCREATITIS

Usually associated with alcoholism (in over half of all patients), chronic pancreatitis can also follow hyperparathyroidism, hyperlipemia or, infrequently, gallstones, trauma, peptic ulcer, posttraumatic stricture, pancreas division, and hereditary or familial pancreatitis. Inflammation and fibrosis cause progressive pancreatic insufficiency and eventually destroy the pancreas.

### Symptoms
Chronic pancreatitis is usually associated with constant dull pain with occasional exacerbations, malabsorption, severe weight loss, and hyperglycemia (leading to diabetic symptoms). Relevant diagnostic measures include patient history, abdominal X-rays or computed tomography scans showing pancreatic calcification, elevated erythrocyte sedimentation rate, and examination of stools for steatorrhea.

### Treatment
The severe pain of chronic pancreatitis often requires large doses of analgesics or narcotics: Addiction may be common. Treatment also includes a low-fat diet and oral administration of pancreatic enzymes, such as pancreatin or pancrelipase to control steatorrhea, insulin or oral antidiabetic agents to curb hyperglycemia and, occasionally, surgical repair of biliary or pancreatic ducts, or the sphincter of Oddi to reduce pressure and promote the flow of pancreatic juice. The prognosis is good if the patient can avoid alcohol but poor if he can't.

to the bowel may cause ileus. Renal failure may occur as a result of severe hypovolemia.

If pancreatitis damages the islets of Langerhans, complications may include diabetes mellitus and enzyme deficiency. (See *Chronic pancreatitis.*) Fulminant pancreatitis causes massive hemorrhage and total destruction of the pancreas, resulting in diabetic acidosis, shock, or coma.

**Diagnosis**
Clinical presentation along with combined laboratory and radiographic findings form the basis for diagnosis. A careful patient history (especially for alcoholism) and physical examination are the first steps in diagnosis, but the retroperitoneal position of the pancreas makes physical assessment difficult.

Dramatically elevated serum amylase levels — frequently over 500 units — confirm pancreatitis and rule out perforated peptic ulcer, acute cholecystitis, appendicitis, and bowel infarction or obstruction. Persistent elevation of serum amylase levels may indicate pancreatic necrosis, pseudocyst, or abscess.

Similarly dramatic elevations of amylase are also found in urine, ascites, or pleural fluid. Characteristically, amylase levels return to normal 48 hours after onset of pancreatitis, despite continuing symptoms. Supportive laboratory values include:
• increased serum lipase levels, which rise more slowly than serum amylase
• white blood cell counts that range from 8,000 to 20,000/µl, with increased polymorphonuclear leukocytes
• elevated glucose levels — as high as 500 to 900 mg/dl, indicating hyperglycemia.

The following other tests may be used to diagnose pancreatitis:

or infected pancreatic necrosis, and later, pancreatic pseudocyst may also occur. Proximity of the inflamed pancreas

- *Abdominal X-rays* show dilation of the small or large bowel or calcification of the pancreas.
- *Chest X-rays* show left-sided pleural effusion.
- *Abdominal computed tomography scan* with contrast is the most sensitive noninvasive test used to confirm the diagnosis of pancreatitis.

## Treatment

The goal of therapy is to maintain circulation and fluid volume. Treatment measures must also relieve pain and decrease pancreatic secretions. In 90% of patients with acute pancreatitis, the disease occurs as a mild self-limiting illness and requires simple supportive care alone. In the remaining 10% of patients, the disease can evolve into a severe form of acute pancreatitis with significant complications, a lengthy duration of illness, and a significant mortality rate.

### Emergency measures

Emergency treatment for shock (which is the most common cause of death in early-stage pancreatitis) consists of vigorous I.V. replacement of electrolytes and proteins.

Metabolic acidosis that develops secondary to hypovolemia and impaired cellular perfusion requires vigorous fluid volume replacement.

Drug treatment choices may include morphine sulfate for pain; diazepam for restlessness and agitation; and antibiotics for documented bacterial infections.

Specific metabolic complications, such as hypokalemia, hypocalcemia, hemorrhage, and coagulopathy, must be treated with appropriate replacement products, such as potassium chloride, I.V. calcium gluconate or chloride, red blood cells, and fresh frozen plasma. Hyperglycemia and glycosuria are manifestations of altered carbohydrate metabolism. Treatment consists of careful titration of glucose and insulin to maintain a euglycemic state.

### After the emergency

After the emergency phase, continuing I.V. therapy should provide adequate electrolytes and protein solutions. If the patient is unable to resume oral feedings, total parenteral nutrition may be necessary. Nonstimulating enteral feedings may be safer because of the decreased risk of infection and maintenance of normal physiology.

Surgery for acute pancreatitis is reserved for specific complications and to correct an anatomic problem. Surgery is usually required for patients with necrotizing pancreatitis to debride devitalized tissue and to provide external drainage. Debridement is often required on multiple occasions, usually at 24- to 48-hour intervals, until the necrotic tissue is replaced by a granulating wound.

## Special considerations

- Acute pancreatitis is a life-threatening emergency. Provide meticulous supportive care and continuous monitoring of vital systems.
- Monitor vital signs and pulmonary artery pressure closely.
- Monitor fluid intake and output and electrolyte levels.
- Assess for crackles, rhonchi, decreased breath sounds, or respiratory failure.
- Observe for signs of calcium deficiency — tetany, cramps, carpopedal spasm, and seizures.
- Administer analgesics, as needed, to relieve the patient's pain and anxiety.
- Observe for adverse reactions to antibiotics: nephrotoxicity with aminoglycosides; pseudomembranous enterocolitis with clindamycin; and blood dyscrasias with chloramphenicol.

• Monitor for complications due to total parenteral nutrition, such as sepsis, hypokalemia, overhydration, and metabolic acidosis.

• Observe for fever, cardiac irregularities, changes in arterial blood gas measurements, and deep respirations (signs of sepsis).

# PANIC DISORDER

Characterized by recurrent episodes of intense apprehension, terror, and impending doom, panic disorder represents anxiety in its most severe form. Initially unpredictable, these panic attacks may come to be associated with specific situations or tasks. The disorder often exists concurrently with agoraphobia. Equal numbers of men and women are affected by panic disorder alone, whereas panic disorder with agoraphobia occurs about twice as often in women.

Panic disorder typically has an onset in late adolescence or early adulthood, often in response to a sudden loss. It also may be triggered by severe separation anxiety experienced during early childhood.

Without treatment, panic disorder can persist for years, with alternating exacerbations and remissions. The patient with panic disorder is at high risk for a psychoactive substance abuse disorder: He may resort to alcohol or anxiolytics in an attempt to relieve his fear.

## Causes
Like other anxiety disorders, panic disorder may stem from a combination of physiologic and psychological factors. For example, some theorists emphasize the role of stressful events or unconscious conflicts that occur early in childhood.

Recent evidence indicates that alterations in brain biochemistry, especially in norepinephrine, serotonin, and gamma-aminobutyric acid activity, may also contribute to panic disorder.

## Signs and symptoms
The symptoms of panic disorder are intensely uncomfortable. The patient with panic disorder typically complains of repeated episodes of unexpected apprehension, fear, and intense discomfort. These panic attacks may last for minutes or hours and leave the patient shaken, fearful, and exhausted. They occur several times a week, sometimes even daily. Because the attacks occur spontaneously, without exposure to a known anxiety-producing situation, the patient often worries between attacks about when the next episode will occur.

Physical examination of the patient during a panic attack may reveal signs of intense anxiety, such as hyperventilation, tachycardia, trembling, and profuse sweating. He may also complain of difficulty breathing, digestive disturbances, and chest pain.

## Diagnosis
For characteristic findings in patients with this condition, see *Diagnosing panic disorder.*

Because many medical conditions can mimic panic disorder, additional tests may be ordered to rule out an organic basis for the symptoms. For example, tests for serum glucose levels rule out hypoglycemia, studies of urine catecholamines and vanillylmandelic acid rule out pheochromocytoma, and thyroid function tests rule out hyperthyroidism.

Urine and serum toxicology tests may reveal the presence of psychoactive substances that can precipitate panic at-

---

# DIAGNOSING PANIC DISORDER

The diagnosis of panic disorder is confirmed when the patient meets the criteria established in the *DSM-IV.*

**Panic attack**
A discrete period of intense fear or discomfort in which at least four of the following symptoms develop abruptly and reach a peak within 10 minutes:
• palpitations, pounding heart, or tachycardia
• sweating
• trembling or shaking
• shortness of breath or smothering sensations
• feeling of choking
• chest pain or discomfort
• nausea or abdominal distress
• dizziness or faintness
• depersonalization or derealization
• fear of losing control or going crazy
• fear of dying
• numbness or tingling sensations (paresthesia)
• hot flashes or chills.

**Panic disorder without agoraphobia**
• The person experiences recurrent unexpected panic attacks and at least one of the attacks has been followed by 1 month (or more) of one (or more) of the following:
– persistent concern about having additional attacks
– worry about the implications of the attack or its consequences

– a significant change in behavior related to the attacks.
• The panic attacks aren't due to the direct physiologic effects of a substance or a general medical condition.
• The panic attacks aren't better accounted for by another mental disorder, such as social phobia, specific phobia, obsessive-compulsive disorder, posttraumatic stress disorder, or separation anxiety disorder.

**Panic disorder with agoraphobia**
• The person experiences recurrent unexpected panic attacks and at least one of the attacks has been followed by 1 month (or more) of one (or more) of the following:
– persistent concern about having additional attacks
– worry about the implications of the attack or its consequences
– a significant change in behavior related to the attacks.
• The person exhibits agoraphobia.
• The panic attacks aren't due to the direct physiologic effects of a substance or a general medical condition.
• The panic attacks aren't better accounted for by another mental disorder, such as social phobia, specific phobia, obsessive-compulsive disorder, posttraumatic stress disorder, or separation anxiety disorder.

---

tacks, including barbiturates, caffeine, and amphetamines.

## Treatment
Panic disorder may respond to behavioral therapy, supportive psychotherapy, or drug therapy, singly or in combination. Behavioral therapy works best when agoraphobia accompanies panic disorder because the identification of anxiety-inducing situations is easier.

Psychotherapy commonly uses cognitive techniques to enable the patient to view anxiety-provoking situations more realistically and to recognize panic symptoms as a misinterpretation of essentially harmless physical sensations.

Drug therapy includes antianxiety drugs, such as diazepam, alprazolam, and clonazepam, and beta blockers such as propranolol to provide symptomatic relief. Antidepressants, including tricyclic antidepressants, selective serotonin reuptake inhibitors, and monoamine oxidase inhibitors, are also effective.

### Special considerations

• Stay with the patient until the attack subsides. If left alone, he may become even more anxious.

▶ CLINICAL TIP Maintain a calm, serene approach. Statements such as "I won't let anything here hurt you" and "I'll stay with you" can assure the patient that you're in control of the immediate situation.

• Avoid giving him insincere expressions of reassurance.

• The patient's perceptual field may be narrowed, and excessive stimuli may cause him to feel overwhelmed. Dim bright lights or raise dim lights as necessary.

• If the patient loses control, move him to a smaller, quieter space.

• The patient may be so overwhelmed that he cannot follow lengthy or complicated instructions. Speak in short, simple sentences, and slowly give one direction at a time. Avoid giving lengthy explanations and asking too many questions.

• Allow the patient to pace around the room (provided he isn't belligerent) to help expend energy. Show him how to take slow, deep breaths if he's hyperventilating.

• Avoid touching the patient until you've established rapport. Unless he trusts you, he may be too stimulated or frightened to find touch reassuring.

• Administer medication as necessary.

• During and after a panic attack, encourage the patient to express his feelings. Discuss his fears and help him identify situations or events that trigger the attacks.

• Teach the patient relaxation techniques, and explain how he can use them to relieve stress or avoid a panic attack.

• Review with the patient any adverse effects of the drugs he'll be taking. Caution him to notify the doctor before discontinuing the medication because abrupt withdrawal could cause severe symptoms.

• Encourage the patient and his family to use community resources such as the Anxiety Disorders Association of America.

# PARKINSON'S DISEASE

Named for James Parkinson, the English doctor who wrote the first accurate description of the disease in 1817, Parkinson's disease (also known as shaking palsy) characteristically produces progressive muscle rigidity, akinesia, and involuntary tremor. Deterioration is a progressive process. Death may result from complications, such as aspiration pneumonia or some other infection.

Parkinson's disease, one of the most common crippling diseases in the United States, affects men more often than women. According to current statistics, it strikes 1 in every 100 people over age 60. Because of increased longevity, this amounts to roughly 60,000 new cases diagnosed annually in the United States alone. Secondary to the aging of the population, an increase in cases is predicted.

### Causes

Although the cause of Parkinson's disease is unknown, study of the extrapyramidal brain nuclei (corpus striatum, globus pallidus, substantia nigra) has established that a dopamine deficiency prevents affected brain cells from performing their normal inhibitory function within the central nervous system.

> CLINICAL TIP More research on the pathogenesis of Parkinson's disease focuses on damage to the substantia nigra from oxidative stress. Oxidative stress is believed to cause alterations in brain iron content, impair mitochondrial function, alter antioxidant and protective systems, reduce glutathione, and damage lipids, proteins, and deoxyribonucleic acid.

### Signs and symptoms

The cardinal symptoms of Parkinson's disease are muscle rigidity and akinesia, and an insidious tremor that begins in the fingers (unilateral pill-roll tremor), increases during stress or anxiety, and decreases with purposeful movement and sleep.

Muscle rigidity results in resistance to passive muscle stretching, which may be uniform (lead-pipe rigidity) or jerky (cogwheel rigidity). Akinesia causes the patient to walk with difficulty (gait lacks normal parallel motion and may be retropulsive or propulsive).

Parkinson's disease also produces a high-pitched, monotone voice; drooling; a masklike facial expression; loss of posture control (the patient walks with body bent forward); and dysarthria, dysphagia, or both. Occasionally, akinesia may also cause oculogyric crises (eyes are fixed upward, with involuntary tonic movements) or blepharospasm (eyelids are completely closed). Parkinson's disease itself doesn't impair the intellect, but a coexisting disorder such as arteriosclerosis may.

### Diagnosis

Generally, laboratory data are of little value in identifying Parkinson's disease; diagnosis is based on the patient's age and history and on the characteristic clinical picture. However, urinalysis may support the diagnosis by revealing decreased dopamine levels.

A conclusive diagnosis is possible only after ruling out other causes of tremor, involutional depression, cerebral arteriosclerosis, and, in patients under age 30, intracranial tumors, Wilson's disease, or phenothiazine or other drug toxicity.

### Treatment

Because there's no cure for Parkinson's disease, the primary aim of treatment is to relieve symptoms and keep the patient functional as long as possible. Treatment consists of drugs, physical therapy and, in severe disease states unresponsive to drugs, stereotactic neurosurgery.

#### Drug therapy

Drug therapy usually includes levodopa, a dopamine replacement that is most effective during early stages. It's given in increasing doses until symptoms are relieved or adverse effects appear. Because adverse effects can be serious, levodopa is frequently given in combination with carbidopa to halt peripheral dopamine synthesis.

When levodopa proves ineffective or too toxic, alternative drug therapy includes anticholinergics such as trihexyphenidyl; antihistamines such as diphenhydramine; and amantadine, an antiviral agent. Selegiline, an enzyme-inhibiting agent, allows conservation of dopamine and enhances the therapeutic effect of levodopa.

> CLINICAL TIP Research on the oxidative stress theory has caused a controversy in drug therapy for Parkinson's disease. Whereas levodopa/carbidopa has traditionally been a first-line drug in management, it has been associated with an acceleration of the disease process. Selegiline followed by

levodopa/carbidopa may provide increased protection.

### Stereotactic neurosurgery

When drug therapy fails, stereotactic neurosurgery may be an alternative. In this procedure, electrical coagulation, freezing, radioactivity, or ultrasound destroys the ventrolateral nucleus of the thalamus to prevent involuntary movement. This is most effective in young, otherwise healthy persons with unilateral tremor or muscle rigidity. Neurosurgery can only *relieve* symptoms.

### Physical therapy

Individually planned physical therapy complements drug treatment and neurosurgery to maintain normal muscle tone and function. Appropriate physical therapy includes both active and passive range-of-motion exercises, routine daily activities, walking, and baths and massage to help relax muscles.

### Special considerations

• Effectively caring for the patient with Parkinson's disease requires careful monitoring of drug treatment, emphasis on teaching self-reliance, and generous psychological support.

• Monitor drug treatment so dosage can be adjusted to minimize adverse effects.

• If the patient has surgery, watch for signs of hemorrhage and increased intracranial pressure by frequently checking level of consciousness and vital signs.

• Encourage independence. The patient with excessive tremor may achieve partial control of his body by sitting on a chair and using its arms to steady himself. Remember that fatigue may cause him to depend more on others.

• Scheduling meals around time of maximum drug efficiency will help minimize complications and promote good nutrition.

• Help the patient overcome problems related to eating and elimination. For example, if he has difficulty eating, offer supplementary or small, frequent meals to increase caloric intake.

• Help establish a regular bowel routine by encouraging the patient to drink at least 2,000 ml of liquids daily and eat high-bulk foods. He may need an elevated toilet seat to assist him from a standing to a sitting position.

• Give the patient and family emotional support. Teach them about the disease, its progressive stages, and drug adverse effects.

• Show the family how to prevent pressure ulcers and contractures by proper positioning. Explain that the patient should avoid high-protein meals (this impairs levodopa effects) and explain household safety measures to prevent accidents.

• Instruct the patient and family on proper food consistency, correct positioning, and swallowing strategies to decrease dysphagia.

• Help the patient and family express their feelings and frustrations about the progressively debilitating effects of the disease.

• Establish long- and short-term treatment goals, and be aware of the patient's need for intellectual stimulation and diversion.

• To obtain more information, refer the patient and family to the National Parkinson Foundation or the United Parkinson Foundation.

# PEDICULOSIS

Pediculosis is caused by parasitic forms of lice: *Pediculus humanus* var. *capitis* causes pediculosis capitis (head lice); *Pediculus humanus* var. *corporis* causes pediculosis corporis (body lice); and *Phthirus pubis* causes pediculosis pubis (crab lice). These lice feed on human blood and lay their eggs (nits) in body hairs or clothing fibers.

After the nits hatch, the lice must feed within 24 hours or die; they mature in about 2 to 3 weeks. When a louse bites, it injects a toxin into the skin that produces mild irritation and a purpuric spot. Repeated bites cause sensitization to the toxin, leading to more serious inflammation. Treatment can effectively eliminate lice.

## Causes

*P. humanus* var. *capitis* (most common species) feeds on the scalp and, rarely, in the eyebrows, eyelashes, and beard. This form of pediculosis is caused by overcrowded conditions and poor personal hygiene, and commonly affects children, especially girls. It spreads through shared clothing, hats, combs, and hairbrushes.

*P. humanus* var. *corporis* lives in the seams of clothing, next to the skin, leaving only to feed on blood. Common causes include prolonged wearing of the same clothing (which might occur in cold climates), overcrowding, and poor personal hygiene. It spreads through shared clothing and bedsheets.

*P. pubis* is primarily found in pubic hairs, but this species may extend to the eyebrows, eyelashes, and axillary or body hair. Pediculosis pubis is transmitted through sexual intercourse or by contact with clothes, bedsheets, or towels harboring lice.

### Signs and symptoms

Clinical features vary with the cause.

### Pediculosis capitis

Signs and symptoms of pediculosis capitis include itching; excoriation (with severe itching); matted, foul-smelling, lusterless hair (in severe cases); occipital and cervical lymphadenopathy; and a rash on the trunk probably due to sensitization. Adult lice migrate from the scalp and deposit oval gray-white nits on hair shafts.

### Pediculosis corporis

Pediculosis corporis initially produces small red papules (usually on the shoulders, trunk, or buttocks). Later wheals (probably a sensitivity reaction) may develop. Untreated pediculosis corporis may lead to vertical excoriations and ultimately to dry, discolored, thickly encrusted, scaly skin, with bacterial infection and scarring. In severe cases, headache, fever, and malaise may accompany cutaneous symptoms.

### Pediculosis pubis

Pediculosis pubis causes skin irritation from scratching, which is usually more obvious than the bites. Small gray-blue spots (maculae caeruleae) may appear on the thighs or upper body.

## Diagnosis

Pediculosis is visible on physical examination as follows:
- *pediculosis capitis:* oval grayish nits that can't be shaken loose like dandruff (the closer the nits are to the end of the hair shaft, the longer the infection has been present, because the ova are laid close to the scalp)
- *pediculosis corporis:* characteristic skin lesions; nits found on clothing
- *pediculosis pubis:* nits attached to pubic hairs, which feel coarse and grainy to the touch.

## Treatment

The type of pediculosis dictates the treatment.

### *Pediculosis capitis*

Treatment consists of permethrin cream rinse rubbed into the hair and rinsed after 10 minutes. A single treatment should be sufficient. Alternatives include pyrethrins and lindane shampoo.

➤ CLINICAL TIP A fine-tooth comb dipped in vinegar removes nits from hair; washing hair with ordinary shampoo removes crustations.

### *Pediculosis corporis*

Pediculosis corporis requires bathing with soap and water to remove lice from the body; in severe infestation, treatment with lindane cream may be necessary. Lice may be removed from clothes by washing them in hot water, ironing, or dry-cleaning. Storing clothes for more than 30 days or placing them in dry heat of 140° F (60° C) kills lice. If clothes can't be washed or changed, application of 10% lindane powder is effective.

### *Pediculosis pubis*

Treatment of pediculosis pubis includes shampooing with lindane shampoo for 4 minutes. Treatment should be repeated in 1 week. Clothes and bedsheets must be laundered to prevent reinfestation.

### Special considerations

• Instruct patients how to use the creams, ointments, powders, and shampoos that can eliminate lice. To prevent self-infestation, avoid prolonged contact with the patient's hair, clothing, and bedsheets.

• Ask the patient with pediculosis pubis for a history of recent sexual contacts, so that they can be examined and treated.

• To prevent the spread of pediculosis to other hospitalized persons, examine all high-risk patients on admission, especially the elderly who depend on others for care, those admitted from nursing homes, or persons living in crowded conditions.

# PELVIC INFLAMMATORY DISEASE

Pelvic inflammatory disease (PID) is any acute, subacute, recurrent, or chronic infection of the oviducts and ovaries, with adjacent tissue involvement. It includes inflammation of the cervix (cervicitis), uterus (endometritis), fallopian tubes (salpingitis), and ovaries (oophoritis), which can extend to the connective tissue lying between the broad ligaments (parametritis).

Early diagnosis and treatment prevents damage to the reproductive system. Untreated PID may cause infertility and may lead to potentially fatal septicemia, pulmonary emboli, and shock.

### Causes

PID can result from infection with aerobic or anaerobic organisms. The aerobic organism *Neisseria gonorrhoeae* is its most common cause because it most readily penetrates the bacteriostatic barrier of cervical mucus.

Normally, cervical secretions have a protective and defensive function. Therefore conditions or procedures that alter or destroy cervical mucus impair this bacteriostatic mechanism and allow bacteria present in the cervix or vagina to ascend into the uterine cavity; such procedures include conization or cauterization of the cervix.

Uterine infection can also follow the transfer of contaminated cervical mucus into the endometrial cavity by instrumentation. Consequently, PID can follow insertion of an intrauterine device (IUD), use of a biopsy curet or of an irrigation catheter, or tubal insufflation. Other predisposing factors include abortion, pelvic surgery, and infection during or after pregnancy.

Bacteria may also enter the uterine cavity through the bloodstream or from drainage from a chronically infected fallopian tube, a pelvic abscess, a ruptured appendix, diverticulitis of the sigmoid colon, or other infectious foci.

The most common bacteria found in cervical mucus are staphylococci, streptococci, diphtheroids, chlamydiae, and coliforms, including *Pseudomonas* and *Escherichia coli.*

Uterine infection can result from any one or several of these organisms or may follow the multiplication of normally nonpathogenic bacteria in an altered endometrial environment. Bacterial multiplication is most common during parturition, because the endometrium is atrophic, quiescent, and not stimulated by estrogen.

### Signs and symptoms
Clinical features of PID vary with the affected area but generally include a profuse, purulent vaginal discharge, sometimes accompanied by low-grade fever and malaise (particularly if gonorrhea is the cause). The patient experiences lower abdomen pain; movement of the cervix or palpation of the adnexa may be extremely painful. (See *Forms of pelvic inflammatory disease,* page 628.)

### Diagnosis
Diagnostic tests generally include:
- *Gram stain* of secretions from the endocervix or cul-de-sac, Culture and sensitivity testing aids selection of the appropriate antibiotic. Urethral and rectal secretions may also be cultured.
- *ultrasonography* to identify an adnexal or uterine mass. (X-rays seldom identify pelvic masses.)

- *culdocentesis* to obtain peritoneal fluid or pus for culture and sensitivity testing.

In addition, patient history is significant. In general, PID is associated with recent sexual intercourse, IUD insertion, childbirth, or abortion.

### Treatment
To prevent progression of PID, antibiotic therapy begins immediately after culture specimens are obtained. Such therapy can be reevaluated as soon as laboratory test results are available (usually after 24 to 48 hours). Infection may become chronic if treated inadequately.

The guidelines of the Centers for Disease Control and Prevention (CDC) for outpatient treatment include a single dose of cefoxitin plus probenecid given concurrently or a single dose of ceftriaxone. Each of these regimens is given with doxycycline for 14 days.

The CDC guidelines for inpatient treatment include doxycycline alone or a combination of clindamycin and gentamicin.

Development of a pelvic abscess necessitates adequate drainage. A ruptured abscess is life-threatening. If this complication develops, the patient may need a total abdominal hysterectomy with bilateral salpingo-oophorectomy.

### Special considerations
- After establishing that the patient has no drug allergies, administer antibiotics and analgesics as necessary.
- Check for fever. If it persists, carefully monitor fluid intake and output for signs of dehydration.
- Watch for abdominal rigidity and distention, possible signs of developing peritonitis. Provide frequent perineal care if vaginal drainage occurs.
- To prevent a recurrence, explain the nature and seriousness of PID, and en-

# FORMS OF PELVIC INFLAMMATORY DISEASE

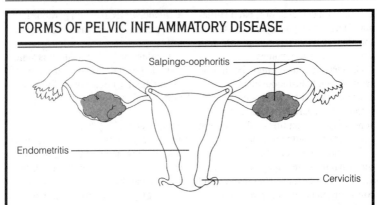

Salpingo-oophoritis

Endometritis

Cervicitis

| CAUSE AND CLINICAL FEATURES | DIAGNOSTIC FINDINGS |
|---|---|

### Salpingo-oophoritis
- *Acute:* sudden onset of lower abdominal and pelvic pain, usually following menses; increased vaginal discharge; fever; malaise; lower abdominal pressure and tenderness; tachycardia; pelvic peritonitis
- *Chronic:* recurring acute episodes

- Blood studies show leukocytosis or normal white blood cell (WBC) count.
- X-ray may show ileus.
- Pelvic exam reveals extreme tenderness.
- Smear of cervical or periurethral gland exudate shows gram-negative intracellular diplococci.

### Cervicitis
- *Acute:* purulent, foul-smelling vaginal discharge; vulvovaginitis, with itching or burning; red, edematous cervix; pelvic discomfort; sexual dysfunction; metrorrhagia; infertility; spontaneous abortion
- *Chronic:* cervical dystocia, laceration or eversion of the cervix, ulcerative vesicular lesion (when cervicitis results from herpes simplex virus II)

- Cultures for *N. gonorrhoeae* are positive (more than 90% of patients).
- Cytologic smears may reveal severe inflammation.
- If cervicitis isn't complicated by salpingitis, WBC count normal or slightly elevated; erythrocyte sedimentation rate (ESR) elevated.
- In *acute cervicitis,* cervical palpation reveals tenderness.
- In *chronic cervicitis,* causative organisms are usually staphylococci or streptococci.

### Endometritis
(generally postpartum or postabortion)
- *Acute:* mucopurulent or purulent vaginal discharge oozing from the cervix; edematous, hyperemic endometrium, possibly leading to ulceration and necrosis (with virulent organisms); lower abdominal pain and tenderness; fever; rebound pain; abdominal muscle spasm; thrombophlebitis of uterine and pelvic vessels (in severe forms)
- *Chronic:* recurring acute episodes (increasingly common because of widespread use of intrauterine devices)

- In severe infection, palpation may reveal boggy uterus.
- Uterine and blood samples positive for causative organism, usually staphylococcus.
- WBC count and ESR are elevated.

courage the patient to comply with the treatment regimen.

- Stress the need for the patient's sexual partner to be examined and, if necessary, treated for infection.
- Because PID may cause painful intercourse, advise the patient to consult with her doctor about sexual activity.

➤ CLINICAL TIP  To prevent infection after minor gynecologic procedures, such as dilatation and curettage, tell the patient to immediately report any fever, increased vaginal discharge, or pain. After such procedures, instruct her to avoid douching and intercourse for at least 7 days.

# PEPTIC ULCERS

Peptic ulcer is a disruption in the gastric or duodenal mucosa when normal defense mechanisms are overwhelmed or impaired by acid or pepsin. Ulcers are circumscribed lesions that extend through the muscularis mucosa. Ulcers occur five times more commonly on the duodenum.

Duodenal ulcers occur most between the ages of 30 and 55. Gastric ulcers occur more commonly between the ages of 55 and 70.

## Causes

Researchers recognize three major causes of peptic ulcer disease: infection with *Helicobacter pylori,* use of nonsteroidal anti-inflammatory drugs (NSAIDs), and pathologic hypersecretory states such as Zollinger-Ellison syndrome.

*H. pylori* is the cause of the majority of duodenal and gastric ulcers, excluding those associated with NSAIDs. Following treatment with standard therapies, 70% to 85% of patients will have

a documented recurrence (by endoscopy) within 1 year.

How *H. pylori* produces an ulcer isn't clear, but the disorder can be cured. Gastric acid, which was considered a primary cause, now appears mainly to contribute to the consequences of infection. Ongoing studies should soon unveil the full mechanism of ulcer formation.

Other causes include use of certain drugs, for example, salicylates and other NSAIDs, which encourage ulcer formation by inhibiting the secretion of prostaglandins (the substances that suppress ulceration). Certain illnesses, such as pancreatitis, hepatic disease, Crohn's disease, Zollinger-Ellison syndrome, and preexisting gastritis, are also known causes.

### Predisposing factors

Ulcers are more common in smokers and chronic users of NSAIDs. Diet and alcohol don't appear to contribute to the development of peptic ulcer disease. It's unclear whether emotional stress is a contributing factor.

## Signs and symptoms

Symptoms vary with the type of ulcer.

### Gastric ulcers

Gastric ulcers are usually signaled by pain that worsens (becomes more intense) with eating. Nausea or anorexia may occur.

### Duodenal ulcers

Duodenal ulcers produce epigastric pain that is gnawing, dull, aching, or "hunger-like." Pain is relieved by food or antacids and usually recurs 2 to 4 hours later. Weight loss or vomiting is usually a sign of malignancy or gastric outlet obstruction.

➤ CLINICAL TIP  If pain changes from rhythmic to constant or radiates, ulcer penetration into the pancreas or perforation may have occurred.

Well-localized midepigastric pain (relieved by food), weight gain (because the patient eats to relieve discomfort), and a peculiar sensation of hot water bubbling in the back of the throat are other reported signs.

Exacerbations tend to recur several times a year, then fade into remission. Vomiting and other digestive disturbances are rare.

### Complications
Both kinds of ulcers may be asymptomatic or may penetrate the pancreas and cause severe back pain. Other complications of peptic ulcers include perforation, hemorrhage, and pyloric obstruction.

### Diagnosis
Patients with dyspepsia may have an upper GI series to diagnose peptic ulcers. For patients with confirmed gastric ulcers, an upper endoscopy should be performed within 8 to 12 weeks to distinguish between benign and malignant disease. An endoscopy should also be performed in patients with GI bleeding to identify areas of ulceration. In patients with a history of peptic ulcer disease, *H. pylori* may be diagnosed with urease breath testing or serologic testing. *H. pylori* can also be diagnosed by biopsy via upper endoscopy.

Other tests may disclose occult blood in the stools and decreased hemoglobin and hematocrit values from GI bleeding.

### Treatment
*H. pylori* can be treated with a number of triple-combination therapy regimens. The most effective agents include clarithromycin, metronidazole, amoxicillin, tetracycline, and proton pump inhibitors. However, none of these drugs are effective in eradication as a monotherapy.

Current recommendations include treating every patient at least once to eradicate *H. pylori* because the infection may occur even with other causes, such as NSAID use. Initial treatment includes tetracycline, bismuth subsalicylate, and metronidazole. Amoxicillin may be tried as an alternative treatment.

Pharmacologic treatments include antisecretory agents, such as proton pump inhibitors and histamine 2 ($H_2$)-receptor antagonists. Proton pump inhibitors (such as omeprazole or lansoprazole) work by binding the acid-secreting enzyme hydrogen/potassium ATPase by inactivating it. $H_2$-receptor antagonists (such as cimetidine, ranitidine, famotidine, and nizatidine) inhibit histamine binding to $H_2$ receptors on the gastric parietal cell, which in turn decreases acid secretion. Drug therapy, which protects the mucosa, includes prostaglandin analogs (misoprostol) and antacids. Prostaglandin analogs may be given to patients taking NSAIDs to suppress ulceration.

GI bleeding may be treated by giving $H_2$-receptor antagonists I.V. as a continuous infusion. Upper endoscopy is preferred as a diagnostic tool when GI bleeding is present. An injection of epinephrine or saline to surround the ulcer can be performed at endoscopy to stop the bleeding. Cautery may also be used for hemostasis.

Surgery is indicated for perforation of the ulcer, continued bleeding despite medical treatment, and suspected malignancy. Surgical procedures for peptic ulcers and gastric outlet obstruction include:

● *vagotomy and pyloroplasty:* severing one or more branches of the vagus nerve to reduce hydrochloric acid secretion and refashioning the pylorus to create a larger lumen and facilitate gastric emptying

• *distal subtotal gastrectomy* (with or without vagotomy): excising the antrum of the stomach, thereby removing the hormonal stimulus of the parietal cells, followed by anastomosis of the remainder of the stomach to the duodenum or the jejunum.

**Special considerations**

Management of peptic ulcers requires administration of medications, focus on patient education, and appropriate postoperative care.

• Administer medications as directed.
• Observe for adverse reactions to $H_2$-receptor antagonists and omeprazole (such as dizziness, fatigue, rash, and mild diarrhea).
• Advocate the use of antacids. Those patients with a history of cardiac disease, or who follow a sodium-restricted diet should be instructed to take only those antacids that contain low amounts of sodium.
• Advise the patient to avoid NSAIDs.
• Warn the patient to avoid stressful situations, excessive intake of coffee, and ingestion of alcoholic beverages during exacerbations of peptic ulcer disease. Counsel the patient to enroll in a smoking cessation program.
• Educate the patient about the potential adverse effects of antibiotic therapy in the treatment of *H. pylori,* which include nausea, vomiting, and diarrhea.
• Discuss with the patient various methods of testing for *H. pylori* infection.

After gastric surgery:
• Maintain patency of the nasogastric (NG) tube. Don't manipulate the tube. If it isn't functioning, notify the surgeon.
• Monitor intake and output. Record NG tube drainage.
• Assess for bowel sounds.

• Maintain patient on nothing-by-mouth status until the NG tube is removed or clamped.
• Replace fluids and electrolytes. Assess for signs of dehydration, sodium deficiency, and metabolic alkalosis, which may occur secondary to gastric suction.
• Monitor for possible complications: hemorrhage; shock; iron, folate, or vitamin $B_{12}$ deficiency anemia (from malabsorption or continued blood loss); and dumping syndrome (weakness, nausea, flatulence, diarrhea, distention, and palpitations within 30 minutes after a meal).
• To avoid dumping syndrome, advise the patient to sit upright up to 2 hours after eating; to drink fluids *between* meals rather than with meals; to avoid eating large amounts of carbohydrates; and to eat four to six small, high-protein, low-carbohydrate meals throughout the day.

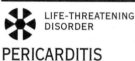 LIFE-THREATENING DISORDER

# PERICARDITIS

Pericarditis is an inflammation of the pericardium, the fibroserous sac that envelops, supports, and protects the heart. It occurs in both acute and chronic forms. Acute pericarditis can be fibrinous or effusive, with purulent, serous, or hemorrhagic exudate; chronic constrictive pericarditis is characterized by dense fibrous pericardial thickening. The prognosis depends on the underlying cause but is generally good in acute pericarditis, unless constriction occurs.

**Causes**

Common causes of this disease include:
• bacterial, fungal, or viral infection (infectious pericarditis)

- neoplasms (primary, or metastases from lungs, breasts, or other organs)
- high-dose radiation to the chest
- uremia
- hypersensitivity or autoimmune disease, such as acute rheumatic fever (most common cause of pericarditis in children), systemic lupus erythematosus, and rheumatoid arthritis
- postcardiac injury, such as myocardial infarction (MI, which later causes an autoimmune reaction [Dressler's syndrome] in the pericardium), trauma, or surgery that leaves the pericardium intact but causes blood to leak into the pericardial cavity
- drugs, such as hydralazine or procainamide
- idiopathic factors (most common in acute pericarditis).

Less common causes include aortic aneurysm with pericardial leakage and myxedema with cholesterol deposits in the pericardium.

### Signs and symptoms

Clinical features vary in the acute and chronic form.

*Acute pericarditis*

In acute pericarditis, a sharp and often sudden pain usually starts over the sternum and radiates to the neck, shoulders, back, and arms. However, unlike the pain of MI, pericardial pain is often pleuritic, increasing with deep inspiration and decreasing when the patient sits up and leans forward, pulling the heart away from the diaphragmatic pleurae of the lungs.

Pericardial effusion, the major complication of acute pericarditis, may produce effects of heart failure — such as dyspnea, orthopnea, and tachycardia — as well as ill-defined substernal chest pain and a feeling of fullness in the chest.

If the fluid accumulates rapidly, cardiac tamponade may occur, resulting in pallor, clammy skin, hypotension, pulsus paradoxus (a decrease in systolic blood pressure ≥10 mm Hg during slow inspiration), neck vein distention and, eventually, cardiovascular collapse and death.

*Chronic pericarditis*

Chronic constrictive pericarditis causes a gradual increase in systemic venous pressure and produces symptoms similar to those of chronic right heart failure (fluid retention, ascites, hepatomegaly).

### Diagnosis

Because pericarditis often coexists with other conditions, diagnosis of acute pericarditis depends on typical clinical features and elimination of other possible causes.

> CLINICAL TIP  A classic symptom, the pericardial friction rub, is a grating sound heard as the heart moves. It can usually be auscultated best during forced expiration, while the patient leans forward or is on his hands and knees in bed.

Pericardial friction rub may have up to three components, corresponding to the timing of atrial systole, ventricular systole, and the rapid-filling phase of ventricular diastole, Occasionally, it's heard only briefly or not at all. Nevertheless, its presence, together with other characteristic features, is diagnostic of acute pericarditis.

In addition, if acute pericarditis has caused very large pericardial effusions, the physical examination reveals increased cardiac dullness and diminished or absent apical impulse and distant heart sounds. In patients with chronic pericarditis, acute inflammation or effusions don't occur — only restricted cardiac filling.

Laboratory results reflect inflammation and may identify its cause:

• normal or elevated white blood cell count, especially in infectious pericarditis

• elevated erythrocyte sedimentation rate

• slightly elevated cardiac enzyme levels with associated myocarditis

• culture of pericardial fluid obtained by open surgical drainage or cardiocentesis (sometimes identifies a causative organism in bacterial or fungal pericarditis).

Electrocardiography shows the following changes in acute pericarditis: elevation of ST segments in the standard limb leads and most precordial leads without significant changes in QRS morphology that occur with MI, atrial ectopic rhythms such as atrial fibrillation, and diminished QRS complex in pericardial effusion.

Other pertinent laboratory studies include blood urea nitrogen level to check for uremia, antistreptolsyin O titers to detect rheumatic fever, and a purified protein derivative skin test to check for tuberculosis. In pericardial effusion, echocardiography is diagnostic when it shows an echo-free space between the ventricular wall and the pericardium.

## Treatment

The goal of treatment is to relieve symptoms and manage underlying systemic disease.

### Bed rest and drug therapy

In acute idiopathic pericarditis, post-MI pericarditis, and postthoracotomy pericarditis, treatment consists of bed rest as long as fever and pain persist and nonsteroidal anti-inflammatory drugs, such as aspirin and indomethacin, to relieve pain and reduce inflammation.

If these drugs fail to relieve symptoms, corticosteroids may be used. Although corticosteroids produce rapid and effective relief, they must be used cautiously because episodes may recur when therapy is discontinued.

Infectious pericarditis that results from disease of the left pleural space, mediastinal abscesses, or septicemia requires antibiotics (possibly by direct pericardial injection), surgical drainage, or both. Cardiac tamponade may require pericardiocentesis. Signs of tamponade include pulsus paradoxus, neck vein distention, dyspnea, and shock.

### Pericardectomy

Recurrent pericarditis may necessitate partial pericardectomy, which creates a "window" that allows fluid to drain into the pleural space. In constrictive pericarditis, total pericardectomy to permit adequate filling and contraction of the heart may be necessary. Treatment must also include management of rheumatic fever, uremia, tuberculosis, and other underlying disorders.

## Special considerations

• Provide complete bed rest.

• Assess pain in relation to respiration and body position to distinguish pericardial pain from myocardial ischemic pain.

• Place the patient in an upright position to relieve dyspnea and chest pain. Provide analgesics and oxygen, and reassure the patient with acute pericarditis that his condition is temporary and treatable.

• Monitor the patient for signs of cardiac compression or cardiac tamponade, possible complications of pericardial effusion. Signs include decreased blood pressure, increased central venous pressure, and pulsus paradoxus. Because cardiac tamponade requires immediate treatment, keep a pericardiocentesis set handy whenever pericardial effusion is suspected.

• Explain tests and treatments to the patient. If surgery is necessary, he should learn deep breathing and coughing exercises beforehand. Postoperative care is similar to that given after cardiothoracic surgery.

# PERIRECTAL ABSCESS AND FISTULA

A perirectal abscess is a localized collection of pus caused by inflammation of the soft tissue outside the anal verge. Such inflammation may produce a fistula in ano — an abnormal opening in the anal skin — that may communicate with the rectum. Men are affected by this disease three times as often as women.

## Causes

The inflammatory process that leads to abscess may begin with an abrasion or tear in the lining of the anal canal, rectum, or perianal skin, and subsequent infection by *Escherichia coli,* staphylococci, or streptococci. Such trauma may result from injections for treatment of internal hemorrhoids, enema-tip abrasions, puncture wounds from ingested eggshells or fishbones, or insertion of foreign objects.

Other preexisting lesions include infected anal fissure, infections from the anal crypt through the anal gland, ruptured anal hematoma, prolapsed thrombotic internal hemorrhoids, and septic lesions in the pelvis, such as acute appendicitis, acute salpingitis, and diverticulitis. Systemic illnesses that may cause abscesses include ulcerative colitis and Crohn's disease. However, many abscesses develop without preexisting lesions. Other causes include trauma, malignancy, radiation, infectious dermatitis, and an immunocompromised state.

As the abscess produces more pus, a fistula may form in the soft tissue beneath the muscle fibers of the sphincters (especially the external sphincter), usually extending into the perianal skin. The internal (primary) opening of the abscess or fistula is usually near the anal glands and crypts; the external (secondary) opening, in the perianal skin.

## Signs and symptoms

Characteristics are throbbing pain and tenderness at the site of the abscess and painful swelling that is exacerbated by defecation. A hard, painful lump develops on one side, preventing comfortable sitting.

## Diagnosis

Perirectal abscess is detectable on physical examination:

• *Perianal abscess* is a red, tender, localized, oval swelling close to the anus. Sitting or coughing increases pain, and pus may drain from the abscess. Digital examination reveals no abnormalities.

• *Ischiorectal abscess* involves the entire perianal region on the affected side of the anus. The only symptom of this large erythematous, indurated, tender mass at the buttock may be pain. It's tender but may not produce drainage. Digital rectal examination reveals a tender induration bulging into the anal canal.

CLINICAL TIP A flexible sigmoidoscopy should be performed at a later date on these patients to rule out carcinoma or inflammatory bowel disease.

• *Submucous or high intermuscular abscess* may produce a dull, aching pain in the rectum, tenderness and, occasionally, induration. Digital examination reveals a smooth swelling of the upper part of the anal canal or lower rectum.

• *Pelvirectal abscess* (rare) produces fever, malaise, and myalgia but no local anal or external rectal signs or pain. Digital examination reveals a tender mass high in the pelvis, perhaps extending into one of the ischiorectal fossae.

If the abscess drains by forming a fistula, the pain usually subsides and the major signs become pruritic drainage and subsequent perianal irritation.

> CLINICAL TIP   Pain and discharge are symptoms of fistula development and when the external or secondary opening has closed.

The external opening of a fistula generally appears as a pink or red, elevated, discharging sinus or ulcer on the skin near the anus. Depending on the infection's severity, the patient may have chills, fever, nausea, vomiting, and malaise. Digital rectal examination may reveal a palpable indurated tract and a drop or two of pus on palpation. The internal opening may be palpated as a depression or ulcer in the midline anteriorly or at the dentate line posteriorly. To identify an internal opening, an examination under anesthesia should be performed.

Flexible sigmoidoscopy, barium studies, and colonoscopy should be performed to rule out underlying conditions.

## Treatment

Perirectal abscesses require surgical incision and drainage. The area may be explored to  identify a fistula tract, and a fistulotomy may be performed at a later date. Fistulas require a fistulotomy — removal of the fistula tract and associated granulation tissue — under general, spinal, or caudal anesthesia. If the fistula tract is epithelialized, treatment requires fistulectomy —

removal of the fistulous tract — followed by insertion of drains, which are gradually removed over time.

## Special considerations

After incision and drainage:
• Provide adequate medication for pain relief.
• Examine the wound frequently to assess proper healing, which should progress from the inside out. Healing should be complete in 4 to 5 weeks for perianal fistulas; in 12 to 16 weeks for deeper wounds.
• Inform the patient that complete recovery takes time. Offer encouragement.
• Stress the importance of perianal cleanliness.
• Dispose of soiled dressings properly.
• Be alert for the first postoperative bowel movement. The patient may suppress the urge to defecate because of anticipated pain; the resulting constipation increases pressure at the wound site. Such a patient may benefit from a stool-softening laxative.

---

LIFE-THREATENING DISORDER

# PERITONITIS

---

Peritonitis is an acute or chronic inflammation of the peritoneum, the membrane that lines the abdominal cavity and covers the visceral organs. Inflammation may extend throughout the peritoneum or may be localized as an abscess.

Peritonitis commonly decreases intestinal motility and causes intestinal distention with gas. Mortality is 10%, with death usually resulting from bowel obstruction; the mortality was much higher before the introduction of antibiotics.

## Causes

Although the GI tract normally contains bacteria, the peritoneum is sterile. In peritonitis, however, bacteria invade the peritoneum. Generally, such infection results from inflammation and perforation of the GI tract, allowing bacterial invasion. Usually, this is a result of appendicitis, diverticulitis, peptic ulcer, ulcerative colitis, volvulus, strangulated obstruction, abdominal neoplasm, or a penetrating wound.

Peritonitis may also result from chemical inflammation, as in rupture of the fallopian tube or the bladder; perforation of a gastric ulcer; or released pancreatic enzymes.

In both chemical and bacterial inflammation, accumulated fluids containing protein and electrolytes make the transparent peritoneum opaque, red, inflamed, and edematous. Because the peritoneal cavity is so resistant to contamination, such infection is often localized as an abscess instead of disseminated as a generalized infection.

## Signs and symptoms

The key symptom of peritonitis is sudden, severe, and diffuse abdominal pain that tends to intensify and localize in the area of the underlying disorder.

> CLINICAL TIP   Direct or rebound tenderness may be elicited over an area affected by diverticulitis.

Pain may be accompanied by anorexia, nausea, vomiting, and altered bowel habits (particularly constipation). For instance, if appendicitis causes the rupture, pain eventually localizes in the lower right quadrant. The patient often displays weakness, pallor, excessive sweating, and cold skin as a result of excessive loss of fluid, electrolytes, and protein into the abdominal cavity.

Decreased intestinal motility and paralytic ileus result from the effect of bacterial toxins on the intestinal muscles.

Intestinal obstruction causes nausea, vomiting, and abdominal rigidity.

### Other clinical characteristics

Typical features include hypotension, tachycardia, signs of dehydration (oliguria, thirst, dry swollen tongue, pinched skin), acutely tender abdomen associated with rebound tenderness, temperature of 103° F (39.4° C) or higher, and hypokalemia. Inflammation of the diaphragmatic peritoneum may cause shoulder pain and hiccups.

Abdominal distention and resulting upward displacement of the diaphragm may decrease respiratory capacity. Typically, the patient with peritonitis tends to breathe shallowly and move as little as possible to minimize pain.

## Diagnosis

Severe abdominal pain in a patient with direct or rebound tenderness suggests peritonitis. Abdominal X-rays showing edematous and gaseous distention of the small and large bowel support the diagnosis. In the case of perforation of a visceral organ, the radiography film shows air in the abdominal cavity.

Other tests include the following:
● *Chest X-ray* may show elevation of the diaphragm.
● *Blood studies* reveal leukocytosis (> 20,000/µl).
● *Paracentesis* reveals bacteria, exudate, blood, pus, or urine.
● *Laparotomy* may be necessary to identify the underlying cause.

## Treatment

Early treatment of GI inflammatory conditions and preoperative and postoperative antibiotic therapy help prevent peritonitis. After peritonitis develops, emergency treatment must combat infection, restore intestinal motility, and replace fluids and electrolytes.

*Antibiotics and supplementary treatment*

Empiric antibiotic therapy usually includes administration of cefoxitin with an aminoglycoside or penicillin G and clindamycin with an aminoglycoside, depending on the infecting organisms. To decrease peristalsis and prevent perforation, the patient should receive nothing by mouth; I.V. fluids are administered. Other supportive measures include preoperative and postoperative administration of analgesia and nasogastric (NG) decompression.

*Surgery*

When peritonitis results from perforation, surgery is necessary. The aim of surgery is to eliminate the source of infection by evacuating the spilled contents and repairing any organ perforation.

**Special considerations**

• Monitor vital signs, fluid intake and output, and the amount of NG drainage or vomitus.
• Place the patient in semi-Fowler's position to facilitate pulmonary toileting.
• Encourage the patient to deep-breathe, cough effectively, and use an incentive spirometer.
• Teach splinting of the incision to facilitate pulmonary toileting.
• Ambulate the patient on the first postoperative day.
• Counteract mouth and nose dryness due to fever and NG intubation with regular cleaning and lubrication.

After surgery to evacuate the peritoneum:
• Maintain parenteral fluid and electrolyte administration as ordered. Accurately record fluid intake and output, including NG and incisional drainage.
• Place the patient in Fowler's position to promote drainage (through drainage tube) by gravity.

• Encourage and assist ambulation as ordered, usually on the first postoperative day.
• Observe for signs of dehiscence (the patient may complain that "something gave way") and abscess formation (persistent abdominal tenderness and fever).
• Frequently assess for peristaltic activity by listening for bowel sounds and evaluating for passage of flatus, bowel movements, and soft abdomen.
• When peristalsis returns and temperature and pulse rate are normal or when NG output diminishes (< 200 ml/24 hr), the NG tube is removed.
• Gradually decrease parenteral fluids and increase oral intake.

# PERNICIOUS ANEMIA

A megaloblastic anemia, pernicious anemia is characterized by decreased gastric production of hydrochloric acid and deficiency of intrinsic factor (IF), a substance normally secreted by the parietal cells of the gastric mucosa that is essential for vitamin $B_{12}$ absorption. The resulting deficiency of vitamin $B_{12}$ causes serious neurologic, gastric, and intestinal abnormalities. Untreated pernicious anemia may lead to permanent neurologic disability and death.

Pernicious anemia primarily affects people of northern European ancestry; in the United States, it's most common in New England and the Great Lakes region because of ethnic concentrations. It's rare in children, blacks, and Asians. Onset typically occurs between the ages of 50 and 60; incidence rises with increasing age.

**Causes**

Familial incidence of pernicious anemia suggests a genetic predisposition.

Significantly higher incidence in patients with immunologically related diseases, such as thyroiditis, myxedema, and Graves' disease, seems to support a widely held theory that an inherited autoimmune response causes gastric mucosal atrophy and, therefore, deficiency of hydrochloric acid and IF.

Deficiency of IF impairs vitamin $B_{12}$ absorption. The resultant vitamin $B_{12}$–deficiency inhibits cell growth, particularly of red blood cells (RBCs), leading to insufficient and deformed RBCs with poor oxygen-carrying capacity. It also impairs myelin formation, causing neurologic damage. Iatrogenic induction can follow partial gastrectomy.

### Signs and symptoms

Characteristically, pernicious anemia has an insidious onset but eventually causes an unmistakable triad of symptoms: weakness, sore tongue, and numbness and tingling in the extremities. The lips, gums, and tongue appear markedly bloodless. Hemolysis-induced hyperbilirubinemia may cause faintly jaundiced sclera and pale to bright yellow skin. In addition, the patient may become highly susceptible to infection, especially of the genitourinary tract.

#### *GI symptoms*

Gastric mucosal atrophy and decreased hydrochloric acid production disturb digestion and lead to nausea, vomiting, anorexia, weight loss, flatulence, diarrhea, and constipation. Gingival bleeding and tongue inflammation may hinder eating and intensify anorexia.

#### *CNS symptoms*

Nerve demyelination caused by vitamin $B_{12}$ deficiency initially affects the peripheral nerves but gradually extends to the spinal cord. Consequently, the neurologic effects of pernicious anemia may include neuritis, weakness in extremities, peripheral numbness and paresthesia, disturbed position sense, lack of coordination, ataxia, impaired fine finger movement, positive Babinski's and Romberg's signs, light-headedness, optic muscle atrophy, loss of bowel and bladder control, impotence (in males), and altered vision (diplopia, blurred vision), taste, and hearing (tinnitus).

The effects of pernicious anemia on the nervous system may also produce irritability, poor memory, headache, depression, and delirium. Although some of these symptoms are temporary, irreversible central nervous system changes may have occurred before treatment is initiated.

#### *Cardiovascular symptoms*

Increasingly fragile cell membranes induce widespread destruction of RBCs, resulting in low hemoglobin (Hb) levels. The impaired oxygen-carrying capacity of the blood secondary to lowered Hb leads to weakness, fatigue, and light-headedness. Compensatory increased cardiac output results in palpitations, wide pulse pressure, dyspnea, orthopnea, tachycardia, premature beats and, eventually, heart failure.

### Diagnosis

A positive family history, typical ethnic heritage, and results of blood studies, bone marrow aspiration, gastric analysis, and the Schilling test establish the diagnosis of pernicious anemia. Laboratory screening must rule out other anemias with similar symptoms, such as folic acid deficiency anemia, because treatment differs.

Diagnosis must also rule out vitamin $B_{12}$ deficiency resulting from malabsorption due to GI disorders, gastric surgery, radiation, or drug therapy.

Blood study results that suggest pernicious anemia include:

• decreased Hb (4 to 5 g/dl) and decreased RBC count

• increased mean corpuscular volume (> 120/µl); because larger-than-normal RBCs *each* contain increased amounts of Hb; mean corpuscular Hb concentration is also increased

• possible low white blood cell and platelet counts and large, malformed platelets

• serum vitamin $B_{12}$–assay levels < 0.1 mcg/ml

• elevated serum lactate dehydrogenase levels.

Bone marrow aspiration reveals erythroid hyperplasia (crowded red bone marrow), with increased numbers of megaloblasts but few normally developing RBCs. Gastric analysis shows absence of free hydrochloric acid after histamine or pentagastrin injection.

### Schilling test

In the Schilling test, the definitive test for pernicious anemia, the patient receives a small oral dose (0.5 to 2 mcg) of radioactive vitamin $B_{12}$ after fasting for 12 hours. A larger dose (1 mg) of nonradioactive vitamin $B_{12}$ is given I.M. 2 hours later, as a parenteral flush, and the radioactivity of a 24-hour urine specimen is measured.

About 7% of the radioactive $B_{12}$ dose is excreted in the first 24 hours; persons with pernicious anemia excrete less than 3%. (In pernicious anemia, the vitamin remains unabsorbed and is passed in the stool.) When the Schilling test is repeated with IF added, the test shows normal excretion of vitamin $B_{12}$.

### Serologic tests

Important serologic findings may include IF antibodies and antiparietal cell antibodies.

### Treatment

Early parenteral vitamin $B_{12}$ replacement can reverse pernicious anemia, minimize complications, and possibly prevent permanent neurologic damage.

### Vitamin $B_{12}$ replacement

An initial high dose of parenteral vitamin $B_{12}$ causes rapid RBC regeneration. Within 2 weeks, Hb should rise to normal, and the patient's condition should markedly improve. Because rapid cell regeneration increases the patient's iron and folate requirements, concomitant iron and folic acid replacement is necessary to prevent iron deficiency anemia.

After the patient's condition improves, the vitamin $B_{12}$ dosage can be decreased to maintenance levels and given monthly. Because such injections must be continued for life, patients should learn self-administration of vitamin $B_{12}$.

### Other measures

If anemia causes extreme fatigue, the patient may require bed rest until Hb rises. If Hb is dangerously low, he may need blood transfusions, digoxin, a diuretic, and a low-sodium diet for heart failure. Most important is the replacement of vitamin $B_{12}$ to control the condition that led to this failure. Antibiotics help combat accompanying infections.

### Special considerations

• Supportive measures minimize the risk of complications and speed recovery. Patient and family teaching can promote compliance with lifelong vitamin $B_{12}$ replacement.

• If the patient has severe anemia, plan activities, rest periods, and necessary diagnostic tests to conserve his energy. Monitor pulse rate often; tachycardia means his activities are too strenuous.

• To ensure accurate Schilling test results, make sure that all urine over a

24-hour period is collected and that the specimens are uncontaminated.

● Warn the patient to guard against infections, and tell him to report signs of infection promptly, especially pulmonary and urinary tract infections, because the patient's weakened condition may increase susceptibility.

● Provide a well-balanced diet, including foods high in vitamin $B_{12}$ (meat, liver, fish, eggs, and milk). Offer between-meal snacks, and encourage the family to bring favorite foods from home.

● Because a sore mouth and tongue make eating painful, ask the dietitian to avoid giving the patient irritating foods. If these symptoms make talking difficult, supply a pad and pencil or some other aid to facilitate nonverbal communication; explain this problem to the family. Provide diluted mouthwash or, with severe conditions, swab the patient's mouth with tap water or warm saline solution.

● Warn the patient with a sensory deficit not to use a heating pad because it may cause burns.

● If the patient is incontinent, establish a regular bowel and bladder routine. After the patient is discharged, a visiting nurse should follow up on this schedule and make adjustments as needed.

● If neurologic damage causes behavioral problems, assess mental and neurologic status often; if necessary, give tranquilizers as ordered, and apply a jacket restraint at night.

● Stress that vitamin $B_{12}$ replacement isn't a permanent cure and that these injections must be continued for life, even after symptoms subside.

➤ CLINICAL TIP To prevent pernicious anemia, emphasize the importance of vitamin $B_{12}$ supplements for patients who have had extensive gastric resections or who follow strict vegetarian diets.

# PERSONALITY DISORDERS

Defined as individual traits that reflect chronic, inflexible, and maladaptive patterns of behavior, personality disorders cause social discomfort and impair social and occupational functioning. Although no statistics document the number of cases of personality disorder, these disorders are known to be widespread. Most patients with a personality disorder don't receive treatment; when they do, they're typically managed as outpatients.

According to the classification system of the *Diagnostic and Statistical Manual of Mental Disorders,* 4th edition, *(DSM-IV),* personality disorders fall on Axis II. Knowing the features of personality disorders helps provide a fuller picture of the patient and a more accurate diagnosis. For example, many features characteristic of personality disorders are apparent during an episode of another mental disorder (such as a major depressive episode in a patient with compulsive personality features).

Personality disorders typically begin before or during adolescence and early adulthood and persist throughout adult life. The prognosis is variable.

### Causes
Only recently have personality disorders been categorized in detail, and research continues to identify their causes. Various theories attempt to explain the origin of personality disorders.

● Biological theories hold that these disorders may stem from chromosomal and neuronal abnormalities or head trauma.

● Social theories hold that the disorders reflect learned responses, having much to do with reinforcement, modeling, and aversive stimuli as contributing factors.

● Psychodynamic theories hold that personality disorders reflect deficiencies in ego and superego development and are related to poor mother-child relationships that are characterized by unresponsiveness, overprotectiveness, or early separation.

### Signs and symptoms

Each specific personality disorder produces characteristic signs and symptoms, which may vary among patients and within the same patient at different times. In general, the history of the patient with a personality disorder will reveal long-standing difficulties in interpersonal relationships, ranging from dependency to withdrawal, and in occupational functioning, with effects ranging from compulsive perfectionism to intentional sabotage.

The patient with a personality disorder may show any degree of self-confidence, ranging from no self-esteem to arrogance. Convinced that his behavior is normal, he avoids responsibility for its consequences, often resorting to projections and blame.

### Diagnosis

For characteristic findings in patients with this condition, see *Diagnosing personality disorders,* pages 642 to 644.

### Treatment

Personality disorders are difficult to treat. Successful therapy requires a trusting relationship in which the therapist can use a direct approach. The type of therapy chosen depends on the patient's symptoms.

Drug therapy is ineffective but may be used to relieve acute anxiety and depression. Family and group therapy usually are effective.

Hospital inpatient milieu therapy can be effective in crisis situations and possibly for long-term treatment of borderline personality disorders. Inpatient treatment is controversial, however, because most patients with personality disorders don't comply with extended therapeutic regimens; for such patients, outpatient therapy may be more useful.

### Special considerations

● Provide consistent care. Take a direct, involved approach to ensure the patient's trust. Keep in mind that many of these patients don't respond well to interviews, whereas others are charming and convincing.

> **CLINICAL TIP** Coordinating care with other health care providers is extremely important to provide consistent expectations and interactions.

● Teach the patient social skills, and reinforce appropriate behavior.

● Encourage expression of feelings, self-analysis of behavior, and accountability for actions.

Specific care measures vary with the particular personality disorder.

#### *Paranoid personality disorder*

● Avoid situations that threaten the patient's autonomy.

● Approach the patient in a straightforward and candid manner, adopting a professional, rather than a casual or friendly, attitude. Remember that remarks intended to be humorous are easily misinterpreted by the paranoid patient.

● Provide a supportive and nonjudgmental environment in which the patient can safely explore and verbalize his feelings.

#### *Schizoid personality disorder*

● Remember that the schizoid patient needs close human contact but is easily overwhelmed. Respect the patient's

# DIAGNOSING PERSONALITY DISORDERS

The diagnosis of a recognized personality disorder is made when a patient's symptoms match the following relevant diagnostic criteria put forth in the *DSM-IV.*

### Paranoid personality disorder

The person must exhibit a pervasive and unwarranted tendency, beginning by early adulthood and present in various contexts, to interpret the actions of people as deliberately demeaning or threatening, as indicated by at least four of the following:

- The person suspects, without sufficient basis, that he's being exploited, deceived, or harmed by others.
- The person questions without justification the loyalty or trustworthiness of friends or associates.
- The person is reluctant to confide in others because of unwarranted fear that the information will be used against him.
- The person finds hostile or evil meanings in benign remarks.
- The person bears grudges or is unforgiving of insults or slights.
- The person is easily slighted and quick to react with anger or to counterattack.
- The person questions without justification the fidelity of a spouse or sexual partner.

The symptoms don't occur exclusively during the course of schizophrenia or other psychotic disorders and aren't the direct physiologic effect of a general medical condition.

### Schizoid personality disorder

The patient must exhibit a pervasive detachment from social relations, and the range of emotions is restricted in interpersonal settings, as indicated by at least four or more of the following:

- The person has no desire or enjoyment of close relationships, including family.
- The person chooses solitary activities.
- The person has little or no interest in sexual activity with others.

- The person finds pleasure in few activities.
- The person has few, if any, close friends other than first-degree relatives.
- The person is indifferent to praise or criticism.
- The person is emotionally cold and detached, showing little expression.

The symptoms don't occur exclusively during the course of schizophrenia, or other psychotic disorders, and aren't due to the direct physiological effect of a general medical condition.

### Borderline personality disorder

This pervasive pattern of instability of interpersonal relationships, self-image, and affect and marked impulsivity, beginning by early adulthood and present in various contexts, is indicated by at least five of the following features:

- The person makes frantic efforts to avoid real or imagined abandonment (excluding suicidal or self-mutilating behavior).
- The person has a pattern of unstable and intense interpersonal relationships characterized by alternating extremes of overidealization and devaluation.
- The person has an identity disturbance — a markedly and persistently unstable self-image or sense of self.
- The person shows impulsiveness in at least two areas that are potentially self-damaging, such as spending, sexual activity, substance abuse, shoplifting, reckless driving, and binge eating (excluding suicidal or self-mutilating behavior).
- The person engages in recurrent suicidal threats, gestures, or behavior or in self-mutilating behavior.

## DIAGNOSING PERSONALITY DISORDERS *(continued)*

• The person has affective instability resulting from marked mood reactivity (for example, depression, irritability, or anxiety lasting usually a few hours and seldom more than a few days).
• The person has chronic feelings of emptiness or boredom.
• The person has inappropriate intense anger or difficulty controlling anger.
• The person has transient, stress-related paranoid ideation or severe dissociative symptoms.

### Histrionic personality disorder
This pervasive pattern of excessive emotionality and attention-seeking behavior, beginning by early adulthood and present in various contexts, is indicated by at least four of the following:
• The person is uncomfortable in situations in which he is not the center of attention.
• The person's interaction with others is often characterized by inappropriately sexually seductive or provocative behavior.
• The person displays rapidly shifting and shallow expression of emotions.
• The person consistently uses physical appearance to draw attention to himself.
• The person has a style of speech that is excessively impressionistic and lacking in detail.
• The person shows self-dramatization, theatricality, and exaggerated emotional expression.
• The person is suggestible (easily influenced by others or circumstances).
• The person considers relationships to be more intimate than they actually are.

### Narcissistic personality disorder
This pervasive pattern of grandiosity, need for admiration, and lack of empathy, beginning by early adulthood and present in various contexts, is indicated by at least five of the following:

• The person has a grandiose sense of self-importance.
• The person is preoccupied with fantasies of unlimited success, power, brilliance, beauty, or ideal love.
• The person believes that he is special and unique and can only be understood by, or should associate with, other special or high-status people (or institutions).
• The person requires excessive admiration.
• The person has a sense of entitlement (an unreasonable expectation of especially favorable treatment or automatic compliance with his expectations).
• The person is interpersonally exploitive, taking advantage of others to achieve his own ends.
• The person lacks empathy.
• The person is often envious of others or believes that others are envious of him.
• The person shows arrogant, naughty behaviors or attitudes.

### Avoidant personality disorder
This pervasive pattern of social inhibition, feelings of inadequacy, and hypersensitivity to negative evaluation, beginning by early adulthood and present in a variety of contexts, is indicated by at least four of the following:
• The person avoids social or occupational activities that involve significant interpersonal contact because of fears of criticism, disapproval, or rejection.
• The person is unwilling to get involved with people unless he's certain that they will like him.
• The person shows restraint within intimate relationships because of the fear of being shamed or ridiculed.
• The person is preoccupied with being criticized or rejected in social situations.
• The person's feelings of inadequacy inhibit him in new interpersonal situations.

*(continued)*

## DIAGNOSING PERSONALITY DISORDERS *(continued)*

• The person views himself as socially inept, personally unappealing, or inferior to others.
• The person is unusually reluctant to take personal risks or to engage in any new activities because they may prove embarrassing.

### Dependent personality disorder

This pervasive and excessive need to be taken care of that leads to submissive and clinging behavior and fears of separation, beginning by early adulthood and present in a variety of contexts, is indicated by at least five of the following:
• The person has difficulty making everyday decisions without an excessive amount of advice or reassurance from others.
• The person needs others to assume responsibility for most major areas of his life.
• The person has difficulty expressing disagreement with others because of fear of loss of support or approval (excluding realistic fears of retribution).
• The person has difficulty initiating projects or doing things on his own (because of a lack of self-confidence in his judgment or abilities rather than a lack of motivation or energy).
• The person goes to excessive lengths to obtain nurture and support from others, to the point of volunteering to do things that are unpleasant.
• The person feels uncomfortable or helpless when alone because of exaggerated fears of inability to care for himself.
• The person urgently seeks another relationship as a source of care and support when a close relationship ends.

• The person is unrealistically preoccupied with fears of being left to take care of himself.

### Obsessive-compulsive personality disorder

This pervasive pattern of preoccupation with orderliness, perfectionism, and mental and interpersonal control at the expense of flexibility, openness, and efficiency, beginning by early adulthood and present in a variety of contexts, is indicated by at least four of the following:
• The person is preoccupied with details, rules, lists, order, organization, or schedules to the extent that the core point of the activity is lost.
• The person shows perfectionism that interferes with task completion.
• The person is excessively devoted to work and productivity to the exclusion of leisure activities and friendships (not accounted for by obvious economic need).
• The person exhibits overconscientiousness, scrupulousness, and inflexibility about matters of morality, ethics, or values (not accounted for by cultural or religious identification).
• The person can't discard worn-out or worthless objects even when they have no sentimental value.
• The person is reluctant to delegate tasks or to work with others unless they submit exactly to his way of doing things.
• The person adopts a miserly spending style toward self and others: money is viewed as something to be hoarded in preparation for future catastrophes.
• The person shows rigidity and stubbornness.

need for privacy, and slowly build a trusting, therapeutic relationship so that he finds more pleasure than fear in relating to you.

• Give the patient plenty of time to express his feelings. Keep in mind that if you push him to do so before he's ready, he may retreat.

### Borderline personality disorder

- Encourage the patient to take responsibility for himself. Don't attempt to rescue him from the consequences of his actions.
- Don't try to solve problems that the patient can solve himself.
- Maintain a consistent approach in all interactions with the patient, and ensure that other staff members do so as well.
- Recognize that the patient may idolize some staff members and devalue others.
- Don't take sides in the patient's disputes with other staff members.

### Histrionic personality disorder

- Give the patient choices in care strategies, and incorporate his wishes into the treatment plan as much as possible. By increasing his sense of self-control, you'll reduce his anxiety.
- Deal with the patient in a professional way. He may be uncomfortable with a casual approach.

### Narcissistic personality disorder

- Respond positively to the patient's sense of entitlement. A critical attitude may cause him to become even more demanding and difficult.
- Focus on positive traits or on feelings of pain, loss, or rejection.

### Avoidant personality disorder

- Assess for signs of depression. Impaired social interaction increases the risk of affective disorders.
- Establish a trusting relationship with the patient. Be aware that he may become dependent on the few staff members whom he believes he can trust.
- Make sure that the patient has plenty of time to prepare for all upcoming procedures. This patient can't handle surprises well.

- Inform the patient when you will and will not be available if he needs assistance.

### Dependent personality disorder

- Initially, give the patient explicit directives, rather than ask him to make decisions. Later, encourage him to make easy decisions, such as what to wear or which television program to watch. Continue to provide support and reassurance as his decision-making ability improves.

### Obsessive-compulsive personality disorder

- Allow the patient to participate in his own treatment plan by offering choices whenever possible.
- Adopt a professional approach in your interactions with the patient. Avoid informality; this patient expects strict attention to detail. (See also "Obsessive-Compulsive disorder" entry.)

# PHARYNGITIS

The most common throat disorder, pharyngitis is an acute or chronic inflammation of the pharynx. It is widespread among adults who live or work in dusty or very dry environments, use their voices excessively, habitually use tobacco or alcohol, or suffer from chronic sinusitis, persistent coughs, or allergies.

## Causes

Pharyngitis is usually caused by a virus. The most common viral agents are rhinovirus, coronavirus, adenovirus, influenza, and parainfluenza viruses. The most common bacterial cause is group A beta-hemolytic streptococci. Other common causes include *Mycoplasma* and *Chlamydia*.

## Signs and symptoms

Pharyngitis produces a sore throat and slight difficulty in swallowing. Swallowing saliva is usually more painful than swallowing food. Pharyngitis may also cause the sensation of a lump in the throat as well as a constant, aggravating urge to swallow. Associated features may include mild fever, headache, muscle and joint pain, coryza, and rhinorrhea. Uncomplicated pharyngitis usually subsides in 3 to 10 days.

## Diagnosis

Physical examination of the pharynx reveals generalized redness and inflammation of the posterior wall and red, edematous mucous membranes studded with white or yellow follicles. Exudate is usually confined to the lymphoid areas of the throat, sparing the tonsillar pillars. Bacterial pharyngitis usually produces a large amount of exudate.

A throat culture may be performed to identify bacterial organisms that may be the cause of the inflammation.

## Treatment

The focus for treatment of acute and chronic pharyngitis varies.

### Acute pharyngitis

In acute viral pharyngitis, treatment is usually symptomatic, and consists mainly of rest, warm saline gargles, throat lozenges containing a mild anesthetic, plenty of fluids, and analgesics as needed. If the patient can't swallow fluids, hospitalization may be required for I.V. hydration.

Suspected bacterial pharyngitis requires rigorous treatment with penicillin or another broad-spectrum antibiotic because *Streptococcus* is the chief infecting organism. Antibiotic therapy should continue for 48 hours until culture results are back.

If the culture (or a rapid strep test) is positive for group A beta-hemolytic streptococci, or if bacterial infection is suspected despite negative culture results, penicillin therapy should be continued for 10 days. This is to prevent the sequelae of acute rheumatic fever.

### Chronic pharyngitis

In chronic pharyngitis, treatment requires the same supportive measures as acute pharyngitis but with greater emphasis on eliminating the underlying cause, such as an allergen. Preventive measures include adequate humidification and avoiding excessive exposure to air conditioning. In addition, the patient should be urged to stop smoking.

## Special considerations

- Administer analgesics and warm saline gargles as appropriate.
- Encourage the patient to drink plenty of fluids. Monitor intake and output scrupulously, and watch for signs of dehydration. Assess skin turgor, mucous membranes and, in young children, tearing.

  **CLINICAL TIP** Encourage intake of cool fluids to soothe the patient's throat. Also have the patient take normal-size swallows, not sips.
- Provide meticulous mouth care to prevent dry lips and oral pyoderma, and maintain a restful environment.
- Elevate the patient's head with three or four pillows.
- Obtain throat cultures, and administer antibiotics as required. If the patient has acute bacterial pharyngitis, emphasize the importance of completing the full course of antibiotic therapy.
- Teach the patient with chronic pharyngitis how to minimize sources of throat irritation in the environment, such as using a bedside humidifier.
- Refer the patient to a self-help group to stop smoking, if appropriate.

# PHENYLKETONURIA

Phenylketonuria (PKU) is an inborn error in phenylalanine metabolism that results in the accumulation of high serum levels of the enzyme phenylalanine in the blood. When left untreated, it results in cerebral damage and mental retardation.

## Causes

PKU is transmitted by an autosomal recessive gene. Patients with this disorder have insufficient hepatic phenylalanine hydroxylase, an enzyme that acts as a catalyst in the conversion of phenylalanine to tyrosine. As a result, phenylalanine and its metabolites accumulate in the blood, eventually causing mental retardation if left untreated. The exact biochemical mechanism that causes this retardation is unclear.

In the United States, this disorder occurs in 1 in approximately 14,000 births. (About 1 person in 60 is an asymptomatic carrier.) The gene is most common in Ireland, Scotland, Belgium, and West Germany and is rare in Blacks, Asians, Native Americans, Finns, and Ashkenazi Jews.

## Signs and symptoms

An infant with undiagnosed and untreated PKU appears normal at birth but by 4 months begins to show signs of arrested brain development, including mental retardation and, later, personality disturbances (schizoid and antisocial personality patterns and uncontrollable temper). Such a child may have a lighter complexion than unaffected siblings and often has blue eyes. He may also have microcephaly; eczematous skin lesions or dry, rough skin; and a musty (mousy) odor due to skin and urinary excretion of phenylacetic acid. Approximately 80% of these children have abnormal EEG patterns, and about one-third have seizures, usually beginning between ages 6 and 12 months.

Children with PKU show a precipitous decrease in IQ in their first year, are usually hyperactive and irritable, and exhibit purposeless, repetitive motions. They have increased muscle tone and an awkward gait.

Although blood phenylalanine levels are near normal at birth, they begin to rise within a few days. By the time they reach significant levels (approximately 30 mg/dl), cerebral damage has begun. Such irreversible damage probably is complete by age 2 or 3. However, early detection and treatment can minimize cerebral damage, and children under strict dietary control can lead normal lives.

## Diagnosis

Most states require screening for PKU at birth; the Guthrie screening test on a capillary blood sample (bacterial inhibition assay) reliably detects PKU. However, because phenylalanine levels may be normal at birth, the infant should be reevaluated after he has received dietary protein for 24 to 48 hours. The common practice of discharging new mothers from the hospital within 24 hours of delivery has resulted in failure to detect some infants with PKU. For this reason, some states now require a minimum hospital stay of 48 hours after a vaginal delivery.

Adding a few drops of 10% ferric chloride solution to a wet diaper is another method of detecting PKU. If the area turns a deep, bluish green, phenylpyruvic acid is present in the urine.

Detection of elevated blood levels of phenylalanine and the presence of phenylpyruvic acid in the infant's urine confirm the diagnosis. (Urine should also be tested 4 to 6 weeks after birth because urinary levels of phenylpyruvic acid vary with the amount of protein ingested.)

## Treatment

Treatment consists of restricting dietary intake of the amino acid phenylalanine to keep phenylalanine blood levels between 3 and 9 mg/dl. Because most natural proteins contain 5% phenylalanine, they must be limited in the child's diet. An enzymatic hydrolysate of casein, such as Lofenalac powder or Progestimil powder, is substituted for milk in the diets of affected infants. This milk substitute contains a minimal amount of phenylalanine, normal amounts of other amino acids, and added amounts of carbohydrate and fat. Dietary restrictions should probably continue throughout life.

The special diet for PKU calls for careful monitoring. Because the body doesn't make phenylalanine, overzealous dietary restriction can induce phenylalanine deficiency, producing lethargy, anorexia, anemia, rashes, and diarrhea.

## Special considerations

In caring for a child with PKU, it's especially important to teach both the parents and child about this disease and to provide emotional support and counseling. (Psychological and emotional problems may result from the difficult dietary restrictions.)

● Emphasize to the child and his parents the critical importance of adhering to the special diet. The child must avoid breads, cheese, eggs, flour, meat, poultry, fish, nuts, milk, legumes, aspartame, and other foods.

&gt; CLINICAL TIP Referral to a dietician trained to assist with this disorder is important.

● Inform the parents that the child will need frequent tests for urine phenylpyruvic acid and blood phenylalanine levels to evaluate the diet's effectiveness.

● As the child grows older and is supervised less closely, his parents will have less control over what he eats. As a result, deviation from the restricted diet becomes more likely, as does the risk of brain damage. Encourage the parents to allow the child some choices in the kinds of low-protein foods he wants to eat; this will help make him feel trusted and more responsible.

● Teach the parents about normal physical and mental growth and development so that they can recognize any developmental delay that may point to excessive phenylalanine intake.

To prevent this disorder:

● Infants should be routinely screened for PKU because detection of the disorder and control of phenylalanine intake soon after birth can prevent severe mental retardation.

&gt; CLINICAL TIP Refer phenylketonuric females who reach reproductive age for genetic counseling because recent research indicates that their offspring may have a higher-than-normal incidence of brain damage, mental retardation, microcephaly, and major congenital malformations, especially of the heart and central nervous system. Such damage may be minimized with a low-phenylalanine diet before conception and during pregnancy, but even patients under good control remain at increased risk for offspring with multiple anomalies and mental retardation.

# PHEOCHROMOCYTOMA

A pheochromocytoma is a chromaffin-cell tumor of the adrenal medulla that secretes an excessive amount of the catecholamines epinephrine and norepinephrine, which results in severe hypertension, increased metabolism, and hyperglycemia. This disorder is potentially fatal, but the prognosis is generally good with treatment.

## Causes
According to some estimates, about 0.1% of newly diagnosed patients with hypertension have pheochromocytoma. Although this tumor is usually benign, it may be malignant in as many as 10% of these patients. It affects all races and both sexes, occurring primarily between the ages of 30 and 40. A pheochromocytoma may result from an inherited autosomal dominant trait.

## Signs and symptoms
The cardinal sign of pheochromocytoma is persistent or paroxysmal hypertension. Common clinical effects include palpitations, tachycardia, headache, diaphoresis, pallor, warmth or flushing, paresthesia, tremor, excitation, fright, nervousness, feelings of impending doom, abdominal pain, tachypnea, nausea, and vomiting.

➤ CLINICAL TIP  The combination of episodic headache, diaphoresis, and palpitations with severely high blood pressure should increase suspicion of pheochromocytoma.

Postural hypotension and paradoxical response to antihypertensive drugs are common, as are associated glycosuria, hyperglycemia, and hypermetabolism. Patients with hypermetabolism may show marked weight loss, but some patients with pheochromocytomas are obese.

### Frequency of episodes
Symptomatic episodes may recur as seldom as once every 2 months or as often as 25 times a day. They may occur spontaneously or may follow certain precipitating events, such as postural change, exercise, laughing, smoking, induction of anesthesia, urination, change in environmental or body temperature, administration of certain medications, or intra-arterial radiographic contrast media.

Often, pheochromocytoma is diagnosed during pregnancy, when uterine pressure on the tumor induces more frequent attacks; such attacks can prove fatal for both mother and fetus as a result of hypertension and vasoconstriction, which can cause cerebrovascular accident, acute pulmonary edema, cardiac arrhythmias, or hypoxia. In such patients, the risk of spontaneous abortion is high, but most fetal deaths occur during labor or immediately after birth.

## Diagnosis
A history of acute episodes of hypertension, headache, sweating, and tachycardia — particularly in a patient with hyperglycemia, glycosuria, and hypermetabolism — strongly suggests pheochromocytoma. A patient who has intermittent attacks may have no symptoms during a latent phase.

The tumor is rarely palpable; when it is, palpation of the surrounding area may induce an acute attack and help confirm the diagnosis. Generally, diagnosis depends on laboratory findings.

Increased urinary excretion of total free catecholamines and their metabolites, vanillylmandelic acid (VMA) and metanephrine, as measured by analysis of a 24-hour urine specimen, confirms pheochromocytoma.

Labile blood pressure necessitates urine collection during a hypertensive episode and comparison of this specimen with a baseline specimen. Direct assay of total plasma catecholamines shows levels 10 to 50 times higher than normal.

Provocative tests with glucagon and phentolamine suggest the diagnosis.

However, they may precipitate a hypertensive crisis, so they're rarely used. The clonidine suppression test will cause decreased plasma catecholamine levels in normal patients but no change in those with pheochromocytoma.

Angiography demonstrates an adrenal medullary tumor (but may precipitate a hypertensive crisis). Adrenal venography, computed tomography scan, or magnetic resonance imaging helps localize the tumor.

## Treatment

Surgical removal of the tumor is the treatment of choice. To decrease blood pressure, alpha-adrenergic blockers or metyrosine is given from 1 to 2 weeks before surgery. A beta-adrenergic blocker (propranolol) may also be used after achieving alpha blockade.

Postoperatively, I.V. fluids, plasma volume expanders, vasopressors and, possibly, transfusions may be required for hypotension. Persistent hypertension in the immediate postoperative period can occur.

If surgery isn't feasible, alpha and beta-adrenergic blockers — such as phenoxybenzamine and propranolol, respectively — are beneficial in controlling catecholamine effects and preventing attacks.

Management of an acute attack or hypertensive crisis requires I.V. phentolamine (push or drip) or nitroprusside to normalize blood pressure.

## Special considerations
• To ensure the reliability of urine catecholamine measurements, make sure the patient avoids foods high in vanillin (such as coffee, nuts, chocolate, and bananas) for 2 days before urine collection of VMA.
• Also, be aware of possible drug therapy that may interfere with the accurate determination of VMA (such as guaife-

nesin and salicylates). Collect the urine in a special container, with hydrochloric acid, that has been prepared by the laboratory.
• Obtain blood pressure readings often because transient hypertensive attacks are possible. Tell the patient to report headaches, palpitations, diaphoresis, nervousness, or other symptoms of an acute attack.
• If hypertensive crisis develops, monitor blood pressure and heart rate every 2 to 5 minutes until blood pressure stabilizes at an acceptable level.
• Check blood for glucose, and watch for weight loss from hypermetabolism.
• After surgery, blood pressure may rise or fall sharply. Keep the patient quiet; provide a private room, if possible, because excitement may trigger a hypertensive episode.
• Postoperative hypertension is common because the stress of surgery and manipulation of the adrenal gland stimulate secretion of catecholamines. Because this excess secretion causes profuse sweating, keep the room cool, and change the patient's clothing and bedding often.
• If the patient receives phentolamine, monitor blood pressure closely. Observe and record adverse effects: dizziness, hypotension, tachycardia. The first 24 to 48 hours immediately after surgery are the most critical because blood pressure can drop drastically.
• If the patient is receiving vasopressors I.V., check blood pressure every 3 to 5 minutes, and regulate the drip to maintain a safe pressure. Arterial pressure lines facilitate constant monitoring.
• Watch for abdominal distention and return of bowel sounds.
• Check dressings and vital signs for indications of hemorrhage (increased pulse rate, decreased blood pressure,

cold and clammy skin, pallor, unresponsiveness).

● Give analgesics for pain as required, but monitor blood pressure carefully because many analgesics, especially meperidine, can cause hypotension. Opiates can also precipitate hypertensive crisis.

● If autosomal dominant transmission of pheochromocytoma is suspected, the patient's family should also be evaluated for this condition.

# PHOBIAS

Defined as a persistent and irrational fear of a specific object, activity, or situation, a phobia results in a compelling desire to avoid the perceived hazard. The patient recognizes that his fear is out of proportion to any actual danger, but he can't control it or explain it away.

Three types of phobias exist: *agoraphobia,* the fear of being alone or of open space; *social,* the fear of embarrassing oneself in public; and *specific,* the fear of a single, specific object, such as animals or heights.

Seven percent of all Americans suffer from a phobic disorder. In fact, phobias are the most common psychiatric disorders in women and the second most common in men. More men than women experience social phobias, whereas agoraphobia and specific phobias are more common in women.

A social phobia typically begins in late childhood or early adolescence; a specific phobia usually begins in childhood. Most phobic patients have no family history of psychiatric illness, including phobias.

Both agoraphobia and social phobia tend to be chronic, but new treatments are improving the prognosis. A specific phobia usually resolves spontaneously as the child matures.

## Causes

A phobia develops when anxiety about an object or a situation compels the patient to avoid it. The precise cause of most phobias is unknown. Psychoanalytic theory holds that the phobia is actually repression and displacement of an internal conflict. Behavior theorists view phobia as a stimulus-response reflex, avoiding a situation or object that causes anxiety.

## Signs and symptoms

The phobic patient typically reports signs of severe anxiety when confronted with the feared object or situation. A patient with agoraphobia, for example, may complain of dizziness, a sensation of falling, a feeling of unreality (depersonalization), loss of bladder or bowel control, vomiting, or cardiac distress when he leaves home or crosses a bridge. Similarly, a patient who fears flying may report that he begins to sweat, his heart pounds, and he feels panicky and short of breath when he's on an airplane.

A patient who routinely avoids the object of his phobia may report a loss of self-esteem and feelings of weakness, cowardice, or ineffectiveness. If he hasn't mastered the phobia, he also may exhibit signs of mild depression.

## Diagnosis

For characteristic findings in this condition, see *Diagnosing phobias,* pages 652 and 653.

## Treatment

The effectiveness of treatment depends on the severity of the patient's phobia. Because phobic behavior may never be completely cured, the goal of treatment is to help the patient function effectively.

# DIAGNOSING PHOBIAS

The diagnosis of all three types of phobias is based on criteria put forth in the *DSM-IV.*

### Agoraphobia
Fear of being in places or situations from which escape might be difficult or embarrassing or in which help might be unavailable if an unexpected or situationally predisposed panic attack or paniclike symptoms occur. Agoraphobic fears typically involve characteristic clusters of situations that include being outside the home alone, being in a crowd or standing in a line, being on a bridge, or traveling in a bus, train, or automobile.
• The situations are avoided or endured with marked distress or with anxiety about having a panic attack or paniclike symptoms, or they require the presence of a companion.
• The anxiety or phobic avoidance is not better accounted for by another mental disorder, such as social phobia, specific phobia, obsessive-compulsive disorder, posttraumatic stress disorder, or separation anxiety disorder.

### Social phobia
A persistent fear of one or more social or performance situations in which the person is exposed to unfamiliar people or possible scrutiny by others. The person fears that he may act in a way that will be humiliating or embarrassing.
• Exposure to the feared social situation almost invariably provokes anxiety, which may take the form of a situationally bound or situationally predisposed panic attack.
• The person recognizes that the fear is excessive or unreasonable.
• The feared social or performance situations are avoided or endured with intense anxiety or distress.
• The avoidance, anxious anticipation, or distress in the feared social or performance situation interferes with the person's normal routine, occupational functioning, or social activities or relationships, or there is marked distress about having the phobia.
• In individuals under age 18, the duration is at least 6 months.
• The fear or avoidance isn't due to the direct physiologic effects of a substance or a general medical condition and isn't better accounted for by another mental disorder.
• If the person has a general medical condition or another mental disorder, the person's social fear is unrelated to the medical or mental condition.

---

Antianxiety and antidepressant drugs may help relieve symptoms in patients with agoraphobia.

Systematic desensitization, a behavioral therapy, may be more effective than drugs, especially if it includes encouragement, instruction, and suggestion.

In some cities, phobia clinics and group therapy are available. People who have recovered from phobias can often help other phobic patients.

### Special considerations
• Provide for the patient's safety and comfort, and monitor fluid and food intake as needed. Certain phobias may inhibit food or fluid intake, disturb hygiene, and disrupt the patient's ability to rest.
• No matter how illogical the patient's phobia seems, avoid the urge to trivialize his fears. Remember that this behavior represents an essential coping mechanism.

CLINICAL TIP  The person realizes that the fear is irrational. Don't attempt to talk him out of it.
• Ask the patient how he normally copes with the fear. When he's able to face the fear, encourage him to verbalize and ex-

However, don't force insight. Challenging the patient may aggravate his anxiety or lead to panic attacks.

● Teach the patient specific relaxation techniques, such as listening to music and meditating.

● Suggest ways to channel the patient's energy and relieve stress (such as running and creative activities).

# PITUITARY TUMORS

Constituting 10% of intracranial neoplasms, pituitary tumors originate most often in the anterior pituitary (adenohypophysis). They occur in adults of both sexes, usually during the third and fourth decades of life. The three tissue types of pituitary tumors are chromophobe adenoma (90%), basophil adenoma, and eosinophil adenoma.

The prognosis is fair to good, depending on the extent to which the tumor spreads beyond the sella turcica.

## Causes
Although the exact cause is unknown, a predisposition to pituitary tumors may be inherited through an autosomal dominant trait. Pituitary tumors aren't malignant in the strict sense, but because their growth is invasive, they're considered a neoplastic disease.

Chromophobe adenoma may be associated with production of corticotropin, melanocyte-stimulating hormone, growth hormone, and prolactin; basophil adenoma, with evidence of excess corticotropin production and, consequently, with signs of Cushing's syndrome; and eosinophil adenoma, with excessive growth hormone.

---

**Specific phobia**
Marked and persistent fear that is excessive or unreasonable and cued by the presence or anticipation of a specific object or situation.

● Exposure to the phobic stimulus almost invariably provokes an immediate anxiety response, which may take the form of a situationally bound or situationally predisposed panic attack.

● The person recognizes that the fear is excessive or unreasonable.

● The person avoids the situation or endures it with intense anxiety or distress.

● The avoidance, anxious anticipation, or distress in the feared situation significantly interferes with the person's normal routine, job, social activities, or relationships, or there is marked distress about having the phobia.

● In individuals under age 18, the duration is at least 6 months.

● The anxiety, panic attacks, or phobic avoidance associated with the specific object or situation isn't better accounted for by another mental disorder, such as obsessive-compulsive disorder, posttraumatic stress disorder, separation anxiety disorder, social phobia, panic disorder with agoraphobia, or agoraphobia without a history of panic disorder.

---

plore his personal strengths and resources with you.

● Don't let the patient withdraw completely. If an agoraphobic patient is being treated as an outpatient, suggest small steps to overcome his fears, such as planning a brief shopping trip with a supportive family member or friend.

● In social phobias, the patient fears criticism. Encourage him to interact with others, and provide continuous support and positive reinforcement.

● Support participation in psychotherapy, including desensitization therapy.

## TRANSSPHENOIDAL PITUITARY SURGERY

Placement of bivalve speculum and rongeur for pituitary gland removal.

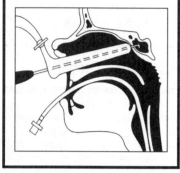

## Signs and symptoms

As pituitary adenomas grow, they replace normal glandular tissue and enlarge the sella turcica, which houses the pituitary gland. The resulting pressure on adjacent intracranial structures produces typical clinical manifestations.

### Neurologic features

• Frontal headache
• Visual symptoms, beginning with blurring and progressing to field cuts (hemianopias) and then unilateral blindness
• Cranial nerve involvement (III, IV, VI) from lateral extension of the tumor, resulting in strabismus; double vision, with compensating head tilting and dizziness; conjugate deviation of gaze; nystagmus; lid ptosis; and limited eye movements
• Increased intracranial pressure (secondary hydrocephalus)
• Personality changes or dementia, if the tumor breaks through to the frontal lobes
• Seizures

• Rhinorrhea, if the tumor erodes the base of the skull
• Pituitary apoplexy secondary to hemorrhagic infarction of the adenoma. Such hemorrhage may lead to both cardiovascular and adrenocortical collapse.

### Endocrine features

• Hypopituitarism, to some degree, in all patients with adenoma, becoming more obvious as the tumor replaces normal gland tissue; symptoms include amenorrhea, decreased libido and impotence in men, skin changes (waxy appearance, decreased wrinkles, and pigmentation), loss of axillary and pubic hair, lethargy, weakness, increased fatigability, intolerance to cold, and constipation (because of decreased corticotropin and thyrotropin production)
• Addisonian crisis, precipitated by stress and resulting in nausea, vomiting, hypoglycemia, hypotension, and circulatory collapse
• Diabetes insipidus, resulting from extension to the hypothalamus
• Prolactin-secreting adenomas (in 70% to 75%), with amenorrhea and galactorrhea; growth hormone–secreting adenomas, with acromegaly; and corticotropin-secreting adenomas, with Cushing's syndrome.

## Diagnosis

• *Skull X-rays* with tomography show enlargement of the sella turcica or erosion of its floor; if growth hormone secretion predominates, X-rays show enlarged paranasal sinuses and mandible, thickened cranial bones, and separated teeth.
• *Carotid angiography* shows displacement of the anterior cerebral and internal carotid arteries if the tumor mass is enlarging; it also rules out intracerebral aneurysm.

• *Computed tomography scan* may confirm the existence of the adenoma and accurately depict its size.

• *Cerebrospinal fluid analysis* may show increased protein levels.

• *Endocrine function tests* may contribute helpful information, but results are often ambiguous and inconclusive.

### Treatment

Surgical options include transfrontal removal of large tumors impinging on the optic apparatus and transsphenoidal resection for smaller tumors confined to the pituitary fossa. (see *Transsphenoidal pituitary surgery.*) Radiation is the primary treatment for small, nonsecretory tumors that don't extend beyond the sella turcica and for patients who may be poor postoperative risks; otherwise, it's an adjunct to surgery.

Postoperative treatment includes hormone replacement with cortisone, thyroid, and sex hormones; correction of electrolyte imbalance; and, as necessary, insulin therapy.

Drug therapy may include bromocriptine, an ergot derivative that shrinks prolactin-secreting and growth hormone–secreting tumors. Cyproheptadine, an antiserotonin drug, can reduce increased corticosteroid levels in the patient with Cushing's syndrome.

Adjuvant radiotherapy is used when only partial removal of the tumor is possible. Cryohypophysectomy (freezing the area with a probe inserted by transsphenoidal route) is a promising alternative to surgical dissection of the tumor.

### Special considerations

• Conduct a comprehensive health history and physical assessment to establish the onset of neurologic and endocrine dysfunction and provide baseline data for later comparison.

> **CLINICAL TIP**
>
> ## POSTCRANIOTOMY CARE
>
> • Monitor vital signs (especially level of consciousness), and perform a baseline neurologic assessment from which to plan further care and assess progress.
> • Maintain the patient's airway; suction as necessary.
> • Monitor intake and output carefully.
> • Give the patient nothing by mouth for 24 to 48 hours to prevent aspiration and vomiting, which increases intracranial pressure.
> • Observe for cerebral edema, bleeding, and cerebrospinal fluid leakage.
> • Provide a restful, quiet environment.

• Make sure the patient and family understand that the patient needs lifelong evaluations and, possibly, hormone replacement.

• Reassure the patient that some of the distressing physical and behavioral signs and symptoms caused by pituitary dysfunction (for example, altered sexual drive, impotence, infertility, loss of hair, and emotional lability) will disappear with treatment.

• Maintain a safe, clutter-free environment for the visually impaired or acromegalic patient. Reassure him that he'll probably recover his sight.

• Position patients who have undergone supratentorial or transsphenoidal hypophysectomy with the head of the bed elevated about 30 degrees to promote venous drainage from the head and reduce cerebral edema. (See *Postcraniotomy care.*)

• Place the patient on his side to allow drainage of secretions and prevent aspiration.

• Withhold oral fluids, which can cause vomiting and subsequent increased intracranial pressure.

• Don't allow a patient who's had transsphenoidal surgery to blow his nose.

• Watch for cerebrospinal fluid drainage from the nose. Monitor for signs of infection from the contaminated upper respiratory tract.

• Make sure the patient understands that he'll lose his sense of smell.

• Regularly compare the patient's postoperative neurologic status with your baseline assessment.

• Monitor intake and output to detect fluid and electrolyte imbalances.

• Before discharge, encourage the patient to wear a medical identification bracelet or necklace that identifies his hormone deficiencies and their proper treatment.

# PLACENTA PREVIA

In placenta previa, the placenta is implanted in the lower uterine segment, where it encroaches on the internal cervical os. This disorder, one of the most common causes of bleeding during the second half of pregnancy, occurs in approximately 1 in 200 pregnancies, more commonly in multigravidas than in primigravidas. Generally, termination of pregnancy is necessary when placenta previa is diagnosed in the presence of heavy maternal bleeding. Maternal prognosis is good if hemorrhage can be controlled; fetal prognosis depends on gestational age and amount of blood lost.

## Causes

In placenta previa, the placenta may cover all (total, complete, or central), part (partial or incomplete), or a fraction (margin or low-lying) of the internal cervical os. (See *Three types of placenta previa.*) The degree of placenta previa depends largely on the extent of cervical dilation at the time of examination because the dilating cervix gradually uncovers the placenta. Although the specific cause of placenta previa is unknown, factors that may affect the site of the placenta's attachment to the uterine wall include:

• defective vascularization of the decidua

• multiple pregnancy (the placenta requires a larger surface for attachment)

• previous uterine surgery

• multiparity

• advanced maternal age.

In placenta previa, the lower segment of the uterus fails to provide as much nourishment as the fundus. The placenta tends to spread out, seeking the blood supply it needs, and becomes larger and thinner than normal. Eccentric insertion of the umbilical cord often develops, for unknown reasons. Hemorrhage occurs as the internal cervical os effaces and dilates, tearing the uterine vessels.

## Signs and symptoms

Placenta previa usually produces painless third-trimester bleeding (often the first complaint). Various malpresentations occur because of the placenta's location and interfere with proper descent of the fetal head. (The fetus remains active, however, with good heart tones.) Complications of placenta previa include shock or maternal and fetal death.

## Diagnosis

Special diagnostic measures that confirm placenta previa include:

## THREE TYPES OF PLACENTA PREVIA

Low marginal implanta-
tion — A small placental
edge can be felt
through the internal os.

Partial placenta previa —
The placenta partially
caps the internal os.

Total placenta previa —
The internal os is cov-
ered entirely.

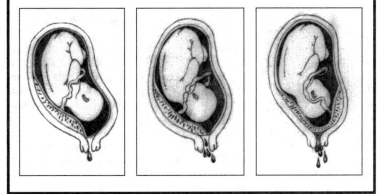

- *transvaginal ultrasound scanning* for placental position
- *pelvic examination* (under a double setup because of the likelihood of hemorrhage), performed only immediately before delivery to confirm the diagnosis. In most cases, only the cervix is visualized.

### Treatment

Treatment of placenta previa is designed to assess, control, and restore blood loss; to deliver a viable infant; and to prevent coagulation disorders. Immediate therapy includes starting an I.V. line using a large-bore catheter; drawing blood for hemoglobin and hematocrit as well as type and crossmatching; initiating external electronic fetal monitoring; monitoring maternal blood pressure, pulse rate, and respirations; and assessing the amount of vaginal bleeding.

If the fetus is premature, following determination of the degree of placen-

ta previa and necessary fluid and blood replacement, treatment consists of careful observation to allow the fetus more time to mature. If clinical evaluation confirms total placenta previa, the patient is usually hospitalized because of the increased risk of hemorrhage. As soon as the fetus is sufficiently mature, or in case of intervening severe hemorrhage, immediate delivery by cesarean section may be necessary. Vaginal delivery is considered only when bleeding is minimal and the placenta previa is marginal, or when labor is rapid. Because of the possibility of fetal blood loss through the placenta, a pediatric team should be on hand during such delivery to immediately assess and treat neonatal shock, blood loss, and hypoxia.

Complications of placenta previa necessitate appropriate and immediate intervention.

### Special considerations

• If the patient shows active bleeding because of placenta previa, a primary nurse should be assigned for continuous monitoring of maternal blood pressure, pulse rate, respirations, central venous pressure, intake and output, amount of vaginal bleeding, and fetal heart tones. Electronic monitoring of fetal heart tones is recommended.

• Prepare the patient and her family for a possible cesarean section and the birth of a premature infant. Thoroughly explain postpartum care, so the patient and her family know what measures to expect.

• Provide emotional support during labor.

➤ CLINICAL TIP Because of the infant's prematurity, the patient may not be given analgesics, so labor pain may be intense. Reassure her of her progress throughout labor, and keep her informed of the fetus's condition. Although neonatal death is a possibility, continued monitoring and prompt management reduce this prospect.

# PLEURAL EFFUSION AND EMPYEMA

Pleural effusion is an excess of fluid in the pleural space. Normally, this space contains a small amount of extracellular fluid that lubricates the pleural surfaces. Increased production or inadequate removal of this fluid results in pleural effusion. Empyema is the accumulation of pus and necrotic tissue in the pleural space. Blood (hemothorax) and chyle (chylothorax) may also collect in this space.

### Causes

The balance of osmotic and hydrostatic pressures in parietal pleural capillaries normally results in fluid movement into the pleural space. Balanced pressures in visceral pleural capillaries promote reabsorption of this fluid.

#### *Transudative pleural effusion*

Excessive hydrostatic pressure or decreased osmotic pressure can cause excessive amounts of fluid to pass across intact capillaries. The result is a transudative pleural effusion, an ultrafiltrate of plasma containing low concentrations of protein. Such effusions frequently result from heart failure, hepatic disease with ascites, peritoneal dialysis, hypoalbuminemia, and disorders resulting in overexpanded intravascular volume.

#### *Exudative pleural effusion*

Exudative pleural effusions result when capillaries exhibit increased permeability with or without changes in hydrostatic and colloid osmotic pressures, allowing protein-rich fluid to leak into the pleural space.

Exudative pleural effusions occur with tuberculosis, subphrenic abscess, pancreatitis, bacterial or fungal pneumonitis or empyema, malignancy, pulmonary embolism with or without infarction, collagen disease (lupus erythematosus and rheumatoid arthritis), myxedema, and chest trauma.

#### *Empyema*

Usually associated with infection in the pleural space, empyema may be idiopathic or may be related to pneumonitis, carcinoma, perforation, or esophageal rupture.

### Signs and symptoms

Patients with pleural effusion characteristically display symptoms relating to the underlying pathology. Most patients with large effusions, particularly those with underlying pulmonary disease, complain of dyspnea. Those with effusions associated with pleurisy complain of pleuritic chest pain. Other clinical features depend on the cause of the effusion. Patients with empyema also develop fever and malaise.

### Diagnosis

Chest X-ray shows radiopaque fluid in dependent regions. Auscultation of the chest reveals decreased breath sounds; percussion detects dullness over the effused area, which doesn't change with respiration. These tests verify pleural effusion. However, diagnosis also requires other tests to distinguish transudative from exudative effusions and to help pinpoint the underlying disorder.

The most useful test is thoracentesis, in which analysis of aspirated pleural fluid shows:

• *transudative effusions:* lactate dehydrogenase (LD) levels < 200 IU and protein levels < 3 g/dl

• *exudative effusions:* ratio of protein in pleural fluid to serum ≥ 0.5, LD in pleural fluid ≥ 200 IU, and ratio of LD in pleural fluid to LD in serum ≥ 0.6

• *empyema:* acute inflammatory white blood cells and microorganisms

• *empyema or rheumatoid arthritis:* extremely decreased pleural fluid glucose levels.

In addition, if a pleural effusion results from esophageal rupture or pancreatitis, fluid amylase levels are usually higher than serum levels. Aspirated fluid may be tested for lupus erythematosus cells, antinuclear antibodies, and neoplastic cells. It may also be analyzed for color and consistency; acid-fast bacillus, fungal, and bacterial cultures; and triglycerides (in chylothorax). Cell analysis shows leukocytosis in empyema. Negative tuberculin skin test strongly rules against tuberculosis as the cause. In exudative pleural effusions in which thoracentesis isn't definitive, pleural biopsy may be done; it's particularly useful for confirming tuberculosis or malignancy.

### Treatment

Depending on the amount of fluid present, symptomatic effusion may require thoracentesis to remove fluid or careful monitoring of the patient's own reabsorption of the fluid. Hemothorax requires drainage to prevent fibrothorax formation.

Treatment of empyema requires insertion of one or more chest tubes after thoracentesis to allow drainage of purulent material and possibly decortication (surgical removal of the thick coating over the lung) or rib resection to allow open drainage and lung expansion. Empyema also requires parenteral antibiotics. Associated hypoxia requires oxygen administration.

### Special considerations

• Explain thoracentesis to the patient. Before the procedure, tell the patient to expect a stinging sensation from the local anesthetic and a feeling of pressure when the needle is inserted.

• Instruct the patient to tell you immediately if he feels uncomfortable or has trouble breathing during the procedure.

• Reassure the patient during thoracentesis. Remind him to breathe normally and to avoid sudden movements, such as coughing or sighing. Monitor vital signs, and watch for syncope.

➤ CLINICAL TIP  If fluid is removed too quickly, the patient may suffer bradycardia, hypotension, pain, pulmonary edema, or even cardiac arrest. Watch for respiratory distress or pneumothorax (sudden onset of dyspnea, cyanosis) after thoracentesis.

- Administer oxygen and, in empyema, antibiotics.
- Encourage the patient to do deep breathing exercises to promote lung expansion. Use an incentive spirometer to promote deep breathing.
- Provide meticulous chest tube care, and use aseptic technique for changing dressings around the tube insertion site in empyema.
- Ensure chest tube patency by watching for bubbles in the underwater seal chamber.
- Record the amount, color, and consistency of any tube drainage.
- Because weeks of such drainage are usually necessary to obliterate the space, make visiting nurse referrals for patients who will be discharged with the tube in place.
- If pleural effusion was a complication of pneumonia or influenza, advise the patient to seek prompt medical attention for chest colds.

# PLEURISY

Also known as pleuritis, pleurisy is inflammation of the visceral and parietal pleurae that line the inside of the thoracic cage and envelop the lungs.

## Causes
Pleurisy develops as a complication of pneumonia, tuberculosis, viruses, systemic lupus erythematosus, rheumatoid arthritis, uremia, Dressler's syndrome, cancer, pulmonary infarction, and chest trauma.

Pleuritic pain is caused by the inflammation or irritation of sensory nerve endings in the parietal pleura. As the lungs inflate and deflate, the visceral pleura covering the lungs moves against the fixed parietal pleura lining the pleur-

al space, causing pain. This disorder usually begins suddenly.

## Signs and symptoms
Sharp, stabbing pain that increases with respiration may be so severe that it limits movement on the affected side during breathing. Dyspnea also occurs. Other symptoms vary according to the underlying pathologic process.

## Diagnosis
Auscultation of the chest reveals a characteristic *pleural friction rub* — a coarse, creaky sound heard during late inspiration and early expiration, directly over the area of pleural inflammation. Palpation over the affected area may reveal coarse vibration.

## Treatment
Generally symptomatic treatment includes anti-inflammatory agents, analgesics, and bed rest. Severe pain may require an intercostal nerve block of two or three intercostal nerves. Pleurisy with pleural effusion calls for thoracentesis as both a therapeutic and a diagnostic measure.

## Special considerations
- Stress the importance of bed rest and plan your care to allow the patient as much uninterrupted rest as possible.
- Administer antitussives and pain medication as necessary, but be careful not to overmedicate.
- If the pain requires a narcotic analgesic, warn the patient about to be discharged to avoid overuse because such medication depresses coughing and respiration.
- Encourage the patient to cough. To minimize pain, apply firm pressure at the pain site during coughing exercises.

# PNEUMOCYSTIS CARINII PNEUMONIA

Because of its association with human immunodeficiency virus (HIV) infection, *Pneumocystis carinii* pneumonia (PCP), an opportunistic infection, has increased in incidence since the 1980s. Before the advent of PCP prophylaxis, this disease was the first clue in about 60% of patients that HIV infection was present.

PCP occurs in up to 90% of HIV-infected patients in the United States at some point during their lifetime. It is the leading cause of death in these patients. Disseminated infection doesn't occur.

PCP also is associated with other immunocompromised conditions, including organ transplantation, leukemia, and lymphoma.

## Causes

*P. carinii,* the cause of PCP, usually is classified as a protozoan, although some investigators consider it more closely related to fungi. The organism exists as a saprophyte in the lungs of humans and various animals.

Part of the normal flora in most healthy people, *P. carinii* becomes an aggressive pathogen in the immunocompromised patient. Impaired cell-mediated (T-cell) immunity is thought to be more important than impaired humoral (B-cell) immunity in predisposing the patient to PCP, but the immune defects involved are poorly understood.

The organism invades the lungs bilaterally and multiplies extracellularly. As the infestation grows, alveoli fill with organisms and exudate, impairing gas exchange. The alveoli hypertrophy and thicken progressively, eventually leading to extensive consolidation.

The primary transmission route seems to be air, although the organism is already resident in most people. The incubation period probably lasts for 4 to 8 weeks.

## Signs and symptoms

The patient typically has a history of an immunocompromising condition (such as HIV infection, leukemia, or lymphoma) or procedure (such as organ transplantation).

PCP begins insidiously with increasing shortness of breath and a nonproductive cough. Anorexia, generalized fatigue, and weight loss may follow. Although the patient may have hypoxemia and hypercapnia, he may not exhibit significant symptoms. He may, however, have a low-grade, intermittent fever.

Other signs and symptoms include tachypnea, dyspnea, accessory muscle use for breathing, crackles (in about one-third of patients), and decreased breath sounds (in advanced pneumonia). Cyanosis may appear with acute illness; pulmonary consolidation develops later.

## Diagnosis

● *Histologic studies* confirm *P. carinii.* In patients with HIV infection, initial examination of a first-morning sputum specimen (induced by inhaling an ultrasonically dispersed saline mist) may be sufficient; however, this technique usually is ineffective in patients without HIV infection.

● *Fiber-optic bronchoscopy* remains the most commonly used study to confirm PCP. Invasive procedures, such as transbronchial biopsy and open lung biopsy, are performed less commonly.

● *Chest X-ray* may show slowly progressing, fluffy infiltrates and occasionally nodular lesions or a spontaneous pneumothorax, but these findings must be differentiated from findings in other types of pneumonia or adult respiratory distress syndrome.

● *Gallium scan* may show increased uptake over the lungs even when the chest X-ray appears relatively normal.

● *Arterial blood gas (ABG) studies* detect hypoxia and an increased alveolar-arterial gradient.

## Treatment

PCP may respond to drug therapy with cotrimoxazole or pentamidine isethionate. Because of immune system impairment, many patients who also have HIV experience severe adverse reactions to drug therapy. These reactions include bone marrow suppression, thrush, fever, hepatotoxicity, and anaphylaxis. Nausea, vomiting, and rashes are common. Diphenhydramine may be prescribed to treat the latter effects and leucovorin may reduce bone marrow suppression (and may be used prophylactically in patients with HIV infection).

Pentamidine may be administered I.V. or in aerosol form. I.V. pentamidine is associated with a high incidence of severe toxic effects. The inhaled form usually is well tolerated. However, inhaled pentamidine may not effectively reach the lung apices. Adverse reactions associated with inhalation include metallic taste, pharyngitis, cough, bronchospasm, shortness of breath, rhinitis, and laryngitis.

Supportive measures, such as oxygen therapy, mechanical ventilation, adequate nutrition, and fluid balance, are important adjunctive therapies.

> **CLINICAL TIP** Oral or I.V. morphine sulfate solution may reduce the respiratory rate and anxiety, thereby enhancing oxygenation.

## Special considerations

● Implement universal precautions to prevent contagion.

● Frequently assess the patient's respiratory status, and monitor ABG levels every 4 hours.

● Administer oxygen therapy as necessary. Encourage the patient to ambulate and to perform deep-breathing exercises and incentive spirometry to facilitate effective gas exchange.

● Administer antipyretics, as required, to relieve fever.

● Monitor intake and output and daily weight to evaluate fluid balance. Replace fluids as necessary.

● Give antimicrobial drugs as required. Never give pentamidine I.M. because it can cause pain and sterile abscesses. Administer the I.V. drug form slowly over 60 minutes to reduce the risk of hypotension.

● Monitor the patient for adverse reactions to antimicrobial drugs. If he's receiving cotrimoxazole, watch for nausea, vomiting, rash, bone marrow suppression, thrush, fever, hepatotoxicity, and anaphylaxis. If he's receiving pentamidine, watch for cardiac arrhythmias, hypotension, dizziness, azotemia, hypocalcemia, and hepatic disturbances.

● Provide diversional activities and coordinate health care team activities to allow adequate rest periods between procedures.

● Teach the patient energy conservation techniques as well.

● Supply nutritional supplements as needed. Encourage the patient to eat a high-calorie, protein-rich diet. Offer small, frequent meals if the patient can't tolerate large amounts of food.

● Reduce anxiety by providing a relaxing environment, eliminating excessive environmental stimuli, and allowing ample time for meals.

- Give emotional support and help the patient identify and use meaningful support systems.
- Instruct the patient about the medication regimen, especially about possible adverse effects.
- If the patient will require oxygen therapy at home, explain that an oxygen concentrator may be most effective.

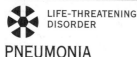

LIFE-THREATENING DISORDER

# PNEUMONIA

An acute infection of the lung parenchyma, pneumonia often impairs gas exchange. The prognosis is generally good for people who have normal lungs and adequate host defenses before the onset of pneumonia; however, pneumonia is the sixth leading cause of death in the United States.

## Causes

Pneumonia can be classified in several ways:

- *Microbiologic etiology* — Pneumonia can be viral, bacterial, fungal, protozoal, mycobacterial, mycoplasmal, or rickettsial in origin.
- *Location* — Bronchopneumonia involves distal airways and alveoli; lobular pneumonia, part of a lobe; and lobar pneumonia, an entire lobe.
- *Type* — Primary pneumonia results from inhalation or aspiration of a pathogen; it includes pneumococcal and viral pneumonia. Secondary pneumonia may follow initial lung damage from a noxious chemical or other insult (superinfection), or may result from hematogenous spread of bacteria from a distant focus. (See *Types of pneumonia,* pages 664 to 667.)

### Predisposing factors

Predisposing factors for bacterial and viral pneumonia include chronic illness and debilitation, cancer (particularly lung cancer), abdominal and thoracic surgery, atelectasis, common colds or other viral respiratory infections, chronic respiratory disease (chronic obstructive pulmonary disease [COPD], asthma, bronchiectasis, cystic fibrosis), influenza, smoking, malnutrition, alcoholism, sickle cell disease, tracheostomy, exposure to noxious gases, aspiration, and immunosuppressant therapy.

Predisposing factors for aspiration pneumonia include old age, debilitation, nasogastric tube feedings, impaired gag reflex, poor oral hygiene, and decreased level of consciousness.

## Signs and symptoms

The five cardinal symptoms of early bacterial pneumonia are coughing, sputum production, pleuritic chest pain, shaking chills, and fever. Physical signs vary widely, ranging from diffuse, fine rales to signs of localized or extensive consolidation and pleural effusion.

Complications include hypoxemia, respiratory failure, pleural effusion, empyema, lung abscess, and bacteremia, with spread of infection to other parts of the body resulting in meningitis, endocarditis, and pericarditis.

## Diagnosis

Clinical features, chest X-ray showing infiltrates, and sputum smear demonstrating acute inflammatory cells support this diagnosis. Positive blood cultures in patients with pulmonary infiltrates strongly suggest pneumonia produced by the organisms isolated from the blood cultures.

Pleural effusions, if present, should be tapped and fluid analyzed for evidence of infection in the pleural space.

*(Text continues on page 666.)*

## TYPES OF PNEUMONIA

| TYPE | SIGNS AND SYMPTOMS |
|------|--------------------|
| **VIRAL** | |
| **Influenza** (prognosis poor even with treatment; 50% mortality) | • Cough (initially nonproductive; later, purulent sputum), marked cyanosis, dyspnea, high fever, chills, substernal pain and discomfort, moist crackles, frontal headache, myalgia<br>• Death results from cardiopulmonary collapse. |
| **Adenovirus** (insidious onset; generally affects young adults) | • Sore throat, fever, cough, chills, malaise, small amounts of mucoid sputum, retrosternal chest pain, anorexia, rhinitis, adenopathy, scattered crackles, and rhonchi |
| **Respiratory syncytial virus (RSV)** (most prevalent in infants and children) | • Listlessness, irritability, tachypnea with retraction of intercostal muscles, slight sputum production, fine moist crackles, fever, severe malaise and, possibly, cough or croup |
| **Measles (rubeola)** | • Fever, dyspnea, cough, small amounts of sputum, coryza, skin rash, and cervical adenopathy |
| **Chickenpox** (varicella) (uncommon in children, but present in 30% of adults with varicella) | • Cough, dyspnea, cyanosis, tachypnea, pleuritic chest pain, hemoptysis, and rhonchi 1 to 6 days after onset of rash |
| **Cytomegalovirus (CMV)** | • Difficult to distinguish from other nonbacterial pneumonias<br>• Fever, cough, shaking chills, dyspnea, cyanosis, weakness, and diffuse crackles<br>• Occurs in neonates as devastating multisystemic infection; in normal adults resembles mononucleosis; in immunocompromised hosts, varies from clinically inapparent to devastating infection |
| **BACTERIAL** | |
| **Streptococcus** (*Diplococcus pneumoniae*) | • Sudden onset of a single, shaking chill, and sustained temperature of 102° to 104° F (38.9° to 40° C), often preceded by upper respiratory tract infection |

| DIAGNOSIS | TREATMENT |
|---|---|
| • *Chest X-ray:* diffuse bilateral bronchopneumonia from hilus<br>• *WBC count:* normal to slightly elevated<br>• *Sputum smears:* no specific organisms | • *Supportive:* for respiratory failure, endotracheal intubation and ventilator assistance; for fever, hypothermia blanket or antipyretics; for influenza A, amantadine or rimantadine |
| • *Chest X-ray:* patchy distribution of pneumonia, more severe than indicated by physical examination<br>• *WBC count:* normal to slightly elevated | • Treat symptoms only.<br>• Mortality low, usually clears with no residual effects |
| • *Chest X-ray:* patchy bilateral consolidation<br>• *WBC count:* normal to slightly elevated | • *Supportive:* humidified air, oxygen, antimicrobials often given until viral etiology confirmed, aerosolized ribavirin<br>• Complete recovery in 1 to 3 weeks |
| • *Chest X-ray:* reticular infiltrates, sometimes with hilar lymph node enlargement<br>• *Lung tissue* specimen: characteristic giant cells | • *Supportive:* bed rest, adequate hydration, antimicrobials, assisted ventilation, if necessary |
| • *Chest X-ray:* shows more extensive pneumonia than indicated by physical examination, and bilateral, patchy, diffuse, nodular infiltrates<br>• *Sputum analysis:* predominant mononuclear cells and characteristic intranuclear inclusion bodies with skin rash confirm diagnosis | • *Supportive:* adequate hydration, oxygen therapy in critically ill patients<br>• Therapy with I.V. acyclovir |
| • *Chest X-ray:* in early stages, variable patchy infiltrates; later, bilateral, nodular, and more predominant in lower lobes<br>• *Percutaneous aspiration of lung tissue, transbronchial biopsy or open lung biopsy:* microscopic examination shows intranuclear and cytoplasmic inclusions; virus can be cultured from lung tissue | • *Supportive:* adequate hydration and nutrition, oxygen therapy, bed rest<br>• Generally, benign and self-limiting in mononucleosis-like form<br>• In immunosuppressed patients, disease is more severe and may be fatal, ganciclovir or foscarnet treatment warranted |
| • *Chest X-ray:* areas of consolidation, often lobar<br>• *WBC count:* elevated<br>• *Sputum culture:* may show gram-positive *S. pneumoniae;* this organism not always recovered | • *Antimicrobial therapy:* macrolide for 7 to 10 days. Such therapy begins after obtaining culture specimen but without waiting for results. |

*(continued)*

## TYPES OF PNEUMONIA *(continued)*

| TYPE | SIGNS AND SYMPTOMS |
|------|--------------------|
| **BACTERIAL** *(continued)* | |
| **Klebsiella** | • Fever and recurrent chills; cough producing rusty, bloody, viscous sputum (currant jelly); cyanosis of lips and nail beds due to hypoxemia; shallow, grunting respirations<br>• Likely in patients with chronic alcoholism, pulmonary disease, and diabetes |
| **Staphylococcus** | • Temperature of 102° to 104° F (38.9° to 40° C), recurrent shaking chills, bloody sputum, dyspnea, tachypnea, and hypoxemia<br>• Should be suspected with viral illness, such as influenza or measles, and in patients with cystic fibrosis |
| **ASPIRATION** | |
| Results from vomiting and aspiration of gastric or oropharyngeal contents into trachea and lungs | • Noncardiogenic pulmonary edema may follow damage to respiratory epithelium from contact with stomach acid<br>• Crackles, dyspnea, cyanosis, hypotension, and tachycardia<br>• May be subacute pneumonia with cavity formation, or lung abscess may occur if foreign body is present |

Occasionally, a transtracheal aspirate of tracheobronchial secretions or bronchoscopy with brushings or washings may be done to obtain material for smear and culture. The patient's response to antimicrobial therapy also provides important evidence of the presence of pneumonia.

### Treatment

Antimicrobial therapy varies with the causative agent. Therapy should be reevaluated early in the course of treatment.

Supportive measures include humidified oxygen therapy for hypoxia, mechanical ventilation for respiratory failure, a high-calorie diet and adequate fluid intake, bed rest, and an analgesic to relieve pleuritic chest pain. Patients with severe pneumonia on mechanical ventilation may require positive endexpiratory pressure to facilitate adequate oxygenation.

### Special considerations

Correct supportive care can increase patient comfort, avoid complications, and speed recovery.

Throughout the illness:
• Maintain a patent airway and adequate oxygenation. Measure arterial blood gas levels, especially in hypoxic patients. Administer supplemental oxygen if partial pressure of arterial oxygen is less than 60 mm Hg. Patients with underlying chronic lung disease should be given oxygen cautiously.
• Teach the patient how to cough and perform deep-breathing exercises to

| DIAGNOSIS | TREATMENT |
|---|---|
| • *Chest X-ray:* typically, but not always, consolidation in the upper lobe that causes bulging of fissures<br>• *WBC count:* elevated<br>• *Sputum culture and Gram stain:* may show gram-negative cocci *(Klebsiella)* | • *Antimicrobial therapy:* an aminoglycoside and a cephalosporin |
| • *Chest X-ray:* multiple abscesses and infiltrates; high incidence of empyema<br>• *WBC count:* elevated<br>• *Sputum culture and Gram stain:* may show gram-positive staphylococci | • *Antimicrobial therapy:* nafcillin or oxacillin for 14 days if staphylococci are penicillinase producing<br>• Chest tube drainage of empyema |
| • *Chest X-ray:* locates areas of infiltrates, which suggest diagnosis | • *Antimicrobial therapy:* penicillin G or clindamycin<br>• *Supportive:* oxygen therapy, suctioning, coughing, deep breathing, adequate hydration |

clear secretions, and encourage him to do so often.

• In severe pneumonia that requires endotracheal intubation or tracheostomy with or without mechanical ventilation, provide thorough respiratory care and suction often, using sterile technique, to remove secretions.

• Obtain sputum specimens as needed, by suction if the patient can't produce specimens independently. Collect specimens in a sterile container and deliver them promptly to the microbiology laboratory.

• Administer antibiotics as necessary, and pain medication as needed; record the patient's response to medications. Fever and dehydration may require I.V. fluids and electrolyte replacement.

• Maintain adequate nutrition to offset high caloric utilization secondary to infection. Ask the dietary department to provide a high-calorie, high-protein diet consisting of soft, easy-to-eat foods. Encourage the patient to eat.

• As necessary, supplement oral feedings with nasogastric tube feedings or parenteral nutrition. Monitor fluid intake and output.

• Provide a quiet, calm environment for the patient, with frequent rest periods.

• To control the spread of infection, dispose of secretions properly. Tell the patient to sneeze and cough into a disposable tissue; tape a waxed bag to the side of the bed for used tissues.

To prevent pneumonia:
- Advise the patient to avoid using antibiotics indiscriminately during minor viral infections because this may result in upper airway colonization with antibiotic-resistant bacteria. If the patient then develops pneumonia, the organisms producing the pneumonia may require treatment with more toxic antibiotics.
- Encourage annual influenza vaccination and Pneumovax for high-risk patients, such as those with COPD, chronic heart disease, or sickle cell disease.
- Urge all bedridden and postoperative patients to perform deep-breathing and coughing exercises frequently. Position such patients properly to promote full aeration and drainage of secretions.

▶ CLINICAL TIP   To prevent aspiration during nasogastric tube feedings, elevate the patient's head, check the tube's position, and administer the formula slowly. Don't give large volumes at one time; this could cause vomiting. If the patient has an endotracheal tube, inflate the tube cuff. Keep the patient's head elevated for at least 30 minutes after the feeding. Check for residual formula at 4- to 6-hour intervals.

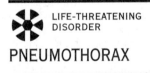

LIFE-THREATENING
DISORDER

# PNEUMOTHORAX

In pneumothorax, air or gas accumulates between the parietal and visceral pleurae. The amount of air or gas trapped in the intrapleural space determines the degree of lung collapse.

In a tension pneumothorax, the air in the pleural space is under higher pressure than air in adjacent lung and vascular structures. Without prompt treatment, a tension or a large pneumothorax results in fatal pulmonary and circulatory impairment.

## Causes

The type of pneumothorax varies with the cause.

### Spontaneous pneumothorax

Usually occurring in otherwise healthy adults ages 20 to 40, spontaneous pneumothorax may be caused by air leakage from ruptured congenital blebs adjacent to the visceral pleural surface, near the apex of the lung. It may also result from an emphysematous bulla that ruptures during exercise or coughing or from tubercular, pneumocystic, or malignant lesions that erode into the pleural space. Spontaneous pneumothorax may also occur in interstitial lung disease, such as eosinophilic granuloma or lymphangiomyomatosis.

### Traumatic pneumothorax

This type of pneumothorax may result from insertion of a central venous line, thoracic surgery, or a penetrating chest injury, such as a gunshot or knife wound, or it may follow a transbronchial biopsy. It may also occur during thoracentesis or a closed pleural biopsy. When traumatic pneumothorax follows a penetrating chest injury, it frequently coexists with hemothorax (blood in the pleural space).

### Tension pneumothorax

In tension pneumothorax, positive pleural pressure develops as a result of any of the causes of traumatic pneumothorax. When air enters the pleural space through a tear in lung tissue and is unable to leave by the same vent, each inspiration traps air in the pleural space, resulting in positive pleural pressure. This in turn causes collapse of the ipsilateral lung and marked impairment of venous return, which can severely compromise cardiac output and may cause a mediastinal shift. Decreased filling of the great veins of the chest results in diminished cardiac output and lowered blood pressure.

### Open or closed pneumothorax

Pneumothorax can also be classified as open or closed. In open pneumothorax (usually the result of trauma), air flows between the pleural space and the outside of the body. In closed pneumothorax, air reaches the pleural space directly from the lung.

### Signs and symptoms

The cardinal features of pneumothorax are sudden, sharp, pleuritic pain (exacerbated by movement of the chest, breathing, and coughing); asymmetrical chest wall movement; shortness of breath; and cyanosis. In moderate to severe pneumothorax, profound respiratory distress may develop, with signs of tension pneumothorax: weak and rapid pulse, pallor, neck vein distention, and anxiety. Tension pneumothorax produces the most severe respiratory symptoms; a spontaneous pneumothorax that releases only a small amount of air into the pleural space may cause no symptoms.

### Diagnosis

Sudden, sharp chest pain and shortness of breath suggest pneumothorax. Chest X-ray showing air in the pleural space and, possibly, mediastinal shift confirms this diagnosis. In the absence of a definitive chest X-ray, physical examination occasionally reveals:

• *on inspection:* overexpansion and rigidity of the affected chest side; in tension pneumothorax, neck vein distention with hypotension and tachycardia

• *on palpation:* crackling beneath the skin, indicating subcutaneous emphy-

sema (air in tissue) and decreased vocal fremitus

• *on percussion:* hyperresonance on the affected side

• *on auscultation:* decreased or absent breath sounds over the collapsed lung.

If the pneumothorax is significant, arterial blood gas findings include pH less than 7.35, partial pressure of arterial oxygen less than 80 mm Hg, and partial pressure of arterial carbon dioxide above 45 mm Hg.

### Treatment

Treatment is conservative for spontaneous pneumothorax in which no signs of increased pleural pressure (indicating tension pneumothorax) appear, lung collapse is less than 30%, and the patient shows no signs of dyspnea or other indications of physiologic compromise.

Such treatment consists of bed rest; careful monitoring of blood pressure, pulse rate, and respirations; oxygen administration; and, possibly, needle aspiration of air with a large-bore needle attached to a syringe.

If more than 30% of the lung is collapsed, treatment to reexpand the lung includes placing a thoracostomy tube in the second or third intercostal space in the midclavicular line, connected to an underwater seal or low suction pressures.

Recurring spontaneous pneumothorax may be treated by instilling a sclerosing agent through a thoracostomy tube or during thoracostomy. Thoracotomy and pleurectomy are also procedures to prevent recurrence by causing the lung to adhere to the parietal pleura. Traumatic and tension pneumothoraces require chest tube drainage; traumatic pneumothorax may also require surgical repair.

## Special considerations

● Watch for pallor, gasping respirations, and sudden chest pain. Carefully monitor vital signs at least every hour for indications of shock, increasing respiratory distress, or mediastinal shift. Listen for breath sounds over both lungs. Falling blood pressure and rising pulse and respiration rates may indicate tension pneumothorax, which could be fatal without prompt treatment.

● After the chest tube is in place, encourage the patient to cough and breathe deeply (at least once an hour) to facilitate lung expansion.

● In the patient undergoing chest tube drainage, watch for continuing air leakage (bubbling), indicating that the lung defect has failed to close; this may require surgery.

● Watch for increasing subcutaneous emphysema by checking around the neck or at the tube insertion site for crackling beneath the skin.

● If the patient is on a ventilator, watch for difficulty in breathing in time with the ventilator, as well as pressure changes on ventilator gauges.

● Change dressings around the chest tube insertion site as necessary. Be careful not to reposition or dislodge the tube.

➤ CLINICAL TIP  If the tube dislodges, place a petrolatum gauze dressing over the opening immediately to prevent rapid lung collapse.

● Monitor vital signs frequently after thoracotomy. Also, for the first 24 hours, assess respiratory status by checking breath sounds hourly.

● Observe the chest tube site for leakage, and note the amount and color of drainage.

● Walk the patient as appropriate (usually on the first postoperative day) to facilitate deep inspiration and lung expansion.

● Reassure the patient, and explain what pneumothorax is, what causes it, and all diagnostic tests and procedures.

● Make the patient as comfortable as possible. (The patient with pneumothorax is usually most comfortable sitting upright.)

# POLYCYSTIC KIDNEY DISEASE

An inherited disorder, polycystic kidney disease is characterized by multiple, bilateral, grapelike clusters of fluid-filled cysts that grossly enlarge the kidneys, compressing and eventually replacing functioning renal tissue. This disease appears in two distinct forms.

The infantile form causes stillbirth or early neonatal death. A few infants with this disease survive for 2 years and then develop fatal renal, heart, or respiratory failure.

The adult form begins insidiously but usually becomes obvious between the ages of 30 and 50; rarely, it causes no symptoms until the patient is in his seventies. In the adult form, renal deterioration is more gradual but, as in the infantile form, progresses relentlessly to fatal uremia.

The prognosis in adults is extremely variable. Progression may be slow, even after symptoms of renal insufficiency appear. However, after uremic symptoms develop, polycystic kidney disease is usually fatal within 4 years unless the patient receives treatment with dialysis, a kidney transplant, or both.

## Causes

Although both types of polycystic kidney disease are genetically transmitted, the incidence in two distinct age-groups and different inheritance patterns suggest two unrelated disorders. The infantile type appears to be inherited as an autosomal recessive trait; the adult type, as an autosomal dominant trait. Both types affect males and females equally.

**Signs and symptoms**
Clinical features vary with the form of disease.

*Infantile form*
The newborn with infantile polycystic disease may have pronounced epicanthal folds, a pointed nose, a small chin, and floppy, low-set ears (Potter facies). Signs of respiratory distress and heart failure may be evident. Eventually, he develops uremia and renal failure. Accompanying hepatic fibrosis may cause portal hypertension and bleeding varices to develop as well.

*Adult form*
Adult polycystic kidney disease is often asymptomatic while the patient is in his thirties and forties but may induce nonspecific symptoms, such as hypertension, polyuria, and urinary tract infection. Later, the patient develops overt symptoms related to the enlarging kidney mass, such as lumbar pain, widening girth, and a swollen or tender abdomen. Such abdominal pain is usually worsened by exertion and relieved by lying down.

In advanced stages, this disease may cause recurrent hematuria, life-threatening retroperitoneal bleeding resulting from a ruptured cyst, proteinuria, and colicky abdominal pain from the ureteral passage of clots or calculi. Generally, about 10 years after symptoms appear, progressive compression of kidney structures by the enlarging mass produces renal failure and uremia.

POLYCYSTIC KIDNEY

**Diagnosis**
A family history and a physical examination revealing large bilateral, irregular masses in the flanks strongly suggest polycystic kidney disease. In advanced stages, grossly enlarged and palpable kidneys make the diagnosis obvious. (See *Polycystic kidney.*) In patients with these findings, the following laboratory results are typical:

• *Excretory urography* or *retrograde uteropyelography* reveals enlarged kidneys, with elongation of pelvis, flattening of the calyces, and indentations caused by cysts. Excretory urography of the newborn shows poor excretion of contrast medium.

• *Ultrasonography, tomography,* and *radioisotope scans* show kidney enlargement and presence of cysts. *Computed tomography* and *magnetic resonance imaging* demonstrate multiple areas of cystic damage.

• *Urinalysis* and *creatinine clearance tests* — nonspecific tests that evaluate renal function — indicate abnormalities.

➤ CLINICAL TIP  Diagnosis must rule out the presence of renal tumors.

## Treatment

Polycystic kidney disease can't be cured. The primary goal of treatment is preserving renal parenchyma and preventing infectious complications. Management of secondary hypertension will also help prevent rapid deterioration in function. Progressive renal failure requires treatment similar to that for other types of renal disease, including dialysis or, rarely, a kidney transplant.

### Asymptomatic stage

When adult polycystic kidney disease is discovered in the asymptomatic stage, careful monitoring is required, including urine cultures and creatinine clearance tests every 6 months. When a urine culture detects infection, prompt and vigorous antibiotic treatment is needed (even when the patient is asymptomatic).

### Progressive renal impairment

As renal impairment progresses, selected patients may undergo dialysis, transplantation, or both. Cystic abscess or retroperitoneal bleeding may require surgical drainage; intractable pain (a rare symptom) may also require surgery. However, because this disease affects both kidneys, nephrectomy usually isn't recommended because it increases the risk of infection in the remaining kidney.

## Special considerations

- Because polycystic kidney disease is usually relentlessly progressive, comprehensive patient teaching and emotional support are essential.
- Refer the young adult patient or the parents of infants with polycystic kidney disease for genetic counseling. Such parents will probably have many questions about the risk to other offspring.
- Provide supportive care to minimize any associated symptoms. Carefully assess the patient's lifestyle and his physical and mental status; determine how rapidly the disease is progressing. Use this information to plan individualized care.
- Acquaint yourself with all aspects of end-stage renal disease, including dialysis and transplantation, so you can provide appropriate care and patient teaching as the disease progresses.
- Explain all diagnostic procedures to the patient or to his family if the patient is an infant. Before beginning excretory urography or other procedures that use an iodine-based contrast medium, determine whether the patient has ever had an allergic reaction to iodine or shellfish. Even if the patient has no history of allergy, watch for an allergic reaction after performing the procedures.
- Administer antibiotics for urinary tract infection. Stress to the patient the need to take the medication exactly as prescribed, even if symptoms are minimal or absent.

# POLYCYTHEMIA, SECONDARY

Also known as reactive polycythemia, secondary polycythemia is a disorder characterized by excessive production of circulating red blood cells (RBCs) due to hypoxia, tumor, or disease. It occurs in approximately 2 out of every 100,000 people living at or near sea level; incidence rises among persons living at high altitudes.

## Causes

Secondary polycythemia may result from increased production of erythropoietin. This hormone, which is possibly produced and secreted in the kidneys, stimulates bone marrow production of RBCs. Increased production may

be a compensatory physiologic response to hypoxemia, which may result from:
- chronic obstructive pulmonary disease (COPD)
- hemoglobin (Hb) abnormalities (such as carboxyhemoglobinemia, which is seen in heavy smokers)
- heart failure (causing a decreased ventilation-perfusion ratio)
- right-to-left shunting of blood in the heart (as in transposition of the great vessels)
- central or peripheral alveolar hypoventilation (as in barbiturate intoxication or pickwickian syndrome)
- low oxygen content at high altitudes.

Increased production of erythropoietin may also be an inappropriate (pathologic) response to renal disease (such as renal vascular impairment, renal cysts, or hydronephrosis), to central nervous system disease (such as encephalitis and parkinsonism), to neoplasms (such as renal tumors, uterine myomas, or cerebellar hemangiomas), or to endocrine disorders (such as Cushing's syndrome, Bartter's syndrome, or pheochromocytomas).

Rarely, secondary polycythemia results from a recessive genetic trait.

### Signs and symptoms
In the hypoxic patient, suggestive physical findings include ruddy cyanotic skin, emphysema, hypoxemia without hepatosplenomegaly, or hypertension. Clubbing of the fingers may occur if the underlying disease is cardiovascular. When the cause isn't hypoxemia, secondary polycythemia is usually an incidental finding during treatment for an underlying disease.

### Diagnosis
Laboratory findings for secondary polycythemia include increased RBC mass (increased hematocrit, hemoglobin, mean corpuscular volume, and mean corpuscular Hb), urinary erythropoietin, and blood histamine, with decreased or normal arterial oxygen saturation.

Bone marrow biopsies reveal hyperplasia confined to the erythroid series. Unlike polycythemia vera, secondary polycythemia isn't associated with leukocytosis or thrombocytosis.

### Treatment
The goal of treatment is correction of the underlying disease or environmental condition. In severe secondary polycythemia where altitude is a contributing factor, relocation may be advisable. If secondary polycythemia has produced hazardous hyperviscosity of the blood or if the patient doesn't respond to treatment for the primary disease, reduction of blood volume by phlebotomy or pheresis may be effective.

Emergency phlebotomy is indicated for prevention of impending vascular occlusion or before emergency surgery. In the latter case, it's usually advisable to remove excess RBCs and reinfuse the patient's plasma.

➤ CLINICAL TIP  Because a patient with polycythemia has an increased risk of hemorrhage during and after surgery, elective surgery should be avoided until polycythemia is controlled. Generally, secondary polycythemia disappears when the primary disease is corrected.

### Special considerations
- Keep the patient as active as possible to decrease the risk of thrombosis due to increased blood viscosity.
- Reduce calorie and sodium intake to counteract the tendency to hypertension.
- Before and after phlebotomy, check blood pressure with the patient lying down. After the procedure, give approximately 24 oz (720 ml) of water or

juice. To prevent syncope, have him sit up for about 5 minutes before walking.
• Emphasize the importance of regular blood studies (every 2 to 3 months), even after the disease is controlled.
• Teach the patient and family about the underlying disorder. Help them understand its relationship to polycythemia and the measures needed to control both.
• Teach the patient to recognize symptoms of recurring polycythemia, and emphasize the importance of reporting them promptly.

# POLYCYTHEMIA, SPURIOUS

Spurious polycythemia has many other names, including relative polycythemia, stress erythrocytosis, stress polycythemia, benign polycythemia, Gaisböck's syndrome, and pseudopolycythemia. Spurious polycythemia is characterized by increased hematocrit and normal or decreased red blood cell (RBC) total mass; it results from decreasing plasma volume and subsequent hemoconcentration. This disease usually affects middle-aged people and occurs more often in men than in women.

## Causes

There are three possible causes of spurious polycythemia.

### Dehydration

Conditions that promote severe fluid loss decrease plasma levels and lead to hemoconcentration. Such conditions include persistent vomiting or diarrhea, burns, adrenocortical insufficiency, aggressive diuretic therapy, decreased fluid intake, diabetic acidosis, and renal disease.

### Hemoconcentration due to stress

Nervous stress leads to hemoconcentration by an unknown mechanism (possibly by temporarily decreasing circulating plasma volume or vascular redistribution of erythrocytes). This form of erythrocytosis (chronically elevated hematocrit) is particularly common in middle-aged men who are chronic smokers and have type A personalities (tense, hard-driving, anxious).

### High-normal RBC mass and low-normal plasma volume

In many patients, an increased hematocrit merely reflects a normally high red cell mass and low plasma volume. This is particularly common in patients who are nonsmokers, are not obese, and have no history of hypertension.

Other factors that may be associated with spurious polycythemia include hypertension, thromboembolitic disease, elevated serum cholesterol and uric acid levels, and familial tendency.

## Signs and symptoms

The patient with spurious polycythemia usually has no specific symptoms but may have vague complaints, such as headaches, dizziness, and fatigue. Less commonly, he may develop diaphoresis, dyspnea, and claudication.

Typically, the patient has a ruddy appearance, a short neck, slight hypertension, and a tendency to hypoventilate when recumbent. He shows no associated hepatosplenomegaly but may have cardiac or pulmonary disease.

## Diagnosis

Hemoglobin and hematocrit levels and RBC count are elevated; RBC mass, arterial oxygen saturation, and bone marrow are normal. Plasma volume may be decreased or normal. Hypercholesterolemia, hyperlipidemia, or hyperuricemia may be present.

Spurious polycythemia is distinguishable from polycythemia vera by its characteristic normal RBC mass, elevated hematocrit, and absence of leukocytosis.

## Treatment

The principal goals of treatment are to correct dehydration and to prevent life-threatening thromboembolism. Rehydration with appropriate fluids and electrolytes is the primary therapy for spurious polycythemia secondary to dehydration. Therapy must also include appropriate measures to prevent continuing fluid loss.

### Special considerations

• During rehydration, carefully monitor intake and output to maintain fluid and electrolyte balance.
• To prevent thromboemboli in predisposed patients, suggest regular exercise and a low-cholesterol diet. Antilipemics may also be necessary. Reduced calorie intake may be required for the obese patient.
• Whenever appropriate, suggest counseling about the patient's work habits and lack of relaxation. If the patient is a smoker, make sure he understands how important it is that he stop smoking. Then, refer him to a smoking cessation program if necessary.
• Emphasize the need for follow-up examinations every 3 to 4 months after leaving the hospital.
• Thoroughly explain spurious polycythemia, all diagnostic measures, and therapy.

CLINICAL TIP The hard-driving person predisposed to spurious polycythemia is likely to be more inquisitive and anxious than the average patient. Answer his questions honestly, but take care to reassure him that he can effectively control symptoms by complying with the prescribed treatment.

# POLYCYTHEMIA VERA

Polycythemia vera (also known as primary polycythemia, erythremia, polycythemia rubra vera, splenomegalic polycythemia, or Vaquez-Osler disease) is a chronic myeloproliferative disorder characterized by increased red blood cell (RBC) mass, leukocytosis, thrombocytosis, and increased hemoglobin concentration, with normal or increased plasma volume. It usually occurs between the ages of 40 and 60, most commonly among males of Jewish ancestry; it rarely affects children or blacks and doesn't appear to be familial.

The prognosis depends on age at diagnosis, the treatment used, and complications. Mortality is high if polycythemia is untreated or is associated with leukemia or myeloid metaplasia.

## Causes

In polycythemia vera, uncontrolled and rapid cellular reproduction and maturation cause proliferation or hyperplasia of all bone marrow cells (panmyelosis). The cause of such uncontrolled cellular activity is unknown, but it is probably due to a multipotential stem cell defect.

## Signs and symptoms

Increased RBC mass results in hyperviscosity and inhibits blood flow to microcirculation. Subsequently, increased viscosity, diminished velocity, and thrombocytosis promote intravascular thrombosis.

### Progressive features

In early stages, polycythemia vera usually produces no symptoms. (Increased hematocrit may be an incidental finding.) However, as altered circulation secondary to increased RBC mass produces hypervolemia and hyperviscosity, the patient may complain of a feeling of fullness in the head, headache, dizziness, and other symptoms, depending on the body system affected. (See *Clinical features of polycythemia vera.*). Hyperviscosity may lead to thrombosis of smaller vessels with ruddy cyanosis of the nose and clubbing of the digits.

### Complication
Paradoxically, hemorrhage is a complication of polycythemia vera. It may be due to defective platelet function or to hyperviscosity and the local effects from excess RBCs exerting pressure on distended venous and capillary walls.

### Diagnosis
Laboratory studies confirm polycythemia vera by showing increased RBC mass and normal arterial oxygen saturation in association with splenomegaly or two of the following: thrombocytosis, leukocytosis, elevated leukocyte alkaline phosphatase level, or elevated serum vitamin $B_{12}$ or unbound $B_{12}$-binding capacity.

Another common finding is increased uric acid production, leading to hyperuricemia and hyperuricuria. Other laboratory results include increased blood histamine, decreased serum iron concentration, and decreased or absent urinary erythropoietin. Bone marrow biopsy reveals panmyelosis.

### Treatment
Phlebotomy can reduce RBC mass promptly. The frequency of phlebotomy and the amount of blood removed each time depend on the patient's condition. Typically, 350 to 500 ml of blood can be removed every other day until the hematocrit is reduced to the low-normal range.

After repeated phlebotomies, the patient develops iron deficiency, which stabilizes RBC production and reduces the need for phlebotomy. Pheresis permits the return of plasma to the patient, diluting the blood and reducing hypovolemic symptoms.

Phlebotomy doesn't reduce the white blood cell or platelet count and won't control the hyperuricemia associated with marrow cell proliferation.

For severe symptoms, myelosuppressive therapy may be used. In the past, radioactive phosphorus ($^{32}P$) or chemotherapeutic agents, such as melphalan, busulfan, or chlorambucil, could usually control the disease. However, these agents may cause leukemia and should be reserved for older patients and those with problems uncontrolled by phlebotomy.

The current preferred myelosuppressive agent is hydroxyurea, which isn't associated with leukemia. Patients who have had previous thrombotic problems should be considered for myelosuppressive therapy.

### Special considerations
• Check blood pressure, pulse rate, and respirations prior to and during phlebotomy.
• During phlebotomy, make sure the patient is lying down comfortably to prevent vertigo and syncope.
• Stay alert for tachycardia, clamminess, or complaints of vertigo. If these effects occur, the procedure should be stopped.
• Immediately after phlebotomy, check blood pressure and pulse rate. Have the patient sit up for about 5 minutes before allowing him to walk; this prevents vasovagal attack or orthostatic hypotension. Also, administer 24 oz (720 ml) of juice or water.
• Tell the patient to watch for and report any symptoms of iron deficiency

# CLINICAL FEATURES OF POLYCYTHEMIA VERA

| SYMPTOMS | CAUSES |
|---|---|
| **Eye, ear, nose, and throat** | |
| • Visual disturbances (blurring, diplopia, scotoma, engorged veins of fundus and retina) and congestion of conjunctiva, retina, retinal veins, oral mucous membrane | • Hypervolemia and hyperviscosity |
| • Epistaxis or gingival bleeding | • Engorgement of capillary beds |
| **Central nervous system** | |
| • Headache or fullness in the head, lethargy, weakness, fatigue, syncope, tinnitus, paresthesia of digits, and impaired mentation | • Hypervolemia and hyperviscosity |
| **Cardiovascular** | |
| • Hypertension | • Hypervolemia and hyperviscosity |
| • Intermittent claudication, thrombosis and emboli, angina, thrombophlebitis | • Hypervolemia, thrombocytosis, and vascular disease |
| • Hemorrhage | • Engorgement of capillary beds |
| **Skin** | |
| • Pruritus (especially after hot bath) | • Basophilia (secondary histamine release) |
| • Urticaria | • Altered histamine metabolism |
| • Ruddy cyanosis | • Hypervolemia and hyperviscosity due to congested vessels, increased oxyhemoglobin, and reduced hemoglobin |
| • Night sweats | • Hypermetabolism |
| • Ecchymosis | • Hemorrhage |
| **Gastrointestinal and hepatic** | |
| • Epigastric distress | • Hypervolemia and hyperviscosity |
| • Early satiety and fullness | • Hepatosplenomegaly |
| • Peptic ulcer pain | • Gastric thrombosis and hemorrhage |
| • Hepatosplenomegaly | • Congestion, extramedullary hemopoiesis, and myeloid metaplasia |
| • Weight loss | • Hypermetabolism |
| **Respiratory** | |
| • Dyspnea | • Hypervolemia and hyperviscosity |
| **Musculoskeletal** | |
| • Joint symptoms | • Increased urate production secondary to nucleoprotein turnover |

(pallor, weight loss, weakness, glossitis).

• Keep the patient active and ambulatory to prevent thrombosis. If bed rest is absolutely necessary, prescribe a daily program of both active and passive range-of-motion exercises.

• Watch for complications: hypervolemia, thrombocytosis, and signs of an impending cerebrovascular accident (decreased sensation, numbness, transitory paralysis, fleeting blindness, headache, and epistaxis).

• Regularly examine the patient closely for bleeding. Tell him which bleeding sites are most common (such as the nose, gingiva, and skin) so he can check for bleeding. Advise him to report any abnormal bleeding promptly.

• To compensate for increased uric acid production, give additional fluids, administer allopurinol, and alkalinize the urine to prevent uric acid calculi.

• If the patient has symptomatic splenomegaly, suggest or provide small, frequent meals, followed by a rest period, to prevent nausea and vomiting.

• Report acute abdominal pain immediately; it may signal splenic infarction, renal calculi, or abdominal organ thrombosis.

During myelosuppressive treatment:

• Monitor complete blood count (CBC) and platelet count before and during therapy. Warn an outpatient who develops leukopenia that his resistance to infection is low; advise him to avoid crowds and watch for the symptoms of infection.

• If leukopenia develops in a hospitalized patient who needs reverse isolation, follow hospital guidelines. If thrombocytopenia develops, tell the patient to watch for signs of bleeding (blood in urine, nosebleeds, black stools).

• Tell the patient about possible adverse effects (nausea, vomiting, and risk of infection) of alkylating agents.

➤ CLINICAL TIP   Alopecia may follow the use of busulfan, cyclophosphamide, and uracil mustard. Sterile hemorrhagic cystitis may follow the use of cyclophosphamide (forcing fluids can prevent it).

• Watch for adverse reactions. If nausea and vomiting occur, begin antiemetic therapy and adjust the patient's diet.

During treatment with $^{32}$P:

• Take a blood sample for CBC and platelet count before beginning treatment. *(Note:* Use of $^{32}$P requires radiation precautions to prevent contamination.)

• Have the patient lie down during I.V. administration (to facilitate the procedure and prevent extravasation) and for 15 to 20 minutes afterward.

# PORPHYRIAS

Porphyrias are metabolic disorders that affect the biosynthesis of heme (a component of hemoglobin) and cause excessive production and excretion of porphyrins or their precursors. Porphyrins, which are present in all protoplasm, figure prominently in energy storage and utilization. Classification of porphyrias depends on the site of excessive porphyrin production; they may be erythropoietic (erythroid cells in bone marrow), hepatic (in the liver), or erythrohepatic (in bone marrow and liver). (See *Types of porphyria.*) An acute episode of intermittent hepatic porphyria may cause fatal respiratory paralysis. In the other forms of porphyrias, the prognosis is good with proper treatment.

# TYPES OF PORPHYRIA

| PORPHYRIA | SIGNS AND SYMPTOMS | TREATMENT |
|---|---|---|
| **ERYTHROPOIETIC PORPHYRIA** | | |
| **Günther's disease**<br>• Usual onset before age 5 | • Red urine (earliest, most characteristic sign); severe cutaneous photosensitivity leading to vesicular or bullous eruptions on exposed areas and, eventually, scarring and ulceration<br>• Hypertrichosis<br>• Brown-stained or red-stained teeth<br>• Splenomegaly, hemolytic anemia | • Beta-carotene by mouth to prevent photosensitivity reactions<br>• Anti-inflammatory ointments<br>• Prednisone to reverse anemia<br>• Packed red calls to inhibit erythropoiesis and excreted porphyrins<br>• Hemin for recurrent attacks<br>• Splenectomy for hemolytic anemia<br>• Topical dihydroxyacetone and sunscreen filter |
| **ERYTHROHEPATIC PORPHYRIA** | | |
| **Protoporphyria**<br>• Usually affects children<br>• Occurs most often in males | • Photosensitive dermatitis<br>• Hemolytic anemia<br>• Chronic hepatic disease | • Avoidance of causative factors<br>• Beta-carotene to reduce photosensitivity |
| **Toxic-acquired porphyria**<br>• Usually affects children<br>• Significant mortality | • Acute colicky pain<br>• Anorexia, nausea, vomiting<br>• Neuromuscular weakness<br>• Behavioral changes<br>• Seizures, coma | • Chlorpromazine I.V. to relieve pain and GI symptoms<br>• Avoidance of lead exposure |
| **HEPATIC PORPHYRIA** | | |
| **Acute intermittent porphyria**<br>• Most common form<br>• Affects females most often, usually between the ages of 15 and 40 | • Colicky abdominal pain with fever, general malaise, and hypertension<br>• Peripheral neuritis, behavioral changes, possibly leading to frank psychosis<br>• Respiratory paralysis can occur | • Chlorpromazine I.V. to relieve abdominal pain and control psychic abnormalities<br>• Avoidance of barbiturates, alcohol, and fasting<br>• Hemin for recurrent attacks<br>• High-carbohydrate diet |

*(continued)*

## TYPES OF PORPHYRIA *(continued)*

| PORPHYRIA | SIGNS AND SYMPTOMS | TREATMENT |
|---|---|---|
| **HEPATIC PORPHYRIA** *(continued)* | | |
| **Variegate porphyria**<br>• Usual onset between the ages of 30 and 50<br>• Occurs almost exclusively among South African whites<br>• Affects males and females equally | • Skin lesions, extremely fragile skin in exposed areas<br>• Hypertrichosis<br>• Hyperpigmentation<br>• Abdominal pain during acute attack<br>• Neuropsychiatric manifestations | • High carbohydrate diet<br>• Avoidance of sunlight, or wearing protective clothing when avoidance isn't possible<br>• Hemin for recurrent attacks |
| **Porphyria cutanea tarda**<br>• Most frequent in men between the ages of 40 and 60<br>• Highest incidence in South Africans | • Facial pigmentation<br>• Red-brown urine<br>• Photosensitive dermatitis<br>• Hypertrichosis | • Avoidance of precipitating factors, such as alcohol and estrogens<br>• Phlebotomy at 2-week intervals to lower serum iron level |
| **Hereditary coproporphyria**<br>• Rare<br>• Affects males and females equally | • Asymptomatic or mild neurologic, abdominal, or psychiatric symptoms | • High-carbohydrate diet<br>• Avoidance of barbiturates<br>• Hemin for recurrent attacks |

## Causes

Porphyrias are inherited as autosomal dominant traits, except for Günther's disease (autosomal recessive trait) and toxic-acquired porphyria (usually from ingestion of or exposure to lead). Menstruation often precipitates acute porphyria in premenopausal women.

## Signs and symptoms

Porphyrias are generally marked by photosensitivity, acute abdominal pain, and neuropathy. Hepatic porphyrias may produce a complex syndrome marked by distinct neurologic and hepatic dysfunction:

• Neurologic symptoms include chronic brain syndrome, peripheral neuropathy and autonomic effects, tachycardia, labile hypertension, severe colicky lower abdominal pain, and constipation.

• During an acute attack, fever, leukocytosis, and fluid and electrolyte imbalance may occur.

• Structural hepatic effects include fatty infiltration of the liver, hepatic siderosis, and focal hepatocellular necrosis.

• Skin lesions may cause itching and burning, erythema, and altered pigmentation and edema in areas exposed to light. Some chronic skin changes include milia (white papules on the dorsal aspects of the hands) and hirsutism on the upper cheeks and periorbital areas.

## Diagnosis

Generally, diagnosis requires screening tests for porphyrins or their precursors (such as aminolevulinic acid [ALA] and porphobilinogen [PBG]) in urine, stool, or blood or, occasionally, skin biopsy. A urinary lead level of 0.2 mg/L confirms toxic-acquired porphyria.

Other laboratory values may include increased serum iron levels in porphyria cutanea tarda; leukocytosis, syndrome of inappropriate antidiuretic hormone, and elevated bilirubin and alkaline phosphatase levels in acute intermittent porphyria.

## Treatment

Treatment for porphyrias includes avoiding overexposure to the sun and using beta-carotene to reduce photosensitivity. Hemin (an enzyme-inhibitor derived from processed red blood cells) is given to control recurrent attacks of acute intermittent porphyria, Günther's disease, variegate porphyria, and hereditary coproporphyria. A high-carbohydrate diet decreases urinary excretion of ALA and PBG, with restricted fluid intake to inhibit release of antidiuretic hormone.

## Special considerations

- Warn the patient to avoid excessive sun exposure, use a sunscreen when outdoors, and take a beta-carotene supplement to reduce photosensitivity.
- Encourage a high-carbohydrate diet.
- Administer beta-carotene and hemin as ordered.

# POSTTRAUMATIC STRESS DISORDER

Posttraumatic stress disorder refers to a persistent psychological disturbance that occurs following a traumatic event. This disorder can follow almost any distressing event, including a natural or manmade disaster, physical or sexual abuse, or an assault or a rape.

Psychological trauma accompanies the physical trauma and involves intense fear and feelings of helplessness and loss of control. Posttraumatic stress disorder can be acute, chronic, or delayed. When the precipitating event is of human design, the disorder is more severe and more persistent. Onset can occur at any age, even during childhood.

## Causes

Posttraumatic stress disorder occurs in response to an extremely distressing event, including a serious threat of harm to the patient or his family, such as war, abuse, or violent crime. It may be triggered by sudden destruction of his home or community by a bombing, fire, flood, tornado, earthquake, or similar disaster. It may also occur after the patient witnesses the death or serious injury of another person by torture, in a death camp, by natural disaster, or by a motor vehicle or airplane crash.

Preexisting psychopathology can predispose some patients to this disorder, but anyone can develop it, especially if the stressor is extreme.

## Signs and symptoms

The psychosocial history of a patient with posttraumatic stress disorder may reveal early life experiences, interpersonal factors, military experiences, or other incidents that suggest the precipitating event. Typically, the patient may report that his symptoms began immediately or soon after the trauma, although they may not develop until months or years later. In such a case, avoidance symptoms usually have been present during the latency period.

Symptoms include pangs of painful emotion and unwelcome thoughts; intrusive memories; dissociative episodes (flashbacks); a traumatic reexperiencing of the event; difficulty falling or staying asleep, frequent nightmares of the traumatic event, and aggressive outbursts on awakening; emotional numbing (diminished or constricted response); and chronic anxiety or panic attacks (with physical signs and symptoms).

The patient may display rage and survivor guilt, use of violence to solve problems, depression and suicidal thoughts, and phobic avoidance of situations that arouse memories of the traumatic event (such as hot weather and tall grasses for the Vietnam veteran).

Other symptoms include memory impairment or difficulty concentrating and feelings of detachment or estrangement that destroy interpersonal relationships. Some have physical symptoms, fantasies of retaliation, and substance abuse.

### Diagnosis

For characteristic findings in patients with this condition, see *Diagnosing posttraumatic stress disorder.*

### Treatment

The goals of treatment for posttraumatic stress disorder include reducing the target symptoms, preventing chronic disability, and promoting occupational and social rehabilitation.

#### Specific treatments

Effective treatment may emphasize behavioral techniques (such as relaxation therapy to decrease anxiety and induce sleep or progressive desensitization). Antianxiety and antidepressant drugs or psychotherapy (supportive, insight, or cathartic) may minimize the risks of dependency and chronicity.

#### Support groups

Such groups are highly effective and are provided through many Veterans Administration centers and crisis clinics. These groups provide a forum in which victims of this disorder can work through their feelings with others who have had similar conflicts.

Group settings are appropriate for most degrees of symptoms presented. Some group programs include spouses and families in their treatment process. Rehabilitation programs in physical, social, and occupational areas also are available for victims of chronic posttraumatic stress disorder.

Many patients need treatment for depression, alcohol or drug abuse, or medical conditions before psychological healing can take place. Treatment for this disorder may be complex, and the prognosis varies.

### Special considerations

- Encourage the patient with posttraumatic stress disorder to express his grief, complete the mourning process, and develop coping skills to relieve anxiety and desensitize him to the memories of the traumatic event.
- Keep in mind that such a patient tends to sharply test your commitment and interest. Therefore, first examine your feelings about the event (war or other trauma) so you won't react with disdain and shock. Such reactions hamper the working relationship with the patient and reinforce his typically poor self-image and sense of guilt.
- Know and practice crisis intervention techniques as appropriate in posttraumatic stress disorder.

# DIAGNOSING POSTTRAUMATIC STRESS DISORDER

The diagnosis of posttraumatic stress disorder is made when the patient's signs and symptoms meet the following criteria documented in the *DSM-IV*:

• The person was exposed to a traumatic event in which both of the following occurred:

— the person experienced, witnessed, or was confronted with an event or events that involved actual or threatened death or serious injury, or a threat to the physical integrity of self or others.

— the person's response involved intense fear, helplessness, or horror (in children, the response may be expressed by disorganized or agitated behavior).

• The person persistently reexperiences the traumatic event in at least one of the following ways:

— recurrent and intrusive distressing recollections of the event, including images, thoughts, or perceptions

— recurrent distressing dreams of the event

— acting or feeling as if the traumatic event were recurring (includes a sense of reliving the experience, illusions, hallucinations, and dissociative episodes that occur even when awakening or intoxicated)

— intense psychological distress at exposure to internal or external cues that symbolize or resemble an aspect of the traumatic event.

• The person persistently avoids stimuli associated with the traumatic event and experiences numbing of general responsiveness (not present before the traumatic event), as indicated by at least three of the following:

— efforts to avoid thoughts or feelings associated with the trauma

— efforts to avoid activities, places, or people that arouse recollections of the trauma

— inability to recall an important aspect of the traumatic event

— markedly diminished interest in significant activities

— feeling of detachment or estrangement from other individuals

— restricted range of affect, for example, inability to love others

— sense of foreshortened future.

• The person has persistent symptoms of increased arousal (not present before the trauma), as indicated by at least two of the following:

— difficulty falling or staying asleep

— irritability or outbursts of anger

— difficulty concentrating

— hypervigilance

— exaggerated startle response.

• The disturbance must be of at least 1 month's duration.

• The disturbance causes clinically significant distress or impairment in the patient's social, occupational, or other important areas of functioning.

---

CLINICAL TIP   Establish trust by accepting the patient's current level of functioning and assuming a positive, consistent, honest, and nonjudgmental attitude toward the patient.

• Provide encouragement as the patient shows a commitment to work on his problem.

• Deal constructively with the patient's displays of anger.

• Encourage joint assessment of angry outbursts (identify how anger escalates and explore preventive measures that family members can take to regain control).

• Provide a safe, staff-monitored room in which the patient can safely deal with urges to commit physical violence or self-abuse through displacement (such as pounding and throwing clay or destroying selected items).

- Encourage the patient to move from physical to verbal expressions of anger.
- Help the patient relieve shame and guilt precipitated by real actions (such as killing or mutilation) that violated a consciously held moral code.
- Help the patient put his behavior into perspective, recognize his isolation and self-destructive behavior as forms of atonement, learn to forgive himself, and accept forgiveness from others.
- Refer the patient to a clergyman as appropriate.
- Provide for group therapy with other victims for peer support and forgiveness, or refer the patient to such a support group.
- Refer the patient to appropriate community resources.

# POTASSIUM IMBALANCE

Potassium, a cation that is the dominant cellular electrolyte, facilitates contraction of both skeletal and smooth muscles — including myocardial contraction — and figures prominently in nerve impulse conduction, acid-base balance, enzyme action, and cell-membrane function. Because serum potassium level has such a narrow range (3.5 to 5 mEq/L), a slight deviation in either direction can produce profound clinical consequences.

Paradoxically, both hypokalemia (potassium deficiency) and hyperkalemia (potassium excess) can lead to muscle weakness and flaccid paralysis because both create an ionic imbalance in neuromuscular tissue excitability. Both conditions also diminish excitability and conduction rate of the heart muscle, which may lead to cardiac arrest.

## Causes

There are a number of possible causes of potassium imbalance.

### *Hypokalemia*

Because many foods contain potassium, hypokalemia rarely results from a dietary deficiency. Instead, potassium loss results from:
- excessive GI or urinary losses, such as vomiting, gastric suction, diarrhea, dehydration, anorexia, or chronic laxative abuse
- trauma (injury, burns, or surgery), in which damaged cells release potassium, which enters serum or extracellular fluid to be excreted in the urine
- chronic renal disease, with tubular potassium wasting
- certain drugs, especially potassium-wasting diuretics, steroids, and certain sodium-containing antibiotics (carbenicillin)
- acid-base imbalances, which cause potassium shifting into cells without true depletion in alkalosis
- prolonged potassium-free I.V. therapy
- hyperglycemia, causing osmotic diuresis and glycosuria
- Cushing's syndrome, primary hyperaldosteronism, excessive ingestion of licorice, and severe serum magnesium deficiency.

### *Hyperkalemia*

Generally, hyperkalemia results from the kidneys' inability to excrete excessive amounts of potassium infused I.V. or administered orally; from decreased urine output, renal dysfunction, or renal failure; or from the use of potassium-sparing diuretics, such as triamterene, by patients with renal disease. It may also result from any injuries or conditions that release cellular potassium or favor its retention, such as burns, crushing injuries, failing renal function,

## CLINICAL FEATURES OF POTASSIUM IMBALANCE

| DYSFUNCTION | HYPOKALEMIA | HYPERKALEMIA |
|---|---|---|
| Cardiovascular | • Dizziness, hypotension, arrhythmias, electrocardiogram (ECG) changes (flattened T waves, elevated U waves, depressed ST segment), cardiac arrest (with serum potassium levels < 2.5 mEq/L) | • Tachycardia and later bradycardia, ECG changes (tented and elevated T waves, widened QRS, prolonged PR interval, flattened or absent P waves, depressed ST segment), cardiac arrest (with levels > 7 mEq/L) |
| Gastrointestinal | • Nausea and vomiting, anorexia, diarrhea, abdominal distention, paralytic ileus or decreased peristalsis | • Nausea, diarrhea, abdominal cramps |
| Musculoskeletal | • Muscle weakness and fatigue, leg cramps | • Muscle weakness, flaccid paralysis |
| Genitourinary | • Polyuria | • Oliguria, anuria |
| CNS | • Malaise, irritability, confusion, mental depression, speech changes, decreased reflexes, respiratory paralysis | • Hyperreflexia progressing to weakness, numbness, tingling, and flaccid paralysis |
| Acid-base balance | • Metabolic alkalosis | • Metabolic acidosis |

adrenal gland insufficiency, dehydration, or diabetic acidosis.

### Signs and symptoms
See *Clinical features of potassium imbalance.*

### Diagnosis
• *Hypokalemia:* serum potassium levels < 3.5 mEq/L.
• *Hyperkalemia:* serum potassium levels > 5 mEq/L.

Additional tests may be necessary to determine the underlying cause of the imbalance.

### Treatment
Potassium imbalances are treated as follows.

#### Hypokalemia
Replacement therapy with potassium chloride (I.V. or by mouth) is the primary treatment of hypokalemia. When diuresis is necessary, spironolactone, a potassium-sparing diuretic, may be administered concurrently with a potassium-wasting diuretic to minimize potassium loss.

Hypokalemia can be prevented by giving a maintenance dose of potassium I.V. to patients who may not take anything by mouth and to others predisposed to potassium loss.

### Hyperkalemia

For management of hyperkalemia, rapid infusion of 10% calcium gluconate decreases myocardial irritability and temporarily prevents cardiac arrest but doesn't correct serum potassium excess; it's also contraindicated in patients receiving a digitalis glycoside.

As an emergency measure, sodium bicarbonate I.V. increases pH and causes potassium to shift back into the cells. Insulin and 10% to 50% glucose I.V. also move potassium back into cells. Infusions should be followed by dextrose 5% in water because infusion of 10% to 15% glucose will stimulate secretion of endogenous insulin.

Sodium polystyrene sulfonate (Kayexalate) with 70% sorbitol produces exchange of sodium ions for potassium ions in the intestine. Hemodialysis or peritoneal dialysis also aids in removal of excess potassium.

### Special considerations

For hypokalemia:
- Check serum potassium and other electrolyte levels in patients who are likely to develop a potassium imbalance and in those requiring potassium replacement; they risk overcorrection to hyperkalemia.
- Assess intake and output carefully.

➤ CLINICAL TIP  Remember, the kidneys excrete 80% to 90% of ingested potassium. Never give supplementary potassium to a patient whose urine output is less than 600 ml/day. Also, measure GI loss from suctioning or vomiting.

- Administer slow-release potassium or dilute oral potassium supplements in 4 oz (120 ml) or more of water or other fluid to reduce gastric and small-bowel irritation.

- Determine the patient's chloride level. As appropriate, give a potassium chloride supplement, if the level is low; potassium gluconate, if it's normal.
- Give I.V. potassium only after it's diluted in solution; potassium is very irritating to vascular, subcutaneous, and fatty tissues and may cause phlebitis or tissue necrosis if it infiltrates.
- Infuse potassium slowly (no more than 20 mEq/L/hour) to prevent hyperkalemia. *Never* administer it by I.V. push or bolus; it may cause cardiac arrest.
- Carefully monitor patients receiving a digitalis glycoside because hypokalemia will enhance its action and may produce signs of digitalis toxicity (anorexia, nausea, vomiting, blurred vision, and arrhythmias).
- To prevent hypokalemia, instruct patients (especially those predisposed to hypokalemia due to long-term diuretic therapy) to include in their diet foods rich in potassium — oranges, bananas, tomatoes, dark green leafy vegetables, milk, dried fruits, apricots, and peanuts.
- Monitor cardiac rhythm, and be alert for irregularities.

For hyperkalemia:
- As in hypokalemia, frequently monitor serum potassium and other electrolyte levels, and carefully record intake and output.
- Administer sodium polystyrene sulfonate orally or rectally (by retention enema). Watch for signs of hypokalemia with prolonged use and for clinical effects of hypoglycemia (muscle weakness, syncope, hunger, diaphoresis) with repeated insulin and glucose treatment.
- Watch for signs of hyperkalemia in predisposed patients, especially those with decreased urine output or those receiving oral or I.V. potassium supplements.

➤ CLINICAL TIP  Administer up to 20 mEq/L of potassium chloride per hour; check the I.V. infusion site for signs of phlebitis or infiltration of potassium into tissues.

• Before giving a blood transfusion, check to see how long ago the blood was donated; older blood cell hemolysis releases potassium. Infuse only *fresh* blood for patients with average to high serum potassium levels.

• Watch for cardiac arrhythmias.

# PREMATURE RUPTURE OF THE MEMBRANES

Premature rupture of the membranes (PROM) is a spontaneous break or tear in the amniochorial sac before onset of regular contractions, resulting in progressive cervical dilation. PROM occurs in nearly 10% of all pregnancies over 20 weeks' gestation, and labor usually starts within 24 hours; over 80% of these infants are mature. The latent period (between membrane rupture and labor onset) is generally brief when the membranes rupture near term; when the infant is premature, this period is prolonged, which increases the risk of mortality from maternal infection (amnionitis, endometritis), fetal infection (pneumonia, septicemia), and prematurity.

## Causes

Although the cause of PROM is unknown, malpresentation and contracted pelvis commonly accompany the rupture. Predisposing factors may include:

• poor nutrition and hygiene and lack of proper prenatal care

• incompetent cervix (perhaps as a result of abortions)

• increased intrauterine tension due to hydramnios or multiple pregnancies

• defects in the amniochorial membranes' tensile strength

• uterine infection.

## Signs and symptoms

Typically, PROM causes blood-tinged amniotic fluid containing vernix particles to gush or leak from the vagina. Maternal fever, fetal tachycardia, and foul-smelling vaginal discharge indicate infection.

## Diagnosis

Characteristic passage of amniotic fluid confirms PROM. Physical examination shows amniotic fluid in the vagina. Examination of this fluid helps determine appropriate management. For example, aerobic and anaerobic cultures and a Gram stain from the cervix reveal pathogenic organisms and indicate uterine or systemic infection. The alkaline pH of fluid collected from the posterior fornix turns nitrazine paper deep blue. (The presence of blood can give a false-positive result.) If a smear of fluid is placed on a slide and allowed to dry, it takes on a fernlike pattern due to the high sodium and protein content of amniotic fluid.

Staining the fluid with Nile blue sulfate reveals two categories of cell bodies. Blue-stained bodies represent shed fetal epithelial cells, while orange-stained bodies originate in sebaceous glands. Incidence of prematurity is low when more than 20% of cells stain orange.

Physical examination also determines the presence of multiple pregnancies. Fetal presentation and size should be assessed by abdominal palpation (Leopold's maneuvers).

Other data determine the fetus's gestational age:

• *historical:* date of last menstrual period, quickening

• *physical:* initial detection of unamplified fetal heart sound, measurement of fundal height above the symphysis, ultrasound measurements of fetal biparietal diameter

• *chemical:* tests on amniotic fluid, such as the lecithin-sphingomyelin (L/S) ratio (an L/S ratio > 2.0 indicates pulmonary maturity); foam stability (shake test) also indicates fetal pulmonary maturity.

## Treatment

Treatment for PROM depends on fetal age and the risk of infection. In a term pregnancy, if spontaneous labor and vaginal delivery aren't achieved within a relatively short time (usually within 24 hours after the membranes rupture), induction of labor with oxytocin is usually required; if induction fails, cesarean delivery is usually necessary. Cesarean hysterectomy is recommended with gross uterine infection.

Management of a preterm pregnancy of less than 34 weeks is controversial. However, with advances in technology, a conservative approach to PROM has now been proven effective. With a preterm pregnancy of 28 to 34 weeks, treatment includes hospitalization and observation for signs of infection (maternal leukocytosis or fever, and fetal tachycardia) while awaiting fetal maturation. If clinical status suggests infection, baseline cultures and sensitivity tests are appropriate. If these tests confirm infection, labor must be induced, followed by I.V. administration of antibiotics. A culture should also be made of gastric aspirate or a swabbing from the infant's ear because antibiotic therapy may be indicated for the newborn as well. In such deliveries, have resuscitative equipment available to treat neonatal distress.

## Special considerations

• Teach the patient in the early stages of pregnancy how to recognize PROM. Make sure she understands that amniotic fluid doesn't always gush; it may leak slowly.

➤ CLINICAL TIP  Stress that the patient *must* report PROM immediately because prompt treatment may prevent dangerous infection.

• Warn the patient not to engage in sexual intercourse or to douche after the membranes rupture.

• Before physical examination in suspected PROM, explain all diagnostic tests and clarify any misunderstandings the patient may have. During the examination, stay with the patient and provide reassurance. Such examination requires sterile gloves and sterile lubricating jelly. *Don't* use iodophor antiseptic solution because it discolors nitrazine paper and makes pH determination impossible.

• After the examination, provide proper perineal care. Send fluid samples to the laboratory promptly because bacteriologic studies need immediate evaluation to be valid. If labor starts, observe the mother's contractions, and monitor vital signs every 2 hours. Watch for signs of maternal infection (fever, abdominal tenderness, and changes in amniotic fluid, such as foul odor or purulence) and fetal tachycardia. (Fetal tachycardia may precede maternal fever.) Report such signs immediately.

# PREMENSTRUAL SYNDROME

Characterized by varying symptoms, premenstrual syndrome (PMS) appears 7 to 14 days before menses and usually subsides with its onset. The effects of PMS range from minimal discomfort to severe, disruptive symptoms and can include nervousness, irritability, depression, and multiple somatic complaints.

Researchers believe that 70% to 90% of women experience PMS at some time during their childbearing years, usually between the ages of 25 and 45.

### Causes

The biological theories offered to explain the cause of PMS include such conditions as a progesterone deficiency in the luteal phase of the menstrual cycle and vitamin deficiencies.

Failure to identify a specific disorder with a specific mechanism suggests that PMS represents a variety of manifestations triggered by normal physiologic hormonal changes.

### Signs and symptoms

Clinical effects vary widely among patients and may include any combination of the following:

• *behavioral* — mild to severe personality changes, nervousness, hostility, irritability, agitation, sleep disturbances, fatigue, lethargy, and depression

• *somatic* — breast tenderness or swelling, abdominal tenderness or bloating, joint pain, headache, edema, diarrhea or constipation, and exacerbations of skin problems (such as acne or rashes), respiratory problems (such as asthma), or neurologic problems (such as seizures).

### Diagnosis

The patient history shows typical symptoms related to the menstrual cycle. To help ensure an accurate history, the patient may be asked to record menstrual symptoms and body temperature on a calendar for 2 to 3 months before diagnosis.

Estrogen and progesterone blood levels may be evaluated to help rule out hormonal imbalance. A psychological evaluation is also recommended to rule out or detect an underlying psychiatric disorder.

### Treatment

Education and reassurance that PMS is a real physiologic syndrome are important parts of treatment. Because treatment is predominantly symptomatic, each patient must learn to cope with her own individual set of symptoms.

Treatment may include diuretics, antidepressants, vitamins such as B complex, progestins, prostaglandin inhibitors, and nonsteroidal anti-inflammatory drugs. For effective treatment, the patient may have to maintain a diet that's low in simple sugars, caffeine, and salt.

### Special considerations

• Inform the patient that self-help groups exist for women with PMS; if appropriate, help her contact such a group.

• Obtain a complete patient history to help identify any emotional problems that may contribute to PMS. If necessary, refer the patient for psychological counseling.

• If possible, discuss ways in which the patient can modify her lifestyle, such as making changes in her diet and avoiding stimulants and alcohol.

CLINICAL TIP Suggest that the patient seek further medical consultation if symptoms are severe and interfere with her normal lifestyle.

# PRESSURE ULCERS

Pressure ulcers, commonly called pressure sores or bedsores, are localized areas of cellular necrosis that occur most often in the skin and subcutaneous (S.C.) tissue over bony prominences. These ulcers may be superficial, caused by local skin irritation with subsequent surface maceration, or deep, originating in underlying tissue. Deep lesions often go undetected until they penetrate the skin; but, by then, they've usually caused S.C. damage.

## Causes

Most pressure ulcers are caused by pressure, particularly over bony prominences, that interrupts normal circulatory function, leading to ischemia of the underlying structures of skin, fat, and muscles. The intensity and duration of such pressure govern the severity of the ulcer; pressure exerted over an area for a moderate period (1 to 2 hours) produces tissue ischemia and increased capillary pressure, leading to edema and multiple small-vessel thromboses. An inflammatory reaction gives way to ulceration and necrosis of ischemic cells. In turn, necrotic tissue predisposes to bacterial invasion and subsequent infection.

The patient's position determines the pressure exerted on the tissues. For example, if the head of the bed is elevated, or the patient assumes a slumped position, gravity pulls his weight downward and forward. This shearing force causes deep ulcers due to ischemic changes in the muscles and S.C. tissues, and occurs most often over the sacrum and ischial tuberosities.

Predisposing conditions for pressure ulcers include altered mobility, inadequate nutrition (leading to weight loss and subsequent reduction of S.C. tissue and muscle bulk), and a breakdown in skin or S.C. tissue (as a result of edema, incontinence, fever, pathologic conditions, or obesity).

## Signs and symptoms

Pressure ulcers commonly develop over bony prominences. Early features of superficial lesions are shiny, erythematous changes over the compressed area, caused by localized vasodilation when pressure is relieved. Superficial erythema progresses to small blisters or erosions and, ultimately, to necrosis and ulceration. (See *Pressure points: Common sites of pressure ulcers.*)

An inflamed area on the skin's surface may be the first sign of underlying damage when pressure is exerted between deep tissue and bone. Bacteria in a compressed site cause inflammation and, eventually, infection, which leads to further necrosis. A foul-smelling, purulent discharge may seep from a lesion that penetrates the skin from beneath. Infected, necrotic tissue prevents healthy granulation of scar tissue; a black eschar may develop around and over the lesion.

## Diagnosis

Pressure ulcers are obvious on physical examination. Wound culture and sensitivity testing of the exudate in the ulcer identify infecting organisms and antibiotics that may be needed. If severe hypoproteinemia is suspected, total serum protein values and serum albumin studies may be appropriate.

## Treatment

Successful treatment must relieve pressure on the affected area, keep the area clean and dry, and promote healing. (See *Special aids for preventing and treating pressure ulcers,* page 692.)

## Special considerations

• During each shift, check the skin of bedridden patients for possible changes in color, turgor, temperature, and sen-

# PRESSURE POINTS: COMMON SITES OF PRESSURE ULCERS

Pressure ulcers may develop in any of these 16 pressure points. To prevent sores, reposition the patient frequently, and carefully check for any change in the patient's skin tone.

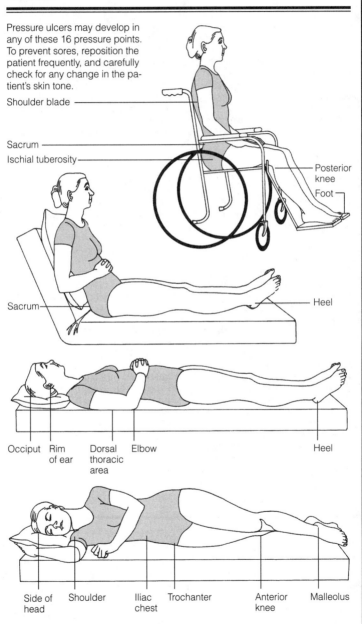

Shoulder blade

Sacrum

Ischial tuberosity

Posterior knee

Foot

Sacrum

Heel

Occiput   Rim of ear   Dorsal thoracic area   Elbow   Heel

Side of head   Shoulder   Iliac chest   Trochanter   Anterior knee   Malleolus

# SPECIAL AIDS FOR PREVENTING AND TREATING PRESSURE ULCERS

Aids for pressure ulcers include relief devices and topical agents.

## Pressure relief aids

• *Gel flotation pads* disperse pressure over a greater skin surface area; convenient and adaptable for home and wheelchair use.

• *Alternating pressure mattress* contains tubelike sections, running lengthwise, that deflate and reinflate, changing areas of pressure. Use mattress with a single untucked sheet because layers of linen decrease its effectiveness.

• *Convoluted foam mattress* minimizes area of skin pressure with its alternating areas of depression and elevation: soft, elevated foam areas cushion skin; depressed areas relieve pressure. This mattress should be used with a single, loosely tucked sheet and is adaptable for home and wheelchair use. If the patient is incontinent, cover mattress with the provided plastic sleeve.

• *Spanco mattress* has polyester fibers with silicon tubes to decrease pressure without limiting the patient's position. It has no weight limitation.

• *Sheepskin* is soft, dry, absorbent, and easy to clean. It should be in direct contact with the patient's skin. It's available in sizes to fit elbows and heels and is adaptable to home use.

• *Clinitron bed* supports the patient at a subcapillary pressure point and provides a warm, relaxing, therapeutic airflow. The bed is filled with beads that move when the air flows. It eliminates friction and maceration.

• *Low air-loss beds,* such as Flexicare and Accucare, slow the drying of any saline soaks, and elderly patients often experience less disorientation than with high air-loss beds. The head of the bed can be elevated so there's less chance of aspiration, especially in patients who require tube feeding. Patients can get out of bed more easily and can be moved more easily on low air-loss surfaces.

## Topical agents

• Gentle soap
• Dakins solution
• Zinc oxide cream
• Absorbable gelatin sponge
• Granulated sugar (mechanical irritant to enhance granulation)
• Dextranomer (inert, absorbing beads)
• Karaya gum patches
• Topical antibiotics *(only* when infection is confirmed by culture and sensitivity tests)
• Silver sulfadiazine cream (antimicrobial agent) for necrotic areas
• Water vapor–permeable dressings
• Duoderm, Tegaderm dressings

## Skin-damaging agents to avoid

• Harsh alkali soaps
• Alcohol-based products (can cause vasoconstriction)
• Tincture of benzoin (may cause painful erosions)
• Hexachlorophene (may irritate the central nervous system)
• Petroleum gauze

sation. Examine an existing ulcer for any change in size or degree of damage. When using pressure relief aids or topical agents, explain their function to the patient.

• Prevent pressure ulcers by repositioning the bedridden patient at least every 2 hours around the clock. To minimize the effects of a shearing force, use a footboard and don't raise the head of the bed to an angle exceeding 60 degrees. Also, use a draw or pull sheet to turn the patient or to pull him up. Keep the patient's knees slightly flexed for short periods. Perform passive range-of-motion exercises, or encourage the patient to do active exercises if possible.

• To prevent pressure ulcers in immobilized patients, use pressure relief aids on their beds.

• Provide meticulous skin care. Keep the skin clean and dry without the use of harsh soaps. Gently massaging the skin around the affected area — not on it — promotes healing. Rub moisturizing lotions into the skin thoroughly to prevent maceration of the skin surface. Change bed linens frequently for patients who are diaphoretic or incontinent. Use a fecal incontinence bag for incontinent patients.

• Clean open lesions with a 3% solution of hydrogen peroxide or normal saline solution. Dressings, if needed, should be porous and lightly taped to healthy skin. Debridement of necrotic tissue may be necessary to allow healing. One method is to apply open wet dressings and allow them to dry on the ulcer. Removal of the dressings mechanically debrides exudate and necrotic tissue. Other methods include surgical debridement with a fine scalpel blade and chemical debridement using proteolytic enzyme agents.

• Encourage adequate intake of food and fluids to maintain body weight and promote healing. Consult with the dietary department to provide a diet that promotes granulation of new tissue. Encourage the debilitated patient to eat frequent, small meals that include protein and calorie-rich supplements. Assist weakened patients with their meals.

# PROCTITIS

Proctitis is an acute or chronic inflammation of the rectal mucosa. The prognosis is good unless massive bleeding occurs.

## Causes

Contributing factors include chronic constipation, habitual laxative use, emotional upset, radiation (especially for cancer of the cervix and of the uterus), endocrine dysfunction, rectal injury, rectal medications, bacterial infections, allergies (especially to milk), vasomotor disturbance that interferes with normal muscle control, and food poisoning.

## Signs and symptoms

Key symptoms include tenesmus, constipation, a feeling of rectal fullness, and left abdominal cramps. The patient feels an intense urge to defecate, which produces a small amount of stool that may contain blood and mucus.

## Diagnosis

In acute proctitis, sigmoidoscopy shows edematous, bright-red or pink rectal mucosa that's thick, shiny, friable, and possibly ulcerated. In chronic proctitis, sigmoidoscopy shows thickened mucosa, loss of vascular pattern, and stricture of the rectal lumen. Other supportive tests include biopsy to rule out carcinoma and a bacteriologic examination. A detailed patient history is essential.

## Treatment

Primary treatment eliminates the underlying cause (fecal impaction, laxatives, or other medications). Soothing enemas or steroid (hydrocortisone) suppositories or enemas may be helpful if proctitis is due to radiation. Tranquilizers may be appropriate for the patient with emotional stress.

### Special considerations

● Tell the patient to watch for and report bleeding and other persistent symptoms.

● Fully explain proctitis and its treatment to help the patient understand the disorder and prevent its recurrence.

● As appropriate, offer emotional support and reassurance during rectal examinations and treatment.

# PROSTATIC CANCER

Prostatic cancer is the second most common neoplasm found in men over age 50. Adenocarcinoma is its most common form; sarcoma occurs only rarely. Most prostatic carcinomas originate in the posterior prostate gland; the rest originate near the urethra.

Malignant prostatic tumors seldom result from the benign hyperplastic enlargement that commonly develops around the prostatic urethra in elderly men. Prostatic cancer seldom produces symptoms until it's advanced.

### Causes

Although androgens regulate prostate growth and function and may also speed tumor growth, no definite link between increased androgen levels and prostatic cancer has been found. When primary prostatic lesions metastasize, they typically invade the prostatic capsule and spread along the ejaculatory ducts in the space between the seminal vesicles or perivesicular fascia.

Prostatic cancer accounts for about 18% of all cancers. Incidence is highest in Blacks and lowest in Asians. Incidence also increases with age more rapidly than any other cancer.

### Signs and symptoms

Manifestations of prostatic cancer appear only in the advanced stages (See *Staging prostatic cancer.*) and include difficulty initiating a urinary stream, dribbling, urine retention, unexplained cystitis and, rarely, hematuria.

### Diagnosis

A digital rectal examination that reveals a small, hard nodule may help diagnose prostatic cancer. The American Cancer Society advises a yearly digital examination for men over age 40, a yearly blood test to detect prostate-specific antigen (PSA) in men over age 50, and ultrasonography if abnormal results are found.

Biopsy confirms the diagnosis. PSA levels will be elevated in all, and serum acid phosphatase levels will be elevated in two-thirds of men with metastatic prostatic cancer. Therapy aims to return the serum acid phosphatase level to normal; a subsequent rise points to recurrence. Magnetic resonance imaging, computed tomography scan, and excretory urography may also aid the diagnosis.

CLINICAL TIP Elevated alkaline phosphatase levels and a positive bone scan point to bone metastasis.

### Treatment

Management of prostatic cancer depends on clinical assessment, tolerance of therapy, expected life span, and the stage of the disease. Treatment must be chosen carefully because prostatic cancer usually affects older men, who commonly have coexisting disorders, such as hypertension, diabetes, or cardiac disease.

Therapy varies with each stage of the disease and generally includes radia-

# STAGING PROSTATIC CANCER

The American Joint Committee on Cancer recognizes the TNM (tumor, node, metastasis) cancer staging system for assessing prostatic cancer.

### Primary tumor
**TX** — primary tumor can't be assessed
**T0** — no evidence of primary tumor
**T1** — tumor an incidental histologic finding
**T1a** — three or fewer microscopic foci of cancer
**T1b** — more than three microscopic foci of cancer
**T2** — tumor limited to the prostate gland
**T2a** — tumor less than 1.5 cm in greatest dimension, with normal tissue on at least three sides
**T2b** — tumor larger than 1.5 cm in greatest dimension or present in more than one lobe
**T3** — unfixed tumor extends into the prostatic apex or into or beyond the prostatic capsule, bladder neck, or seminal vesicle
**T4** — tumor fixed or invades adjacent structures not listed in T3

### Regional lymph nodes
**NX** — regional lymph nodes can't be assessed
**N0** — no evidence of regional lymph node metastasis
**N1** — metastasis in a single lymph node, 2 cm or less in greatest dimension
**N2** — metastasis in a single lymph node, between 2 and 5 cm in greatest dimension, or metastasis to several lymph nodes, none more than 5 cm in greatest dimension
**N3** — metastasis in a lymph node, more than 5 cm in greatest dimension

### Distant metastasis
**MX** — distant metastasis can't be assessed
**M0** — no known distant metastasis
**M1** — distant metastasis

### Staging categories
Prostatic cancer progresses from mild to severe as follows
**Stage 0 or Stage I** — T1a, N0, M0; T2a, N0, M0
**Stage II** — T1b, N0, M0; T21b, N0, M0
**Stage III** — T3, N0, M0
**Stage IV** — T4, N0, M0; any T, N1, M0; any T, N2, M0; any T, N3, M0; any T, any N, M1

---

tion, prostatectomy, orchiectomy to reduce androgen production, and hormone therapy with synthetic estrogen (diethylstilbestrol [DES]) and antiandrogens such as cyproterone, megestrol, and flutamide. Radical prostatectomy is usually effective for localized lesions.

Radiation therapy is used to cure some locally invasive lesions and to relieve pain from metastatic bone involvement. A single injection of the radionuclide strontium-89 is also used to treat pain caused by bone metastasis.

If hormone therapy, surgery, and radiation therapy aren't feasible or suc-

cessful, chemotherapy (using combinations of cyclophosphamide, doxorubicin, fluorouracil, cisplatin, etoposide, and vindesine) may be tried. However, current drug therapy offers little benefit. Combining several treatment methods may be most effective.

### Special considerations
Care should emphasize psychological support, postoperative care, and treatment of radiation adverse effects.

Before prostatectomy:
● Explain the expected aftereffects of surgery (such as impotence and incon-

tinence) and radiation. Discuss tube placement and dressing changes.

• Teach the patient to do perineal exercises 1 to 10 times an hour. Have him squeeze his buttocks together, hold this position for a few seconds, then relax.

After prostatectomy or suprapubic prostatectomy:

• Regularly check the dressing, incision, and drainage systems for excessive bleeding; watch the patient for signs of bleeding (pallor, falling blood pressure, rising pulse rate) and infection.

• Maintain adequate fluid intake.

• Give antispasmodics, as necessary, to control postoperative bladder spasms. Also give analgesics as needed.

• Urinary incontinence is common after surgery; keep the patient's skin clean, dry, and free of drainage and urine.

• Encourage perineal exercises within 24 to 48 hours after surgery.

• Provide meticulous catheter care — especially if a three-way catheter with a continuous irrigation system is in place. Check the tubing for kinks and blockages, especially if the patient reports pain. Warn him not to pull on the catheter.

After transurethral prostatic resection:

• Watch for signs of urethral stricture (dysuria, decreased force and caliber of urinary stream, and straining to urinate) and for abdominal distention (from urethral stricture or catheter blockage). Irrigate the catheter as needed.

After perineal prostatectomy:

• Avoid taking a rectal temperature or inserting any kind of rectal tube. Provide pads to absorb urine leakage, a rubber ring for the patient to sit on, and sitz baths for pain and inflammation.

After perineal or retropubic prostatectomy:

• Explain that urine leakage after catheter removal is normal and will subside.

• When a patient receives hormonal therapy, watch for adverse effects. Gynecomastia, fluid retention, nausea, and vomiting are common with DES. Thrombophlebitis may also occur, especially with DES.

After radiation therapy:

• Watch for common adverse effects: proctitis, diarrhea, bladder spasms, and urinary frequency. Internal radiation usually results in cystitis in the first 2 to 3 weeks.

• Urge the patient to drink at least 2,000 ml of fluid daily.

• Provide analgesics and antispasmodics as ordered.

# PROSTATITIS

An inflammation of the prostate gland, prostatitis may be acute or chronic. Acute prostatitis most often results from gram-negative bacteria and is easy to recognize and treat. However, chronic prostatitis, the most common cause of recurrent urinary tract infection (UTI) in men, is less easy to recognize. As many as 35% of men over age 50 have chronic prostatitis.

## Causes

About 80% of bacterial prostatitis cases result from infection by *Escherichia coli;* the rest, from infection by *Klebsiella, Enterobacter, Proteus, Pseudomonas, Streptococcus,* or *Staphylococcus.* These organisms probably spread to the prostate by the bloodstream or from ascending urethral infection, invasion of rectal bacteria via lymphatics, reflux of infected bladder urine into prostate ducts or, less commonly, infrequent or excessive sexual intercourse or such procedures as cystoscopy or catheterization. Chronic prostatitis usually results from bacterial invasion from the urethra.

## Signs and symptoms

Acute prostatitis begins with fever, chills, low back pain, myalgia, perineal fullness, and arthralgia. Urination is frequent and urgent. Dysuria, nocturia, and urinary obstruction may also occur. The urine may appear cloudy. When palpated rectally, the prostate is tender, indurated, swollen, firm, and warm.

Chronic bacterial prostatitis sometimes produces no symptoms but usually elicits the same urinary symptoms as the acute form but to a lesser degree. UTI is a common complication. Other possible signs include painful ejaculation, hemospermia, persistent urethral discharge, and sexual dysfunction.

## Diagnosis

Although a urine culture can often identify the causative infectious organism and characteristic rectal examination findings suggest prostatitis, firm diagnosis depends on a comparison of urine cultures of specimens obtained by the Meares and Stamey technique. This test requires four specimens:
• one collected when the patient starts voiding (voided bladder one — VB1)
• another specimen collected midstream (VB2)
• another specimen collected after the patient stops voiding and the doctor massages the prostate to produce secretions (expressed prostate secretions; EPS)
• a final voided specimen (VB3).
A significant increase in colony count in the prostatic specimens confirms prostatitis.

## Treatment

Appropriate treatment includes drug therapy and support measures. Surgery may be necessary if drug therapy is unsuccessful.

### Drug therapy

Systemic antibiotic therapy is the treatment of choice for acute prostatitis. Cotrimoxazole is given orally and, if the pathogen is sensitive to it, continued for about 30 days. If sepsis is likely, I.V. cotrimoxazole or I.V. gentamicin plus ampicillin may be given until sensitivity test results are known.

If test results and clinical response are favorable, parenteral therapy continues for 48 hours to 1 week; then an oral agent is substituted for 30 more days. In chronic prostatitis due to *E. coli,* cotrimoxazole is usually given for at least 6 weeks.

### Support measures

Supportive therapy includes bed rest, adequate hydration, and administration of analgesics, antipyretics, sitz baths, and stool softeners as necessary. In symptomatic chronic prostatitis, regular massage of the prostate is most effective. Regular ejaculation may help promote drainage of prostatic secretions. Anticholinergics and analgesics may help relieve nonbacterial prostatitis symptoms. Alpha-adrenergic blockers and muscle relaxants may relieve prostatodynia.

### Surgery

If drug therapy is unsuccessful, treatment may include transurethral resection of the prostate, which requires removal of all infected tissue. However, this procedure is usually not performed on young adults because it may cause retrograde ejaculation and sterility. Total prostatectomy is curative but may cause impotence and incontinence.

## Special considerations

• Ensure bed rest and adequate hydration. Provide stool softeners and administer sitz baths as required.

• As necessary, prepare to assist with suprapubic needle aspiration of the bladder or a suprapubic cystostomy.

• Emphasize the need for strict adherence to the prescribed drug regimen. Instruct the patient to drink at least 8 glasses of water a day. Have him report adverse drug reactions (rash, nausea, vomiting, fever, chills, and GI irritation).

# PROTEIN-CALORIE MALNUTRITION

One of the most prevalent and serious depletion disorders, protein-calorie malnutrition (PCM) occurs as marasmus (protein-calorie deficiency), characterized by growth failure and wasting, and as kwashiorkor (protein deficiency), characterized by tissue edema and damage. Both forms vary from mild to severe and may be fatal, depending on accompanying stress (particularly sepsis or injury) and duration of deprivation. PCM increases the risk of death from pneumonia, chickenpox, or measles.

## Causes

Both marasmus (nonedematous PCM) and kwashiorkor (edematous PCM) are common in underdeveloped countries and in areas where dietary amino acid content is insufficient to satisfy growth requirements. Kwashiorkor typically occurs at about age 1, after infants are weaned from breast milk to a protein-deficient diet of starchy gruels or sugar water, but it can develop at any time during the formative years. Marasmus affects infants ages 6 to 18 months as a result of breast-feeding failure or a debilitating condition such as chronic diarrhea.

In industrialized countries, PCM may occur secondary to chronic metabolic disease that decreases protein and calorie intake or absorption, or trauma that increases protein and calorie requirements. In the United States, PCM is estimated to occur to some extent in 50% of surgical and 48% of medical patients. Those who aren't allowed anything by mouth for an extended period are at high risk of developing PCM. Conditions that increase protein-calorie requirements include severe burns and injuries, systemic infections, and cancer (accounts for the largest group of hospitalized patients with PCM). Conditions that cause defective utilization of nutrients include malabsorption syndrome, short-bowel syndrome, and Crohn's disease.

## Signs and symptoms

Children with chronic PCM are small for their chronological age and tend to be physically inactive, mentally apathetic, and susceptible to frequent infections. Anorexia and diarrhea are common.

In acute PCM, children are small, gaunt, and emaciated, with no adipose tissue. Skin is dry and "baggy," and hair is sparse and dull brown or reddish yellow. Temperature is low; pulse rate and respirations, slowed. Such children are weak, irritable, and usually hungry, although they may have anorexia, with nausea and vomiting.

Unlike marasmus, chronic kwashiorkor allows the patient to grow in height, but adipose tissue diminishes as fat metabolizes to meet energy demands. Edema often masks severe muscle wasting; dry, peeling skin and hepatomegaly are common. Patients with secondary PCM show signs similar to marasmus, primarily loss of adipose tissue and lean body mass, lethargy, and edema. Severe secondary PCM may cause loss of immunocompetence.

## Diagnosis

Clinical appearance, dietary history, and anthropometry confirm PCM. If the patient doesn't suffer from fluid retention, weight change over time is the best index of nutritional status.

The following factors support the diagnosis:

• height and weight less than 80% of standard for the patient's age and sex, and below-normal arm circumference and triceps skinfold

• serum albumin level < 2.8 g/dl (normal: 3.3 to 4.3 g/dl)

• urinary creatinine (24-hour) level is used to show lean body mass status by relating creatinine excretion to height and ideal body weight, to yield creatinine-height index

• skin tests with standard antigens to indicate degree of immunocompromise by determining reactivity expressed as a percentage of normal reaction

• moderate anemia.

## Treatment

The aim of treatment is to provide sufficient proteins, calories, and other nutrients for nutritional rehabilitation and maintenance. When treating severe PCM, restoring fluid and electrolyte balance parenterally is the initial concern. A patient who shows normal absorption may receive enteral nutrition after anorexia has subsided. When possible, the preferred treatment is oral feeding of high-quality protein foods, especially milk, and protein-calorie supplements. A patient who is unwilling or unable to eat may require supplementary feedings through a nasogastric tube or total parenteral nutrition (TPN) through a central venous catheter. Accompanying infection must also be treated, preferably with antibiotics that do not inhibit protein synthesis. Cautious realimentation is essential to prevent complications from overloading the compromised metabolic system.

## Special considerations

• Encourage the patient with PCM to consume as much nutritious food and beverage as possible (it's often helpful to "cheer him on" as he eats). Assist the patient to eat if necessary. Cooperate closely with the dietitian to monitor intake, and provide acceptable meals and snacks.

• If TPN is necessary, observe strict aseptic technique when handling catheters, tubes, and solutions and during dressing changes.

• Watch for PCM in patients who have been hospitalized for a prolonged period, have had no oral intake for several days, or have cachectic disease.

• To help eradicate PCM in developing countries, encourage prolonged breast-feeding, educate mothers about their children's needs, and provide supplementary foods as needed.

CLINICAL TIP  If the older patient is anorectic, consider asking family members and other visitors to bring in special foods from home that may improve the patient's appetite. In addition, encouraging the family to collaborate on feeding a dependent patient can help promote his recovery, enhance his feelings of well-being, and stimulate him to eat more.

LIFE-THREATENING DISORDER

# PSEUDOMEMBRANOUS ENTEROCOLITIS

An acute inflammation and necrosis of the small and large intestines, pseudomembranous enterocolitis usually affects the mucosa but may extend into submucosa and, rarely, other layers. Marked by severe diarrhea, this rare condition is generally fatal in 1 to 7 days from severe dehydration and from toxicity, peritonitis, or perforation.

## Causes

Pseudomembranous enterocolitis is thought to be caused by a change in the flora of the colon and an overgrowth of a toxin-producing strain of *Clostridium difficile.*

Pseudomembranous enterocolitis has occurred postoperatively in debilitated patients who undergo abdominal surgery or patients who have been treated with broad-spectrum antibiotics. Ampicillin, clindamycin, and cephalosporins are suspected as causative factors. Immunocompromised patients (such as individuals with cystic fibrosis, neurologic disease, liver and renal disease, diabetes mellitus, malnutrition, and hematologic disorders) are at increased risk for this disease. Whatever the cause, necrosed mucosa is replaced by a pseudomembrane filled with staphylococci, leukocytes, mucus, fibrin, and inflammatory cells.

## Signs and symptoms

Pseudomembranous enterocolitis begins suddenly with copious watery diarrhea, abdominal pain, and fever. Diarrhea, with or without blood, and abdominal pain may occur within 48 hours after administration of the drug. Signs and symptoms may begin with mild to moderate watery diarrhea with lower abdominal cramping. As the disease progresses, the patient may have profuse watery diarrhea with up to 30 stools per day and abdominal pain. Low-grade fever, along with abdominal tenderness and leukocytosis, occurs.

In a small number of presenting patients, colitis will develop with bradycardia, fever, abdominal pain, and distention. Serious complications may be associated with this disorder. They include such conditions as severe dehydration, electrolyte imbalance, hypotension, shock, and colonic perforation.

## Diagnosis

In this disorder, diagnosis is often difficult because of the abrupt onset of enterocolitis and the emergency situation it creates, so consideration of patient history is essential. A rectal biopsy through sigmoidoscopy confirms pseudomembranous enterocolitis. Stool cultures can identify *C. difficile.*

## Treatment

A patient who is receiving broad-spectrum antibiotic therapy requires immediate discontinuation of the antibiotics. If possible, medications that slow peristalsis should be avoided. Effective treatment usually includes orally administered metronidazole (250 mg). Oral vancomycin is usually given for severe or resistant cases, but this is costly.

Supportive treatment must maintain fluid and electrolyte balance and combat hypotension and shock with pressors, such as dopamine and levarterenol.

## Special considerations

● Monitor vital signs, skin color, and level of consciousness. Be alert for signs of shock.

● Record fluid intake and output, including fluid lost in stools. Watch for dehydration (poor skin turgor, sunken eyes, and decreased urine output).

● Check serum electrolyte levels daily, and watch for clinical signs of hypokalemia, especially malaise and a weak, rapid, irregular pulse.

➤ CLINICAL TIP Excessive diarrhea may cause excoriation and skin breakdown. To decrease excoriation and facilitate drainage measurement, insert a rectal tube or large indwelling catheter (inserted but not inflated) into the rectum and attach it to a drainage bag to gravity as ordered.

---

**LIFE-THREATENING DISORDER**

# *PSEUDOMONAS* INFECTIONS

---

*Pseudomonas* is a small gram-negative bacillus that produces nosocomial infections, superinfections of various parts of the body, and a rare disease called melioidosis. This bacillus is also associated with bacteremia, endocarditis, and osteomyelitis in drug addicts.

In local *Pseudomonas* infections, treatment is usually successful and complications rare. However, in patients with poor immunologic resistance — premature infants, the elderly, or those with debilitating disease, burns, or wounds — septicemic *Pseudomonas* infections are serious and sometimes fatal.

## Causes

The most common species of *Pseudomonas* is *P. aeruginosa*. Other species that typically cause disease in humans include *P. maltophilia, P. cepacia, P. fluorescens, P. testosteroni, P. acidovorans, P. alcaligenes, P. stutzeri, P. putrefaciens,* and *P. putida.*

These organisms are frequently found in hospital liquids that have been allowed to stand for a long time, such as benzalkonium chloride, hexachlorophene soap, saline solution, penicillin, water in flower vases, and fluids in incubators, humidifiers, and respiratory therapy equipment.

In elderly patients, *Pseudomonas* infection usually enters through the genitourinary tract; in infants, through the umbilical cord, skin, and GI tract.

## Signs and symptoms

The most common infections associated with *Pseudomonas* include skin infections (such as burns and pressure ulcers), urinary tract infections, infant epidemic diarrhea and other diarrheal illnesses, bronchitis, pneumonia, bronchiectasis, meningitis, corneal ulcers, mastoiditis, otitis externa, otitis media, endocarditis, and bacteremia.

Drainage in these infections has a distinct, sickly sweet odor and a greenish-blue pus that forms a crust on wounds. Other symptoms depend on the site of infection. For example, when it invades the lungs, *Pseudomonas* causes pneumonia with fever, chills, and a productive cough.

## Diagnosis

Diagnosis requires isolation of the *Pseudomonas* organism in blood, spinal fluid, urine, exudate, or sputum culture.

## Treatment

In the debilitated or otherwise vulnerable patient with clinical evidence of *Pseudomonas* infection, treatment should begin immediately, without waiting for results of laboratory tests. Antibiotic treatment includes aminoglycosides, such as gentamicin or tobramycin, combined with a *Pseudomonas*-sensitive penicillin, such as carbenicillin disodium or ticarcillin. An alternative combination is amikacin and a similar penicillin. Such combination therapy is necessary because *Pseudomonas* quickly becomes resistant to carbenicillin alone.

▶ CLINICAL TIP  In bacteremia, an aminoglycoside and beta-lactam with anti-*Pseudomonal* activity increases survival rates.

In urinary tract infections, carbenicillin indanyl sodium can be used alone if the organism is susceptible and the infection doesn't have systemic effects; it is excreted in the urine and builds up high urine levels that prevent resistance.

Local *Pseudomonas* infections or septicemia secondary to wound infection requires 1% acetic acid irrigations, topical application of colistimethate sodium and polymyxin B, and debridement or drainage of the infected wound.

### Special considerations

• Observe and record the character of wound exudate and sputum.

• Before administering antibiotics, ask the patient about a history of allergies, especially to penicillin.

➤ CLINICAL TIP  If combinations of carbenicillin or ticarcillin and an aminoglycoside are ordered, schedule the doses 1 hour apart (carbenicillin and ticarcillin may decrease the antibiotic effect of the aminoglycoside). *Don't give both antibiotics through the same administration set.*

• Monitor the patient's renal function (urine output, blood urea nitrogen, specific gravity, urinalysis, creatinine) during treatment with aminoglycosides.

• Protect immunocompromised patients from exposure to this infection. Attention to hand washing and aseptic techniques prevent further spread.

• To prevent *Pseudomonas* infection, maintain proper endotracheal and tracheostomy suctioning technique: Use strict sterile technique when caring for I.V. lines, catheters, and other tubes; dispose of suction bottle contents properly; and label and date solution bottles and change them frequently, according to policy.

# PSORIASIS

This chronic, recurrent disease is marked by epidermal proliferation. Its lesions, which appear as erythematous papules and plaques covered with silver scales, vary widely in severity and distribution. Psoriasis affects about 21% of the population in the United States.

Although this disorder often affects young adults, it may strike at any age, including infancy. Psoriasis is characterized by recurring partial remissions and exacerbations. Flare-ups are often related to specific systemic and environmental factors but may be unpredictable; they can usually be controlled with therapy.

### Causes

The tendency to develop psoriasis is genetically determined. Researchers have discovered a significantly higher-than-normal incidence of certain human leukocyte antigens (HLA) in families with psoriasis, suggesting a possible immune disorder. Onset of the disease is also influenced by environmental factors.

Trauma can trigger the isomorphic effect or Koebner's phenomenon, in which lesions develop at sites of injury. Infections, especially those resulting from beta-hemolytic streptococci, may cause a flare-up of guttate (drop-shaped) lesions. Other contributing factors include pregnancy, endocrine changes, climate (cold weather tends to exacerbate psoriasis), and emotional stress.

Generally, a skin cell takes 14 days to move from the basal layer to the stratum corneum, where after 14 days of normal wear and tear, it's sloughed off. The life cycle of a normal skin cell is 28 days, compared to only 4 days for a psoriatic skin cell. This markedly short-ened cycle doesn't allow time for the cell to mature. Consequently, the stratum corneum becomes thick and flaky, producing the cardinal manifestations of psoriasis.

### Signs and symptoms

The most common complaint of the patient with psoriasis is itching and occasional pain from dry, cracked, encrusted lesions.

### *Plaques*

Psoriatic lesions are erythematous and usually form well-defined plaques, sometimes covering large areas of the body (See *Viewing psoriasis.*) Such lesions most commonly appear on the scalp, chest, elbows, knees, back, and buttocks.

The plaques consist of characteristic silver scales that either flake off easily or can thicken, covering the lesion. Removal of psoriatic scales frequently produces fine bleeding points (Auspitz sign). Occasionally, small guttate lesions appear, either alone or with plaques; these lesions are typically thin and erythematous, with few scales.

Widespread involvement of scales and erythema is called exfoliative or erythrodermic psoriasis. In about 60% of patients, psoriasis spreads to the fingernails, producing small indentations or pits and yellow or brown discoloration. In some cases, the accumulation of thick, crumbly debris under the nail causes it to separate from the nailbed (onycholysis).

### *Pustular psoriasis*

Rarely, psoriasis becomes pustular, taking one of two forms. In localized pustular psoriasis, pustules appear on the palms and soles and remain sterile until opened. In generalized pustular (Von Zumbusch) psoriasis, which often oc-

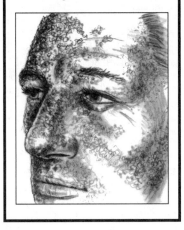

## VIEWING PSORIASIS

In this patient with psoriasis, plaques consisting of silver scales cover a large area of the face.

curs with fever, leukocytosis, and malaise, groups of pustules coalesce to form lakes of pus on red skin. These pustules also remain sterile until opened and commonly involve the tongue and oral mucosa.

### *Arthritic symptoms*

Some patients with psoriasis develop arthritic symptoms, usually in one or more joints of the fingers or toes, in the larger joints, or sometimes in the sacroiliac joints, which may progress to spondylitis. Such patients may complain of morning stiffness. Joint symptoms show no consistent linkage to the course of the cutaneus manifestations of psoriasis; they demonstrate remissions and exacerbations similar to those of rheumatoid arthritis.

### Diagnosis

Diagnosis depends on patient history, appearance of the lesions and, if needed, the results of skin biopsy. Typically, serum uric acid level is elevated in severe cases, due to accelerated nucleic acid degradation, but indications of gout are absent. HLA-Cw6, B-13, and Bw-57 may be present in early-onset familial psoriasis.

## Treatment

Appropriate treatment depends on the type of psoriasis, the extent of the disease and the patient's response to it, and what effect the disease has on the patient's lifestyle. No permanent cure exists, and all methods of treatment are palliative.

### UVB exposure

Methods to retard rapid cell production include exposure to ultraviolet light (UVB or natural sunlight) to the point of minimal erythema. Tar preparations or crude coal tar itself may be applied to affected areas about 15 minutes before exposure or may be left on overnight and wiped off the next morning.

A thin layer of petroleum jelly may be applied before UVB exposure (the most common treatment for generalized psoriasis). Exposure time can increase gradually. Outpatient or day treatment with UVB avoids long hospitalizations and prolongs remission.

### Drug therapy

Steroid creams and ointments are useful to control psoriasis. A potent fluorinated steroid works well, except on the face and intertriginous areas. These creams require application two times a day, preferably after bathing to facilitate absorption, and overnight use of occlusive dressings, such as plastic wrap, plastic gloves or booties, or a vinyl exercise suit (under direct medical or nursing supervision).

Small, stubborn plaques may require intralesional steroid injections. Anthralin ointment or paste mixture may be used for well-defined plaques but must not be applied to unaffected areas because it causes injury and stains normal skin. Apply petroleum jelly around the affected skin before applying anthralin. Often used concurrently with steroids, anthralin is applied at night and steroids during the day. A new topical agent is calcipotriene ointment, a vitamin $D_3$ analogue.

> **CLINICAL TIP** Calcipotriene treatment also works best when alternated with a topical steroid, as noted above with anthralin.

### Goeckerman, Ingram, and PUVA

In a patient with severe chronic psoriasis, the Goeckerman regimen — which combines tar baths and UVB treatments — may help achieve remission and clear the skin in 3 to 5 weeks. The Ingram technique is a variation of this treatment, using anthralin instead of tar. A therapy called PUVA combines administration of psoralens with exposure to high-intensity UVA.

### Other treatments

As a last resort, a cytotoxin, usually methotrexate, may help severe, refractory psoriasis. Acitretin, a retinoid compound, is effective in treating extensive cases of psoriasis. However, because this drug is a strong teratogen, it is unsafe for use in women of childbearing age. Cyclosporine, an immunosuppressant, may be used in resistive cases.

Low-dose antihistamines, oatmeal baths, emollients, and open wet dressings may help relieve pruritus. Aspirin and local heat help alleviate the pain of psoriatic arthritis; severe cases may require nonsteroidal anti-inflammatory drugs.

Therapy for psoriasis of the scalp consists of a tar shampoo followed by application of a steroid lotion. No effective topical treatment exists for psoriasis of the nails.

**Special considerations**
● Design your care to include patient teaching and careful monitoring for adverse effects of therapy.
● Make sure the patient understands his prescribed therapy; provide written instructions to avoid confusion.
● Teach correct application of prescribed ointments, creams, and lotions. A steroid cream, for example, should be applied in a thin film and rubbed gently into the skin until the cream disappears.
● Warn the patient never to put an occlusive dressing over anthralin. Suggest use of mineral oil, then soap and water, to remove anthralin.
● Caution the patient to avoid scrubbing his skin vigorously, to prevent Koebner's phenomenon. If a medication has been applied to the scales to soften them, suggest the patient use a soft brush to remove them.
● Watch for adverse reactions, especially allergic reactions to anthralin, atrophy and acne from steroids, and burning, itching, nausea, and squamous cell epitheliomas from PUVA.
● Initially evaluate the patient on methotrexate weekly, then monthly for red blood cell, white blood cell, and platelet counts because cytotoxins may cause hepatic or bone marrow toxicity. Liver biopsy may be done to assess the effects of methotrexate.
● Caution the patient receiving PUVA therapy to stay out of the sun on the day of treatment, and to protect his eyes with sunglasses that screen UVA for 24 hours after treatment. Tell him to wear goggles during exposure to this light.

● Be aware that psoriasis can cause psychological problems. Assure the patient that psoriasis is not contagious, and although exacerbations and remissions occur, they're controllable with treatment. However, be sure he understands there is no cure.
● Because stressful situations tend to exacerbate psoriasis, help the patient learn to cope with these situations.
● Explain the relationship between psoriasis and arthritis, but point out that psoriasis causes no other systemic disturbances.
● Refer all patients to the National Psoriasis Foundation, which provides information and directs patients to local chapters.

# PSORIATIC ARTHRITIS

Psoriatic arthritis is a rheumatoid-like joint disease associated with psoriasis of skin and nails. Although the arthritis component of this syndrome may be clinically indistinguishable from rheumatoid arthritis, the rheumatoid nodules are absent, and serologic tests for rheumatoid factor are negative. Some patients develop a more asymmetrical oligoarthritis affecting large or small joints. Psoriatic arthritis usually is mild, with intermittent flare-ups, but in rare cases it may progress to crippling arthritis mutilans. This disease affects both men and women equally; onset usually occurs between the ages of 30 and 35.

CLINICAL TIP  To help differentiate between psoriatric and rheumatoid arthritis, keep in mind that in psoriatic arthritis, the disease may be asymmetrical, psoriasis is present, and bone erosion with areas of "fluffy" new bone growth may be seen on X-ray films. Rheumatoid arthritis, however, is usually symmetrical, and X-ray studies don't show new bone formation.

## Causes

Evidence suggests that predisposition to psoriatic arthritis is hereditary; 20% to 50% of patients are HLA-B27–positive. However, onset may be precipitated by streptococcal infection or trauma.

## Signs and symptoms

Psoriatic lesions usually precede the arthritic component, but once the full syndrome is established, joint and skin lesions may recur simultaneously. Arthritis may involve one joint or several joints asymmetrically or symmetrically. Spinal involvement occurs in some patients. Peripheral joint involvement is most common in the distal interphalangeal joints of the hands, which have a characteristic sausage-like appearance. Nail changes include pitting, transverse ridges, onycholysis, keratosis, yellowing, and destruction. The patient may experience general malaise, fever, and eye involvement.

## Diagnosis

Inflammatory arthritis in a patient with psoriatic skin lesions suggests psoriatic arthritis. X-rays confirm joint involvement and show:
- marginal erosion at interphalangeal joints with areas of thin, "fluffy" new bone formation
- "whittling" of the distal end of the terminal phalanges
- "pencil-in-cup" deformity of the distal interphalangeal joints
- relative absence of osteoporosis
- sacroiliitis
- atypical spondylitis with syndesmophyte formation, resulting in hyperostosis and paravertebral ossification, which may lead to vertebral fusion.

Blood studies indicate negative rheumatoid factor and elevated erythrocyte sedimentation rate and uric acid levels.

## Treatment

In mild psoriatic arthritis, treatment is supportive and consists of immobilization through joint rest or splints, isometric exercises, paraffin baths, heat therapy, and aspirin and other nonsteroidal anti-inflammatory drugs. Some patients respond well to low-dose systemic corticosteroids; topical steroids may help control skin lesions. Gold salts, cyclosporin, sulfasalazines, and—most commonly—methotrexate therapy are effective in treating both the articular and cutaneous effects of psoriatic arthritis. Antimalarials may be used with caution because they can provoke exfoliative dermatitis.

## Special considerations

- Explain the disease and its treatment to the patient and his family.
- Reassure the patient that psoriatic plaques aren't contagious. Avoid showing revulsion at the sight of psoriatic patches—doing so will only reinforce the patient's fear of rejection.
- Encourage exercise, particularly swimming, to maintain strength and range of motion.
- Teach the patient how to apply skin care products and medications correctly; explain possible adverse effects.
- Stress the importance of adequate rest and protection of affected joints.
- Encourage regular, moderate exposure to the sun.
- Refer the patient to the Arthritis Foundation for self-help and support groups.

## LIFE-THREATENING DISORDER

# PULMONARY EDEMA

In pulmonary edema, fluid accumulates in the extravascular spaces of the lung. In cardiogenic pulmonary edema, fluid accumulation results from elevations in pulmonary venous and capillary hydrostatic pressures. A common complication of cardiac disorders, pulmonary edema can occur as a chronic condition or develop quickly and rapidly become fatal.

## Causes

Pulmonary edema usually results from left ventricular failure due to arteriosclerotic, hypertensive, cardiomyopathic, or valvular cardiac disease. In such disorders, the compromised left ventricle requires increased filling pressures to maintain adequate output; these pressures are transmitted to the left atrium, pulmonary veins, and pulmonary capillary bed.

This increased pulmonary capillary hydrostatic force promotes transudation of intravascular fluids into the pulmonary interstitium, decreasing lung compliance and interfering with gas exchange. Other factors that may predispose a person to pulmonary edema include:

• infusion of excessive volumes of I.V. fluids

• decreased serum colloid osmotic pressure as a result of nephrosis, extensive burns, hepatic disease, or nutritional deficiency

• impaired lung lymphatic drainage from Hodgkin's disease or obliterative lymphangitis after radiation

• mitral stenosis and left atrial myxoma, which impair left atrial emptying

• pulmonary veno-occlusive disease.

## Signs and symptoms

Symptoms vary with the stage of pulmonary edema.

### Early symptoms

The early symptoms of pulmonary edema reflect interstitial fluid accumulation and diminished lung compliance: dyspnea on exertion, paroxysmal nocturnal dyspnea, orthopnea, and coughing. Clinical features include tachycardia, tachypnea, dependent crackles, neck vein distention, and a diastolic ($S_3$) gallop.

### Later symptoms

With severe pulmonary edema, the alveoli and bronchioles may fill with fluid and intensify the early symptoms. Respiration becomes labored and rapid, with more diffuse crackles and coughing productive of frothy, bloody sputum. Tachycardia increases and arrhythmias may occur. Skin becomes cold, clammy, diaphoretic, and cyanotic. Blood pressure falls and pulse becomes thready as cardiac output falls.

Symptoms of severe heart failure with pulmonary edema may also include depressed level of consciousness and confusion.

## Diagnosis

Clinical features of pulmonary edema permit a working diagnosis. The following tests are also helpful:

• *Arterial blood gas (ABG) analysis* usually shows hypoxia; partial pressure of arterial carbon dioxide varies. Both profound respiratory alkalosis and acidosis may occur. Metabolic acidosis occurs when cardiac output is low.

• *Chest X-ray* shows diffuse haziness of the lung fields and, often, cardiomegaly and pleural effusions.

• *Pulmonary artery catheterization* helps identify left ventricular failure by showing elevated pulmonary artery wedge pressures. This helps to rule out adult respiratory distress syndrome — in which pulmonary wedge pressure is usually normal.

**Treatment**

In pulmonary edema, treatment is designed to reduce extravascular fluid, to improve gas exchange and myocardial function and, if possible, to correct the underlying disorder.

Administration of high concentrations of oxygen by a cannula, a face mask and, if the patient fails to maintain an acceptable partial pressure of arterial oxygen, assisted ventilation improves oxygen delivery to the tissues and usually improves acid-base disturbances.

Diuretics — furosemide and bumetanide, for example — promote diuresis, which in turn helps to mobilize extravascular fluid.

Treatment of myocardial dysfunction includes a digitalis glycoside or pressor agents to increase cardiac contractility, antiarrhythmics (particularly when arrhythmias are associated with decreased cardiac output) and, occasionally, arterial vasodilators, such as nitroprusside, which decrease peripheral vascular resistance, preload, and afterload.

Other treatment includes morphine to reduce anxiety and dyspnea and to dilate the systemic venous bed, promoting blood flow from the pulmonary circulation to the periphery.

**Special considerations**

• Carefully monitor the vulnerable patient for early signs of pulmonary edema, especially tachypnea, tachycardia, and abnormal breath sounds. Check for peripheral edema, which may also indicate that fluid is accumulating in pulmonary tissue.

• Administer oxygen as necessary.

• Monitor vital signs every 15 to 30 minutes while administering nitroprusside in dextrose 5% in water by I.V. drip.

> **CLINICAL TIP** Protect nitroprusside from light by wrapping the bottle or bag with aluminum foil.

• Watch for arrhythmias in patients receiving a digitalis glycoside and for marked respiratory depression in those receiving morphine.

• Assess the patient's condition frequently, and record his response to treatment.

• Monitor ABG levels, oral and I.V. fluid intake, urine output and, in the patient with a pulmonary artery catheter, pulmonary end-diastolic and wedge pressures. Check the cardiac monitor often.

---

**LIFE-THREATENING DISORDER**

# PULMONARY EMBOLISM AND INFARCTION

---

The most common pulmonary complication in hospitalized patients, pulmonary embolism is an obstruction of the pulmonary arterial bed by a dislodged thrombus or foreign substance. It strikes an estimated 6 million adults each year in the United States, resulting in 100,000 deaths.

Although pulmonary infarction may be so mild as to be asymptomatic, massive embolism (more than 50% obstruction of pulmonary arterial circulation) and infarction can be rapidly fatal.

## Causes

Pulmonary embolism generally results from dislodged thrombi originating in the leg veins. More than half of such thrombi arise in the deep veins of the legs and are usually multiple.

Other less common sources of thrombi are the pelvic veins, renal veins, hepatic vein, right heart, and upper extremities. Such thrombus formation results directly from vascular wall damage, venostasis, or hypercoagulability of the blood.

### Rare causes

Rarely, the emboli contain air, fat, amniotic fluid, talc (from drugs intended for oral administration that are injected I.V. by addicts), or tumor cells. Thrombi may embolize spontaneously during clot dissolution or may be dislodged during trauma, sudden muscular action, or a change in peripheral blood flow.

Rarely, pulmonary infarction (tissue death) may evolve from pulmonary embolism. Pulmonary infarction develops more frequently when pulmonary embolism occurs in patients with chronic cardiac or pulmonary disease. However if the embolus obstructs a large vessel, bronchial circulation may provide an inadequate oxygen supply to the lung supplied by the occluded vessel.

### Risk factors

Predisposing factors to pulmonary embolism include:
- long-term immobility
- chronic pulmonary disease
- heart failure or atrial fibrillation
- thrombophlebitis, polycythemia vera, thrombocytosis, autoimmune hemolytic anemia, and sickle cell disease
- varicose veins and vascular injury
- recent surgery
- advanced age
- pregnancy

- lower extremity fractures or surgery
- burns
- obesity
- malignancy
- use of oral contraceptives.

## Signs and symptoms

Total occlusion of the main pulmonary artery is rapidly fatal; smaller or fragmented emboli produce symptoms that vary with the size, number, and location of the emboli. Usually, the first symptom of pulmonary embolism is dyspnea, which may be accompanied by anginal or pleuritic chest pain.

Other clinical features include tachycardia, productive cough (sputum may be blood-tinged), low-grade fever, and pleural effusion. Less common signs include massive hemoptysis, splinting of the chest, leg edema and, with a large embolus, cyanosis, syncope, and distended neck veins.

In addition, pulmonary embolism may cause pleural friction rub and signs of circulatory collapse (weak, rapid pulse; hypotension) and hypoxia (restlessness).

## Diagnosis

The patient history reveals any predisposing conditions for pulmonary embolism. The following diagnostic tests are also helpful:

- *Chest X-ray* helps to rule out other pulmonary diseases; it also shows areas of atelectasis, elevated diaphragm and pleural effusion, prominent pulmonary artery and, occasionally, the characteristic wedge-shaped infiltrate suggestive of pulmonary infarction.

- *Lung scan* shows perfusion defects in areas beyond occluded vessels; however, it doesn't rule out microemboli.

- *Pulmonary angiography* is the most definitive test but requires a skilled angiographer and radiologic equipment; it also poses some risk to the patient.

Its use depends on the uncertainty of the diagnosis and the need to avoid unnecessary anticoagulant therapy in high-risk patients.

• *Electrocardiography (ECG)* is inconclusive but helps distinguish pulmonary embolism from myocardial infarction. In extensive embolism, the ECG may show right axis deviation; right bundle-branch block; tall, peaked P waves; depression of ST segments and T-wave inversions (indicating right heart strain); and supraventricular tachyarrhythmias.

• *Auscultation* occasionally reveals a right ventricular $S_3$ gallop and increased intensity of the pulmonic component of $S_2$. Also, crackles and a pleural rub may be heard at the site of embolism.

• *Arterial blood gas (ABG) analysis* showing decreased partial pressure of arterial oxygen and carbon dioxide are characteristic but don't always occur.

If pleural effusion is present, thoracentesis may rule out empyema, which indicates pneumonia.

## Treatment

In pulmonary embolism, treatment is designed to maintain adequate cardiovascular and pulmonary function during resolution of the obstruction and to prevent recurrence of embolic episodes.

### Oxygen and anticoagulants

Because most emboli resolve within 10 to 14 days, treatment consists of oxygen therapy, as needed, and anticoagulation with heparin to inhibit new thrombus formation. Heparin therapy is monitored by daily coagulation studies (partial thromboplastin time [PTT]).

### Drug therapy

Patients with massive pulmonary embolism and shock may need fibrinolytic therapy with urokinase, streptokinase, or alteplase to enhance fibrinolysis of the pulmonary emboli and remaining thrombi. Emboli that cause hypotension may require the use of vasopressors. Treatment of septic emboli requires antibiotics, not anticoagulants, and evaluation for the infection's source, particularly endocarditis.

### Surgery

Interruption of the inferior vena cava is used for patients who can't take anticoagulants, who have recurrent emboli during anticoagulant therapy, or who have been treated with thrombolytic agents or pulmonary thromboendarterectomy.

Surgery (which shouldn't be done without angiographic evidence of pulmonary embolism) consists of vena caval ligation, plication, or insertion of a device (umbrella filter) to filter blood returning to the heart and lungs. To prevent postoperative venous thromboembolism, a combination of heparin and dihydroergotamine may be given.

## Special considerations

• Give oxygen by nasal cannula or mask. Check ABG levels in the event of fresh emboli or worsening dyspnea.

• Be prepared to provide endotracheal intubation with assisted ventilation if breathing is severely compromised.

• Administer heparin, as needed, through I.V. push or continuous drip. Monitor coagulation studies daily. Effective heparin therapy raises PTT to approximately 1½ to 2½ times normal.

• Watch closely for nosebleed, petechiae, and other signs of abnormal bleeding; check stools for occult blood. Tell the patient to prevent bleeding by shaving with an electric razor and by brushing his teeth with a soft toothbrush.

• After the patient is stable, encourage him to move about frequently, and assist with isometric and range-of-motion exercises.

• Check pedal pulses, temperature, and color of feet to detect venostasis. *Never* vigorously massage the patient's legs.

• Help the patient walk as soon as possible after surgery to prevent venostasis.

• Maintain adequate nutrition and fluid balance to promote healing.

• Note frequent pleuritic chest pain so that analgesics can be prescribed.

• Use incentive spirometry to assist in deep breathing. Provide tissues and a bag for easy disposal of expectorations.

• Warn the patient not to cross his legs; this promotes thrombus formation.

• Most patients need treatment with an oral anticoagulant (warfarin) for 4 to 6 months after a pulmonary embolism.

CLINICAL TIP   Advise patients taking anticoagulants to watch for signs of bleeding (bloody stools, blood in urine, large ecchymoses), to take the prescribed medication exactly as ordered, and to avoid taking any additional medication (even for headaches or colds) or changing doses of medication without consulting their doctors.

• Stress the importance of follow-up laboratory tests (prothrombin time) to monitor anticoagulant therapy.

• To prevent pulmonary emboli, encourage early ambulation in patients predisposed to this condition. With close medical supervision, low-dose heparin may be useful prophylactically.

# PULMONARY HYPERTENSION

Pulmonary hypertension occurs when pulmonary artery pressure (PAP) rises above normal and isn't attributable to the effects of aging or altitude. There is no definitive set of values used to diagnose pulmonary hypertension, but the National Institutes of Health requires that the resting mean PAP measures 25 mm Hg or more.

*Primary,* or *idiopathic, pulmonary hypertension* is rare, occurring most often in women between the ages of 20 and 40; pregnant women have the highest mortality. *Secondary pulmonary hypertension* results from existing cardiac or pulmonary disease. The prognosis depends on the severity of the underlying disorder.

## Causes

Primary pulmonary hypertension begins as hypertrophy of the small pulmonary arteries. The medial and intimal muscle layers of these vessels thicken, decreasing distensibility and increasing resistance. This disorder then progresses to vascular sclerosis and obliteration of small vessels. Because this form of pulmonary hypertension occurs in association with collagen diseases, it is thought to result from altered immune mechanisms.

Usually, pulmonary hypertension is secondary to hypoxemia from an underlying disease process, including:

• *alveolar hypoventilation* from chronic obstructive pulmonary disease (most common cause in the United States), sarcoidosis, diffuse interstitial pneumonia, pulmonary metastasis, and certain diseases such as scleroderma.

These diseases may cause pulmonary hypertension through alveolar destruction and increased pulmonary vascular resistance. Other disorders that cause alveolar hypoventilation without lung tissue damage include obesity, kyphoscoliosis, and obstructive sleep apnea.

• *vascular obstruction* from pulmonary embolism, vasculitis, and disorders that cause obstructions of small or large pulmonary veins, such as left atrial myxoma, idiopathic veno-occlusive disease, fibrosing mediastinitis, and mediastinal neoplasm,

• *primary cardiac disease,* which may be congenital or acquired. Congenital defects that cause left-to-right shunting of blood—such as patent ductus arteriosus, or atrial or ventricular septal defect—increase blood flow into the lungs and consequently raise pulmonary vascular pressure.

Acquired cardiac disease, such as rheumatic valvular disease and mitral stenosis, increases pulmonary venous pressure by restricting blood flow returning to the heart.

### Signs and symptoms

Most patients complain of increasing dyspnea on exertion, weakness, syncope, and fatigability. Many also show signs of right heart failure, including peripheral edema, ascites, neck vein distention, and hepatomegaly. Other clinical effects vary according to the underlying disorder.

### Diagnosis

Characteristic diagnostic findings in patients with pulmonary hypertension include the following:

• *auscultation:* abnormalities associated with the underlying disorder

• *arterial blood gas (ABG) analysis:* hypoxemia (decreased partial pressure of oxygen)

• *electrocardiography:* in right ventricular hypertrophy, shows right axis deviation and tall or peaked P waves in inferior leads

• *cardiac catheterization:* increased PAP—pulmonary systolic pressure above 30 mm Hg; pulmonary artery wedge pressure (PAWP) increased if the underlying cause is left atrial myxoma, mitral stenosis, or left ventricular failure—otherwise normal

• *pulmonary angiography:* detects filling defects in pulmonary vasculature, such as those that develop in patients with pulmonary emboli

• *pulmonary function tests:* in underlying obstructive disease, may show decreased flow rates and increased residual volume; in underlying restrictive disease, total lung capacity may decrease.

### Treatment

Appropriate treatment usually includes oxygen therapy to decrease hypoxemia and resulting pulmonary vascular resistance. For patients with right heart failure, treatment also includes fluid restriction, digitalis glycosides to increase cardiac output, and diuretics to decrease intravascular volume and extravascular fluid accumulation. An important goal of treatment is correction of the underlying cause.

➤ CLINICAL TIP   Patients with primary pulmonary hypertension usually respond to epoprostenol ($PGI_2$) as a continuous home infusion.

### Special considerations

• Pulmonary hypertension requires keen observation and careful monitoring, as well as skilled supportive care.

• Administer oxygen therapy as required, and observe the response. Be alert for signs of increasing dyspnea so that treatment can be adjusted accordingly.

• Monitor ABG levels for acidosis and hypoxemia. Watch for changes in level of consciousness.

• When caring for a patient with right heart failure, especially one receiving diuretics, record weight daily, carefully measure intake and output, and explain all medications and diet restrictions.

• Check for increasing neck vein distention, which may indicate fluid overload.

• Monitor vital signs, especially blood pressure and heart rate. Watch for hypotension and tachycardia. If the patient has a pulmonary artery catheter, check PAP and PAWP as required and watch for any changes.

• Before discharge, help the patient adjust to the limitations imposed by this disorder.

• Advise against overexertion and suggest frequent rest periods between activities.

• Refer the patient to the social services department if special equipment, such as oxygen equipment, is needed for home use.

• Make sure the patient understands the prescribed diet and medications.

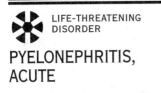

LIFE-THREATENING
DISORDER

# PYELONEPHRITIS, ACUTE

One of the most common renal diseases, acute pyelonephritis (also known as acute infective tubulointerstitial nephritis) is a sudden inflammation caused by bacteria that primarily affects the interstitial area and the renal pelvis or, less often, the renal tubules. With treatment and continued follow-up, the prognosis is good and extensive permanent damage is rare.

## Causes

Acute pyelonephritis results from bacterial infection of the kidneys. Infecting bacteria usually are normal intestinal and fecal flora that grow readily in urine. The most common causative organism is *Escherichia coli,* but *Proteus, Pseudomonas, Staphylococcus aureus,* and *Streptococcus faecalis* may also cause such infections.

Typically, the infection spreads from the bladder to the ureters, then to the kidneys, as in vesicoureteral reflux. Vesicoureteral reflux may result from congenital weakness at the junction of the ureter and the bladder. (See *Chronic pyelonephritis,* page 714.)

Bacteria refluxed to intrarenal tissues may create colonies of infection within 24 to 48 hours. Infection may also result from instrumentation (such as catheterization, cystoscopy, or urologic surgery), from a hematogenic infection (as in septicemia or endocarditis), or possibly from lymphatic infection.

Pyelonephritis may also result from an inability to empty the bladder (for example, in patients with neurogenic bladder), urinary stasis, or urinary obstruction due to tumors, strictures, or benign prostatic hyperplasia.

Pyelonephritis occurs more often in females, probably because of a shorter urethra and the proximity of the urinary meatus to the vagina and the rectum (both of which allow bacteria to reach the bladder more easily) and a lack of the antibacterial prostatic secretions produced in the male.

### Risk factors

Incidence increases with age and is higher in the following groups:

• *sexually active women* — increased risk of bacterial contamination from intercourse.

• *pregnant women* — about 5 % develop asymptomatic bacteriuria; if untreated, about 40% develop pyelonephritis.

• *diabetics* — neurogenic bladder causes incomplete emptying and urinary stasis; glycosuria may support bacterial growth in the urine.

## CHRONIC PYELONEPHRITIS

Chronic pyelonephritis is a persistent kidney inflammation that can scar the kidneys and may lead to chronic renal failure. Its etiology may be bacterial, metastatic, or urogenous. This disease is most common in patients who are predisposed to recurrent acute pyelonephritis, such as those with urinary obstructions or vesicoureteral reflux especially in late stages, hypertension. Uremia rarely develops from chronic pyelonephritis unless structural abnormalities exist in the excretory system. Bacteriuria may be intermittent. When no bacteria are found in the urine, diagnosis depends on excretory urography (renal pelvis may appear small and flattened) and renal biopsy.

### Clinical features
Patients with chronic pyelonephritis may have a childhood history of unexplained fevers or bedwetting. Signs and symptoms may include flank pain, anemia, low urine specific gravity, proteinuria, leukocytes in urine and,

### Treatment
Effective treatment of chronic pyelonephritis requires control of hypertension, elimination of the existing obstruction (when possible), and long-term antimicrobial therapy.

---

• *people with other renal diseases* — increased susceptibility resulting from compromised renal function.

### Signs and symptoms
Typical clinical features include urgency, frequency, burning during urination, dysuria, nocturia, and hematuria (usually microscopic but may be gross). Urine may appear cloudy and have an ammoniacal or fishy odor. Other common symptoms include a temperature of 102° F (38.9° C) or higher, shaking chills, flank pain, anorexia, and general fatigue.

These symptoms characteristically develop rapidly over a few hours or a few days. Although these symptoms may disappear within days, even without treatment, residual bacterial infection is likely and may cause later recurrence of symptoms.

### Diagnosis
Diagnosis requires urinalysis and culture. Typical findings include:

• *pyuria* (pus in urine) — urine sediment reveals the presence of leukocytes singly, in clumps, and in casts; and, possibly, a few red blood cells

• *significant bacteriuria* — more than 100,000 organisms/µl of urine revealed in urine culture

• *low specific gravity* and *osmolality* — resulting from a temporarily decreased ability to concentrate urine

• *slightly alkaline urine pH*

• *proteinuria, glycosuria,* and *ketonuria* — less common.

X-rays also help in the evaluation of acute pyelonephritis. X-rays of the kidneys-ureters-bladder may reveal calculi, tumors, or cysts in the kidneys and the urinary tract. Excretory urography may show asymmetrical kidneys.

### Treatment
Effective treatment centers on antibiotic therapy appropriate to the specific infecting organism after identification by urine culture and sensitivity studies.

### Antibiotic therapy

*S. faecalis* requires treatment with ampicillin, penicillin G, or vancomycin. *S. aureus* requires penicillin G or, if resistance develops, a semisynthetic penicillin, such as nafcillin, or a cephalosporin. *E. coli* may be treated with sulfisoxazole, nalidixic acid, and nitrofurantoin; *Proteus,* with ampicillin, sulfisoxazole, nalidixic acid, and a cephalosporin; and *Pseudomonas,* with gentamicin, tobramycin, and carbenicillin.

When the infecting organism can't be identified, therapy usually consists of a broad-spectrum antibiotic, such as ampicillin or cephalexin. If the patient is pregnant, antibiotics must be prescribed cautiously. Urinary analgesics such as phenazopyridine are also appropriate.

Symptoms may disappear after several days of antibiotic therapy. Although urine usually becomes sterile within 48 to 72 hours, the course of such therapy is 10 to 14 days.

### Follow-up treatment

Follow-up treatment includes reculturing urine 1 week after drug therapy stops, then periodically for the next year to detect residual or recurring infection. Most patients with uncomplicated infections respond well to therapy and don't suffer reinfection.

CLINICAL TIP   In infection from obstruction or vesicoureteral reflux, antibiotics may be less effective; treatment may then necessitate surgery to relieve the obstruction or correct the anomaly. Patients at high risk of recurring urinary tract and kidney infections — such as those with prolonged use of an indwelling urinary catheter or maintenance antibiotic therapy — require long-term follow-up.

---

TEACHING CHECKLIST

## PREVENTING ACUTE PYELONEPHRITIS

Review these teaching points with your patient to help prevent acute pyelonephritis.

• Instruct female patients to prevent bacterial contamination by wiping the perineum from front to back after defecation.
• Advise routine checkups for patients with a history of urinary tract infections.
• Teach patients to recognize signs of infection, such as cloudy urine, burning on urination, urgency, and frequency, especially when accompanied by a low-grade fever.

---

### Special considerations

• Administer antipyretics for fever.
• Force fluids to achieve urine output of more than 2,000 ml/day. This helps to empty the bladder of contaminated urine. Don't encourage intake of more than 3 L, because this may decrease the effectiveness of the antibiotics.
• Provide an acid-ash diet to prevent calculus formation.
• Teach proper technique for collecting a clean-catch urine specimen. Be sure to refrigerate or culture a urine specimen within 30 minutes of collection to prevent overgrowth of bacteria.
• Stress the need to complete prescribed antibiotic therapy, even after symptoms subside. Encourage long-term follow-up care for high-risk patients.
• For patient-teaching information on disease prevention, see *Preventing acute pyelonephritis.*

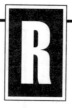

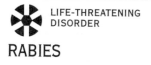
# RABIES

Usually transmitted by an animal bite, rabies (hydrophobia) is an acute central nervous system (CNS) infection caused by a ribonucleic acid virus.

If the bite is on the face, the risk of developing rabies is about 60%; on the upper extremities, 15% to 40%; and on the lower extremities, about 10%. In the United States, dog vaccinations have reduced rabies transmission to humans. Wild animals, such as skunks, foxes, and bats, account for 70% of rabies cases.

If symptoms occur, rabies is almost always fatal. Treatment soon after a bite, however, may prevent fatal CNS invasion.

## Causes

Generally, the rabies virus is transmitted to a human through the bite of an infected animal that introduces the virus through the skin or mucous membrane. The virus begins to replicate in the striated muscle cells at the bite site.

It next spreads up the nerve to the CNS and replicates in the brain. Finally, it moves through the nerves into other tissues, including the salivary glands. Occasionally, airborne droplets and in-fected tissue transplants can transmit the virus.

## Signs and symptoms

Clinical features are progressive.

### Local and prodromal symptoms

Typically, after an incubation period of 1 to 3 months, rabies produces local or radiating pain or burning, a sensation of cold, pruritus, and tingling at the bite site. It also produces prodromal symptoms, such as a slight fever (100° to 102° F [37.8° to 38.9° C]), malaise, headache, anorexia, nausea, sore throat, and persistent loose cough.

After this, the patient begins to show nervousness, anxiety, irritability, hyperesthesia, photophobia, sensitivity to loud noises, pupillary dilation, tachycardia, shallow respirations, and excessive salivation, lacrimation, and perspiration.

### Excitation and hydrophobia

About 2 to 10 days after onset of prodromal symptoms, a phase of excitation begins. It's characterized by agitation, marked restlessness, anxiety and apprehension, and cranial nerve dysfunction that causes ocular palsies, strabismus, asymmetrical pupillary dilation or constriction, absence of corneal reflexes, weakness of facial muscles, and hoarseness. Severe systemic symptoms include tachycardia or brachycardia, cyclic respirations, urinary retention, and a temperature of about 103° F (39.4° C).

About 50% of affected patients exhibit hydrophobia (literally, "fear of water"), during which forceful, painful pharyngeal muscle spasms expel liquids from the mouth and cause dehydration, and possibly apnea, cyanosis, and death. Difficulty swallowing causes frothy saliva to drool from the patient's mouth.

Eventually, even the sight, mention, or thought of water causes uncontrollable pharyngeal muscle spasms and excessive salivation. Between episodes of excitation and hydrophobia, the patient commonly is cooperative and lucid.

### Terminal phase

After about 3 days, excitation and hydrophobia subside and the progressively paralytic, terminal phase of this illness begins. The patient experiences gradual, generalized, flaccid paralysis that ultimately leads to peripheral vascular collapse, coma, and death.

### Diagnosis

Because rabies is fatal unless treated promptly, always suspect rabies in any person who suffers an unprovoked animal bite until you can prove otherwise.

Virus isolation from the patient's saliva or throat and examination of his blood for fluorescent rabies antibody (FRA) are considered the tests that provide the most definitive diagnosis. Other results typically include an elevated white blood cell count, with increased polymorphonuclear and large mononuclear cells, and elevated urinary glucose, acetone, and protein levels.

Confinement of the suspected animal for 10 days of observation by a veterinarian also helps support this diagnosis. If the animal appears rabid, it should be killed and its brain tissue tested for FRA and Negri bodies (oval or round

---

> **CLINICAL TIP**
>
> ## FIRST AID IN ANIMAL BITES
>
> - Immediately wash the bite vigorously with soap and water for at least 10 minutes to remove the animal's saliva.
> - Flush the wound with a viricidal agent, followed by a clear-water rinse.
> - Apply a sterile dressing.
> - If possible, don't suture the wound and don't immediately stop the bleeding (unless it's massive), because blood flow helps to clean the wound.
> - Question the patient about the bite. Ask if he provoked the animal (if so, chances are it's not rabid) and if he can identify it or its owner (the animal may be confined for observation).
> - Consult local health authorities for treatment information.

---

masses that conclusively confirm rabies).

### Treatment

The patient requires wound treatment and immunization as soon as possible after exposure.

Thoroughly wash all bite wounds and scratches with soap and water. (See *First aid in animal bites.*)

Check the patient's immunization status, and administer tetanus-diphtheria prophylaxis, if needed. Take measures to control bacterial infection. If the wound requires suturing, special treatment and suturing techniques must be used to allow proper wound drainage.

**CLINICAL TIP** Antiserum is infiltrated locally if the wound is sutured.

After rabies exposure, a patient who hasn't been immunized before must receive passive immunization with rabies immune globulin (RIg) and active immunization with human diploid cell vaccine (HDCV) as soon as possible. If the patient has received HDCV before and has an adequate rabies antibody titer, he doesn't need RIg immunization, just an HDCV booster.

**Special considerations**

• When injecting the rabies vaccine, rotate injection sites on the upper arm or thigh. Watch for and treat symptoms of redness, itching, pain, and tenderness at the injection site.

• Cooperate with public health authorities to determine the vaccination status of the animal. If the animal is proven rabid, help identify others at risk.

• If rabies develops, provide aggressive supportive care (even after onset of coma) to make probable death less agonizing.

• Monitor cardiac and pulmonary function continuously.

• Isolate the patient. Wear a gown, gloves, and protection for the eyes and mouth when handling saliva and articles contaminated with saliva. Take precautions to avoid being bitten by the patient during the excitation phase.

• Keep the room dark and quiet.

• Establish communication with the patient and his family. Provide psychological support to help them cope with the patient's symptoms and probable death.

• To help prevent this dreaded disease, stress the need for vaccination of household pets that may be exposed to rabid wild animals. Warn people not to try to touch wild animals, especially if they appear ill or overly docile (a possible sign of rabies).

• Recommend prophylactic rabies vaccine to high-risk people, such as farm workers, forest rangers, spelunkers (cave explorers), and veterinarians.

# RAPE TRAUMA SYNDROME

The term "rape" refers to illicit sexual intercourse without consent. It's a violent assault in which sex is used as a weapon. Rape inflicts varying degrees of physical and psychological trauma.

Rape trauma syndrome occurs during the period following the rape or attempted rape. It refers to the victim's short-term and long-term reactions and to the methods she uses to cope with this trauma.

In the United States, a rape is reported every 7 minutes (200 per day, 62,500 per year). Incidence of reported rape is highest in large cities and is rising. However, possibly more than 90% of assaults are never reported.

Known victims of rape range from age 2 months to 97 years. The age-group most affected is 10- to 19-year-olds; the average victim's age is 13½. About 1 out of 7 reported rapes involves a prepubertal child.

Over 50% of rapes occur in the home; about one-third of these involve a male intruder who forces his way into a home. Approximately half the time, the victim has some casual acquaintance with the attacker. Most rapists are ages 15 to 24. Usually, the attack is planned.

In most cases, the rapist is a man and the victim is a woman. However, rapes do occur between persons of the same sex, especially in prisons, schools, hospitals, and other institutions.

Children are also often victims of rape; most of the time these cases involve manual, oral, or genital contact with the child's genitalia. Usually, the rapist is a member of the child's family. In rare instances, a man or child is sexually abused by a woman.

The prognosis is good if the rape victim receives physical and emotional support and counseling to help her deal with her feelings. Victims who articulate their feelings are able to cope with fears, interact with others, and return to normal routines faster than those who don't.

### Causes

Some of the cultural, sociologic, and psychological factors that contribute to rape include increasing exposure to sex, permissiveness, cynicism about relationships, feelings of anger, and powerlessness amid social pressures.

The rapist often has feelings of violence or hatred toward women or sexual problems, such as impotence or premature ejaculation. Often he feels socially isolated and unable to form warm, loving relationships. Some rapists may be psychopaths who need violence for physical pleasure, no matter how it affects their victims; others rape to satisfy a need for power. Some were abused as children.

### Signs and symptoms

A physical examination (including a pelvic examination by a gynecologist) will probably show signs of physical trauma, especially if the assault was prolonged. Depending on specific body areas attacked, a patient may have a sore throat, mouth irritation, difficulty swallowing, ecchymoses, or rectal pain and bleeding.

If additional physical violence accompanied the rape, the victim may have hematomas, lacerations, bleeding, severe internal injuries, and hemorrhage, and if the rape occurred outdoors, she may suffer from exposure. X-rays may reveal fractures. The patient may have injuries severe enough to require hospitalization.

### Assessment

● When a rape victim arrives in the emergency department, assess her physical injuries. If she isn't *seriously* injured, allow her to remain clothed and take her to a private room where she can talk with you or a counselor before the necessary physical examination.

● Remember, immediate reactions to rape differ and include crying, laughing, hostility, confusion, withdrawal, or outward calm; often anger and rage don't surface until later. During the assault, the victim may have felt demeaned, helpless, and afraid for her life; afterward, she may feel ashamed, guilty, shocked, and vulnerable, and have a sense of disbelief and lowered self-esteem.

● Offer support and reassurance. Help her explore her feelings; listen, convey trust and respect, and remain nonjudgmental. Don't leave her alone unless she asks you to.

● Being careful to upset the victim as little as possible; obtain an accurate history of the rape, pertinent to physical assessment.

**◗ CLINICAL TIP** Remember, your notes may be used as evidence if the rapist is tried.

● Record the victim's statements in the first person, using quotation marks. Also document objective information provided by others.

● Never speculate as to what may have happened or record subjective impressions or thoughts.

● Include in your notes the time the victim arrived at the hospital, the date and time of the alleged rape, and the time the victim was examined. Ask the victim about allergies to penicillin and other drugs, if she has had recent illnesses (especially venereal disease), if she was pregnant before the attack, the date of her last menstrual period, and details of her obstetric-gynecologic history.

• Thoroughly explain the examination she'll have, and tell her why it's necessary (to rule out internal injuries and obtain a specimen for venereal disease testing). Obtain her informed consent for treatment and for the police report. Allow her some control, if possible; for instance, ask her if she's ready to be examined or if she'd rather wait a bit.

• Before the examination, ask the victim whether she douched, bathed, or washed before coming to the hospital. Note this on her chart. Have her change into a hospital gown, and place her clothing in *paper bags. (Never* use plastic bags, because secretions and seminal stains will mold, destroying valuable evidence.) Label each bag and its contents.

• Tell the victim she may urinate, but warn her not to wipe or otherwise clean the perineal area. If the patient wishes, ask a counselor to stay with her throughout the examination. This examination is typically very distressing for the rape victim. Reassure her and allow her as much control as possible.

• Throughout the examination, provide support and reassurance, and carefully label all possible evidence. Before the victim's pelvic area is examined, take vital signs, and if the patient is wearing a tampon, remove it, wrap it, and label it as evidence.

• During the examination, make sure all specimens collected, including those for semen and gonorrhea, receive careful labeling. Include the patient's name, the doctor's name, and the location from which the specimen was obtained. List all specimens in your notes.

• If the case comes to trial, specimens will be used for evidence, so accuracy is essential. Most emergency departments have "rape kits" with containers for specimens. Carefully collect and label fingernail scrapings and foreign material obtained by combing the victim's pubic hair; these also provide valuable evidence. Note to whom these specimens are given.

• For a male victim, be especially alert for injury to the mouth, perineum, and anus. Obtain a pharyngeal specimen for a gonorrhea culture and rectal aspirate for acid phosphatase or sperm analysis.

• Photographs of the patient's injuries will also be taken. This may be delayed for a day or repeated when bruises and ecchymoses are more apparent.

• Most states require hospitals to report rape. The patient may not press charges and may not assist the police. If the patient does not go to the hospital, she may not report the rape.

• If the police interview the patient in the hospital, be supportive and encourage her to recall details of the rape. Your kindness and empathy are invaluable.

• The patient may also want you to call her family. Help her to verbalize anticipation of her family's response.

## Treatment

The rape victim should receive supportive care and protection against venereal disease and, if she wishes, against pregnancy.

Antibiotics are given to prevent venereal disease. To prevent pregnancy as a result of the rape, the patient may be given the "morning-after pill" (Ovral) within 72 hours of the assault. If a pregnancy test is negative, two pills are given and the dose is repeated in 12 hours. Menses follows in 3 to 4 days. Or she may wait 3 to 4 weeks and undergo a dilatation and curettage or a vacuum aspiration to abort a pregnancy.

If the patient has vulvar lacerations and hair cuts, the area will be cleaned and the lacerations repaired after all the evidence is obtained. Topical use of ice packs may reduce vulvar swelling.

All victims of rape should be offered testing for human immunodeficiency virus infection and receive medical counseling and follow-up. Testing for hepatitis B and C should be considered and prophylaxis given.

Recovery from rape, which may be prolonged, consists of the acute phase (immediate reaction) and the reorganization phase. During the acute phase, physical aspects include pain, loss of appetite, and wound healing; emotional reactions typically include shaking, crying, and mood swings. Feelings of grief, anger, fear, or revenge may color the victim's social interactions.

Counseling helps the victim identify her coping mechanisms. She may relate more easily to a counselor of the same sex.

During the reorganization phase, which usually begins a week after the rape and may last months or years, the victim is concerned with restructuring her life. Initially, she often has nightmares in which she's powerless; later dreams show her gradually gaining more control. When she's alone, she may also suffer from "daymares" — frightening thoughts about the rape. She may have reduced sexual desire or may develop fear of intercourse or mistrust of men.

**Special considerations**

• Because cultures can't detect gonorrhea or syphilis for 5 to 6 days after the rape, stress the importance of returning for follow-up venereal disease testing.

• If the patient receives DES, explain its possible adverse effects.

• Legal proceedings during this time force the victim to relive the trauma, leaving her feeling lonely and isolated, perhaps even temporarily halting her emotional recovery. To help her cope, encourage her to write her thoughts, feelings, and reactions in a daily diary.

➤ CLINICAL TIP    Refer the victim to organizations such as Women Organized Against Rape or a local rape crisis center for assistance and counseling.

# RAYNAUD'S DISEASE

One of several primary arteriospastic disorders, Raynaud's disease is characterized by episodic vasospasm in the small peripheral arteries and arterioles, precipitated by exposure to cold or stress. This condition occurs bilaterally and usually affects the hands or, less often, the feet.

Raynaud's disease is most prevalent in women, particularly between puberty and age 40. A benign condition, it requires no specific treatment and has no serious sequelae.

Raynaud's phenomenon, however, a condition often associated with several connective tissue disorders — such as scleroderma, systemic lupus erythematosus, and polymyositis — has a progressive course, leading to ischemia, gangrene, and amputation. Differentiating the two disorders is difficult because some patients who experience mild symptoms of Raynaud's disease for several years may later develop overt connective tissue disease — most commonly scleroderma.

**Causes**

Although the cause is unknown, several theories account for the reduced digital blood flow: intrinsic vascular wall hyperactivity to cold, increased vasomotor tone resulting from sympathetic stimulation, and antigen antibody immune response (the most probable theory, because abnormal immunologic test results accompany Raynaud's phenomenon).

### Signs and symptoms

After exposure to cold or stress, the skin on the fingers typically blanches, then becomes cyanotic before changing to red and before changing from cold to normal temperature. Numbness and tingling may also occur. These symptoms are relieved by warmth.

In longstanding disease, trophic changes such as sclerodactyly, ulcerations, or chronic paronychia may result. Although it's extremely uncommon, minimal cutaneous gangrene necessitates amputation of one or more phalanges.

### Diagnosis

Clinical criteria that establish Raynaud's disease include skin color changes induced by cold or stress; bilateral involvement; absence of gangrene or, if present, minimal cutaneous gangrene; normal arterial pulses; and a patient history of clinical symptoms of longer than 2 years' duration. The diagnosis must also rule out secondary disease processes, such as chronic arterial occlusive or connective tissue disease.

### Treatment

Initially, treatment consists of avoidance of cold, mechanical, or chemical injury; cessation of smoking; and reassurance that symptoms are benign.

Because adverse drug effects, especially from vasodilators, may be more bothersome than the disease itself, drug therapy is reserved for unusually severe symptoms. Such therapy may include phenoxybenzamine or reserpine.

➤ CLINICAL TIP  Low doses (30 mg) of sustained-release nifedipine may be given.

When conservative treatment fails to prevent ischemic ulcers, sympathectomy may be helpful; fewer than a quarter of patients require this procedure.

### Special considerations

• Warn against exposure to the cold. Tell the patient to wear mittens or gloves in cold weather or when handling cold items or defrosting the freezer.
• Advise the patient to avoid stressful situations and to stop smoking.
• Instruct the patient to inspect the skin frequently and to seek immediate care for signs of skin breakdown or infection.
• Teach the patient about drugs, their use, and their adverse effects.
• Provide psychological support and reassurance to allay the patient's fear of amputation and disfigurement.

# RENAL CALCULI

Although renal calculi (kidney stones) may form anywhere in the urinary tract, they usually develop in the renal pelvis or the calyces of the kidneys. Such formation follows precipitation of substances normally dissolved in the urine (calcium oxalate, calcium phosphate, magnesium ammonium phosphate or, occasionally, urate or cystine).

Renal calculi vary in size and may be solitary or multiple. They may remain in the renal pelvis or enter the ureter and may damage renal parenchyma; large calculi cause pressure necrosis. In certain locations, calculi cause obstruction, with resultant hydronephrosis, and tend to recur.

Among Americans, renal calculi develop in 1 in 1,000 people, are more common in men (especially those ages 30 to 50) than in women, and are rare in blacks and children. They're particularly prevalent in certain geographic areas, such as the southeastern United States ("stone belt"), possibly because a hot climate promotes dehydration or because of regional dietary habits.

## Causes

Although the exact cause of renal calculi is unknown, predisposing factors include the following:

• *Dehydration* and resultant decreased urine production concentrates calculus-forming substances.

• *Infection* in tissue provides a site for calculus development; pH changes provide a favorable medium for calculus formation (especially for magnesium ammonium phosphate or calcium phosphate calculi); infected calculi (usually magnesium ammonium phosphate or staghorn calculi) may develop if bacteria serve as the nucleus in calculus formation. Such infections may promote destruction of renal parenchyma.

• *Obstruction* can result from urinary stasis (as in immobility from spinal cord injury), which allows calculus constituents to collect and adhere, forming calculi. Obstruction also promotes infection, which, in turn, compounds the obstruction.

• *Metabolic factors* that can predispose to renal calculi include hyperparathyroidism, renal tubular acidosis, elevated uric acid (usually with gout), defective metabolism of oxalate, genetic defect in metabolism of cystine, and excessive intake of vitamin D or dietary calcium.

## Signs and symptoms

Clinical effects vary with size, location, and etiology of the calculi.

### Pain

The key symptom, pain usually results from obstruction; large, rough calculi

occlude the opening to the ureter and increase the frequency and force of peristaltic contractions. The pain of classic renal colic travels from the costovertebral angle to the flank, to the suprapubic region and external genitalia.

The intensity of this pain fluctuates and may be excruciating at its peak. If calculi are in the renal pelvis and calyces, pain may be more constant and dull. Back pain (from calculi that produce an obstruction within a kidney) and severe abdominal pain (from calculi traveling down a ureter) may also occur. Nausea and vomiting usually accompany severe pain.

### Accompanying signs

Other associated signs include fever, chills, hematuria (when calculi abrade a ureter), abdominal distention, pyuria and, rarely, anuria (from bilateral obstruction or unilateral obstruction in the patient with one kidney).

## Diagnosis

The clinical picture in conjunction with the following diagnostic tests allows a diagnosis:

• *Kidney-ureter-bladder X-rays* reveal most renal calculi.

• *Calculus analysis* shows mineral content.

• *Excretory urography* confirms the diagnosis and determines size and location of calculi.

• *Kidney ultrasonography,* an easily performed noninvasive, nontoxic test, detects obstructive changes, such as unilateral or bilateral hydronephrosis.

• *Urine culture* of midstream specimen may indicate urinary tract infection.

• *Urinalysis* may be normal or may show increased specific gravity and acid or alkaline pH suitable for different types of stone formation. Other urinalysis findings include hematuria (gross or microscopic), crystals (urate, calcium, or

TEACHING CHECKLIST

## PREVENTING RECURRENCE OF RENAL CALCULI

Before discharge, your patient needs to learn how to prevent a recurrence of renal calculi. Teach him to:

- follow the prescribed dietary and medication regimens closely
- increase fluid intake
- check his urine pH, if appropriate, and keep a daily record
- report symptoms of acute obstruction (pain and inability to void) immediately.

cystine), casts, and pyuria with or without bacteria and white blood cells.

- A *24-hour urine collection* is evaluated for calcium oxalate, phosphorus, and uric acid excretion levels.
- *Serial blood calcium and phosphorus levels* detect hyperparathyroidism and show an increased calcium level in proportion to the normal level of serum protein.
- *Blood protein level* determines level of free calcium unbound to protein.
- *Blood chloride* and bicarbonate levels may show renal tubular acidosis.
- *Increased blood uric acid levels* may indicate gout as the cause.

Diagnosis must rule out appendicitis, cholecystitis, peptic ulcer, and pancreatitis as potential sources of pain.

### Treatment

Because 90% of renal calculi are smaller than 5 mm in diameter, treatment usually consists of measures to promote their natural passage. Along with vigorous hydration, such treatment includes antimicrobial therapy (varying with the cultured organism) for infection; analgesics, such as meperidine, for pain; and diuretics to prevent urinary stasis and further calculus formation. (Thiazides decrease calcium excretion into the urine.)

Prophylaxis to prevent calculus formation includes a low-calcium diet for absorptive hypercalciuria, parathyroidectomy for hyperparathyroidism, and allopurinol and urinary alkalynization for uric acid calculi.

Calculi too large for natural passage may require surgical removal. When a calculus is in the ureter, a cystoscope may be inserted through the urethra and the calculus manipulated with catheters or retrieval instruments. A small-diameter telescope, the ureteroscope, may be inserted through the ureter to remove stones from the ureter and kidney. Extraction of calculi from other areas (kidney calyx, renal pelvis) rarely may necessitate a flank or lower abdominal approach.

Percutaneous ultrasonic lithotripsy and extracorporeal shock-wave lithotripsy shatter the calculus into fragments for removal by suction or natural passage. To prevent recurrence of calculi, the patient will also need teaching before discharge. (See *Preventing recurrence of renal calculi.*)

### Special considerations

- To aid diagnosis, maintain a 24- to 48-hour record of urine pH, with nitrazine pH paper; strain all urine through gauze or a tea strainer; and save all solid material recovered for analysis.
- To facilitate spontaneous passage, encourage the patient to walk, if possible. To help prevent future stones, promote sufficient intake of fluids to maintain a urine output of 3 to 4 L/day (urine should be very diluted and colorless).

➤ CLINICAL TIP Use caution in patients with a cardiac history be-

cause they may not tolerate these large volumes of fluid.
- To help acidify urine, offer fruit juices, particularly cranberry juice. If the patient can't drink the required amount of fluid, supplemental I.V. fluids may be given. Record intake and output and daily weight to assess fluid status and renal function.
- Stress the importance of proper diet and compliance with drug therapy. For example, if the patient's stone is caused by a hyperuricemic condition, advise the patient or whoever prepares his meals which foods are high in purine.
- If surgery is necessary, provide reassurance. The patient is apt to be fearful, especially if surgery includes removal of a kidney, so emphasize that the body can adapt well to having one kidney. If he is to have an abdominal or flank incision, teach deep-breathing and coughing exercises.
- After surgery, the patient will probably have an indwelling urinary catheter or a nephrostomy tube in place. Unless one of his kidneys was removed, expect bloody drainage from the catheter.
- Check dressings regularly for bloody drainage, and know how much drainage to expect. Watch closely for signs of suspected hemorrhage (excessive drainage, rising pulse rate). Use sterile technique when changing dressings or providing catheter care.
- Watch for signs of infection (rising fever, chills), and give antibiotics as needed.
- To prevent pneumonia, encourage frequent position changes, and ambulate the patient as soon as possible. Have him hold a small pillow over the operative site to splint the incision and thereby facilitate deep-breathing and coughing exercises.

**LIFE-THREATENING DISORDER**

# RENAL FAILURE, ACUTE

Obstruction, reduced circulation, and renal parenchymal disease can all cause the sudden interruption of kidney function. Acute renal failure is usually reversible with medical treatment; otherwise, it may progress to end-stage renal disease, uremic syndrome, and death.

## Causes
Acute renal failure can be classified as prerenal, intrinsic (or parenchymal), and postrenal.

### Prerenal failure
Diminished blood flow to the kidneys causes prerenal failure. Such decreased flow may result from hypovolemia, shock, embolism, blood loss, sepsis, pooling of fluid in ascites or burns, and cardiovascular disorders, such as heart failure, arrhythmias, and tamponade.

### Intrinsic renal failure
Parenchymal, or intrinsic, renal failure results from damage to the kidneys themselves, usually resulting from acute tubular necrosis. Such damage may also result from acute poststreptococcal glomerulonephritis, systemic lupus erythematosus, polyarteritis nodosa, vasculitis, sickle-cell disease, bilateral renal vein thrombosis, nephrotoxins, ischemia, renal myeloma, and acute pyelonephritis.

### Postrenal failure
Bilateral obstruction of urinary outflow results in postrenal failure. Its multiple causes include kidney stones, clots, papillae from papillary necrosis, tumors,

benign prostatic hyperplasia, strictures, and urethral edema from catheterization.

## Signs and symptoms

Acute renal failure is a critical illness. Its early signs are oliguria, azotemia and, rarely, anuria. Electrolyte imbalances, metabolic acidosis, and other severe effects follow as the patient becomes increasingly uremic and renal dysfunction disrupts other body systems:

- *GI* — anorexia, nausea, vomiting, diarrhea or constipation, stomatitis, bleeding, hematemesis, dry mucous membranes, uremic breath
- *central nervous system (CNS)* — headache, drowsiness, irritability, confusion, peripheral neuropathy, seizures, coma
- *cutaneous* — dryness, pruritus, pallor, purpura; rarely, uremic frost
- *cardiovascular* — early in the disease, hypotension; later, hypertension, arrhythmias, fluid overload, heart failure, systemic edema, anemia, altered clotting mechanisms
- *respiratory* — Kussmaul's respirations, pulmonary edema.

Fever and chills indicate infection, a common complication.

## Diagnosis

The patient's history may include a disorder that can cause renal failure. Blood test results indicating intrinsic acute renal failure include elevated blood urea nitrogen, serum creatinine, and potassium levels and low blood pH, bicarbonate, hematocrit (HCT), and hemoglobin (Hb) levels.

Urine specimens show casts, cellular debris, decreased specific gravity and, in glomerular diseases, proteinuria and urine osmolality close to serum osmolality. The urine sodium level is less than 20 mEq/L if oliguria results from

decreased perfusion, more than 40 mEq/L if it results from an intrinsic problem.

Other studies include renal ultrasonography, kidney-ureter-bladder radiography, cautious use of excretory urography, renal scan, retrograde pyelography, and nephrotomography.

## Treatment

Supportive measures include a diet high in calories and low in protein, sodium, and potassium, with supplemental vitamins and restricted fluids. Meticulous electrolyte monitoring is essential to detect hyperkalemia.

If hyperkalemia occurs, acute therapy may include dialysis, hypertonic glucose and insulin infusions, and sodium bicarbonate — all administered I.V — and sodium polystyrene sulfonate, given orally or by enema, to remove potassium from the body.

If measures fail to control uremic symptoms, hemodialysis or peritoneal dialysis may be necessary.

## Special considerations

- Measure and record intake and output, including all body fluids, such as wound drainage, nasogastric output, and diarrhea. Weigh the patient daily.
- Assess HCT and Hb levels and replace blood components as needed. *Don't* use whole blood if the patient is prone to heart failure and can't tolerate extra fluid volume.
- Monitor vital signs. Watch closely for any signs of pericarditis (pleuritic chest pain, tachycardia, pericardial friction rub), inadequate renal perfusion (hypotension), and acidosis.
- Maintain proper electrolyte balance. Strictly monitor potassium levels.

➤ CLINICAL TIP  Monitor for hyperkalemia. Symptoms include malaise, anorexia, paresthesia, muscle weakness, and electrocardiogram changes (tall, peaked T waves; widening QRS segment; and disappearing P waves). Don't give medications containing potassium.

• Assess the patient frequently, especially during emergency treatment to lower potassium levels. If the patient receives hypertonic glucose and insulin infusions, monitor potassium levels. If you give sodium polystyrene sulfonate rectally, make sure the patient doesn't retain it and become constipated to prevent bowel perforation.

• Maintain nutritional status. Provide a high-calorie, low-protein, low-sodium, low-potassium diet, with vitamin supplements. Give the patient with anorexia small, frequent meals.

• Use aseptic technique; the patient with acute renal failure is highly susceptible to infection. Don't allow personnel with upper respiratory tract infections to care for the patient.

• Prevent complications of immobility by encouraging frequent coughing and deep breathing and by performing passive range-of-motion exercises. Help the patient walk as soon as possible. Add lubricating lotion to the patient's bathwater to combat skin dryness.

• Provide good mouth care frequently for dry mucous membranes. If stomatitis occurs, the patient may need an antibiotic solution. Have the patient swish the solution around in his mouth before swallowing.

• Monitor for GI bleeding by applying the guaiac test to all stools. Administer medications carefully, especially antacids and stool softeners.

• Use appropriate safety measures, such as side rails and restraints; the patient with CNS involvement may be dizzy or confused.

• Provide emotional support to the patient and his family. Reassure them by clearly explaining all procedures.

• During peritoneal dialysis, position the patient carefully. Elevate the head of the bed to reduce pressure on the diaphragm and aid respiration. Be alert for signs of infection (cloudy drainage, elevated temperature) and bleeding.

• If pain occurs, reduce the amount of dialysate. Monitor the blood glucose level of the patient with diabetes periodically, and administer insulin as needed. Watch for complications, such as peritonitis, atelectasis, hypokalemia, pneumonia, and shock.

• If the patient requires hemodialysis, check the blood access site (arteriovenous fistula, subclavian or femoral catheter) every 2 hours for patency and signs of clotting. Don't use the arm with the shunt or fistula for taking blood pressures or drawing blood. Weigh the patient before beginning dialysis.

• During dialysis, monitor vital signs, clotting times, blood flow, the function of the vascular access site, and arterial and venous pressures. Watch for complications, such as septicemia, embolism, hepatitis, and rapid fluid and electrolyte loss.

• After dialysis, monitor vital signs and the vascular access site, weigh the patient, and watch for signs of fluid and electrolyte imbalances.

• Follow universal precautions when handling all blood and body fluids.

LIFE-THREATENING DISORDER

# RENAL FAILURE, CHRONIC

Although chronic renal failure is usually the result of a gradually progressive loss of renal function, it occasionally results from a rapidly progressive disease of sudden onset. Few symptoms develop until after more than 75% of glomerular filtration is lost; then, the remaining normal parenchyma deteriorates progressively, and symptoms worsen as renal function decreases.

If this condition continues unchecked, uremic toxins accumulate and produce potentially fatal physiologic changes in all major organ systems. If the patient can tolerate it, maintenance dialysis or kidney transplantation can sustain life.

## Causes

Chronic renal failure may result from:
- *chronic glomerular disease* such as glomerulonephritis
- *chronic infections,* such as chronic pyelonephritis or tuberculosis
- *congenital anomalies* such as polycystic kidneys
- *vascular diseases,* such as renal nephrosclerosis or hypertension
- *obstructive processes* such as calculi
- *collagen diseases* such as systemic lupus erythematosus
- *nephrotoxic agents* such as long-term aminoglycoside therapy
- *endocrine diseases* such as diabetic neuropathy.

Such conditions gradually destroy the nephrons and eventually cause irreversible renal failure. Similarly, acute renal failure that fails to respond to treatment becomes chronic renal failure.

Chronic renal failure may progress through the following stages:
- reduced renal reserve (glomerular filtration rate [GFR] 40 to 70 ml/minute)
- renal insufficiency (GFR 20 to 40 ml/minute)
- renal failure (GFR 10 to 20 ml/minute)
- end-stage renal disease (GFR < 10 ml/minute).

## Signs and symptoms

Chronic renal failure produces major changes in all body systems.

### Renal and urologic changes

Initially, salt-wasting and consequent hyponatremia produce hypotension, dry mouth, loss of skin turgor, listlessness, fatigue, and nausea. Later, somnolence and confusion develop.

As the number of functioning nephrons decreases, so does the kidneys' capacity to excrete sodium, resulting in salt retention and overload. Accumulation of potassium causes muscle irritability, then muscle weakness as the potassium level continues to rise.

Fluid overload and metabolic acidosis also occur. Urine output decreases; urine is very dilute and contains casts and crystals.

### Cardiovascular changes

Renal failure leads to hypertension and arrhythmias, including life-threatening ventricular tachycardia or fibrillation. Other effects include cardiomyopathy, uremic pericarditis, pericardial effusion with possible cardiac tamponade, heart failure, and peripheral edema.

### Respiratory changes

Pulmonary changes include reduced pulmonary macrophage activity with increased susceptibility to infection, pulmonary edema, pleuritic pain, pleural friction rub and effusions, and uremic pleuritis and uremic lung (or uremic pneumonitis). Dyspnea from heart failure also occurs, as do Kussmaul's respirations as a result of acidosis.

### GI changes

Inflammation and ulceration of GI mucosa cause stomatitis, gum ulceration and bleeding and, possibly, parotitis, esophagitis, gastritis, duodenal ulcers, lesions on the small and large bowel, uremic colitis, pancreatitis, and proctitis. Other GI symptoms include a metallic taste in the mouth, uremic fetor (ammonia smell to breath), anorexia, nausea, and vomiting.

### Cutaneous changes

Typically, the skin is pallid, yellowish bronze, dry, and scaly. Other cutaneous symptoms include severe itching; purpura; ecchymoses; petechiae; uremic frost (most often in critically ill or terminal patients); thin, brittle fingernails with characteristic lines; and dry, brittle hair that may change color and fall out easily.

### Neurologic changes

Restless leg syndrome, one of the first signs of peripheral neuropathy, causes pain, burning, and itching in the legs and feet, which may be relieved by voluntarily shaking, moving, or rocking them. Eventually, this condition progresses to paresthesia and motor nerve dysfunction (usually bilateral footdrop) unless dialysis is initiated.

Other signs and symptoms include muscle cramping and twitching, shortened memory and attention span, apathy, drowsiness, irritability, confusion, coma, and seizures. Electroencephalogram changes indicate metabolic encephalopathy.

### Endocrine changes

Common endocrine abnormalities include stunted growth patterns in children (even with elevated growth hormone levels), infertility and decreased libido in both sexes, amenorrhea and cessation of menses in women, and impotence and decreased sperm production in men. Other changes include increased aldosterone secretion (related to increased renin production) and impaired carbohydrate metabolism (causing increased blood glucose levels similar to those found in diabetes mellitus).

### Hematopoietic changes

Anemia, decreased red blood cell (RBC) survival time, blood loss from dialysis and GI bleeding, mild thrombocytopenia, and platelet defects occur. Other problems include increased bleeding and clotting disorders, demonstrated by purpura, hemorrhage from body orifices, easy bruising, ecchymoses, and petechiae.

### Skeletal changes

Calcium-phosphorus imbalance and consequent parathyroid hormone imbalances cause muscle and bone pain, skeletal demineralization, pathologic fractures, and calcifications in the brain, eyes, gums, joints, myocardium, and blood vessels. Arterial calcification may produce coronary artery disease. In children, renal osteodystrophy (renal rickets) may develop.

### Diagnosis

Clinical assessment, a history of chronic progressive debilitation, and gradual deterioration of renal function as determined by creatinine clearance tests lead to a diagnosis of chronic renal failure.

The following laboratory findings also aid in diagnosis:

• *Blood studies* show elevated blood urea nitrogen, serum creatinine, and potassium levels; decreased arterial pH and bicarbonate; and low hemoglobin (Hb) and hematocrit (HCT).

• *Urine specific gravity* becomes fixed at 1.010; urinalysis may show proteinuria, glycosuria, erythrocytes, leukocytes, and casts, depending on the etiology.

• *X-ray studies* include kidney-ureter-bladder radiography, excretory urography, nephrotomography, renal scan, and renal arteriography.

• *Kidney biopsy* allows histologic identification of underlying pathology.

## Treatment
Conservative treatment aims to correct specific symptoms.

### Diet
A low-protein diet reduces the production of end-products of protein metabolism that the kidneys can't excrete. (A patient receiving continuous peritoneal dialysis should receive a high-protein diet.)

A high-calorie diet prevents ketoacidosis and the negative nitrogen balance that results in catabolism and tissue atrophy. Such a diet also restricts sodium and potassium.

### Fluid status
Maintaining fluid balance requires careful monitoring of vital signs, weight changes, and urine volume (if present). Loop diuretics such as furosemide (if some renal function remains) and fluid restriction can reduce fluid retention. Digitalis glycosides may be used to mobilize edema fluids; antihypertensives, especially ACE inhibitors, can be used to control blood pressure and associated edema.

### Treatment for GI and blood problems
Antiemetics taken before meals may relieve nausea and vomiting; cimetidine, omeprazole, or ranitidine may decrease gastric irritation. Methylcellulose or docusate can help prevent constipation.

Treatment may also include regular stool analysis (guaiac test) to detect occult blood and, as needed, cleansing enemas to remove blood from the GI tract.

Anemia necessitates iron and folate supplements; severe anemia requires infusion of fresh frozen packed cells or washed packed cells. However, transfusions relieve anemia only temporarily. Synthetic erythropoietin (epoetin alfa) may be given to stimulate the division and differentiation of cells within the bone marrow to produce RBCs. Androgen therapy (testosterone or nandrolone) may increase RBC production.

### Drug therapy, surgery, and dialysis
Drug therapy often relieves associated symptoms: an antipruritic, such as trimeprazine or diphenhydramine, for itching and aluminum hydroxide gel to lower serum phosphate levels.

CLINICAL TIP Be alert for aluminum toxicity, a potential adverse effect of aluminum hydroxide.

The patient may also benefit from supplementary vitamins (particularly B vitamins and vitamin D) and essential amino acids.

Careful monitoring of serum potassium levels is necessary to detect hyperkalemia. Emergency treatment for severe hyperkalemia includes dialysis therapy and administration of 50% hypertonic glucose I.V., regular insulin, calcium gluconate I.V., sodium bicarbonate I.V., and cation exchange resins such as sodium polystyrene sulfonate. Cardiac tamponade resulting from pericardial effusion may require emergency pericardial tap or surgery.

Blood gas measurements may indicate acidosis; intensive dialysis and thoracentesis can relieve pulmonary edema and pleural effusions.

Hemodialysis or peritoneal dialysis (particularly continuous ambulatory peritoneal dialysis and continuous cyclic peritoneal dialysis) can help control most manifestations of end-stage renal disease. (See *Continuous ambulatory peritoneal dialysis.*) Altering dialyzing bath fluids can correct fluid and electrolyte disturbances. However, anemia, peripheral neuropathy, cardiopulmonary

## CONTINUOUS AMBULATORY PERITONEAL DIALYSIS

Continuous ambulatory peritoneal dialysis is an increasingly useful alternative to hemodialysis in patients with renal failure. Using the peritoneum as a dialysis membrane, it allows almost uninterrupted exchange of dialysis solution.

With this method, four to six exchanges of fresh dialysis solution are infused each day. The approximate dwell-time for the daytime exchanges is 5 hours; for the overnight exchange the dwell-time is 8 to 10 hours. After each dwell-time, the patient removes the dialyzing solution by gravity drainage.

This form of dialysis offers the unique advantages of a simple, easily taught procedure and allows the patient independence from a special treatment center.

In this procedure, a Tenckhoff catheter is surgically implanted in the abdomen, just below the umbilicus. A bag of dialysis solution is aseptically attached to the tube, and the fluid is allowed to flow into the peritoneal cavity. (This takes about 10 minutes.)

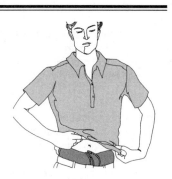

The fluid is then drained out of the peritoneal cavity through gravity flow by unrolling the bag and suspending it below the pelvis. (Drainage takes about 20 minutes.) After it drains, the patient aseptically connects a new bag of dialyzing solution and fills the peritoneal cavity again. He repeats this procedure four to six times per day.

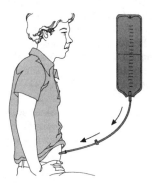

The dialyzing fluid remains in the peritoneal cavity for about 4 to 6 hours. During this time, the bag may be rolled up and placed under a shirt or blouse, and the patient can go about normal activities while dialysis takes place.

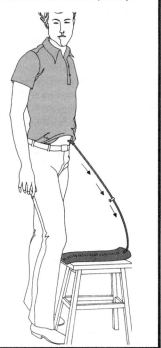

and GI complications, sexual dysfunction, and skeletal defects may persist.

Maintenance dialysis itself may produce complications, such as protein wasting, refractory ascites, and dialysis dementia. A kidney transplant may eventually be the treatment of choice for some patients with end-stage renal disease.

**Special considerations**
• Provide good skin care. Bathe the patient daily, using superfatted soaps, oatmeal baths, and skin lotion to ease pruritus. Give good perineal care, using mild soap and water. Pad the side rails to guard against ecchymoses. Turn the patient often, and use a convoluted foam mattress to prevent skin breakdown.
• Provide good oral hygiene. Brush the patient's teeth often with a soft brush or sponge tip to reduce breath odor. Hard candy and mouthwash minimize bad taste in the mouth and alleviate thirst.
• Offer small, palatable meals that are also nutritious; try to provide favorite foods within dietary restrictions. Encourage intake of high-calorie foods. Instruct the outpatient to avoid high-sodium, high-protein, and high-potassium foods.
• Encourage adherence to fluid and protein restrictions. To prevent constipation, stress the need for exercise and sufficient dietary fiber.
• Watch for hyperkalemia. Observe for cramping of the legs and abdomen and diarrhea. As potassium levels rise, watch for muscle irritability and a weak pulse rate. Monitor the electrocardiogram for indications of hyperkalemia — tall, peaked T waves; widening QRS segment; prolonged PR interval; and disappearance of P waves.
• Assess hydration status carefully. Check for jugular vein distention and auscultate the lungs for crackles. Measure daily intake and output carefully, including all drainage, vomitus, diarrhea, and blood loss. Record daily weight, presence or absence of thirst, axillary sweat, dryness of tongue, hypertension, and peripheral edema.
• Monitor for bone and joint complications. Prevent pathologic fractures by turning the patient carefully and ensuring his safety. Provide passive range-of-motion exercises for the bedridden patient.
• Encourage deep breathing and coughing to prevent pulmonary congestion. Listen often for crackles, rhonchi, and decreased lung sounds. Be alert for clinical effects of pulmonary edema (dyspnea, restlessness, crackles). Administer diuretics and other medications as needed.
• Maintain strict aseptic technique. Use a micropore filter during I.V. therapy. Watch for signs of infection (listlessness, high fever, leukocytosis). Urge the outpatient to avoid contact with infected persons during the cold and flu season.
• Carefully observe and document seizure activity. Infuse sodium bicarbonate for acidosis and sedatives or anticonvulsants for seizures. Pad the side rails and keep an oral airway and suction setup at bedside. Assess neurologic status periodically, and check for Chvostek's and Trousseau's signs, indicators of low serum calcium levels.
• Observe for signs of bleeding. Watch for prolonged bleeding at puncture sites and at the vascular access site used for hemodialysis. Monitor Hb and HCT, and check stools, urine, and vomitus for blood.
• Watch for signs of pericarditis, such as a pericardial friction rub and chest pain. Also, watch for the disappearance of friction rub, with a drop of 15 to 20 mm Hg in blood pressure during inspiration (paradoxical pulse) — an early sign of pericardial tamponade.

• Schedule medications carefully. Give iron before meals, aluminum hydroxide gels after meals, and antiemetics, as necessary, a half hour before meals. Administer antihypertensives at appropriate intervals.

• If the patient requires a rectal infusion of sodium polystyrene sulfonate for dangerously high potassium levels, apply an emollient to soothe the perianal area. Be sure the sodium polystyrene sulfonate enema is expelled; otherwise, it will cause constipation and won't lower potassium levels.

• Recommend antacid cookies as an alternative to aluminum hydroxide gels needed to bind GI phosphate.

If the patient requires dialysis:

• Prepare the patient by fully explaining the procedure. Be sure that he understands how to protect and care for the arteriovenous shunt, fistula, or other vascular access.

• Check the vascular access site every 2 hours for patency and the extremity for adequate blood supply and intact nervous function (temperature, pulse rate, capillary refill, and sensation).

• If a fistula is present, feel for a thrill and listen for a bruit. Use a gentle touch to avoid occluding the fistula. Note signs of possible clotting.

• Don't use the arm with the vascular access site to take blood pressure readings, draw blood, or give injections; these procedures may rupture the fistula or cause scarring that occludes blood flow.

• Withhold the 6 a.m. (or morning) dose of antihypertensive on the morning of dialysis, and instruct the outpatient to do the same.

• Check the patient's hepatitis antigen status. If it's positive, he's a carrier of hepatitis B, and stool, needle, blood, and excretion precautions should be instituted.

• Monitor Hb and HCT. Assess the patient's tolerance of his levels; some individuals are more sensitive to lower levels than others. Instruct the anemic patient to conserve energy and to rest frequently.

• After dialysis, check for disequilibrium syndrome, a result of sudden correction of blood chemistry abnormalities. Symptoms range from a headache to seizures. Also, check for excessive bleeding from the dialysis site. Apply a pressure dressing or absorbable gelatin sponge as indicated. Monitor blood pressure carefully after dialysis.

• A patient undergoing dialysis is under a great deal of stress, as is his family. Refer them to appropriate counseling agencies for assistance in coping with chronic renal failure.

---

LIFE-THREATENING
DISORDER

# RENAL INFARCTION

---

Renal blood vessel occlusion results in renal infarction — the formation of a coagulated, necrotic area in one or both kidneys. The location and size of the infarction depend on the site of vascular occlusion. Most commonly, infarction affects the renal cortex but it can extend into the medulla. (See *Sites of renal infarction,* page 734.) Residual renal function after infarction depends on the extent of the damage from the infarction.

**Causes**
In 75% of patients, renal infarction results from renal artery embolism secondary to mitral stenosis, infective endocarditis, atrial fibrillation, microthrombi in the left ventricle, rheumatic

## SITES OF RENAL INFARCTION

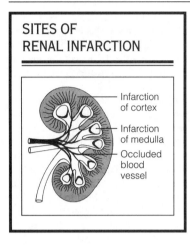

- Infarction of cortex
- Infarction of medulla
- Occluded blood vessel

valvular disease, or recent myocardial infarction.

The embolism reduces the rate of blood flow to renal tissue and leads to ischemia. The rate and degree of blood flow reduction determine whether the insult will be acute or chronic as arterial narrowing progresses.

Less common causes of renal infarction are atherosclerosis, with or without thrombus formation; and thrombus from flank trauma, sickle cell anemia, scleroderma, and arterionephrosclerosis.

### Signs and symptoms

Although renal infarction may be asymptomatic, typical symptoms include severe upper abdominal pain or gnawing flank pain and tenderness, costovertebral tenderness, fever, anorexia, nausea, and vomiting. When arterial occlusion causes infarction, the affected kidney is small and not palpable.

Renovascular hypertension, a frequent complication that may occur several days after infarction, results from reduced blood flow, which stimulates the renin-angiotensin mechanism.

### Diagnosis

A history of predisposing cardiovascular disease or other factors in a patient with typical clinical features strongly suggests renal infarction. A firm diagnosis requires the appropriate laboratory tests:

- *Urinalysis* reveals proteinuria and microscopic hematuria.
- *Urine enzyme levels,* especially lactate dehydrogenase (LD) and alkaline phosphatase, are often elevated as a result of tissue destruction.
- *Blood studies* may reveal elevated serum enzyme levels, especially aspartate aminotransferase, alkaline phosphatase, and LD. Blood studies may also reveal leukocytosis and an increased erythrocyte sedimentation rate.
- *Excretory urography* shows diminished or absent excretion of contrast dye, indicating vascular occlusion or urethral obstruction.
- *Isotopic renal scan,* a noninvasive technique, demonstrates absent or reduced blood flow to the kidneys.
- *Renal arteriography* provides absolute proof of an existing infarction but is used as a last resort because it's a high-risk procedure.

### Treatment

Infection in the infarcted area or significant hypertension may require surgical repair of the occlusion or nephrectomy. Surgery to establish collateral circulation to the area can relieve renovascular hypertension.

Persistent hypertension may respond to antihypertensives and a low-sodium diet. Additional treatments may include administration of intra-arterial streptokinase, lysis of blood clots, catheter embolectomy, and heparin therapy.

### Special considerations

• Assess the degree of renal function and offer supportive care to maintain homeostasis.

• Monitor intake and output, vital signs (particularly blood pressure), electrolyte levels, and daily weight.

➤ CLINICAL TIP   Watch for signs of fluid overload, such as dyspnea, tachycardia, pulmonary edema, and electrolyte imbalances.

• Carefully explain all diagnostic procedures.

• Provide reassurance and emotional support for the patient and family.

• Encourage the patient to return for a follow-up examination, which usually includes excretory urography or a renal scan to assess regained renal function.

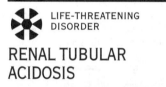

LIFE-THREATENING
DISORDER

# RENAL TUBULAR ACIDOSIS

A syndrome of persistent dehydration, hyperchloremia, hypokalemia, metabolic acidosis, and nephrocalcinosis, renal tubular acidosis (RTA) results from the kidneys' inability to conserve bicarbonate. This disorder occurs as distal RTA (Type I, or classic RTA) or proximal RTA (Type II). The prognosis is usually good but depends on the severity of renal damage that precedes treatment.

### Causes

Metabolic acidosis usually results from renal excretion of bicarbonate. However, metabolic acidosis associated with RTA results from a defect in the kidneys' normal tubular acidification of urine.

### Distal RTA

Type I RTA results from an inability of the distal tubule to secrete hydrogen ions against established gradients across the tubular membrane. This results in decreased excretion of titratable acids and ammonium, increased loss of potassium and bicarbonate in the urine, and systemic acidosis.

Prolonged acidosis causes mobilization of calcium from bone and eventually hypercalciuria, predisposing to the formation of renal calculi.

Distal RTA may be classified as primary or secondary:

• *Primary distal RTA* may occur sporadically or through a hereditary defect and is most prevalent in females, older children, adolescents, and young adults.

• *Secondary distal RTA* has been linked to many renal or systemic conditions, such as starvation, malnutrition, hepatic cirrhosis, and several genetically transmitted disorders.

### Proximal RTA

Type II RTA results from defective reabsorption of bicarbonate in the proximal tubule. This causes bicarbonate to flood the distal tubule, which normally secretes hydrogen ions, and leads to impaired formation of titratable acids and ammonium for excretion. Ultimately, metabolic acidosis results.

Proximal RTA occurs in two forms:

• In *primary proximal RTA,* the reabsorptive defect is idiopathic and is the only disorder present.

• In *secondary proximal RTA,* the reabsorptive defect may be one of several defects and results from proximal tubular cell damage from a disease such as Fanconi's syndrome.

### Signs and symptoms

In infants, RTA produces anorexia, vomiting, occasional fever, polyuria, dehydration, growth retardation, apathy, weakness, tissue wasting, constipation, nephrocalcinosis, and rickets.

In children and adults, RTA may lead to urinary tract infection, rickets, and growth problems. Possible complications of RTA include nephrocalcinosis and pyelonephritis.

### Diagnosis

Demonstration of impaired acidification of urine with systemic metabolic acidosis confirms distal RTA. Demonstration of bicarbonate wasting from impaired reabsorption confirms proximal RTA.

Other relevant laboratory results show:

• decreased serum bicarbonate, pH, potassium, and phosphorus levels
• increased serum chloride and alkaline phosphatase levels
• alkaline pH, with low titratable acids and ammonium content in urine; and increased urinary bicarbonate and potassium levels, with low specific gravity.

In later stages, X-rays may show nephrocalcinosis.

### Treatment

Supportive treatment for patients with RTA requires replacement of those substances being abnormally excreted, especially bicarbonate. It may include sodium bicarbonate tablets or Shohl's solution to control acidosis, oral potassium for dangerously low potassium levels, and vitamin D for bone disease. If pyelonephritis occurs, treatment may include antibiotics as well.

Treatment for renal calculi secondary to nephrocalcinosis varies and may include supportive therapy until the calculi pass or until surgery for severe obstruction is performed.

### Special considerations

• Urge compliance with all medication instructions. Inform the patient and his family that the prognosis for RTA and bone lesion healing is directly related to the adequacy of treatment.
• Monitor laboratory values, especially potassium levels, for hypokalemia.
• Test urine for pH and strain it for calculi.
• If rickets develops, explain the condition and its treatment to the patient and his family.
• Teach the patient how to recognize signs and symptoms of calculi (hematuria and low abdominal or flank pain). Advise him to report such signs and symptoms immediately.
• Instruct the patient with low potassium levels to eat foods with a high potassium content, such as bananas and baked potatoes. Orange juice is also high in potassium.
• Because RTA may be caused by a genetic defect, encourage family members to seek genetic counseling or screening for this disorder.

 LIFE-THREATENING DISORDER

# RENAL VEIN THROMBOSIS

Clotting in the renal vein results in renal congestion, engorgement and, possibly, infarction. Renal vein thrombosis may affect both kidneys and may occur in an acute or chronic form.

Chronic thrombosis usually impairs renal function, causing nephrotic syndrome. Abrupt onset of thrombosis that causes extensive damage may precipitate rapidly fatal renal infarction.

If thrombosis affects both kidneys, the prognosis is poor. However, less severe thrombosis that affects only one kidney or gradual progression that allows development of collateral circulation may preserve partial renal function.

## Causes

Renal vein thrombosis often results from a tumor that obstructs the renal vein (usually hypernephroma).

Other causes include thrombophlebitis of the inferior vena cava (may result from abdominal trauma) or blood vessels of the legs, heart failure, and periarteritis. In infants, renal vein thrombosis usually follows diarrhea that causes severe dehydration.

Chronic renal vein thrombosis is often a complication of other glomerulopathic diseases, such as amyloidosis, systemic lupus erythematosus, diabetic nephropathy, and membranoproliferative glomerulonephritis.

### Signs and symptoms

Clinical features of renal vein thrombosis vary with the speed of onset.

Rapid onset of venous obstruction produces severe lumbar pain and tenderness in the epigastric region and the costovertebral angle. Other characteristic features include fever, leukocytosis, pallor, hematuria, proteinuria, peripheral edema and, when the obstruction is bilateral, oliguria and other uremic signs. The kidneys enlarge and become easily palpable. Hypertension is unusual but may develop.

Gradual onset causes symptoms of nephrotic syndrome. Peripheral edema is possible, but pain is generally absent. Other clinical signs include proteinuria, hypoalbuminemia, and hyperlipemia.

Infants with this disease have enlarged kidneys, oliguria, and renal insufficiency that may progress to acute or chronic renal failure.

### Diagnosis

• *Excretory urography* provides reliable diagnostic evidence. In acute renal vein thrombosis, the kidneys appear enlarged and excretory function diminishes. The contrast medium seems to "smudge" necrotic renal tissue. In chronic thrombosis, this test may show ureteral indentations that result from collateral venous channels.

• *Renal arteriography* and a *kidney biopsy* may confirm the diagnosis.

• *Urinalysis* reveals gross or microscopic hematuria, proteinuria (more than 2 g/day in chronic disease), casts, and oliguria.

• *Blood studies* show leukocytosis, hypoalbuminemia, and hyperlipidemia.

• *Venography* confirms thrombosis.

• *Magnetic resonance imaging* holds promise for diagnosis of thrombosis.

### Treatment

Gradual thrombosis that affects only one kidney responds best to treatment. Anticoagulant therapy may prove helpful, especially if used long-term.

Surgery must be performed within 24 hours of thrombosis but even then has limited success because thrombi often extend into the small veins. Extensive intrarenal bleeding may necessitate nephrectomy.

Patients who survive abrupt thrombosis with extensive renal damage develop nephrotic syndrome and require treatment for renal failure, such as dialysis and possible transplantation. Some infants with renal vein thrombosis recover completely after heparin therapy or surgery; others suffer irreversible kidney damage.

### Special considerations

• Assess renal function regularly. Monitor vital signs, intake and output, daily weight, and electrolytes.

• Administer diuretics for edema, and enforce dietary restrictions, such as limited sodium and potassium intake.

• Monitor closely for signs of pulmonary emboli (chest pain, dyspnea).
• If heparin is given by constant I.V. infusion, frequently monitor partial thromboplastin time to determine the patient's response to it. Dilute the drug; administer it by infusion pump or controller so the patient receives the least amount necessary.
• During anticoagulant therapy, watch for signs of bleeding, such as tachycardia, hypotension, hematuria, bleeding from the nose or gums, ecchymoses, petechiae, and black, tarry stools.
• Instruct the patient on maintenance warfarin therapy to use an electric razor and a soft toothbrush and to avoid trauma. Suggest that he wear a medical identification bracelet and tell him to avoid aspirin, which aggravates bleeding tendencies. Stress the need for close medical follow-up.

LIFE-THREATENING
DISORDER

# RESPIRATORY ACIDOSIS

An acid-base disturbance characterized by reduced alveolar ventilation and manifested by hypercapnia (partial pressure of arterial carbon dioxide [$Paco_2$,] greater than 45 mm Hg), respiratory acidosis can be acute (from a sudden failure in ventilation) or chronic (as in long-term pulmonary disease). The prognosis depends on the severity of the underlying disturbance, as well as the patient's general clinical condition.

## Causes

Several factors predispose the patient to respiratory acidosis:
• *Drugs:* Narcotics, anesthetics, hypnotics, and sedatives decrease the sensitivity of the respiratory center.

• *Central nervous system (CNS) trauma:* Medullary injury may impair ventilatory drive.
• *Chronic metabolic alkalosis:* Respiratory compensatory mechanisms attempt to normalize pH by decreasing alveolar ventilation.
• *Neuromuscular disease* (such as myasthenia gravis, Guillain-Barré syndrome, and poliomyelitis): Failure of respiratory muscles to respond properly to respiratory drive reduces alveolar ventilation.

In addition, respiratory acidosis can result from airway obstruction or parenchymal lung disease, which interferes with alveolar ventilation, or from chronic obstructive pulmonary disease (COPD), asthma, severe adult respiratory distress syndrome, chronic bronchitis, large pneumothorax, extensive pneumonia, or pulmonary edema.

Hypoventilation compromises excretion of carbon dioxide produced through metabolism. The retained carbon dioxide then combines with water to form an excess of carbonic acid, decreasing the blood pH. As a result, the concentration of hydrogen ions in body fluids, which directly reflects acidity, increases.

## Signs and symptoms

Acute respiratory acidosis produces CNS disturbances that reflect changes in the pH of cerebrospinal fluid rather than increased carbon dioxide levels in cerebral circulation.

Effects range from restlessness, confusion, and apprehension to somnolence, with a fine or flapping tremor (asterixis), or coma. The patient may complain of headaches and exhibit dyspnea and tachypnea with papilledema and depressed reflexes. Unless the patient is receiving oxygen, hypoxemia accompanies respiratory acidosis.

This disorder may also cause cardiovascular abnormalities, such as tachycardia, hypertension, atrial and ventricular arrhythmias and, in severe acidosis, hypotension with vasodilation (bounding pulses and warm periphery).

**Diagnosis**

The following arterial blood gas (ABG) levels confirm respiratory acidosis: a $Paco_2$ exceeding the normal level of 45 mm Hg, pH usually below the normal range of 7.35 to 7.45, and a bicarbonate level that's normal in the acute stage but elevated in the chronic stage.

**Treatment**

Effective treatment of respiratory acidosis is designed to correct the underlying source of alveolar hypoventilation. Significantly reduced alveolar ventilation may require mechanical ventilation until the underlying condition can be treated.

In COPD, treatment includes bronchodilators, oxygen, corticosteroids and, frequently, antibiotics; drug therapy for conditions such as myasthenia gravis; removal of foreign bodies from the airway; antibiotics for pneumonia; dialysis or charcoal to remove toxic drugs; and correction of metabolic alkalosis. An elevated $Paco_2$ may persist in a patient with COPD despite optimal treatment.

**Special considerations**

• Closely monitor the patient's blood pH level.

➤ CLINICAL TIP   If the pH level drops below 7.15, profound CNS and cardiovascular deterioration may result, requiring administration of I.V. sodium bicarbonate.

• Be alert for critical changes in the patient's respiratory, CNS, and cardiovascular functions. Also watch closely for variations in ABG values and electrolyte status. Maintain adequate hydration.

• If acidosis requires mechanical ventilation, maintain a patent airway and provide adequate humidification. Perform tracheal suctioning regularly and vigorous chest physiotherapy if needed. Continuously monitor ventilator settings and respiratory status.

• To prevent respiratory acidosis, closely monitor patients with COPD and chronic carbon dioxide retention for signs of acidosis. Also, administer oxygen at low flow rates and closely monitor all patients who receive narcotics and sedatives.

• Instruct the patient who has received a general anesthetic to turn, cough, and perform deep-breathing exercises frequently to prevent the onset of respiratory acidosis.

---

✦ **LIFE-THREATENING DISORDER**

# RESPIRATORY ALKALOSIS

---

Caused by alveolar hyperventilation, respiratory alkalosis is a condition marked by a decrease in partial pressure of arterial carbon dioxide ($Paco_2$,) to below 35 mm Hg. Uncomplicated respiratory alkalosis leads to a decrease in hydrogen ion concentration, which causes elevated blood pH. Hypocapnia occurs when the elimination of carbon dioxide by the lungs exceeds the production of carbon dioxide at the cellular level.

**Causes**

Respiratory alkalosis can result from pulmonary or nonpulmonary causes:

• *Pulmonary* causes include pneumonia, interstitial lung disease, pulmonary vascular disease, and acute asthma.

• *Nonpulmonary* causes include anxiety, fever, aspirin toxicity, metabolic acidosis, CNS disease (inflammation or tumor), sepsis, hepatic failure, and pregnancy.

**Signs and symptoms**

The cardinal sign of respiratory alkalosis is deep, rapid breathing, possibly exceeding 40 breaths/minute and much like the Kussmaul's respirations that characterize diabetic acidosis.

Such hyperventilation usually leads to CNS and neuromuscular disturbances, such as light-headedness or dizziness (from below-normal carbon dioxide levels that decrease cerebral blood flow), agitation, circumoral and peripheral paresthesias, carpopedal spasms, twitching (possibly progressing to tetany), and muscle weakness. Severe respiratory alkalosis may cause cardiac arrhythmias that fail to respond to conventional treatment, seizures, or both.

**Diagnosis**

Arterial blood gas (ABG) analysis confirms respiratory alkalosis and rules out respiratory compensation for metabolic acidosis. Findings include a $Paco_2$ below 35 mm Hg, a pH that's elevated in proportion to the fall in $Paco_2$ in the acute stage but that drops toward normal in the chronic stage, and a bicarbonate level that's normal in the acute stage but below normal in the chronic stage.

**Treatment**

The goal of treatment is to eradicate the underlying condition — for example, removal of ingested toxins, treatment of fever or sepsis, and treatment of CNS disease.

> **CLINICAL TIP** In severe respiratory alkalosis, the patient may be instructed to breathe into a paper bag, which helps relieve acute anxiety and increases carbon dioxide levels.

Prevention of hyperventilation in patients receiving mechanical ventilation requires monitoring ABG values and adjusting dead space or minute ventilation volume.

**Special considerations**

• Watch for and report any changes in neurologic, neuromuscular, or cardiovascular functions.

• Remember that twitching and cardiac arrhythmias may be associated with alkalemia and electrolyte imbalances. Monitor ABG and serum electrolyte levels closely, watching for any variations.

---

�֍ LIFE-THREATENING DISORDER

# RESPIRATORY DISTRESS SYNDROME

Also called hyaline membrane disease, respiratory distress syndrome (RDS) is the most common cause of neonatal mortality. In the United States alone, it causes the death of 40,000 neonates every year. If untreated, RDS is fatal within 72 hours of birth in up to 14% of neonates weighing less than 5½ lb (2,500 g).

RDS occurs almost exclusively in neonates born before the 37th week of gestation (in 60% of those born before the 28th week). It occurs more often in neonates of diabetic mothers, those delivered by cesarean section, and those delivered suddenly after antepartum hemorrhage.

Aggressive management using mechanical ventilation can improve the prognosis, but a few neonates who survive have bronchopulmonary dysplasia. Mild RDS slowly subsides after 3 days.

## Causes

Although the airways and alveoli of a neonate's respiratory system are present by the 27th week of gestation, the intercostal muscles are weak and the alveoli and capillary blood supply are immature. In RDS, the premature neonate develops widespread alveolar collapse because of lack of surfactant, a lipoprotein present in alveoli and respiratory bronchioles.

Surfactant normally lowers surface tension and aids in maintaining alveolar patency, preventing collapse, particularly at end expiration. But a deficiency results in widespread atelectasis, which leads to inadequate alveolar ventilation with shunting of blood through collapsed areas of lung, causing hypoxia and acidosis.

### Signs and symptoms

Although a neonate with RDS may breathe normally at first, he usually develops rapid, shallow respirations within minutes or hours of birth, with intercostal, subcostal, or sternal retractions; nasal flaring; and audible expiratory grunting. This grunting is a natural compensatory mechanism designed to produce positive end-expiratory pressure (PEEP) and prevent further alveolar collapse.

The neonate may also display hypotension, peripheral edema, and oliguria; in severe disease, apnea, bradycardia, and cyanosis (from hypoxemia, left-to-right shunting through the foramen ovale, or right-to-left shunting through atelectatic regions of the lung). Other clinical features include pallor,

frothy sputum, and low body temperature as a result of an immature nervous system and the absence of subcutaneous fat.

### Diagnosis

Although signs of respiratory distress in a premature neonate during the first few hours of life strongly suggest RDS, the following tests are necessary to confirm the diagnosis:

● *Chest X-ray* may be normal for the first 6 to 12 hours (in 50% of neonates with RDS) but later shows a fine reticulonodular pattern.

● *Arterial blood gas (ABG) analysis* shows decreased partial pressure of arterial oxygen ($Pao_2$); normal, decreased, or increased partial pressure of arterial carbon dioxide ($Paco_2$); and decreased pH (from respiratory or metabolic acidosis or both).

● *Chest auscultation* reveals normal or diminished air entry and crackles (rare in early stages).

When a cesarean section is necessary before the 36th week of gestation, amniocentesis allows determination of the lecithin-sphingomyelin ratio, which helps to assess prenatal lung development and the risk of RDS.

### Treatment

An infant with RDS requires vigorous respiratory support. Warm, humidified, oxygen-enriched gases are administered by oxygen hood or, if such treatment fails, by mechanical ventilation. Severe cases may require mechanical ventilation with PEEP or continuous positive airway pressure (CPAP), administered by a tightly fitting face mask or, when necessary, endotracheal (ET) intubation.

Treatment also includes:

● a radiant infant warmer or isolette for thermoregulation

• I.V. fluids and sodium bicarbonate to control acidosis and maintain fluid and electrolyte balance
• tube feedings or total parenteral nutrition if the neonate is too weak to eat
• administration of surfactant by an ET tube.

**Special considerations**
• Closely monitor ABG levels as well as fluid intake and output. If the neonate has an umbilical catheter (arterial or venous), check for arterial hypotension or abnormal central venous pressure.
• Watch for such complications as infection, thrombosis, or decreased circulation to the legs.
• If the neonate has a transcutaneous $Pao_2$ monitor (an accurate method for determining $Pao_2$), change the site of the lead placement every 2 to 4 hours to avoid burning the skin.
• Weigh the neonate once or twice daily. To evaluate his progress, assess skin color, rate and depth of respirations, severity of retractions, nostril flaring, frequency of expiratory grunting, frothing at the lips, and restlessness.
• Regularly assess the effectiveness of oxygen or ventilator therapy. Evaluate every change in the fraction of inspired oxygen and PEEP or CPAP by monitoring oxygen saturation or ABG levels. Be sure to adjust PEEP or CPAP as indicated, based on findings.

➤ CLINICAL TIP When the neonate is on mechanical ventilation, watch carefully for signs of barotrauma (increase in respiratory distress or subcutaneous emphysema) and accidental disconnection from the ventilator. Check ventilator settings frequently.

Be alert for signs of complications of PEEP or CPAP therapy, such as decreased cardiac output, pneumothorax, and pneumomediastinum. Mechanical ventilation increases the risk of infection in premature neonates, so preventive measures are essential.

• As needed, arrange for follow-up care with a neonatal ophthalmologist to check for retinal damage.
• Teach the parents about their neonate's condition and, if possible, let them participate in his care (using aseptic technique) to encourage normal parent-infant bonding. Advise parents that full recovery may take up to 12 months. When the prognosis is poor, prepare the parents for the neonate's impending death and offer emotional support.
• Help reduce mortality in RDS by detecting respiratory distress early. Recognize intercostal retractions and grunting, especially in a premature neonate, as signs of RDS, and make sure the neonate receives immediate treatment.

# RESPIRATORY SYNCYTIAL VIRUS INFECTION

A subgroup of the myxoviruses resembling paramyxovirus causes respiratory syncytial virus (RSV) infection. RSV is the leading cause of lower respiratory tract infections in infants and young children; it's the major cause of pneumonia, tracheobronchitis, and bronchiolitis in this age-group and a suspected cause of the fatal respiratory diseases of infancy.

**Causes and incidence**
Antibody titers seem to indicate that few children under age 4 escape contracting some form of RSV, even if it's mild. In fact, RSV is the only viral disease that has its maximum impact during the first few months of life (incidence of RSV bronchiolitis peaks at age 2 months).

This virus creates annual epidemics that occur during the late winter and early spring in temperate climates and during the rainy season in the tropics. The organism is transmitted from person to person by respiratory secretions and has an incubation period of 4 to 5 days.

Reinfection is common, producing milder symptoms than the primary infection. School-age children, adolescents, and young adults with mild reinfections are probably the source of infection for infants and young children.

### Signs and symptoms

Clinical features of RSV infection vary in severity, ranging from mild coldlike symptoms to bronchiolitis or bronchopneumonia and, in a few patients, severe, life-threatening lower respiratory tract infections. Generally, symptoms include coughing, wheezing, malaise, pharyngitis, dyspnea, and inflamed mucous membranes in the nose and throat.

Otitis media is a common complication of RSV in infants. RSV has also been identified in patients with a variety of central nervous system disorders, such as meningitis and myelitis.

### Diagnosis

The following clinical findings and epidemiologic information aid in the diagnosis:

- Cultures of nasal and pharyngeal secretions may show RSV; however, the virus is very labile, so cultures aren't always reliable.
- Serum antibody titers may be elevated, but before age 6 months, maternal antibodies may impair test results.
- Two serologic techniques that aid in diagnosis are indirect immunofluorescence and the enzyme-linked immunosorbent assay (ELISA).

- Chest X-rays help detect pneumonia.

### Treatment

Among the goals of treatment are support of respiratory function, maintenance of fluid balance, and relief of symptoms.

### Special considerations

- Monitor respiratory status. Observe the rate and pattern; watch for nasal flaring or retraction, cyanosis, pallor, and dyspnea; and auscultate for wheezing, rhonchi, or other signs of respiratory distress. Monitor arterial blood gas values.
- Maintain a patent airway, and be especially watchful when the patient has periods of acute dyspnea. Perform percussion and provide drainage and suction when necessary. Provide a high-humidity atmosphere. Semi-Fowler's position may help prevent aspiration of secretions.

> **CLINICAL TIP** The head of the bed or crib may be elevated to help prevent aspiration of secretions.

- Monitor intake and output carefully. Observe for signs of dehydration such as decreased skin turgor. Encourage the patient to drink plenty of high-calorie fluids, and administer I.V. fluids as needed.
- Promote bed rest, allowing for as much uninterrupted rest as possible.
- Hold and cuddle infants; talk to and play with toddlers. Offer diversional activities suitable to the child's condition and age. Foster parental visits and cuddling. Restrain a child only as necessary.
- Impose contact isolation. Enforce strict handwashing, because RSV may be transmitted from fomites.
- Staff members with respiratory illnesses shouldn't care for infants.

# RETINAL DETACHMENT

When the sensory retina splits from the retinal pigment epithelium (RPE), retinal detachment occurs, creating a subretinal space. This space then fills with fluid, called subretinal fluid. Retinal detachment usually involves only one eye, but may involve the other eye later.

Surgical reattachment is often successful. However, the prognosis for good vision depends on the area of the retina that's been affected.

## Causes

Any retinal tear or hole allows the liquid vitreous to seep between the retinal layers, separating the retina from its choroidal blood supply. In adults, retinal detachment usually results from degenerative changes of aging, which cause a spontaneous retinal hole.

Predisposing factors include myopia, cataract surgery, and trauma. Perhaps the influence of trauma explains why retinal detachment is twice as common in males.

Retinal detachment may also result from seepage of fluid into the subretinal space (because of inflammation, tumors, or systemic diseases) or from traction that's placed on the retina by vitreous bands or membranes (from proliferative diabetic retinopathy, posterior uveitis, or a traumatic intraocular foreign body).

Retinal detachment is rare in children, but occasionally can develop as a result of retinopathy of prematurity, tumors (retinoblastomas), or trauma. It can also be inherited, usually in association with myopia.

## Signs and symptoms

Initially, the patient may complain of floating spots and recurrent flashes of light. But as detachment progresses, gradual, painless vision loss may be described as a veil, curtain, or cobweb that eliminates a portion of the visual field.

## Diagnosis

Ophthalmoscopy after full pupil dilation allows diagnosis. Examination shows the usually transparent retina as gray and opaque; in severe detachment, it reveals folds in the retina and a ballooning out of the area. Indirect ophthalmoscopy is used to search for retinal tears. Ultrasonography is performed if the lens is opaque.

## Treatment

Depending on the location and severity of the detachment, treatment may include restriction of eye movements and complete bed rest to prevent further detachment.

A hole in the peripheral retina can be treated with cryothermy; in the posterior portion, with laser therapy. Retinal detachment usually requires scleral buckling to reattach the retina and, possibly, replacement of the vitreous with oil, air, gas, or silicone.

## Special considerations

● Provide emotional support; the patient may be distraught because of his decreased vision.

● To prepare for surgery, wash the patient's face with no-tears shampoo. Administer antibiotics and cycloplegic-mydriatic eyedrops.

● Postoperatively, instruct the patient to lie in the position that facilitates the gas or oil to tamponade the retina. This may be a prone position. Discourage straining during defecation, bending down, and hard coughing, sneezing, or vomiting, which can raise intraocular pressure. Antiemetics may be indicated. Discourage activities that may cause bumping the eye.

• After removing the protective patch, gently clean the eye with cycloplegic eyedrops and steroid-antibiotic eyedrops.

• Use cold compresses to decrease swelling (postoperative edema) and pain.

• Administer analgesics such as acetaminophen as needed, noting persistent pain.

• Teach the patient how to instill eyedrops properly, and emphasize compliance and follow-up care.

➤ CLINICAL TIP   Encourage wearing dark glasses to compensate for sensitivity to light.

# REYE'S SYNDROME

An acute childhood illness, Reye's syndrome causes fatty infiltration of the liver with concurrent hyperammonemia, encephalopathy, and increased intracranial pressure (ICP). In addition, fatty infiltration of the kidneys, brain, and myocardium may occur.

Reye's syndrome affects children from infancy to adolescence and occurs equally in boys and girls. It affects Whites over age 1 more often than Blacks.

The prognosis depends on the severity of central nervous system depression. Previously, mortality was as high as 90%. Today, ICP monitoring and, consequently, early treatment of increased ICP, along with other treatment measures, have cut mortality to about 20%. Death is usually a result of cerebral edema or respiratory arrest. Comatose patients who survive may have residual brain damage.

## Causes

Reye's syndrome almost always follows within 1 to 3 days of an acute viral infection, such as an upper respiratory infection, type B influenza, or varicella (chickenpox). Incidence often rises during influenza outbreaks and may be linked to aspirin use.

In Reye's syndrome, damaged hepatic mitochondria disrupt the urea cycle, which normally changes ammonia to urea for its excretion from the body. This results in hyperammonemia, hypoglycemia, and an increase in serum short-chain fatty acids, leading to encephalopathy. Simultaneously, fatty infiltration is found in renal tubular cells, neuronal tissue, and muscle tissue, including the heart.

## Signs and symptoms

The severity of the child's signs and symptoms varies with the degree of encephalopathy and cerebral edema. In any case, Reye's syndrome develops in five stages.

After the initial viral infection, a brief recovery period follows when the child doesn't seem seriously ill. A few days later, he develops intractable vomiting, lethargy, rapidly changing mental status (mild to severe agitation, confusion, irritability, delirium), hyperactive reflexes, and rising blood pressure, respiratory rate, and pulse rate.

Reye's syndrome often progresses to coma. As the coma deepens, seizures develop, followed by decreased tendon reflexes and, frequently, respiratory failure.

Increased ICP, a serious complication, results from cerebral edema. Such edema may develop as a result of acidosis, increased cerebral metabolic rate, and an impaired autoregulatory mechanism.

# STAGES OF TREATMENT FOR REYE'S SYNDROME

| SIGNS AND SYMPTOMS | BASELINE TREATMENT | BASELINE INTERVENTION |
|---|---|---|
| **Stage I** Vomiting, lethargy, hepatic dysfunction | • To decrease intracranial pressure (ICP) and brain edema, give I.V. fluids at two-thirds of the maintenance dose. Also give an osmotic diuretic or furosemide. <br> • To treat hypoprothrombinemia, give vitamin K; if vitamin K is unsuccessful, give fresh frozen plasma. <br> • Monitor serum ammonia and blood glucose levels and plasma osmolality every 4 to 8 hours to check progress. | • Monitor vital signs and check level of consciousness for increasing lethargy. Take vital signs more often as the patient's condition deteriorates. <br> • Monitor fluid intake and output to prevent fluid overload. Maintain urine output at 1 ml/kg/hour, plasma osmolality at 290 mOsm, and blood glucose at 150 mg/dl. (Goal: Keep glucose levels high, osmolality normal to high, and ammonia levels low.) Also restrict protein. |
| **Stage II** Hyperventilation, delirium, hepatic dysfunction, hyperactive reflexes | • Continue baseline treatment. | • Maintain seizure precautions. <br> • Watch closely for any signs of coma that require invasive or supportive therapy such as intubation. <br> • Keep head of bed at a 30-degree angle. |
| **Stage III** Coma, hyperventilation, decorticate rigidity, hepatic dysfunction | • Continue baseline and seizure treatment. <br> • Monitor ICP with a subarachnoid screw or other invasive device. <br> • Provide endotracheal intubation and mechanical ventilation to control partial pressure of carbon dioxide ($Pco_2$). A paralyzing agent, such as pancuronium I.V., may help maintain ventilation. <br> • Give mannitol I.V. or glycerol by nasogastric tube. | • Monitor ICP (should be < 20 mm Hg before suctioning) or give a barbiturate I.V. as needed; hyperventilate the patient as necessary. <br> • When ventilating the patient, maintain $Pco_2$ between 25 and 30 mm Hg and $Po_2$ between 80 and 100 mm hg <br> • Closely monitor cardiovascular status with a pulmonary artery catheter or central venous pressure line. <br> • Give good skin and mouth care and perform range-of-motion exercises. |
| **Stage IV** Deepening coma; decerebrate rigidity; large, fixed pupils; minimal hepatic dysfunction | • Continue baseline and supportive care. <br> • If all previous measures fail, some pediatric centers use barbiturate coma, decompressive craniotomy, hypothermia, or an exchange transfusion. | • Check patient for loss of reflexes and signs of flaccidity. <br> • Give the family the extra support they need, considering their child's poor prognosis. |

## STAGES OF TREATMENT FOR REYE'S SYNDROME *(continued)*

| SIGNS AND SYMPTOMS | BASELINE TREATMENT | BASELINE INTERVENTION |
|---|---|---|
| **Stage V** Seizures, loss of deep tendon reflexes, flaccidity, respiratory arrest, ammonia level > 300 mg/dl | • Continue baseline and supportive care. | • Help the family to face the patient's impending death. |

### Diagnosis

A history of a recent viral disorder with typical clinical features strongly suggests Reye's syndrome. An increased serum ammonia level, abnormal clotting studies, and hepatic dysfunction confirm it.

Testing the serum salicylate level rules out aspirin overdose. Absence of jaundice, despite increased liver transaminase levels, rules out acute hepatic failure and hepatic encephalopathy.

Abnormal test results may include the following:

• *Liver-function studies* show aspartate aminotransferase and alanine aminotransferase elevated to twice normal levels; bilirubin is usually normal.

• *Liver biopsy* reveals fatty droplets uniformly distributed throughout cells.

• *Cerebrospinal fluid (CSF) analysis* reveals a white blood cell count of less than 10; with coma, CSF pressure increases.

• *Coagulation studies* result in prolonged prothrombin and partial thromboplastin times.

• *Blood values* show elevated serum ammonia levels; normal or, in 15% of cases, low serum glucose levels; and increased serum fatty acid and lactate levels.

### Treatment and special considerations

The stage of the syndrome dictates the type of treatment necessary. (See *Stages of treatment for Reye's syndrome.*)

Advise parents to give nonsalicylate analgesics and antipyretics such as acetaminophen. Refer parents to the National Reye's Syndrome Foundation for more information.

# RHEUMATIC FEVER AND RHEUMATIC HEART DISEASE

Often recurrent, acute rheumatic fever is a systemic inflammatory disease of childhood that follows a group A beta-hemolytic streptococcal infection. Rheumatic heart disease refers to the cardiac manifestations of rheumatic fever, and includes pancarditis (myocarditis, pericarditis, and endocarditis) during the early acute phase, and chronic valvular disease later.

Long-term antibiotic therapy can minimize recurrence of rheumatic fever, reducing the risk of permanent cardiac damage and eventual valvular deformity. However, severe pancarditis occasionally produces fatal heart failure during the acute phase. Of the patients who survive this complication, about 20% die within 10 years.

## Causes

Rheumatic fever appears to be a hypersensitivity reaction to a group A beta-hemolytic streptococcal infection, in which antibodies manufactured to combat streptococci react and produce characteristic lesions at specific tissue sites, especially in the heart and joints. Because very few people (about 0.3%) with streptococcal infections ever contract rheumatic fever, altered host resistance must be involved in its development or recurrence.

Although rheumatic fever tends to run in families, this may merely reflect contributing environmental factors. For example, in lower socioeconomic groups, incidence is highest in children between ages 5 and 15, probably as a result of malnutrition and crowded living conditions.

This disease strikes most often during cool, damp weather in the winter and early spring. In the United States, it's most common in the northern states.

## Signs and symptoms

In 95% of patients, rheumatic fever characteristically follows a streptococcal infection that appeared a few days to 6 weeks earlier. A temperature of at least 100.4° F (38° C) occurs.

### Joint pain

Most patients complain of migratory joint pain or polyarthritis. Swelling, redness, and signs of effusion usually accompany such pain, which most commonly affects the knees, ankles, elbows, or hips.

### Skin lesions and nodules

In 5% of patients (generally those with carditis), rheumatic fever causes skin lesions such as erythema marginatum. This nonpruritic, macular, transient rash gives rise to red lesions with blanched centers.

Rheumatic fever may also produce firm, movable, nontender, subcutaneous nodules about 3 mm to 2 cm in diameter, usually near tendons or bony prominences of joints (especially the elbows, knuckles, wrists, and knees) and less often on the scalp and backs of the hands. These nodules persist for a few days to several weeks and, like erythema marginatum, often accompany carditis.

### Chorea

Later, rheumatic fever may cause transient chorea, which develops up to 6 months after the original streptococcal infection.

Mild chorea may produce hyperirritability, a deterioration in handwriting, or an inability to concentrate. Severe chorea causes purposeless, nonrepetitive, involuntary muscle spasms; poor muscle coordination; and weakness. Chorea always resolves without residual neurologic damage.

### Carditis

The most destructive effect of rheumatic fever is carditis, which develops in up to 50% of patients. It may affect the endocardium, myocardium, pericardium, or the heart valves.

Pericarditis causes a pericardial friction rub and, occasionally, pain and effusion. Myocarditis produces characteristic lesions called Aschoff's bodies (in the acute stages) and cellular swelling and fragmentation of interstitial collagen, leading to formation of a progressively fibrotic nodule and interstitial scars.

Endocarditis causes valve leaflet swelling, erosion along the lines of leaflet closure, and blood, platelet, and fibrin deposits, which form beadlike vegetations. Endocarditis affects the mitral valve most often in females; the aortic valve most often in males. In both sexes, endocarditis affects the tricuspid valves occasionally and the pulmonic valve only rarely.

Severe rheumatic carditis may cause heart failure with dyspnea, upper right quadrant pain, tachycardia, tachypnea, significant mitral and aortic murmurs, and a hacking, nonproductive cough.

The most common of such murmurs include:

- a systolic murmur of mitral insufficiency (high-pitched, blowing, holosystolic, loudest at apex, possibly radiating to the anterior axillary line)
- a midsystolic murmur caused by stiffening and swelling of the mitral leaflet
- occasionally, a diastolic murmur of aortic insufficiency. Valvular disease may eventually result in chronic valvular stenosis and insufficiency, including mitral stenosis and insufficiency and aortic insufficiency. In children, mitral insufficiency remains the major sequela of rheumatic heart disease.

## Diagnosis

Recognition of one or more of the classic symptoms (carditis, polyarthritis, chorea, erythema marginatum, or subcutaneous nodules) and a detailed patient history allow diagnosis. The following laboratory data support the diagnosis:

- *White blood cell count* and *erythrocyte sedimentation rate* may be elevated (during the acute phase); blood studies show slight anemia from suppressed erythropoiesis during inflammation.

- *C-reactive protein* is positive (especially during the acute phase).
- *Cardiac enzyme levels* may be increased in severe carditis.
- *Antistreptolysin O titer* is elevated in 95% of patients within 2 months of onset.
- *Electrocardiography* changes aren't diagnostic, but the PR interval is prolonged in 20% of patients.
- *Chest X-rays* show normal heart size (except with myocarditis, heart failure, or pericardial effusion).
- *Echocardiography* helps evaluate valvular damage, chamber size, and ventricular function.
- *Cardiac catheterization* evaluates valvular damage and left ventricular function in severe cardiac dysfunction.

## Treatment

Effective management eradicates the streptococcal infection, relieves symptoms, and prevents recurrence, reducing the chance of permanent cardiac damage.

### Treatment in acute phase

During the acute phase, treatment includes penicillin or (for patients with penicillin hypersensitivity) erythromycin. Salicylates such as aspirin relieve fever and minimize joint swelling and pain; if carditis is present or salicylates fail to relieve pain and inflammation, corticosteroids may be used.

Supportive treatment requires strict bed rest for about 5 weeks during the acute phase with active carditis, followed by a progressive increase in physical activity, depending on clinical and laboratory findings and the response to treatment.

### Preventive treatment

After the acute phase subsides, a monthly I.M. injection of penicillin G benzathine or daily doses of oral sulfadiazine or penicillin G may be used to prevent recurrence. Such preventive treatment usually continues for 5 to 10 years.

### Surgery and other measures

Heart failure necessitates continued bed rest and diuretics. Severe mitral or aortic valvular dysfunction causing persistent heart failure requires corrective valvular surgery, including commissurotomy (separation of the adherent, thickened leaflets of the mitral valve), valvuloplasty (inflation of a balloon within a valve), or valve replacement (with a prosthetic valve). Corrective valvular surgery is rarely necessary before late adolescence.

### Special considerations

- Teach the patient and family about this disease and its treatment.
- Before giving penicillin, ask the parents if the child has ever had a hypersensitivity reaction to it. Even if the patient has never had a reaction to penicillin, warn that such a reaction is possible.
- Tell the child's parents to stop the drug and immediately report the development of a rash, fever, chills, or other signs of allergy *at any time* during penicillin therapy.
- Instruct the parents to watch for and report early signs of heart failure, such as dyspnea and a hacking, nonproductive cough.
- Stress the need for bed rest during the acute phase and suggest appropriate, physically undemanding diversions.
- After the acute phase, encourage family and friends to spend as much time as possible with the child to minimize boredom. Advise the parents to secure a tutor to help the child keep up with schoolwork during his long convalescence.
- Help the parents overcome any guilt they may feel about their child's illness.

Tell them that failure to seek treatment for streptococcal infection is common, because this illness often seems no worse than a cold.

- If the child has severe carditis, help parents prepare for permanent changes in the child's lifestyle.
- Warn the parents to watch for and immediately report signs of recurrent streptococcal infection — sudden sore throat, diffuse throat redness and oropharyngeal exudate, swollen and tender cervical lymph glands, pain on swallowing, a temperature of 101° to 104° F (38.3° to 40° C), headache, and nausea. Urge them to keep the child away from people with respiratory tract infections.

➤ CLINICAL TIP Explain the importance of good dental hygiene in preventing gingival infection.

- Make sure the child and his family understand the need to comply with prolonged antibiotic therapy and follow-up care and the need for additional antibiotics during dental surgery.
- Arrange for a visiting nurse to oversee home care if necessary.

# RHEUMATOID ARTHRITIS

A chronic, systemic inflammatory disease, rheumatoid arthritis (RA) primarily attacks peripheral joints and surrounding muscles, tendons, ligaments, and blood vessels. Partial remissions and unpredictable exacerbations mark the course of this potentially crippling disease.

RA occurs worldwide, striking women three times more often than men. It it can occur at any age but 80% of patients develop RA between ages 35 and 50. RA affects more than 6.5 million people in the United States alone.

This disease usually requires lifelong treatment and, sometimes, surgery. In most patients, it follows an intermittent course and allows normal activity, although 10% suffer total disability from severe articular deformity, associated extra-articular symptoms, or both. The prognosis worsens with the development of nodules, vasculitis, and high titers of rheumatoid factor (RF).

## Causes

What causes the chronic inflammation characteristic of RA isn't known. One theory states that abnormal immune activation (occurring in a genetically susceptible individual) leads to inflammation, complement activation, and cell proliferation within joints and tendon sheaths. Although no single environmental factor has been found to be a consistent and reproducible cause of this response, infection (viral or bacterial), hormonal factors, and lifestyle factors may all influence disease onset.

Some RA patients develop an IgM antibody against their body's own IgG, which is called the rheumatoid factor (RF). Increased production of this antibody may also play a role in genetic inflammation.

### Pathogenesis

Much more is known about the pathogenesis of RA than about its causes. If unarrested, the inflammatory process within the joints occurs in four stages.

In the first stage, synovitis develops from congestion and edema of the synovial membrane and joint capsule. Infiltration by lymphocytes, macrophages, and neutrophils perpetuates the local inflammatory response. These cells, as well as fibroblast-like synovial cells, produce enzymes that help to degrade bone and cartilage. Formation of pannus — thickened layers of granulation tissue — marks the onset of the second stage. Pannus covers and invades cartilage and eventually destroys the joint capsule and bone.

Progression to the third stage is characterized by fibrous ankylosis — fibrous invasion of the pannus and scar formation that occludes the joint space. Bone atrophy and malalignment cause visible deformities and disrupt the articulation of opposing bones, causing muscle atrophy and imbalance and, possibly, partial dislocations or subluxations.

In the fourth stage, fibrous tissue calcifies, resulting in bony ankylosis and total immobility.

## Signs and symptoms

RA usually develops insidiously and initially produces nonspecific symptoms. These include fatigue, malaise, anorexia, persistent low-grade fever, weight loss, lymphadenopathy, and vague articular symptoms.

### Specific symptoms

As the disease progresses, more specific localized articular symptoms develop, frequently in the fingers at the proximal interphalangeal (PIP), metacarpophalangeal (MCP), and metatarsophalangeal joints. These symptoms usually occur bilaterally and symmetrically and may extend to the wrists, knees, elbows, and ankles.

The affected joints stiffen after inactivity, especially on rising in the morning. The fingers may assume a spindle shape from marked edema and congestion in the joints. The joints become tender and painful, at first only when the patient moves them, but eventually even at rest. They often feel hot to the touch. Ultimately, joint function is diminished. Deformities are common if active disease continues.

PIP joints may develop flexion deformities or become hyperextended. MCP joints may swell dorsally, and volar subluxation and stretching of tendons may pull the fingers to the ulnar side ("ulnar drift").

The fingers may become fixed in a characteristic "swan's neck" appearance or "boutonniere" deformity. The hands appear foreshortened, the wrists boggy; carpal tunnel syndrome from synovial pressure on the median nerve causes paresthesia in the fingers.

> CLINICAL TIP  Early intervention, under the guidance of an occupational therapist, with splinting and joint protection devices can effectively delay the progression of joint deformities.

### Extra-articular signs

The most common extra-articular finding is the gradual appearance of rheumatoid nodules — subcutaneous, round or oval, nontender masses. These are seen in 20% of RA patients who are RF-positive. They usually appear on pressure areas such as the elbows, hands, or Achilles tendon.

Vasculitis can lead to skin lesions, leg ulcers, and multiple systemic complications. Peripheral neuropathy may produce numbness or tingling in the feet or weakness and loss of sensation in the fingers. Stiff, weak, or painful muscles are common.

Other common extra-articular effects include pericarditis, pulmonary nodules or fibrosis, pleuritis, scleritis, and episcleritis.

### Other complications

Another complication is destruction of the odontoid process, part of the second cervical vertebra. With $C_1$ or $C_2$ instability and subluxation, spinal cord compression may occur, particularly in patients with longstanding deforming RA. Upper motor neuron signs, such as a positive Babinski's sign and muscle weakness, may also develop.

RA can also cause temporomandibular joint disease, which impairs chewing and causes earaches. Other extra-articular findings may include infection, osteoporosis, myositis, cardiopulmonary lesions, lymphadenopathy, and peripheral neuritis.

### Diagnosis

Typical clinical features suggest RA, with a firm diagnosis supported by laboratory and other test results:

● *X-rays* in early stages show bone demineralization and soft-tissue swelling; later, loss of cartilage and narrowing of joint spaces; and finally, cartilage and bone destruction and erosion, subluxations, and deformities.

● *RF* is positive in 75% to 80% of patients, as indicated by a titer of 1:160 or higher.

● *Synovial fluid analysis* shows increased volume and turbidity but decreased viscosity and elevated WBC counts (often greater than 10,000/ul).

● *Serum protein electrophoresis* may show elevated serum globulin levels.

● *Erythrocyte sedimentation rate* and *C-reactive protein* are elevated in 85% to 90% of patients (may be useful to monitor response to therapy because elevation frequently parallels disease activity).

● *Complete blood count* usually shows moderate anemia, slight leukocytosis, and thrombocytosis.

### Treatment

Salicylates, particularly aspirin, are the mainstay of RA therapy, because they decrease inflammation and relieve joint pain. Other useful medications include nonsteroidal anti-inflammatory agents (such as indomethacin, fenoprofen, and ibuprofen), antimalarials (hydroxychloroquine), sulfasalazine, gold salts, penicillamine, and corticosteroids (prednisone). (See *Drug therapy for arthritis.*)

# DRUG THERAPY FOR ARTHRITIS

| DRUG AND ADVERSE EFFECTS | CLINICAL CONSIDERATIONS |
|---|---|
| **Aspirin**<br>• Prolonged bleeding time; GI disturbances, including nausea, dyspepsia, anorexia nervosa, ulcers, and hemorrhage; hypersensitivity reactions ranging from urticaria to anaphylaxis; salicylism (mild toxicity: tinnitus, dizziness; moderate toxicity: restlessness, hyperpnea, delirium, marked lethargy; severe toxicity: coma, seizures, severe hyperpnea) | • Don't use in patients with GI ulcers, bleeding, or hypersensitivity or in neonates<br>• Give with food, milk, antacid, or a large glass of water to reduce GI adverse effects.<br>• Monitor salicylate level. Remember that toxicity can develop rapidly in febrile, dehydrated children.<br>• Teach patient to reduce dose, one tablet at a time, if tinnitus occurs.<br>• Teach patient to watch for signs of bleeding, such as bruising, melena, and petechiae. |
| **Fenoprofen, ibuprofen, naproxen, piroxicam, sulindac, and tolmetin**<br>• Prolonged bleeding time, central nervous system abnormalities (headache, drowsiness, restlessness, dizziness, tremor); GI disturbances, including hemorrhage and peptic ulcer; increased blood urea nitrogen and liver enzyme levels | • Don't use in patients with renal disease, in asthmatics with nasal polyps, or in children.<br>• Use cautiously in GI disorders and cardiac disease or when patient is allergic to other nonsteroidal anti-inflammatory drugs.<br>• Give with milk or meals to reduce GI adverse effects.<br>• Tell patient that drug's effect may be delayed for 2 to 3 weeks.<br>• Monitor kidney, liver, and auditory functions in long-term therapy. Stop drugs if abnormalities develop<br>• Use cautiously in elderly patients; they may experience severe GI bleeding without warning. |
| **Hydroxychloroquine**<br>• Blood dyscrasias, GI irritation, corneal opacities, and keratopathy or retinopathy | • Contraindicated in patients with retinal or visual field changes.<br>• Use cautiously in patients with hepatic disease, alcoholism, glucose-6-phosphate dehydrogenase deficiency, or psoriasis.<br>• Perform complete blood count (CBC) and liver function tests before therapy and during chronic therapy. Patient should also have regular ophthalmologic examination.<br>• Tell patient to take drug with food or milk<br>• Warn patient that dizziness may occur. |
| **Gold (oral and parenteral)**<br>• Dermatitis, pruritus, rash, stomatitis, nephrotoxicity, and blood dyscrasias; with oral form, GI distress and diarrhea | • Watch for adverse effects. Observe for nitritoid reaction (flushing, fainting, sweating).<br>• Check urine for blood and albumin before each dose If positive, drug may need to be withheld. Stress the need for regular follow-up, including blood and urine testing. |

DRUG THERAPY FOR ARTHRITIS *(continued)*

| DRUG AND ADVERSE EFFECTS | CLINICAL CONSIDERATIONS |
|---|---|
| **Gold (oral and parenteral)** *(continued)* | • To avoid local nerve irritation, mix drug well and give deep I.M. injection in buttock<br>• Advise patient not to expect improvement for 3 to 6 months.<br>• Instruct patient to report rash, bruising, bleeding, hematuria, or oral ulcers. |
| **Methotrexate**<br>• Tubular necrosis, bone marrow depression, leukopenia, thrombocytopenia, pulmonary interstitial infiltrates, stomatitis, hyperuricemia, rash, pruritus, dermatitis, alopecia, diarrhea, dizziness, cirrhosis, and hepatic fibrosis | • Don't give to breast-feeding or pregnant women or to alcoholic patients.<br>• Monitor uric acid (UA) levels, CBC, and liver function tests.<br>• Monitor intake and output.<br>• Warn patient to report any unusual bleeding (especially GI) or bruising promptly.<br>• Warn patient to avoid alcohol.<br>• Advise patient to follow prescribed regimen. |
| **Sulfasalazine**<br>• Nausea, vomiting, abdominal pains, rash, bone marrow suppression, headache, and hypersensitivity reaction | • Give in divided doses.<br>• Don't give to patients with known sulfa allergy.<br>• Monitor CBC, UA, and liver enzymes.<br>• Caution patient not to take sulfasalazine at same time as antacids, which interfere with absorption. |
| **Cyclosporine**<br>• Nephrotoxicity (rise in blood urea nitrogen [BUN] and creatinine levels), hypertension, bone marrow suppression, nausea, vomiting, paresthesias, and bone pain | • Avoid use in patients with preexisting hypertension or renal disease.<br>• Monitor blood pressure closely.<br>• Monitor BUN and creatinine levels.<br>• Be aware that levels of cyclosporine may be increased by other medications that are metabolized by the liver. |
| **Prednisone**<br>• Hyperglycemia, hypertension, fluid retention and weight gain, acne, cataracts, dyspepsia, muscle weakness, osteoporosis, mental status changes, insomnia, psychosis | • Give as an initial high dose to suppress inflammation, followed by slow tapering to the lowest possible dose.<br>• Advise patient not to stop the drug suddenly because this can lead to adrenal insufficiency.<br>• Monitor glucose levels and blood pressure. |

Immunosuppressants, such as methotrexate, cyclosporine, and azathioprine, are also therapeutic. They are being used more commonly in early disease.

Supportive measures include 8 to 10 hours of sleep every night, frequent rest periods between daily activities, and splinting to rest inflamed joints. A physical therapy program, including range-of-motion exercises and carefully individualized therapeutic exercises, forestalls loss of joint function.

Application of heat relaxes muscles and relieves pain. Moist heat usually works best for patients with chronic disease. Ice packs are effective during acute episodes.

### Treatment in advanced disease

Advanced disease may require synovectomy, joint reconstruction, or total joint arthroplasty. (See *When arthritis requires surgery,* page 756.)

Useful surgical procedures in RA include metatarsal head and distal ulnar resectional arthroplasty, insertion of a Silastic prosthesis between MCP and PIP joints, and arthrodesis (joint fusion). Arthrodesis sacrifices joint mobility for stability and relief of pain.

Synovectomy (removal of destructive, proliferating synovium, usually in the wrists, knees, and fingers) may halt or delay the course of this disease. Osteotomy (the cutting of bone or excision of a wedge of bone) can realign joint surfaces and redistribute stresses.

Tendons may rupture spontaneously, requiring surgical repair. Tendon transfers may prevent deformities or relieve contractures.

### Special considerations

● If the patient requires knee or hip arthroplasty, provide appropriate teaching and postoperative care.
● Assess all joints carefully. Look for deformities, contractures, immobility,

and inability to perform everyday activities.
● Monitor vital signs, and note weight changes, sensory disturbances, and level of pain. Administer analgesics, and watch for adverse effects.
● Give meticulous skin care. Check for rheumatoid nodules, as well as pressure ulcers and breakdowns from immobility, vascular impairment, corticosteroid treatment, or improper splinting. Use lotion or cleansing oil, not soap, for dry skin.
● Explain all diagnostic tests and procedures. Tell the patient to expect multiple blood samples to allow a firm diagnosis and accurate monitoring of therapy.
● Monitor the duration, not the intensity, of morning stiffness, because duration more accurately reflects the severity of the disease. Encourage the patient to take hot showers or baths at bedtime or in the morning to reduce the need for pain medication.
● Apply splints carefully and correctly. Observe for pressure ulcers if the patient is in traction or wearing splints.
● Explain the nature of RA. Make sure the patient and his family understand that RA is a chronic disease that requires major changes in lifestyle. Emphasize that there are no miracle cures, despite claims to the contrary.
● Encourage a balanced diet, but make sure the patient understands that special diets won't cure RA. Stress the need for weight control because obesity adds further stress to joints.
● Urge the patient to perform activities of daily living, such as dressing and feeding himself. (Supply easy-to-open cartons, lightweight cups, and unpackaged silverware.) Allow the patient enough time to calmly perform these tasks.
● Provide emotional support. Remember that the patient with chronic illness

# WHEN ARTHRITIS REQUIRES SURGERY

Arthritis severe enough to necessitate total knee or total hip arthroplasty calls for comprehensive preoperative teaching and postoperative care.

### Before surgery
- Explain preoperative and surgical procedures. Show the patient the prosthesis to be used if available.
- Teach the patient postoperative exercises (such as isometrics), and supervise his practice. Also, teach deep-breathing and coughing exercises that will be necessary after surgery.
- Explain that total hip or knee arthroplasty requires frequent range-of-motion exercises of the leg after surgery; total knee arthroplasty requires frequent leg-lift exercises.
- Show the patient how to use a trapeze to move himself about in bed after surgery, and make sure he has a fracture bedpan handy.
- Tell the patient what kind of dressings to expect after surgery. After total knee arthroplasty, the patient's knee may be placed in a constant-passive-motion device to increase postoperative mobility and prevent emboli. After total hip arthroplasty, he'll have an abduction pillow between the legs to help keep the hip prosthesis in place.

### After surgery
- Closely monitor and record vital signs. Watch for complications, such as steroid crisis and shock in patients receiving steroids. Monitor distal leg pulses often, marking them with a waterproof marker to make them easier to find.
- As soon as the patient awakens, make sure he can perform active dor-

siflexion. Supervise isometric exercises every 2 hours. After total hip arthroplasty, check traction for pressure areas and keep the head of the bed raised between 30 and 45 degrees.
- Change or reinforce dressings as needed, using aseptic technique. Check wounds for hematoma, excessive drainage, color changes, or foul odor—all possible signs of hemorrhage or infection. (Wounds on rheumatoid arthritis patients may heal slowly.) Avoid contaminating dressings while helping the patient use the urinal or bedpan.
- Administer blood replacement products, antibiotics, and pain medication as needed. Monitor serum electrolyte levels, hemoglobin, and hematocrit.
- Have the patient turn, cough, and deep-breathe every 2 hours; then percuss his chest.
- After total knee arthroplasty, keep the patient's leg extended and slightly elevated.
- After total hip arthroplasty, keep the patient's hip in abduction to prevent dislocation. Watch for any inability to rotate the hip or bear weight on it, increased pain, or a leg that appears shorter—all may indicate dislocation.
- As soon as allowed, help the patient get out of bed and sit in a chair, keeping his weight on the unaffected side. When he's ready to walk, consult with the physical therapist for walking instruction and aids.

easily becomes depressed, discouraged, and irritable. Encourage the RA patient to discuss his fears concerning dependency, sexuality, body image, and self-esteem. Refer him to an appropriate social service agency as needed.

- Discuss sexual aids: alternative positions, pain medication, and moist heat to increase mobility.
- Before discharge, make sure the patient knows how and when to take his

prescribed medication and how to recognize its possible adverse effects.

• Teach the patient how to stand, walk, and sit correctly: upright and erect. Tell him to sit in chairs with high seats and armrests; he'll find it easier to get up from a chair if his knees are lower than his hips. If he doesn't own a chair with a high seat, recommend putting blocks of wood under the legs of a favorite chair. Suggest an elevated toilet seat.

• Instruct the patient to pace daily activities, resting for 5 to 10 minutes out of each hour and alternating sitting and standing tasks. Adequate sleep is important, and so is correct sleeping posture. He should sleep on his back on a firm mattress and should avoid placing a pillow under his knees, which encourages flexion deformity.

• Teach the patient to avoid putting undue stress on joints and to use the largest joint available for a given task; to support weak or painful joints as much as possible; to avoid positions of flexion and promote positions of extension; to hold objects parallel to the knuckles as briefly as possible; to always use his hands toward the center of his body; and to slide—not lift—objects whenever possible.

• Enlist the aid of the occupational therapist to teach how to simplify activities and protect arthritic joints. Stress the importance of shoes with proper support.

• Suggest dressing aids—long-handled shoehorn, reacher, elastic shoelaces, zipper-pull, and buttonhook—and helpful household items, such as easy-to-open drawers, a hand-held shower nozzle, handrails, and grab bars.

• Suggest wearing mittens to the patient who has trouble maneuvering fingers into gloves. Tell him to dress while in a sitting position as often as possible.

• Refer the patient to the Arthritis Foundation for more information on coping with RA.

# ROSEOLA INFANTUM

Also called exanthema subitum, roseola infantum is an acute, benign, presumably viral infection. It usually affects infants and young children (ages 6 months to 3 years).

Roseola affects boys and girls alike. It occurs year-round but is most prevalent in the spring and fall. Overt roseola, the most common exanthem in infants under age 2, affects 30% of all children; inapparent roseola (febrile illness without a rash) may affect the rest.

Characteristically, it first causes a high fever and then a rash that accompanies an abrupt drop to normal temperature. (See *Incubation and duration of common rash-producing infections,* page 758.)

## Causes and incidence
The mode of transmission isn't known. Only rarely does an infected child transmit roseola to a sibling.

## Signs and symptoms
After a 10- to 15-day incubation period, the infant with roseola develops an abruptly rising, unexplainable fever and, sometimes, seizures. Temperature peaks at 103° to 105° F (39.4° to 40.6° C) for 3 to 5 days, then drops suddenly. In the early febrile period, the infant may be anorexic, irritable, and listless but doesn't seem particularly ill.

Simultaneously with an abrupt drop in temperature, a maculopapular, nonpruritic rash develops, which blanches on pressure. The rash is profuse on the infant's trunk, arms, and neck, and is

## INCUBATION AND DURATION OF COMMON RASH-PRODUCING INFECTIONS

| INFECTION | INCUBATION (DAYS) | DURATION (DAYS) |
|---|---|---|
| Roseola | 10 to 15 | 3 to 6 |
| Varicella | 10 to 14 | 7 to 14 |
| Rubeola | 13 to 17 | 5 |
| Rubella | 6 to 18 | 3 |
| Herpes simplex | 2 to 12 | 7 to 21 |

mild on the face and legs. It fades within 24 hours. Although possible, complications are extremely rare.

### Diagnosis
Diagnosis requires observation of the typical rash that appears about 48 hours after fever subsides.

### Treatment
Because roseola is self-limiting, treatment is supportive and symptomatic: antipyretics to lower fever and, if necessary, anticonvulsants to relieve seizures.

### Special considerations
• Teach parents how to lower their infant's fever by giving tepid baths, keeping him in lightweight clothes, and maintaining normal room temperature. Stress the need for adequate fluid intake. Strict bed rest and isolation are unnecessary.
• Tell parents that a short febrile convulsion will not cause brain damage. Explain that convulsions will cease after fever subsides and that phenobarbital is likely to cause drowsiness; parents should call immediately if it causes stupor.

# RUBELLA

Commonly called German measles, rubella is an acute, mildly contagious viral disease that produces a distinctive 3-day rash and lymphadenopathy. It occurs most often among children ages 5 to 9, adolescents, and young adults.

Worldwide in distribution, rubella flourishes during the spring (particularly in big cities), and epidemics occur sporadically. This disease is self-limiting, and the prognosis is excellent.

### Causes
The rubella virus is transmitted through contact with the blood, urine, stools, or nasopharyngeal secretions of infected persons and possibly by contact with contaminated articles of clothing. Transplacental transmission, especially in the first trimester of pregnancy, can cause serious birth defects.

Humans are the only known hosts for the rubella virus. The period of communicability lasts from about 10 days before until 5 days after the rash appears.

## Signs and symptoms

In children, after an incubation period of from 16 to 18 days, an exanthematous, maculopapular rash erupts abruptly. In adolescents and adults, prodromal symptoms — headache, anorexia, malaise, low-grade fever, coryza, lymphadenopathy and, sometimes, conjunctivitis — are the first symptoms. Suboccipital, postauricular, and postcervical lymph node enlargement is a hallmark of rubella.

### *Short-term rash*

Typically, the rubella rash begins on the face. This maculopapular eruption spreads rapidly, often covering the trunk and extremities within hours. Small, red, petechial macules on the soft palate (Forschheimer spots) may precede or accompany the rash.

By the end of the second day, the facial rash begins to fade, but the rash on the trunk may be confluent and may be mistaken for scarlet fever. The rash continues to fade in the downward order in which it appeared. The rash generally disappears on the third day, but it may persist for 4 or 5 days — sometimes accompanied by mild coryza and conjunctivitis.

The rapid appearance and disappearance of the rubella rash distinguishes it from rubeola. Rubella can occur without a rash, but this is rare. Low-grade fever (99° to 101° F [37.2° to 38.3° C]) may accompany the rash, but it usually doesn't persist after the first day of the rash; rarely, temperature may reach 104° F (40° C).

## Complications

Complications seldom occur in children with rubella, but when they do, they often appear as hemorrhagic problems such as thrombocytopenia. Young women, however, often experience transient joint pain or arthritis, usually just as the rash is fading. Fever may then recur. These complications usually subside spontaneously within 5 to 30 days.

## Diagnosis

The rubella rash, lymphadenopathy, other characteristic signs, and a history of exposure to infected people usually permit clinical diagnosis without laboratory tests. However, cell cultures of the throat, blood, urine, and cerebrospinal fluid can confirm the virus' presence. Convalescent serum that shows a fourfold rise in antibody titers confirms the diagnosis.

## Treatment

Because the rubella rash is self-limiting and only mildly pruritic, it doesn't require topical or systemic medication. Treatment consists of aspirin for fever and joint pain. Bed rest isn't necessary, but the patient should be isolated until the rash disappears.

Immunization with live-virus vaccine RA27/3, the only rubella vaccine available in the United States, is necessary for prevention and appears to be more immunogenic than previous vaccines. The rubella vaccine should be given with measles and mumps vaccines at age 15 months to decrease the cost and the number of injections needed.

## Special considerations

• Make the patient with active rubella as comfortable as possible. Give children books to read or games to play to keep them occupied.

• Explain why respiratory isolation is necessary. Make sure the patient understands how important it is to avoid exposing pregnant women to this disease.

• Report confirmed cases of rubella to local public health officials.

When giving the rubella vaccine:

• Obtain a history of allergies, especially to neomycin. If the patient has this allergy or has had a reaction to immunization in the past, check with the doctor before giving the vaccine.

• Ask women of childbearing age if they're pregnant. If they are or think they may be, *don't* give the vaccine.

➤ CLINICAL TIP Warn women who receive rubella vaccine to use an effective means of birth control for at least 3 months after immunization.

• Give the vaccine at least 3 months after any administration of immune globulin or blood, which could have antibodies that neutralize the vaccine.

• Don't vaccinate any immunocompromised patients, patients with immunodeficiency diseases, or those receiving immunosuppressive, radiation, or corticosteroid therapy. Instead, administer immune serum globulin to prevent or reduce infection in susceptible patients.

• After giving the vaccine, observe for signs of anaphylaxis for at least 30 minutes. Keep epinephrine 1:1,000 handy.

• Warn about possible mild fever, slight rash, transient arthralgia (in adolescents), and arthritis (in elderly patients). Suggest aspirin or acetaminophen for fever.

• Advise the patient to apply warmth to the injection site for 24 hours after immunization (to help the body absorb the vaccine). If swelling persists after the initial 24 hours, suggest a cold compress to promote vasoconstriction and prevent antigenic cyst formation.

# RUBEOLA

Also known as measles or morbilli, rubeola is an acute, highly contagious paramyxovirus infection. It is one of the most common and the most serious of all communicable childhood diseases.

In temperate zones, incidence is highest in late winter and early spring. Before the availability of measles vaccine, epidemics occurred every 2 to 5 years in large urban areas. Use of the vaccine has reduced the occurrence of measles during childhood; as a result, measles is becoming more prevalent in adolescents and adults. (See *Administering measles vaccine.*)

In the United States, the prognosis is usually excellent. However, measles is a major cause of death in children in underdeveloped countries.

## Causes

Measles is spread by direct contact or by contaminated airborne respiratory droplets. The portal of entry is the upper respiratory tract.

## Signs and symptoms

Incubation is from 10 to 14 days.

### Prodromal phase

Initial symptoms begin and greatest communicability occurs during a prodromal phase beginning about 11 days after exposure to the virus. This phase lasts from 4 to 5 days; symptoms include fever, photophobia, malaise, anorexia, conjunctivitis, coryza, hoarseness, and hacking cough.

At the end of the prodrome, Koplik's spots, the hallmark of the disease, appear. These spots look like tiny, bluish gray specks surrounded by a red halo.

## ADMINISTERING MEASLES VACCINE

Generally, one bout of measles renders immunity (a second infection is extremely rare and may represent misdiagnosis); infants under age 4 months may be immune because of circulating maternal antibodies.

Under normal conditions, measles vaccine isn't administered to children younger than age 15 months. However, during an epidemic, infants as young as 6 months may receive the vaccine; they must be reimmunized at age 15 months.

An alternative approach calls for administration of gamma globulin to infants between ages 6 and 15 months who are likely to be exposed to measles.

### Special considerations
• Warn the patient or his parents that possible adverse effects of the vaccine include anorexia, malaise, rash, mild thrombocytopenia or leukopenia, and fever. Explain that the vaccine may produce slight reactions, usually within 7 to 10 days.
• Ask the patient about known allergies, especially to neomycin (each dose contains a small amount). However, a patient who's allergic to eggs may receive the vaccine because it contains only minimal amounts of albumin and yolk components.
• Avoid giving the vaccine to a pregnant woman (ask for the date of her last menstrual period). Warn women receiving the vaccine to avoid pregnancy for at least 3 months after vaccination.
• Don't vaccinate children with untreated tuberculosis, immunodeficiencies, leukemia, or lymphoma or those receiving immunosuppressives. If such children are exposed to the virus, recommend that they receive gamma globulin. (Gamma globulin won't prevent measles but will lessen its severity.)
• Older unimmunized children who have been exposed to measles for more than 5 days may also require gamma globulin. Be sure to immunize them 3 months later.
• Delay vaccination for 8 to 12 weeks after administration of whole blood, plasma, or gamma globulin because measles antibodies in these components may neutralize the vaccine.
• Watch for signs of anaphylaxis for 30 minutes after vaccination. Keep epinephrine 1:1,000 handy.
• Advise application of a warm compress to the vaccination site to facilitate absorption of the vaccine. If swelling occurs within 24 hours after vaccination, tell the patient to apply cold compresses to promote vasoconstriction and to prevent antigenic cyst formation.

They appear on the oral mucosa opposite the molars and occasionally bleed.

### Progressive symptoms
About 5 days after Koplik's spots appear, temperature rises sharply, spots slough off, and a slightly pruritic rash appears. This characteristic rash starts as faint macules behind the ears and on the neck and cheeks.

These macules become papular and erythematous, rapidly spreading over the entire face, neck, eyelids, arms, chest, back, abdomen, and thighs. When the rash reaches the feet (2 to 3 days later), it begins to fade in the same sequence it appeared, leaving a brownish discoloration that disappears in 7 to 10 days.

The disease climax occurs 2 to 3 days after the rash appears and is marked by a temperature of 103° to 105° F (39.4° to 40.6° C), severe cough, rhinorrhea, and puffy, red eyes. About 5 days after the rash appears, other symptoms disappear and communicability ends.

Symptoms are usually mild in patients with partial immunity (conferred by administration of gamma globulin) or infants with transplacental antibodies. More severe symptoms and complications are more likely to develop in young infants, adolescents, adults, and immunocompromised patients than in young children.

Atypical measles may appear in patients who received the killed measles vaccine. These patients are acutely ill with a fever and maculopapular rash that's most obvious in the arms and legs, or with pulmonary involvement and no skin lesions.

### *Complications*
Severe infection may lead to secondary bacterial infection and to autoimmune reaction or organ invasion by the virus, resulting in otitis media, pneumonia, and encephalitis. Subacute sclerosing panencephalitis (SSPE), a rare and invariably fatal complication, may develop several years after measles. SSPE is less common in patients who have received the measles vaccine.

### Diagnosis
Measles results in distinctive clinical features, especially the pathognomonic Koplik's spots. Mild measles may resemble rubella, roseola infantum, enterovirus infection, toxoplasmosis, and drug eruptions; laboratory tests are required for a differential diagnosis.

If necessary, measles virus may be isolated from the blood, nasopharyngeal secretions, and urine during the febrile period. Serum antibodies appear within 3 days after onset of the rash and reach peak titers 2 to 4 weeks later.

### Treatment
Therapy consists of bed rest, relief of symptoms, and respiratory isolation throughout the communicable period. Vaporizers and a warm environment help reduce respiratory irritation, but cough preparations and antibiotics are generally ineffective; antipyretics can reduce fever. Treatment must also combat complications.

### Special considerations
• Teach parents the importance of immunizing their children against measles, and follow appropriate procedures when giving the vaccine.
• Teach parents supportive measures, and stress the need for isolation, plenty of rest, and increased fluid intake. Advise them to cope with photophobia by darkening the room or providing sunglasses and to reduce fever with antipyretics and tepid sponge baths.
• Warn parents to watch for and report the early signs and symptoms of complications, such as encephalitis, otitis media, and pneumonia.
• Children at home should be kept out of school for at least 4 days after the rash appears.

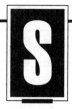

# SALMONELLOSIS

A common infection in the United States, salmonellosis is caused by gram-negative bacilli of the genus *Salmonella,* a member of the Enterobacteriaceae family. It occurs as enterocolitis, bacteremia, localized infection, typhoid, or paratyphoid fever. (See *Clinical variants of salmonellosis,* page 764.) Nontyphoidal forms usually produce mild to moderate illness with low mortality.

Typhoid, the most severe form of salmonellosis, usually lasts from 1 to 4 weeks. Mortality is about 3% in persons who are treated and 10% in those untreated, usually as a result of intestinal perforation or hemorrhage, cerebral thrombosis, toxemia, pneumonia, or acute circulatory failure.

An attack of typhoid confers lifelong immunity, although the patient may become a carrier. Most typhoid patients are under age 30; most carriers are women over age 50. Incidence of typhoid in the United States is increasing as a result of travelers returning from endemic areas.

Enterocolitis and bacteremia are common (and more virulent) among infants, elderly people, and people already weakened by other infections; paratyphoid fever is rare in the United States.

Salmonellosis occurs 20 times more often in patients with acquired immunodeficiency syndrome. Features are increased incidence of bacteremia, inability to identify the infection source, and tendency of the infection to recur after therapy is stopped.

## Causes

Of an estimated 1,700 serotypes of *Salmonella,* 10 cause the diseases most common in the United States; all 10 can survive for weeks in water, ice, sewage, or food. Nontyphoidal salmonellosis generally follows the ingestion of contaminated or inadequately processed foods, especially eggs, chicken, turkey, and duck. Proper cooking reduces the risk of contracting salmonellosis.

Other causes include contact with infected people or animals or ingestion of contaminated dry milk, chocolate bars, or drugs of animal origin. Salmonellosis may occur in children under age 5 from fecal-oral spread.

Typhoid results most frequently from drinking water contaminated by excretions of a carrier.

## Signs and symptoms

Clinical manifestations of salmonellosis vary but usually include fever, abdominal pain, and severe diarrhea with enterocolitis. Headache, increasing fever, and constipation are more common with typhoidal infection.

# CLINICAL VARIANTS OF SALMONELLOSIS

| VARIANT | CAUSE | CLINICAL FEATURES |
|---|---|---|
| Enterocolitis | Any species of non-typhoidal Salmonella, but usually *S. enteritidis*. Incubation period of 6 to 48 hours. | Mild to severe abdominal pain, diarrhea, sudden fever up to 102° F (38.8° C), nausea, vomiting; usually self-limiting but may progress to enteric fever (resembling typhoid), local abscesses (usually abdominal), dehydration, septicemia. |
| Paratyphoid | *S. paratyphi* and *S. schottmülleri* (formerly *S. paratyphi* B). Incubation period of 3 weeks or more. | Fever and transient diarrhea, generally resembles typhoid but less severe |
| Bacteremia | Any Salmonella species, but most commonly *S. choleraesius*. Incubation period varies. | Fever, chills, anorexia, weight loss (without GI symptoms), joint pains |
| Localized infections | Usually follows bacteremia caused by Salmonella species. | Site of localization determines symptoms; localized abscesses may cause osteomyelitis, endocarditis, bronchopneumonia, pyelonephritis, and arthritis. |
| Typhoid fever | *S. typhi* enters GI tract and invades the bloodstream via the lymphatics, setting up intracellular sites. During this phase, infection of biliary tract leads to intestinal seeding with millions of bacilli. Involved lymphoid tissues (especially Peyer's patches in ilium) enlarge, ulcerate, and necrose, resulting in hemorrhage. Incubation period of usually 1 to 2 weeks. | Symptoms of enterocolitis may develop within hours of ingestion of *S. typhi;* they usually subside before onset of typhoid symptoms. *First week:* gradually increasing fever, anorexia, myalgia, malaise, headache *Second week:* remittent fever up to 104° F (40°C) usually in the evening, chills, diaphoresis, weakness, delirium, increasing abdominal pain and distention, diarrhea or constipation, cough, moist crackles, tender abdomen with enlarged spleen, maculopapular rash (especially on abdomen) *Third week:* persistent fever, increasing fatigue and weakness; usually subsides at end of third week, although relapses may occur *Complications:* intestinal perforation or hemorrhage, abscesses, thrombophlebitis, cerebral thrombosis, pneumonia, osteomyelitis, myocarditis, acute circulatory failure, chronic carrier state |

## Diagnosis

Generally, diagnosis depends on isolation of the organism in a culture, particularly blood (in typhoid, paratyphoid, and bacteremia) or feces (in enterocolitis, paratyphoid, and typhoid). Other appropriate culture specimens include urine, bone marrow, pus, and vomitus.

In endemic areas, clinical symptoms of enterocolitis allow a working diagnosis before cultures are positive. Presence of *S. typhi* in stools 1 or more years after treatment indicates that the patient is a carrier, which is true of 3% of patients.

Widal's test, an agglutination reaction against somatic and flagellar antigens, may suggest typhoid with a fourfold rise in titer. However, drug use or hepatic disease can also increase these titers and invalidate test results.

Other supportive laboratory values may include transient leukocytosis during the first week of typhoidal salmonellosis, leukopenia during the third week, and leukocytosis in local infection.

## Treatment

Antimicrobial therapy for typhoid, paratyphoid, and bacteremia depends on the organism's sensitivity. It may include amoxicillin, chloramphenicol and, in severely toxemic patients, cotrimoxazole, ciprofloxacin, or ceftriaxone. Localized abscesses may also need surgical drainage.

Enterocolitis requires a short course of antibiotics only if it causes septicemia or prolonged fever. Other treatments include bed rest and replacement of fluids and electrolytes. Camphorated opium tincture, kaolin with pectin, diphenoxylate hydrochloride, codeine, or small doses of morphine may be necessary to relieve diarrhea and control cramps in patients who must remain active.

## Special considerations

● Follow standard precautions. Always wash your hands thoroughly before and after any contact with the patient, and advise other hospital personnel to do the same. Teach the patient to use proper hand-washing technique, especially after defecating and before eating or handling food. Wear gloves and a gown when disposing of feces or fecally contaminated objects.

● Continue standard precautions until three consecutive stool cultures are negative — the first one 48 hours after antibiotic treatment ends, followed by two more at 24-hour intervals.

● Observe the patient closely for indications of bowel perforation: sudden pain in the lower right abdomen, possibly after one or more rectal bleeding episodes; sudden fall in temperature or blood pressure; and rising pulse rate.

● During acute infection, allow the patient as much rest as possible. Raise the side rails and use other safety measures because the patient may become delirious.

● The patient should have a room close to the nurses' station so he can be checked on often. Use a room deodorizer (preferably electric) to minimize odor from diarrhea and to provide a comfortable atmosphere for rest.

● Accurately record intake and output. Maintain adequate I.V. hydration. When the patient can tolerate oral feedings, encourage high-calorie fluids such as milk shakes. Watch for constipation.

● Provide good skin and mouth care. Turn the patient frequently, and perform mild passive exercises as indicated. Apply mild heat to the abdomen to relieve cramps.

CLINICAL TIP *Don't* administer antipyretics because they mask fever and may lead to possible hypothermia. Instead, to promote heat loss through the skin without causing shivering (which keeps fever high by vasoconstriction), apply tepid, wet towels (don't use alcohol or ice) to the patient's groin and axillae. To promote heat loss by vasodilation of peripheral blood vessels, use additional wet towels on the arms and legs, wiping with long, vigorous strokes.

• After draining the abscesses of a joint, provide heat, elevation, and passive range-of-motion exercises to decrease swelling and maintain mobility.

• If the patient has positive stool cultures on discharge, tell him to use a different bathroom than other family members if possible (while he's on antibiotics); to wash his hands afterwards; and to avoid preparing uncooked foods, such as salads, for family members.

• To prevent salmonellosis, advise prompt refrigeration of meat and cooked foods (avoid keeping them at room temperature for any prolonged period), and teach the importance of proper hand washing. Advise those at high risk of contracting typhoid (laboratory workers, travelers) to seek vaccination.

# SARCOIDOSIS

A multisystemic, granulomatous disorder, sarcoidosis characteristically produces lymphadenopathy, pulmonary infiltration, and skeletal, liver, eye, or skin lesions. It occurs most often in young adults (ages 20 to 40). In the United States, sarcoidosis occurs predominantly among blacks and affects twice as many women as men.

Acute sarcoidosis usually resolves within 2 years. Chronic, progressive sarcoidosis, which is uncommon, is associated with pulmonary fibrosis and progressive pulmonary disability.

## Causes

Although the cause of sarcoidosis is unknown, the following possible causes have been considered:

• *hypersensitivity response* (possibly from a T-cell imbalance) to such agents as atypical mycobacteria, fungi, and pine pollen

• *genetic predisposition* (suggested by a slightly higher incidence of sarcoidosis within the same family)

• *chemicals,* such as zirconium or beryllium, can lead to illnesses resembling sarcoidosis, suggesting an extrinsic cause for this disease.

## Signs and symptoms

Initial signs of sarcoidosis include arthralgia (in the wrists, ankles, and elbows), fatigue, malaise, and weight loss. Other clinical features vary according to the extent and location of fibrosis:

• *respiratory* — breathlessness, cough (usually nonproductive), substernal pain; complications in advanced pulmonary disease include pulmonary hypertension and cor pulmonale

• *cutaneous* — erythema nodosum, subcutaneous skin nodules with maculopapular eruptions, extensive nasal mucosal lesions

• *ophthalmic* — anterior uveitis (common); glaucoma, blindness (rare)

• *lymphatic* — bilateral hilar and right paratracheal lymphadenopathy and splenomegaly

• *musculoskeletal* — muscle weakness, polyarthralgia, pain, punched-out lesions on phalanges

• *hepatic* — granulomatous hepatitis, usually asymptomatic

• *genitourinary* — hypercalciuria

• *cardiovascular* — arrhythmias (premature beats, bundle branch block, or complete heart block); cardiomyopathy (rare)

• *central nervous system (CNS)* — cranial or peripheral nerve palsies, basilar meningitis, seizures, pituitary and hypothalamic lesions producing diabetes insipidus.

## Diagnosis

Typical clinical features with appropriate laboratory data and X-ray findings suggest sarcoidosis. A positive Kveim-Siltzbach skin test supports the diagnosis.

In this test, the patient receives an intradermal injection of an antigen prepared from human sarcoidal spleen or lymph nodes from patients with sarcoidosis. If the patient has active sarcoidosis, granuloma develops at the injection site in 2 to 6 weeks. This reaction is considered positive when a biopsy of the skin at the injection site shows discrete epitheloid cell granuloma.

Other relevant findings include the following:

• *Chest X-ray* shows bilateral hilar and right paratracheal adenopathy with or without diffuse interstitial infiltrates; occasionally large nodular lesions are present in lung parenchyma.

• *Lymph node, skin,* or *lung biopsy* reveals noncaseating granulomas with negative cultures for mycobacteria and fungi.

• *Other laboratory data* infrequently reveal increased serum calcium, mild anemia, leukocytosis, or hyperglobulinemia.

• *Pulmonary function tests* show decreased total lung capacity and compliance and decreased diffusing capacity.

• *Arterial blood gas (ABG) analysis* shows decreased partial pressure of arterial oxygen.

Negative tuberculin skin test, fungal serologies, and sputum cultures for mycobacteria and fungi, as well as negative biopsy cultures, help rule out infection.

## Treatment

Asymptomatic sarcoidosis requires no treatment. However, sarcoidosis that causes ocular, respiratory, CNS, cardiac, or systemic symptoms (such as fever and weight loss) requires treatment with systemic or topical steroids, as does sarcoidosis that produces hypercalcemia or destructive skin lesions. Such therapy is usually continued for 1 to 2 years, but some patients may need lifelong therapy.

Other treatment includes a low-calcium diet and avoidance of direct exposure to sunlight in patients with hypercalcemia.

## Special considerations

• Watch for and report any complications. Be aware of any abnormal laboratory results (anemia, for example) that could alter patient care.

• For the patient with arthralgia, administer analgesics as needed. Record signs of progressive muscle weakness.

• Provide a nutritious, high-calorie diet and plenty of fluids. If the patient has hypercalcemia, suggest a low-calcium diet. Weigh the patient regularly to detect weight loss.

• Monitor respiratory function. Check chest X-rays for the extent of lung involvement; note and record any bloody sputum or increase in sputum. If the patient has pulmonary hypertension or end-stage cor pulmonale, check ABG values, watch for arrhythmias, and administer oxygen as needed.

• Because steroids may induce or worsen diabetes mellitus, perform fingerstick glucose tests at least every 12 hours at the beginning of steroid therapy. Also, watch for other adverse effects of steroids, such as fluid retention, electrolyte imbalance (especially hypokalemia), moon face, hypertension, and personality change.

➤ CLINICAL TIP During or after steroid withdrawal (particularly in association with infection or other types of stress), watch for vomiting, orthostatic hypotension, hypoglycemia, restlessness, anorexia, malaise, and fatigue. Remember that the patient on long-term or high-dose steroid therapy is vulnerable to infection.

• When preparing the patient for discharge, stress the need for compliance with prescribed steroid therapy and regular, careful follow-up examinations and treatment.

• Refer the patient with failing vision to community support and resource groups and the American Foundation for the Blind if necessary.

# SCABIES

An age-old skin infection, scabies results from infestation with *Sarcoptes scabiei* var. *hominis* (itch mite), which provokes a sensitivity reaction. It occurs worldwide, is predisposed by overcrowding and poor hygiene, and can be endemic.

## Causes

Mites can live their entire life cycles in the skin of humans, causing chronic infection. The female mite burrows into the skin to lay her eggs, from which larvae emerge to copulate and then reburrow under the skin.

Transmission of scabies occurs through skin or sexual contact. The adult mite can survive without a human host for only 2 or 3 days.

## Signs and symptoms

Typically, scabies causes itching that intensifies at night. Characteristic lesions take many forms but are usually excoriated and may appear as erythematous nodules.

Burrows are threadlike lesions approximately ⅜″ long and generally occur between fingers, on flexor surfaces of the wrists, on elbows, in axillary folds, at the waistline, on nipples in females, and on genitalia in males. In infants, the burrows may appear on the head and neck.

Intense scratching can lead to severe excoriation and secondary bacterial infection. Itching may become generalized secondary to sensitization.

## Diagnosis

A drop of mineral oil placed over the burrow, followed by superficial scraping and examination of expressed material under a low-power microscope, may reveal the mite, ova, or mite feces. However, excoriation or inflammation of the burrow often makes such identification difficult.

If diagnostic tests offer no positive identification of the mite and if scabies is still suspected (for example, close contacts of the patient also report itching), skin clearing that occurs after a therapeutic trial of a pediculicide confirms the diagnosis.

## Treatment

Generally, treatment of scabies consists of application of a pediculicide — permethrin cream or lindane lotion — in a thin layer over the entire skin surface. The pediculicide is left on for 8 to 12 hours. To make certain that all areas have been treated, this application should be repeated in approximately 1 week.

Another pediculicide, crotamiton cream, may be applied on 5 consecutive nights but is not as effective. Widespread bacterial infections require systemic antibiotics.

Persistent pruritus (from mite sensitization or contact dermatitis) may develop from repeated use of pediculicides rather than from continued infection. An antipruritic emollient or topical steroid can reduce itching; intralesional steroids may resolve erythematous nodules.

**Special considerations**
- Instruct the adult patient to apply permethrin cream or lindane lotion at bedtime from the neck down, covering the entire body. The cream or lotion should be washed off in 8 to 12 hours. Contaminated clothing and linens must be washed in hot water or dry-cleaned.
- Tell the patient not to apply lindane lotion if skin is raw or inflamed. Advise the patient to report any skin irritation or hypersensitivity reaction immediately, to discontinue using the drug, and to wash it off thoroughly.
- Suggest that family members and other close contacts of the patient be checked for possible symptoms and be treated if necessary.
- If a hospitalized patient has scabies, prevent transmission to other patients: Practice good hand-washing technique or wear gloves when touching the patient, observe wound and skin precautions for 24 hours after treatment with a pediculicide, gas autoclave blood pressure cuffs before using them on other patients, isolate linens until the patient is noninfectious, and thoroughly disinfect the patient's room after discharge.

# SCHIZOAFFECTIVE DISORDER

Patients who show concurrent symptoms of both mood disorders (bipolar or depressive types) and psychotic disorder are given the diagnosis of schizoaffective disorder. Onset is usually during young adulthood. The chronic symptoms are typically fewer and less severe than among those patients with schizophrenia.

**Causes**
Schizoaffective disorder may result from a combination of physiologic and psychological causes. The specific cause is unknown at this time.

**Signs and symptoms**
The patient must show clear symptoms of schizophrenia. During both the active and residual phases of the illness, symptoms of mood disturbance must also occur. These symptoms may not be caused by substance abuse or by a medical condition. Patients may experience difficulty functioning in the workplace. They have a restricted range of social contacts and may also have difficulty performing self-care.

**Diagnosis**
According to the *Diagnostic and Statistical Manual of Mental Disorders,* 4th edition *(DSM-IV)* classification, a schizoaffective disorder is diagnosed if the patient's symptoms meet the following criteria:
- The patient experiences a period of uninterrupted illness in which there is a major depressive episode (with depressed mood), a manic episode, or a mixed episode, concurrent with symptoms of schizophrenia.

• During the same period of illness, there are delusions or hallucinations for at least 2 weeks in the absence of prominent mood symptoms.

• The patient experiences symptoms of the mood episode and they are present for a substantial portion of the total duration of the active and residual periods of the illness.

• The illness of the patient is not due to direct physiologic effects of a substance (drug abuse, medication) or a general medical condition.

The schizoaffective disorder may be a specific type:

• In the *bipolar type*, the disturbance includes a manic or a mixed episode, or a manic or a mixed episode plus a major depressive episode.

• In the *depressive type*, the disturbance includes only major depressive episodes.

## Treatment

As is indicated by the symptoms, treatment must focus on both psychotic and mood disorders. Antipsychotics are used to control the symptoms of schizophrenia. Antidepressant and antimanic medications are used for the mood disorder. Psychotherapy can be useful to help the patient understand the nature of the illness and the necessity of ongoing treatment. Support groups increase socialization and provide safe opportunities to build interpersonal skills. The family should be encouraged to attend a support group to understand the illness better and to learn ways they can be supportive of the patient.

➤ CLINICAL TIP   Strategies that work with patients who have a mood disorder may not be appropriate for someone who also has a thought disorder. Gauge the extent of the thought disorder before you develop a plan of treatment.

## Special considerations

• As symptoms subside, encourage the patient to assume responsibility for personal care.

• Provide emotional support, maintain a calm environment, and set realistic goals for the behavior.

• Collaborate with other staff members to provide consistent responses to the patient's manipulative or acting-out behaviors.

• Watch for early signs of frustration, and intervene appropriately to prevent acting out.

• If the patient is hitting and behavior is unacceptable, calmly tell him so. Tell him that the staff will move him to a quiet area and will help him control his behavior.

• If the patient is taking lithium, tell the patient and the family to discontinue the drug and notify the doctor if signs of toxicity (diarrhea, abdominal cramps, vomiting, unsteadiness, drowsiness, muscle weakness, polyuria, or tremors) occur.

• If the patient is having trouble expressing his feelings, encourage him to talk about them or write them down.

• Record behavior and conversations.

• Institute suicide precautions as indicated by the hospital policy.

• Attend to the patient's physical needs if he is too depressed to take care of himself (hygiene, meals, physical activity, sleep).

• Speak slowly and allow ample time for the patient to respond because thinking and reactions may be sluggish.

• Affirm the patient by listening attentively and respectfully, preventing interruptions, and avoiding judgmental responses.

• Provide a structured routine, including noncompetitive activities, to build the patient's self-confidence and encourage interaction with others.

• Urge the patient to join group activities and to socialize.

# SCHIZOPHRENIA

This disorder is characterized by disturbances (for at least 6 months) in thought content and form, perception, affect, sense of self, volition, interpersonal relationships, and psychomotor behavior. The *Diagnostic and Statistical Manual of Mental Disorders,* 4th edition *(DSM-IV),* recognizes paranoid, disorganized, catatonic, undifferentiated, and residual schizophrenia.

Schizophrenia affects 1% to 2% of the U.S. population and is equally prevalent in both sexes. Onset of symptoms usually occurs during adolescence or early adulthood.

The disorder produces varying degrees of impairment. Up to one-third of patients with schizophrenia have just one psychotic episode and no more. Some patients have no disability between periods of exacerbation; others need continuous institutional care. The prognosis worsens with each episode.

## Causes

Schizophrenia may result from a combination of genetic, biological, cultural, and psychological factors.

### Genetic evidence

Some evidence supports a genetic predisposition. Close relatives of persons with schizophrenia are up to 50 times more likely to develop schizophrenia; the closer the degree of biological relatedness, the higher the risk.

### Biochemical theory

The most widely accepted biochemical hypothesis holds that schizophrenia results from excessive activity at dopaminergic synapses. Other neurotransmitter alterations may also contribute to schizophrenic symptoms. In addition, patients with schizophrenia have structural abnormalities of the frontal and temporolimbic systems.

### Other causes

Numerous psychological and sociocultural causes, such as disturbed family and interpersonal patterns, also have been proposed. Schizophrenia occurs more often among people from lower socioeconomic groups, possibly the result of downward social drift, lack of upward socioeconomic mobility, and high stress levels that may stem from poverty, social failure, illness, and inadequate social resources. Higher incidence also is linked to low birth weight.

## Signs and symptoms

Schizophrenia is associated with a variety of abnormal behaviors; therefore, signs and symptoms vary widely, depending on the type and phase (prodromal, active, or residual) of the illness.

Watch for these signs and symptoms:
• ambivalence — coexisting strong positive and negative feelings, leading to emotional conflict
• apathy
• clang associations — words that rhyme or sound alike used in an illogical, nonsensical manner, for instance, "It's the rain, train, pain"
• concrete associations — inability to form or understand abstract thoughts
• delusions — false ideas or beliefs accepted as real by the patient. Delusions of grandeur, persecution, and reference (distorted belief regarding the relation between events and oneself, such as a belief that television programs address the patient on a personal level) are common in schizophrenia. Also common

are feelings of being controlled, somatic illness, and depersonalization.

• echolalia — meaningless repetition of words or phrases

• echopraxia — involuntary repetition of movements observed in others

• flight of ideas — rapid succession of incomplete and unconnected ideas

• hallucinations — false sensory perceptions with no basis in reality; usually visual or auditory but may also be olfactory, gustatory, or tactile

• illusions — false sensory perceptions with some basis in reality, such as a car's backfiring mistaken for a gunshot

• loose associations — rapid shifts among unrelated ideas

• magical thinking — a belief that thoughts or wishes can control others or events

• neologisms — bizarre words that have meaning only for the patient

• poor interpersonal relationships

• regression — return to an earlier developmental stage

• thought blocking — sudden interruption in the patient's train of thought

• withdrawal — disinterest in objects, people, or surroundings

• word salad — illogical word groupings, such as "She had a star, barn, plant."

## Diagnosis

After complete physical and psychiatric examinations rule out an organic cause of symptoms, such as an amphetamine-induced psychosis, a diagnosis of schizophrenia is made if the patient's symptoms match those in the *DSM-IV.* (See *Diagnosing schizophrenia.*)

## Treatment

In schizophrenia, treatment focuses on meeting the physical and psychosocial needs of the patient, based on his previous level of adjustment and his response to various interventions. Treatment may combine drug therapy, long-term psychotherapy for the patient and his family, psychosocial rehabilitation, vocational counseling, and the use of community resources.

### *Antipsychotic drugs*

The primary treatment for more than 30 years, antipsychotic drugs (also called neuroleptic drugs) appear to work by blocking postsynaptic dopamine receptors. These drugs reduce the incidence of psychotic symptoms, such as hallucinations and delusions, and relieve anxiety and agitation.

Other psychiatric drugs, such as antidepressants and anxiolytics, may control associated signs and symptoms.

Certain antipsychotic drugs are associated with numerous adverse reactions, some of which are irreversible. Most experts agree that patients who are withdrawn, isolated, or apathetic show little improvement after antipsychotic drug treatment.

High-potency antipsychotics include fluphenazine, haloperidol, thiothixene, and trifluoperazine. Loxapine, molindone, and perphenazine are intermediate in potency, and chlorpromazine and thioridazine are low-potency agents.

Haloperidol decanoate, fluphenazine decanoate, and fluphenazine enanthate are depot formulations that are implanted I.M. once or twice a week to once a month; this method allows gradual release of the drug. A new antipsychotic, risperidone, also is reported to be effective.

Clozapine, which differs chemically from other antipsychotic drugs, may be prescribed for severely ill patients who fail to respond to standard treatment. This agent effectively controls a wider range of psychotic signs and symptoms without the usual adverse effects. However, clozapine can cause drowsiness, sedation, excessive salivation, tachy-

# DIAGNOSING SCHIZOPHRENIA

The following criteria described in the *DSM-IV* are used to diagnose a person with schizophrenia.

## Characteristic symptoms

A person with schizophrenia has two or more of the following symptoms (each present for a significant time during a 1-month period — or less if successfully treated):

- delusions
- hallucinations
- disorganized speech
- grossly disorganized or catatonic behavior
- negative symptoms (such as flat affect or poverty of speech).

The diagnosis requires only one of these characteristic symptoms if the person's delusions are bizarre or if hallucinations consist of a voice issuing a running commentary on the person's behavior or thoughts, or two or more voices conversing.

## Social and occupational dysfunction

For a significant period since the onset of the disturbance, one or more major areas of functioning (such as work, interpersonal relations, or self-care) are markedly below the level achieved before the onset. When the disturbance begins in childhood or adolescence, the dysfunction takes the form of failure to achieve the expected level of interpersonal or academic development.

## Duration

Continuous signs of the disturbance persist for at least 6 months. The 6-month period must include at least 1 month of symptoms (or less if signs and symptoms have been successfully treated) that match the characteristic symptoms and may include periods of prodromal or residual symptoms.

During the prodromal or residual period, signs of the disturbance may be manifested by only negative symptoms or by two or more characteristic symptoms in a less severe form.

## Schizoaffective and mood disorder exclusion

Schizoaffective disorder and mood disorder with psychotic features have been ruled out for these reasons: either no major depressive, manic, or mixed episodes have occurred concurrently with the active-phase symptoms *or*, if mood disorder episodes have occurred during active-phase symptoms, their total duration has been brief relative to the duration of the active and residual periods.

## Substance and general medical condition exclusion

The disturbance is not the result of the direct physiologic effects of a substance or a general medical condition.

## Relationship to a pervasive developmental disorder

If the person has a history of autistic disorder or another pervasive developmental disorder, the additional diagnosis of schizophrenia is appropriate only if prominent delusions or hallucinations also are present for at least 1 month (less if successfully treated).

---

cardia, dizziness, and seizures, as well as agranulocytosis.

A potentially fatal blood disorder, agranulocytosis is characterized by a low white blood cell count and pronounced neutropenia. Routine blood monitoring is essential to detect the estimated 1% to 2% of all patients taking clozapine who develop agranulocytosis. If caught in the early stages, this disorder is reversible.

*Psychotherapy*

Clinicians disagree about the effectiveness of psychotherapy in treating schizophrenia. Some consider it a useful adjunct to drug therapy.

Others suggest that psychosocial rehabilitation, education, and social skills training are more effective for chronic schizophrenia. In addition to improving understanding of the disorder, these methods teach the patient and his family coping strategies, effective communication techniques, and social skills.

Because schizophrenia typically disrupts the family, family therapy may be helpful to reduce guilt and disappointment as well as improve acceptance of the patient and his bizarre behavior.

### Special considerations

● Assess the patient's ability to carry out activities of daily living, paying special attention to his nutritional status. Monitor his weight if he isn't eating.

➤ CLINICAL TIP Schizophrenia affects the family's level of functioning as well as the patient's. Supportive care for both is vital.

● If the patient thinks that his food is poisoned, let him fix his own food when possible or offer foods in closed containers that he can open. If you give liquid medication in a unit-dose container, allow the patient to open the container.

● Maintain a safe environment, minimizing stimuli. Administer prescribed medications to decrease symptoms and anxiety. Use physical restraints according to your facility's policy to ensure the patient's safety and that of others.

● Adopt an accepting and consistent approach with the patient. Short, repeated contacts are best until trust has been established.

● Avoid promoting dependence. Reward positive behavior to help the patient improve his level of functioning.

● Engage the patient in reality-oriented activities that involve human contact, such as inpatient social skills training groups, outpatient day care, and sheltered workshops.

● Provide reality-based explanations for distorted body images or hypochondriacal complaints. Explain to the patient that his private language, autistic inventions, or neologisms are not understood. Set limits on inappropriate behavior.

● If the patient is hallucinating, explore the content of the hallucinations. If he hears voices, find out if he believes that he must do what they command. Explore the emotions connected with the hallucinations, but don't argue about them. If possible, change the subject.

● Teach the patient techniques that interrupt the hallucinations (listening to an audiocassette player, singing out loud, or reading out loud).

● Don't tease or joke with a schizophrenic patient. Choose words and phrases that are unambiguous and clearly understood. For instance, a patient who's told "That procedure will be done on the floor" may become frightened, thinking he'll need to lie down on the floor.

● If the patient expresses suicidal thoughts, institute suicide precautions. Document his behavior and your actions.

● If the patient expresses homicidal thoughts (for example, "I have to kill my mother"), institute homicidal precautions. Notify appropriate facility personnel and the potential victim. Document the patient's comments and the names of those who were notified.

● Don't touch the patient without telling him first exactly what you're going to do — for example, "I'm going to put this cuff on your arm so I can take your blood pressure."

• If necessary, postpone procedures that require physical contact with facility personnel until the patient is less suspicious or agitated.

• Remember, institutionalization may produce symptoms and handicaps that are not part of the patient's illness, so evaluate symptoms carefully.

• Mobilize community resources to provide a support system for the patient. Ongoing support is essential to his mastery of social skills.

• Encourage compliance with the medication regimen to prevent a relapse. Also, monitor the patient carefully for adverse reactions to drug therapy, including drug-induced parkinsonism, acute dystonia, akathisia, tardive dyskinesia, and malignant neuroleptic syndrome. Document all such reactions.

• Help the patient explore possible connections between anxiety and stress and the exacerbation of symptoms.

For catatonic schizophrenia:

• Assess for physical illness. Remember that the mute patient won't complain of pain or physical symptoms; if he's in a bizarre posture, he's at risk for pressure ulcers or decreased circulation to a body area.

• Meet the patient's physical needs for adequate food, fluid, exercise, and elimination; provide urinary catheterization and enemas as needed.

• Provide range-of-motion exercises for the patient or help him walk every 2 hours.

• Prevent physical exhaustion and injury during periods of hyperactivity.

• Tell the patient directly, specifically, and concisely which procedures need to be done. For example, you might say to the patient, "It's time to go for a walk. Let's go." Don't offer the negativistic patient a choice.

• Spend some time with the patient even if he's mute and unresponsive. The patient is acutely aware of his environment even though he seems not to be. Your presence can be reassuring and supportive.

• Verbalize for the patient the message that his nonverbal behavior seems to convey; encourage him to do so as well.

• Offer reality orientation. You might say, "The leaves on the trees are turning colors and the air is cooler. It's fall!" Emphasize reality in all contacts to reduce distorted perceptions.

• Stay alert for violent outbursts; if they occur, get help promptly to ensure the patient's safety and your own.

For paranoid schizophrenia:

• When the patient is newly admitted, minimize his contact with the facility staff.

• Don't crowd the patient physically or psychologically; he may strike out to protect himself.

• Be flexible; allow the patient some control. Approach him in a calm and unhurried manner. Let him talk about anything he wishes initially, but keep the conversation light and social, and avoid entering into power struggles.

• Respond to the patient's condescending attitudes (arrogance, put-downs, sarcasm, or open hostility) with neutral remarks.

• Don't let the patient put you on the defensive, and don't take his remarks personally. If he tells you to leave him alone, do leave, but return soon. Brief contacts with the patient may be most useful at first.

• Don't make attempts to combat the patient's delusions with logic. Instead, respond to feelings, themes, or underlying needs — for example, "It seems you feel you've been treated unfairly" (persecution).

• Be honest and dependable. Don't threaten the patient or make promises that you can't fulfill.

• If the patient is taking clozapine, stress the importance of returning weekly to the facility or an outpatient setting to have his blood monitored.

• Teach the patient the importance of complying with the medication regimen. Tell him to report any adverse reactions instead of discontinuing the drug. If he takes a slow-release formulation, make sure that he understands when to return for his next dose.

• Involve the patient's family in his treatment. Teach them how to recognize an impending relapse, and suggest ways to manage symptoms, such as tension, nervousness, insomnia, decreased ability to concentrate, and apathy.

# SCOLIOSIS

Scoliosis, a lateral curvature of the spine may be found in the thoracic, lumbar, or thoracolumbar spinal segment. The curve may be convex to the right (more common in thoracic curves) or to the left (more common in lumbar curves). Rotation of the vertebral column around its axis occurs and may cause rib cage deformity Scoliosis is often associated with kyphosis (humpback) and lordosis (swayback).

## Causes

Scoliosis may be functional or structural. Functional (postural) scoliosis usually results from poor posture or a discrepancy in leg lengths, not fixed deformity of the spinal column. In structural scoliosis, curvature results from a deformity of the vertebral bodies.

Structural scoliosis may be one of three types:

• *Congenital scoliosis* is usually related to a congenital defect, such as wedge vertebrae, fused ribs or vertebrae, or hemivertebrae.

• *Paralytic or musculoskeletal scoliosis* develops several months after asymmetrical paralysis of the trunk muscles from polio, cerebral palsy, or muscular dystrophy.

• *Idiopathic scoliosis* (the most common form) may be transmitted as an autosomal dominant or multifactoral trait. This form appears in a previously straight spine during the growing years.

Idiopathic scoliosis can be classified as infantile, which affects mostly male infants between birth and age 3 and causes left thoracic and right lumbar curves; juvenile, which affects both sexes between ages 4 and 10 and causes varying types of curvature; or adolescent, which generally affects girls between age 10 and achievement of skeletal maturity and causes varying types of curvature.

## Signs and symptoms

The most common curve in functional or structural scoliosis arises in the thoracic segment, with convexity to the right, and compensatory curves (S curves) in the cervical segment above and the lumbar segment below, both with convexity to the left. As the spine curves laterally, compensatory curves develop to maintain body balance and mark the deformity.

Scoliosis rarely produces subjective symptoms until it's well established; when symptoms do occur, they include backache, fatigue, and dyspnea. Because many teenagers are shy about their bodies, their parents suspect that something is wrong only after they notice uneven hemlines, pant legs that appear unequal in length, or subtle physical signs like one hip appearing higher than the other.

Untreated scoliosis may result in pulmonary insufficiency (curvature may decrease lung capacity), back pain, degenerative arthritis of the spine, disk disease, and sciatica.

### Diagnosis

Anterior, posterior, and lateral spinal X-rays, taken with the patient standing upright and bending, confirm scoliosis and determine the degree of curvature (Cobb method) and flexibility of the spine. (See *Cobb method for measuring angle of curvature*.) A scoliometer can also be used to measure the angle of trunk rotation.

A physical examination reveals unequal shoulder heights, elbow levels, and heights of the iliac crests. Muscles on the convex side of the curve may be rounded; those on the concave side, flattened, producing asymmetry of paraspinal muscles.

### *Treatment*

The severity of the deformity and potential spine growth determine appropriate treatment, which may include such noninvasive measures as close observation, exercise, or a brace. For more serious deformity, surgery or a combination of methods may be needed. To be most effective, treatment should begin early, when spinal deformity is still subtle.

### *Noninvasive measures*

A curve of less than 25 degrees is mild and can be monitored by X-rays and an examination every 3 months. An exercise program that includes sit-ups, pelvic tilts, spine hyperextension, push-ups, and breathing exercises may strengthen torso muscles and prevent curve progression. A heel lift also may help.

A curve of 30 to 50 degrees requires management with spinal exercises and a brace. (Transcutaneous electrical nerve

## COBB METHOD FOR MEASURING ANGLE OF CURVATURE

The Cobb method measures the angle of curvature in scoliosis.

The top vertebra in the curve (T6 in the illustration) is the uppermost vertebra whose upper face tilts toward the curve's concave side. The bottom vertebra in the curve (T12) is the lowest vertebra whose lower face tilts toward the curve's concave side.

The angle at which perpendicular lines drawn from the upper face of the top vertebra and the lower face of the bottom vertebra intersect is the angle of the curve.

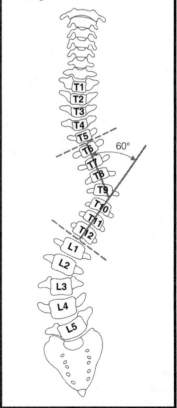

stimulation may be used as an alternative.)

A brace halts progression in most patients but doesn't reverse the established curvature. Such devices passively strengthen the patient's spine by applying asymmetric pressure to skin, muscles, and ribs. Braces can be adjusted as the patient grows and can be worn until bone growth is complete.

### Surgery

A curve of 40 degrees or more requires surgery (spinal fusion with instrumentation) because a lateral curve continues to progress at the rate of 1 degree a year even after skeletal maturity.

➤ CLINICAL TIP  Some surgeons prescribe Cotrel dynamic traction for 7 to 10 days for preoperative preparation. This traction consists of a belt-pulley-weight system. While in traction, the patient should exercise for 10 minutes every hour, increasing muscle strength while keeping the vertebral column immobile.

Surgery corrects lateral curvature by posterior spinal fusion and internal stabilization with a Harrington rod. A distraction rod on the concave side of the curve "jacks" the spine into a straight position and provides an internal splint. A Cotrel-Dubousset rod system may also be used.

An alternative procedure, anterior spinal fusion with Dwyer or Zielke instrumentation, corrects curvature with vertebral staples and an anterior stabilizing cable. Some spinal fusions may require postoperative immobilization in a brace.

Postoperatively, periodic checkups are required for several months to monitor stability of the correction.

### Special considerations

● Keep in mind that scoliosis often affects adolescent girls, who are likely to find activity limitations and treatment with orthopedic appliances distressing. Therefore, provide emotional support, along with meticulous skin and cast care, and patient teaching.

If the patient needs a brace:
● Enlist the help of a physical therapist, a social worker, and an orthotist (orthopedic appliance specialist). Before the patient goes home, explain what the brace does and how to care for it (how to check the screws for tightness and pad the uprights to prevent excessive wear on clothing). Suggest that loose-fitting, oversized clothes be worn for greater comfort.
● Tell the patient to wear the brace 23 hours a day and to remove it only for bathing and exercise. While she's still adjusting to the brace, tell her to lie down and rest several times a day.
● Suggest a soft mattress if a firm one is uncomfortable.
● To prevent skin breakdown, advise the patient not to use lotions, ointments, or powders on areas where the brace contacts the skin. Instead, suggest that she use rubbing alcohol or tincture of benzoin to toughen the skin. Tell her to keep the skin dry and clean and to wear a snug T-shirt under the brace.
● Advise the patient to increase activities gradually and to avoid strenuous sports. Emphasize the importance of conscientiously performing prescribed exercises. Recommend swimming during the 1 hour out of the brace but strongly warn against diving.
● Instruct the patient to turn her whole body, instead of just her head, when looking to the side. To make reading easier, tell her to hold the book so she can look straight ahead at it instead of down. If she finds this difficult, help her to obtain prism glasses.

If the patient needs traction or a cast before surgery:

• Explain these procedures to the patient and family. Remember that application of a body cast can be traumatic because it's done on a special frame and the patient's head and face are covered throughout the procedure.

• Check the skin around the cast edge daily. Keep the cast clean and dry and edges of the cast "petaled" (padded). Warn the patient not to insert anything under the cast or let anything get under it and to immediately report cracks in the cast, pain, burning, skin breakdown, numbness, or odor.

• Before surgery, assure the patient and family that she'll have adequate pain control postoperatively. Check sensation, movement, color, and blood supply in all extremities to detect neurovascular deficit, a serious complication following spinal surgery.

After corrective surgery:

• Check neurovascular status every 2 to 4 hours for the first 48 hours, then several times a day. Logroll the patient often.

• Measure intake, output, and urine specific gravity to monitor effects of blood loss, which is often substantial.

• Monitor abdominal distention and bowel sounds.

• Encourage deep-breathing exercises to avoid pulmonary complications.

• Give analgesics as needed, especially before any activity.

• Promote active range-of-motion (ROM) arm exercises to help maintain muscle strength. Remember that any exercise, even brushing the hair or teeth, is helpful.

• Encourage the patient to perform quadriceps-setting, calf-pumping, and active ROM exercises of ankles and feet.

• Watch for skin breakdown and signs of cast syndrome. Teach the patient how to recognize these signs.

• Remove antiembolism stockings for at least 30 minutes daily.

• Offer emotional support to help prevent depression, which may result from altered body image and immobility. Encourage the patient to wear her own clothes, wash her hair, and use makeup.

• If the patient is being discharged with a Harrington rod and cast and must have bed rest, arrange for a social worker and a visiting nurse to provide home care. Before discharge, make sure the patient understands activity limitations.

• If you work in a school, screen children routinely for scoliosis during physical examinations.

# SEPTIC ARTHRITIS

A medical emergency, septic (infectious) arthritis is caused by bacterial invasion of a joint, resulting in inflammation of the synovial lining. If the organisms enter the joint cavity, effusion and pyogenesis follow, with eventual destruction of bone and cartilage.

Septic arthritis can lead to ankylosis and even fatal septicemia. However, prompt antibiotic therapy and joint aspiration or drainage cures most patients.

## Causes

In most cases of septic arthritis, bacteria spread from a primary site of infection, usually in adjacent bone or soft tissue, through the bloodstream to the joint.

Common infecting organisms include four strains of gram-positive cocci — *Staphylococcus aureus, Streptococcus pyogenes, Streptococcus pneumoniae,* and *Streptococcus viridans* — and two strains of gram-negative cocci — *Neisseria gonorrhoeae* and *Haemophilus influenzae.* Various gram-negative bacilli — *Escherichia coli, Salmonella,* and

*Pseudomonas,* for example—also cause infection.

Anaerobic organisms such as gram-positive cocci usually infect adults and children over age 2. *H. influenzae* most often infects children under age 2.

### Risk factors

Various factors can predispose a person to septic arthritis. Any concurrent bacterial infection (of the genitourinary or the upper respiratory tract, for example) or serious chronic illness (such as cancer, renal failure, rheumatoid arthritis, systemic lupus erythematosus, diabetes, or cirrhosis) heightens susceptibility. Consequently, alcoholics and elderly people run a higher risk of developing septic arthritis.

Of course, susceptibility increases with diseases that depress the autoimmune system or with prior immunosuppressive therapy. I.V. drug abuse (by heroin addicts, for example) can also cause septic arthritis.

Other predisposing factors include recent articular trauma, joint surgery, intra-articular injections, and local joint abnormalities.

### Signs and symptoms

Acute septic arthritis begins abruptly, causing intense pain, inflammation, and swelling of the affected joint, with low-grade fever. It usually affects a single joint. It most often develops in the large joints but can strike any joint, including the spine and small peripheral joints.

CLINICAL TIP  Systemic signs of inflammation may not appear in some patients. Migratory polyarthritis sometimes precedes localization of the infection. If the bacteria invade the hip, pain may occur in the groin, upper thigh, or buttock, or may be referred to the knee.

### Diagnosis

Identifying the causative organism in a Gram stain or culture of synovial fluid or a biopsy of synovial membrane confirms septic arthritis. Joint fluid analysis shows gross pus or watery, cloudy fluid of decreased viscosity, usually with 50,000/μl or more white blood cells (WBCs), primarily neutrophils.

When synovial fluid culture is negative, a positive blood culture may confirm the diagnosis. Synovial fluid glucose is often low compared with a simultaneous 6-hour postprandial blood glucose test.

Other diagnostic measures include the following:

● *X-rays* can show typical changes as early as 1 week after initial infection—distention of joint capsules, for example, followed by narrowing of joint space (indicating cartilage damage) and erosions of bone (joint destruction).

● *Radioisotope joint scan* for less accessible joints (such as spinal articulations) may help detect infection or inflammation but isn't itself diagnostic.

● *C-reactive protein* may be elevated, as well as *WBC count,* with many polymorphonuclear cells; *erythrocyte sedimentation rate* is increased.

● *Two sets of positive culture* and *Gram stain smears* of skin exudates, sputum, urethral discharge, stools, urine, or nasopharyngeal smear confirm septic arthritis.

● *Lactic assay* can distinguish septic from nonseptic arthritis.

### Treatment

Antibiotic therapy should begin promptly; it may be modified when sensitivity results become available.

### Antibiotic therapy

Penicillin G is effective against infections caused by *S. aureus, S. pyogenes, S. pneumoniae, S. viridans,* and *N. gon-*

*orrhoeae.* A penicillinase-resistant penicillin, such as nafcillin, is recommended for penicillin G-resistant strains of *S. aureus;* ampicillin, for *H. influenzae;* gentamicin, for gram-negative bacilli.

Medication selection requires drug sensitivity studies of the infecting organism. Bioassays or bactericidal assays of synovial fluid and bioassays of blood may confirm clearing of the infection.

### Other measures
Treatment of septic arthritis requires monitoring of progress through frequent analysis of joint fluid cultures, synovial fluid WBC counts, and glucose determinations.

Codeine or propoxyphene can be given for pain if needed. (Aspirin causes a misleading reduction in swelling, hindering accurate monitoring of progress.) The affected joint can be immobilized with a splint or traction until movement can be tolerated.

Needle aspiration (arthrocentesis) to remove grossly purulent joint fluid should be repeated daily until fluid appears normal. If excessive fluid is aspirated or the WBC count remains elevated, open surgical drainage (usually arthrotomy with lavage of the joint) may be necessary for resistant infection or chronic septic arthritis.

### Surgery
Late reconstructive surgery is warranted only for severe joint damage and only after all signs of active infection have disappeared, which usually takes several months. In some cases, the recommended procedure may be arthroplasty or joint fusion.

Prosthetic replacement remains controversial; it may exacerbate the infection. However, it has helped patients with damaged femoral heads or acetabula.

### Special considerations
• Practice strict aseptic technique with all procedures. Prevent contact between immunosuppressed patients and infected patients.
• Watch for signs of joint inflammation: heat, redness, swelling, pain, or drainage. Monitor vital signs and fever pattern. Remember that corticosteroids mask signs of infection.
• Check splints or traction regularly. Keep the joint in proper alignment, but avoid prolonged immobilization. Start passive range-of-motion exercises immediately, and progress to active exercises as soon as the patient can move the affected joint and put weight on it.
• Monitor pain levels and medicate accordingly, especially before exercise (remember that the pain of septic arthritis is easy to underestimate). Administer analgesics and narcotics for acute pain and heat or ice packs for moderate pain.
• Carefully evaluate the patient's condition after joint aspiration. Provide emotional support throughout the diagnostic tests and procedures, which should be previously explained to the patient. Warn the patient before the first aspiration that it will be *extremely* painful.

LIFE-THREATENING DISORDER

# SEPTIC SHOCK

Second only to cardiogenic shock as the leading cause of shock death, septic shock (usually a result of bacterial infection) causes inadequate blood perfusion and circulatory collapse. It occurs most often among hospitalized patients, especially men over age 40 and women ages 25 to 45.

About 25% of patients who develop gram-negative bacteremia go into shock. Unless vigorous treatment begins promptly, preferably before symptoms fully develop, septic shock rapidly progresses to death (often within a few hours) in up to 80% of these patients.

## Causes

In two-thirds of patients, septic shock results from infection with gram-negative bacteria: *Escherichia coli, Klebsiella, Enterobacter, Proteus, Pseudomonas,* and *Bacteroides;* in others, from gram-positive bacteria: *Streptococcus pneumoniae, Streptococcus pyogenes,* and *Actinomyces.* Infections with viruses, rickettsiae, chlamydiae, and protozoa may be complicated by shock.

These organisms produce septicemia in persons whose resistance is already compromised by an existing condition. Infection also results from transplantation of bacteria from other areas of the body through surgery, I.V. therapy, and catheters.

Septic shock often occurs in patients hospitalized for primary infection of the genitourinary, biliary, GI, and gynecologic tracts. Other predisposing factors include immunodeficiency, advanced age, trauma, burns, diabetes mellitus, cirrhosis, and disseminated cancer.

## Signs and symptoms

Indications of septic shock vary according to the stage of the shock, the organism causing it, and the age of the patient.
- *Early stage:* oliguria, sudden fever (over 101° F [38.3° C]), chills, nausea, vomiting, diarrhea, and prostration.
- *Late stage:* restlessness, apprehension, irritability, thirst from decreased cerebral tissue perfusion, tachycardia, and tachypnea. Hypotension, altered level of consciousness, and hyperventilation may be the *only* signs among infants and elderly people.

Hypothermia and anuria are common late signs. Complications of septic shock include disseminated intravascular coagulation (DIC), renal failure, heart failure, GI ulcers, and abnormal hepatic function.

## Diagnosis

Observation of one or more typical signs (fever, confusion, nausea, vomiting, hyperventilation) in a patient suspected of having an infection suggests septic shock and necessitates immediate treatment.

In the early stages, arterial blood gas (ABG) analysis indicates respiratory alkalosis (low partial pressure of carbon dioxide [$P_{CO_2}$], low or normal bicarbonate [$HCO_3^-$] level, and high pH). As shock progresses, metabolic acidosis develops, with hypoxemia indicated by decreasing $P_{CO_2}$ (which may increase as respiratory failure ensues), as well as decreasing partial pressure of oxygen, $HCO_3^-$, and pH levels.

The following laboratory tests support the diagnosis and determine the treatment:
- blood cultures to isolate the organism
- decreased platelet count and leukocytosis (15,000 to 30,000/μl)
- increased blood urea nitrogen and creatinine levels and decreased creatinine clearance
- abnormal prothrombin and partial thromboplastin time
- simultaneous measurement of urine and plasma osmolalities for renal failure (urine osmolality below 400 milliosmoles, with a ratio of urine to plasma below 1.5)
- decreased central venous pressure (CVP), pulmonary artery wedge pressure (PAWP), and cardiac output. (In

early septic shock, cardiac output increases.)

● electrocardiogram demonstrating ST-segment depression, inverted T waves, and arrhythmias resembling myocardial infarction.

## Treatment

The first goal of treatment is to monitor and reverse shock through volume expansion.

### Fluid infusion

I.V. fluids are administered, and a pulmonary artery catheter is inserted to check pulmonary circulation and PAWP. Administration of whole blood or plasma can then raise the PAWP to a satisfactory level of 14 to 18 mm Hg.

A respirator may be necessary for proper ventilation to overcome hypoxia. A urinary catheter allows accurate measurement of hourly urine output.

### Antibiotic therapy

Treatment also requires immediate administration of I.V. antibiotics to control the infection. Depending on the organism, the antibiotic combination usually includes an aminoglycoside, such as gentamicin or tobramycin for gram-negative bacteria, combined with a penicillin, such as carbenicillin or ticarcillin.

Sometimes treatment includes a cephalosporin, such as cefazolin, and nafcillin for suspected staphylococcal infection instead of carbenicillin or ticarcillin. Therapy may also include chloramphenicol for nonsporulating anaerobes (*Bacteroides*), although it may cause bone marrow depression, and clindamycin, which may produce pseudomembranous enterocolitis.

Appropriate anti-infectives for other causes of septic shock depend on the suspected organism. Other measures to combat infections include surgery to drain and excise abscesses and debridement.

### Other drug therapy

If shock persists after fluid infusion, treatment with vasopressors, such as dopamine, maintains adequate blood perfusion in the brain, liver, GI tract, kidneys, and skin. Other treatment includes I.V. bicarbonate to correct acidosis and I.V. corticosteroids, which may improve blood perfusion and increase cardiac output.

## Special considerations

● Determine which of your patients are at high risk for developing septic shock. Know the signs of impending septic shock, but don't rely solely on technical aids to judge the patient's status. Consider any change in mental status and urine output as significant as a change in CVP.

● Carefully maintain the pulmonary artery catheter. Check ABG values for adequate oxygenation or gas exchange, watching for any changes.

● Keep accurate intake and output records. Maintain adequate urine output (0.5 to 1 ml/kg/hour) and systolic pressure. Be careful to avoid fluid overload.

● Monitor serum gentamicin level, and administer drugs.

● Watch closely for complications of septic shock: DIC (abnormal bleeding), renal failure (oliguria, increased specific gravity), heart failure (dyspnea, edema, tachycardia, distended neck veins), GI ulcers (hematemesis, melena), and hepatic abnormalities (jaundice, hypoprothrombinemia, and hypoalbuminemia).

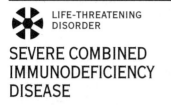

# SEVERE COMBINED IMMUNODEFICIENCY DISEASE

Both cell-mediated (T-cell) and humoral (B-cell) immunity are deficient or absent in severe combined immunodeficiency disease (SCID). This results in susceptibility to infection from all classes of microorganisms during infancy.

At least three types of SCID exist: *reticular dysgenesis,* the most severe type, in which the hematopoietic stem cell fails to differentiate into lymphocytes and granulocytes; *Swiss-type agammaglobulinemia,* in which the hematopoietic stem cell fails to differentiate into lymphocytes alone; and *enzyme deficiency,* such as adenosine deaminase (ADA) deficiency, in which the buildup of toxic products in the lymphoid tissue causes damage and subsequent dysfunction.

SCID affects more males than females; its estimated incidence is 1 in every 100,000 to 500,000 births. Most untreated patients die from infection within 1 year of birth.

## Causes
SCID is usually transmitted as an autosomal recessive trait, although it may be X-linked. In most cases, the genetic defect seems associated with failure of the stem cell to differentiate into T and B lymphocytes.

Many molecular defects, such as mutation of the kinase ZAP-70, can cause SCID. X-linked SCID results from a mutation of a subunit of the interleukin-2 (IL-2), IL-4, and IL-7 receptors. Less commonly, it results from an enzyme deficiency.

## Signs and symptoms
An extreme susceptibility to infection becomes obvious in the infant with SCID in the first months of life. The infant fails to thrive and develops chronic otitis, sepsis, watery diarrhea (associated with *Salmonella* or *Escherichia coli*), recurrent pulmonary infections (usually caused by *Pseudomonas,* cytomegalovirus, or *Pneumocystis carinii*), persistent oral candidiasis (sometimes with esophageal erosions), and possibly fatal viral infections (such as chickenpox).

*P. carinii* pneumonia usually strikes a severely immunodeficient infant in the first 3 to 5 weeks of life. Onset is typically insidious, with gradually worsening cough, low-grade fever, tachypnea, and respiratory distress. A chest X-ray characteristically shows bilateral pulmonary infiltrates.

## Diagnosis
Clinical indications point to the diagnosis. Most infants with SCID suffer recurrent overwhelming infections within 1 year of birth. Some are diagnosed after a severe reaction to vaccination.

Defective humoral immunity is difficult to detect before an infant is 5 months old. Before age 5 months, even normal infants have very small amounts of the serum immunoglobulins (Ig) IgM and IgA, and normal IgG levels merely reflect maternal IgG. However, severely diminished or absent T-cell number and function and lymph node biopsy showing absence of lymphocytes can confirm the diagnosis of SCID.

## Treatment
Restoring immune response and preventing infection are the first goals of

treatment. Histocompatible bone marrow transplant is the only satisfactory treatment available to correct immunodeficiency.

Because bone marrow cells must be matched according to human leukocyte antigen and mixed leukocyte culture, the most common donors are histocompatible siblings. But bone marrow transplant can produce a potentially fatal graft-versus-host (GVH) reaction, so newer methods of bone marrow transplant that eliminate GVH reaction (such as lectin separation and the use of monoclonal antibodies) are being evaluated.

Fetal thymus and liver transplants have achieved limited success. Administration of immune globulin may also play a role in treatment. Some SCID infants have received long-term protection by being isolated in a completely sterile environment. However, this approach isn't effective if the infant already has had recurring infections.

Gene therapy is being used for ADA deficiency.

**Special considerations**

• Monitor the infant constantly for early signs of infection; if infection develops, provide prompt and aggressive drug therapy.

• Watch for adverse effects of any medications given. Avoid vaccinations, and give only irradiated blood products if the patient needs a transfusion.

• Explain all procedures, medications, and precautions to the parents.

• Although SCID infants must remain in strict protective isolation, try to provide a stimulating atmosphere to promote growth and development. Encourage parents to visit their child often, to hold him, and to bring him toys that can be easily sterilized.

• Maintain a normal daily and nightly routine, and talk to the child as much as possible. If the parents can't visit, call them often to report on their infant's condition.

• Refer parents for genetic counseling. Refer parents and siblings for psychological and spiritual counseling to help them cope with the child's inevitable long-term illness and early death.

• For assistance in coping with the financial burden of the child's long-term hospitalization, refer the parents to social services.

# SICKLE CELL ANEMIA

A congenital hemolytic anemia that occurs primarily, but not exclusively, in blacks, sickle cell anemia results from a defective hemoglobin (Hb) molecule (hemoglobin S) that causes red blood cells (RBCs) to roughen and become sickle-shaped. Such cells impair circulation, resulting in chronic ill health (fatigue, dyspnea on exertion, swollen joints), periodic crises, long-term complications, and premature death.

Sickle cell anemia is most common in tropical Africans and in people of African descent; about 1 in 10 blacks carries the abnormal gene. If two such carriers have offspring, there is a 1 in 4 (25%) chance that each child will have the disease. Overall, 1 in every 400 to 600 black children has sickle cell anemia.

This disease also occurs in Puerto Rico, Turkey, India, the Middle East, and the Mediterranean, as well as in other populations. The defective Hb gene may have persisted in areas where malaria is endemic because the heterozygous sickle cell trait provides re-

## SICKLE CELL TRAIT

This relatively benign condition results from heterozygous inheritance of the abnormal hemoglobin S (Hb S) gene from one parent, while receiving one normal Hb gene from the other parent. Like sickle cell anemia, this condition is most common in blacks. Sickle cell trait never progresses to sickle cell anemia.

In persons with sickle cell trait (also called carriers), 20% to 40% of their total Hb is Hb S; the rest is normal.

Such carriers usually have no symptoms. They have normal Hb and hematocrit values and can expect a normal life span. Nevertheless, they must avoid situations that provoke hypoxia because these occasionally cause a sickling crisis similar to that in sickle cell anemia.

Genetic counseling is essential for sickle cell carriers. If two sickle cell carriers marry, each of their children has a 25% chance of inheriting sickle cell anemia.

*Altered cells*

The abnormal Hb S found in RBCs of patients with sickle cell anemia becomes insoluble whenever hypoxia occurs. As a result, these RBCs become rigid, rough, and elongated, forming a crescent, or sickle, shape. Such sickling can produce hemolysis (cell destruction).

In addition, these altered cells tend to pile up in capillaries and smaller blood vessels, making the blood more viscous. Normal circulation is impaired, causing pain, tissue infarctions, and swelling. Such blockage causes anoxic changes that lead to further sickling and obstruction.

### Signs and symptoms

Characteristically, sickle cell anemia produces tachycardia, cardiomegaly, systolic and diastolic murmurs, pulmonary infarctions (which may result in cor pulmonale), chronic fatigue, unexplained dyspnea or dyspnea on exertion, hepatomegaly, jaundice, pallor, joint swelling, aching bones, chest pains, ischemic leg ulcers (especially around the ankles), and increased susceptibility to infection.

Such symptoms usually don't develop until after age 6 months, because large amounts of fetal Hb protect infants for the first few months after birth. Low socioeconomic status and related problems, such as poor nutrition and education, may delay diagnosis and supportive treatment.

Infection, stress, dehydration, and conditions that provoke hypoxia — strenuous exercise, high altitude, unpressurized aircraft, cold, and vasoconstrictive drugs — may all provoke periodic crisis. Four types of crises can occur: painful, aplastic, acute sequestration, or hemolytic.

sistance to malaria and is actually beneficial.

Penicillin prophylaxis can decrease morbidity and mortality from bacterial infections. Half of such patients die by their early twenties; few live to middle age.

### Causes

Sickle cell anemia results from homozygous inheritance of the Hb S gene, which causes substitution of the amino acid valine for glutamic acid in the B Hb chain. Heterozygous inheritance of this gene results in sickle cell trait, usually an asymptomatic condition. (See *Sickle cell trait.*)

### Painful crisis

Also called a vaso-occlusive crisis or infarctive crisis, painful crisis is the most common crisis and the hallmark of this disease. It usually appears periodically after age 5.

A painful crisis results from blood vessel obstruction by rigid, tangled sickle cells, which causes tissue anoxia and possible necrosis. It's characterized by severe abdominal, thoracic, muscular, or bone pain and possibly increased jaundice, dark urine, or a low-grade fever.

Autosplenectomy, in which splenic damage and scarring is so extensive that the spleen shrinks and becomes impalpable, occurs in patients with long-term disease. This can lead to increased susceptibility to *Streptococcus pneumoniae* sepsis, which can be fatal without prompt treatment.

After the crisis subsides (in 4 days to several weeks), infection may develop, causing such signs as lethargy, sleepiness, fever, and apathy.

### Aplastic crisis

Also called megaloblastic crisis, aplastic crisis results from bone marrow depression and is associated with infection, usually viral. It's characterized by pallor, lethargy, sleepiness, dyspnea, possible coma, markedly decreased bone marrow activity, and RBC hemolysis.

### Acute sequestration crisis

In infants between 8 months and 2 years old, an acute sequestration crisis may cause sudden massive entrapment of RBCs in the spleen and liver. This rare crisis causes lethargy and pallor; if untreated, it commonly progresses to hypovolemic shock and death.

### Hemolytic crisis

Quite rare, hemolytic crisis usually occurs in patients who have glucose-6-phosphate dehydrogenase deficiency with sickle cell anemia. It probably results from complications of sickle cell anemia, such as infection, rather than from the disorder itself.

Hemolytic crisis causes liver congestion and hepatomegaly as a result of degenerative changes. It worsens chronic jaundice, although increased jaundice doesn't always point to a hemolytic crisis.

### Indicators of crisis

Suspect any of these crises in a sickle cell anemia patient with pale lips, tongue, palms, or nail beds; lethargy; listlessness; sleepiness, with difficulty awakening; irritability; severe pain; temperature over 104° F (40° C); or a fever of 100° F (37.8° C) that persists for 2 days.

### Long-term complications

Sickle cell anemia also causes long-term complications. Typically, such a child is small for his age, and puberty is delayed. (However, fertility isn't impaired). If he reaches adulthood, his body build tends to be spiderlike — narrow shoulders and hips, long extremities, curved spine, barrel chest, and elongated skull.

An adult usually has complications with organ infarction, such as retinopathy and nephropathy. Premature death commonly results from infection or repeated occlusion of small blood vessels and consequent infarction or necrosis of major organs. For example, cerebral blood vessel occlusion causes cerebrovascular accident.

## Diagnosis

A positive family history and typical clinical features suggest sickle cell anemia. Hb electrophoresis showing Hb S or other hemoglobinopathies can confirm it. Electrophoresis should be done on umbilical cord blood samples at birth to provide sickle cell disease screening for all neonates at risk.

Additional laboratory studies show a low RBC count, elevated white blood cell and platelet counts, decreased erythrocyte sedimentation rate, increased serum iron level, decreased RBC survival, and reticulocytosis. Hb may be low or normal.

During early childhood, palpation may reveal splenomegaly, but as the child grows older, the spleen shrinks.

## Treatment
Prophylactic penicillin is given before age 4 months. If the patient's Hb drops suddenly or if his condition deteriorates rapidly, a transfusion of packed RBCs is needed.

In a sequestration crisis, treatment may include sedation, administration of analgesics, blood transfusion, oxygen administration, and large amounts of oral and I.V. fluids. A good antisickling agent isn't available yet; the most commonly used drug, sodium cyanate, has many adverse effects.

## Special considerations
During a painful crisis:
• Apply warm compresses to painful areas and cover the child with a blanket. (Never use cold compresses; this aggravates the condition.)
• Administer an analgesic-antipyretic, such as aspirin or acetaminophen.
• Encourage bed rest, and place the patient in a sitting position. If dehydration or severe pain occurs, hospitalization may be necessary.
• Give antibiotics when appropriate.
• Suggest biofeedback techniques, which may be helpful.
• If the patient is an adolescent or adult male, warn him that he may have sudden, painful episodes of priapism. Explain that such episodes are common and, if prolonged, can have serious re-

productive consequences. Advise the patient to report the occurrence of such episodes.

During remission:
• Advise the patient to avoid tight clothing that restricts circulation.
• Warn against strenuous exercise, vasoconstricting medications, cold temperatures (including drinking large amounts of ice water and swimming), unpressurized aircraft, high altitude, and other conditions that provoke hypoxia.
• Stress the importance of normal childhood immunizations, meticulous wound care, good oral hygiene, regular dental checkups, and a balanced diet as safeguards against infection.
• Emphasize the need for prompt treatment of infection.
• Stress the need to increase fluid intake to prevent dehydration resulting from impaired ability to concentrate urine. Tell parents to encourage such a child to drink more fluids, especially in the summer, by offering milk shakes, ice pops, and eggnog.
• Encourage normal mental and social development in the child by warning parents against being overprotective. Although the child must avoid strenuous exercise, he can enjoy most everyday activities.
• Refer parents of children with sickle cell anemia for genetic counseling to answer their questions about the risk to future offspring. Recommend screening of other family members to determine if they're heterozygote carriers. These parents may also need psychological counseling to cope with guilt feelings. In addition, suggest they join an appropriate community support group. (See *Coping with sickle cell anemia*.)

During pregnancy or surgery:
➤ CLINICAL TIP   Women with sickle cell anemia may be a poor obstetric risk, and their use of oral con-

traceptives is risky. Refer them for birth control counseling by a gynecologist. If women with sickle cell anemia do become pregnant, they should maintain a balanced diet and may benefit from a folic acid supplement.

• During general anesthesia, make sure the patient has optimal ventilation to prevent hypoxic crisis. Provide a preoperative transfusion of packed RBCs as needed.

# SIDEROBLASTIC ANEMIAS

Sideroblastic anemias, a group of heterogenous disorders, produce a common defect — failure to use iron in hemoglobin (Hb) synthesis, despite the availability of adequate iron stores. These anemias may be hereditary or acquired; the acquired form, in turn, can be primary or secondary.

Hereditary sideroblastic anemia often responds to treatment with pyridoxine. Correction of the secondary acquired form depends on the causative disorder; the primary acquired (idiopathic) form, however, resists treatment and usually proves fatal within 10 years after onset of complications or a concomitant disease.

## Causes

Hereditary sideroblastic anemia appears to be transmitted by X-linked inheritance, occurring mostly in young males; females are carriers and usually show no signs of this disorder.

The acquired form may be secondary to ingestion of, or exposure to, toxins, such as alcohol and lead, or to drugs, such as isoniazid and chloramphenicol. It can also occur as a complication of other diseases, such as rheumatoid

---

> **TEACHING CHECKLIST**
>
> ## COPING WITH SICKLE CELL ANEMIA
>
> Before discharge, the patient must learn how to live with sickle cell anemia. Review with both the patient and his family the need to:
>
> • eat a well-balanced, healthy diet
> • keep up-to-date on immunizations
> • get adequate rest
> • take all medications as prescribed
> • drink plenty of fluids
> • contact health care providers at the first sign of infection or pain
> • keep telephone numbers for health care providers handy
> • plan ahead for emergencies
> • contact national support groups, local groups, or genetic counselors for up-to-date information on treatment and research.

---

arthritis, lupus erythematosus, multiple myeloma, tuberculosis, and severe infections.

The primary acquired form, known as refractory anemia with ringed sideroblasts, is most common in elderly people. It's often associated with thrombocytopenia or leukopenia as part of a myelodysplastic syndrome.

In sideroblastic anemia, normoblasts fail to use iron to synthesize Hb. As a result, iron is deposited in the mitochondria of normoblasts, which are then called ringed sideroblasts.

## Signs and symptoms

Sideroblastic anemias usually produce nonspecific clinical effects, which may exist for several years before being identified. Such effects include anorexia, fatigue, weakness, dizziness, pale skin and mucous membranes and, occasionally, enlarged lymph nodes.

Heart and liver failure may develop from excessive iron accumulation in these organs, causing dyspnea, exertional angina, slight jaundice, and hepatosplenomegaly. Hereditary sideroblastic anemia is associated with increased GI absorption of iron, causing signs of hemosiderosis. Additional symptoms in secondary sideroblastic anemia depend on the underlying cause.

## Diagnosis

Ringed sideroblasts on microscopic examination of bone marrow aspirate, stained with Prussian blue or alizarin red dye, confirm the diagnosis.

Microscopic examination of blood shows hypochromic or normochromic, and slightly macrocytic, erythrocytes. Red blood cell (RBC) precursors may be megaloblastic, with anisocytosis (abnormal variation in RBC size) and poikilocytosis (abnormal variation in RBC shape).

Unlike iron deficiency anemia, sideroblastic anemia lowers Hb and raises serum iron and transferrin levels. In turn, faulty Hb production raises urobilinogen and bilirubin levels. Platelet and leukocyte levels remain normal, but thrombocytopenia or leukopenia occasionally occurs.

## Treatment

The underlying cause determines the type of treatment.

### Hereditary form

Hereditary sideroblastic anemia usually responds to several weeks of treatment with high doses of pyridoxine (vitamin $B_6$).

### Primary acquired form

Elderly patients with sideroblastic anemia — most commonly the primary ac-

quired form — are less likely to improve quickly and are more likely to develop serious complications. Deferoxamine may be used to treat chronic iron overload in selected patients.

Carefully cross-matched transfusions (providing needed Hb) or high doses of androgens are effective palliative measures for some patients with the primary acquired form of sideroblastic anemia. However, this form is essentially refractory to treatment and usually leads to death from acute leukemia or from respiratory or cardiac complications.

➤ CLINICAL TIP  Some patients with sideroblastic anemia may benefit from phlebotomy to prevent hemochromatosis. Phlebotomy steps up the rate of erythropoiesis and uses up excess iron stores; thus, it reduces serum and total-body iron levels.

### Secondary acquired form

The acquired secondary form generally subsides after the causative drug or toxin is removed or the underlying condition is adequately treated. Folic acid supplements may also be beneficial when concomitant megaloblastic nuclear changes in RBC precursors are present.

## Special considerations

• Administer medications as needed. Teach the patient the importance of continuing prescribed therapy, even after he begins to feel better.

• Provide frequent rest periods if the patient becomes easily fatigued.

• If phlebotomy is scheduled, explain the procedure thoroughly to help reduce anxiety. If this procedure must be repeated frequently, provide a high-protein diet to help replace the protein lost during phlebotomy. Encourage the patient to follow a similar diet at home.

• Always inquire about the possibility of exposure to lead in the home (especially for children) or on the job.
• Identify patients who abuse alcohol; refer them for appropriate therapy.

# SILICOSIS

A progressive disease characterized by nodular lesions, silicosis frequently progresses to fibrosis. It's the most common form of pneumoconiosis.

Silicosis can be classified according to the severity of pulmonary disease and the rapidity of its onset and progression; it usually occurs as a simple asymptomatic illness.

Acute silicosis develops after 1 to 3 years in workers (sandblasters, tunnel workers) exposed to very high concentrations of respirable silica. Accelerated silicosis appears after an average of 10 years of exposure to lower concentrations of free silica. Chronic silicosis develops after 20 or more years of exposure to lower concentrations of free silica.

The prognosis is good, unless the disease progresses into the complicated fibrotic form, which causes respiratory insufficiency and cor pulmonale and is associated with pulmonary tuberculosis.

## Causes

Silicosis results from the inhalation and pulmonary deposition of respirable crystalline silica dust, mostly from quartz.

The danger to the worker depends on the concentration of dust in the atmosphere, the percentage of respirable free silica particles in the dust, and the duration of exposure. Respirable particles are less than 10 microns in diameter, but the disease-causing particles deposited in the alveolar space are usually 1 to 3 microns in diameter.

Industrial sources of silica in its pure form include the manufacture of ceramics (flint) and building materials (sandstone). It occurs in mixed form in the production of construction materials (cement); it's found in powder form (silica flour) in paints, porcelain, scouring soaps, and wood fillers and in the mining of gold, coal, lead, zinc, and iron.

Foundry workers, boiler scalers, and stonecutters are all exposed to silica dust. All are at high risk of developing silicosis.

## Pathophysiology

Nodules result when alveolar macrophages ingest silica particles, which they are unable to process. As a result, the macrophages die and release proteolytic enzymes into the surrounding tissue. The subsequent inflammation attracts other macrophages and fibroblasts into the region to produce fibrous tissue and wall off the reaction.

The resulting nodule has an onion-skin appearance when viewed under a microscope. Nodules develop adjacent to terminal and respiratory bronchioles, concentrate in the upper lobes, and are frequently accompanied by bullous changes throughout both lungs.

If the disease doesn't progress, minimal physiologic disturbances occur, with no disability. Occasionally, however, the fibrotic response accelerates, engulfing and destroying large areas of the lung (progressive massive fibrosis or conglomerate lesions). Fibrosis may continue despite termination of exposure to dust.

## Signs and symptoms

Silicosis initially may be asymptomatic or it may produce dyspnea on exertion, often attributed to being "out of shape" or "slowing down."

## Progressive features

If the disease progresses to the chronic and complicated stage, dyspnea on exertion worsens, and other signs — usually tachypnea and an insidious, dry cough that's most pronounced in the morning — appear. Progression to the advanced stage causes dyspnea on minimal exertion, worsening cough, and pulmonary hypertension, which in turn leads to right ventricular failure and cor pulmonale.

Patients with silicosis have a high incidence of active tuberculosis, which should be considered when evaluating a patient with this disease. Central nervous system changes — confusion, lethargy, and a decrease in the rate and depth of respiration as partial pressure of carbon dioxide increases — also occur in advanced silicosis.

## Other features

Other clinical features include malaise, disturbed sleep, and hoarseness.

> CLINICAL TIP The severity of these symptoms may not correlate with chest X-ray findings or the results of pulmonary function studies.

## Diagnosis

Patient history reveals occupational exposure to silica dust. Physical examination is normal in simple silicosis; in chronic silicosis with conglomerate lesions, it may reveal decreased chest expansion, diminished intensity of breath sounds, areas of hyporesonance and hyperresonance, fine to medium crackles, and tachypnea.

In simple silicosis, chest X-rays show small, discrete, nodular lesions distributed throughout both lung fields but typically concentrated in the upper lung zones; the hilar lung nodes may be enlarged and exhibit "eggshell" calcification. In complicated silicosis, X-rays show one or more conglomerate masses of dense tissue.

Pulmonary function studies yield the following results:

● *Forced vital capacity (FVC)* is reduced in complicated silicosis.

● *Forced expiratory volume in 1 second (FEV$_1$)* is reduced in obstructive disease (emphysematous areas of silicosis); it's also reduced in complicated silicosis, but the ratio of FEV$_1$ to FVC is normal or high.

● *Maximum voluntary ventilation* is reduced in both restrictive and obstructive diseases.

● *Diffusing capacity of the lung for carbon monoxide* is reduced when fibrosis destroys alveolar walls and obliterates pulmonary capillaries or when fibrosis thickens the alveolar capillary membrane.

In addition, arterial blood gas studies show the following:

● *Partial pressure of oxygen* is normal in simple silicosis; it may be significantly decreased when the patient breathes room air in the late stages of chronic or complicated disease.

● *Partial pressure of carbon dioxide* is normal in early stages but may decrease because of hyperventilation; it may increase as a restrictive pattern develops, particularly if the patient is hypoxic and has severe impairment of alveolar ventilation.

## Treatment

The goal of treatment is to relieve respiratory symptoms, to manage hypoxia and cor pulmonale, and to prevent respiratory tract irritation and infections. Treatment also includes careful observation for the development of tuberculosis.

Respiratory symptoms may be relieved through daily use of bronchodilating aerosols and increased fluid intake (at least 3 L daily). Steam inhalation and chest physiotherapy techniques, such as controlled coughing and segmental bronchial drainage with chest percussion and vibration, help clear secretions.

In severe cases, oxygen may be administered by cannula or mask (1 to 2 L/minute) for the patient with chronic hypoxia or by mechanical ventilation if arterial oxygen can't be maintained above 40 mm Hg. Respiratory infections require prompt administration of antibiotics.

### Special considerations

• Teach the patient to prevent infections by avoiding crowds and people with respiratory infections and by receiving influenza and pneumococcal vaccines.
• Increase the patient's exercise tolerance by encouraging regular activity. Advise the patient to plan his daily activities to decrease the work of breathing; he should pace himself, rest often, and generally move slowly through his daily routine.

# SINUSITIS

Inflammation of the paranasal sinuses may be acute, subacute, chronic, allergic, or hyperplastic.

Acute sinusitis usually results from the common cold and lingers in subacute form in only about 10% of patients. Chronic sinusitis follows persistent bacterial infection; allergic sinusitis accompanies allergic rhinitis; hyperplastic sinusitis is a combination of purulent acute sinusitis and allergic sinusitis or rhinitis. The prognosis is good for all types.

### Causes

Sinusitis usually results from viral or bacterial infection. The bacteria responsible for acute sinusitis are usually pneumococci, other streptococci, *Haemophilus influenzae,* and *Moraxella catarrhalis.* Staphylococci and gram-negative bacteria are more likely to occur in chronic cases or in patients in intensive care.

> CLINICAL TIP On rare occasions, fungi can also be an etiologic factor. *Aspergillus fumigatus* is the fungus most frequently associated with sinus disease.

Predisposing factors include any condition that interferes with drainage and ventilation of the sinuses, such as chronic nasal edema, deviated septum, viscous mucus, nasal polyps, allergic rhinitis, nasal intubation, nasogastric tubes, or debilitation related to chemotherapy, malnutrition, diabetes, blood dyscrasias, chronic use of steroids, or immunodeficiency.

Bacterial invasion commonly occurs from the conditions listed above or after a viral infection. It may also result from swimming in contaminated water.

### Signs and symptoms

Features vary with sinusitis type.

#### *Acute sinusitis*

The primary symptom of acute sinusitis is nasal congestion, followed by a gradual buildup of pressure in the affected sinus. For 24 to 48 hours after onset, nasal discharge may be present and later may become purulent. Associated symptoms include malaise, sore throat, headache, low-grade fever (temperature of 99° to 99.5° F [37.2° to 37.5° C]), malodorous breath, painless morning periorbital swelling, and a sense of facial fullness.

Characteristic pain depends on the affected sinus: maxillary sinusitis caus-

## SURGERY FOR CHRONIC AND HYPERPLASTIC SINUSITIS

### For maxillary sinusitis
• Nasal window procedure creates an opening in the sinus, allowing secretions and pus to drain through the nose.
• Caldwell-Luc procedure removes diseased mucosa in the maxillary sinus through an incision under the upper lip.

### For chronic ethmoid sinusitis
• Ethmoidectomy removes all infected tissue through an external or intranasal incision into the ethmoidal sinus.

### For sphenoid sinusitis
• External ethmoidectomy removes infected ethmoidal sinus tissue through a crescent-shaped incision, beginning under the inner eyebrow and extending along the side of the nose.

### For chronic frontal sinusitis
• Frontoethmoidectomy removes infected frontal sinus tissue through an extended external ethmoidectomy.
• Osteoplastic flap drains the sinuses through an incision across the skull, behind the hairline.

es pain over the cheeks and upper teeth; ethmoid sinusitis, pain over the eyes; frontal sinusitis, pain over the eyebrows; and sphenoid sinusitis (rare), pain behind the eyes.

### Subacute sinusitis
Purulent nasal drainage that continues for longer than 3 weeks after an acute infection subsides suggests subacute sinusitis. Other clinical features of the subacute form include a stuffy nose, vague facial discomfort, fatigue, and a nonproductive cough.

### Other types
The effects of chronic sinusitis are similar to those of acute sinusitis, but the chronic form causes continuous mucopurulent discharge.

The effects of allergic sinusitis are the same as those of allergic rhinitis. In both conditions, the prominent symptoms are sneezing, frontal headache, watery nasal discharge, and a stuffy, burning, itchy nose.

In hyperplastic sinusitis, bacterial growth on the diseased tissue causes pronounced tissue edema. Thickening of the mucosal lining, as well as the development of mucosal polyps, combine to produce chronic stuffiness of the nose in addition to headaches.

### Diagnosis
The following measures are useful:
• *Nasal examination* reveals inflammation and pus.
• *Sinus X-rays* reveal cloudiness in the affected sinus, air and fluid, and any thickening of the mucosal lining.
• *Antral puncture* promotes drainage of purulent material. It may also be used to provide a specimen for culture and sensitivity testing of the infecting organism but is rarely done.
• *Ultrasonography* and *computed tomography (CT) scan* aid in diagnosing suspected complications. CT scans are more sensitive than routine X-rays in detecting sinusitis.

### Treatment
Effective treatment depends on the type of sinusitis.

## Acute sinusitis

In acute sinusitis, local decongestants usually are tried before systemic decongestants; steam inhalation may also be helpful. Local application of heat may help to relieve pain and congestion.

Antibiotics are necessary to combat purulent or persistent infection. (The patient should be aware that allergic reactions to penicillin can occur.) Amoxicillin, ampicillin, and amoxicillin-clavulanate potassium are usually the antibiotics of choice; question the patient about any known allergy to penicillin. Sinusitis is a deep-seated infection, so antibiotics should be given for 2 to 3 weeks.

## Subacute sinusitis

In subacute sinusitis, antibiotics and decongestants may be helpful.

## Other types

Treatment of allergic sinusitis must include treatment of allergic rhinitis — administration of antihistamines, identification of allergens by skin testing, and desensitization by immunotherapy. Severe allergic symptoms may require treatment with corticosteroids and epinephrine.

In chronic sinusitis and hyperplastic sinusitis, antihistamines, antibiotics, and a steroid nasal spray may relieve pain and congestion. If irrigation fails to relieve symptoms, one or more sinuses may require surgery. (See *Surgery for chronic and hyperplastic sinusitis*, page 794.)

## Special considerations

• Enforce bed rest, and encourage the patient to drink plenty of fluids to promote drainage. Don't elevate the head of the bed more than 30 degrees.

• To relieve pain and promote drainage, apply warm compresses continuously, or four times daily for 2-hour intervals. In addition, give analgesics and antihistamines as needed.

• Watch for complications, such as vomiting, chills, fever, edema of the forehead or eyelids, blurred or double vision, and personality changes.

• If surgery is necessary, tell the patient what to expect postoperatively: A nasal packing will be in place for 12 to 24 hours after surgery, he'll have to breathe through his mouth, and he won't be able to blow his nose. After surgery, monitor for excessive drainage or bleeding and watch for complications.

• To prevent edema and promote drainage, place the patient in semi-Fowler's position. To relieve edema and pain and to minimize bleeding, apply ice compresses or a rubber glove filled with ice chips over the nose and iced saline gauze over the eyes. Continue these measures for 24 hours.

• Frequently change the mustache dressing or drip pad, and record the consistency, amount, and color of drainage (expect scant, bright red, and clotty drainage).

• Because the patient will be breathing through his mouth, provide meticulous mouth care.

• Tell the patient that even after the packing is removed, nose blowing may cause bleeding and swelling. If the patient is a smoker, instruct him not to smoke for at least 2 or 3 days after surgery.

• Instruct the patient to finish the prescribed antibiotics, even if his symptoms disappear.

➤ CLINICAL TIP Vasoconstrictive nose drops and spray are associated with rebound edema if used for more than 5 to 7 days.

# SJÖGREN'S SYNDROME

The second most common autoimmune rheumatic disorder after rheumatoid arthritis (RA), Sjögren's syndrome (SS) is characterized by diminished lacrimal and salivary gland secretion (sicca complex). SS occurs mainly in women (90% of patients); its mean age of occurrence is 50.

SS may be a primary disorder or may be associated with a connective tissue disorder, such as RA, scleroderma, systemic lupus erythematosus, or polymyositis. In some patients, the disorder is limited to the exocrine glands (glandular SS); in others, it also involves other organs, such as the lungs and kidneys (extraglandular SS).

## Causes

The cause of SS is unknown. Most likely, genetic and environmental factors contribute to its development. Viral or bacterial infection or perhaps exposure to pollen may trigger SS in a genetically susceptible individual.

Tissue damage results from infiltration by lymphocytes or from the deposition of immune complexes. Lymphocytic infiltration may be classified as benign lymphoma, malignant lymphoma, or pseudolymphorna (nonmalignant, but tumorlike aggregates of lymphoid cells).

## Signs and symptoms

About 50% of patients with SS have confirmed RA and a history of slowly developing sicca complex. However, some seek medical help for rapidly progressive and severe oral and ocular dryness, often accompanied by periodic parotid gland enlargement.

### Ocular effects

Ocular dryness (xerophthalmia) leads to foreign body sensation (gritty, sandy eye), redness, burning, photosensitivity, eye fatigue, itching, and mucoid discharge. The patient may also complain of a film across his field of vision.

### Oral effects

Oral dryness (xerostomia) leads to difficulty swallowing and talking; abnormal taste or smell sensation, or both; thirst; ulcers of the tongue, buccal mucosa, and lips (especially at the corners of the mouth); and severe dental caries. Dryness of the respiratory tract leads to epistaxis, hoarseness, chronic nonproductive cough, recurrent otitis media, and increased incidence of respiratory infections.

### Other features

Other effects may include dyspareunia and pruritus (associated with vaginal dryness), generalized itching, fatigue, recurrent low-grade fever, and arthralgia or myalgia.

> **CLINICAL TIP** Lymphadenopathy is relatively common in patients with SS, but persistent, firm lymph node enlargement may be the first sign of malignant transformation. Patients with primary SS have a 44 times greater relative risk of lymphoma than does the general population.

Specific extraglandular findings in SS include interstitial pneumonitis; interstitial nephritis, which results in renal tubular acidosis in 25% of patients; Raynaud's phenomenon (20%); arthritis and arthralgias (60%); peripheral neuropathy (2% to 5%); and vasculitis, usually limited to the skin and characterized by palpable purpura on the legs (5% to 10%).

About 50% of patients show evidence of hypothyroidism related to autoimmune thyroid disease. A few patients develop systemic necrotizing vasculitis.

## Diagnosis

A patient with SS has at least two of the following conditions: xerophthalmia, xerostomia (with a salivary gland biopsy showing lymphocytic infiltration), and an associated autoimmune or lymphoproliferative disorder.

### Tests to rule out other causes

Diagnosis must rule out other causes of oral and ocular dryness, including sarcoidosis, endocrine disorders, anxiety or depression, and effects of therapy such as radiation to the head and neck. Over 200 commonly used drugs also produce dry mouth.

In patients with salivary gland enlargement and severe lymphoid infiltration, the diagnosis must rule out cancer.

### Laboratory tests

Laboratory values include an elevated erythrocyte sedimentation rate in most patients, mild anemia and leukopenia in 30%, and hypergammaglobulinemia in 50%. Autoantibodies are also common, including SSA (anti-Ro) and SSB (anti-La), which are antinuclear and antisalivary duct antibodies. From 75% to 90% of patients test positive for rheumatoid factor; 90%, for antinuclear antibodies.

### Other tests

Other tests help support this diagnosis. Schirmer's tearing test and slit-lamp examination with rose bengal dye are used to measure eye involvement. Salivary gland involvement is evaluated by measuring the volume of parotid saliva and by secretory sialography and salivary scintigraphy. A lower lip biopsy shows salivary gland infiltration by lymphocytes.

## Treatment

Usually symptomatic, treatment includes conservative measures to relieve ocular or oral dryness.

### Symptomatic treatment

Mouth dryness can be relieved by using a methylcellulose swab or spray and by drinking plenty of fluids, especially at meals. New agents for treatment of salivary hypofunction, such as pilocarpine hydrochloride or bromnexine, may be useful. Meticulous oral hygiene is essential, including regular flossing, brushing, and fluoride treatment at home and frequent dental checkups.

Instillation of artificial tears as often as every half hour prevents eye damage (corneal ulcerations, corneal opacifications) from insufficient tear secretion.

➤ CLINICAL TIP  Artificial tears, whose drops are thicker and more viscous, require less frequent application but may cause blurring or leave residue on eyelashes.

Some patients may also benefit from instillation of an eye ointment at bedtime, or from twice-a-day sustained-release cellulose capsules.

If an eye infection develops, antibiotics should be given immediately; topical steroids should be avoided.

### Other measures

Other treatment measures vary with associated extraglandular findings. Parotid gland enlargement requires local heat and analgesics; arthritis and arthralgias, hydroxychloroquine or nonsteroidal anti-inflammatory drugs; pulmonary and renal interstitial disease, corticosteroids; accompanying lymphoma, a combination of chemotherapy, surgery, and radiation.

## Special considerations

● Advise the patient to avoid drugs that decrease saliva production, such as atropine derivatives, antihistamines, anticholinergics, and antidepressants

● If mouth lesions make eating painful, suggest high-protein, high-calorie liquid supplements to prevent malnutrition. Advise the patient to avoid sugar, which contributes to dental caries, and tobacco, alcohol, and spicy, salty, or highly acidic foods, which cause mouth irritation. Adequate dental hygiene after meals can also decrease the frequency of dental caries.

CLINICAL TIP  Saliva flow can be stimulated by use of sugar-free, highly flavored lozenges (such as lemon drops).

● Suggest the use of sunglasses to protect the patient's eyes from dust, wind, and strong light. Moisture chamber spectacles may also be helpful.

● Because dry eyes are more susceptible to infection, advise the patient to keep his face clean and to avoid rubbing his eyes.

● To help relieve respiratory dryness, stress the need to humidify home and work environments. Suggest normal saline solution drops or aerosolized spray for nasal dryness. Advise the patient to avoid prolonged hot showers and baths and to use moisturizing lotions to help ease dry skin. Suggest using a vaginal lubricant.

● Refer the patient to the Sjögren's Syndrome Foundation for additional information and support.

LIFE-THREATENING DISORDER

# SKULL FRACTURES

Skull fractures may be simple (closed) or compound (open) and may or may not displace bone fragments. Skull fractures are further described as linear, comminuted, or depressed. A linear fracture is a common hairline break, without displacement of structures; a comminuted fracture splinters or crushes the bone into several fragments; a depressed fracture pushes the bone toward the brain.

CLINICAL TIP  Because possible damage to the brain is the first concern, rather than the fracture itself, a skull fracture is considered a neurosurgical condition.

In children, the skull's thinness and elasticity allow a depression without a fracture (a linear fracture across a suture line increases the possibility of epidural hematoma).

Skull fractures are also classified according to location, such as a cranial vault fracture; a basilar fracture is at the base of the skull and involves the cribriform plate and the frontal sinuses. Because of the danger of grave cranial complications and meningitis, basilar fractures are usually far more serious than vault fractures.

## Causes

Like concussions and cerebral contusions or lacerations, skull fractures invariably result from a traumatic blow to the head. Motor vehicle accidents, bad falls, and severe beatings (especially in children) top the list of causes.

## Signs and symptoms

Skull fractures are often accompanied by scalp wounds — abrasions, contusions, lacerations, or avulsions. If the scalp has been lacerated or torn away, bleeding may be profuse because the scalp contains many blood vessels.

Bleeding can occasionally be heavy enough to induce hypovolemic shock. The patient may also be in shock from other injuries or from medullary failure in severe head injuries.

Linear fractures that are associated only with concussion don't produce loss of consciousness. They require evaluation, but not definitive treatment.

A fracture that results in cerebral contusion or laceration, however, may cause the classic signs of brain injury: agitation and irritability, loss of consciousness, changes in respiratory pattern (labored respirations), abnormal deep tendon reflexes, and altered pupillary and motor response.

If the patient with a skull fracture remains conscious, he's apt to complain of a persistent, localized headache. A skull fracture also may result in cerebral edema, which may cause compression of the reticular activating system, cutting off the normal flow of impulses to the brain and resulting in possible respiratory distress. The patient may experience an altered level of consciousness (LOC), progressing to unconsciousness or even death.

When jagged bone fragments pierce the dura mater or the cerebral cortex, skull fractures may cause subdural, epidural, or intracerebral hemorrhage or hematoma. With the resulting space-occupying lesions, clinical findings may include hemiparesis, unequal pupils, dizziness, seizures, projectile vomiting, decreased pulse and respiratory rates, and progressive unresponsiveness.

Sphenoidal fractures may also damage the optic nerve, causing blindness. Temporal fractures may cause unilateral deafness or facial paralysis.

Symptoms reflect the severity and extent of the head injury. However, some elderly patients may have cortical brain atrophy, with more space for brain swelling under the cranium, and consequently may not show signs of increased intracranial pressure (ICP) until it's very high.

A vault fracture often produces soft-tissue swelling near the fracture, making it hard to detect without a computed tomography (CT) scan.

A basilar fracture often produces hemorrhage from the nose, pharynx, or ears; blood under the periorbital skin ("raccoon's eyes") and under the conjunctiva; and Battle's sign (supramastoid ecchymosis), sometimes with bleeding behind the eardrum. This type of fracture may also cause cerebrospinal fluid (CSF) or even brain tissue to leak from the nose or ears.

Depending on the extent of brain damage, the patient with a skull fracture may suffer residual effects, such as seizure disorders (epilepsy), hydrocephalus, and organic brain syndome. Children may develop headaches, giddiness, easy fatigability, neuroses, and behavior disorders.

## Diagnosis

Suspect brain injury in all patients with a skull fracture until clinical evaluation proves otherwise. Every suspected skull injury calls for a thorough history of the trauma and a CT scan to attempt to locate the fracture. (Keep in mind that vault fractures often aren't visible or palpable.)

A fracture also requires a neurologic examination to check cerebral function (mental status and orientation to time, place, and person), LOC, pupillary response, motor function, and deep tendon reflexes.

Using reagent strips, the draining nasal or ear fluid should be tested for CSF. The tape will turn blue if CSF is present; it won't change in the presence of blood alone. However, the tape will also turn blue if the patient is hyperglycemic.

The patient's bedsheets may show the halo sign — a blood-tinged spot surrounded by a lighter ring — from leakage of CSF.

Brain damage can be assessed through a CT scan and magnetic resonance imaging, which disclose intracranial hemorrhage from ruptured blood vessels and swelling. Expanding lesions contraindicate lumbar puncture.

## Treatment
Effective treatment depends on the type and severity of the fracture.

### Linear fractures
Although occasionally even a simple linear skull fracture can tear an underlying blood vessel or cause a CSF leak, linear fractures generally require only supportive treatment, including mild analgesics (such as acetaminophen), and cleaning and debridement of any wounds after injection of a local anesthetic.

If the patient with a skull fracture has not lost consciousness, he should be observed in the emergency room for at least 4 hours. After this observation period, if vital signs are stable and if the neurosurgeon concurs, the patient can be discharged. At this time, the patient should be given an instruction sheet to follow for 24 to 48 hours of observation at home.

### Vault and basilar fractures
More severe vault fractures, especially depressed fractures, usually require a craniotomy to elevate or remove fragments that have been driven into the brain and to extract foreign bodies and necrotic tissue, thereby reducing the risk of infection and further brain damage. Other treatments for severe vault fractures include antibiotic therapy and, in profound hemorrhage, blood transfusions.

Basilar fractures call for immediate prophylactic antibiotics to prevent the onset of meningitis from CSF leaks as well as close observation for secondary hematomas and hemorrhages. Surgery may be necessary.

In addition, basilar and vault fractures often require dexamethasone I.V. or I.M. to reduce cerebral edema and minimize brain tissue damage.

### Special considerations
- Establish and maintain a patent airway; nasal airways are contraindicated in patients with possible basilar skull fractures. Intubation may be necessary.
- Suction the patient through the mouth, not the nose, to prevent the introduction of bacteria in case a CSF leak is present.
- Be sure to obtain a complete history of the trauma from the patient, his family, any eyewitnesses, and ambulance personnel.
- Ask whether the patient lost consciousness and, if so, for how long. The patient will need further diagnostic tests, including a complete neurologic examination, a CT scan, and other studies.
- Check for abnormal reflexes such as Babinski's reflex.
- Look for CSF draining from the patient's ears, nose, or mouth. Check bed linens for CSF leaks and look for a halo sign. If the patient's nose is draining

CSF, wipe it — *don't let him blow it.* If an ear is draining, cover it lightly with sterile gauze — *don't pack it.*

• Position the patient with a head injury so secretions can drain properly. Elevate the head of the bed 30 degrees if intracerebral injury is suspected.

• Cover scalp wounds carefully with a sterile dressing; control any bleeding as necessary.

• Take seizure precautions, but don't restrain the patient. Agitated behavior may stem from hypoxia or increased ICP, so check for these symptoms. Speak in a calm, reassuring voice, and touch the patient gently. Don't make any sudden, unexpected moves.

• Don't give the patient narcotics or sedatives because they may depress respirations, increase carbon dioxide levels, lead to increased ICP, and mask changes in neurologic status. Give acetaminophen or another mild analgesic for pain.

When a skull fracture requires surgery:

• Obtain consent, as needed, to shave the patient's head. Explain that you're performing this procedure to provide a clean area for surgery. Type and cross-match blood. Obtain baseline laboratory studies, such as a complete blood count, serum electrolyte studies, and urinalysis.

• After surgery, monitor vital signs and neurologic status frequently (usually every 5 minutes until the patient is stable, and then every 15 minutes for 1 hour), watching for any changes in LOC. Because skull fractures and brain injuries heal slowly, don't expect dramatic postoperative improvement.

• Monitor intake and output frequently, and maintain patency of the indwelling urinary catheter. Take special care with fluid intake. Hypotonic fluids (even dextrose 5% in water) can increase

cerebral edema. Their use should be restricted; give them only as needed.

• If the patient is unconscious, provide parenteral nutrition. (Remember, the patient may regurgitate and aspirate food if you use a nasogastric tube for feedings.)

If the fracture doesn't require surgery:

• Wear sterile gloves to examine the scalp laceration. With your finger, probe the wound for foreign bodies and a palpable fracture. Gently clean lacerations and the surrounding area. Cover with sterile gauze. The patient may need suturing.

• Provide emotional support for the patient and his family. Explain the need for procedures to reduce the risk of brain injury.

• Before discharge, instruct the patient's family to watch closely for changes in mental status, LOC, or respirations and to relieve the patient's headache with acetaminophen. Tell them to return him to the hospital immediately if his LOC decreases, if his headache persists after several doses of mild analgesics, if he vomits more than once, or if weakness develops in his arms or legs.

• Teach the patient and his family how to care for his scalp wound. Emphasize the need to return for suture removal and follow-up evaluation.

# SNAKEBITES, POISONOUS

Each year, poisonous snakes bite about 7,000 people in the United States, resulting in about 20 deaths. Such bites are most common during summer afternoons in grassy or rocky habitats. Poisonous snakebites are medical emergencies. With prompt, correct treatment, they need not be fatal.

## Causes

The only poisonous snakes in the United States are pit vipers (Crotalidae) and coral snakes (Elapidae). Pit vipers include rattlesnakes, water moccasins (cottonmouths), and copperheads. They have a pitted depression between their eyes and nostrils and two fangs, ¾″ to 1¼″ (2 to 3 cm) long. Because fangs may break off or grow behind old ones, some snakes may have one, three, or four fangs.

Because coral snakes are nocturnal and placid, their bites are less common than pit viper bites; pit vipers are also nocturnal but are more active. The fangs of coral snakes are short but have teeth behind them. Coral snakes have distinctive red, black, and yellow bands (yellow bands always border red ones), tend to bite with a chewing motion, and may leave multiple fang marks, small lacerations, and much tissue destruction.

## Signs and symptoms

Most snakebites happen on the arms and legs, below the elbow or knee. Bites to the head or trunk are most dangerous, but any bite into a blood vessel is dangerous, regardless of location.

Most pit viper bites that result in envenomation cause immediate and progressively severe pain and edema (the entire extremity may swell within a few hours), local elevation in skin temperature, fever, skin discoloration, petechiae, ecchymoses, blebs, blisters, bloody wound discharge, and local necrosis.

Because pit viper venom is neurotoxic, pit viper bites may cause local and facial numbness and tingling, fasciculation and twitching of skeletal muscles, seizures (especially in children),

extreme anxiety, difficulty speaking, fainting, weakness, dizziness, excessive sweating, occasional paralysis, mild to severe respiratory distress, headache, blurred vision, marked thirst and, in severe envenomation, coma and death. Pit viper venom may also impair coagulation and cause hematemesis, hematuria, melena, bleeding gums, and internal bleeding. Other symptoms of pit viper bites include tachycardia, lymphadenopathy, nausea, vomiting, diarrhea, hypotension, and shock.

The reaction to coral snakebite is usually delayed—sometimes up to several hours. These snakebites cause little or no local tissue reaction (local pain, swelling, or necrosis). However, because coral snake venom is neurotoxic, a reaction can progress swiftly, producing such effects as local paresthesia, drowsiness, nausea, vomiting, difficulty swallowing, marked salivation, dysphonia, ptosis, blurred vision, miosis, respiratory distress and possible respiratory failure, loss of muscle coordination and, possibly, shock with cardiovascular collapse and death.

## Diagnosis

The patient's history and account of the injury, observation of fang marks, snake identification (when possible), and progressive symptoms of envenomation all point to poisonous snakebite. Laboratory test results help identify the extent of envenomation and provide guidelines for supportive treatment.

Abnormal test results in poisonous snakebites may include the following:
• prolonged bleeding time and partial thromboplastin time
• decreased hemoglobin and hematocrit values
• sharply decreased platelet count (less than 200,000/µl)
• urinalysis disclosing hematuria

- increased white blood cell count in victims who develop an infection (the mouth of a snake typically contains gram-negative bacteria)
- pulmonary edema as shown on chest X-ray
- possibly tachycardia and ectopic heartbeats on the electrocardiogram (usually necessary only in cases of severe envenomation for a patient over age 40)
- possibly abnormal EEG findings in cases of severe envenomation.

**Treatment**

Prompt, appropriate first aid can reduce venom absorption and prevent severe symptoms.

- If possible, identify the snake, but don't waste time trying to find it.
- Place the victim in the supine position to slow venom metabolism and absorption.
- Don't give the victim any food, beverage, or medication orally.
- Authorities disagree about what constitutes appropriate prehospital care. Some recommend against placing a constrictive tourniquet (band) on the affected limb unless the victim is far from a medical facility.
- Whether you apply a tourniquet or not, immediately immobilize the victim's affected limb below heart level, and instruct the victim to remain as quiet as possible.
- If a tourniquet is applied, the victim or the person applying the tourniquet should check the victim's distal pulses regularly and loosen the tourniquet slightly as needed to maintain circulation.

❯ CLINICAL TIP Remember that the goal of applying a tourniquet is to obstruct lymphatic drainage, not blood flow. The use of a tourniquet in prehospital care is controversial.

- Once indicated, apply the tourniquet so that it's slightly constrictive, obstructing only lymphatic and superficial venous blood flow. Apply the band about 4″ (10 cm) above the fang marks or just above the first joint proximal to the bite. The tourniquet should be loose enough to allow a finger between the band and the skin. Once the tourniquet is in place, do not remove it until the victim is examined by a doctor.

*Caution*: Do not apply a tourniquet if more than 30 minutes have elapsed since the bite. Keep in mind also that total tourniquet time should not exceed *2* hours and that the use of a tourniquet should not delay antivenin administration. *Remember:* Loss of a limb is possible if a tourniquet is too tight or if tourniquet time is too long.

- If the patient is more than 30 minutes away from a facility, wash the skin over the fang marks. Within 1 hour of a pit viper bite, make an incision through the fang marks about ½″ (1.27 cm) long and ⅛″ (3 mm) deep. Be especially careful if the bite is on the hand, where blood vessels and tendons are close to the skin surface.

Using a bulb syringe — or, if no other means is available, mouth suction — apply suction for up to *2* hours in the absence of antivenin administration.

*Remember:* An incision and suction are effective only in pit viper bites and only within 1 hour of the bite and if transport time to an emergency facility would exceed 30 minutes. Mouth suction is contraindicated if the rescuer has oral ulcers, if the victim is close to a medical facility, or if antivenin can be given promptly.

- Never give the victim alcoholic drinks or stimulants because they speed venom absorption. Never apply ice to a snakebite because it will increase tissue damage.

• Record the signs and symptoms of progressive envenomation and when they develop. Most snakebite victims are hospitalized for only 24 to 48 hours. Treatment usually consists of antivenin administration, but minor snakebites may not require antivenin. Other treatments include tetanus toxoid or tetanus immune globulin; various broad-spectrum antibiotics; and, depending on respiratory status, severity of pain, and the type of snakebite, acetaminophen, codeine, morphine, or meperidine. (Narcotics are contraindicated in coral snakebites.)

Necrotic snakebites usually need surgical debridement after 3 or 4 days. Intense, rapidly progressive edema requires fasciotomy within 2 or 3 hours of the bite; extreme envenomation may require amputation of the limb and subsequent reconstructive surgery, rehabilitation, and physical therapy.

**Special considerations**

When the patient arrives at the hospital, immobilize the extremity if this hasn't already been done. If a tight tourniquet has been applied within the past hour, apply a loose tourniquet proximally and remove the first tourniquet. Release the second tourniquet gradually during antivenin administration as ordered. A sudden release of venom into the bloodstream can cause cardiorespiratory collapse, so keep emergency equipment handy.

• On a flow sheet, document vital signs, level of consciousness, skin color, swelling, respiratory status, a description of the bite and surrounding area, and symptoms. Monitor vital signs every 15 minutes, and check for a pulse in the affected limb.

• Start an I.V. line with a large-bore needle for antivenin administration. Severe bites that result in coagulotoxic signs and symptoms may require two I.V. lines: one for antivenin and one for blood products.

• Before antivenin administration, obtain a patient history of allergies and other medical problems. Perform hypersensitivity tests, as ordered and assist with desensitization as needed. During antivenin administration, keep epinephrine, oxygen, and vasopressors available to combat anaphylaxis from horse serum.

• Give packed red blood cells, I.V. fluids and, possibly, fresh frozen plasma or platelets as ordered, to counteract coagulotoxicity and maintain blood pressure.

• If the patient develops respiratory distress and requires endotracheal intubation or a tracheotomy, provide good tracheostomy care.

• Give analgesics as needed. *Do not give narcotics to victims of coral snakebites.* Clean the snakebite using sterile technique. Open, debride, and drain any blebs and blisters because they may contain venom. Change dressings daily.

• If the patient requires hospitalization for more than 48 hours, position him carefully to avoid contractures. Perform passive exercises until the fourth day after the bite; after that, perform active exercises and give whirlpool treatments as ordered.

# SODIUM IMBALANCE

Sodium is the major cation (90%) in extracellular fluid; potassium, the major cation in intracellular fluid. During repolarization, the sodium-potassium pump continually shifts sodium into the cells and potassium out of the cells; during depolarization, it does the reverse.

Sodium cation functions include maintaining tonicity and concentration of extracellular fluid, acid-base balance (reabsorption of sodium ions and excretion of hydrogen ions), nerve conduction and neuromuscular function, glandular secretion, and water balance.

The body requires only 2 to 4 g of sodium daily. However, most Americans consume 6 to 10 g daily (mostly sodium chloride, as table salt), excreting excess sodium through the kidneys and skin.

A low-sodium diet or excessive use of diuretics may induce hyponatremia (decreased serum sodium concentration); dehydration may induce hypernatremia (increased serum sodium concentration).

## Causes

Sodium imbalance can result from several causes.

### Hyponatremia

One of the main causes of hyponatremia is excessive GI loss of water and electrolytes. This can result from vomiting, suctioning, or diarrhea; excessive perspiration or fever; potent diuretics; or use of tap-water enemas.

When such losses decrease circulating fluid volume, increased secretion of antidiuretic hormone (ADH) promotes maximum water reabsorption, which further dilutes serum sodium. These factors are especially likely to cause hyponatremia when combined with too much electrolyte-free water intake.

Excessive drinking of water, infusion of I.V. dextrose in water without other solutes, malnutrition or starvation, and a low-sodium diet can also cause hyponatremia, usually in combination with one of the other causes.

Trauma, surgery (wound drainage), and burns, which cause sodium to shift into damaged cells, can lead to decreased serum sodium levels, as can adrenal gland insufficiency (Addison's disease), hypoaldosteronism, and cirrhosis of the liver with ascites.

Syndrome of inappropriate antidiuretic hormone secretion (SIADH), resulting from brain tumor, cerebrovascular accident, pulmonary disease, or neoplasm with ectopic ADH production, can lead to hyponatremia also. Certain drugs, such as chlorpropamide and clofibrate, may produce an SIADH-like syndrome.

### Hypernatremia

Decreased water intake can cause hypernatremia. When severe vomiting and diarrhea cause water loss that exceeds sodium loss, serum sodium levels rise, but overall extracellular fluid volume decreases.

Other causes include excess adrenocortical hormones, as in Cushing's syndrome, and ADH deficiency (diabetes insipidus). Salt intoxication — an uncommon cause — may result from excessive ingestion of table salt.

## Signs and symptoms

Sodium imbalance has profound physiologic effects and can induce severe central nervous system, cardiovascular, and GI abnormalities. (See *Clinical effects of sodium imbalance,* page 806.)

For example, hyponatremia may result in renal dysfunction or, if serum sodium loss is abrupt or severe, seizures; hypernatremia may produce pulmonary edema, circulatory disorders, and decreased level of consciousness.

## Diagnosis

Hyponatremia is defined as a serum sodium level less than 135 mEq/L; hy-

## CLINICAL EFFECTS OF SODIUM IMBALANCE

| SYSTEM | HYPONATREMIA | HYPERNATREMIA |
| --- | --- | --- |
| Central nervous system | • Anxiety, headaches, muscle twitching and weakness, seizures | • Fever, agitation, restlessness, seizures |
| Cardiovascular | • Hypotension; tachycardia; with severe deficit, vasomotor collapse, thready pulse | • Hypertension, tachycardia, pitting edema, excessive weight gain |
| GI | • Nausea, vomiting, abdominal cramps | • Rough, dry tongue; intense thirst |
| Genitourinary | • Oliguria or anuria | • Oliguria |
| Respiratory | • Cyanosis with severe deficiency | • Dyspnea, respiratory arrest, and death (from dramatic rise in osmotic pressure) |
| Cutaneous | • Cold, clammy skin; decreased skin turgor | • Flushed skin; dry, sticky mucous membranes |

pernatremia, as a serum sodium level greater than 145 mEq/L. However, additional laboratory studies are necessary to determine etiology and differentiate between a true deficit and an apparent deficit resulting from sodium shift or from hypervolemia or hypovolemia.

In true hyponatremia, supportive values include urine sodium greater than 100 mEq/24 hours, with low serum osmolality; in true hypernatremia, urine sodium is less than 40 mEq/24 hours, with high serum osmolality.

### Treatment

The type of treatment varies with the severity of the imbalance.

#### Hyponatremia

Treatment for mild hyponatremia usually consists of restricted electrolyte-free water intake when it results from hemodilution, SIADH, or conditions such as congestive heart failure, cirrhosis of the liver, and renal failure. If fluid restriction alone fails to normalize serum sodium levels, demeclocycline or lithium, which blocks ADH action in the renal tubules, can be used to promote water excretion.

In extremely rare instances of severe symptomatic hyponatremia, when the serum sodium level falls below 110 mEq/L, treatment may include an infusion of 3% or 5% saline solution.

Treatment with saline infusion requires careful monitoring of venous pressure to prevent potentially fatal circulatory overload. The aim of treatment of secondary hyponatremia is to correct the underlying disorder.

## Hypernatremia

Primary treatment of hypernatremia is administration of salt-free solutions (such as dextrose in water) to return serum sodium levels to normal, followed by infusion of 0.45% sodium chloride to prevent hyponatremia.

Other measures include a sodium-restricted diet and discontinuation of drugs that promote sodium retention.

### Special considerations

For hyponatremia:
● Watch for extremely low serum sodium and accompanying serum chloride levels. Monitor urine specific gravity and other laboratory results. Record fluid intake and output accurately, and weigh the patient daily.
● During administration of isosmolar or hyperosmolar saline solution, watch closely for signs of hypervolemia (dyspnea, crackles, engorged neck or hand veins). Note conditions that may cause excessive sodium loss — diaphoresis, prolonged diarrhea or vomiting, or severe burns.
● Refer the patient receiving a maintenance dosage of diuretics to a dietitian for instruction about dietary sodium intake.
● To prevent hyponatremia, administer isosmolar solutions.

For hypernatremia:
● Measure serum sodium levels every 6 hours or at least daily. Monitor vital signs for changes, especially for rising pulse rate. Watch for signs of hypervolemia, especially in the patient receiving I.V. fluids.
● Record fluid intake and output accurately, checking for body fluid loss. Weigh the patient daily.
● Obtain a drug history to check for drugs that promote sodium retention.
● Explain the importance of sodium restriction, and teach the patient how to plan a low-sodium diet. Closely monitor the serum sodium levels of high-risk patients.

# SOMATIZATION DISORDER

When multiple recurrent signs and symptoms of several years' duration suggest that physical disorders exist without a verifiable disease or pathophysiologic condition to account for them, somatization disorder is present.

The typical patient with somatization disorder usually undergoes repeated medical examinations and diagnostic testing that — unlike the symptoms themselves — can be potentially dangerous or debilitating. However, unlike the hypochondriac, she's not preoccupied with the belief that she has a specific disease.

Somatization disorder usually is chronic, with exacerbations during times of stress.

> ◢ CLINICAL TIP  The patient's signs and symptoms are involuntary, and she consciously wants to feel better. Nonetheless, she's seldom entirely symptom-free.

Signs and symptoms usually begin in adolescence; rarely, in the 20s. This disorder primarily affects women; it's seldom diagnosed in men.

### Causes

Both genetic and environmental factors contribute to the development of somatization disorder.

### Signs and symptoms

A patient with somatization disorder presents physical complaints in a dramatic, vague, or exaggerated way, of-

## DIAGNOSING SOMATIZATION DISORDER

The diagnosis of somatization disorder is made when the patient's symptoms match the diagnostic criteria in the *Diagnostic and Statistical Manual of Mental Disorders,* 4th edition, as follows.

• The patient has a history of many physical complaints, beginning before age 30 and persisting for several years, that result in the patient seeking treatment or in the patient experiencing significant social, occupational, or other impairment.

• The patient has a selection of symptoms as follows (with individual symptoms occurring at any time during the disturbance):

—Pain: a history of pain related to at least four different sites or functions (head, abdomen, back, joints, arms and legs, chest, rectum, menstruation, sexual intercourse, or urination)

—GI upset: a history of at least two GI symptoms other than pain (vomiting other than during pregnancy, nausea, bloating, diarrhea, intolerance of different foods)

—Sexual symptoms: a history of at least one sexual or reproductive symptom other than pain—for example, sexual indifference, erectile or ejaculatory dysfunction, irregular menses, excessive menstrual bleeding, vomiting throughout pregnancy

—Pseudoneurologic symptoms: a history of at least one symptom or deficit suggesting a neurologic condition not limited to pain (for example, conversion symptoms, such as impaired coordination or balance, paralysis or localized weakness, difficulty swallowing or lump in the throat, aphonia, urine retention, hallucinations, loss of touch or pain sensation, double vision, blindness, deafness, seizures; dissociative symptoms such as amnesia; or loss of consciousness other than fainting).

• A thorough investigation discloses that either the above symptoms cannot be fully explained by a known general medical condition or the direct effects of a substance or, if a related general medical condition exists, the physical complaints or resulting impairments exceed what would be expected from the history, physical examination, and diagnostic findings.

• The symptoms are not intentionally produced or feigned (as in factitious disorder or malingering).

---

ten as part of a complicated medical history in which many medical diagnoses have been considered.

An important clue to this disorder is a history of multiple medical evaluations by different doctors at different institutions — sometimes simultaneously — without significant findings. The patient usually appears anxious and depressed.

Common physical complaints include:

• conversion or pseudoneurologic signs and symptoms (for example, paralysis or blindness)

• GI discomfort (abdominal pain, nausea, or vomiting)

• female reproductive difficulties (such as painful menstruation) or male reproductive difficulties (such as erectile dysfunction)

• psychosexual problems (such as sexual indifference)

• chronic pain (such as back pain)

• cardiopulmonary symptoms (chest pain, dizziness, or palpitations).

The patient typically relates her current complaints and previous evaluations in great detail. She may be quite knowledgeable about tests, procedures, and medical jargon.

Attempts to explore areas other than her medical history may cause noticeable anxiety. She tends to disparage previous health care professionals and previous treatments, often with the comment, "Everyone thinks I'm imagining these things."

Ongoing assessment should focus on new signs or symptoms or any change in old ones to avoid missing a developing physical disorder.

### Diagnosis

The *Diagnostic and Statistical Manual of Mental Disorders*, 4th edition, details the characteristics of patients with this condition. (See *Diagnosing somatization disorder*.)

Diagnostic tests rule out physical disorders that cause vague and confusing symptoms, such as hyperparathyroidism, porphyria, multiple sclerosis, and systemic lupus erythematosus. In addition, multiple physical signs and symptoms that appear for the first time late in life usually stem from physical disease, rather than somatization disorder.

### Treatment

The goal of treatment is to help the patient learn to live with her signs and symptoms. After diagnostic evaluation has ruled out organic causes, the patient should be told that she has no serious illness currently but will receive care for her genuine distress and ongoing medical attention for her symptoms.

The most important aspect of treatment is a continuing supportive relationship with a health care provider who acknowledges the patient's signs and symptoms and is willing to help her live with them. The patient should have regularly scheduled appointments to review her complaints and the effectiveness of her coping strategies.

The patient with somatization disorder seldom acknowledges any psychological aspect of her illness and rejects psychiatric treatment.

### Special considerations

• Acknowledge the patient's symptoms, and support her efforts to function and cope despite distress. Don't characterize her signs and symptoms as imaginary. Do tell her the results of tests and their significance.

• Emphasize the patient's strengths (for example, "It's good that you can still work with this pain"). Gently point out the time relationship between stress and physical symptoms.

• Help the patient manage stress. Typically, her relationships are linked to her signs and symptoms; relieving them can impair her interactions with others.

• Help the patient's family understand the patient's need for troublesome signs and symptoms.

# SPINAL CORD DEFECTS

Various malformations of the spine — including spina bifida, meningocele, and myelomeningocele — result from defective embryonic neural tube closure during the first trimester of pregnancy. Generally, these defects occur in the lumbosacral area, but they are occasionally found in the sacral, thoracic, and cervical areas.

Spina bifida occulta is the most common and least severe spinal cord defect. It's characterized by incomplete closure of one or more vertebrae without protrusion of the spinal cord or meninges.

However, in more severe forms of spina bifida, incomplete closure of one or more vertebrae causes protrusion of the spinal contents in an external sac or cystic lesion.

In spina bifida with meningocele, this sac contains meninges and cerebrospinal fluid (CSF). In spina bifida with myelomeningocele (meningomyelocele), this sac contains meninges, CSF, and a portion of the spinal cord or nerve roots distal to the conus medullaris.

Spina bifida is relatively common and affects about 5% of the population. In the United States, about 12,000 neonates each year are born with some form of spina bifida; spina bifida with myelomeningocele is less common than spina bifida occulta and spina bifida with meningocele. Incidence is highest in persons of Welsh or Irish ancestry.

The prognosis varies with the degree of accompanying neurologic deficit. It's worst in patients with large open lesions, neurogenic bladders (which predispose to infection and renal failure), or total paralysis of the legs.

➤ CLINICAL TIP  Because such features are usually absent in spina bifida occulta and meningocele, the prognosis is better than in myelomeningocele, and many patients with these conditions can lead normal lives.

## Causes
Normally, about 20 days after conception, the embryo develops a neural groove in the dorsal ectoderm. This groove rapidly deepens, and the two edges fuse to form the neural tube.

By about day 23, this tube is completely closed except for an opening at each end. Theoretically, if the posterior portion of this neural tube fails to close by the fourth week of gestation,

or if it closes but then splits open from a cause such as an abnormal increase in CSF later in the first trimester, a spinal defect results.

Viruses, radiation, and other environmental factors may be responsible for such defects. However, spinal cord defects occur more often in offspring of women who have previously had children with similar defects, so genetic factors may also be responsible.

## Signs and symptoms
Indications vary depending on the type of defect.

### Spina bifida occulta
Although overt signs may be absent, spina bifida occulta is often accompanied by a depression or dimple, tuft of hair, soft fatty deposits, port wine nevi, or a combination of these abnormalities on the skin over the spinal defect.

Spina bifida occulta doesn't usually cause neurologic dysfunction but occasionally is associated with foot weakness or bowel and bladder disturbances. Such disturbances are especially likely during rapid growth phases, when the spinal cord's ascent within the vertebral column may be impaired by its abnormal adherence to other tissues.

### Meningocele and myelomeningocele
A saclike structure protrudes over the spine in both meningocele and myelomeningocele.

Like spina bifida occulta, meningocele rarely causes neurologic deficit. But myelomeningocele, depending on the level of the defect, causes permanent neurologic dysfunction, such as flaccid or spastic paralysis and bowel and bladder incontinence.

Associated disorders include trophic skin disturbances (ulcerations, cyanosis), clubfoot, knee contractures, and hydrocephalus (in about 90% of patients). Mental retardation, Arnold-Chiari syndrome (in which part of the brain protrudes into the spinal canal), and curvature of the spine can also occur.

## Diagnosis

The diagnosis varies with the type of defect.

### Spina bifida occulta

Although often overlooked, spina bifida occulta is occasionally palpable, and a spinal X-ray can show the bone defect. Myelography can differentiate it from other spinal abnormalities, especially spinal cord tumors.

### Meningocele and myelomeningocele

Meningocele and myelomeningocele are obvious on examination; transillumination of the protruding sac can sometimes distinguish between them. (In meningocele, it typically transilluminates; in myelomeningocele, it does not.)

In myelomeningocele, a pinprick examination of the legs and trunk shows the level of sensory and motor involvement; skull X-rays, cephalic measurements, and a computed tomography scan demonstrate associated hydrocephalus.

Other appropriate laboratory tests in patients with myelomeningocele include urinalysis, urine cultures, and tests for renal function starting in the neonatal period and continuing at regular intervals.

Although amniocentesis can detect only open defects, such as myelomeningocele and meningocele, this procedure is recommended for all pregnant women who have previously had children with spinal cord defects; these women are at an increased risk for having children with similar defects. If these defects are present, amniocentesis shows increased alpha-fetoprotein levels by 14 weeks' gestation.

Ultrasonography can also detect or confirm the presence and extent of neural tube defects.

## Treatment

Spina bifida occulta usually requires no treatment. Treatment of meningocele consists of surgical closure of the protruding sac and continual assessment of growth and development.

Treatment of myelomeningocele requires repair of the sac and supportive measures to promote independence and prevent further complications. Surgery doesn't reverse neurologic deficits. A shunt may be needed to relieve associated hydrocephalus.

If the patient has a severe spinal defect, short- and long-term treatment will require a team approach, including a neurosurgeon, orthopedist, urologist, nurse, social worker, occupational and physical therapists, and parents.

### Rehabilitation

In children or adults, rehabilitation measures may include:

• waist supports, long leg braces, walkers, crutches, and other orthopedic appliances

• diet and bowel training to manage fecal incontinence

• neurogenic bladder management to reduce urinary stasis, possibly intermittent catheterization, and antispasmodics, such as bethanechol or propantheline. In severe cases, insertion of an artificial urinary sphincter is often successful; a urinary diversion is used as a last resort to preserve kidney function.

## Special considerations

Before surgery for meningocele or myelomeningocele:

## DISCHARGE TEACHING IN SPINAL CORD DEFECTS

Before discharge, review the following points with parents of children with spinal cord defects:

• Teach parents how to recognize such early signs of complications as hydrocephalus, pressure ulcers, and urinary tract infections (UTIs). Also show them how to provide psychological support to the child and encourage a positive attitude.

• Encourage parents to begin training their child in a toileting routine by age 3. Emphasize the need for increased fluid intake to prevent UTIs. Teach intermittent catheterization and conduit hygiene as needed.

• Explain to parents how to prevent constipation and bowel obstruction. Stress the need for increased fluid intake, a high-bulk diet, exercise, and use of a stool softener (if prescribed). Teach parents to empty their child's bowel by exerting slight pressure on the abdomen, telling the child to bear down, and giving a glycerin suppository as needed.

• Teach parents to recognize developmental lags early (a possible result of hydrocephalus). If the child does fall behind, stress the importance of follow-up IQ assessment to help plan realistic educational goals. The child may need to attend a school with special facilities. Also, stress the need for stimulation to ensure maximum mental development. Help parents plan activities appropriate to their child's age and abilities.

• Prevent local infection by cleaning the defect gently with sterile saline solution or other solutions. Inspect the defect often for signs of infection, and cover it with sterile dressings moistened with sterile saline solution. Don't use ointments on the defect; they may cause skin maceration.

• Prevent skin breakdown by placing sheepskin or a foam pad under the infant. Keep skin clean, and apply lotion to knees, elbows, chin, and other pressure areas. Give antibiotics as needed.

• Handle the infant carefully. Hold and cuddle him, but avoid placing pressure on the sac. When holding him on your lap, position him on his abdomen, and teach the parents to do the same.

• Usually, the infant can't wear a diaper or a shirt until after surgical correction because it will irritate the sac, so keep him warm in an infant Isolette. Position him on his abdomen with the head of the bed slightly elevated to prevent contamination of the sac with urine or feces.

• Provide adequate time for parent-child bonding if possible.

• Measure head circumference daily, and watch for signs of hydrocephalus and meningeal irritation, such as fever or nuchal rigidity. Be sure to mark the spot so you get accurate readings.

• Minimize contractures with passive range-of-motion exercises and casting. To prevent hip dislocation, abduct the hips with a pad between the knees or with sandbags and ankle rolls.

• Monitor intake and output. Watch for decreased skin turgor, dryness, or other signs of dehydration. Provide meticulous skin care to genitals and buttocks to prevent infection.

• Ensure adequate nutrition.

After surgical repair of the defect:

- Watch for hydrocephalus, which often follows such surgery. Measure the child's head circumference.
- Monitor vital signs often. Watch for signs of shock (decreased blood pressure, tachycardia, lethargy), infection (malaise, elevated temperature, alteration in feeding pattern), and increased intracranial pressure (projectile vomiting).
- Frequently assess the infant's fontanels. Remember that before age 2, infants don't show typical signs of increased intracranial pressure because suture lines aren't fully closed. The most telling sign is bulging fontanels.
- Change the dressing regularly, and watch for any signs of drainage, wound rupture, or infection.
- If leg casts have been applied to treat deformities, watch for signs that the child is outgrowing the cast. Check distal pulses to ensure adequate circulation. Petal the edges of the cast to prevent softening and skin irritation. Use a cool-air blow-dryer to dry skin under the cast. Periodically check for foul odor and other indications of skin breakdown.
- Help parents work through their feelings of guilt, anger, and helplessness.
- Teach parents how to cope with their infant's problems and successfully meet long-range treatment goals. (See *Discharge teaching in spinal cord defects*.)
- Refer parents for genetic counseling, and suggest that amniocentesis be performed in future pregnancies. For more information and names of support groups, refer parents to the Spina Bifida Association of America.

�֍ LIFE-THREATENING
DISORDER

# SPINAL INJURIES

Aside from spinal cord damage, spinal injuries include fractures, contusions, and compressions of the vertebral column, usually the result of trauma to the head or neck. The real danger lies in possible spinal cord damage. Spinal fractures most commonly occur in the 5th, 6th, and 7th cervical, 12th thoracic, and first lumbar vertebrae.

## Causes

Most serious spinal injuries result from motor vehicle accidents, falls, diving into shallow water, and gunshot wounds; less serious injuries, from lifting heavy objects and minor falls. Spinal dysfunction may also result from hyperparathyroidism and neoplastic lesions.

## Signs and symptoms

The most obvious symptom of spinal injury is muscle spasm and back pain that worsens with movement. In cervical fractures, pain may produce point tenderness; in dorsal and lumbar fractures, it may radiate to other body areas such as the legs.

If the injury damages the spinal cord, clinical effects range from mild paresthesia to quadriplegia and shock. After milder injuries, such symptoms may be delayed for several days or weeks.

▶ CLINICAL TIP Because the diaphragm is innervated by cervical levels 1 to 4, damage to this level will result in respiratory compromise. Also, be aware of edema at levels C5 to C7, which may expand up into these areas, resulting in problems.

## Complications

The following are complications of spinal injuries: autonomic dysreflexia, spinal shock, and neurogenic shock.

### Autonomic dysreflexia

Also known as autonomic hyperreflexia, autonomic dysreflexia is a serious medical condition that occurs after resolution of spinal shock. Emergency recognition and management is a must. Suspect autonomic dysreflexia in the patient with a history of spinal cord trauma at level T6 and above who exhibits cold or goose-fleshed skin below the lesion level, bradycardia, and hypertension. The hypertension is generally accompanied by severe, pounding headache. Some dyreflexia is caused by noxious stimuli, most commonly a distended bladder or skin lesion. Treatment focuses on eliminating the stimulus; rapid identification and removal may avoid the need for pharmacologic control of the headache and hypertension.

### Spinal shock

Spinal shock is the loss of autonomic, reflex, motor, and sensory activity below the level of the cord lesion. It occurs secondary to damage of the spinal cord. Signs of spinal shock include flaccid paralysis, loss of deep tendon and perianal reflexes, and loss of motor and sensory function. Until spinal shock has resolved (usually 1 to 6 weeks after injury), the extent of actual cord damage cannot be assessed. The earliest indicator of spinal shock resolution is the return of reflex activity.

### Neurogenic shock

This temporary loss of autonomic function below the level of injury produces cardiovascular changes. Signs of neurogenic shock include orthostatic hypotension, bradycardia, and loss of the ability to sweat below the level of the lesion. This abnormal vasomotor response occurs secondary to disruption of sympathetic impulses from the brain stem to the thoracolumbar area and is seen most frequently in cervical cord injury.

## Diagnosis

Typically, a diagnosis is based on the patient history, the physical examination, X-rays and, possibly, lumbar puncture, computed tomography (CT) scan, and magnetic resonance imaging (MRI):

• *Patient history* may reveal trauma, a metastatic lesion, an infection that could produce a spinal abscess, or an endocrine disorder.

• *Physical examination* (including a neurologic evaluation) locates the level of injury and detects cord damage.

• *Spinal X-rays,* the most important diagnostic measure, locate the fracture.

• *Lumbar puncture* may show increased cerebrospinal fluid pressure from a lesion or trauma in spinal compression.

• *CT scan* or *MRI* can locate the spinal mass.

## Treatment

The primary treatment after spinal injury is immediate immobilization to stabilize the spine and prevent cord damage; other treatment is supportive. Cervical injuries require immobilization, using sandbags on both sides of the patient's head, a hard cervical collar, or skeletal traction with skull tongs or a halo device. When patients show clinical evidence of cord injury, high doses of methylprednisone are started.

### Supportive treatment

Treatment of stable lumbar and dorsal fractures consists of bed rest on firm support (such as a bed board), analgesics, and muscle relaxants until the fracture stabilizes (usually 10 to 12 weeks). Later treatment includes exercises to strengthen the back muscles and a back brace or corset to provide support while walking.

An unstable dorsal or lumbar fracture requires a plaster cast, a turning frame and, in severe fracture, laminectomy and spinal fusion.

### Other treatment

When the damage results in compression of the spinal column, neurosurgery may relieve the pressure. If the cause of compression is a metastatic lesion, chemotherapy and radiation may relieve it. Surface wounds accompanying the spinal injury require tetanus prophylaxis unless the patient has had recent immunization.

### Special considerations

- In all spinal injuries, suspect cord damage until proven otherwise.
- During the initial assessment and X-rays, immobilize the patient on a firm surface, with sandbags on both sides of his head. Tell him not to move; avoid moving him, because hyperflexion can damage the cord.
- If you must move the patient, get at least one other member of the staff to help you logroll him to avoid disturbing body alignment.
- Throughout the assessment, offer comfort and reassurance. Remember, the fear of possible paralysis will be overwhelming. Allow a family member who isn't too distraught to accompany the patient and talk to him quietly and calmly.
- If the injury requires surgery, administer prophylactic antibiotics. Catheterize the patient to avoid urine retention, and monitor defecation patterns to avoid impaction.

- Explain traction methods to the patient and his family, and reassure them that traction devices don't penetrate the brain. If the patient has a halo or skull-tong traction device, clean pin sites daily, trim hair short, and provide analgesics for persistent headaches.
- During traction, turn the patient often to prevent pneumonia, embolism, and skin breakdown; perform passive range-of-motion exercises to maintain muscle tone. If available, use a Circ-Olectric bed or Stryker frame to facilitate turning and to avoid spinal cord injury.
- Turn the patient on his side during feedings to prevent aspiration. Create a relaxed atmosphere at mealtimes.
- Suggest appropriate diversionary activities to fill your patient's hours of immobility.
- Watch closely for neurologic changes. Changes in skin sensation and loss of muscle strength could point to pressure on the spinal cord, possibly as a result of edema or shifting bone fragments.
- If damage occurred to the spinal cord, involve a rehabilitation specialist as soon as possible to assist with a detailed and personal plan of care.
- Before discharge, instruct the patient about continuing analgesics or other medication, and stress the importance of regular follow-up examinations.
- To help prevent a spinal injury from becoming a spinal cord injury, educate fire fighters, police officers, paramedics, and the general public about the proper way to handle such injuries.

# SPINAL NEOPLASMS

A spinal neoplasm is any one of many tumor types that are similar to intracranial tumors and involve the spinal cord or its roots. If untreated, they can eventually cause paralysis.

Primary spinal neoplasms originate in the meningeal coverings, the parenchyma of the cord or its roots, the intraspinal vasculature, or the vertebrae. They can also occur as metastatic foci from primary tumors.

## Causes

Primary spinal cord tumors may be extramedullary (occurring outside the spinal cord) or intramedullary (occurring within the cord itself). Extramedullary tumors may be intradural (meningiomas and schwannomas), which account for 60% of all primary spinal cord neoplasms, or extradural (metastatic tumors from breasts, lungs, prostate, leukemia, or lymphomas), which account for 25% of these neoplasms.

Intramedullary tumors, or gliomas (astrocytomas or ependymomas), are comparatively rare, accounting for only about 10% of tumors. In children, they're low-grade astrocytomas.

Spinal cord tumors are rare compared with intracranial tumors (ratio of 1:4). They occur with equal frequency in men and women, with the exception of meningiomas, which occur most often in women. Spinal cord tumors can occur anywhere along the length of the cord or its roots.

## Signs and symptoms

Extramedullary tumors produce symptoms by pressing on nerve roots, the spinal cord, and spinal vessels; intramedullary tumors, by destroying the parenchyma and compressing adjacent areas. Because intramedullary tumors may extend over several spinal cord segments, their symptoms are more variable than those of extramedullary tumors.

The following clinical effects are likely with all spinal cord neoplasms:

• *Pain* is most severe directly over the tumor, radiates around the trunk or down the limb on the affected side, and is unrelieved by bed rest.

• *Motor symptoms* include asymmetrical spastic muscle weakness, decreased muscle tone, exaggerated reflexes, and a positive Babinski's sign. If the tumor is at the level of the cauda equina, muscle flaccidity, muscle wasting, weakness, and progressive diminution in tendon reflexes are characteristic.

• *Sensory deficits* include contralateral loss of pain, temperature, and touch sensation (Brown-Séquard syndrome). These losses are less obvious to the patient than functional motor changes. Caudal lesions invariably produce paresthesias in the nerve distribution pathway of the involved roots.

• *Bladder symptoms* vary according to the stage of the tumor. Early signs include incomplete emptying or difficulty with the urinary stream, which is usually unnoticed or ignored. Urine retention is an inevitable late sign with cord compression. Cauda equina tumors cause bladder and bowel incontinence from flaccid paralysis.

• *Constipation* can also occur.

## Diagnosis

Several tests aid in diagnosis:

• *Spinal tap* shows clear yellow cerebrospinal fluid (CSF) as a result of increased protein levels if the flow is completely blocked. If the flow is partially blocked, protein levels rise, but the fluid is only slightly yellow in proportion to the CSF protein level. A Papanicolaou smear of the CSF may show malignant cells of metastatic carcinoma.

- *X-rays* show distortions of the intervertebral foramina, changes in the vertebrae, collapsed areas in the vertebral body, and localized enlargement of the spinal canal, indicating an adjacent block.
- *Myelography* identifies the level of the lesion by outlining it if the tumor is causing partial obstruction; it shows anatomic relationship of the tumor to the cord and the dura. If the obstruction is complete, the injected dye can't flow past the tumor.

*Note:* This study is dangerous if cord compression is nearly complete because withdrawal or escape of CSF will actually allow the tumor to exert greater pressure against the cord.

- *Radioisotope bone scan* demonstrates metastatic invasion of the vertebrae by showing a characteristic increase in osteoblastic activity.
- *Computed tomography scan* shows cord compression and tumor location.
- *Frozen section biopsy* at surgery identifies the tissue type.

**Treatment**

Spinal cord tumors usually require decompression or radiation. Laminectomy is indicated for primary tumors that produce spinal cord or cauda equina compression; it's *not* usually indicated for metastatic tumors.

If the tumor is slowly progressive, or if it's treated before the cord degenerates from compression, symptoms are likely to disappear, and complete restoration of function is possible. In a patient with metastatic carcinoma or lymphoma who suddenly experiences complete transverse myelitis with spinal shock, functional improvement is unlikely, even with treatment, and his outlook is ominous.

If the patient has incomplete paraplegia of rapid onset, emergency surgical decompression may save cord function. Steroid therapy minimizes cord edema until surgery can be performed. Partial removal of intramedullary gliomas, followed by radiation, may alleviate symptoms for a short time.

Metastatic extradural tumors can be controlled with radiation, analgesics and, in the case of hormone-mediated tumors (breast and prostate), appropriate hormone therapy.

Transcutaneous electrical nerve stimulation (TENS) may control radicular pain from spinal cord tumors and is a useful alternative to narcotic analgesics. In TENS, an electrical charge is applied to the skin to stimulate large-diameter nerve fibers and thereby inhibit transmission of pain impulses through small-diameter nerve fibers.

**Special considerations**

- On your first contact with the patient, perform a complete neurologic evaluation to obtain baseline data for planning future care and evaluating changes in his clinical status.
- Provide psychological support. Help the patient and his family to understand and cope with the diagnosis, treatment, potential disabilities, and necessary changes in lifestyle.
- After laminectomy, check neurologic status frequently and watch for signs of infection. Administer analgesics, and aid the patient in early walking.
- Take safety precautions for the patient with impaired sensation and motor deficits. Use side rails if the patient is bedridden; if he's not, encourage him to wear flat shoes, and remove scatter rugs and clutter to prevent falls.
- Make sure the patient receives appropriate rehabilitation, including bowel and bladder retraining.
- Administer steroids and antacids for cord edema after radiation therapy. Mon-

itor for sensory or motor dysfunction, which indicates the need for more steroids.

• Enforce bed rest for the patient with vertebral body involvement until he can safely walk; body weight alone can cause cord collapse and cord laceration from bone fragments.

• Logroll and position the patient on his side every 2 hours to prevent pressure ulcers and other complications of immobility.

• If the patient is to wear a back brace, make sure he wears it whenever he gets out of bed.

# SPRAINS AND STRAINS

A *sprain* is a complete or incomplete tear in the supporting ligaments surrounding a joint that usually follows a sharp twist. A *strain* is an injury to a muscle or tendinous attachment. Both usually heal without surgical repair.

## Signs and symptoms
Sprains and strains cause varying signs and symptoms.

### *Sprains*
A sprain causes local pain (especially during joint movement), swelling, loss of mobility (which may not occur until several hours after the injury), and a black-and-blue discoloration from blood extravasating into surrounding tissues. A sprained ankle is the most common joint injury.

### *Strains*
A strain may be acute (an immediate result of vigorous muscle overuse or overstress) or chronic (a result of repeated overuse).

An acute strain causes a sharp, transient pain (the patient may say he heard a snapping noise) and rapid swelling. When severe pain subsides, the muscle is tender; after several days, ecchymoses appear.

A chronic strain causes stiffness, soreness, and generalized tenderness. These conditions appear several hours after the injury.

## Diagnosis
A history of recent injury or chronic overuse, clinical findings, and an X-ray to rule out fractures establish the diagnosis.

## Treatment
Effective treatment differs for sprains and strains.

### *Sprains*
Sprains call for control of pain and swelling and immobilization of the injured joint to promote healing. Immediately after the injury, elevating the joint above the level of the heart and intermittently applying ice for 12 to 48 hours controls swelling. A towel between the ice pack and the skin prevents cold injuries.

An immobilized sprain usually heals in 2 to 3 weeks, and the patient can then gradually resume normal activities. Occasionally, however, torn ligaments don't heal properly and cause recurrent dislocation, necessitating surgical repair.

Some athletes may request immediate surgical repair to hasten healing; to prevent sprains, they may tape their wrists and ankles before sports activities.

### *Strains*
Acute strains require analgesics and application of ice for up to 48 hours, then

heat. Complete muscle rupture may require surgery.

Chronic strains usually don't need treatment, but heat application, nonsteroidal anti-inflammatory drugs (such as ibuprofen), or an analgesic-muscle relaxant can relieve discomfort.

**Special considerations**
• For sprains, immobilize the joint, using an elastic bandage or cast or, if the sprain is severe, a soft cast or splint. Depending on the severity of the injury, an analgesic may be necessary.

➤ CLINICAL TIP If the patient has a sprained ankle, make sure he receives crutch gait training. Because patients with sprains seldom require hospitalization, provide patient teaching.
• Tell the patient with a sprain to elevate the joint for 48 to 72 hours after the injury (while sleeping, the joint can be elevated with pillows) and to apply ice intermittently for 12 to 48 hours.
• If an elastic bandage has been applied, teach the patient to reapply it by wrapping from below to above the injury, forming a figure eight. For a sprained ankle, apply the bandage from the toes to midcalf. Tell the patient to remove the bandage before going to sleep and to loosen it if it causes the leg to become pale, numb, or painful.
• Instruct the patient to call if pain worsens or persists. An additional X-ray may detect a fracture originally missed.

# SQUAMOUS CELL CARCINOMA

Arising from the keratinizing epidermal cells, squamous cell carcinoma of the skin is an invasive tumor with metastatic potential. It occurs most often in fair-skinned white men over age 60. Outdoor employment and residence in a sunny, warm climate (southwestern United States and Australia, for example) greatly increase the risk of developing squamous cell carcinoma.

**Causes**
Predisposing factors associated with squamous cell carcinoma include overexposure to the sun's ultraviolet rays and the presence of premalignant lesions (such as actinic keratosis or Bowen's disease).

Other predisposing factors include X-ray therapy, ingestion of herbicides containing arsenic, chronic skin irritation and inflammation, exposure to local carcinogens (such as tar and oil), and hereditary diseases (such as xeroderma pigmentosum and albinism). Rarely, squamous cell carcinoma may develop on the site of smallpox vaccination, psoriasis, or chronic discoid lupus erythematosus.

**Signs and symptoms**
Squamous cell carcinoma commonly develops on the skin of the face, the ears, the dorsa of the hands and forearms, and other sun-damaged areas. Lesions on sun-damaged skin tend to be less invasive and less likely to metastasize than lesions on unexposed skin.

Notable exceptions to this tendency are squamous cell lesions on the lower lip and the ears. These are almost invariably markedly invasive metastatic lesions with a generally poor prognosis.

Transformation from a premalignant lesion to squamous cell carcinoma may begin with induration and inflammation of the preexisting lesion. When squamous cell carcinoma arises from nor-

# STAGING SQUAMOUS CELL CARCINOMA

The American Joint Committee on Cancer uses the following tumor, node, metastasis (TNM) system for staging squamous cell carcinoma.

### Primary tumor
*TX* — primary tumor can't be assessed
*T0* — no evidence of primary tumor
*Tis* — carcinoma in situ
*T1* — tumor 2 cm or less in greatest dimension
*T2* — tumor between 2 and 5 cm in greatest dimension
*T3* — tumor > 5 cm in greatest dimension
*T4* — tumor invades deep extradermal structures (such as cartilage, skeletal muscle, or bone)

### Regional lymph nodes
*NX* — regional lymph nodes can't be assessed
*N0* — no evidence of regional lymph node involvement
*N1* — regional lymph node involvement

### Distant metastasis
*MX* — distant metastasis can't be assessed
*M0* — no known distant metastasis
*M1* — distant metastasis

### Staging categories
Squamous cell carcinoma progresses from mild to severe as follows:
*Stage 0* — Tis, N0, M0
*Stage I* — T1, N0, M0
*Stage II* — T2, N0, M0; T3, N0, M0
*Stage III* — T4, N0, M0; any T, N1, M0
*Stage IV* — any T, any N, M1

mal skin, the nodule grows slowly on a firm, indurated base.

If untreated, this nodule eventually ulcerates and invades underlying tissues. Metastasis can occur to the regional lymph nodes, producing characteristic systemic symptoms of pain, malaise, fatigue, weakness, and anorexia. (See *Staging squamous cell carcinoma*.)

## Diagnosis
An excisional biopsy provides a definitive diagnosis of squamous cell carcinoma. Other appropriate laboratory tests depend on systemic symptoms.

## Treatment
The size, shape, location, and invasiveness of a squamous cell tumor and the condition of the underlying tissue determine the treatment method used.

Premalignant lesions respond well to treatment. (See *Treating actinic keratoses*.) A deeply invasive tumor may require a combination of techniques.

All the major treatment methods have excellent cure rates; the prognosis is usually better with a well-differentiated lesion than with a poorly differentiated one in an unusual location.

Depending on the lesion, treatment may consist of:
• wide surgical excision
• electrodesiccation and curettage (which offer good cosmetic results for small lesions)
• radiation therapy (generally for elderly or debilitated patients)
• chemosurgery (reserved for resistant or recurrent lesions).

## Special considerations
• Establish a standard routine for changing the patient's dressing. This helps the

patient and family learn how to care for the wound.

• Keep the wound dry and clean.

• Tell the patient to use lip screens to protect the lips from sun damage.

➤ CLINICAL TIP Try to control odor with balsam of Peru, yogurt flakes, oil of cloves, or other odor-masking substances, even though they are often ineffective for long-term use. Topical or systemic antibiotics also temporarily control odor and eventually alter the lesion's bacterial flora.

• Be prepared for other problems that accompany a metastatic disease (pain, fatigue, weakness, anorexia).

• To prevent squamous cell carcinoma, tell the patient to avoid excessive sun exposure and wear protective clothing (hats, long sleeves).

• Instruct the patient to periodically examine the skin for precancerous lesions and have any removed promptly.

• Advise the patient to use sunscreen containing para-aminobenzoic acid, benzophenone, and zinc oxide. He should apply these agents 30 to 60 minutes before sun exposure.

---

# STAPHYLOCOCCAL INFECTIONS

---

Staphylococci are coagulase-negative *(Staphylococcus epidermidis)* or coagulase-positive *(Staphylococcus aureus)* gram-positive bacteria. Coagulase-negative staphylococci grow abundantly as normal flora on skin, but they can also cause boils, abscesses, and carbuncles. In the upper respiratory tract, they are usually nonpathogenic but can cause serious infections. Pathogenic strains of staphylococci are found in many adult carriers — usually on the nasal mucosa, axilla, or groin. Sometimes, carriers shed staphylococci, infecting themselves or other susceptible people. Coagulase-positive staphylococci tend to form pus; they cause many types of infections.

For specific information on different types of staphylococcal infections, see *Comparing staphylococcal infections,* pages 822 to 827.

*(Text continues on page 828.)*

---

## TREATING ACTINIC KERATOSES

A useful drug for treating actinic keratoses, fluorouracil is available in different strengths (1%, 2%, and 5%) as a cream or solution.

Local application causes stinging and burning, followed by erythema, vesiculation, erosion, superficial ulceration, necrosis, and re-epithelialization. The 5% solution induces the most severe inflammatory response but provides complete involution of the lesions with little recurrence.

### Special considerations

• Keep fluorouracil away from eyes, scrotum, or mucous membranes.

• Warn the patient to avoid excessive sun exposure during treatment because sun intensifies the inflammatory reaction.

• Continue application of fluorouracil until the lesions reach the ulcerative and necrotic stages (2 to 4 weeks); then consider application of a corticosteroid preparation as an anti-inflammatory agent.

• Possible adverse effects include postinflammatory hyperpigmentation. Complete healing occurs within 1 to 2 months.

## COMPARING STAPHYLOCOCCAL INFECTIONS

| PREDISPOSING FACTORS | SIGNS AND SYMPTOMS | DIAGNOSIS |
| --- | --- | --- |

### Bacteremia
- Infected surgical wounds
- Abscesses
- Infected I.V. or intra-arterial catheter sites or catheter tips
- Infected vascular grafts or prostheses
- Infected pressure ulcers
- Osteomyelitis
- Parenteral drug abuse
- Source unknown (primary bacteremia)
- Cellulitis
- Burns
- Immunosuppression
- Debilitating diseases, such as chronic renal insufficiency and diabetes
- Infective endocarditis (coagulase-positive staphylococci) and subacute bacterial endocarditis (coagulase-negative staphylococci)
- Cancer (leukemia) or neutrophil nadir after chemotherapy or radiation

- Fever (high fever with no obvious source in children under age 1), shaking chills, tachycardia
- Cyanosis or pallor
- Confusion, agitation, stupor
- Skin microabscesses
- Joint pain
- Complications: shock; acute bacterial endocarditis (in prolonged infection; indicated by new or changing systolic murmur); retinal hemorrhages; splinter hemorrhages under nails and small, tender red nodes on pads of fingers and toes (Osler's nodes); abscess formation in skin, bones, lungs, brain, and kidneys; pulmonary emboli if tricuspid valve is infected
- Prognosis poor in patients over age 60 or with chronic illness

- Blood cultures (two to four samples from different sites at different times): growing staphylococci and leukocytosis (usually 12,000 white blood cells [WBCs]/µl), with shift to the left of polymorphonuclear leukocytes (70% to 90% neutrophils)
- Urinalysis shows microscopic hematuria.
- Erythrocyte sedimentation rate (ESR) elevated, especially in chronic or subacute bacterial endocarditis
- Severe anemia or thrombocytopenia (possible)
- Prolonged partial thromboplastin time and prothrombin time; low fibrinogen and platelet counts, and low factor assays; possible disseminated intravascular coagulation
- Cultures of urine, sputum, and draining skin lesions may identify primary infection site. So may chest X-rays and scans of lungs, liver, abdomen, and brain.
- Echocardiogram may show heart valve vegetation.

## TREATMENT

- Semisynthetic penicillins (oxacillin, nafcillin) or cephalosporins (cefazolin) given I.V.
- Vancomycin I.M. for those with penicillin allergy or methicillin-resistant organism
- Possibly, probenecid given to partially prevent urinary excretion of penicillin and to prolong blood levels
- I.V. fluids to reverse shock
- Removal of infected catheter or foreign body
- Surgery

## SPECIAL CONSIDERATIONS

- *S. aureus* bacteremia can be fatal within 12 hours. Be especially alert for it in debilitated patients with I.V. catheters or in those with a history of drug abuse.
- Administer antibiotics on time to maintain adequate blood levels, but give them slowly, using the prescribed amount of diluent, to prevent thrombophlebitis.
- Watch for signs of penicillin allergy, especially pruritic rash (possible anaphylaxis). Keep epinephrine 1:1,000 and resuscitation equipment handy. Monitor vital signs, urine output, and mental state for signs of shock.
- Obtain cultures carefully, and observe for clues to the primary site of infection. Never refrigerate blood cultures; it delays identification of organisms by slowing their growth.
- Impose wound and skin precautions if the primary site of infection is draining. Special blood precautions are not necessary because the number of organisms present, even in fulminant bacteremia, is minimal.
- Obtain peak and trough levels of vancomycin to determine the adequacy of treatment.

*(continued)*

## COMPARING STAPHYLOCOCCAL INFECTIONS *(continued)*

| PREDISPOSING FACTORS | SIGNS AND SYMPTOMS | DIAGNOSIS |
|---|---|---|
| **Pneumonia**<br>• Immune deficiencies, especially in elderly people and in children under age 2<br>• Chronic lung diseases and cystic fibrosis<br>• Malignant tumors<br>• Antibiotics that kill normal respiratory flora but spare *S. aureus*<br>• Viral respiratory infections, especially influenza<br>• Hematogenous (blood-borne) bacteria spread to the lungs from primary sites of infections (such as heart valves, abscesses, and pulmonary emboli)<br>• Recent bronchial or endotracheal suctioning or intubation | • High temperature: adults, 103° to 105° F (39.4° to 40.6° C); children, 101° F (38.3° C)<br>• Cough, with purulent, yellow, or bloody sputum<br>• Dyspnea, crackles, and decreased breath sounds<br>• Pleuritic pain<br>• In infants: mild respiratory infection that suddenly worsens: irritability, anxiety, dyspnea, anorexia, vomiting, diarrhea, spasms of dry coughing, marked tachypnea, expiratory grunting, sternal retractions, and cyanosis<br>• Complications: necrosis, lung abscess, pyopneumothorax; empyema; pneumatocele; shock, hypotension, oliguria or anuria, cyanosis, loss of consciousness | • WBC count elevated (15,000 to 40,000/µl in adults; 15,000 to 20,000/µl in children), with predominance of polymorphonuclear leukocytes<br>• Sputum Gram stain: mostly gram-positive cocci in clusters, with many polymorphonuclear leukocytes<br>• Sputum culture: mostly coagulase-positive staphylococci<br>• Chest X-rays: usually patchy infiltrates<br>• Arterial blood gas analysis: hypoxia and respiratory acidosis |
| **Enterocolitis**<br>• Broad-spectrum antibiotics (tetracycline, chloramphenicol, or neomycin) or aminoglycosides (tobramycin, streptomycin, or kanamycin) as prophylaxis for bowel surgery or treatment of hepatic coma<br>• Usually occurs in elderly people but also in neonates (associated with staphylococcal skin lesions) | • Sudden onset of profuse, watery diarrhea usually 2 days to several weeks after start of antibiotic therapy, I.V. or by mouth<br>• Nausea, vomiting, abdominal pain and distention<br>• Hypovolemia and dehydration (decreased skin turgor, hypotension, fever) | • Stool Gram stain: many gram-positive cocci and polymorphonuclear leukocytes, with few gram-negative rods<br>• Stool culture: *S. aureus*<br>• Sigmoidoscopy: mucosal ulcerations<br>• Blood studies: leukocytosis, moderately increased blood urea nitrogen level, and decreased serum albumin level |

| TREATMENT | SPECIAL CONSIDERATIONS |
|---|---|
| • Semisynthetic penicillins (oxacillin, nafcillin) or cephalosporins given I.V.<br>• Vancomycin I.V. for those with penicillin allergy or methicillin-resistant organisms<br>• Isolation until sputum shows minimal numbers of *S. aureus* (about 24 to 72 hours after starting antibiotics) | • Use masks with isolated patient because staphylococci from lungs spread by air as well as direct contact. Use gown and gloves only when handling contaminated respiratory secretions. Use respiratory isolation precautions.<br>• Keep the door to the patient's room closed. Don't store extra supplies in his room. Empty suction bottles carefully. Place any articles containing sputum (such as tissues and clothing) in a sealed plastic bag. Mark them "contaminated," and dispose of them promptly by incineration.<br>• When obtaining sputum specimens, make sure you're collecting thick sputum, not saliva. The presence of epithelial cells (found in the mouth, not lungs) indicates a poor specimen.<br>• Administer antibiotics strictly on time, but slowly. Watch for signs of penicillin allergy and for signs of infection at I.V sites. Change the I.V site at least every third day.<br>• Perform frequent chest physical therapy. Do chest percussion and postural drainage after intermittent positive pressure breathing treatments. Concentrate on consolidated areas (revealed by X-rays or auscultation). |
| • Broad-spectrum antibiotics discontinued<br>• Possibly, antistaphylococcal agents such as vancomycin by mouth<br>• Normal flora replenished with yogurt | • Monitor vital signs frequently to prevent shock. Force fluids to correct dehydration.<br>• Know serum electrolyte levels. Measure and record bowel movements when possible. Check serum chloride level for alkalosis (hypochloremia).<br>• Collect serial stool specimens for Gram stain, and culture for diagnosis and for evaluating effectiveness of treatment.<br>• Observe enteric precautions.<br>• Consider reporting requirements, especially in a group situation such as a nursing home. |

*(continued)*

## COMPARING STAPHYLOCOCCAL INFECTIONS *(continued)*

| PREDISPOSING FACTORS | SIGNS AND SYMPTOMS | DIAGNOSIS |
|---|---|---|
| **Osteomyelitis**<br>• Hematogenous organisms<br>• Skin trauma<br>• Infection spreading from adjacent joint or other infected tissues<br>• *S. aureus* bacteremia<br>• Orthopedic surgery or trauma<br>• Cardiothoracic surgery<br>• Usually occurs in growing bones, especially femur and tibia, of children under age 12<br>• More common in males | • Abrupt onset of fever — usually 101° F (38.3° C); shaking chills; pain and swelling over infected area; restlessness; headache<br>• About 20% of children develop a chronic infection if not properly treated. | • Possible history of prior trauma to involved area<br>• Positive bone and pus cultures (and blood cultures in about 50% of patients)<br>• X-ray changes apparent after 2nd or 3rd week<br>• ESR elevated with leukocyte shift to the left |
| **Food poisoning**<br>• Enterotoxin produced by toxigenic strains of *S. aureus* in contaminated food (second most common cause of food poisoning in United States) | • Anorexia, nausea, vomiting, diarrhea, and abdominal cramps 1 to 6 hours after ingestion of contaminated food<br>• Symptoms usually subside within 18 hours, with complete recovery in 1 to 3 days. | • Clinical findings sufficient<br>• Stool cultures usually negative for *S. aureus* |
| **Skin infections**<br>• Decreased resistance<br>• Burns or pressure ulcers<br>• Decreased blood flow<br>• Possibly skin contamination from nasal discharge<br>• Foreign bodies<br>• Underlying skin diseases, such as eczema and acne<br>• Common in persons with poor hygiene living in crowded quarters | • Cellulitis — diffuse, acute inflammation of soft tissue (no drainage)<br>• Pus-producing lesions in and around hair follicles (folliculitis)<br>• Boil-like lesions (furuncles and carbuncles) extend from hair follicles to subcutaneous tissues. These painful, red, indurated lesions are I to 2 cm in diameter and have a purulent yellow discharge.<br>• Small macule or skin bleb that may develop into vesicle containing pus (bullous impetigo); common in school-age children<br>• Mild or spiking fever<br>• Malaise | • Clinical findings and analysis of pus cultures if sites are draining<br>• Cultures of nondraining cellulitis taken from the margin of the reddened area by infiltration with 1 ml sterile saline solution and immediate fluid aspiration |

| TREATMENT | SPECIAL CONSIDERATIONS |
|---|---|
| • Surgical debridement<br>• Prolonged antibiotic therapy (4 to 8 weeks)<br>• Vancomycin I.V. for patients with penicillin allergy or methicillin-resistant organisms | • Identify the infected area, and mark it on the care plan.<br>• Check the penetration wound from which the organism originated for evidence of present infection.<br>• Severe pain may render the patient immobile. If so, perform passive range-of-motion exercises. Apply heat as needed, and elevate the affected part. (Extensive involvement may require casting until the infection subsides.)<br>• Before such procedures as surgical debridement, warn the patient to expect some pain. Explain that drainage is essential for healing, and that he will continue to receive analgesics and antibiotics after surgery. |
| • No treatment necessary unless dehydration becomes a problem (usually in infants and elderly); then, I.V. therapy may be necessary to replace fluids. | • Obtain a complete history of symptoms, recent meals, and other known cases of food poisoning.<br>• Monitor vital signs, fluid balance, and serum electrolyte levels.<br>• Check for dehydration if vomiting is severe or prolonged, and for decreased blood pressure.<br>• Observe and report the number and color of stools. |
| • Topical ointments; bacitracin-neomycin-polymyxin or gentamicin<br>• P.O. cloxacillin, dicloxacillin, or erythromycin; I.V. oxacillin or nafcillin for severe infection; I.V. vancomycin for oxacillin-resistant organisms<br>• Application of heat to reduce pain<br>• Surgical drainage<br>• Identification and treatment of sources of reinfection (nostrils, perineum)<br>• Cleaning and covering the area with moist, sterile dressings | • Identify the site and extent of infection.<br>• Keep lesions clean with saline solution and peroxide irrigations as ordered. Cover infections near wounds or genitourinary tract with gauze pads. Keep pressure off the site to facilitate healing.<br>• Be alert for the extension of skin infections.<br>• Severe infection or abscess may require surgical drainage. Explain the procedure to the patient. Determine if cultures will be taken, and be ready to collect a specimen.<br>• Impetigo is contagious. Isolate the patient and alert his family. Use secretion precautions for all draining lesions. |

# STAPHYLOCOCCAL SCALDED SKIN SYNDROME

A severe skin disorder, staphylococcal scalded skin syndrome (SSSS) is marked by epidermal erythema, peeling, and superficial necrosis that give the skin a scalded appearance. SSSS is most prevalent in infants ages 1 to 3 months but may develop in children; it's rare in adults.

This disease follows a consistent pattern of progression, and most patients recover fully. Mortality is 2% to 3%, with death usually resulting from complications of fluid and electrolyte loss, sepsis, and involvement of other body systems.

## Causes

The causative organism in SSSS is Group 2 *Staphylococcus aureus*, primarily phage type 71. Predisposing factors may include impaired immunity and renal insufficiency — present to some extent in the normal neonate because of immature development of these systems.

## Signs and symptoms

SSSS can often be traced to a prodromal upper respiratory tract infection, possibly with concomitant purulent conjunctivitis. Cutaneous changes progress through three stages.

### Erythema

In the first stage, erythema becomes visible, usually around the mouth and other orifices, as well as body fold areas, and may spread in widening circles over the entire body surface. The skin becomes tender; Nikolsky's sign (sloughing of the skin when friction is applied) may appear.

### Exfoliation

About 24 to 48 hours later, exfoliation occurs. In the more common, localized form of this disease, superficial erosions and minimal crusting develop, generally around body orifices, and may spread to exposed areas of the skin.

In the more severe forms of this disease, large, flaccid bullae erupt and may spread to cover extensive areas of the body. These bullae eventually rupture, revealing denuded skin.

### Desquamation

In this final stage, affected areas dry up and powdery scales form. Normal skin replaces these scales in 5 to 7 days.

## Diagnosis

Careful observation of the three-stage progression of this disease allows diagnosis. Results of exfoliative cytology and a biopsy aid in the differential diagnosis, ruling out erythema multiforme and drug-induced toxic epidermal necrolysis, both of which are similar to SSSS.

> CLINICAL TIP  A blood culture is necessary to rule out sepsis.

## Treatment

Systemic antibiotics, usually penicillinase-resistant penicillin, treat the underlying infection. Replacement measures maintain fluid and electrolyte balance.

## Special considerations

• Provide special care for the neonate if required, including placement in a warming infant incubator to maintain body temperature and provide isolation.
• Carefully monitor intake and output to assess fluid and electrolyte balance.

In severe cases, I.V. fluid replacement may be necessary.

● Check vital signs. Be especially alert for a sudden rise in temperature, indicating sepsis, which requires prompt, aggressive treatment.

● Maintain skin integrity. Remember to use strict aseptic technique to preclude secondary infection, especially during the exfoliative stage, because of open lesions.

● To prevent friction and sloughing of the patient's skin, leave affected areas uncovered or loosely covered. Place cotton between fingers and toes that are severely affected to prevent webbing.

● Administer warm baths and soaks during the recovery period. Gently debride exfoliated areas.

● Reassure parents that complications are rare and residual scars are unlikely.

# STOMATITIS AND OTHER ORAL INFECTIONS

A common infection, stomatitis — inflammation of the oral mucosa — may extend to the buccal mucosa, lips, and palate. It may occur alone or as part of a systemic disease.

There are two main types: acute herpetic stomatitis and aphthous stomatitis. Acute herpetic stomatitis is common and mild. Aphthous stomatitis is common in young girls and female adolescents.

Acute herpetic stomatitis is usually short-lived and easily recognized; however, it may be severe and, in neonates, may be generalized and potentially fatal. Aphthous stomatitis usually heals spontaneously, without a scar, in 10 to 14 days.

Other oral infections include gingivitis, periodontitis, Vincent's angina, and glossitis. (See *Oral infections,* pages 830 and 831.)

## Causes

Acute herpetic stomatitis results from herpes simplex virus. The cause of aphthous stomatitis is unclear.

## Signs and symptoms

Acute herpetic stomatitis begins with burning mouth pain. In immunocompromised individuals, reactivation of the herpes simplex virus infection may be frequent and severe. Gums are swollen and bleed easily, and the mucous membranes are extremely tender. Papulovesicular ulcers appear in the mouth and throat and eventually become punched-out lesions with reddened areolae. The small vesicles rupture and form scales. Another common finding is submaxillary lymphadenitis.

Pain usually disappears from 2 to 4 days before healing of ulcers is complete.

A patient with aphthous stomatitis will typically report burning, tingling, and slight swelling of the mucous membrane. Single or multiple, small round ulcers with whitish centers and red borders appear and heal at one site but then appear at another. The painful stage lasts 7 to 10 days, with healing complete in 1 to 3 weeks.

## Diagnosis

Physical examination allows diagnosis. In Vincent's angina, a smear of ulcer exudate allows identification of the causative organism.

## Treatment and special considerations

For acute herpetic stomatitis, treatment is conservative. For local symptoms, management includes warm-water mouth rinses (antiseptic mouthwashes are contraindicated because they're ir-

# ORAL INFECTIONS

| DISEASE AND CAUSES | SIGNS AND SYMPTOMS | TREATMENT |
|---|---|---|
| **Gingivitis** (inflammation of the gingiva) • Early sign of hypovitaminosis, diabetes, blood dyscrasias • Occasionally related to use of oral contraceptives | • Inflammation with painless swelling, redness, change of normal contours, bleeding, and periodontal pocket (gum detachment from teeth) | • Removal of irritating factors (calculus, faulty dentures) • Good oral hygiene, regular dental checkups, vigorous chewing • Oral or topical corticosteroids |
| **Periodontitis** (progression of gingivitis; inflammation of the oral mucosa) • Early sign of hypovitaminosis, diabetes, blood dyscrasias • Occasionally related to use of oral contraceptives • Dental factors: calculus, poor oral hygiene, malocclusion. Major cause of tooth loss after middle age | • Acute onset of bright red gum inflammation, painless swelling of interdental papillae, easy bleeding • Loosening of teeth, typically without inflammatory symptoms, progressing to loss of teeth and alveolar bone • Acute systemic infection (fever, chills) | • Scaling, root planing, and curettage for infection control • Periodontal surgery to prevent recurrence • Good oral hygiene, regular dental checkups, vigorous chewing |
| **Vincent's angina** (trench mouth, necrotizing ulcerative gingivitis) • Fusiform bacillus or spirochete infection • Predisposing factors: stress, poor oral hygiene, insufficient rest, nutritional deficiency, smoking | • Sudden onset: painful, superficial bleeding; gingival ulcers (rarely, on buccal mucosa) covered with a gray-white membrane • Ulcers become punched-out lesions after slight pressure or irritation • Malaise, mild fever, excessive salivation, bad breath, pain on swallowing or talking, enlarged submaxillary lymph nodes | • Removal of devitalized tissue with ultrasonic cavitron • Antibiotics (penicillin or oral erythromycin) for infection • Analgesics as needed • Hourly mouth rinses (equal parts hydrogen peroxide and warm water) • Soft, nonirritating diet; rest; no smoking • With treatment, improvement within 24 hours |

*(continued)*

## ORAL INFECTIONS *(continued)*

| DISEASE AND CAUSES | SIGNS AND SYMPTOMS | TREATMENT |
|---|---|---|
| **Glossitis** (tongue inflammation) • Streptococcal infection • Irritation or injury, jagged teeth, ill-fitting dentures, biting during convulsions, alcohol, spicy foods, smoking, sensitivity to toothpaste or mouthwash • Vitamin B deficiency, anemia • Skin conditions: lichen planus, erhythema multiforme, pemiphigus vulgaris | • Reddened ulcerated or swollen tongue (may obstruct airway) • Painful chewing and swallowing • Painful tongue without inflammation | • Treatment of underlying cause • Topical anesthetic mouthwash or systemic analgesics (aspirin or acetaminophen) for painful lesions • Good oral hygiene, regular dental check-ups, vigorous chewing • Avoidance of alcohol and hot, cold, or spicy foods |

ritating) and a topical anesthetic to relieve mouth ulcer pain.

➤ CLINICAL TIP   A course of acyclovir (200 to 800 mg, 5 times daily for 7 to 14 days) may shorten the course and reduce postherpetic pain.

Supplementary treatment includes bland or liquid diet and, in severe cases, I.V. fluids to maintain hydration, and bed rest.

For aphthous stomatitis, primary treatment is application of a topical anesthetic. Effective long-term treatment requires alleviation or prevention of precipitating factors.

# STRABISMUS

Also called squint, heterotropia, crosseye, or walleye, strabismus is a condition of eye malalignment that results from the absence of normal, parallel, or coordinated eye movement. In children, it may be concomitant, in which the degree of deviation doesn't vary with the direction of gaze; inconcomitant, in which the degree of deviation varies with the direction of gaze; congenital (present at birth or during the first 6 months); or acquired (present during the first 2½ years).

Strabismus can also be latent (phoria), apparent when the child is tired or sick, or manifest (tropia). Tropias are categorized into four types: esotropia (eyes deviate inward), exotropia (eyes deviate outward), hypertropia (eyes deviate upward), and hypotropia (eyes deviate downward). (See *Viewing esotropia,* page 832.)

Strabismus affects about 2% of the population. Incidence of strabismus is higher in patients with central nervous system (CNS) disorders, such as cerebral palsy, mental retardation, and Down syndrome.

The prognosis for correction varies with the timing of treatment and the onset of the disease. Muscle imbalances

## VIEWING ESOTROPIA

In esotropia, medial deviation occurs.

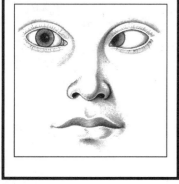

may be corrected by glasses, patching, or surgery, depending on the cause. However, residual defects in vision and extraocular muscle alignment may persist even after treatment.

### Causes

Strabismus is frequently inherited, but its cause is unknown. Controversy exists over whether or not amblyopia ("lazy eye") causes or results from strabismus. In adults, strabismus may result from trauma.

Strabismic amblyopia is characterized by a loss of central vision in one eye that typically results in esotropia (from fixation in the dominant eye and suppression of images in the deviating eye). Strabismic amblyopia may result from hyperopia (farsightedness) or anisometropia (unequal refractive power).

Esotropia may result from muscle imbalance and may be congenital or acquired. In accommodative esotropia, the child's attempt to compensate for the farsightedness affects the convergent reflex, and the eyes cross.

Malalignment of the eyes leads to suppression of vision in one of the eyes. It causes amblyopia if it develops early in life, before bifoveal fixation is established.

### Signs and symptoms

Malalignment of the eyes can be detected by external eye examination when deviation is obvious or by observation of the corneal light reflex in the center of the pupils.

In addition, strabismus causes diplopia and other visual disturbances, which is often the reason the patient seeks medical help.

### Diagnosis

Parents of children with strabismus will typically seek medical advice. Older persons with strabismus commonly seek treatment to correct double vision, to improve appearance because of changes caused by thyroid ophthalmopathy (thyroid eye disease), or following eye injury. A careful, detailed patient history is essential not only for the diagnosis, but also for the prognosis and treatment of strabismus.

The following ophthalmologic tests help diagnose strabismus:

• *Visual acuity test* evaluates the degree of visual defect.

• *Hirschberg's method* detects malalignment. The patient fixes his gaze on a light at a distance of about 13″ (33 cm) as the examiner observes the light decentered in the deviating eye.

• *Retinoscopy* determines refractive error. This is usually done with pupils dilated.

• *Maddox rods test* assesses specific muscle involvement.

• *Convergence test* shows the distance at which convergence is sustained.

• *Duction test* reveals limitations of eye movement.

- *Cover-uncover test* demonstrates eye deviation and the rate of recovery to original alignment.
- *Alternate-cover test* shows intermittent or latent deviation.

A neurologic examination determines whether the condition is muscular or neurologic in origin. It should be performed if the onset of strabismus is sudden or if the CNS is involved.

➤ CLINICAL TIP  Deviation of an eye is the second most common symptom in a child with retinoblastoma. Therefore, an acquired strabismus should always be checked.

### Treatment

Initial treatment depends on the type of strabismus. For strabismic amblyopia, therapy includes patching the normal eye and prescribing corrective glasses to keep the eye straight and to counteract farsightedness (especially in accommodative esotropia).

Surgery is often necessary for cosmetic and psychological reasons to correct strabismus that results from basic esotropia or residual accommodative esotropia after correction with glasses.

Timing of surgery varies with individual circumstances. For example, a 6-month-old infant with equal visual acuity and a large esotropia will have the deviation corrected surgically. But a child with unequal visual acuity and an acquired deviation will have the affected eye patched until visual acuity is equal, *then* undergo surgery.

Surgical correction includes recession (moving the muscle posteriorly from its original insertion) or resection (shortening the muscle). A recent surgical procedure uses an adjustable suture.

Possible complications include overcorrection or undercorrection, slipped muscle, and perforation of the globe. Postoperative therapy may include patching the affected eye and applying combination antibiotic-steroid eyedrops. Eye exercises and corrective glasses may still be necessary; surgery may have to be repeated.

### Special considerations

- Postoperatively, discourage the child from rubbing his eyes.
- Gently wipe the child's tears, which will be serosanguineous. Reassure his parents that this is normal.
- Administer antiemetics if necessary.
- Apply antibiotic or steroid combination eye drops to the affected eye postoperatively if ordered. Teach the patient or his parents how to instill the drops.
- Because this surgery is usually a 1-day procedure, most patients are discharged after they recover from anesthesia. Encourage compliance with recommended follow-up care.

# STREPTOCOCCAL INFECTIONS

Streptococci are small gram-positive bacteria, spherical to ovoid in shape and linked together in pairs of chains. Several species occur as part of normal human flora in the respiratory, GI, and genitourinary tracts. Although researchers have identified 21 species of streptococci, three classes — groups A, B, and D — cause most of the infections. Organisms belonging to groups A and B beta-hemolytic streptococci are associated with a characteristic pattern of human infections. Most disorders due to group D streptococcus are caused by *Enterococcus faecalis* (formerly called *Streptococcus faecalis*) or *Streptococcus bovis*.

Clinically, there are three states of streptococcal infection: carrier, acute, and delayed nonsuppurative complications. In the carrier state, the patient is infected with a disease-causing species of streptococci without evidence of infection. In the acute form, streptococci invade the tissues and cause physical symptoms. In the delayed nonsuppurative complications state, specific complications associated with streptococcal infection occur. These include the

---

# COMPARING STREPTOCOCCAL INFECTIONS

| CAUSES AND INCIDENCE | SIGNS AND SYMPTOMS |
|---|---|

### *STREPTOCOCCUS PYOGENES* (GROUP A STREPTOCOCCUS)

**Streptococcal pharyngitis (strep throat)**

- Accounts for 95% of all cases of bacterial pharyngitis
- Most common in children ages 5 to 10 from October to April
- Spread by direct person-to-person contact via droplets of saliva or nasal secretions
- Organism usually colonizes throats of persons with no symptoms; up to 20% of school children may be carriers. Pets may also be carriers.

- After 1- to 5-day incubation period: temperature of 101° to 104° F (38.3° to 40° C), sore throat with severe pain on swallowing, beefy red pharynx, tonsillar exudate, edematous tonsils and uvula, swollen glands along the jaw line, generalized malaise and weakness, occasional abdominal discomfort
- Up to 40% of small children have symptoms too mild for diagnosis.
- Fever abates in 3 to 5 days; nearly all symptoms subside within a week.

**Scarlet fever (scarlatina)**

- Usually follows streptococcal pharyngitis; may follow wound infections or puerperal sepsis
- Caused by streptococcal strain that releases an erythrogenic toxin
- Most common in children ages 2 to 10
- Spread by inhalation or direct contact

- Streptococcal sore throat, fever, strawberry tongue, fine erythematous rash that blanches on pressure and resembles sunburn with goosebumps
- Rash usually appearing first on upper chest, then spreads to neck, abdomen, legs, and arms, sparing soles and palms; flushed cheeks; pallor around mouth
- Skin sheds during convalescence.

**Erysipelas**

- Occurs primarily in infants and adults over age 30
- Usually follows strep throat
- Exact mode of spread to skin unknown

- Sudden onset, with reddened, swollen, raised lesions (skin looks like an orange peel), usually on face and scalp, bordered by areas that often contain easily ruptured blebs filled with yellow-tinged fluid. Lesions sting and itch. Lesions on the trunk, arms, or legs usually affect incision or wound sites.
- Other symptoms: vomiting, fever, headache, cervical lymphadenopathy, sore throat

inflammatory state of acute rheumatic fever, chorea, and glomerulonephritis. If complications occur, they usually appear about 2 weeks after the acute illness, but they may be evident after a nonsymptomatic illness.

For information on the most common types of streptococcal infections, see *Comparing streptococcal infections.*

*(Text continues on page 840.)*

| DIAGNOSIS | COMPLICATIONS | TREATMENT AND SPECIAL CONSIDERATIONS |
|---|---|---|
| • Clinically indistinguishable from viral pharyngitis<br>• Throat culture shows group A beta-hemolytic streptococci (carriers have positive throat culture)<br>• Elevated white blood cell (WBC) count<br>• Serology shows a fourfold rise in streptozyme titers during convalescence. | • Acute otitis media or acute sinusitis occurs most frequently.<br>• Rarely, bacteremic spread may cause arthritis, endocarditis, meningitis, osteomyelitis, or liver abscess.<br>• Poststreptococcal sequelae: acute rheumatic fever or acute glomerulonephritis<br>• Reye's syndrome | • Penicillin or erythromycin, analgesics, and antipyretics<br>• Stress the need for bed rest and isolation from other children for 24 hours after antibiotic therapy begins. Patient should finish prescription, even if symptoms subside; abscess, glomerulonephritis, and rheumatic fever can occur.<br>• Tell the patient not to skip doses and to properly dispose of soiled tissues. |
| • Characteristic rash and strawberry tongue<br>• Culture and Gram stain show *S. pyogenes* from nasopharynx.<br>• Granulocytosis | • Although rare, complications may include high fever, arthritis, jaundice, pneumonia, pericarditis, and peritonsillar abscess. | • Penicillin or erythromycin<br>• Isolation for first 24 hours<br>• Carefully dispose of purulent discharge.<br>• Stress the need for prompt and complete antibiotic treatment. |
| • Typical reddened lesions<br>• Culture taken from edge of lesions shows group A beta-hemolytic streptococci.<br>• Throat culture is almost always positive for group A beta-hemolytic streptococci. | • Untreated lesions on trunk, arms, or legs may involve large body areas and lead to death. | • Penicillin or erythromycin I.V. or by mouth<br>• Cold packs, analgesics (aspirin and codeine for local discomfort), topical anesthetics<br>• Prevention: prompt treatment of streptococcal infections, and drainage and secretion precautions |

*(continued)*

## COMPARING STREPTOCOCCAL INFECTIONS *(continued)*

| CAUSES AND INCIDENCE | SIGNS AND SYMPTOMS |
|---|---|

*STREPTOCOCCUS PYOGENES* **(GROUP A STREPTOCOCCUS)** *(continued)*

### Impetigo (streptococcal pyoderma)

● Common in poor children ages 2 to 5 in hot, humid weather; high rate of familial spread
● Predisposing factors: close contact in schools, overcrowded living quarters, poor skin hygiene, minor skin trauma
● May spread by direct contact, environmental contamination, or arthropod vector

● Small macules rapidly develop into vesicles, then become pustular and encrusted, causing pain, surrounding erythema, regional adenitis, cellulitis, and itching. Scratching spreads infection.
● Lesions commonly affect the face, heal slowly, and leave depigmented areas.

### Streptococcal gangrene (necrotizing fasciitis)

● More common in elderly patients with arteriosclerotic vascular disease or diabetes
● Predisposing factors: surgery, wounds, skin ulcers, diabetes, peripheral vascular disease
● Spread by direct contact

● Mimics gas gangrene; within 72 hours of onset, patient shows red-streaked, painful skin lesions with dusky red surrounding tissue. Bullae with yellow or reddish black fluid develop and rupture.
● Other signs and symptoms: fever, tachycardia, lethargy, prostration, disorientation, hypotension, jaundice, hypovolemia, severe pain followed by anesthesia (due to nerve destruction)

*STREPTOCOCCUS AGALACTIAE* **(GROUP B STREPTOCOCCUS)**

### Neonatal streptococcal infections

● Incidence of early-onset infection (age 5 days or less): 2/1,000 live births
● Incidence of late-onset infection (age 7 days to 3 months): 1/1,000 live births
● Spread by vaginal delivery or hands of nursery staff
● Predisposing factors: maternal genital tract colonization, membrane rupture over 24 hours before delivery, crowded nursery

● Early onset: bacteremia, pneumonia, and meningitis; mortality from 14% for neonates over 1,500 g at birth to 61% for neonates under 1,500 g at birth
● Late onset: bacteremia with meningitis, fever, and bone and joint involvement; mortality 15% to 20%
● Other signs and symptoms, such as skin lesions, depend on the site affected.

| DIAGNOSIS | COMPLICATIONS | TREATMENT AND SPECIAL CONSIDERATIONS |
|---|---|---|
| • Characteristic lesions with honey-colored crust<br>• Culture and Gram stain of swabbed lesions show *S. pyogenes*. | • Septicemia (rare)<br>• Ecthyma, a form of impetigo with deep ulcers | • Penicillin I.V. or by mouth, or erythromycin, or antibiotic ointments<br>• Frequent washing of lesions with antiseptics, such as povidone-iodine or antibacterial soap, followed by thorough drying<br>• Isolation of patient with draining wounds<br>• Prevention: good hygiene and proper wound care |
| • Culture and Gram stain usually show *S. pyogenes* from early bullous lesions and commonly from blood. | • Extensive necrotic sloughing<br>• Bacteremia, metastatic abscesses, and death<br>• Thrombophlebitis, when lower extremities are involved | • Immediate, wide, deep surgery of all necrotic tissues<br>• High-dose penicillin I.V.<br>• Good preoperative skin preparation, aseptic surgical and suturing technique |
| • Isolation of group B streptococcus from blood, cerebrospinal fluid (CSF), or skin<br>• Chest X-ray shows massive infiltrate similar to that of respiratory distress syndrome or pneumonia. | • Overwhelming pneumonia, sepsis, and death | • Penicillin or ampicillin and an aminoglycoside I.V.<br>• Patient isolation is unnecessary unless open draining lesion is present, but careful hand washing is essential. If draining lesion is present, take drainage and secretion precautions.<br>• Vaccine in development |

*(continued)*

## COMPARING STREPTOCOCCAL INFECTIONS *(continued)*

| CAUSES AND INCIDENCE | SIGNS AND SYMPTOMS |
|---|---|

*STREPTOCOCCUS AGALACTIAE* (GROUP B STREPTOCOCCUS) *(continued)*

### Adult group B streptococcal infection

- Most adult infections occur in postpartum women, usually in the form of endometritis or wound infection following cesarean section.
- Incidence of group B streptococcal endometritis: 1.3/1,000 live births

- Fever, malaise, uterine tenderness
- Change in lochia

*STREPTOCOCCUS PNEUMONIAE* (GROUP D STREPTOCOCCUS)

### Pneumococcal pneumonia

- Accounts for 70% of all cases of bacterial pneumonia
- More common in men, elderly people, Blacks, and Native Americans, in winter and early spring
- Spread by air and contact with infective secretions
- Predisposing factors: trauma, viral infection, underlying pulmonary disease, overcrowded living quarters, chronic diseases, immunodeficiency
- Among the 10 leading causes of death in the United States

- Sudden onset with severe shaking chills, temperature of 102° to 105° F (38.9° to 40.6° C), bacteremia, cough (with thick, scanty, blood-tinged sputum) accompanied by pleuritic pain
- Malaise, weakness, and prostration common
- Tachypnea, anorexia, nausea, and vomiting less common
- Severity of pneumonia usually due to host's cellular defenses, not bacterial virulence

### Otitis media

- About 76% to 95% of all children have otitis media at least once. *S. pneumoniae* causes half of these cases.

- Ear pain, ear drainage, hearing loss, fever, lethargy, irritability
- Other possible symptoms: vertigo, nystagmus, tinnitus

### Meningitis

- Can follow bacteremic pneumonia, mastoiditis, sinusitis, skull fracture, or endocarditis
- Mortality (30% to 60%) highest in infants and in elderly patients

- Fever, headache, nuchal rigidity, vomiting, photophobia, lethargy, coma, wide pulse pressure, bradycardia

| DIAGNOSIS | COMPLICATIONS | TREATMENT AND SPECIAL CONSIDERATIONS |
|---|---|---|
| • Isolation of group B streptococcus from blood or infection site | • Bacteremia followed by meningitis or endocarditis | • Ampicillin or penicillin I.V.<br>• Careful observation for symptoms of infection following delivery<br>• Drainage and secretion precautions |
| • Gram stain of sputum shows gram-positive diplococci; culture shows *S. pneumoniae.*<br>• Chest X-ray shows lobular consolidation in adults; bronchopneumonia in children and in elderly patients<br>• Elevated WBC count<br>• Blood cultures often positive for *S. pneumoniae* | • Pleural effusion occurs in 25% of patients<br>• Pericarditis (rare)<br>• Lung abscess (rare)<br>• Bacteremia<br>• Disseminated intravascular coagulation<br>• Death possible if bacteremia is present<br>• Recurrent attacks may cause hearing loss. | • Penicillin or erythromycin I.V. or I.M.<br>• Monitor and support respirations as needed. Record sputum color and amount.<br>• Prevent dehydration.<br>• Avoid sedatives and narcotics to preserve cough reflex.<br>• Carefully dispose of all purulent drainage. (Respiratory isolation is unnecessary.) Advise high-risk patients to receive vaccine and to avoid infected persons. |
| • Fluid in middle ear<br>• Isolation of *S. pneumoniae* from aspirated fluid if necessary | • Persistent hearing deficits, seizures, hemiparesis, or other nerve deficits<br>• Encephalitis | • Amoxicillin or ampicillin and analgesics<br>• Tell patient to report lack of response to therapy after 72 hours. |
| • Isolation of *S. pneumoniae* from CSF or blood culture<br>• Increased CSF cell count and protein level; decreased CSF glucose level<br>• Computed tomography scan of head<br>• EEG | • Embolization<br>• Pulmonary infarction<br>• Osteomyelitis | • Penicillin I.V. or chloramphenicol<br>• Monitor closely for neurologic changes.<br>• Watch for symptoms of septic shock, such as acidosis and tissue hypoxia. |

*(continued)*

COMPARING STREPTOCOCCAL INFECTIONS *(continued)*

| CAUSES AND INCIDENCE | SIGNS AND SYMPTOMS |
|---|---|

***STREPTOCOCCUS PNEUMONIAE* (GROUP D STREPTOCOCCUS)** *(continued)*

**Endocarditis**
- Group D streptococci (enterococci) causes 10% to 20% of all bacterial endocarditis.
- Most common in elderly patients and in those who abuse I.V. substances
- Often follows bacteremia from an obvious source, such as a wound infection or I.V. insertion site infection
- Most cases are subacute.

- Weakness, fatigability, weight loss, fever, night sweats, anorexia, arthralgia, splenomegaly, new systolic murmur

---

LIFE-THREATENING
DISORDER

# SUDDEN INFANT DEATH SYNDROME

A medical mystery of early infancy, sudden infant death syndrome (SIDS) — commonly called crib death — kills apparently healthy infants, usually between ages 4 weeks and 7 months, for reasons that remain unexplained, even after an autopsy. Typically, parents put the infant to bed and later find him dead, often with no indications of a struggle or distress of any kind.

Some infants may have had signs of a cold, but such symptoms are usually absent. SIDS has occurred throughout history, all over the world, and in all climates.

## Causes

SIDS accounts for 7,500 to 8,000 deaths annually in the United States, making it one of the leading causes of infant death. Most of these deaths occur during the winter, in poor families, and among underweight babies and those born to mothers under age 20.

Although infants who die from SIDS often appear healthy, research suggests that many may have had undetected abnormalities such as an immature respiratory system and respiratory dysfunction. In fact, the current thinking is that SIDS may result from an abnormality in the control of ventilation, which causes prolonged apneic periods with profound hypoxemia and serious cardiac arrhythmias.

Bottle-feeding instead of breast-feeding and advanced parental age *don't* cause SIDS.

## Signs and symptoms

Although parents find some victims wedged in crib corners or with blankets wrapped around their heads, autopsies rule out suffocation as the cause of death. Even when frothy, blood-tinged sputum is found around the infant's mouth or on the crib sheets, an autop-

| DIAGNOSIS | COMPLICATIONS | TREATMENT AND SPECIAL CONSIDERATIONS |
|---|---|---|
| • Anemia, increased erythrocyte sedimentation rate and serum immunoglobulin level, and positive blood culture for group D streptococcus<br>• Echocardiogram shows vegetation on valves. | • Embolization<br>• Pulmonary infarction<br>• Osteomyelitis | • Penicillin for *Streptococcus bovis* (non-enterococcal group D streptococci)<br>• Penicillin or ampicillin and an aminoglycoside for enterococcal group D streptococci |

sy shows a patent airway, so aspiration of vomitus is not the cause of death.

Typically, SIDS babies don't cry out and show no signs of having been disturbed in their sleep, although their positions or tangled blankets may suggest movement just before death, perhaps from terminal spasm.

Depending on how long the infant has been dead, a SIDS baby may have a mottled complexion, with extreme cyanosis of the lips and fingertips, or pooling of blood in the legs and feet that may be mistaken for bruises. Pulse and respirations are absent, and the infant's diaper is wet and full of stools.

### Diagnosis
An autopsy rules out other causes of death. Characteristic histologic findings on autopsy include small or normal adrenal glands and petechiae over the visceral surfaces of the pleura, within the thymus (which is enlarged), and in the epicardium.

An autopsy also reveals extremely well-preserved lymphoid structures and certain pathologic characteristics that suggest chronic hypoxemia, such as increased pulmonary artery smooth muscle. Examination also shows edematous, congestive lungs fully expanded in the pleural cavities, liquid (not clotted) blood in the heart, and curd from the stomach inside the trachea.

### Treatment
If the parents bring the infant to the emergency department, the doctor will decide whether to try to resuscitate him. An "aborted SIDS" is an infant who is found apneic and is successfully resuscitated. Such an infant, or any infant who had a sibling stricken by SIDS, should be tested for infantile apnea. If tests are positive, a home apnea monitor may be recommended.

Because most infants can't be resuscitated, however, treatment focuses on emotional support for the family

### Special considerations
• Make sure that both parents are present when the child's death is announced. The parents may lash out at emergency department personnel, the

babysitter, or anyone else involved in the child's care — even at each other. Stay calm and let them express their feelings. Reassure them that they were not to blame.

• Let the parents see the baby in a private room. Allow them to express their grief in their own way. Stay in the room with them if appropriate. Offer to call clergy, friends, or relatives.

• After the parents and family have recovered from their initial shock, explain the necessity for an autopsy to confirm the diagnosis of SIDS (in some states, this is mandatory). At this time, provide the family with some basic facts about SIDS and encourage them to give their consent for the autopsy. Make sure they receive the autopsy report promptly.

• Find out whether there is a local counseling and information program for SIDS parents. Participants in such a program will contact the parents, ensure that they receive the autopsy report promptly, put them in touch with a professional counselor, and maintain supportive telephone contact.

• Find out whether there is a local SIDS parents' group; such a group can provide significant emotional support. Contact the National Sudden Infant Death Foundation for information about such local groups.

• If your hospital's policy is to assign a public health nurse to the family, she will provide the continuing reassurance and assistance the parents will need.

➤ CLINICAL TIP If the parents decide to have another child, make sure they receive information and counseling to help them deal with the pregnancy and the first year of the new infant's life.

# SYNDROME OF INAPPROPRIATE ANTIDIURETIC HORMONE SECRETION

Excessive release of antidiuretic hormone (ADH) disturbs fluid and electrolyte balance in syndrome of inappropriate antidiuretic hormone secretion (SIADH). The excessive ADH causes an inability to excrete dilute urine, retention of free water, expansion of extracellular fluid volume, and hyponatremia.

SIADH occurs secondary to diseases that affect the osmoreceptors (supraoptic nucleus) of the hypothalamus. The prognosis depends on the underlying disorder and response to treatment.

## Causes

The most common cause of SIADH is small cell carcinoma of the lung, which secretes excessive levels of ADH or vasopressin-like substances. Other neoplastic diseases — such as pancreatic and prostatic cancer, Hodgkin's disease, and thymoma — may also trigger SIADH.

Less common causes include:

• *central nervous system disorders* — brain tumor or abscess, cerebrovascular accident, head injury, and Guillain-Barré syndrome

• *pulmonary disorders* — pneumonia, tuberculosis, lung abscess, and positive-pressure ventilation

• *drugs* — chlorpropamide, vincristine, cyclophosphamide, carbamazepine, clofibrate, metoclopramide, and morphine

• *miscellaneous conditions* — psychosis and myxedema.

## Signs and symptoms

SIADH may produce weight gain despite anorexia, nausea, and vomiting; muscle weakness; restlessness; and possibly seizures and coma. Edema is rare unless water overload exceeds 4 L because much of the free-water excess is within cellular boundaries.

## Diagnosis

A complete medical history revealing positive water balance may suggest SIADH. Serum osmolality less than 280 mOsm/kg of water and low serum sodium confirm it. Urine osmolality is greater than plasma osmolality.

Supportive laboratory values include high urine sodium secretion (more than 20 mEq/L) without diuretics. In addition, diagnostic studies show normal renal function and no evidence of dehydration.

## Treatment

Symptomatic treatment begins with restricted water intake (500 to 1,000 ml/day). With severe water intoxication, administration of 200 to 300 ml of 3% saline solution may be necessary to raise the serum sodium level.

When possible, treatment should include correction of the underlying cause of SIADH. If SIADH results from cancer, success in alleviating water retention may be obtained by surgical resection, irradiation, or chemotherapy.

If fluid restriction is ineffective, demeclocycline may be helpful by blocking the renal response to ADH.

## Special considerations

• Closely monitor and record intake and output, vital signs, and daily weight. Follow serum sodium levels.

• Observe for restlessness, irritability, seizures, heart failure, and unresponsiveness resulting from hyponatremia and water intoxication.

• To prevent water intoxication, explain to the patient and his family why he *must* restrict his intake.

# SYPHILIS

A chronic, infectious, sexually transmitted disease, syphilis begins in the mucous membranes and quickly becomes systemic, spreading to nearby lymph nodes and the bloodstream. This disease, when untreated, is characterized by progressive stages: primary, secondary, latent, and late (formerly called tertiary).

About 34,000 cases of syphilis, in primary and secondary stages, are reported annually in the United States. Incidence is highest among urban populations, especially in persons between ages 15 and 39, drug users, and those infected with the human immunodeficiency virus (HIV).

Untreated syphilis leads to crippling or death, but the prognosis is excellent with early treatment.

## Causes

Infection from the spirochete *Treponema pallidum* causes syphilis. Transmission occurs primarily through sexual contact during the primary, secondary, and early latent stages of infection. Prenatal transmission from an infected mother to her fetus is also possible. (See *Prenatal syphilis*, page 844.)

## Signs and symptoms

Each stage produces distinctive signs and symptoms.

# PRENATAL SYPHILIS

A woman can transmit syphilis transplacentally to her unborn child throughout pregnancy. This type of syphilis is often called congenital, but prenatal is a more accurate term. Approximately 50% of infected fetuses die before or shortly after birth. The prognosis is better for those who develop overt infection after age 2.

### Signs and symptoms
The neonate with prenatal syphilis may appear healthy at birth but usually develops characteristic lesions — vesicular, bullous eruptions, often on the palms and soles — 3 weeks later. Shortly afterward, a maculopapular rash similar to that in secondary syphilis may erupt on the face, mouth, genitalia, palms, or soles. Condylomata lata often occur around the anus.

Lesions may erupt on the mucous membranes of the mouth, pharynx, and nose. When the infant's larynx is affected, his cry becomes weak and forced. If the nasal mucous membranes are involved, he may also develop nasal discharge, which can be slight and mucopurulent or copious with blood-tinged pus.

Visceral and bone lesions, liver or spleen enlargement with ascites, and nephrotic syndrome may also develop.

Late prenatal syphilis becomes apparent after age 2; it may be identifiable only through blood studies or may cause unmistakable syphilitic changes: screwdriver-shaped central incisors, deformed molars or cusps, thick clavicles, saber shins, bowed tibias, nasal septum perforation, eighth cranial nerve deafness, and neurosyphilis.

### Diagnosis
In the neonate with prenatal syphilis, Venereal Disease Research Laboratory titer, if reactive at birth, stays the same or rises, indicating active disease. The infant's titer drops in 3 months if the mother has received effective prenatal treatment. An absolute diagnosis necessitates a dark-field examination of umbilical vein blood or lesion drainage.

### Treatment
An infant with abnormal cerebrospinal fluid (CSF) may be treated with aqueous crystalline penicillin G, I.M. or I.V. (50,000 units/kg of body weight/day divided in two doses for at least 10 days), or aqueous penicillin G procaine I.M. (50,000 units/kg of body weight/day for at least 10 days). An infant with normal CSF may be treated with a single injection of penicillin G benzathine (50,000 units/kg of body weight).

When caring for a child with prenatal syphilis, record the extent of the rash, and watch for signs of systemic involvement, especially laryngeal swelling, jaundice, and decreasing urine output.

*Primary syphilis*
After an incubation period that generally lasts about 3 weeks, symptoms of primary syphilis develop.

Initially, one or more chancres (small, fluid-filled lesions) erupt on the genitalia; others may erupt on the anus, fingers, lips, tongue, nipples, tonsils, or eyelids. These chancres, which are usually painless, start as papules and then erode; they have indurated, raised edges and clear bases.

Chancres typically disappear after 3 to 6 weeks, even when untreated. They are usually associated with regional lymphadenopathy (unilateral or bilateral). In women, chancres are frequently overlooked because they often develop on internal structures—the cervix or the vaginal wall.

### Secondary syphilis

The development of symmetrical mucocutaneous lesions and general lymphadenopathy signals the onset of secondary syphilis, which may develop within a few days or up to 8 weeks after the onset of initial chancres.

The rash of secondary syphilis can be macular, papular, pustular, or nodular. Lesions are of uniform size, well defined, and generalized. Macules often erupt between rolls of fat on the trunk and on the arms, palms, soles, face, and scalp. In warm, moist areas (perineum, scrotum, vulva, between rolls of fat), the lesions enlarge and erode, producing highly contagious, pink, or grayish-white lesions (condylomata lata).

Mild constitutional symptoms of syphilis appear in the second stage and may include headache, malaise, anorexia, weight loss, nausea, vomiting, sore throat and, possibly, slight fever. Alopecia may occur, with or without treatment, and is usually temporary. Nails become brittle and pitted.

### Latent syphilis

Although no clinical symptoms occur in latent syphilis, it produces a reactive serologic test for syphilis. Because infectious mucocutaneous lesions may reappear when infection is of less than 4 years' duration, early latent syphilis is considered contagious.

Approximately two-thirds of patients remain asymptornatic in the late latent stage until death. The rest develop characteristic late-stage symptoms.

### Late syphilis

The final, destructive, but noninfectious stage of the disease, late syphilis has three subtypes, any or all of which may affect the patient: late benign syphilis, cardiovascular syphilis, and neurosyphilis.

The lesions of late benign syphilis develop between 1 and 10 years after infection. They may appear on the skin, bones, mucous membranes, upper respiratory tract, liver, or stomach.

The typical lesion is a gumma—a chronic, superficial nodule or deep, granulomatous lesion that is solitary, asymmetrical, painless, and indurated. Gummas can be found on any bone, particularly the long bones of the legs, and in any organ.

If late syphilis involves the liver, it can cause epigastric pain, tenderness, enlarged spleen, and anemia; if it involves the upper respiratory tract, it may cause perforation of the nasal septum or the palate. In severe cases, late benign syphilis results in destruction of bones or organs, which eventually causes death.

Cardiovascular syphilis develops about 10 years after the initial infection in approximately 10% of patients with late, untreated syphilis. It causes fibrosis of elastic tissue of the aorta and leads to aortitis, most often in the ascending and transverse sections of the aortic arch. Cardiovascular syphilis may be asymptomatic or may cause aortic regurgitation or aneurysm.

Symptoms of neurosyphilis develop in about 8% of patients with late, untreated syphilis and appear from 5 to 35 years after infection. These clinical effects consist of meningitis and widespread central nervous system damage that may include general paresis, personality changes, and arm and leg weakness.

### Diagnosis

Identifying *T. pallidum* from a lesion on a dark-field examination provides immediate diagnosis of syphilis. This method is most effective when moist lesions are present, as in primary, secondary, and prenatal syphilis.

The fluorescent treponemal antibody-absorption test identifies antigens of *T. pallidum* in tissue, ocular fluid, cerebrospinal fluid (CSF), tracheobronchial secretions, and exudates from lesions. This is the most sensitive test available for detecting syphilis in all stages. Once reactive, it remains so permanently.

Other appropriate procedures include the following:

• *Venereal Disease Research Laboratory (VDRL) slide test* and *rapid plasma reagin test* detect nonspecific antibodies. Both tests, if positive, become reactive within 1 to 2 weeks after the primary lesion appears or 4 to 5 weeks after the infection begins.

• *CSF examination* identifies neurosyphilis when the total protein level is above 40 mg/100 ml, VDRL slide test is reactive, and CSF cell count exceeds five mononuclear cells/μl.

## Treatment

Administration of penicillin I.M. is the treatment of choice. For early syphilis, treatment may consist of a single injection of penicillin G benzathine I.M. (2.4 million units). Syphilis of more than 1 year's duration should be treated with penicillin G benzathine I.M. (2.4 million units/week for 3 weeks).

Nonpregnant patients who are allergic to penicillin may be treated with oral tetracycline or doxycycline for 15 days for early syphilis; 30 days for late infections. Nonpenicillin therapy for latent or late syphilis should be used only after neurosyphilis has been excluded. Tetracycline is contraindicated in pregnant women.

## Special considerations

• Stress the importance of completing the course of therapy even after symptoms subside.

• Check for a history of drug sensitivity before administering the first dose.

• Practice standard precautions.

• In secondary syphilis, keep lesions clean and dry. If they're draining, dispose of contaminated materials properly.

• In late syphilis, provide symptomatic care during prolonged treatment.

• In cardiovascular syphilis, check for signs of decreased cardiac output (decreased urine output, hypoxia, and decreased sensorium) and pulmonary congestion.

• In neurosyphilis, regularly check level of consciousness, mood, and coherence. Watch for signs of ataxia.

• Urge patients to seek VDRL testing after 3, 6, 12, and 24 months to detect possible relapse. Patients treated for latent or late syphilis should receive blood tests at 6-month intervals for 2 years.

• Be sure to report all cases of syphilis to local public health authorities. Urge the patient to inform sexual partners of his infection so that they can receive treatment also.

• Refer the patient and his sexual partners for HIV testing.

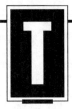

# TAY-SACHS DISEASE

The most common of the lipid storage diseases, Tay-Sachs disease results from a congenital deficiency of the enzyme hexosaminidase A. It's characterized by progressive mental and motor deterioration and is usually fatal before age 5, although some adolescents and adults with variations of hexosaminidase A deficiency have been noted.

## Causes

Tay-Sachs disease (also known as $GM_2$ gangliosidosis) is an autosomal recessive disorder in which the enzyme hexosaminidase A is virtually absent or deficient. This enzyme is necessary for metabolism of gangliosides, water-soluble glycolipids found primarily in central nervous system (CNS) tissues. Without hexosaminidase A, accumulating lipid pigments distend and progressively destroy and demyelinate CNS cells.

Tay-Sachs disease appears in fewer than 100 neonates born each year in the United States. However, it strikes persons of Eastern European Jewish (Ashkenazi) ancestry about 100 times more often than the general population, occurring in about 1 in 3,600 live births in this ethnic group. About 1 in 30 Ashkenazi Jews, French Canadians, and American Cajuns are heterozygous carriers. If two such carriers have children, each of their offspring has a 25% chance of having Tay-Sachs disease.

## Signs and symptoms

A neonate with classic Tay-Sachs disease appears normal at birth, although he may have an exaggerated Moro reflex. By age 3 to 6 months, he becomes apathetic and responds only to loud sounds. His neck, trunk, arm, and leg muscles grow weaker, and soon he can't sit up or lift his head. He has difficulty turning over, can't grasp objects, and has progressive vision loss.

By age 18 months, the infant is usually deaf and blind and has seizures, generalized paralysis, and spasticity. His pupils are dilated and don't react to light. Decerebrate rigidity and a vegetative state follow. The child suffers recurrent bronchopneumonia after age 2 and usually dies before age 5. A child who survives may develop ataxia and progressive motor retardation between ages 2 and 8.

The "juvenile" form of Tay-Sachs disease generally appears between ages 2 and 5 as a progressive deterioration of psychomotor skills and gait. Patients with this type can survive to adulthood.

## Diagnosis

Typical clinical features point to Tay-Sachs disease, but serum analysis showing deficient hexosaminidase A is the key to diagnosis. An ophthalmologic examination showing optic nerve atrophy and a distinctive cherry-red spot on the retina supports the diagnosis. (The cherry-red spot may be absent in the juvenile form.)

Carrier screening is essential for all couples when at least one partner is of Ashkenazi Jewish, French Canadian, or Cajun ancestry and for others with a family history of the disease. A blood test evaluating hexosaminidase A levels can identify carriers. Amniocentesis or chorionic villus sampling can detect hexosaminidase A deficiency in the fetus.

For two-carrier parents, utilizing in-vitro fertilization to achieve pregnancies, preimplantation genetic testing has been attempted with some success. Healthy embryos are transferred to the woman's uterus.

### Treatment

Tay-Sachs disease has no known cure. Supportive treatment includes tube feedings of nutritional supplements, suctioning and postural drainage to remove pharyngeal secretions, skin care to prevent pressure ulcers in bedridden children, and mild laxatives to relieve neurogenic constipation. Anticonvulsants usually fail to prevent seizures. Because these children need constant physical care, many parents have full-time skilled home nursing care or place them in long-term special care facilities.

### Special considerations

Your most important job is to help the family deal with inevitably progressive illness and death.
● Offer carrier testing to all couples from high-risk ethnic groups.
● Refer the parents for genetic counseling, and stress the importance of amniocentesis in future pregnancies. Refer siblings for screening to determine whether they're carriers. If they are carriers and are adults, refer them for genetic counseling, but stress that there is no danger of transmitting the disease to

offspring if they don't marry another carrier.
● Because the parents of an affected child may feel excessive stress or guilt because of the child's illness and the emotional and financial burden it places on them, refer them for psychological counseling if indicated.
● If the parents care for their child at home, teach them how to do suctioning, postural drainage, and tube feeding. Also teach them how to provide good skin care to prevent pressure ulcers.

For more information on this disease, refer parents to the National Tay-Sachs and Allied Diseases Association.

# TENDINITIS AND BURSITIS

A painful inflammation of tendons and of tendon-muscle attachments to bone, *tendinitis* usually occurs in the shoulder rotator cuff, hip, Achilles tendon, or hamstring.

*Bursitis* is a painful inflammation of one or more of the bursae — closed sacs that are lubricated with small amounts of synovial fluid that facilitate the motion of muscles and tendons over bony prominences. Bursitis usually occurs in the subdeltoid, olecranon, trochanteric, calcaneal, or prepatellar bursae.

### Causes

Tendinitis commonly results from trauma (such as strain during sports activity), another musculoskeletal disorder (rheumatic diseases, congenital defects), postural misalignment, abnormal body development, or hypermobility.

Bursitis usually occurs in middle age from recurring trauma that stresses or pressures a joint or from an inflammatory joint disease (rheumatoid arthritis, gout). Chronic bursitis follows attacks of acute bursitis or repeated trauma and infection. Septic bursitis may result from wound infection or from bacterial invasion of skin over the bursa.

## Signs and symptoms
Tendinitis and bursitis have characteristic signs and symptoms.

### Tendinitis
The patient with tendinitis of the shoulder complains of restricted shoulder movement, especially abduction, and localized pain, which is most severe at night and often interferes with sleep. The pain extends from the acromion (the shoulder's highest point) to the deltoid muscle insertion, predominately in the so-called painful arc — that is, when the patient abducts his arm between 50 and 130 degrees. Fluid accumulation causes swelling.

In calcific tendinitis, calcium deposits in the tendon cause proximal weakness and, if calcium erodes into adjacent bursae, acute calcific bursitis.

### Bursitis
In bursitis, fluid accumulation in the bursae causes irritation, inflammation, sudden or gradual pain, and limited movement. Other symptoms vary according to the affected site. Subdeltoid bursitis impairs arm abduction; prepatellar bursitis (housemaid's knee) produces pain when the patient climbs stairs; hip bursitis makes crossing the legs painful.

## Diagnosis
In tendinitis, X-rays may be normal at first but later show bony fragments, osteophyte sclerosis, or calcium deposits. Arthrography is usually normal, with occasional small irregularities on the undersurface of the tendon.

Diagnosis of tendinitis must rule out other causes of shoulder pain, such as myocardial infarction, cervical spondylosis, and tendon tear or rupture.

Significantly, in tendinitis, heat aggravates shoulder pain; in other painful joint disorders, heat usually provides relief.

Localized pain and inflammation and a history of unusual strain or injury 2 to 3 days before onset of pain are the bases for diagnosing bursitis. During early stages, X-rays are usually normal, except in calcific bursitis, in which X-rays may show calcium deposits.

## Treatment
Therapy to relieve pain includes resting the joint (by immobilization with a sling, splint, or cast), systemic analgesics, application of cold or heat, ultrasound, or local injection of an anesthetic and corticosteroids to reduce inflammation.

A mixture of a corticosteroid and an anesthetic, such as lidocaine, generally provides immediate pain relief. Extended-release injections of a corticosteroid, such as triamcinolone or prednisolone, offer longer pain relief. Until the patient is free of pain and able to perform range-of-motion exercises easily, treatment also includes oral anti-inflammatory agents, such as sulindac and indomethacin. Short-term analgesics include codeine, propoxyphene, acetaminophen with codeine and, occasionally, oxycodone.

### Supplementary treatment
Other treatment measures include fluid removal by aspiration, physical therapy to preserve motion and prevent frozen joints (improvement usually follows in 1 to 4 weeks), and heat therapy; for calcific tendinitis, ice packs. Rarely, calcific tendinitis requires surgical removal of calcium deposits.

Long-term control of chronic bursitis and tendinitis may require changes in lifestyle to prevent recurring joint irritation.

**Special considerations**
• Assess the severity of pain and the range of motion to determine effectiveness of the treatment.
• Before injecting corticosteroids or local anesthetics, ask the patient about drug allergies.
• Before intra-articular injection, scrub the patient's skin thoroughly with povidone-iodine or a comparable solution, and shave the injection site if necessary. After the injection, massage the area to ensure penetration through the tissue and joint space. Apply ice intermittently for about 4 hours to minimize pain. Avoid applying heat to the area for 2 days.

Patient teaching is essential. (See *Tendinitis and bursitis tips.*)

# TESTICULAR CANCER

Malignant testicular tumors primarily affect young to middle-aged men and are the most common solid tumor in this group. (In children, testicular tumors are rare.) Most testicular tumors originate in gonadal cells. About 40% are seminomas — uniform, undifferentiated cells resembling primitive gonadal cells. The rest are nonseminomas — tumor cells showing various degrees of differentiation.

The prognosis varies with the cell type and disease stage. When treated with surgery and radiation, almost all patients with localized disease survive beyond 5 years.

**Causes**
The cause of testicular cancer isn't known, but incidence (which peaks between ages 20 and 40) is higher in men with cryptorchidism (even when surgically corrected) and in men whose mothers used diethylstilbestrol during pregnancy. Testicular cancer is rare in nonwhite males and accounts for fewer than 1% of male cancer deaths.

Testicular cancer spreads through the lymphatic system to the para-aortic, iliac, and mediastinal lymph nodes and may metastasize to the lungs, liver, viscera, and bone.

**Signs and symptoms**
The first sign is usually a firm, painless, smooth testicular mass, varying in size and sometimes producing a sense of testicular heaviness. When such a tumor causes chorionic gonadotropin or estrogen production, gynecomastia and nipple tenderness may result.

In advanced stages, signs and symptoms include ureteral obstruction, ab-

## STAGING TESTICULAR CANCER

The tumor, node, metastasis (TNM) staging system adopted by the American Joint Committee on Cancer has established the following stages for testicular cancer.

### Primary tumor
**TX**—primary tumor can't be assessed (this stage is used in the absence of radical orchiectomy)
**T0**—histologic scar or no evidence of primary tumor
**Tis**—intratubular tumor: preinvasive cancer
**T1**—tumor limited to testicles, including the rete testis
**T2**—tumor extends beyond tunica albuginea or into epididymis
**T3**—tumor extends into spermatic cord
**T4**—tumor invades scrotum

### Regional lymph nodes
**NX**—regional lymph nodes can't be assessed
**N0**—no evidence of regional lymph node metastasis
**N1**—metastasis in a single lymph node, 2 cm or less in greatest dimension

**N2**—metastasis in a single lymph node, between 2 and 5 cm in greatest dimension, or metastases to several lymph nodes, none more than 5 cm in greatest dimension
**N3**—metastasis in a lymph node more than 5 cm in greatest dimension

### Distant metastasis
**MX**—distant metastasis unassessible
**M0**—no known distant metastasis
**M1**—distant metastasis

### Staging categories
Testicular cancer progresses as follows:
**Stage 0**—Tis, N0, M0
**Stage I**—T1, N0, M0; T2, N0, M0
**Stage II**—T3, N0, M0; T4, N0, M0
**Stage III**—any T, N1, M0
**Stage IV**—any T, N2, M0; any T, N3, M0; any T, any N, M1

dominal mass, cough, hemoptysis, shortness of breath, weight loss, fatigue, pallor, and lethargy.

### Diagnosis
• Two effective means of detecting a testicular tumor are regular self-examinations and testicular palpation during a routine physical examination.

• Transillumination can distinguish between a tumor (which doesn't transilluminate) and a hydrocele or spermatocele (which does). Follow-up measures should include an examination for gynecomastia and abdominal masses.

• Diagnostic tests include excretory urography to detect ureteral deviation resulting from para-aortic node in-volvement, urinary or serum luteinizing hormone levels, blood tests, lymphangiography, ultrasound, and abdominal computed tomography scan.

Serum alpha-fetoprotein and beta-human chorionic gonadotropin levels, indicators of testicular tumor activity, provide a baseline for measuring response to therapy and determining the prognosis.

• Surgical excision and biopsy of the tumor and testis permits histologic verification of the tumor cell type — essential for effective treatment. Inguinal exploration determines the extent of nodal involvement. (See *Staging testicular cancer*.)

## Treatment

The extent of surgery, radiation, and chemotherapy varies with tumor cell type and stage.

### Surgery

Surgical procedures include orchiectomy and retroperitoneal node dissection. Most surgeons remove the testis, not the scrotum (to allow for a prosthetic implant). Hormone replacement therapy may be needed after bilateral orchiectomy.

### Radiation

The retroperitoneal and homolateral iliac nodes may receive radiation after removal of a seminoma. All positive nodes receive radiation after removal of a nonseminoma. Patients with retroperitoneal extension receive prophylactic radiation to the mediastinal and supraclavicular nodes.

### Chemotherapy

Essential for tumors beyond Stage 0, chemotherapy combinations include bleomycin, etoposide, and cisplatin; cisplatin, vindesine, and bleomycin; cisplatin, vinblastine, and bleomycin; and cisplatin, vincristine, methotrexate, bleomycin, and leucovorin.

Chemotherapy and radiation followed by autologous bone marrow transplantation may help unresponsive patients.

## Special considerations

● Develop a treatment plan that addresses the patient's psychological and physical needs.

Before orchiectomy:

● Reassure the patient that sterility and impotence need not follow unilateral orchiectomy, that synthetic hormones can restore hormonal balance, and that most surgeons don't remove the scrotum. In many cases, a testicular prosthesis can correct anatomic disfigurement.

After orchiectomy:

● For the first day after surgery, apply an ice pack to the scrotum and provide analgesics.

● Check for excessive bleeding, swelling, and signs of infection.

● Provide a scrotal athletic supporter to minimize pain during ambulation.

During chemotherapy:

● Give antiemetics, as needed, for nausea and vomiting. Encourage small, frequent meals to maintain oral intake despite anorexia.

● Establish a mouth care regimen and check for stomatitis. Watch for signs of myelosuppression.

➤ CLINICAL TIP If the patient receives vinblastine, assess for neurotoxicity (peripheral paresthesia, jaw pain, and muscle cramps). If he receives cisplatin, check for ototoxicity.

● To prevent renal damage, encourage increased fluid intake and provide I.V. fluids, a potassium supplement, and diuretics.

✦ LIFE-THREATENING DISORDER

# TETANUS

Lockjaw or tetanus is an acute exotoxin-mediated infection caused by the anaerobic, spore-forming, gram-positive bacillus *Clostridium tetani*. Usually, such infection is systemic; less often, localized.

Tetanus is fatal in up to 60% of non-immunized persons, usually within 10 days of onset. When symptoms develop within 3 days after exposure, the prognosis is poor.

## Causes

Normally, transmission is through a puncture wound that is contaminated by soil, dust, or animal excreta containing *C. tetani,* or by way of burns and minor wounds. After *C. tetani* enters the body, it causes local infection and tissue necrosis. It also produces toxins that then enter the bloodstream and lymphatics and eventually spread to central nervous system tissue.

Tetanus occurs worldwide, but it's more prevalent in agricultural regions and developing countries that lack mass immunization programs. It's one of the most common causes of neonatal deaths in developing countries, where neonates of unimmunized mothers are delivered under unsterile conditions. In such neonates, the unhealed umbilical cord is the portal of entry.

In America, about 75% of all cases occur between April and September.

## Signs and symptoms

The incubation period varies from 3 to 4 weeks in mild tetanus to less than 2 days in severe tetanus. When symptoms occur within 3 days after injury, death is more likely. If tetanus remains localized, signs of onset are spasm and increased muscle tone near the wound.

If tetanus is generalized (systemic), indications include marked muscle hypertonicity, hyperactive deep tendon reflexes, tachycardia, profuse sweating, low-grade fever, and painful, involuntary muscle contractions:
• neck and facial muscles, especially cheek muscles — locked jaw (trismus) and a grotesque, grinning expression called *risus sardonicus*
• somatic muscles — arched-back rigidity (opisthotonos), boardlike abdominal rigidity
• intermittent tonic convulsions lasting several minutes, which may result in

cyanosis and sudden death by asphyxiation.

Despite such pronounced neuromuscular symptoms, cerebral and sensory functions remain normal. Complications include atelectasis, pneumonia, pulmonary emboli, acute gastric ulcers, flexion contractures, and cardiac arrhythmias.

Neonatal tetanus is always generalized. The first clinical sign is difficulty in sucking, which usually appears 3 to 10 days after birth. It progresses to total inability to suck, with excessive crying, irritability, and nuchal rigidity.

## Diagnosis

Frequently, diagnosis must rest on clinical features and a history of trauma and no previous tetanus immunization. Blood cultures and tetanus antibody tests are often negative; only one-third of patients have a positive wound culture. Cerebrospinal fluid pressure may rise above normal. Diagnosis also must rule out meningitis, rabies, phenothiazine or strychnine toxicity, and other conditions that mimic tetanus.

## Treatment

Within 72 hours after a puncture wound, a patient with no previous history of tetanus immunization first requires tetanus immune globulin (TIG) or tetanus antitoxin to confer temporary protection. Next, he needs active immunization with tetanus toxoid. A patient who has not received tetanus immunization within 5 years needs a booster injection of tetanus toxoid.

If tetanus develops despite immediate postinjury treatment, the patient will require airway maintenance and a muscle relaxant, such as diazepam, to decrease muscle rigidity and spasm. If muscle contractions aren't relieved by muscle relaxants, a neuromuscular blocker may be needed. The patient with tetanus needs high-dose antibiotics (penicillin administered I.V., if he's not allergic to it).

**Special considerations**
When caring for the patient with a puncture wound:

● Thoroughly debride and cleanse the injury site with 3% hydrogen peroxide, and check the patient's immunization history. Record the cause of injury. If it's a dog bite, report the case to local public health authorities.

● Before giving penicillin and TIG, antitoxin, or toxoid, obtain an accurate history of allergies to immunizations or penicillin. If the patient has a history of any allergies, keep epinephrine 1:1,000 and resuscitative equipment available.

● Stress the importance of maintaining active immunization with a booster dose of tetanus toxoid every 10 years.

After tetanus develops:

● Maintain an adequate airway and ventilation to prevent pneumonia and atelectasis. Suction often and watch for signs of respiratory distress. Keep emergency airway equipment on hand because the patient may require artificial ventilation or oxygen administration.

● Maintain an I.V. line for medications and emergency care if necessary.

● Monitor electrocardiography frequently for arrhythmias. Accurately record intake and output, and check vital signs often.

● Turn the patient frequently to prevent pressure sores and pulmonary stasis.

● Because even minimal external stimulation provokes muscle spasms, keep the patient's room dark and quiet. Warn visitors not to upset or overly stimulate the patient.

● If urinary retention develops, insert an indwelling urinary catheter.

● Give muscle relaxants and sedatives as ordered, and schedule patient care to coincide with heaviest sedation.

● Insert an artificial airway, if necessary, to prevent tongue injury and maintain airway during spasms.

● Provide adequate nutrition to meet the patient's increased metabolic needs. The patient may need nasogastric feedings or hyperalimentation.

# THROMBOCYTOPENIA

The most common cause of hemorrhagic disorders, thrombocytopenia is characterized by deficiency of circulating platelets. Because platelets play a vital role in coagulation, this disease poses a serious threat to hemostasis.

The prognosis is excellent in drug-induced thrombocytopenia if the offending drug is withdrawn; in such cases, recovery may be immediate. Otherwise, the prognosis depends on response to treatment of the underlying cause. (See *Precautions in thrombocytopenia.*)

**Causes**
Thrombocytopenia may be congenital or acquired; the acquired form is more common. In either case, it usually results from the following:

● decreased or defective production of platelets in the marrow (such as occurs in leukemia, aplastic anemia, or toxicity with certain drugs)

● increased destruction outside the marrow caused by an underlying disorder (such as cirrhosis of the liver, disseminated intravascular coagulation, or severe infection)

● less commonly, sequestration (hypersplenism, hypothermia) or platelet loss.

Acquired thrombocytopenia may result from certain drugs, such as nonsteroidal anti-inflammatory agents, sulfonamides, histamine blockers, alky-

TEACHING CHECKLIST

## PRECAUTIONS IN THROMBOCYTOPENIA

- Warn the patient to avoid aspirin in any form, and other drugs that impair coagulation. Teach him how to recognize aspirin or ibuprofen compounds on labels of over-the-counter remedies.
- Advise the patient to avoid straining at stool or coughing because both can lead to increased intracranial pressure, possibly causing cerebral hemorrhage in the patient with thrombocytopenia. Provide a stool softener to prevent constipation.

- If thrombocytopenia is drug-induced, stress the importance of avoiding the offending drug.
- If the patient must receive long-term steroid therapy, teach him to watch for and report cushingoid symptoms (acne, moon face, hirsutism, buffalo hump, hypertension, girdle obesity, thinning arms and legs, glycosuria, and edema). Emphasize that steroid doses must be discontinued gradually.

---

lating agents, or antibiotic chemotherapeutic agents.

An idiopathic form of thrombocytopenia commonly occurs in children. A transient form may follow viral infections (Epstein-Barr or infectious mononucleosis).

### Signs and symptoms
Thrombocytopenia typically produces a sudden onset of petechiae or ecchymoses in the skin or bleeding into any mucous membrane. Nearly all patients are otherwise asymptomatic, although some may complain of malaise, fatigue, and general weakness.

In adults, large blood-filled bullae characteristically appear in the mouth. In severe thrombocytopenia, hemorrhage may lead to tachycardia, shortness of breath, loss of consciousness, and death.

### Diagnosis
To diagnose thrombocytopenia, obtain a patient history (especially a drug history), a physical examination, and the following laboratory tests:

- *Coagulation tests* reveal a decreased platelet count (in adults, < 100,000/µl), prolonged bleeding time, and normal prothrombin time and partial thromboplastin time.
- If increased destruction of platelets is causing thrombocytopenia, *bone marrow studies* will reveal a greater number of megakaryocytes (platelet precursors) and shortened platelet survival (several hours or days rather than the usual 7 to 10 days).

### Treatment
Effective treatment varies with the underlying cause and may include corticosteroids or immune globulin to increase platelet production. When possible, treatment consists of correction of the underlying cause or, in drug-induced thrombocytopenia, removal of the offending agents. Platelet transfusions are helpful in thrombocytopenia only in treating complications of severe hemorrhage.

## Special considerations

• When caring for the patient with thrombocytopenia, take every possible precaution against bleeding.

• Protect the patient from trauma. Keep the side rails up, and pad them if possible. Promote the use of an electric razor and a soft toothbrush. Avoid invasive procedures, such as venipuncture or urinary catheterization, if possible. When venipuncture is unavoidable, be sure to exert pressure on the puncture site for at least 20 minutes or until the bleeding stops.

• Monitor platelet count daily.

• Test stool for guaiac; dipstick urine and emesis for blood.

• Watch for bleeding (petechiae, ecchymoses, surgical or GI bleeding, menorrhagia).

• During periods of active bleeding, maintain the patient on strict bed rest if necessary.

• When administering platelet concentrate, remember that platelets are extremely fragile, so infuse them quickly. Do not give platelets to a patient with a fever.

• During platelet transfusion, monitor for febrile reaction (flushing, chills, fever, headache, tachycardia, hypertension). HLA-typed platelets may prevent febrile reaction.

> **CLINICAL TIP** A patient with a history of minor reactions may benefit from acetaminophen and diphenhydramine before transfusion.

• During steroid therapy, monitor fluid and electrolyte balance, and watch for infection, pathologic fractures, and mood changes.

• A 1- to 2-hour postplatelet count will aid assessment of response.

# THROMBOPHLEBITIS

An acute condition characterized by inflammation and thrombus formation, thrombophlebitis may occur in deep (intermuscular or intramuscular) or superficial (subcutaneous [S.C.]) veins.

*Deep-vein thrombophlebitis* affects small veins, such as the soleal venous sinuses, or large veins, such as the vena cava, and the femoral, iliac, and subclavian veins. This disorder is frequently progressive, leading to pulmonary embolism, a potentially lethal complication.

*Superficial thrombophlebitis* is usually self-limiting and rarely leads to pulmonary embolism. Thrombophlebitis often begins with localized inflammation alone (phlebitis), but such inflammation rapidly provokes thrombus formation. Rarely, venous thrombosis develops without associated inflammation of the vein (phlebothrombosis).

## Causes

A thrombus occurs when an alteration in the epithelial lining causes platelet aggregation and consequent fibrin entrapment of red blood cells, white blood cells, and additional platelets. Thrombus formation is more rapid in areas where blood flow is slower, due to greater contact between platelets and thrombin accumulation.

The rapidly expanding thrombus initiates a chemical inflammatory process in the vessel epithelium that leads to fibrosis. The enlarging clot may occlude the vessel lumen partially or totally, or it may detach and embolize, to lodge elsewhere in the systemic circulation.

### Deep-vein thrombophlebitis

This type of thrombophlebitis may be idiopathic, but it usually results from endothelial damage, accelerated blood clotting, and reduced blood flow. Predisposing factors are prolonged bed rest, trauma, surgery, childbirth, and use of oral contraceptives such as estrogens.

### Superficial thrombophlebitis

Causes of superficial thrombophlebitis include trauma, infection, I.V. drug abuse, and chemical irritation due to the extensive use of the I.V. route for medications and diagnostic tests.

## Signs and symptoms

In both types of thrombophlebitis, clinical features vary with the site and length of the affected vein. Although deep-vein thrombophlebitis may occur asymptomatically, it may also produce severe pain, fever, chills, malaise and, possibly, swelling and cyanosis of the affected arm or leg.

Superficial thrombophlebitis produces visible and palpable signs, such as heat, pain, swelling, rubor, tenderness, and induration along the length of the affected vein. Extensive vein involvement may cause lymphadenitis.

## Diagnosis

Some patients may display signs of inflammation and, possibly, a positive Homans' sign (pain on dorsiflexion of the foot) during physical examination; others are asymptomatic. Consequently, essential laboratory tests include the following:

• *Doppler ultrasonography* is used to identify reduced blood flow to a specific area and any obstruction to venous flow, particularly in iliofemoral deep-vein thrombophlebitis.

• *Plethysmography* shows decreased circulation distal to affected area; it's more sensitive than ultrasound in detecting deep-vein thrombophlebitis.

• *Phlebography* can show filling defects and diverted blood flow and usually confirms the diagnosis.

Diagnosis must rule out arterial occlusive disease, lymphangitis, cellulitis, and myositis.

Diagnosis of superficial thrombophlebitis is based on physical examination (redness and warmth over affected area, palpable vein, and pain during palpation or compression).

## Treatment

The goals of treatment are to control thrombus development, prevent complications, relieve pain, and prevent recurrence of the disorder. Symptomatic measures include bed rest, with elevation of the affected arm or leg; warm, moist soaks to the affected area; and analgesics.

### Deep-vein thrombophlebitis

After the acute episode of deep-vein thrombophlebitis subsides, the patient may resume activity while wearing antiembolism stockings that were applied before he got out of bed.

Treatment may also include anticoagulants (initially, heparin; later, warfarin) to prolong clotting time. Full anticoagulant dose must be discontinued during any operative period, due to the risk of hemorrhage.

After some types of surgery, especially major abdominal or pelvic operations, prophylactic doses of anticoagulants may reduce the risk of deep-vein thrombophlebitis and pulmonary embolism. For lysis of acute, extensive deep-vein thrombosis, treatment should include streptokinase.

Rarely, deep-vein thrombophlebitis may cause complete venous occlusion, which necessitates venous interruption through simple ligation to vein plication, or clipping. Embolectomy and insertion of a vena caval umbrella or filter may also be done.

### *Superficial thrombophlebitis*
Therapy for severe superficial thrombophlebitis includes an anti-inflammatory drug such as indomethacin, antiembolism stockings, warm soaks, and elevation of the leg.

### Special considerations
● Patient teaching, identification of high-risk patients, and measures to prevent venostasis can prevent deep-vein thrombophlebitis; close monitoring of anticoagulant therapy can prevent serious complications such as internal hemorrhage.
● Enforce bed rest, and elevate the patient's affected arm or leg. If you plan to use pillows for elevating the leg, place them so they support the entire length of the affected leg to prevent possible compression of the popliteal space.
● Apply warm soaks to increase circulation to the affected area and to relieve pain and inflammation. Give analgesics to relieve pain.
● Measure and record the circumference of the affected arm or leg daily, and compare this measurement to the other arm or leg. To ensure accuracy and consistency of serial measurements, mark the skin over the area and measure at the same spot daily.
● Administer heparin I.V. with an infusion monitor or pump to control the flow rate if necessary.

➤ CLINICAL TIP Measure partial thromboplastin time regularly for the patient receiving heparin therapy, and prothrombin time (PT) and International Normalized Ratio (INR) for the patient receiving warfarin (therapeutic anticoagulation values for both

are 1½ to 2 times control values, and INR is 2 to 3 times control values).
● Watch for signs and symptoms of bleeding, such as coffee-ground vomitus, ecchymoses, and black, tarry stools. Encourage the patient to use an electric razor and to avoid medications that contain aspirin.
● Be alert for signs of pulmonary emboli (rales, dyspnea, hemoptysis, sudden changes in mental status, restlessness, and hypotension).
To prepare the patient with thrombophlebitis for discharge:
● Emphasize the importance of follow-up blood studies to monitor anticoagulant therapy.
● If the patient is being discharged on heparin therapy, teach him or his family how to give S.C. injections. If he requires further assistance, arrange for a visiting nurse.
● Tell the patient to avoid prolonged sitting or standing to help prevent recurrence.
● Teach the patient how to properly apply and use antiembolism stockings. Tell him to report any complications such as cold, blue toes.
● To prevent thrombophlebitis in high-risk patients, perform range-of-motion exercises while the patient is on bed rest, use intermittent pneumatic calf massage during lengthy surgical or diagnostic procedures, apply antiembolism stockings postoperatively, and encourage early ambulation.

# THYROID CANCER

Cancer of the thyroid occurs in all age groups, especially in persons who have had radiation treatment to the neck area. Papillary and follicular carcinomas are most common and are usually associated with prolonged survival.

*Papillary carcinoma* accounts for half of all thyroid cancers in adults; it's most common in young adult females and metastasizes slowly. It's the least virulent form of thyroid cancer. *Follicular carcinoma* is less common but more likely to recur and metastasize to the regional nodes and through blood vessels into the bones, liver, and lungs.

*Medullary carcinoma* originates in the parafollicular cells derived from the last branchial pouch and contains amyloid and calcium deposits. It can produce calcitonin, histaminase, corticotropin (producing Cushing's syndrome), and prostaglandin $E_2$ and $F_3$ (producing diarrhea).

This rare form of thyroid cancer is familial, associated with pheochromocytoma, and completely curable when detected before it causes symptoms. Untreated, it progresses rapidly.

Seldom curable by resection, *giant and spindle cell cancer* (anaplastic tumor) resists radiation and metastasizes rapidly.

## Causes

Predisposing factors include radiation exposure, prolonged thyrotropin stimulation (through radiation or heredity), familial predisposition, or chronic goiter.

## Signs and symptoms

The primary signs of thyroid cancer are a painless nodule, a hard nodule in an enlarged thyroid gland, or palpable lymph nodes with thyroid enlargement. Eventually, the pressure of such a nodule or enlargement causes hoarseness, dysphagia, dyspnea, and pain on palpation.

If the tumor is large enough to destroy the gland, hypothyroidism follows, with its typical symptoms of low metabolism (mental apathy and sensitivity to cold). However, if the tumor stimulates excess thyroid hormone production, it induces symptoms of thyrotoxicosis (sensitivity to heat, restlessness, and hyperactivity).

Other clinical features include diarrhea, anorexia, irritability, vocal cord paralysis, and symptoms of distant metastasis.

## Diagnosis

The first clue to thyroid cancer is usually an enlarged, palpable node in the thyroid gland, neck, lymph nodes of the neck, or vocal cords. A patient history of radiation therapy or a family history of thyroid cancer supports the diagnosis. However, tests must rule out nonmalignant thyroid enlargements, which are more common.

• *Thyroid scan* differentiates between functional nodes (rarely malignant) and hypofunctional nodes (commonly malignant) by measuring how readily nodules trap isotopes compared with the rest of the thyroid gland. In thyroid cancer, the scintiscan shows a "cold," nonfunctioning nodule.

• Other tests include needle biopsy, computed tomography scan, ultrasonic scan, chest X-ray, serum alkaline phosphatase, and serum calcitonin assay to diagnose medullary cancer. Calcitonin assay is a reliable clue to silent medullary carcinoma. (See *Staging thyroid cancer,* page 860.)

## Treatment

• Total or subtotal thyroidectomy, with modified node dissection (bilateral or unilateral) on the side of the primary cancer (papillary or follicular cancer)

• Total thyroidectomy and radical neck excision (for medullary, giant, or spindle cell cancer)

• Radiation ($^{131}I$) with external radiation (for inoperable cancer and sometimes postoperatively in lieu of radical neck excision) or alone (for metastasis)

# STAGING THYROID CANCER

The classification and staging systems adopted by the American Joint Committee on Cancer describe thyroid cancer according to the tumor's (T) size and extent at its origin, its invasion of regional (cervical and upper mediastinal) lymph nodes (N), and the disease's metastasis (M) to other structures,

## Primary tumor

*TX* — primary tumor can't be assessed

*T0* — no evidence of primary tumor

*T1* — tumor 1 cm or less in greatest dimension and limited to the thyroid

T2 — tumor > 1 cm but < 4 cm in greatest dimension and limited to the thyroid

*T3* — tumor > 4 cm and limited to the thyroid

*T4* — tumor (any size) extends beyond the thyroid

## Regional lymph nodes

*NX*— regional lymph nodes can't be assessed

*N0* — no evidence of regional lymph node metastasis

*N1* — regional lymph node metastasis

*N1a* — metastasis in ipsilateral cervical nodes

*N1b* — metastasis in bilateral, midline, or contralateral cervical or mediastinal lymph nodes

## Distant metastasis

*MX* — distant metastasis can't be assessed

*M0* — no evidence of distant metastasis

*M1* — distant metastasis

## Staging categories for papillary or follicular cancer

Papillary or follicular cancer progresses from mild to severe as follows:

*Stage I* — any T, any N, M0 (patient under age 45); T1, N0, M0 (patient age 45 or over)

*Stage II* — any T any N, M1 (patient under age 45); T2, N0, M0; T3, N0, M0 (patient age 45 or over)

*Stage III* — T4, N0, M0; any T, N1, M0 (patient age 45 or over)

*Stage IV* — any T, any N, M1 (patient age 45 or over)

## Staging categories for medullary cancer

Medullary cancer progresses from mild to severe as follows:

*Stage I* — T1, N0, M0

*Stage II* — T2, N0, M0; T3, N0, M0; T4, N0, M0

*Stage III* — any T, N1, M0

*Stage IV* — any T, any N, M1

Staging categories for undifferentiated cancer

All cases are Stage IV.

*Stage IV* — any T, any N, any M

---

• Adjunctive thyroid suppression, with exogenous thyroid hormones suppressing thyrotropin production, and simultaneous administration of an adrenergic blocking agent, such as propranolol, increasing tolerance to surgery and radiation

• Chemotherapy for symptomatic, widespread metastasis is limited, but doxorubicin is sometimes beneficial.

## Special considerations

• Before surgery, tell the patient to expect temporary voice loss or hoarseness lasting several days after surgery.

Postoperative care:

• When the patient regains consciousness, keep him in semi-Fowler's position, with his head neither hyperextended nor flexed, to avoid pressure on the suture line. Support the patient's head and neck with sandbags and pillows; when you move him, continue this support with your hands.

- After monitoring vital signs, check the patient's dressing, neck, and back for bleeding. If he complains that the dressing feels tight, loosen it.
- Check serum calcium levels daily; hypocalcemia may develop if parathyroid glands are removed.
- Watch for and report other complications: hemorrhage and shock (elevated pulse rate and hypotension), tetany (carpopedal spasm, twitching, and seizures), thyroid storm (high fever, severe tachycardia, delirium, dehydration, and extreme irritability), and respiratory obstruction (dyspnea, crowing respirations, retraction of neck tissues).
- Keep a tracheotomy set and oxygen equipment handy in case of respiratory obstruction. Use continuous steam inhalation in the patients room until his chest is clear.
- The patient may need I.V. fluids or a soft diet, but many patients can tolerate a regular diet within 24 hours of surgery.
- Care of the patient after extensive tumor and node excision is identical to other radical neck postoperative care.

# THYROIDITIS

Inflammation of the thyroid gland occurs as autoimmune thyroiditis (long-term inflammatory disease), postpartum thyroiditis, subacute granulomatous thyroiditis (self-limiting inflammation), Riedel's thyroiditis (rare, invasive fibrotic process), and miscellaneous thyroiditis (acute suppurative, chronic infective, and chronic noninfective). Thyroiditis is more common in women than in men.

## Causes
*Autoimmune thyroiditis* is due to antibodies to thyroid antigens. It may cause inflammation and lymphocytic infiltration (Hashimoto's thyroiditis). Glandular atrophy and Graves' disease are linked to autoimmune thyroiditis.

*Postpartum thyroiditis* (silent thyroiditis) is another form of autoimmune thyroiditis that occurs in women within 1 year after delivery.

*Subacute granulomatous thyroiditis* usually follows mumps. influenza, coxsackievirus, or adenovirus infection. *Riedel's thyroiditis* is a rare condition of unknown etiology.

*Miscellaneous thyroiditis* results from bacterial invasion of the gland in acute suppurative thyroiditis; tuberculosis, syphilis, actinomycosis, or other infectious agents in the chronic infective form; and sarcoidosis and amyloidosis in chronic noninfective thyroiditis.

## Signs and symptoms
Autoimmune thyroiditis is usually asymptomatic and commonly occurs in women, with peak incidence in middle age. It's the most prevalent cause of spontaneous hypothyroidism.

In subacute granulomatous thyroiditis, moderate thyroid enlargement may follow an upper respiratory tract infection or a sore throat. The thyroid may be painful and tender, and dysphagia may occur.

In Riedel's thyroiditis, the gland enlarges slowly as it is replaced by hard, fibrous tissues. This fibrosis may compress the trachea or the esophagus. The thyroid feels firm.

Clinical effects of miscellaneous thyroiditis are characteristic of pyogenic infection: fever, pain, tenderness, and reddened skin over the gland.

## Diagnosis

Precise diagnosis depends on the type of thyroiditis:

• *autoimmune:* high titers of thyroglobulin and microsomal antibodies present in serum

• *subacute granulomatous:* elevated erythrocyte sedimentation rate, increased thyroid hormone levels, decreased thyroidal radioactive iodine uptake

• *chronic infective and noninfective:* varied findings, depending on underlying infection or other disease.

## Treatment

Appropriate treatment varies with the type of thyroiditis. Drug therapy includes levothyroxine for accompanying hypothyroidism, analgesics and anti-inflammatory drugs for mild subacute granulomatous thyroiditis, propranolol for transient thyrotoxicosis, and steroids for severe episodes of acute inflammation. Suppurative thyroiditis requires antibiotic therapy.

A partial thyroidectomy may be necessary to relieve tracheal or esophageal compression in Riedel's thyroiditis.

## Special considerations

• Before treatment, obtain a patient history to identify underlying diseases that may cause thyroiditis, such as tuberculosis or a recent viral infection.

• Check vital signs, and examine the patient's neck for unusual swelling, enlargement, or redness. Provide a liquid diet if the patient has difficulty swallowing, especially when due to fibrosis. If the neck is swollen, measure and record the circumference daily to monitor progressive enlargement.

• In suppurative thyroiditis, administer antibiotics, and report and record elevations in temperature.

• Instruct the patient to watch for and report signs of hypothyroidism (lethargy, restlessness, sensitivity to cold, forgetfulness, dry skin) — especially if he has Hashimoto's thyroiditis, which often causes hypothyroidism.

• Check for signs of thyrotoxicosis (nervousness, tremor, weakness), which often occur in subacute thyroiditis.

• After thyroidectomy, check vital signs every 15 to 30 minutes until the patient's condition stabilizes. Stay alert for signs of tetany secondary to accidental parathyroid injury during surgery. Keep 10% calcium gluconate available for I.M. use if needed.

• Assess dressings frequently for excessive bleeding. Watch for signs of airway obstruction, such as difficulty talking or increased swallowing; keep tracheotomy equipment handy.

• Explain to the patient that lifelong thyroid hormone replacement therapy is necessary if permanent hypothyroidism occurs. (Many patients will have transient hypothyroidism as the gland recovers from subacute thyroiditis.) Tell the patient to watch for signs of an overdose, such as nervousness and palpitations.

# THYROTOXICOSIS

Thyrotoxicosis is a metabolic imbalance that results from thyroid hormone overproduction or thyroid hormone over-release from the gland. The most common form of thyrotoxicosis is Graves' disease, which increases thyroxine production, enlarges the thyroid gland (goiter), and causes multiple system changes. (See *Other forms of thyrotoxicosis.*)

Incidence of Graves' disease is highest between ages 30 and 40, especially in people with family histories of thyroid abnormalities; only 5% of patients

# OTHER FORMS OF THYROTOXICOSIS

Varied forms of thyrotoxicosis may include the following.

## Toxic adenoma

This small, benign nodule in the thyroid gland that secretes thyroid hormone is a common cause of thyrotoxicosis. The cause of toxic adenoma is unknown. Clinical effects are essentially similar to those of Graves' disease, except that toxic adenoma doesn't induce ophthalmopathy, pretibial myxedema, or acropachy.

Presence of adenoma is confirmed by iodine 131 ($^{131}$I) uptake and a thyroid scan, which show a single hyperfunctioning nodule suppressing the rest of the gland. Treatment includes $^{131}$I therapy or surgery to remove adenoma after antithyroid drugs achieve a euthyroid state.

## Toxic multinodular goiter

Common in the elderly, this form of thyrotoxicosis involves overproduction of thyroid hormone by one or more autonomously functioning nodules within a diffusely enlarged gland.

## Thyrotoxicosis factitia

This form of thyrotoxicosis results from a chronic ingestion of thyroid hormone for thyrotropin suppression in patients with thyroid carcinoma, or from thyroid hormone abuse by persons who are trying to lose weight.

## Functioning metastatic thyroid carcinoma

This rare disease causes excess production of thyroid hormone.

## TSH-secreting pituitary tumor

A pituitary tumor that secretes thyroid-stimulating hormone (TSH) causes overproduction of thyroid hormone.

## Subacute thyroiditis

This is a virus-induced granulomatous inflammation of the thyroid, producing transient thyrotoxicosis associated with fever, pain, pharyngitis, and tenderness in the thyroid gland.

## Silent thyroiditis

Self-limiting, silent thyroiditis is a transient form of thyrotoxicosis, with histologic thyroiditis but no inflammatory symptoms.

---

with thyrotoxicosis are younger than age 15.

With treatment, most patients can lead normal lives. However, thyroid storm — an acute, severe exacerbation of thyrotoxicosis — is a medical emergency that may lead to life-threatening cardiac, hepatic, or renal consequences.

## Causes

Thyrotoxicosis may result from genetic and immunologic factors.

● An increased incidence of this disorder in monozygotic twins points to an inherited factor, probably an autosomal recessive gene.

● This disease occasionally coexists with other endocrine abnormalities, such as diabetes mellitus, thyroiditis, and hyperparathyroidism.

● Thyrotoxicosis may also be caused by the production of autoantibodies (thyroid-stimulating immunoglobulin and thyroid-stimulating hormone [TSH]-binding inhibitory immunoglobulin), possibly because of a defect in suppressor-T-lymphocyte function that allows the formation of autoantibodies.

● In latent thyrotoxicosis, excessive dietary intake of iodine and, possibly, stress can precipitate clinical thyrotoxicosis.

• In a person with inadequately treated thyrotoxicosis, stress — including surgery, infection, toxemia of pregnancy, and diabetic ketoacidosis — can precipitate thyroid storm.

## Signs and symptoms

The classic features of Graves' disease are an enlarged thyroid (goiter), nervousness, heat intolerance, weight loss despite increased appetite, sweating, frequent bowel movements, tremor, and palpitations. Exophthalmos is considered most characteristic but is absent in many patients with thyrotoxicosis.

Many other signs and symptoms are common because thyrotoxicosis profoundly affects virtually every body system:

• *Central nervous system:* difficulty in concentrating because increased thyroxine secretion accelerates cerebral function; excitability or nervousness due to increased basal metabolic rate; fine tremor, shaky handwriting, and clumsiness from increased activity in the spinal cord area that controls muscle tone; emotional instability and mood swings, ranging from occasional outbursts to overt psychosis

• *Skin, hair, and nails:* smooth, warm, flushed skin (patient sleeps with minimal covers and little clothing); fine, soft hair; premature graying and increased hair loss in both sexes; friable nails and onycholysis (distal nail separated from the bed); pretibial myxedema (dermopathy), producing thickened skin; and accentuated hair follicles, raised red patches of skin that are itchy and sometimes painful, with occasional nodule formation. Microscopic examination shows increased mucin deposits.

• *Cardiovascular system:* tachycardia; full, bounding pulse; wide pulse pressure; cardiomegaly; increased cardiac output and blood volume; visible point of maximal impulse; paroxysmal supraventricular tachycardia and atrial fibrillation (especially in elderly people); and, occasionally, a systolic murmur at the left sternal border

• *Respiratory system:* dyspnea on exertion and at rest, possibly from cardiac decompensation and increased cellular oxygen utilization

• *GI system:* excessive oral intake with weight loss; nausea and vomiting due to increased GI motility and peristalsis; increased defecation; soft stools or, with severe disease, diarrhea; and liver enlargement

• *Musculoskeletal system:* weakness (especially in proximal muscles), fatigue, and muscle atrophy; rare coexistence with myasthenia gravis; possibly generalized or localized paralysis associated with hypokalemia; and occasional acropachy (soft-tissue swelling, accompanied by underlying bone changes where new bone formation occurs)

• *Reproductive system:* in females, oligomenorrhea or amenorrhea, decreased fertility, higher incidence of spontaneous abortions; in males, gynecomastia due to increased estrogen levels; in both sexes, diminished libido

• *Eyes:* exophthalmos (produced by the combined effects of accumulation of mucopolysaccharides and fluids in the retroorbital tissues that force the eyeball outward, and of lid retraction that produces the characteristic staring gaze); occasional inflammation of conjunctivae, corneas, or eye muscles; diplopia; and increased tearing.

When thyrotoxicosis escalates to thyroid storm, these symptoms can be accompanied by extreme irritability, hypertension, tachycardia, vomiting, temperature up to 106° F (41.1° C), delirium, and coma.

> CLINICAL TIP  In elderly patients, consider apathetic thyrotoxicosis

in patients who exhibit atrial fibrillation or depression.

## Diagnosis

The diagnosis of thyrotoxicosis usually is straightforward and depends on a careful clinical history and physical examination, a high index of suspicion, and routine hormone determinations. The following tests confirm the disorder:

• *Radioimmunoassay* shows increased serum thyroxine ($T_4$) and triiodothyronine ($T_3$) concentrations.

• *Thyroid scan* reveals increased uptake of radioactive iodine 131 ($^{131}I$) in Graves' disease, and usually in toxic multinodular goiter and toxic adenoma. Radioactive uptake is low in thyroiditis and thyrotoxic factitia. This test is contraindicated if the patient is pregnant.

• *TSH levels* are decreased.

• *Thyroid-releasing hormone (TRH) stimulation test* indicates thyrotoxicosis if the TSH level fails to rise within 30 minutes after the administration of TRH. TRH testing is rarely necessary and is currently done to highly sensitive TSH assays.

• *Ultrasonography* confirms subclinical ophthalmopathy.

## Treatment

A number of approaches are utilized for the treatment of thyrotoxicosis. The primary forms of therapy include antithyroid drugs, $^{131}I$, and surgery. Appropriate treatment depends on the size of the goiter, the causes, the patient's age and parity, and how long surgery will be delayed (if the patient is an appropriate candidate for surgery).

### Antithyroid therapy

Therapy with antithyroid drugs is used for children, young adults, pregnant women, and patients who refuse surgery or $^{131}I$ treatment. Antithyroid drugs are also used to correct the thyrotoxic state in preparation for $^{131}I$ treatment or surgery. Treatment options include the following:

• Thyroid hormone antagonists include propylthiouracil and methimazole, which block thyroid hormone synthesis. Although hypermetabolic symptoms subside within 4 to 8 weeks after such therapy begins, the patient must continue the medication for 6 months to 2 years, in an attempt to achieve remission in Graves' disease.

• Propranolol may be given concomitantly to manage tachycardia and other peripheral effects of excessive hypersympathetic activity. Propranolol blocks the conversion of $T_4$ to the active $T_3$ hormone.

• During pregnancy, antithyroid medication should be kept at the minimum dosage required to keep maternal thyroid function within the high-normal range until delivery and to minimize the risk of fetal hypothyroidism. Propylthiouracil is the preferred agent for the pregnant patient.

Most infants of hyperthyroid mothers are born with mild and transient thyrotoxicosis, caused by placental transfer of thyroid-stimulating immunoglobulins. Neonatal thyrotoxicosis may even necessitate treatment with antithyroid medications and propranolol for 2 to 3 months.

Because thyrotoxicosis is sometimes exacerbated in the puerperal period, continuous control of maternal thyroid function is essential. Approximately 3 to 6 months postpartum, antithyroid drug administration can be gradually tapered and thyroid function reassessed.

The mother receiving low-dose antithyroid treatment may breast-feed as long as the infant's thyroid function is checked periodically. Small amounts of the drug can be found in breast milk.

## *131I*

The treatment of choice for patients not planning to have children is a single oral dose of $^{131}$I. (Patients of reproductive age must give informed consent for this treatment, since small amounts of $^{131}$I concentrate in the gonads.)

During treatment with $^{131}$I, the thyroid gland picks up the radioactive element as it would regular iodine. Subsequently, the radioactivity destroys some of the cells that normally concentrate iodine and produce $T_4$, thus decreasing thyroid hormone production and normalizing thyroid size and function.

In most patients, hypermetabolic symptoms diminish from 6 to 8 weeks after such treatment. However, some patients may require a second dose of $^{131}$I.

> CLINICAL TIP   Patients commonly become permanently hypothyroid after $^{131}$I ablation.

## *Surgery*

Near-total thyroidectomy, which decreases the thyroid gland's capacity for hormone production, is indicated for patients whose thyrotoxicosis has repeatedly relapsed after drug therapy or patients who refuse or aren't candidates for $^{131}$I treatment.

Preoperatively, the patient may receive iodides (Lugol's solution or saturated solution of potassium iodide), antithyroid drugs, and propranolol to help prevent thyroid storm. If euthyroidism isn't achieved, surgery should be delayed, and antithyroid drugs and propranolol should be administered to decrease the systemic effects (such as cardiac arrhythmias) caused by thyrotoxicosis.

After surgery, patients require regular medical supervision for the rest of their lives because they usually develop hypothyroidism, sometimes as long as several years after treatment.

### *Treatment for ophthalmopathy*

Therapy includes local application of topical medications but may require high doses of corticosteroids. A patient with severe exophthalmos that causes pressure on the optic nerve may require external-beam radiation therapy or surgical decompression to lessen pressure on the orbital contents.

### *Treatment for thyroid storm*

This includes administration of an antithyroid drug, propranolol I.V. or by mouth, to block sympathetic effects and conversion of $T_4$ to $T_3$. Corticosteroids also inhibit the conversion of $T_4$ to $T_3$, and an iodide is used to block release of thyroid hormone.

Supportive measures include administration of nutrients, vitamins, fluids, and sedatives.

### Special considerations

Patients with thyrotoxicosis require vigilant care to prevent acute exacerbations and complications.

- Record vital signs and weight.
- Monitor serum electrolytes, and check periodically for hyperglycemia and glycosuria.
- Carefully monitor cardiac function if the patient is elderly or has coronary artery disease. If the heart rate is more than 100 beats/minute, check blood pressure and pulse rate often.
- Check the patient's level of consciousness and urine output.
- If the patient is pregnant, tell her to watch closely during the first trimester for signs of spontaneous abortion (spotting, occasional mild cramps) and report such signs immediately.
- The patient with dyspnea will be most comfortable sitting upright or in high Fowler's position.

• Remember, severe thyrotoxicosis may produce bizarre behavior. Reassure the patient and his family that such behavior will probably subside with treatment. Provide sedatives as necessary, and encourage the patient to verbalize his feelings about changes in body image.

• If iodide is part of the treatment, mix it with milk, juice, or water to prevent GI distress, and administer it through a straw to prevent tooth discoloration.

> CLINICAL TIP Administer preparations containing iodine only after antithyroid drugs have been initiated. Otherwise, the iodine will be utilized by the already overactive gland to make more thyroid hormone and worsen the toxic state.

• Watch for signs of thyroid storm (tachycardia, hyperkinesis, fever, vomiting, hypertension).

• Check intake and output carefully to ensure adequate hydration and fluid balance.

• Closely monitor blood pressure, cardiac rate and rhythm, and temperature. If the patient has a high fever, reduce it with appropriate hypothermic measures. Maintain an I.V. line and give drugs as needed.

• If the patient has exophthalmos or another ophthalmopathy, suggest eye patches to protect his eyes from dryness at night. Moisten the conjunctivae often with isotonic eyedrops. Instruct him to report signs of decreased visual acuity.

• Avoid excessive palpation of the thyroid to avoid precipitating thyroid storm. After thyroidectomy:

• Check often for respiratory distress, and keep a tracheotomy tray at bedside.

• Watch for evidence of hemorrhage into the neck, such as a tight dressing with no blood on it. Change dressings and perform wound care; check the *back* of the dressing for drainage. Keep the patient in semi-Fowler's position, and support his head and neck with sandbags to ease tension on the incision.

• Check for dysphagia or hoarseness from possible laryngeal nerve injury.

• Watch for signs of hypoparathyroidism (tetany, numbness), a complication that results from accidental removal of the parathyroid glands during surgery.

• Stress the importance of regular medical follow-up after discharge because hypothyroidism may develop from 2 to 4 weeks postoperatively.

Drug therapy and $^{131}$I therapy require careful monitoring and comprehensive patient teaching as follows:

• After $^{131}$I therapy, tell the patient not to allow people close to his neck because the radiation is concentrated there. Also, tell patients to keep people away from his bladder area where unabsorbed $^{131}$I accumulates before excretion. These cautions should be maintained for several days. Stress the need for repeated measurement of serum thyroxine levels.

• If the patient is taking propylthiouracil and methimazole, monitor the complete blood count periodically to detect leukopenia, thrombocytopenia, and agranulocytosis. Instruct him to take these medications with meals to minimize GI distress, and to avoid over-the-counter cough preparations because many contain iodine.

• Tell him to report signs of hypersensitivity — fever, enlarged cervical lymph nodes, sore throat, mouth sores, and other signs of blood dyscrasias and any rash or skin eruptions. He should also watch for signs of liver dysfunction, such as jaundice or dark urine.

• Watch the patient taking propranolol for signs of hypotension (dizziness, decreased urine output). Tell him to rise slowly after sitting or lying down to prevent orthostatic hypotension.

## DIAGNOSING TIC DISORDERS

The diagnosis of a tic disorder is based on *DSM-IV* criteria.

### Tourette syndrome
• The patient has had multiple motor tics and one or more vocal tics at some time during the illness, although not necessarily concurrently.
• The tics occur many times a day (usually in bouts) nearly every day or intermittently for more than 1 year.
• The disturbance causes marked distress or significant impairment in social, occupational, or other important areas of functioning.
• Onset occurs before age 18.
• The disturbance isn't the direct physiologic effect of a substance or a general medical condition.

### Chronic motor or vocal tic disorder
• The patient has had single or multiple motor or vocal tics, but not both, at some time during the illness.
• The tics occur many times a day nearly every day or intermittently for more than 1 year. During this time, the person never had a tic-free period exceeding 3 consecutive months.

• The disturbance causes marked distress or significant impairment in social, occupational, or other important areas of functioning.
• Onset occurs before age 18.
• The disturbance isn't the direct physiologic effect of a substance or a general medical condition.
• Criteria have never been met for Tourette syndrome.

### Transient tic disorder
• The patient has single or multiple motor or vocal tics, or both.
• The tics occur many times a day nearly every day for at least 4 weeks, but for no longer than 12 consecutive months.
• The disturbance causes marked distress or significant impairment in social, occupational, or other important areas of functioning.
• Onset occurs before age 18.
• The disturbance is not the direct physiologic effect of a substance or a general medical condition.
• Criteria have never been met for Tourette syndrome or chronic motor or vocal tic disorder.

---

• Instruct the patient receiving antithyroid drugs or [131]I therapy to report any symptoms of hypothyroidism.

# TIC DISORDERS

Including Tourette syndrome, chronic motor or vocal tic disorder, and transient tic disorder, tic disorders are similar pathophysiologically but differ in severity and prognosis. All tic disorders, commonly known simply as tics, are involuntary, spasmodic, recurrent, and purposeless motor movements or vocalizations. These disorders are classified as motor or vocal and as simple or complex.

Tics begin before age 18. All tic disorders are three times more common in boys than in girls. Transient tics usually are self-limiting, but Tourette syndrome follows a chronic course with remissions and exacerbations.

## Causes
Although their exact cause is unknown, tic disorders occur more frequently in certain families, suggesting a genetic cause. Tics commonly develop when a child experiences overwhelming anxiety, usually associated with normal mat-

# STRESS DISORDERS WITH PHYSICAL SIGNS

Besides tic disorders, stress-related disorders that produce physical signs in children include stuttering, functional enuresis, functional encopresis, sleepwalking, and sleep terrors.

## Stuttering

Characterized by abnormal speech rhythms with repetitions and hesitations at the beginning of words, stuttering may involve movements of the respiratory muscles, shoulders, and face. It may be associated with mental dullness, low socioeconomic staus, and a history of birth trauma. However, this disorder most commonly occurs in children of average or superior intelligence who fear they can't meet expectations.

Related problems may include low self-esteem, anxiety, humiliation, and withdrawal from social situations. About 80% of stutterers recover after age 16. Evaluation and treatment by a speech pathologist teaches the stutterer to place equal weight on each syllable in a sentence, how to breathe properly, and how to control anxiety.

## Functional enuresis

This disorder is characterized by intentional or involuntary urination, usually at night (nocturnal enuresis). Considered normal in children until age 3 or 4, functional enuresis occurs in about 40% of children at this age and persists in 10% to age 5, in 5% to age 10, and in 1% of boys to age 18.

Causes may be related to stress, such as the birth of a sibling, the move to a new home, divorce, hospitalization, faulty toilet training (inconsistent, demanding, or punitive), and unrealistic responsibilities. Associated problems include low self-esteem, social withdrawal because of ostracism and ridicule, and anger, rejection, and punishment by caregivers.

Advise parents that a matter-of-fact attitude helps the child learn bladder control without undue stress. If enuresis persists into late childhood, treatment with imipramine may help. Dry-bed therapy may include the use of an alarm (wet bell pad), social motiva-

tion, self-correction of accidents, and positive reinforcement.

## Functional encopresis

Denoted by evacuation of feces into the child's clothes or inappropriate receptacles, functional encopresis is associated with low intelligence, cerebral dysfunction, or other developmental symptoms.

Some children also show inefficient, ineffective gastric motility. Related problems may include repressed anger, withdrawal from peer relationships, and loss of self-esteem.

Treatment involves encouraging the child to come to his parents when he has an "accident." Advise parents to give the child clean clothes without criticism or punishment. Medical examination should rule out any physical disorder. Child, adult, and family therapy may help reduce anger and disappointment over the child's development and improve parenting techniques.

## Sleepwalking and sleep terrors

In sleepwalking, the child calmly rises from bed in a state of altered consciousness and walks around with no subsequent recollection of any dreams. In sleep terrors, he awakes terrified, in a state of clouded consciousness, often unable to recognize parents and familiar surroundings. Visual hallucinations are common.

Sleepwalking is usually a response to an emotional concern. Tell parents to gently "talk" the child back to his bed. If he wakes, they should comfort and support him, not tease him.

Sleep terrors are normal in 2- to 3-year-olds, usually occurring within 30 minutes to 3½ hours of sleep onset. Tachycardia, tachypnea, diaphoresis, dilated pupils, and piloerection are associated with sleep terrors. The child also may fear being alone.

Tell parents to make sure the child has access to them at night. Sleep terrors usually are self-limiting and subside within a few weeks.

uration. Tics may be precipitated or exacerbated by the use of phenothiazines or central nervous system stimulants or by head trauma.

### Signs and symptoms

Assessment findings vary according to the type of tic disorder. Inspection, coupled with the patient's history, may reveal the specific motor or vocal patterns that characterize the tic, as well as the frequency, complexity, and precipitating factors. The patient or his family may report that the tics occur sporadically many times a day.

Note whether certain situations exacerbate the tics. All tic disorders may be exacerbated by stress, and they usually diminish markedly during sleep. The patient also may report that they occur during activities that require concentration, such as reading or sewing.

Determine whether the patient can control the tics. Most patients can, with conscious effort, control them for short periods.

Psychosocial assessment may reveal underlying stressful factors, such as problems with social adjustment, lack of self-esteem, and depression.

### Diagnosis

For characteristic findings in patients with this condition, see *Diagnosing tic disorders,* page 868.

### Treatment

Behavior modification and operant conditioning help treat some tic disorders. Psychotherapy can help the patient uncover underlying conflicts and issues as well as deal with the problems caused by the tics. Tourette syndrome is best treated with medications and psychotherapy.

No medications are helpful in treating transient tics. Haloperidol is the drug of choice for Tourette syndrome.

Pimozide (an oral dopamine-blocking drug) and clonidine are alternative choices. Antianxiety agents may be useful in dealing with secondary anxiety but do not reduce the severity or frequency of the tics.

### Special considerations

● Offer emotional support and help the patient prevent fatigue.
● Suggest that the patient with Tourette syndrome contact the Tourette Syndrome Association for information and support.
● Help the patient identify and eliminate any avoidable stress and learn positive new ways to deal with anxiety.
● Encourage the patient to verbalize his feelings about his illness. Help him understand that the movements are involuntary and that he shouldn't feel guilty or blame himself.
● For more information on other stress disorders, see *Stress disorders with physical signs,* page 869.

# TONSILLITIS

Inflammation of the tonsils, or tonsillitis, can be acute or chronic. The uncomplicated acute form usually lasts 4 to 6 days and commonly affects children between ages 5 and 10. The presence of proven chronic tonsillitis justifies tonsillectomy, the only effective treatment. Tonsils tend to hypertrophy during childhood and atrophy after puberty.

### Causes

Tonsillitis generally results from infection with group A beta-hemolytic streptococci but can result from other bacteria or viruses or from oral anaerobes.

## Signs and symptoms

Acute and chronic tonsillitis have different signs and symptoms.

### *Acute tonsillitis*

The acute form of tonsillitis commonly begins with a mild to severe sore throat. A very young child, unable to complain about a sore throat, may stop eating. Tonsillitis may also produce dysphagia, fever, swelling and tenderness of the lymph glands in the submandibular area, muscle and joint pain, chills, malaise, headache, and pain (frequently referred to the ears).

Excess secretions may elicit the complaint of a constant urge to swallow; the back of the throat may feel constricted. Such discomfort usually subsides after 72 hours.

### *Chronic tonsillitis*

The chronic form of tonsillitis produces a recurrent sore throat and purulent drainage in the tonsillar crypts. Frequent attacks of acute tonsillitis may also occur. Complications include obstruction from tonsillar hypertrophy and peritonsillar abscess.

## Diagnosis

Diagnostic confirmation requires a thorough throat examination that reveals:
• generalized inflammation of the pharyngeal wall
• swollen tonsils that project from between the pillars of the fauces and exude white or yellow follicles
• purulent drainage when pressure is applied to the tonsillar pillars
• possible edematous and inflamed uvula.

Culture may determine the infecting organism and indicate appropriate antibiotic therapy. Leukocytosis is also usually present. Differential diagnosis rules out infectious mononucleosis and diphtheria.

## Treatment

Effective treatment of acute tonsillitis requires rest, adequate fluid intake, administration of aspirin or acetaminophen and, for bacterial infection, antibiotics.

When the causative organism is group A beta-hemolytic streptococcus, penicillin is the drug of choice (another broad-spectrum antibiotic may be substituted). Most oral anaerobes will also respond to penicillin. To prevent complications, antibiotic therapy should continue for 10 to 14 days.

Chronic tonsillitis or the development of complications (obstructions from tonsillar hypertrophy, peritonsillar abscess) may require a tonsillectomy, but only after the patient has been free of tonsillar or respiratory tract infections for 3 to 4 weeks.

## Special considerations

• Despite dysphagia, urge the patient to drink plenty of fluids, especially if he has a fever. Offer a child ice cream and flavored drinks and ices. Suggest gargling to soothe the throat, unless it exacerbates pain. Make sure the patient and parents understand the importance of completing the prescribed course of antibiotic therapy.
• Before tonsillectomy, explain to the adult patient that a local anesthetic prevents pain but allows a sensation of pressure during surgery. Warn the patient to expect considerable throat discomfort and some bleeding postoperatively.
• For the pediatric patient, keep your explanation simple and nonthreatening. Show the child the operating and recovery rooms, and briefly explain the hospital routine. Most facilities allow one parent to stay with the child.

• Advise the patient not to take aspirin or medications containing aspirin for 7 to 10 days before surgery to decrease the risk of bleeding.

• Postoperatively, maintain a patent airway. To prevent aspiration, place the patient on his side.

• Monitor vital signs frequently, and check for bleeding. Be alert for excessive bleeding, increased pulse rate, dropping blood pressure, or frequent swallowing.

• After the patient is fully alert and the gag reflex has returned, allow him to drink water.

• Urge the patient to drink plenty of nonirritating fluids.

> **CLINICAL TIP** Encourage oral intake. Tell the patient to begin with cool liquids; advance to a soft, bland diet as tolerated; and to avoid citrus juices and highly spiced foods.

• Encourage the patient to ambulate and to take frequent deep breaths to prevent pulmonary complications. Give pain medication as needed.

• Before discharge, provide the patient or parents with written instructions on home care. Tell the patient to expect a white scab to form in the throat between 5 and 10 days postoperatively and to report bleeding, ear discomfort, or a fever that lasts longer than 3 days.

• Tell the patient that aspirin and medications containing aspirin are contraindicated postoperatively.

• Instruct the patient to avoid coughing or excessive clearing of the throat, which can irritate the throat and cause increased bleeding.

• Tell the patient that blood-tinged mucus is normal for 5 to 7 days after surgery.

## ✦ LIFE-THREATENING DISORDER

# TOXIC SHOCK SYNDROME

An acute bacterial infection, toxic shock syndrome (TSS) is caused by toxin-producing, penicillin-resistant strains of *Staphylococcus aureus*, such as TSS toxin-1 and staphylococcal enterotoxins B and C. The disease primarily affects menstruating women under age 30 and is associated with continuous use of tampons during the menstrual period.

TSS incidence peaked in the mid-1980s and has since declined, probably because of the withdrawal of high-absorbency tampons from the market.

## Causes

Although tampons are clearly implicated in TSS, their exact role is uncertain. Theoretically, tampons may contribute to development of TSS by:

• introducing *S. aureus* into the vagina during insertion

• absorbing toxin from the vagina

• traumatizing the vaginal mucosa during insertion, thus leading to infection

• providing a favorable environment for the growth of *S. aureus.*

When TSS isn't related to menstruation, it seems to be linked to *S. aureus* infections, such as abscesses, osteomyelitis, and postsurgical infections.

## Signs and symptoms

Typically, TSS produces intense myalgias, fever over 104° F (40° C), vomiting, diarrhea, headache, decreased level of consciousness, rigors, conjunctival hyperemia, and vaginal hyperemia and discharge. Severe hypotension occurs with hypovolemic shock. Within a few hours of onset, a deep red rash develops — especially on the palms and soles — and later desquamates.

Major complications include persistent neuropsychological abnormalities, mild renal failure, rash, and cyanotic arms and legs.

## Diagnosis

A diagnosis of TSS is based on clinical findings and the presence of at least three of the following:

● GI effects, including vomiting and profuse diarrhea

● muscular effects, with severe myalgias or a fivefold or greater increase in creatine kinase

● mucous membrane effects, such as frank hyperemia

● renal involvement with elevated blood urea nitrogen or creatinine levels (at least twice the normal levels)

● liver involvement with elevated bilirubin, alanine aminotransferase, or aspartate aminotransferase levels (at least twice the normal levels)

● blood involvement with signs of thrombocytopenia and a platelet count < 100,000/µl

● central nervous system effects, such as disorientation without focal signs.

In addition, isolation of *S. aureus* from vaginal discharge or lesions helps support the diagnosis. Negative results on blood tests for Rocky Mountain spotted fever, leptospirosis, and measles help rule out these disorders.

## Treatment

TSS is treated with I.V. antistaphylococcal antibiotics that are beta-lactamase–resistant, such as oxacillin and nafcillin. To reverse shock, replace fluids with saline solution and colloids.

➤ CLINICAL TIP Shock that doesn't respond to fluids may necessitate use of pressor agents such as dopamine.

## Special considerations

● Monitor the patient's vital signs frequently.

● Administer antibiotics slowly and strictly on time. Be sure to watch for signs of penicillin allergy.

● Check the patient's fluid and electrolyte balance.

● Obtain specimens of vaginal and cervical secretions for culture of *S. aureus*.

● Tell the patient to avoid using tampons.

● Implement standard precautions.

# TOXOPLASMOSIS

One of the most common infectious diseases, toxoplasmosis results from the protozoa *Toxoplasma gondii*. Distributed worldwide, it's less common in cold or hot arid climates and at high elevations. It usually causes localized infection but may produce significant generalized infection, especially in immunodeficient patients or neonates.

Congenital toxoplasmosis, characterized by lesions in the central nervous system, may result in stillbirth or serious birth defects.

## Causes

*T. gondii* exists in trophozoite forms in the acute stages of infection and in cystic forms (tissue cysts and oocysts) in the latent stages. Ingestion of tissue cysts in raw or undercooked meat (heating, drying, or freezing destroys these cysts) or fecal-oral contamination from infected cats transmits toxoplasmosis. (See *Avoiding toxoplasmosis,* page 874.)

However, toxoplasmosis also occurs in vegetarians who aren't exposed to cats, so other means of transmission may exist.

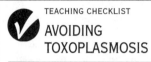

Congenital toxoplasmosis follows transplacental transmission from a chronically infected mother or one who acquired toxoplasmosis shortly before or during pregnancy.

## Signs and symptoms
The following signs and symptoms characterize congenital toxoplasmosis and acquired toxoplasmosis.

### *Congenital toxoplasmosis*
Toxoplasmosis acquired in the first trimester of pregnancy often results in stillbirth. About one-third of neonates who survive have congenital toxoplasmosis. The later in pregnancy maternal infection occurs, the greater the risk of congenital infection in the neonate.

Obvious signs of congenital toxoplasmosis include retinochoroiditis, hydrocephalus or microcephalus, cerebral calcification, seizures, lymphadenopathy, fever, hepatosplenomegaly, jaundice, and rash. Other defects, which may become apparent months or years later, include strabismus, blindness, epilepsy, and mental retardation.

### *Acquired toxoplasmosis*
Acquired toxoplasmosis may cause localized (mild lymphatic) or generalized (fulminating, disseminated) infection. Localized infection produces fever and a mononucleosis-like syndrome (malaise, myalgia, headache, fatigue, sore throat) and lymphadenopathy.

Generalized infection produces encephalitis, fever, headache, vomiting, delirium, seizures, and a diffuse maculopapular rash (except on the palms, soles, and scalp). Generalized infection may lead to myocarditis, pneumonitis, hepatitis, and polymyositis.

## Diagnosis
Identification of *T. gondii* in an appropriate tissue specimen confirms toxoplasmosis. Serologic tests may be useful, and in patients with toxoplasmosis encephalitis, computed tomography and magnetic resonance imaging scans disclose lesions.

## Treatment
Acute disease is treated with sulfonamides and pyrimethamine for about 4 weeks and, possibly, folinic acid to control adverse effects. In patients who also have acquired immunodeficiency syndrome, treatment continues indefinitely.

CLINICAL TIP   No safe, effective treatment exists for chronic toxoplasmosis or toxoplasmosis occurring in the first trimester of pregnancy.

## Special considerations
• When caring for patients with toxoplasmosis, monitor drug therapy carefully and emphasize thorough patient teaching to prevent complications and control spread of the disease.

- Because sulfonamides cause blood dyscrasias and pyrimethamine depresses bone marrow, closely monitor the patient's hematologic values.
- Report all cases of toxoplasmosis to your local public health department.

# TRIGEMINAL NEURALGIA

Also called tic douloureux, trigeminal neuralgia is a painful disorder of one or more branches of the fifth cranial (trigeminal) nerve that produces paroxysmal attacks of excruciating facial pain precipitated by stimulation of a trigger zone.

It occurs mostly in people over age 40, in women more often than men, and on the right side of the face more often than the left. Trigeminal neuralgia can subside spontaneously, with remissions lasting from several months to years.

## Causes

Although the cause remains undetermined, trigeminal neuralgia may:
- reflect an afferent reflex phenomenon located centrally in the brain stem or more peripherally in the sensory root of the trigeminal nerve
- be related to compression of the nerve root by posterior fossa tumors, middle fossa tumors, or vascular lesions (subclinical aneurysm), although such lesions usually produce simultaneous loss of sensation
- occasionally be a manifestation of multiple sclerosis or herpes zoster.

Whatever the cause, the pain of trigeminal neuralgia is probably produced by an interaction or short-circuiting of touch and pain fibers.

## Signs and symptoms

Typically, the patient reports a searing or burning pain that occurs in lightning-like jabs and lasts from 1 to 15 minutes (usually 1 to 2 minutes) in an area innervated by one of the divisions of the trigeminal nerve, primarily the superior mandibular or maxillary division.

The pain rarely affects more than one division, and seldom the first division (ophthalmic) or both sides of the face. It affects the second (maxillary) and third (mandibular) divisions of the trigeminal nerve equally. (See *Trigeminal nerve distribution and function*, page 876.)

These attacks characteristically follow stimulation of a trigger zone, usually by a light touch to a hypersensitive area, such as the tip of the nose, the cheeks, or the gums. Although attacks can occur at any time, they may follow a draft of air, exposure to heat or cold, eating, smiling, talking, or drinking hot or cold beverages.

The frequency of attacks varies greatly, from many times a day to several times a month or year. Between attacks, most patients are free from pain, although some have a constant, dull ache. No patient is ever free from the fear of the next attack.

## Diagnosis

The patient's pain history is the basis for diagnosis, because trigeminal neuralgia produces no objective clinical or pathologic changes. Physical examination shows no impairment of sensory or motor function; indeed, sensory impairment implies a space-occupying lesion as the cause of pain.

Observation during the examination shows the patient favoring (splinting) the affected area. To ward off a painful attack, the patient often holds his face immobile when talking. He may also leave the affected side of his face un-

## TRIGEMINAL NERVE DISTRIBUTION AND FUNCTION

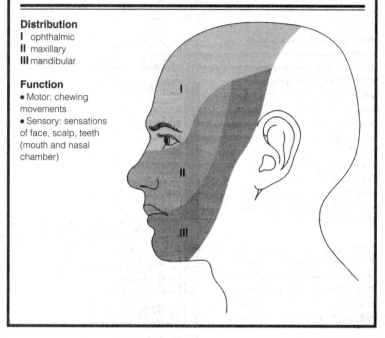

**Distribution**
I ophthalmic
II maxillary
III mandibular

**Function**
● Motor: chewing movements
● Sensory: sensations of face, scalp, teeth (mouth and nasal chamber)

washed and unshaven, or protect it with a coat or shawl.

When asked where the pain occurs, he points to — but never touches — the affected area. Witnessing a typical attack helps to confirm the diagnosis. Rarely, a tumor in the posterior fossa can produce pain that is clinically indistinguishable from trigeminal neuralgia. Skull X-rays, tomography, and computed tomography scan rule out tumors and sinus or tooth infections.

### Treatment
Oral administration of carbamazepine or phenytoin may temporarily relieve or prevent pain. Narcotics may be helpful during the pain episode.

When these medical measures fail or attacks become increasingly frequent or severe, neurosurgical procedures may provide permanent relief. The preferred procedure is percutaneous electrocoagulation of nerve rootlets, under local anesthesia.

New treatments include a percutaneous radio frequency procedure, which causes partial root destruction and relieves pain, and microsurgery for vascular decompression of the trigeminal nerve.

### Special considerations
● Observe and record the characteristics of each attack, including the patient's protective mechanisms.
● Provide adequate nutrition in small, frequent meals at room temperature.
● If the patient is receiving carbamazepine, watch for cutaneous and hemato-

logic reactions (erythematous and pruritic rashes, urticaria, photosensitivity, exfoliative dermatitis, leukopenia, agranulocytosis, eosinophilia, aplastic anemia, thrombocytopenia) and, possibly, urine retention and transient drowsiness.

• For the first 3 months of carbamazepine therapy, complete blood count and liver function should be monitored weekly, then monthly thereafter. Warn the patient to immediately report fever, sore throat, mouth ulcers, easy bruising, or petechial or purpuric hemorrhage.

> **CLINICAL TIP**  Fever, sore throat, mouth ulcers, easy bruising, or petechial or purpuric hemorrhage may signal thrombocytopenia or aplastic anemia and may require discontinuation of drug therapy.

• If the patient is receiving phenytoin, also watch for side effects, including ataxia, skin eruptions, gingival hyperplasia, and nystagmus.

• After resection of the first division of the trigeminal nerve, tell the patient to avoid rubbing his eyes and using aerosol spray. Advise him to wear glasses or goggles outdoors and to blink often.

• After surgery to sever the second or third division, tell the patient to avoid hot foods and drinks, which could burn his mouth, and to chew carefully to avoid biting his mouth.

• Advise the patient to place food in the unaffected side of his mouth when chewing, to brush his teeth and rinse his mouth often, and to see a dentist twice a year to detect cavities. (Cavities in the area of the severed nerve won't cause pain.)

• After surgical decompression of the root or partial nerve dissection, check neurologic and vital signs often.

• Provide emotional support, and encourage the patient to express his fear and anxiety. Promote independence through self-care and maximum phys-ical activity. Reinforce natural avoidance of stimulation (air, heat, cold) of trigger zones (lips, cheeks, gums).

# TRISOMY 18 SYNDROME

Trisomy 18 syndrome (also known as Edwards' syndrome) is the second most common multiple malformation syndrome. Most affected neonates have full trisomy 18, involving an extra (third) copy of chromosome 18 in each cell, but partial trisomy 18 (with varying phenotypes) and translocation types have also been reported. Most neonates with this disorder present with intrauterine growth retardation, congenital heart defects, microcephaly, and other malformations.

Full trisomy 18 syndrome is generally fatal or has an extremely poor prognosis; 30% to 50% of these infants die within the first 2 months of life, and 90% die within the first year. Most surviving patients are profoundly mentally retarded.

## Causes

Most cases of trisomy 18 syndrome are caused by spontaneous meiotic nondisjunction. The risk of chromosomal abnormalities typically increases with maternal age; however, the mean maternal age for this disorder is 32.5. Incidence ranges from 1 in 3,000 to 8,000 neonates, with 3 to 4 females affected for every male.

## Signs and symptoms

Growth retardation begins in utero, and remains significant after birth. Initial hypotonia may soon give way to hypertonia. Common findings include microcephaly and dolichocephaly, micrognathia, genital and perineal abnormalities (including imperforate anus), diaphragmatic hernia, and various renal defects. Congenital heart defects, such as ventricular septal defect, tetralogy of Fallot, transposition of the great vessels, and coarctation of the aorta, occur in 80% to 90% of patients and may be the cause of death in many infants.

Other findings may include a short and narrow nose with upturned nares; unilateral or bilateral cleft lip and palate; low-set, slightly pointed ears; a short neck; a conspicuous clenched hand with overlapping fingers (often seen on ultrasound as well); neural tube defects; omphalocele; cystic hygroma; choroid plexus cysts (also seen in some normal infants); and oligohydramnios.

### Diagnosis

Multiple marker maternal serum screening tests involving different combinations of alpha-fetoprotein, human chorionic gonadotropin, and unconjugated estriol may be abnormal in many pregnant women with an affected fetus; however, these tests are not diagnostic. Fetal ultrasound may reveal varying degrees of abnormalities, but many fetuses have few detectable defects.

Diagnosis should be based on karyotype, done either prenatally (by amniocentesis) or using peripheral blood or skin fibroblasts after birth.

### Treatment

Treatment aims to provide comfort for the infant and emotional support for the parents.

### Special considerations

• Because the neonate's sucking reflex is poor, nutrition is maintained using gavage feedings. Teach parents about home care and feeding techniques.
• Allow adequate time for the parents to bond with and hold their child.

• Refer the parents of an affected child for genetic counseling to explore the cause of the disorder and discuss the risk of recurrence in a future pregnancy.
• Refer the parents to a social worker or grief counselor for additional support if needed.

▶ CLINICAL TIP   Refer the parents to the Support Organization for Trisomy 18, 13, and Related Disorders (S.O.F.T.) National Support Group to allow them interaction with other parents of infants with trisomy 18 and trisomy 13.

❋ LIFE-THREATENING DISORDER

# TUBERCULOSIS

An acute or chronic infection caused by *Mycobacterium tuberculosis,* tuberculosis (TB) is characterized by pulmonary infiltrates, formation of granulomas with caseation, fibrosis, and cavitation. People living in crowded, poorly ventilated conditions are most likely to become infected.

In patients with strains that are sensitive to the usual antitubercular agents, the prognosis is excellent with correct treatment. However, in those with strains that are resistant to two or more of the major antitubercular agents, mortality is 50%.

### Causes

After exposure to *M. tuberculosis,* roughly 5% of infected people develop active tuberculosis within 1 year; in the remainder, microorganisms cause a latent infection. The host's immune system usually controls the tubercle bacillus by killing it or walling it up in a tiny nodule (tubercle). However, the bacillus may lie dormant within the tubercle for years and later reactivate and spread.

### Reactivation risk factors

Although the primary infection site is the lungs, mycobacteria commonly exist in other parts of the body. A number of factors increase the risk of infection reactivation: gastrectomy, uncontrolled diabetes mellitus, Hodgkin's disease, leukemia, silicosis, acquired immunodeficiency syndrome, and treatment with corticosteroids or immunosuppressants.

### Mode of transmission

TB is transmitted by droplet nuclei produced when infected persons cough or sneeze. After inhalation, if a tubercle bacillus settles in an alveolus, infection occurs. Cell-mediated immunity to the mycobacteria, which develops about 3 to 6 weeks later, usually contains the infection and arrests the disease.

### Response to reactivation

If the infection reactivates, the body's response characteristically leads to caseation — the conversion of necrotic tissue to a cheeselike material. The caseum may localize, undergo fibrosis, or excavate and form cavities, the walls of which are studded with multiplying tubercle bacilli. If this happens, infected caseous debris may spread throughout the lungs by the tracheobronchial tree.

Sites of extrapulmonary TB include pleura, meninges, joints, lymph nodes, peritoneum, genitourinary tract, and bowel.

### Signs and symptoms

• In primary infection, after an incubation period of from 4 to 8 weeks, TB is usually asymptomatic but may produce nonspecific symptoms, such as fatigue, weakness, anorexia, weight loss, night sweats, and low-grade fever.

• In reactivation, symptoms may include a cough that produces mucopurulent sputum, occasional hemoptysis, and chest pains.

### Diagnosis

Diagnostic tests include chest X-rays, a tuberculin skin test, and sputum smears and cultures to identify *M. tuberculosis*. The following procedures aid diagnosis:

• *Auscultation* detects crepitant rales, bronchial breath sounds, wheezes, and whispered pectoriloquy.

• *Chest percussion* detects a dullness over the affected area, indicating consolidation or pleural fluid.

• *Chest X-ray* shows nodular lesions, patchy infiltrates (mainly in upper lobes), cavity formation, scar tissue, and calcium deposits; however, it may not be able to distinguish active from inactive TB.

• *Tuberculin skin test* detects TB infection. Intermediate-strength purified protein derivative (PPD) or 5 tuberculin units (0.1 ml) are injected intracutaneously on the forearm.

The test results are read in 48 to 72 hours; a positive reaction (induration of 5 to 15 mm or more, depending on risk factors) develops 2 to 10 weeks after infection in active and inactive TB. However, severely immunosuppressed patients may never develop a positive reaction.

• *Stains and cultures* (of sputum, cerebrospinal fluid, urine, drainage from abscess, or pleural fluid) show heat-sensitive, nonmotile, aerobic, acid-fast bacilli.

### Treatment

Antitubercular therapy with daily oral doses of isoniazid, rifampin, and pyrazinamide (and sometimes ethambutol) for at least 6 months usually cures TB. After 2 to 4 weeks, the disease generally is no longer infectious. The patient can resume his normal lifestyle while taking medication.

Patients with atypical mycobacterial disease or drug-resistant TB may require treatment with second-line drugs, such as capreomycin, streptomycin, para-aminosalicylic acid, cycloserine, amikacin, and quinolone drugs.

**Special considerations**
• Isolate the infectious patient in a quiet, well-ventilated room until he's no longer contagious.
• Teach the patient to cough and sneeze into tissues and to dispose of all secretions properly. Place a covered trash can nearby or tape a waxed bag to the side of the bed for used tissues.
• Instruct the patient to wear a mask when outside his room. Visitors and hospital personnel should wear masks when they are in the patient's room.
• Remind the patient to get plenty of rest and to eat balanced meals. If the patient is anoretic, urge him to eat small meals throughout the day. Record weight weekly.
• Be alert for adverse effects of medications. Because isoniazid sometimes leads to hepatitis or peripheral neuritis, monitor aspartate aminotransferase and alanine aminotransferase levels. To prevent or treat peripheral neuritis, give pyridoxine (vitamin $B_6$).

➤ CLINICAL TIP If the patient receives ethambutol, watch for optic neuritis; if it develops, discontinue the drug. If he receives rifampin, watch for hepatitis and purpura. Also observe the patient for other complications such as hemoptysis.
• Emphasize the importance of regular follow-up examinations, and instruct the patient and his family concerning the signs and symptoms of recurring TB.
• Advise persons who have been exposed to infected patients to receive tuberculin tests and, if necessary, chest X-rays and prophylactic isoniazid.

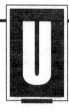

# ULCERATIVE COLITIS

An inflammatory condition that affects the surface of the colon, ulcerative colitis causes friability and erosions with bleeding. The disease more commonly affects the rectum and sigmoid colon. Less frequently, it extends into the splenic flexure, or more proximally extends upward into the entire colon. It rarely affects the small intestine, except for the terminal ileum.

Severity ranges from a mild, localized disorder to a fulminant disease that may lead to a perforated colon, progressing to peritonitis and toxemia.

## Causes

Although the etiology of ulcerative colitis is unknown, it is thought to be related to an autoimmune response. Stress is no longer thought to be a cause of the disease. However, it may precipitate or increase the severity of the attack.

Ulcerative colitis occurs primarily in young adults, especially women; it's also more prevalent among the Jewish population and individuals in higher socioeconomic groups. Onset of symptoms seems to peak in the 15- to 20-year-old age-group, with another peak occurring in the 55- to 60-year-old age-group.

## Signs and symptoms

The hallmark of ulcerative colitis is bloody diarrhea. The intensity of these attacks varies with the extent of inflammation. Patients with mild to moderate disease may experience approximately five or fewer bowel movements per day with intermittent bleeding and mucus production. Individuals may experience left lower quadrant pain relieved by defecation, along with fecal urgency and tenesmus. Patients with more severe disease will have more than five bowel movements per day, which may result in anemia, hypovolemia, and impaired nutrition. Extracolonic manifestations also may be present, including erythema nodosum, pyoderma gangrenosum, episcleritis, thromboembolic events, and arthritis.

Ulcerative colitis may lead to complications affecting the following organs and systems:

• *Blood:* anemia from iron deficiency, coagulation defects due to vitamin K deficiency

• *Skin:* erythema nodosum on the face and arms; pyoderma gangrenosum on the legs and ankles

• *Eye:* uveitis

• *Liver:* pericholangitis, sclerosing cholangitis, cirrhosis, possible cholangiocarcinoma

• *Musculoskeletal:* arthritis, ankylosing spondylitis, loss of muscle mass

• *GI:* strictures, pseudopolyps, stenosis, and perforated colon, leading to peritonitis and toxemia.

> **CLINICAL TIP** The risk of colorectal cancer in patients who have had ulcerative colitis for more than 10 years increases by approximately 1% per year. Also, patients with disease proximal to the sigmoid colon have an increased risk of developing colon carcinomas.

## Diagnosis

- *History* and *physical examination* should include questions regarding frequency of stools, rectal bleeding, cramps, abdominal pain, weight loss, and tenesmus. Peritoneal inflammation should be assessed, as well as volume status and nutritional levels.
- *Sigmoidoscopy* establishes a diagnosis by demonstrating increased mucosal friability, decreased mucosal detail, edema, and erosions. Biopsy can help confirm the diagnosis.
- *Colonoscopy* may be used both to determine the extent of the disease and for cancer surveillance after the patient's flare-up has resolved.

> **CLINICAL TIP** Colonoscopy should not be performed during an acute episode because of the risk of perforation.

- *Stool specimen* should be cultured and analyzed for leukocytes, ova, and parasites.

Other supportive laboratory values include decreased serum levels of potassium, magnesium, hemoglobin, and albumin, as well as leukocytosis and prolonged prothrombin time. Elevated erythrocyte sedimentation rate correlates with the severity of the attack.

## Treatment

The goals of treatment are to relieve symptoms of the acute attack and prevent recurrent attacks, to replace nutritional losses and blood volume, and to prevent complications.

Supportive treatment includes I.V. fluid replacement and a clear-liquid diet. For patients awaiting surgery or showing signs of dehydration and debilitation from excessive diarrhea, total parenteral nutrition rests the intestinal tract, decreases stool volume, and restores positive nitrogen balance. Blood transfusions or iron supplements may be necessary to correct anemia.

### *Drug therapy*

Medications to control inflammation include corticotropin and adrenal corticosteroids, such as prednisone, prednisolone, and hydrocortisone; sulfasalazine, which has anti-inflammatory and antimicrobial properties, may also be used.

Patients with mild to moderate disease may eat a regular diet, excluding caffeinated beverages and gas-producing foods. Fiber supplementation may be used to control diarrhea and rectal symptoms. Antidiarrheal agents (loperamide, atropine [Lomotil], and tincture of opium) should be used only in patients with mild symptoms, not in those with the acute phase of this illness.

Patients with disease primarily affecting the rectum or rectosigmoid should be managed with topical agents such as mesalamine. Topical steroids may be used, but they may be less effective.

Patients with mild to moderate disease extending above the sigmoid colon who fail to improve after 2 to 3 weeks on sulfasalazine or mesalamine should have a corticosteroid added to their regimen.

Severe colitis is usually managed with nothing-by-mouth status and parenteral alimentation. Volumizers and blood should be provided as needed. Surgical consultation should be obtained in all patients with severe disease.

## Surgery

Surgery is recommended for patients who have toxic megacolon or who fail to respond to drugs and supportive measures.

The *ileoanal restorative proctocolectomy* with ileoanal pouch anastomosis is being performed more frequently. This procedure entails performing a total proctocolectomy, creating a pouch from the terminal ileum, and anastomosing the pouch to the anal canal. A temporary ileostomy is created to divert stools and allow the rectal anastomosis to heal. This technique is now more common than total proctocolectomy with ileostomy. The ileostomy is closed in 2 to 3 months.

*Total proctocolectomy (with ileostomy)* provides complete cure of disease. However, the patients' self-image and social interactions may be affected by wearing an external appliance.

*Pouch ileostomy (Kock pouch or continent ileostomy),* in which the surgeon creates a pouch from a small loop of the terminal ileum and a nipple valve from the distal ileum, may be an option. The resulting stoma opens just above the pubic hairline, and the pouch empties periodically through a catheter inserted in the stoma. Patients may experience six or more bowel movements per day. A low-residue diet should be maintained to promote pouch adaptation. Patients may also need bulking agents or antidiarrheals to slow stool output. This procedure is performed less often now than in the past.

A *colectomy* may be performed after 10 years of active ulcerative colitis because of the increased incidence of colon cancer in these patients. Performing a partial colectomy to prevent colon cancer is controversial.

## Special considerations

● Accurately record intake and output, particularly the frequency and volume of stools.

● Watch for signs of dehydration and electrolyte imbalances, specifically signs of hypokalemia (muscle weakness, paresthesia) and hypernatremia (fever, tachycardia, flushed skin, dry tongue).

● Monitor hemoglobin and hematocrit, and transfuse if necessary.

● Provide good mouth care for the patient who is allowed nothing by mouth.

● After each bowel movement, thoroughly clean the skin around the rectum.

● Administer medication. Watch for adverse effects of prolonged corticosteroid therapy (moonface, hirsutism, edema, gastric irritation). Be aware that such therapy may mask infection.

● If the patient needs total parenteral nutrition, change dressings, assess for inflammation at the insertion site, and check blood glucose every 6 hours.

● Take precautionary measures if the patient is prone to bleeding. Watch closely for signs of complications, such as a perforated colon and peritonitis (fever, severe abdominal pain, abdominal rigidity and tenderness, and cool, clammy skin), and toxic megacolon (abdominal distention, decreased bowel sounds).

● Prepare the patient for surgery, and provide teaching related to the care of an ileostomy. Consult the enterostomal therapy nurse for preoperative teaching and stoma marking. Provide a bowel preparation.

● After surgery, provide education regarding ostomy care as well as psychological support. Arrange for the patient to consult an enterostomal therapy nurse.

● Keep the nasogastric tube patent. After removal of the tube, provide a clear-liquid diet. Gradually advance to a low-residue diet as tolerated.

• After a proctocolectomy and ileostomy, provide education regarding ostomy care. Wash the skin around the stoma with soapy water and dry it thoroughly. Apply karaya powder around the base of the stoma to prevent irritation and provide a tight seal. Cut an opening in the ring to fit over the stoma, and secure the pouch to the skin. Empty the pouch when it's one-third full.

• After a pouch ileostomy, uncork the catheter every hour to allow contents to drain. After 10 to 14 days, gradually increase the length of time the catheter is left corked until it can be opened every 3 hours. Then remove the catheter and reinsert it every 3 to 4 hours for drainage. Teach the patient how to insert the catheter and how to take care of the stoma.

• Encourage the patient to have regular physical examinations.

# URINARY TRACT INFECTION, LOWER

Cystitis and urethritis, the two forms of lower urinary tract infection (UTI), are nearly 10 times more common in women than in men and affect approximately 10% to 20% of all women at least once. Lower UTI is also a prevalent bacterial disease in children, with girls also most commonly affected.

In men and children, lower UTIs are frequently related to anatomic or physiologic abnormalities and therefore require extremely close evaluation. UTIs often respond readily to treatment, but recurrence and resistant bacterial flare-up during therapy are possible. (See *Treating and preventing urinary tract infections*.)

## Causes

Most lower UTIs result from ascending infection by a single gram-negative enteric bacterium, such as *Escherichia coli, Klebsiella, Proteus, Enterobacter, Pseudomonas,* or *Serratia.* However, in a patient with neurogenic bladder, an indwelling urinary catheter, or a fistula between the intestine and bladder, lower UTI may result from simultaneous infection with multiple pathogens.

Recent studies suggest that infection results from a breakdown in local defense mechanisms in the bladder that allow bacteria to invade the bladder mucosa and multiply. These bacteria cannot be readily eliminated by normal micturition.

### Bacterial flare-up

During treatment, bacterial flare-up is generally caused by the pathogenic organism's resistance to the prescribed antimicrobial therapy. The presence of even a small number (less than 10,000/ml) of bacteria in a midstream urine sample obtained during treatment casts doubt on the effectiveness of treatment.

### Recurrent UTI

In 99% of patients, recurrent lower UTI results from reinfection by the same organism or from some new pathogen; in the remaining 1%, recurrence reflects persistent infection, usually from renal calculi, chronic bacterial prostatitis, or a structural anomaly that may become a source of infection.

### High incidence in women

The high incidence of lower UTI among women may result from the shortness of the female urethra ($1\frac{1}{4}''$ to $2''$ [3 to 5 cm]), which predisposes women to infection caused by bacteria from the vagina, perineum, rectum, or a sexual partner.

---

TEACHING CHECKLIST

# ✔ TREATING AND PREVENTING URINARY TRACT INFECTIONS

Teach the female patient how to clean the perineum properly and keep the labia separated during voiding to collect a clean, midstream urine specimen. Explain that a noncontaminated midstream specimen is essential for accurate diagnosis.

## Treatment
• Explain the nature and purpose of antimicrobial therapy. Emphasize the importance of completing the prescribed course of therapy or, with long-term prophylaxis, of adhering strictly to ordered dosage.
• Recommend taking nitrofurantoin macrocrystals with milk or a meal to prevent GI distress. If therapy includes phenazopyridine, warn the patient that this drug may turn urine red-orange.
• Urge the patient to drink at least eight glasses of water a day. Stress the need to maintain a consistent fluid intake of about 2,000 ml/day. More or less than this amount may alter the effect of the prescribed antimicrobial.
• Tell the patient that fruit juices, especially cranberry juice, and oral doses of vitamin C may help acidify the urine

and enhance the action of the medication.
• Suggest warm sitz baths for relief of perineal discomfort.

## Prevention
To prevent recurrent infections in men, urge prompt treatment of predisposing conditions such as chronic prostatitis.
  To prevent recurrent infections in women, teach the patient to:
• carefully wipe the perineum from front to back and to clean it thoroughly with soap and water after defecation
• void immediately after sexual intercourse
• drink plenty of fluids
• routinely avoid postponing urination. Recommend frequent comfort stops during long car trips, and stress the need to empty the bladder completely.

---

Men are less vulnerable because their urethras are longer (7¾″ [19.68 cm]) and their prostatic fluid serves as an antibacterial shield. In men and women, infection usually ascends from the urethra to the bladder.

## Signs and symptoms
Lower UTI usually produces urgency, frequency, dysuria, cramps or spasms of the bladder, itching, a feeling of warmth during urination, nocturia, and possibly urethral discharge in males. Inflammation of the bladder wall also causes hematuria and fever.

Other common features include low back pain, malaise, nausea, vomiting,

abdominal pain or tenderness over the bladder area, chills, and flank pain.

## Diagnosis
Characteristic clinical features and a microscopic urinalysis showing red blood cells and white blood cells greater than 10/high-power field suggest lower UTI.
• *A clean, midstream urine specimen* revealing a bacterial count of more than 100,000/ml confirms the diagnosis. Lower counts do not necessarily rule out infection, especially if the patient is voiding frequently, because bacteria require 30 to 45 minutes to reproduce in urine.

Careful midstream, clean-catch collection is preferred to catheterization, which can reinfect the bladder with urethral bacteria.

• *Sensitivity testing* determines the appropriate therapeutic antimicrobial agent.

• *Voiding cystoureterography* or *excretory urography* may detect congenital anomalies that predispose the patient to recurrent UTIs.

• If patient history and physical examination warrant, a blood test or a stained smear of the discharge rules out a sexually transmitted disease.

**Treatment**

Appropriate antimicrobials are the treatment of choice for most initial lower UTIs. A 7- to 10-day course of antibiotic therapy is standard, but recent studies suggest that a single dose of an antibiotic or a 3- to 5-day antibiotic regimen may be sufficient to render the urine sterile. After 3 days of antibiotic therapy, urine culture should show no organisms.

If the urine is not sterile, bacterial resistance has probably occurred, making the use of a different antimicrobial necessary. Single-dose antibiotic therapy with amoxicillin or co-trimoxazole may be effective in women with acute, noncomplicated UTI. A urine culture taken 1 to 2 weeks later indicates whether the infection has been eradicated.

Recurrent infections due to infected renal calculi, chronic prostatitis, or structural abnormality may necessitate surgery; prostatitis also requires long-term antibiotic therapy. In patients without these predisposing conditions, long-term, low-dosage antibiotic therapy is the treatment of choice.

**Special considerations**

• Watch for GI disturbances from antimicrobial therapy.

• If sitz baths are not effective, apply heat sparingly to the perineum, but be careful not to burn the patient. Apply topical antiseptics, such as povidone-iodine ointment, on the urethral meatus as necessary.

• Collect all urine samples for culture and sensitivity testing carefully and promptly.

# UTERINE CANCER

Cancer of the endometrium, or uterine cancer, is the most common gynecologic cancer. It usually affects postmenopausal women between ages 50 and 60; it's uncommon between ages 30 and 40 and extremely rare before age 30. Most premenopausal women who develop uterine cancer have a history of anovulatory menstrual cycles or another hormonal imbalance.

An average of 33,000 new cases of uterine cancer are reported annually; of these, 5,500 are eventually fatal.

**Causes**

Uterine cancer seems linked to several predisposing factors:

• low fertility index and anovulation

• abnormal uterine bleeding

• obesity, hypertension, or diabetes

• familial tendency

• history of uterine polyps or endometrial hyperplasia

• estrogen therapy (still controversial).

Generally, uterine cancer is an adenocarcinoma that metastasizes late, usually from the endometrium to the cervix, ovaries, fallopian tubes, and other peritoneal structures. It may spread to distant organs, such as the lungs and the brain, through the blood or the lymphatic system. Lymph node involvement can also occur. Less common uterine tumors include adenoacanthoma, endometrial stromal sarcoma, lymphosarcoma, mixed mesodermal tumors (including carcinosarcoma), and leiomyosarcoma.

### Signs and symptoms
Uterine enlargement and persistent and unusual premenopausal bleeding, or any postmenopausal bleeding, are the most common indications of uterine cancer. The discharge may at first be watery and blood-streaked but gradually becomes more bloody. Other symptoms, such as pain and weight loss, don't appear until the cancer is well-advanced.

### Diagnosis
Unfortunately, a Pap smear, so useful for detecting cervical cancer, doesn't dependably predict early-stage uterine cancer. Diagnosis of uterine cancer requires endometrial, cervical, and endocervical biopsies. (See *Staging uterine cancer.*)

Negative biopsies call for a fractional dilatation and curettage to determine diagnosis. Positive diagnosis requires the following tests for baseline data and staging:

• multiple cervical biopsies and endocervical curettage to pinpoint cervical involvement

• Schiller's test, staining the cervix and vagina with an iodine solution that turns healthy tissues brown; cancerous tissues resist the stain.

• complete physical examination

• chest X-ray or computed tomography scan

• excretory urography and, possibly, cystoscopy

• complete blood count

• electrocardiography

• proctoscopy or barium enema studies, if bladder and rectal involvement are suspected.

---

## STAGING UTERINE CANCER

The International Federation of Gynecology and Obstetrics defines uterine (endometrial) cancer stages as follows.

**Stage 0** — carcinoma *in situ*
**Stage I** — carcinoma confined to the corpus
**Stage IA** — length of the uterine cavity < 8 cm
**Stage IB** — length of the uterine cavity > 8 cm
  Stage I disease is subgrouped by the following histologic grades of the adenocarcinoma:
• G1 — highly differentiated adenomatous carcinoma
• G2 — moderately differentiated adenomatous carcinoma with partly solid areas
• G3 — predominantly solid or entirely undifferentiated carcinoma
**Stage II** — carcinoma has involved the corpus and the cervix but has not extended outside the uterus
**Stage III** — carcinoma has extended outside the uterus but not outside the true pelvis
**Stage IV** — carcinoma has extended outside the true pelvis or has obviously involved the mucosa of the bladder or rectum
**Stage IVA** — spread of the growth to adjacent organs
**Stage IVB** — spread to distant organs

---

### Treatment
Uterine cancer treatment varies, depending on the extent of the disease.

#### Surgery
Rarely curative, surgery generally involves total abdominal hysterectomy, bilateral salpingo-oophorectomy, or possibly omentectomy with or without

# MANAGING PELVIC EXENTERATION

### Before pelvic exenteration
• Teach the patient about ileal conduit and possible colostomy, and make sure the patient understands that her vagina will be removed.
• To minimize the risk of infection, supervise a rigorous bowel and skin preparation procedure. Decrease the residue in the patient's diet for 48 to 72 hours, then maintain a diet ranging from clear liquids to nothing by mouth. Administer oral or I.V. antibiotics as ordered, and prep skin daily with antibacterial soap.
• Instruct the patient about postoperative procedures: I.V. therapy, central venous pressure catheter, blood drainage system, and an unsutured perineal wound with gauze packing.

### After pelvic exenteration
• Check the stoma, incision, and perineal wound for drainage. Be especially careful to check the perineal wound for bleeding after the packing is removed. Expect red or serosanguineous drainage, but notify the doctor immediately if drainage is excessive, continuously bright red, foul-smelling, or purulent, or if there is bleeding from the conduit.
• Provide excellent skin care because of draining urine and feces. Use warm water and saline solution to clean the skin because soap may be too drying and may increase skin breakdown.

cal removal of diseased parts. (See *Managing pelvic exenteration*.)

### *Radiation therapy*
When the tumor isn't well differentiated, intracavitary or external radiation (or both), given 6 weeks before surgery, may inhibit recurrence and lengthen survival time.

### *Hormonal therapy*
Synthetic progesterones — such as medroxyprogesterone or megestrol — may be administered for systemic disease. Tamoxifen (which produces a 20% to 40% response rate) may be given as a second-line treatment.

### *Chemotherapy*
Varying combinations of cisplatin, doxorubicin, etoposide, and dactinomycin are usually tried when other treatments have failed.

## Special considerations
• Patients with uterine cancer require teaching to help them cope with surgery, radiation, and chemotherapy. Also provide good postoperative care and psychological support.
   Before surgery:
• Reinforce any previous teaching about the surgery, and explain routine tests (such as repeated blood tests the morning after surgery) and postoperative care.
• If the patient will undergo lymphadenectomy *and* total hysterectomy, explain that she'll probably have a blood drainage system for about 5 days after surgery.
• Explain indwelling urinary catheter care.
• Fit the patient with antiembolism stockings for use during and after surgery.
• Make sure the patient's blood has been typed and crossmatched.

pelvic or para-aortic lymphadenectomy.
   Total exenteration involves removal of all pelvic organs, including the vagina, and is done only when the disease is sufficiently contained to allow surgi-

• If the patient is premenopausal, inform her that removal of her ovaries will induce menopause.

After surgery:

• Measure fluid contents of the blood drainage system every 8 hours. Be alert for drainage that exceeds 400 ml/8 hours.

• If the patient has received subcutaneous heparin, continue administration until he's fully ambulatory again. Give prophylactic antibiotics and provide good indwelling urinary catheter care.

• Check vital signs every 4 hours. Watch for any sign of complications, such as bleeding, abdominal distention, severe pain, wheezing, or other breathing difficulties. Provide analgesics.

• Regularly encourage the patient to breathe deeply and cough to help prevent complications. Promote the use of an incentive spirometer once every waking hour to help keep lungs expanded.

• Find out whether the patient is to have internal or external radiation or both. Usually, internal radiation therapy is done first.

If the patient receives internal radiation:

• Explain the internal radiation procedure, answer the patient's questions, and encourage her to express her fears and concerns.

• Explain that internal radiation usually requires a 2- to 3-day hospital stay, bowel preparation, a povidone-iodine vaginal douche, a clear-liquid diet, and nothing taken by mouth the night before the implantation.

• Mention that internal radiation also requires an indwelling urinary catheter.

• Tell the patient that if the procedure is performed in the operating room, she will receive a general anesthetic. She'll be placed in a dorsal position, with her knees and hips flexed and her heels resting in footrests.

If the radioactive source isn't implanted in the operating room, it may be implanted by a member of the radiation team while the patient is in her room.

> **CLINICAL TIP** Remember that safety precautions, including time, distance, and shielding, must be imposed immediately after the radioactive source has been implanted.

• Tell the patient that she'll require a private room.

• Encourage the patient to limit movement while the source is in place. If necessary, administer a tranquilizer to help her relax and remain still. If she prefers, elevate the head of the bed slightly. Make sure she can reach everything she needs (call bell, telephone, water) without stretching or straining.

• Assist the patient in range-of-motion arm exercises (leg exercises and other body movements could dislodge the source). Organize the time you spend with the patient to minimize your exposure to radiation.

• Check the patient's vital signs every 4 hours; watch for skin reaction, vaginal bleeding, abdominal discomfort, or evidence of dehydration.

• Inform visitors of safety precautions and hang a sign listing these precautions on the patient's door.

If the patient receives external radiation:

• Teach the patient and her family about the therapy before it begins. Tell the patient that treatment is usually given 5 days a week for 6 weeks. Warn her not to scrub body areas marked with indelible ink for treatment because it's important to direct treatment to exactly the same area each time.

• Instruct the patient to maintain a high-protein, high-carbohydrate, low-residue diet to reduce bulk and yet maintain calories.

• Administer diphenoxylate with atropine to minimize diarrhea, a possible side effect of pelvic radiation.

• To minimize skin breakdown and reduce the risk of skin infection, tell the patient to keep the treatment area dry, to avoid wearing clothes that rub against the area, and to avoid using heating pads, alcohol rubs, or any skin creams.

• Teach the patient how to use a vaginal dilator to prevent vaginal stenosis and to facilitate vaginal examinations and sexual intercourse.

• Explain that except in total pelvic exenteration, the vagina remains intact and that once she recovers, sexual intercourse is possible.

# UTERINE LEIOMYOMAS

Also called myomas, fibromyomas, and fibroids, uterine leiomyomas are the most common benign tumors in women. These smooth-muscle tumors usually occur in multiples in the uterine corpus, although they may appear on the cervix or on the round or broad ligament.

Uterine leiomyomas are often called fibroids, but this term is misleading because they consist of muscle cells and not fibrous tissue. Uterine leiomyomas occur in 20% to 25% of women of reproductive age and affect three times as many Blacks as Whites. The tumors become malignant (leiomyosarcoma) in only 0.1% of patients.

## Causes

The cause of uterine leiomyomas is unknown, but steroid hormones, including estrogen and progesterone, and several growth factors, including epidermal growth factor, have been implicated as regulators of leiomyoma growth.

Leiomyomas typically arise after menarche and regress after menopause, implicating estrogen as a promoter of leiomyoma growth.

## Signs and symptoms

Leiomyomas may be located within the uterine wall or may protrude into the endometrial cavity or from the serosal surface of the uterus. Most leiomyomas produce no symptoms. The most common symptom is abnormal bleeding, which typically presents clinically as menorrhagia.

Uterine leiomyomas probably do not cause pain directly except when associated with torsion of a pedunculated subserous tumor. Pelvic pressure and impingement on adjacent viscera are common indications for treatment. Various reproductive disorders, including infertility, recurrent spontaneous abortion, and preterm labor, have been attributed to uterine leiomyomas.

## Diagnosis

Clinical findings and the patient history suggest uterine leiomyomas.

• *Blood studies* showing anemia from abnormal bleeding support the diagnosis.

• *Bimanual examination* may reveal an enlarged, firm, nontender, and irregularly contoured uterus.

• *Ultrasonography* allows accurate assessment of the dimensions, number, and location of tumors.

• Other diagnostic procedures include hysterosalpingography, dilatation and curettage, endometrial biopsy, and laparoscopy.

## Treatment

Effective treatment depends on the severity of symptoms, the size and location of the tumors, and the patient's age, parity, pregnancy status, desire to have children, and general health. Treatment options include nonsurgical as well as surgical procedures.

### Nonsurgical treatment
Conservative treatment includes taking serial histories, performing physical assessments at clinically indicated intervals, and administering gonadotropin-releasing hormone (GnRH) analogues. These drugs are capable of rapidly suppressing pituitary gonadotropin release, leading to profound hypoestrogenemia and a 50% reduction in uterine volume.

The peak effects of these GnRH analogues occur in the 12th week of therapy. The benefits are reduction in tumor size before surgery, reduction in intraoperative blood loss, and an increase in preoperative hematocrit.

### Surgery
Surgery includes abdominal, laparoscopic, or hysteroscopic myomectomy for patients who want to preserve fertility. Hysterectomy is the definitive treatment for symptomatic women who have completed childbearing.

### Special considerations
• Tell the patient to report any abnormal bleeding or pelvic pain immediately.
• If a hysterectomy or oophorectomy is indicated, explain the effects of the operation on menstruation, menopause, and sexual activity to the patient.

➤ CLINICAL TIP    Reassure the patient that she won't experience premature menopause if her ovaries are left intact.
• If the patient will undergo multiple myomectomy, make sure she understands that pregnancy is still possible. However, if the uterine cavity is entered during surgery, explain that a cesarean delivery may be necessary.

• In a patient with severe anemia due to excessive bleeding, administer iron and blood transfusions.

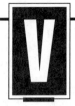

# VALVULAR HEART DISEASE

In valvular heart disease, three types of mechanical disruption can occur: stenosis, or narrowing, of the valve opening; incomplete closure of the valve; or prolapse of the valve. They can result from such disorders as endocarditis (most common), congenital defects, and inflammation, and they can lead to heart failure. (For information about causes, signs and symptoms, and diagnosis, see *Forms of valvular heart disease*.)

Valvular heart disease occurs in varying forms:

● *Mitral insufficiency.* In this form, blood from the left ventricle flows back into the left atrium during systole, causing the atrium to enlarge to accommodate the backflow. As a result, the left ventricle also dilates to accommodate the increased volume of blood from the atrium and to compensate for diminishing cardiac output.

Ventricular hypertrophy and increased end-diastolic pressure result in increased pulmonary artery pressure, eventually leading to left and right ventricular failure.

● *Mitral stenosis.* Narrowing of the valve by valvular abnormalities, fibrosis, or calcification obstructs blood flow from the left atrium to the left ventricle. Consequently, left atrial volume and pressure rise and the chamber dilates.

Greater resistance to blood flow causes pulmonary hypertension, right ventricular hypertrophy, and right ventricular failure. Also, inadequate filling of the left ventricle produces low cardiac output.

● *Mitral valve prolapse (MVP).* One or both valve leaflets protrude into the left atrium. MVP syndrome is the term used when the anatomic prolapse is accompanied by signs and symptoms unrelated to the valvular abnormality.

● *Aortic insufficiency.* Blood flows back into the left ventricle during diastole, causing fluid overload in the ventricle, which dilates and hypertrophies. The excess volume causes fluid overload in the left atrium and, finally, the pulmonary system. Left ventricular failure and pulmonary edema eventually result.

● *Aortic stenosis.* Increased left ventricular pressure tries to overcome the resistance of the narrowed valvular opening. The added workload increases the demand for oxygen, and diminished cardiac output causes poor coronary artery perfusion, ischemia of the left ventricle, and left ventricular failure.

● *Pulmonic insufficiency.* Blood ejected into the pulmonary artery during systole flows back into the right ventricle during diastole, causing fluid overload in the ventricle, ventricular hypertrophy and, finally, right ventricular failure.

*(Text continues on page 896.)*

# FORMS OF VALVULAR HEART DISEASE

| CAUSES AND INCIDENCE | CLINICAL FEATURES | DIAGNOSTIC MEASURES |
|---|---|---|
| **Mitral stenosis**<br>• Results from rheumatic fever (most common cause)<br>• Most common in females<br>• May be associated with other congenital anomalies | • Dyspnea on exertion, paroxysmal nocturnal dyspnea, orthopnea, weakness, fatigue, palpitations<br>• Peripheral edema, jugular vein distention, ascites, hepatomegaly (right ventricular failure in severe pulmonary hypertension)<br>• Crackles, cardiac arrhythmias (atrial fibrillation), signs of systemic emboli<br>• Auscultation that reveals a loud $S_1$ or opening snap and a diastolic murmur at the apex | • Cardiac catheterization: diastolic pressure gradient across valve; elevated left atrial and pulmonary artery wedge pressures (PAWP > 15 mm Hg) with severe pulmonary hypertension and pulmonary artery pressures; elevated right-sided heart pressure, decreased cardiac output (CO); and abnormal contraction of the left ventricle<br>• X-ray: left atrial and ventricular enlargement, enlarged pulmonary arteries, and mitral valve calcification<br>• Echocardiography: thickened mitral valve leaflets, left atrial enlargement<br>• Electrocardiography: left atrial hypertrophy, atrial fibrillation, right ventricular hypertrophy, and right axis deviation |
| **Mitral insufficiency**<br>• Results from rheumatic fever, hypertrophic cardiomyopathy, mitral valve prolapse, myocardial infarction, severe left ventricular failure, or ruptured chordae tendineae<br>• Associated with other congenital anomalies such as transposition of the great arteries<br>• Rare in children without other congenital anomalies | • Orthopnea, dyspnea, fatigue, angina, palpitations<br>• Peripheral edema, jugular vein distention, hepatomegaly (right ventricular failure)<br>• Tachycardia, crackles, pulmonary edema<br>• Auscultation that reveals a holosystolic murmur at apex, possible split $S_2$, and an $S_3$ | • Cardiac catheterization: mitral regurgitation with increased left ventricular end-diastolic volume and pressure, increased atrial pressure and PAWP, and decreased CO<br>• X-ray: left atrial and ventricular enlargement, pulmonary venous congestion<br>• Echocardiography: abnormal valve leaflet motion, left atrial enlargement<br>• Electrocardiography: may show left atrial and ventricular hypertrophy, sinus tachycardia, and atrial fibrillation |

*(continued)*

## FORMS OF VALVULAR HEART DISEASE *(continued)*

| CAUSES AND INCIDENCE | CLINICAL FEATURES | DIAGNOSTIC MEASURES |
|---|---|---|
| **Mitral valve prolapse syndrome**<br>• Cause unknown. Researchers speculate that metabolic or neuroendocrine factors cause constellation of signs and symptoms.<br>• Most commonly affects young women but may occur in both sexes and in all age-groups | • May produce no signs<br>• Chest pain, palpitations, headache, fatigue, exercise intolerance, dyspnea, light-headedness, syncope, mood swings, anxiety, panic attacks<br>• Auscultation that typically reveals a mobile, mid-systolic click, with or without a mid-to-late systolic murmur | • Two-dimensional echocardiography: prolapse of mitral valve leaflets into left atrium<br>• Color-flow Doppler studies: mitral insufficiency<br>• Resting electrocardiography: ST-segment changes, biphasic or inverted T waves in leads II, III, or AVF<br>• Exercise electrocardiography: evaluates chest pain and arrhythmias |
| **Aortic insufficiency**<br>• Results from rheumatic fever, syphilis, hypertension, endocarditis, or may be idiopathic<br>• Associated with Marfan syndrome<br>• Most common in males<br>• Associated with ventricular septal defect, even after surgical closure | • Dyspnea, cough, fatigue, palpitations, angina, syncope<br>• Pulmonary vein congestion, heart failure, pulmonary edema (left ventricular failure), "pulsating" nail beds (Quincke's sign)<br>• Rapidly rising and collapsing pulses (pulsus biferiens), cardiac arrhythmias, wide pulse pressure in severe regurgitation<br>• Auscultation that reveals an $S_3$ and a diastolic blowing murmur at left sternal border<br>• Palpation and visualization of apical impulse in chronic disease | • Cardiac catheterization: reduction in arterial diastolic pressures, aortic regurgitation, other valvular abnormalities, and increased left ventricular end-diastolic pressure<br>• X-ray: left ventricular enlargement, pulmonary vein congestion<br>• Echocardiography: left ventricular enlargement, alterations in mitral valve movement (indirect indication of aortic valve disease), and mitral thickening<br>• Electrocardiography: sinus tachycardia, left ventricular hypertrophy, and left atrial hypertrophy in severe disease |

## FORMS OF VALVULAR HEART DISEASE (continued)

| CAUSES AND INCIDENCE | CLINICAL FEATURES | DIAGNOSTIC MEASURES |
|---|---|---|
| **Aortic stenosis**<br>• Results from congenital aortic bicuspid valve (associated with coarctation of the aorta), congenital stenosis of valve cusps, rheumatic fever, or atherosclerosis in the elderly<br>• Most common in males | • Dyspnea on exertion, paroxysmal nocturnal dyspnea, fatigue, syncope, angina, palpitations<br>• Pulmonary vein congestion, heart failure, pulmonary edema (left ventricular failure)<br>• Diminished carotid pulses, decreased cardiac output, cardiac arrhythmias; may have pulsus alternans<br>• Auscultation that reveals systolic murmur heard at base or in carotids and, possibly, an $S_4$ | • Cardiac catheterization: pressure gradient across valve (indicating obstruction), increased left ventricular end-diastolic pressures<br>• X-ray: valvular calcification, left ventricular enlargement, and pulmonary vein congestion<br>• Echocardiography: thickened aortic valve and left ventricular wall, possibly coexistent with mitral valve stenosis<br>• Electrocardiography: left ventricular hypertrophy |
| **Pulmonic insufficiency**<br>• May be congenital or may result from pulmonary hypertension<br>• May rarely result from prolonged use of pressure monitoring catheter in the pulmonary artery | • Dyspnea, weakness, fatigue, chest pain<br>• Peripheral edema, jugular vein distention, hepatomegaly (right ventricular failure)<br>• Auscultation that reveals diastolic murmur in pulmonic area | • Cardiac catheterization: pulmonary regurgitation, increased right ventricular pressure, and associated cardiac defects<br>• X-ray: right ventricular and pulmonary arterial enlargement<br>• Electrocardiography: right ventricular or right atrial enlargement |
| **Pulmonic stenosis**<br>• Results from congenital stenosis of valve cusp or rheumatic heart disease (infrequent)<br>• Associated with other congenital heart defects such as tetralogy of Fallot | • Asymptomatic or symptomatic with dyspnea on exertion, fatigue, chest pain, syncope<br>• May lead to peripheral edema, jugular vein distention, hepatomegaly (right ventricular failure)<br>• Auscultation that reveals a systolic murmur at the left sternal border, a split $S_2$ with a delayed or absent pulmonic component | • Cardiac catheterization: increased right ventricular pressure, decreased pulmonary artery pressure, and abnormal valve orifice<br>• Electrocardiography: may show right ventricular hypertrophy, right axis deviation, right atrial hypertrophy, and atrial fibrillation |

*(continued)*

## FORMS OF VALVULAR HEART DISEASE *(continued)*

| CAUSES AND INCIDENCE | CLINICAL FEATURES | DIAGNOSTIC MEASURES |
|---|---|---|
| **Tricuspid insufficiency**<br>• Results from right ventricular failure, rheumatic fever and, rarely, trauma and endocarditis<br>• Associated with congenital disorders | • Dyspnea and fatigue<br>• May lead to peripheral edema, jugular vein distention, hepatomegaly, and ascites (right ventricular failure)<br>• Auscultation that reveals possible $S_3$ and systolic murmur at lower left sternal border that increases with inspiration | • Right heart catheterization: high atrial pressure, tricuspid regurgitation, and decreased or normal cardiac output<br>• X-ray: right atrial dilation, right ventricular enlargement<br>• Echocardiography: systolic prolapse of tricuspid valve, right atrial enlargement<br>• Electrocardiography: right atrial or right ventricular hypertrophy, atrial fibrillation |
| **Tricuspid stenosis**<br>• Results from rheumatic fever<br>• May be congenital<br>• Associated with mitral or aortic valve disease<br>• Most common in women | • May be symptomatic with dyspnea, fatigue, syncope<br>• Possibly peripheral edema, jugular vein distention, hepatomegaly, and ascites (right ventricular failure)<br>• Auscultation that reveals diastolic murmur at lower left sternal border that increases with inspiration | • Cardiac catheterization: increased pressure gradient across valve, increased right atrial pressure, decreased cardiac output<br>• X-ray: right atrial enlargement<br>• Echocardiography: leaflet abnormality, right atrial enlargement<br>• Electrocardiography: right atrial hypertrophy, right or left ventricular hypertrophy, and atrial fibrillation |

• *Pulmonic stenosis.* Obstructed right ventricular outflow causes right ventricular hypertrophy, eventually resulting in right ventricular failure.

• *Tricuspid insufficiency.* Blood flows back into the right atrium during systole, decreasing blood flow to the lungs and left side of the heart. Cardiac output also lessens. Fluid overload in the right side of the heart can eventually lead to right ventricular failure.

• *Tricuspid stenosis.* Obstructed blood flow from the right atrium to the right ventricle causes the right atrium to dilate and hypertrophy. Eventually, this leads to right ventricular failure and increases pressure in the vena cava.

## Treatment

Therapy depends on the nature and severity of associated symptoms. For example, heart failure requires digoxin, diuretics, a sodium-restricted diet and, in acute cases, oxygen.

Other measures may include anticoagulant therapy to prevent thrombus formation around diseased or replaced valves, prophylactic antibiotics before and after surgery or dental care, and valvuloplasty. If the patient has severe signs and symptoms that can't be managed medically, open-heart surgery using cardiopulmonary bypass for valve replacement is indicated.

**Special considerations**
- Watch closely for signs of heart failure or pulmonary edema and for adverse effects of drug therapy.
- Teach the patient about diet restrictions, medications, and the importance of consistent follow-up care.
- If the patient undergoes surgery, watch for hypotension, arrhythmias, and thrombus formation. Monitor vital signs, arterial blood gases, intake, output, daily weight, blood chemistries, chest X-rays, and pulmonary artery catheter readings.

# VANCOMYCIN INTERMEDIATELY RESISTANT *STAPHYLOCOCCUS AUREUS*

Vancomycin intermediately resistant *Staphylococcus aureus* (VISA) is a mutation of a bacterium that is spread easily by direct person-to-person contact. It was first discovered in mid-1996 when clinicians found the microbe in a Japanese infant's surgical wound. Similar isolates were reported in Michigan and New Jersey. Both patients had received multiple courses of vancomycin for methicillin-resistant *Staphylococcus aureus* (MRSA) infections.

Another mutation, vancomycin-resistant *Staphylococcus aureus* (VRSA) is fully resistant to vancomycin. Patients most at risk for resistant organisms include:
- patients with a history of taking vancomycin, third-generation cephalosporins, or antibiotics targeted at anaerobic bacteria (such as *Clostridium difficile*)
- patients with indwelling urinary or central venous catheters
- elderly patients, especially those with prolonged or repeated hospital admissions
- patients with cancer or chronic renal failure
- patients undergoing cardiothoracic or intra-abdominal surgery or organ transplants
- patients with wounds with an opening to the pelvic or intra-abdominal area, including surgical wounds, burns, and pressure ulcers
- patients with enterococcal bacteremia, often associated with endocarditis
- patients exposed to contaminated equipment or to a patient with the infecting microbe.

**Causes**
Vancomycin-resistant enterococcus (VRE) and MRSA enter health care facilities through an infected or colonized patient or a colonized health care worker. It's thought that VISA and VRSA are colonized in a similar method. They're spread through direct contact between the patient and caregiver or between patients. They may also be spread through patient contact with contaminated surfaces such as an overbed table. They're capable of living for weeks on surfaces. They've been detected on patient gowns, bed linens, and handrails.

## Signs and symptoms

There are no specific signs or symptoms related to this microbe. The causative agent may be found incidentally when culture results show the organism.

## Diagnosis

Someone with no signs or symptoms of infection is considered colonized if VISA or VRSA can be isolated from stool or a rectal swab. A patient who's colonized is more than 10 times as likely to become infected with the organism (such as through a breach in the immune system) than a patient who isn't.

## Treatment

There is virtually no antibiotic to combat VISA or VRSA. Recently, the Centers for Disease Control and Prevention and the Hospital Infection Control Practices Advisory Committee proposed a two-level system of precautions to simplify isolation for resistant organisms. The first level calls for standard precautions, which incorporate features of universal blood and body fluid precautions and body substance isolation precautions to be used for all patient care. The second level calls for transmission-based precautions, implemented when a particular infection is suspected.

To prevent the spread of VISA and VRSA, some hospitals perform weekly surveillance cultures on at-risk patients in intensive care or oncology units and on patients who have been transferred from a long-term care facility. A colonized patient is then placed in contact isolation until he's culture-negative or discharged. Colonization can last indefinitely; no protocol has been established for the length of time a patient should remain in isolation.

Because no single antibiotic is currently available, the doctor may opt not to treat an infection at all. Instead, he may stop all antibiotics and simply wait for normal bacteria to repopulate and replace the strain. Combinations of various drugs may also be used, depending on the source of the infection.

## Special considerations

● Personnel in contact with an infected patient should wash their hands before and after care of the patient.

▶ CLINICAL TIP   Good hand washing is the most effective way to prevent VISA and VRSA from spreading.

● Use an antiseptic soap such as chlorhexidine; bacteria have been cultured from worker's hands after they've washed with milder soap.

● Maintain contact isolation precautions when in contact with the patient. Provide a private room and dedicated equipment, and disinfect the environment.

● Change gloves when contaminated or when moving from a "dirty" area of the body to a clean one.

● Do not touch potentially contaminated surfaces, such as a bed or bed stand, after removing gown and gloves.

● Be particularly prudent in caring for a patient with an ileostomy, colostomy, or draining wound that is not contained by a dressing.

● Instruct family and friends to wear protective garb when they visit the patient, and teach them how to dispose of the garb.

● Provide teaching and emotional support to the patient and family members.

● Consider grouping infected patients together (known as *cohorting*) and having the same nursing staff care for them.

● Do not lay equipment used on the patient on the bed or bed stand; wipe it with appropriate disinfectant before leaving the room.

● Ensure judicious and careful use of antibiotics. Encourage doctors to limit the use of antibiotics.

- Instruct patients to take antibiotics for the full prescription period, even if they begin to feel better.

# VANCOMYCIN-RESISTANT ENTEROCOCCUS

Vancomycin-resistant enterococcus (VRE) is a mutation of a very common bacterium that is spread easily by direct person-to-person contact. Facilities in more than 40 states have reported VRE, with rates as high as 14% in oncology units of large teaching facilities. Patients most at risk for VRE include:

- immunosuppressed patients or those with severe underlying disease
- patients with a history of taking vancomycin, third-generation cephalosporins, or antibiotics targeted at anaerobic bacteria (such as *Clostridium difficile*)
- patients with indwelling urinary or central venous catheters
- elderly patients, especially those with prolonged or repeated hospital admissions
- patients with cancer or chronic renal failure
- patients undergoing cardiothoracic or intra-abdominal surgery or organ transplants
- patients with wounds with an opening to the pelvic or intra-abdominal area, including surgical wounds, burns, and pressure ulcers
- patients with enterococcal bacteremia, often associated with endocarditis
- patients exposed to contaminated equipment or to a VRE-positive patient.

## Causes

VRE enters health care facilities through an infected or colonized patient or a colonized health care worker. VRE is spread through direct contact between the patient and caregiver or between patients. It can also be spread through patient contact with contaminated surfaces such as an overbed table. It is capable of living for weeks on surfaces. It has been detected on patient gowns, bed linens, and handrails.

## Signs and symptoms

There are no specific signs and symptoms related to VRE. The causative agent may be found incidentally when culture results show the organism.

## Diagnosis

Someone with no signs or symptoms of infection is considered colonized if VRE can be isolated from stool or a rectal swab. Once colonized, a patient is more than 10 times as likely to become infected with VRE, for example, through a breach in the immune system.

## Treatment

There is no specific treatment at this time for eradicating VRE. Recently, the Centers for Disease Control and Prevention and the Hospital Infection Control Practices Advisory Committee proposed a two-level system of precautions to simplify isolation. The first level calls for standard precautions, which incorporate features of universal blood and body fluid precautions and body substance isolation precautions, to be used for all patient care. The second level calls for transmission-based precautions, which are implemented when a particular infection is suspected.

To prevent the spread of VRE, some facilities perform weekly surveillance cultures on at-risk patients on intensive care units or oncology units and on patients who've been transferred from a long-term care facility. Any colonized patient is then placed in contact isolation until culture-negative or until discharged. Colonization can last indefinitely, and no protocol has been established for the length of time a patient should remain in isolation.

Because no single antibiotic currently available can eradicate VRE, the doctor may, in some cases, opt not to treat an infection at all. Instead, he may stop all antibiotics and simply wait for normal bacteria to repopulate and replace the VRE strain. Combinations of various drugs may also be used, depending on the source of the infection.

**Special considerations**
• Hand washing before and after care of the patient is crucial.

> CLINICAL TIP   Good hand washing is the most effective way to prevent VRE from spreading.

• Use an antiseptic soap such as chlorhexidine; bacteria have been cultured from worker's hands after they've washed with milder soap.
• Use contact isolation precautions when in contact with the patient. Provide a private room and dedicated equipment for the patient. Disinfect the environment.
• Change gloves when contaminated or when moving from a "dirty" area of the body to a clean one.
• Do not touch potentially contaminated surfaces, such as a bed or bed stand, after removing gown and gloves.
• Be particularly prudent in caring for a patient with an ileostomy, colostomy, or draining wound that is not contained by a dressing.
• Instruct family and friends to wear protective garb when they visit the patient, and teach them how to dispose of it.
• Provide teaching and emotional support to the patient and family members.

• Consider grouping ("cohorting") infected patients together and having the same nursing staff care for them.
• Do not lay equipment used on the patient on the bed or the bed stand. Wipe equipment with appropriate disinfectant before leaving the room.
• Ensure judicious and careful use of antibiotics. Encourage doctors to limit the use of antibiotics.
• Instruct patients to take antibiotics for the full prescription period, even if they begin to feel better.

# VARICELLA

Also called chickenpox, varicella is a common, acute, and highly contagious infection caused by the herpesvirus varicella-zoster (V-Z), the same virus that, in its latent stage, causes herpes zoster (shingles). It can occur at any age, but it's most common in 2- to 8-year-olds.

Varicella vaccine is effective in preventing chickenpox in up to 90% of recipients. The American Academy of Pediatrics recommends the vaccine for all children and for adolescents and adults who haven't had chickenpox. It is unknown how the vaccine affects shingles.

**Causes**
Congenital varicella may affect infants whose mothers had acute infections in their first or early second trimester. Neonatal infection is rare, probably due to transient maternal immunity. Second attacks are also rare.

Chickenpox is transmitted by direct contact (primarily with respiratory secretions; less often with skin lesions) and indirect contact (air waves). The incubation period lasts from 13 to 17 days. Chickenpox is probably communicable from 1 day before lesions erupt to 6 days after vesicles form (it's most contagious in the early stages of eruption of skin lesions).

Most children recover completely. Potentially fatal complications may affect children receiving corticosteroids, antimetabolites, or other immunosuppressant agents, and those with leukemia, other neoplasms, or immunodeficiency disorders. Congenital and adult varicella may also have severe effects.

This disease occurs worldwide and is endemic in large cities. Outbreaks occur sporadically, usually in areas with large groups of susceptible children. It affects all races and both sexes equally. Seasonal distribution varies; in temperate areas, incidence is higher during late autumn, winter, and spring.

### Signs and symptoms

Chickenpox produces distinctive signs and symptoms, notably a pruritic rash. During the prodromal phase, the patient has slight fever, malaise, and anorexia. Within 24 hours, the rash typically begins as crops of small, erythematous macules on the trunk or scalp that progress to papules and then clear vesicles on an erythematous base (the so-called "dewdrop on a rose petal").

The vesicles become cloudy and break easily; then scabs form. The rash spreads to the face and, rarely, to the extremities. New vesicles continue to appear for 3 to 4 days, so the rash contains a combination of red papules, vesicles, and scabs in various stages. Occasionally, chickenpox also produces shallow ulcers on mucous membranes of the mouth, conjunctivae, and genitalia.

Congenital varicella causes hypoplastic deformity and scarring of a limb, retarded growth, and central nervous system and eye manifestations. In progressive varicella, an immunocompromised patient will have lesions and a high fever for more than 7 days.

### Complications

Severe pruritus with this rash may provoke persistent scratching, which can lead to infection, scarring, impetigo, furuncles, and cellulitis. Rare complications include pneumonia, myocarditis, fulminating encephalitis (Reye's syndrome), bleeding disorders, arthritis, nephritis, hepatitis, and acute myositis.

### Diagnosis

Chickenpox is diagnosed by characteristic clinical signs and usually doesn't require laboratory tests. However, the virus can be isolated from vesicular fluid within the first 3 to 4 days of the rash; Giemsa stain distinguishes V-Z from vaccinia-variola viruses. Serum contains antibodies 7 days after onset.

### Treatment

Patients must remain in strict isolation until all the vesicles and most of the scabs disappear (usually for 1 week after the onset of the rash). Children can go back to school, however, if just a few scabs remain because, at this stage, chickenpox is no longer contagious. Congenital chickenpox requires no isolation.

Generally, treatment consists of the following:

• local or systemic antipruritics
• cool bicarbonate of soda baths
• calamine lotion
• diphenhydramine or another antihistamine
• antibiotics if bacterial infection develops.

Salicylates are contraindicated because of their link with Reye's syndrome.

Susceptible patients may need special treatment. When given up to 72 hours after exposure to varicella, varicella-zoster immune globulin may provide passive immunity. Acyclovir may slow vesicle formation, speed skin healing, and control the systemic spread of infection.

## Special considerations

• Teach the child and his family how to apply topical antipruritic medications correctly. Stress the importance of good hygiene.

• Tell the patient not to scratch the lesions. However, because the need to scratch may be overwhelming, parents should trim the child's fingernails or tie mittens on his hands.

• Warn parents to watch for and immediately report signs of complications. Severe skin pain and burning may indicate a serious secondary infection and require prompt medical attention.

> CLINICAL TIP   A live, attenuated varicella vaccine has been licensed for use in the United States.

• To help prevent chickenpox, don't admit a child exposed to chickenpox to a unit that contains children who receive immunosuppressant agents or who have leukemia or immunodeficiency disorders. A vulnerable child who's been exposed to chickenpox should receive varicella-zoster immune globulin to lessen its severity.

---

# VASCULAR RETINOPATHIES

---

Vascular retinopathies are noninflammatory retinal disorders that result from interference with the blood supply to the eyes. The five distinct types of vascular retinopathy are central retinal artery occlusion, central retinal vein occlusion, diabetic retinopathy, hypertensive retinopathy, and sickle cell retinopathy.

## Causes

When one of the arteries maintaining blood circulation in the retina becomes obstructed, the diminished blood flow causes visual deficits.

### *Central retinal artery occlusion*

This form of vascular retinopathy may be idiopathic or may result from embolism, atherosclerosis, infection, or conditions that retard blood flow, such as carotid occlusion and heart valve vegetations. Central retinal artery occlusion is rare and occurs unilaterally; it affects elderly patients as well as younger patients with valvular disease.

### *Central retinal vein occlusion*

Causes of central retinal vein occlusion include external compression of the retinal vein, trauma, diabetes, thrombosis, granulomatous diseases, generalized and localized infections, glaucoma, and atherosclerosis. This form of vascular retinopathy is most prevalent in elderly patients.

### *Diabetic retinopathy*

This form results from juvenile or adult diabetes. Microcirculatory changes occur more rapidly when diabetes is poorly controlled. About 75% of patients with juvenile diabetes develop retinopathy within 20 years of onset of diabetes.

In adults with diabetes, incidence increases with the duration of diabetes; 80% of patients who have had diabetes for 20 to 25 years develop retinopathy. This condition is a leading cause of acquired adult blindness.

### *Hypertensive retinopathy*

This form results from prolonged hypertensive disease, producing retinal vasospasm, and consequent damage and arteriolar narrowing.

### Sickle cell retinopathy

This form results from impaired ability of the sickled cell to pass through the microvasculature, producing vasocclusion. This results in microaneurysms, chorioretinal infarction, and retinal detachment.

## Signs and symptoms

The following features characterize vascular retinopathy.

### Central retinal artery occlusion

This type of occlusion produces sudden, painless, unilateral loss of vision (partial or complete). It may follow amaurosis fugax or transient episodes of unilateral loss of vision lasting from a few seconds to minutes, probably due to vasospasm.

This condition typically causes permanent loss of vision. However, some patients experience spontaneous resolution within hours and regain partial vision.

### Central retinal vein occlusion

Occlusion of this type causes reduced visual acuity, allowing perception of only hand movement and light. This condition is painless, except when it results in secondary neovascular glaucoma (uncontrolled proliferation of weak blood vessels). Prognosis is poor—5% to 20% of patients with this condition develop secondary glaucoma within 3 to 4 months after occlusion.

### Diabetic retinopathy

*Nonproliferative diabetic retinopathy* produces changes in the lining of the retinal blood vessels that cause the vessels to leak plasma or fatty substances, which decrease or block blood flow (nonperfusion) within the retina. This disorder may also produce microaneurysms and small hemorrhages.

Although nonproliferative retinopathy causes no symptoms in some patients, in others leakage of fluid into the macular region causes significant loss of central visual acuity (necessary for reading and driving) and diminished night vision.

*Proliferative diabetic retinopathy* produces fragile new blood vessels on the disk and elsewhere in the fundus (neovascularization). These vessels can grow into the vitreous and then rupture, causing vitreous hemorrhage with corresponding sudden vision loss.

Scar tissue that may form along the new blood vessels can pull on the retina, causing macular distortion and even retinal detachment.

### Hypertensive retinopathy

Symptoms of hypertensive retinopathy depend on the location of retinopathy. For example, mild visual disturbances, such as blurred vision, result from retinopathy located near the macula.

Without treatment, the prognosis is poor (50% of patients become blind within 5 years). With treatment, the prognosis varies with the severity of the disorder. Severe, prolonged disease eventually produces blindness; mild, prolonged disease, visual defects.

## Diagnosis

Appropriate diagnostic tests depend on the type of vascular retinopathy. (See *Diagnosis of vascular retinopathies,* page 904.) Always include determination of visual acuity and ophthalmoscopic examination.

## Treatment

The following measures are used to treat vascular retinopathy.

### Central retinal artery occlusion

No treatment has been shown to control central retinal artery occlusion.

# DIAGNOSIS OF VASCULAR RETINOPATHIES

In vascular retinopathies, diagnosis varies, depending on the type of retinopathy.

## Central retinal artery occlusion

In central retinal artery occlusion, the patient reports sudden loss of vision.

- *External examination* reveals a marked afferent pupillary defect.
- *Ophthalmoscopy* reveals narrowed retinal arterioles, "boxcarring" or segmentation of the blood column in the arterioles, and may reveal whitening of the retina around the disk (caused by a decreased blood supply) and a cherry red spot in the macula.
- *Physical examination* may reveal elevated blood pressure.
- *Erythrocyte sedimentation rate* may detect giant cell arteritis.
- *Doppler ultrasound* provides carotid artery evaluation.
- *Echocardiogram* and *Holter monitoring* reveal clots from vegetations on a heart valve.
- *Fluorescein angiography* confirms diagnosis.

## Central retinal vein occlusion

- *Ophthalmoscopy (direct or indirect)* shows retinal hemorrhages, retinal vein engorgement, white patches among hemorrhages, and edema around the disk.
- *History* may reveal use of oral contraceptives or diuretics or sudden loss of monocular vision.

- *Physical examination* may detect elevated blood pressure and reveal underlying cause.

## Diabetic retinopathy

- *Indirect ophthalmoscopy* shows retinal changes such as microaneurysms (earliest change), retinal hemorrhages and edema, venous dilation and beading of the vessel, exudates, and vitreous hemorrhage. New blood vessel growth, which leaks lipids and causes edema, and microinfarcts of the nerve fiber layer may also occur.
- *Fluorescein angiography* shows leakage of fluorescein from new blood vessels and differentiates between microaneurysms and true hemorrhages.
- *History* reveals longstanding diabetes and decreased vision.

## Hypertensive retinopathy

- *Ophthalmoscopy (direct or indirect)* shows changes in arteriovenous crossing; cottonwool spots; flame-shaped, silver-wire appearance of narrowed arterioles; nicking of veins where arteries cross them (arteriovenous nicking); hard exudates (lipid deposits); "macular star," flame-shaped hemorrhages; retinal edema; arterial microaneurysms; and swelling of the optic nerve head (disk edema).
- *Physical examination* detects elevated blood pressure.
- *History* reveals decreased vision, occipital headache, and hypertension.

---

However, an attempt is made to release the occlusion into the peripheral circulation.

To reduce intraocular pressure, treatments include immediate ocular massage, anterior chamber paracentesis after anesthetizing the surface with topical cocaine 2% to 4% drops, acetazolamide 500 mg I.V., and inhalation of carbogen (95% oxygen and 5% carbon dioxide) to improve retinal oxygenation. Because inhalation therapy may be given hourly for up to 48 hours, the patient should be hospitalized so vital signs can be monitored.

If the patient is young, the source of the occlusion may be the heart. Echocardiography may be necessary. Treatment in this case is to heparinize the patient.

### Central retinal vein occlusion

Therapy for central retinal vein occlusion may include aspirin, which acts as a mild anticoagulant. Laser photocoagulation can reduce the risk of neovascular glaucoma for some patients whose eyes have widespread capillary nonperfusion.

### Diabetic retinopathy

Treatment of *nonproliferative diabetic retinopathy* is prophylactic. Careful control of blood glucose levels during the first 5 years of the disease may reduce the severity of the retinopathy or delay its onset.

Patients with early symptoms of microaneurysms should have frequent eye examinations (3 to 4 times a year); children with diabetes should have an annual eye examination.

Treatment for *proliferative diabetic retinopathy* is laser photocoagulation, which cauterizes the leaking blood vessels, thereby eliminating the cause of the edema. Laser treatment may be focal (aimed at new blood vessels) or panretinal (placing burns throughout the peripheral retina).

Despite treatment, neovascularization doesn't always regress, and vitreous hemorrhage, with or without retinal detachment, may follow. Vitrectomy is the treatment of choice for vitreous hemorrhage to restore vision.

### Hypertensive retinopathy

Treatment for hypertensive retinopathy includes control of blood pressure with appropriate drugs, diet, and exercise.

### Special considerations

● Arrange for *immediate* ophthalmologic evaluation when a patient complains of sudden, unilateral loss of vision. Blindness may be permanent if treatment is delayed.

● Be sure to monitor a patient's blood pressure if he complains of occipital headache and blurred vision.

● Administer acetazolamide I.V. During inhalation therapy, monitor vital signs carefully. Discontinue therapy if blood pressure fluctuates or if patient develops arrhythmias or disorientation.

● Encourage a patient with diabetes to comply with the prescribed regimen.

● For a patient with hypertensive retinopathy, stress the importance of complying with antihypertensive therapy.

# VASCULITIS

A broad spectrum of disorders, vasculitis is characterized by inflammation and necrosis of blood vessels. Its clinical effects depend on the vessels involved and reflect tissue ischemia caused by blood flow obstruction.

The prognosis is also variable. For example, hypersensitivity vasculitis is usually a benign disorder limited to the skin, but more extensive polyarteritis nodosa can be rapidly fatal.

Vasculitis can occur at any age, except for mucocutaneous lymph node syndrome, which occurs only during childhood. Vasculitis may be a primary disorder or secondary to other disorders, such as rheumatoid arthritis or systemic lupus erythematosus.(See *Types of vasculitis,* pages 906 to 909.)

### Causes

How vascular damage develops in vasculitis isn't well understood. In some cases, it has been associated with a history of serious infectious disease, such as hepatitis B or bacterial endocarditis, and high-dose antibiotic therapy. Four possible mechanisms are currently under investigation.

*(Text continues on page 908.)*

## TYPES OF VASCULITIS

| TYPE | VESSELS INVOLVED | PEAK AGE AT ONSET (YEARS) |
|---|---|---|
| Polyarteritis nodosa (PAN) | Small- to medium-sized arteries throughout body. Lesions tend to be segmental, occur at bifurcations and branchings of arteries, and spread distally to arterioles. In severe cases, lesions circumferentially involve adjacent veins. They do not involve arterioles or venules. | 40 to 60 |
| Allergic angiitis and granulomatosis (Churg-Strauss syndrome) | Small- to medium-sized arteries and small vessels (arterioles, capillaries, and venules), mainly of the lung, kidney, and other organs | 40 to 60 |
| Microscopic polyangiitis | Small- to medium-sized arteries and small vessels (arterioles, capillaries, venules) of lung and kidney (different from PAN, in that smaller vessels are involved) | 40 to 60 |
| Wegener's granulomatosis | Medium- to large-sized vessels of the upper and lower respiratory tract and kidney; may also involve small arteries and veins | 30 to 50 |
| Temporal arteritis | Medium- to large-sized arteries, most commonly branches of the carotid artery; involvement may skip segments | 60 to 75 |
| Takayasu's arteritis (aortic arch syndrome) | Medium- to large-sized arteries, particularly the aortic arch and its branches and, possibly, the pulmonary artery | 15 to 25 |

| MALE: FEMALE RATIO | SIGNS AND SYMPTOMS | DIAGNOSIS |
|---|---|---|
| 2:1 | Hypertension, abdominal pain, myalgias, headache, joint pain, weakness, weight loss, mono- or polyneuropathy | History of symptoms. Elevated BUN and creatinine levels, elevated erythrocyte sedimentation rate (ESR), leukocytosis, anemia, thrombocytosis, depressed C3 complement, rheumatoid factor > 1:60, circulating immune complexes. Tissue biopsy shows necrotizing vasculitis and immune deposits. |
| 2:1 | Resembles polyarteritis nodosa with hallmark of severe pulmonary involvement | History of asthma. Eosinophilia, increased serum Igl; tissue biopsy shows granulomatous inflammation with eosinophilic infiltration. |
| 1.8:1 | Fever, pulmonary congestion, hemoptysis, hematuria, abnormal urine sediment, weight loss, malaise | Usually involves lung and kidneys, elevated ESR; 50% are positive for pANCA. Tissue biopsy shows necrotizing vasculitis without immune deposits or granuloma formation. |
| 1:1 | Fever, pulmonary congestion, cough, malaise, anorexia, weight loss, mild to severe hematuria | Tissue biopsy shows necrotizing vasculitis with granulomatous inflammation. Leukocytosis, elevated ESR, IgA, and IgG; low titer rheumatoid factor; circulating immune complexes: antineutrophil cytoplasmic antibody (cANCA) in more than 90% of patients. Renal biopsy shows focal segmental glomerulonephritis. |
| 1:3 | Fever, myalgia, jaw claudication, visual changes, headache (associated with polymyalgia rheumatica syndrome) | Decreased hemoglobin (Hb); elevated ESR; tissue biopsy shows panarteritis with infiltration of mononuclear cells, giant cells within vessel wall (seen in 50%), fragmentation of internal elastic lamina, and proliferation of intima. |
| 1:9 | Malaise, pallor, nausea, night sweats, arthralgias, anorexia, weight loss, pain or paresthesia distal to affected area, bruits, loss of distal pulses, syncope and, if carotid artery is involved, diplopia and transient blindness. May progress to heart failure or CVA. | Decreased Hb, leukocytosis, positive LE cell preparation, and elevated ESR. Arteriography shows calcification and obstruction of affected vessels. Tissue biopsy shows inflammation of adventitia and intima of vessels and thickening of vessel walls. |

*(continued)*

## TYPES OF VASCULITIS *(continued)*

| TYPE | VESSELS INVOLVED | PEAK AGE AT ONSET (YEARS) |
| --- | --- | --- |
| Hypersensitivity vasculitis | Small vessels, especially of the skin | 30 to 50 |
| Mucocutaneous lymph node syndrome (Kawasaki disease) | Small- to medium-sized vessels, primarily of the lymph nodes; may progress to involve coronary arteries | 1 to 5 |
| Henoch-Schönlein purpura (HSP) | Small vessels (arterioles, venules, capillaries) especially of skin and GI tract | 5 to 20 |
| Behçet's disease | Small vessels, primarily of the mouth and genitalia but also of the eyes, skin, joints, GI tract, and central nervous system | 20 to 25 |

### Excessive antigen theory

This theory holds that vasculitis is initiated by excessive circulating antigen, which triggers the formation of soluble antigen-antibody complexes. These complexes can't be effectively cleared by the reticuloendothelial system and so are deposited in blood vessel walls (Type III hypersensitivity).

Increased vascular permeability associated with release of vasoactive amines by platelets and basophils enhances such deposition. The deposited complexes activate the complement cascade, resulting in chemotaxis of neutrophils, which release lysosomal enzymes. In turn, these enzymes cause vessel damage and necrosis, which may precipitate thrombosis, occlusion, hemorrhage, and ischemia.

### Autoantibody production

An additional factor in certain types of vasculitis is the formation of autoantibodies directed at the body's own cellular and extracellular proteins. Such autoantibodies can lead to activation of inflammatory cells or cytotoxicity (a type II hypersensitivity reaction).

Potential autoantibodies being studied include those directed against cytoplasmic antigens of neutrophils and monocytes (antineutrophil cytoplasmic antibody, known as cANCA or pANCA) or those directed against surface antigens of endothelial cells (antiendothe-

| MALE: FEMALE RATIO | SIGNS AND SYMPTOMS | DIAGNOSIS |
|---|---|---|
| 1:1 | Palpable purpura, papules, nodules, vesicles, bullae, ulcers, or chronic or recurrent urticaria | History of exposure to antigen, such as a microorganism or drug. Tissue biopsy shows leukocytoclastic angiitis, usually in postcapillary venules. |
| 1.5:1 | Fever: nonsuppurative cervical adenitis, edema, congested conjunctivae ' erythema of oral cavity, lips, and palms ' and desquamation of fingertips. May progress to arthritis, myocarditis, pericarditis, MI, and cardiomegaly. | History of symptoms; elevated ESR. Tissue biopsy shows intimal proliferation and infiltration of vessel walls with mononuclear cells. Echocardiography is necessary. |
| 1:1 | Abdominal pain, bloody diarrhea, palpable purpura, and maculopapular rash | History of symptoms; may see elevated serum IgA. Tissue biopsy shows leukocytoclastic vasculitis. |
| 1:1 | Recurrent oral ulcers, eye lesions, genital lesions, and cutaneous lesions | History of symptoms. |

lial cell antibody, or AECA). The exact role of autoantibodies remains unclear.

### Immune response

Another mechanism that may contribute to vascular damage is the cell-mediated (T cell) immune response. In this response, circulating antigen triggers the release of soluble mediators by sensitized lymphocytes, which attracts macrophages.

The macrophages release intracellular enzymes, which cause vascular damage. They can also transform into the epithelioid and multinucleated giant cells that typify the granulomatous vasculitides. Phagocytosis of immune complexes by macrophages enhances granuloma formation.

### Other factors

Atopic individuals can develop vasculitis following exposure to allergens. This type I hypersensitivity reaction can lead to mast cell degranulation, hypereosinophilia, and inflammation, leading to vasculitis.

### Signs, symptoms, and diagnosis

Clinical effects of vasculitis and confirming laboratory procedures depend on the blood vessels involved.

### Treatment

The aim of treatment is to minimize irreversible tissue damage associated with ischemia. In secondary vasculitis, treatment focuses on the underlying disorder. Primary vasculitis is mainly treated with drugs.

Treatment may involve removal of an offending antigen or use of anti-inflammatory or immunosuppressive drugs. For example, antigenic drugs, food, and other environmental substances should be identified and eliminated if possible.

Drug therapy in primary vasculitis frequently involves low-dose cyclophosphamide (2 mg/kg by mouth daily) with daily corticosteroids. In rapidly fulminant vasculitis, cyclophosphamide dosage may be increased to 4 mg/kg daily for the first 2 to 3 days, followed by the regular dose. Prednisone should be given in a dose of 1 mg/kg daily in divided doses for 7 to 10 days, with consolidation to a single morning dose by 2 to 3 weeks.

When the vasculitis appears to be in remission or when prescribed cytotoxic drugs take full effect, corticosteroids are tapered down to a single daily dose and then to an alternate-day schedule for 1 to 2 months, after which steroids are slowly discontinued.

### Special considerations

• Assess for dry nasal mucosa in patients with Wegener's granulomatosis. Instill nose drops to lubricate the mucosa and help diminish crusting. Or irrigate the nasal passages with warm normal saline solution.

• Monitor vital signs. Use a Doppler ultrasonic flowmeter, if available, to auscultate blood pressure in patients with Takayasu's arteritis, whose peripheral pulses are frequently difficult to palpate.

• Monitor intake and output. Check daily for edema. Keep the patient well hydrated (3 L daily) to reduce the risk of hemorrhagic cystitis associated with cyclophosphamide therapy.

• Provide emotional support to help the patient and his family cope with an al-

tered body image — the result of the disorder or its therapy. (For example, Wegener's granulomatosis may be associated with saddle nose, steroids may cause weight gain, and cyclophosphamide may cause alopecia.)

• Teach the patient how to recognize adverse reactions to drugs.

• Monitor the patient's white blood cell count during cyclophosphamide therapy to prevent severe leukopenia.

# VITILIGO

Marked by stark-white skin patches that may cause a serious cosmetic problem, vitiligo results from the destruction and loss of pigment cells. This condition affects about 1% of the U.S. population, usually persons between ages 10 and 30, with peak incidence around age 20.

Vitiligo shows no racial preference, but the distinctive patches are most prominent in blacks. Vitiligo doesn't favor one sex; however, women tend to seek treatment more often than men. Repigmentation therapy, which is widely used in treating vitiligo, may necessitate several summers of exposure to sunlight; the effects of this treatment may not be permanent.

### Causes

Vitiligo is now believed to be an autoimmune disorder. An autoantibody to tyrosinase, the enzyme responsible for melanin synthesis, has been found in most patients.

Some link exists between vitiligo and other autoimmune disorders that it often accompanies — autoimmune thyroiditis, pernicious anemia, Addison's disease, and alopecia areata.

## Signs and symptoms

Vitiligo produces depigmented or stark white patches on the skin; on fair-skinned Whites, these are almost imperceptible. Lesions are usually bilaterally symmetric with sharp borders, which occasionally are hyperpigmented. (See *Depigmented skin*.)

These unique patches generally appear over bony prominences, around orifices (such as the eyes and mouth), within body folds, and at sites of trauma. The hair within these lesions may also turn white. Because hair follicles and certain parts of the eyes also contain pigment cells, vitiligo may be associated with premature gray hair and ocular pigmentary changes.

## Diagnosis

Diagnosing vitiligo requires accurate history of onset and of associated illnesses, family history, and observation of characteristic lesions. Other skin disorders, such as tinea versicolor, must be ruled out.

In fair-skinned patients, Wood's light examination in a darkened room detects vitiliginous patches; depigmented skin reflects the light, and pigmented skin absorbs it. If autoimmune or endocrine disturbances are suspected, laboratory studies (thyroid indexes, for example) are appropriate.

## Treatment

Two main types of treatment — repigmentation therapy and depigmentation therapy — are used for vitiligo.

### Repigmentation therapy

This treatment combines systemic and topical psoralen compounds (trimethylpsoralen or 8-methoxypsoralen) with exposure to sunlight or artificial ultraviolet light, wavelength A (UVA). New pigment rises from hair follicles and appears on the skin as small freckles,

### DEPIGMENTED SKIN

This illustration shows characteristic depigmented skin patches in vitiligo. These patches are usually bilaterally symmetrical, with distinct borders.

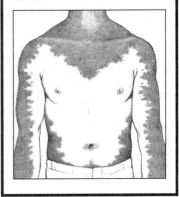

which gradually enlarge and coalesce. Body parts containing few hair follicles (such as the fingertips) may resist this therapy.

Because psoralens and UVA affect the entire skin surface, systemic therapy enhances the contrast between normal skin, which turns darker than usual, and white, vitiliginous skin. Use of sunscreen on normal skin may minimize contrast while preventing sunburn.

### Depigmentation therapy

Patients with vitiligo affecting over 50% of the body surface may benefit from depigmentation therapy. A cream containing 20% monobenzone permanently destroys pigment cells in unaffected areas of the skin and produces a uniform skin tone.

This medication is applied initially to a small area of normal skin once daily to test for unfavorable reactions (contact dermatitis, for example). In the absence of adverse effects, the patient begins applying the cream twice daily. Eventually, the entire skin may be depigmented to achieve a uniform color.

*Note:* Depigmentation is permanent and results in extreme photosensitivity.

### Other measures

Commercial cosmetics may also help deemphasize vitiliginous skin. Some patients have used dyes because these remain on the skin for several days, although the results are not always satisfactory. The newer artificial tanning lotions are now preferred.

Avoidance of exposure to sunlight through the use of screening agents and protective clothing may help minimize lesions.

### Special considerations

● Instruct the patient to use psoralens medications 3 to 4 times weekly. *(Note:* Systemic psoralens should be taken 2 hours before exposure to sun; topical solutions should be applied 30 to 60 minutes before exposure.)

● Warn the patient to use a sunscreen (of highest protection factor) to protect affected and normal skin during exposure and to wear sunglasses after taking the medication. If periorbital areas require exposure, tell the patient to keep eyes closed during treatment.

● Suggest that the patient receiving depigmentation therapy wear protective clothing and use sunscreen (SPF 15 to SPF 30).

● Explain the therapy thoroughly, and allow the patient plenty of time to decide whether to undergo this treatment. Make sure the patient understands that the results of depigmentation are permanent and that he must thereafter protect his skin from the adverse effects of sunlight.

● Caution the patient about buying commercial cosmetics or dyes without try-

ing them first because some may not be suitable.

● Remind patients undergoing repigmentation therapy that exposure to sunlight also darkens normal skin. After being exposed to UVA for the prescribed amount of time, the patient should apply a sunscreen.

● If sunburn occurs, advise the patient to discontinue therapy temporarily and to apply open wet dressings (using thin sheeting) to affected areas for 15 to 20 minutes, 4 or 5 times daily or as necessary for comfort. After application of wet dressings, allow the skin to air-dry. Suggest application of a soothing lubricating cream or lotion while the skin is still slightly moist.

● Reinforce patient teaching with written instructions.

● Be sensitive to the patient's emotional needs, but avoid promoting unrealistic hope for a total cure.

# VOCAL CORD NODULES AND POLYPS

Nodules on the vocal cord result from hypertrophy of fibrous tissue and form at the point where the cords come together forcibly. Vocal cord polyps are swellings on the true vocal cord caused by edema in the lamina propria of the mucous membrane. Nodules and polyps have good prognoses, unless continued voice abuse causes recurrence, with subsequent scarring and permanent hoarseness.

### Causes

Vocal cord nodules and polyps usually result from voice abuse, especially in the presence of infection. Voice abuse results from speaking consistently at the wrong pitch or for a long duration, and

## HOW NODULES CAUSE HOARSENESS

Vocal cord nodules cause hoarseness by inhibiting proper closure of the vocal cords during phonation. The most common site of vocal cord nodules is the point of maximal vibration and impact (junction of the anterior one-third and the posterior two-thirds of the vocal cord).

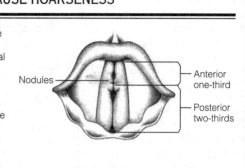

Nodules — Anterior one-third

Posterior two-thirds

using too loud a voice. Many vocal abusers combine all three practices. Consequently, vocal cord nodules and polyps are seen most commonly in teachers, singers, and sports fans, and in energetic children (ages 8 to 12) who continually shout while playing. Polyps are common in adults who smoke, live in dry climates, or have allergies.

### Signs and symptoms

Nodules and polyps inhibit the approximation of vocal cords and produce painless hoarseness. The voice may also develop a breathy or husky quality.

### Diagnosis

Persistent hoarseness suggests vocal cord nodules and polyps; visualization by indirect laryngoscopy confirms it.

• In the patient with vocal cord nodules, laryngoscopy initially shows small red nodes; later, white solid nodes on one or both cords.

• In the patient with polyps, laryngoscopy reveals unilateral or, occasionally, bilateral, sessile, or pedunculated polyps of varying size, anywhere on the vocal cords. (See *How nodules cause hoarseness.*)

### Treatment

Conservative management of small vocal cord nodules and polyps includes humidification, speech therapy (voice rest, training to reduce the intensity and duration of voice production), and treatment of any underlying allergies.

When conservative treatment fails to relieve hoarseness, nodules or polyps require removal under direct laryngoscopy. Microlaryngoscopy may be done for small lesions to avoid injuring the vocal cord surface.

If nodules or polyps are bilateral, excision may be performed in two stages: one cord is allowed to heal before the polyps on the other cord are excised. Two-stage excision prevents laryngeal web, which occurs when epithelial tissue is removed from adjacent cord surfaces and these surfaces grow together.

For children, treatment consists of speech therapy. If possible, surgery should be delayed until the child is old enough to benefit from voice training, or until he can understand the need to abstain from voice abuse.

### Special considerations

• Postoperatively, stress the importance of resting the voice for 10 days to 2 weeks while the vocal cords heal. Provide an alternative means of communication — Magic Slate, pad and pencil, or alphabet board.

• Place a sign over the bed to remind visitors that the patient shouldn't talk. Mark the intercom so other hospital personnel are aware the patient can't answer.

• Minimize the need to speak by trying to anticipate the patient's needs.

• If the patient is a smoker, encourage him to stop smoking entirely or, at the very least, to refrain from smoking during recovery from surgery.

• Use a vaporizer to increase humidity and decrease throat irritation.

• Make sure the patient receives speech therapy after healing, if necessary, because continued voice abuse causes recurrence of growths.

➤ CLINICAL TIP Patients on voice rest are not allowed even to whisper. Whispering involves approximating the vocal cords, which will irritate the cords and increase swelling.

# VOCAL CORD PARALYSIS

Paralysis of the vocal cords results from disease of or injury to the superior or, most often, the recurrent laryngeal nerve.

## Causes

Vocal cord paralysis commonly results from the accidental severing of the recurrent laryngeal nerve or of one of its extralaryngeal branches during thyroidectomy.

Other causes include pressure from an aortic aneurysm or from an enlarged atrium (in patients with mitral stenosis), bronchial or esophageal carcinoma, hypertrophy of the thyroid gland, trauma (such as neck injuries) and intubation, and neuritis due to infections or metallic poisoning. Vocal cord paralysis can also result from hysteria and, rarely, lesions of the central nervous system.

## Signs and symptoms

Unilateral paralysis, the most common form, may cause vocal weakness and hoarseness. Bilateral paralysis typically produces vocal weakness and incapacitating airway obstruction if the cords become paralyzed in the adducted position.

## Diagnosis

Patient history and characteristic features suggest vocal cord paralysis. Visualization by indirect laryngoscopy shows one or both cords fixed in an adducted or partially abducted position and confirms the diagnosis.

## Treatment

In unilateral vocal cord paralysis, treatment consists of injection of Teflon into the paralyzed cord, under direct laryngoscopy. This procedure enlarges the cord and brings it closer to the other cord, which usually strengthens the voice and protects the airway from aspiration.

Thyroplasty also serves to medialize the vocal cord, but in this procedure an implant is placed through a neck incision. The ansa cervicalis nerve transfer allows for reinnervation of the muscles of the vocal cord. Bilateral cord paralysis in an adducted position necessitates tracheotomy.

Alternative treatments for adults include encloscopic arytenoidectomy to open the glottis, and lateral fixation of the arytenoid cartilage through an external neck incision. Excision or fixation of the arytenoid cartilage improves airway patency but produces residual voice impairment. Treatment of hysterical aphonia may include psychotherapy and hypnosis.

### Special considerations

● If the patient chooses direct laryngoscopy and Teflon injection, explain these procedures thoroughly. Tell him these measures will improve his voice but won't restore it to normal. Patients are sometimes placed on voice rest for 24 to 48 hours to reduce stress on the vocal cords, which would increase the edema and might lead to airway obstruction.

> CLINICAL TIP  Do not allow the patient on voice rest even to whisper. Whispering involves approximating the vocal cords, which will irritate the cords and increase swelling.

● Many patients with bilateral cord paralysis prefer to keep a tracheostomy instead of having an arytenoidectomy; their voices are generally better with a tracheostomy alone than after corrective surgery.

● If the patient is scheduled to undergo a tracheotomy, explain the procedure thoroughly, and offer reassurance. Because the procedure is performed under a local anesthetic, the patient may be apprehensive.

● Teach the patient how to suction, clean, and change the tracheostomy tube.

● Reassure the patient that he can still speak by covering the lumen of the tracheostomy tube with his finger or a tracheostomy plug.

● If the patient elects to have an arytenoidectomy, explain the procedure thoroughly. Advise the patient that the tracheostomy will remain in place until the edema has subsided and the airway is patent.

# VOLVULUS

A twisting of the intestine at least 180 degrees on its mesentery, volvulus results in blood vessel compression and ischemia.

### Causes

In volvulus, twisting may result from an anomaly of rotation, an ingested foreign body, or an adhesion; in some cases, however, the cause is unknown. Adhesions are common causes of volvulus in pregnant women. Chronic constipation is thought to be a cause in elderly people.

Volvulus usually occurs in a bowel segment with a mesentery long enough to twist. The most common area, particularly in adults, is the sigmoid; the small bowel is a common site in children. Other common sites include the stomach and cecum. Volvulus secondary to meconium ileus may occur in patients with cystic fibrosis.

### Signs and symptoms

Signs and symptoms of colonic obstruction include nausea, vomiting, cramps, abdominal pain, absence of bowel movements, and failure to pass flatus. Without the appropriate intervention, volvulus can lead to strangulation, ischemia, perforation and, finally, peritonitis.

### Diagnosis

● *Physical examination* may reveal a distended abdomen and tenderness.

● *Abdominal X-rays* may show a markedly dilated sigmoid colon and proximal small bowel and possibly a distended sigmoid loop.

● *Barium enema* may reveal a dilated sigmoid loop with a corkscrew appearance. It may demonstrate retrograde obstruction to the flow of barium at the level of the obstruction. A narrowing with proximal dilation and partial obstruction may also be visible.

• *Upper GI series* shows, in midgut volvulus, obstruction and possibly a twisted contour in a narrow area near the duodenojejunal junction, where barium won't pass.

• *White blood cell count* shows a count > 15,000/μl in strangulation; > 20,000/μl in bowel infarction.

## Treatment

Therapy varies according to the severity and location of the volvulus. For children with midgut volvulus, treatment is surgical. For adults with sigmoid volvulus, a flexible sigmoidoscopy examination is performed to check for infarction, and nonsurgical treatment includes reduction by careful insertion of a sigmoidoscope or a long rectal tube to deflate the bowel.

Success of nonsurgical reduction results in expulsion of flatus and immediate relief of abdominal pain. If the bowel is distended but viable, surgery consists of detorsion (untwisting); a necrotic bowel warrants exploratory laparostomy and resection.

## Special considerations

• After surgical correction of volvulus, monitor vital signs, watching for fever (a sign of sepsis), and tachycardia and hypotension (signs of septic shock).

• Carefully monitor fluid intake and output (including stools), electrolyte values, and complete blood count. Be sure to measure and record drainage from the nasogastric tube and drains.

• Encourage frequent coughing and deep breathing.

• Reposition the patient every 2 hours.

• Encourage ambulation on the day of surgery.

• Keep dressings clean and dry. Record any excessive or unusual drainage.

• Following dressing removal, assess for erythema and wound separation.

• When bowel sounds and peristalsis return, begin oral feedings with clear liquids as ordered. Before removing the nasogastric tube, clamp it for a trial period, and watch for abdominal distention, nausea, or vomiting. Advance to regular diet as tolerated.

• Reassure the patient and family, and explain all diagnostic procedures. If the patient is a child, encourage parents to participate in their child's care to minimize the stress of hospitalization.

# VON WILLEBRAND'S DISEASE

A hereditary bleeding disorder, von Willebrand's disease is characterized by prolonged bleeding time, moderate deficiency of clotting Factor $VIII_{AHF}$ (antihemophilic factor), and impaired platelet function.

This disease commonly causes bleeding from the skin or mucosal surfaces and, in females, excessive uterine bleeding. Bleeding may range from mild and asymptomatic to severe, potentially fatal hemorrhage. Prognosis, however, is usually good.

## Causes

Unlike hemophilia, von Willebrand's disease is inherited as an autosomal dominant trait and occurs more often in females. One theory of pathophysiology holds that mild to moderate deficiency of Factor VIII and defective platelet adhesion prolong coagulation time. Specifically, this results from a deficiency of the von Willebrand factor (VWF), which stabilizes the Factor VIII molecule and is needed for proper platelet function.

Defective platelet function is characterized by:

• decreased agglutination and adhesion at the bleeding site

• reduced platelet retention when filtered through a column of packed glass beads

• diminished ristocetin-induced platelet aggregation.

Recently, an acquired form has been identified in patients with cancer and immune disorders.

### Signs and symptoms

Von Willebrand's disease produces easy bruising, epistaxis, and bleeding from the gums. Severe forms of this disease may cause hemorrhage after laceration or surgery, menorrhagia, and GI bleeding. Excessive postpartum bleeding is uncommon, because Factor VIII levels and bleeding time abnormalities become less pronounced during pregnancy.

Massive soft-tissue hemorrhage and bleeding into joints rarely occur. The severity of bleeding may lessen with age. Bleeding episodes typically occur sporadically — a patient may bleed excessively after one dental extraction but not after another.

### Diagnosis

Diagnosing this disease is difficult, because symptoms are mild, laboratory values are borderline, and Factor VIII levels fluctuate. However, a positive family history and characteristic bleeding patterns and laboratory values help establish diagnosis. Typical laboratory data include:

• prolonged bleeding time (<6 minutes)

• slightly prolonged partial thromboplastin time (>45 seconds)

• absent or reduced levels of Factor VIII-related antigens ($VIII_{AHN}$), and low Factor VIII activity level

• defective *in vitro* platelet aggregation (using the ristocetin coagulation factor assay test)

• normal platelet count and normal clot retraction.

### Treatment

The aims of treatment are to shorten bleeding time by local measures and to replace Factor VIII (and, consequently, VWF) by infusion of cryoprecipitate or blood fractions that are rich in Factor VIII.

During bleeding and before surgery, I.V. infusion of cryoprecipitate or fresh frozen plasma (in quantities sufficient to raise Factor VIII levels to 50% of normal) shortens bleeding time. Desmopressin given parenterally or intranasally is effective in raising serum levels of VWF.

### Special considerations

• Care should include local measures to control bleeding and patient teaching to prevent bleeding, unnecessary trauma, and complications.

• After surgery, monitor bleeding time for 24 to 48 hours, and watch for signs of new bleeding.

• During a bleeding episode, elevate and apply cold compresses and gentle pressure to the bleeding site.

• Refer parents of affected children for genetic counseling.

• Advise the patient to seek medical attention after even minor trauma and before all surgery, to determine whether replacement of blood components is necessary.

• Tell the patient to watch for signs of hepatitis for 6 weeks to 6 months after transfusion.

• Warn against using aspirin and other drugs that impair platelet function.

• Advise the patient who has a severe form to avoid contact sports.

# VULVOVAGINITIS

Inflammation of the vulva (vulvitis) and vagina (vaginitis) is called vulvovaginitis. Because of the proximity of these two structures, inflammation of one usually precipitates inflammation of the other. Vulvovaginitis may occur at any age and affects most females at some time. Prognosis is good with treatment.

## Causes
Common causes of vaginitis (with or without consequent vulvitis) include:
- infection with *Trichomonas vaginalis,* a protozoan flagellate, usually transmitted through sexual intercourse
- infection with *Candida albicans (Monilia),* a fungus that requires glucose for growth. Incidence rises during the secretory phase of the menstrual cycle. Such infection occurs twice as often in pregnant females as in nonpregnant females. It also commonly affects users of oral contraceptives, diabetics, and patients receiving systemic therapy with broad-spectrum antibiotics (incidence may reach 75%).
- infection with *Gardnerella vaginitis,* a gram-negative bacillus
- venereal infection with *Neisseria gonorrhoeae* (gonorrhea), a gram-negative diplococcus
- viral infection with venereal warts (condylomata acuminata) or herpesvirus Type II, usually transmitted by sexual intercourse
- vaginal mucosa atrophy in menopausal women due to decreasing levels of estrogen, which predisposes to bacterial invasion.
  Common causes of vulvitis include:
- parasitic infection *(Phthirus pubis* [crab louse])
- trauma (skin breakdown may lead to secondary infection)
- poor personal hygiene
- chemical irritations, or allergic reactions to hygiene sprays, douches, detergents, clothing, or toilet paper
- vulval atrophy in menopausal women due to decreasing estrogen levels
- retention of a foreign body, such as a tampon or diaphragm.

## Signs and symptoms
- In trichomonal vaginitis, vaginal discharge is thin, bubbly, green-tinged, and malodorous. This infection causes marked irritation and itching, and urinary symptoms, such as burning and frequency.
- Monilia vaginitis produces a thick, white, cottage-cheese–like discharge and red, edematous mucous membranes, with white flecks adhering to the vaginal wall, and is often accompanied by intense itching.
- Hemophilus vaginitis produces a gray, foul-smelling discharge.
- Gonorrhea may produce no symptoms at all, or a profuse, purulent discharge and dysuria.
- Acute vulvitis causes a mild to severe inflammatory reaction, including edema, erythema, burning, and pruritus. Severe pain on urination and dyspareunia may necessitate immediate treatment.
- Herpes infection may cause painful ulceration or vesicle formation during the active phase.
- Chronic vulvitis generally causes relatively mild inflammation, possibly associated with severe edema that may involve the entire perineum.

## Diagnosis
Vaginitis is diagnosed by identification of the infectious organism during microscopic examination of vaginal exudate on a wet slide preparation (a drop

of vaginal exudate placed in normal saline solution).

• In trichomonal infections, the presence of motile, flagellated trichomonads confirms the diagnosis.

• In monilia vaginitis, 10% potassium hydroxide is added to the slide, and microscopic examination seeks "clue cells" (granular epithelial cells); however, diagnosis requires identification of *C. albicans* fungi.

• Gonorrhea necessitates culture of vaginal exudate on Thayer-Martin or Transgrow medium to confirm diagnosis.

Diagnosis of vulvitis or suspected venereal disease may require complete blood count, urinalysis, cytology screening, biopsy of chronic lesions to rule out malignancy, and culture of exudate from acute lesions.

### Treatment
Common therapeutic measures include the following:

• oral metronidazole for the patient with trichomonal vaginitis and for all sexual partners

• topical miconazole 2% or clotrimazole 1% for candidal infection

• metronidazole for *Gardnerella*

• systemic antibiotic therapy for the patient with gonorrhea and for all sexual partners

• doxycycline or erythromycin for chlamydial infection.

Cold compresses or cool sitz baths may provide relief from pruritus in acute vulvitis; severe inflammation may require warm compresses. Other therapy includes avoiding drying soaps, wearing loose clothing to promote air circulation, and applying topical corticosteroids to reduce inflammation.

Chronic vulvitis may respond to topical hydrocortisone or antipruritics and good hygiene (especially in elderly or incontinent patients). Topical estrogen ointments may be used to treat atrophic vulvovaginitis.

No cure currently exists for herpesvirus infections; however, oral and topical acyclovir (Zovirax) decreases the duration and symptoms of active lesions.

### Special considerations
Ask the patient if she has any drug allergies. Stress the importance of taking the medication for the length of time prescribed, even if symptoms subside.

## WOUNDS, OPEN TRAUMA

Open trauma wounds (abrasions, avulsions, crush wounds, lacerations, missile injuries, and punctures) are injuries that commonly result from home, work, or motor vehicle accidents and from acts of violence.

### Signs and symptoms

In all open wounds, assess the extent of injury, vital signs, level of consciousness (LOC), obvious skeletal damage, local neurologic deficits, and general patient condition. Obtain an accurate history of the injury from the patient or witnesses, including such details as the mechanism and time of injury and any treatment already provided. If the injury involved a weapon, notify the police.

Also assess for peripheral nerve damage — a common complication in lacerations and other open trauma wounds, as well as for fractures and dislocations. Signs of peripheral nerve damage vary with location as follows:

• radial nerve — weak forearm dorsiflexion, inability to extend thumb in a hitchhiker's sign

• median nerve — numbness in tip of index finger; inability to place forearm in prone position; weak forearm, thumb, and index finger flexion

• ulnar nerve — numbness in tip of little finger, clawing of hand

• peroneal nerve — footdrop, inability to extend the foot or big toe

• sciatic and tibial nerves — paralysis of ankles and toes, footdrop, weakness in leg, numbness in sole.

Most open wounds require emergency treatment. In those with suspected nerve involvement, however, electromyography, nerve conduction, and electrical stimulation tests can provide more detailed information about possible peripheral nerve damage.

### Treatment

• If hemorrhage occurs, stop bleeding by applying direct pressure on the wound and, if necessary, on arterial pressure points. If the wound is on an extremity, elevate it if possible. Don't apply a tourniquet except in a life-threatening hemorrhage. If you must do so, be aware that resulting lack of perfusion to tissue could require limb amputation. (For a description of types of wounds and specific management, see *Managing open trauma wounds.*)

### Special considerations

• Frequently assess vital signs in patients with major wounds. Be alert for a 20 mm Hg drop in blood pressure and a 20 beat increase in pulse (compare the patient's blood pressure and pulse taken when he's sitting with those taken when he's lying down), increased respiratory rate, decreasing LOC, thirst, and cool, clammy skin — all indicate blood loss and hypovolemic shock.

*(Text continues on page 924.)*

# MANAGING OPEN TRAUMA WOUNDS

| TYPE | CLINICAL ACTION |
|---|---|
| **Abrasion**<br>• Open surface wounds (scrapes) of epidermis and possibly the dermis, resulting from friction; nerve endings exposed<br>• Diagnosis based on scratches, reddish welts, bruises, pain, and history of friction injury | • Obtain a history to distinguish injury from second-degree burn.<br>• Clean the wound gently with topical germicide, and irrigate it. Too vigorous scrubbing of abrasions will increase tissue damage.<br>• Remove all imbedded foreign objects. Apply a local anesthetic if cleaning is very painful.<br>• Apply a light, water-soluble antibiotic cream to prevent infection.<br>• If the wound is severe, apply a loose protective dressing that allows air to circulate.<br>• Administer tetanus prophylaxis if necessary. |
| **Avulsion**<br>• Complete tissue loss that prevents approximation of wound edges, resulting from cutting, gouging, or complete tearing of skin; frequently affects nose tip, earlobe, fingertip, and penis<br>• Diagnosis based on full-thickness skin loss, hemorrhage, pain, history of trauma; X-ray required to rule out bone damage; complete blood count (CBC) before surgery | • Check the patient history for bleeding tendencies and use of anticoagulants.<br>• Record the time of injury to help determine whether tissue is salvageable. Preserve tissue (if available) in cool saline solution for a possible split-thickness graft or flap.<br>• Control hemorrhage with pressure, an absorbable gelatin sponge, or topical thrombin.<br>• Clean the wound gently, irrigate it with saline solution, and debride it if necessary. Cover with a bulky dressing.<br>• Tell the patient to leave the dressing in place until return visit, to keep the area dry, and to watch for signs of infection (pain, fever, redness, swelling).<br>• Administer analgesics and tetanus prophylaxis if necessary. |

*(continued)*

## MANAGING OPEN TRAUMA WOUNDS *(continued)*

| TYPE | CLINICAL ACTION |
|---|---|
| **Crush wound**<br>• Heavy falling object splits skin and causes necrosis along split margins and damages tissue underneath. May look like a laceration.<br>• Diagnosis based on history of trauma, edema, hemorrhage, massive hematomas, damage to surrounding tissues (fractures, nerve injuries, loss of tendon function), shock, pain, history of trauma; X-rays required to determine extent of injury to surrounding structures; CBC and electrolyte count also required | • Check the patient history for bleeding tendencies and use of anticoagulants.<br>• Clean open areas gently with soap and water.<br>• Control hemorrhage with pressure and cold pack.<br>• Apply a dry, sterile bulky dressing; wrap the entire extremity in a compression dressing.<br>• Immobilize the injured extremity, and encourage the patient to rest. Monitor vital signs, and check peripheral pulses and circulation often.<br>• Administer tetanus prophylaxis if necessary.<br>• A severe injury may require I.V. infusion of lactated Ringer's or saline solution with a large-bore catheter as well as surgical exploration, debridement, and repair. |
| **Puncture wound**<br>• Small-entry wounds that probably damage underlying structures, resulting from sharp, pointed objects<br>• Diagnosis based on hemorrhage (rare), deep hematomas (in chest or abdominal wounds), ragged wound edges (in bites), small-entry wound (in very sharp object), pain, and history of trauma; X-rays can detect retention of injuring object | • Check the patient history for bleeding tendencies and use of anticoagulants.<br>• Obtain a description of the injury, including force of entry.<br>• Assess the extent of the injury.<br>• Don't remove impaling objects until the injury has been completely evaluated. (If the eye is injured, call an ophthalmologist immediately.)<br>• Thoroughly clean the injured area with soap and water. Irrigate all minor wounds with saline solution after removing a foreign object.<br>• Unless they're on the face, very large, or gaping, leave human bite wounds open. Apply a dry, sterile dressing to other minor puncture wounds.<br>• Consider antibiotic use in victims of human and animal bites.<br>• Tell the patient to apply warm soaks daily.<br>• Administer tetanus prophylaxis and, if necessary, a rabies vaccine.<br>• Deep wounds that damage underlying tissues may require exploratory surgery; retention of the injuring object requires surgical removal. |

## MANAGING OPEN TRAUMA WOUNDS *(continued)*

| TYPE | CLINICAL ACTION |
|---|---|
| **Laceration**<br>• Open wound, possibly extending into deep epithelium, resulting from penetration with knife or other sharp object or from a severe blow with a blunt object<br>• Diagnosis based on hemorrhage, torn or destroyed tissues, pain, and history of trauma | *In laceration less than 8 hours old and in all lacerations of face and areas of possible functional disability (such as the elbow):*<br>• Apply pressure and elevate the injured extremity to control hemorrhage.<br>• Clean the wound gently with saline solution or water; irrigate with normal saline solution.<br>• As necessary, debride necrotic margins and close the wound, using strips of tape or sutures.<br>• A severe laceration with underlying structural damage may require surgery.<br>*In grossly contaminated lacerations or lacerations more than 8 hours old (except lacerations of face and areas of possible functional disability):*<br>• Administer a broad-spectrum antibiotic for at least a 5-day course.<br>• *Don't* close the wound immediately.<br>• Instruct the patient to elevate the injured extremity for 24 hours after the injury to reduce swelling.<br>• Tell him to keep the dressing clean and dry and to watch for signs of infection.<br>• After 5 to 7 days, close the wound with sutures or a butterfly dressing if it appears uninfected with healthy granulated tissue.<br>• Apply a sterile dressing and splint.<br>*In all lacerations:*<br>• Check the patient history for bleeding tendencies and anticoagulant use.<br>• Determine the approximate time of injury, and estimate the amount of blood lost.<br>• Assess for neuromuscular, tendon, and circulatory damage.<br>• Administer tetanus prophylaxis as needed.<br>• Stress the need for follow-up and suture removal.<br>• If sutures become infected, culture the wound and scrub with surgical soap preparation. Remove some or all sutures, and give a broad-spectrum antibiotic as ordered. Instruct the patient to soak the wound in warm, soapy water for 15 minutes, three times daily, and to return for a follow-up visit every 2 to 3 days until the wound heals.<br>• If the injury is the result of foul play, report it to the police department. |

*(continued)*

## MANAGING OPEN TRAUMA WOUNDS *(continued)*

| TYPE | CLINICAL ACTION |
|---|---|
| **Missile injury**<br>• High-velocity tissue penetration, such as a gunshot wound<br>• Diagnosis based on entry and possibly exit wounds, signs of hemorrhage, shock, pain, and history of trauma; X-rays, CBC, and electrolyte levels required to assess extent of injury and estimate blood loss | • Check the patient history for bleeding tendencies and use of anticoagulants.<br>• Control hemorrhage with pressure if possible. If the injury is near vital organs, use large-bore catheters to start two I.V. lines, using lactated Ringer's solution, normal saline solution, or blood transfusions for volume replacement. Prepare for possible exploratory surgery.<br>• Maintain a patent airway, and monitor for signs of hypovolemia, shock, and cardiac arrhythmias. Check vital signs and neurovascular response often.<br>• Cover a sucking chest wound during exhalation with petroleum gauze and an occlusive dressing.<br>• Clean the wound gently with saline solution or water; debride as necessary.<br>• If damage is minor, apply a dry, sterile dressing.<br>• Administer tetanus prophylaxis if necessary.<br>• Obtain X-rays, to detect retained fragments.<br>• If possible, determine the caliber of the weapon.<br>• Report the injury to the police department. |

• Administer oxygen as ordered.

• Send blood samples to the laboratory for type and crossmatch, complete blood count (including hematocrit and hemoglobin levels), and prothrombin and partial thromboplastin times.

• Prepare the patient for surgery if needed.

• As much as possible, tell the patient about the procedures that he'll undergo (even if he appears unconscious) and provide reassurance.

• Start I.V. lines, using two large-bore catheters, and infuse lactated Ringer's solution, normal saline solution, or whole blood as ordered.

• Insert a central venous pressure line, and place the patient in a modified V position (with his head flat and his legs elevated). If the modified V position doesn't help, the Trendelenburg position may be an alternative.

# APPENDIX, REFERENCES, AND INDEX

# APPENDIX: LESS COMMON DISEASES

The following is an alphabetical list of additional diseases that the practitioner may see in treating patients.

| NAME (other names) | ETIOLOGY | TREATMENT |
|---|---|---|
| Acceleration-deceleration cervical injury (whiplash) | Mild to severe anterior and posterior neck pain resulting from sharp hyperextension and flexion of the neck that damages muscles, ligaments, disks, and nerve tissue. | • Mild analgesics are given to relieve neck pain.<br>• Hot showers or warm compresses to the neck may help relieve pain.<br>• Neck is immobilized with a soft, padded cervical collar for days or weeks. |
| Actinomycosis | Infection caused by gram-positive anaerobic bacillus *Actinomyces israelii,* resulting in painful swellings of granulomatous, suppurative lesions with abscesses commonly on the head, neck, thorax, and abdomen. | • High-dose I.V. penicillin or tetracycline is administered for 3 to 6 weeks, followed by oral penicillin or tetracycline for 1 to 6 months.<br>• Lesions are surgically excised and drained. |
| Adenoid hyperplasia | Enlargement, rather than normal atrophy, of the lymphoid tissue of the nasopharynx in children. Causation unknown but may be hereditary or result from chronic infections or irritations (allergy, congestion). | • Adenoidectomy is performed in symptomatic patients. |
| Adenovirus infection | Acute, self-limiting febrile infection resulting in inflammation of the respiratory or ocular mucous membranes, or both. There are 35 serotypes that cause five major infections; transmitted by direct inoculation into the eye, oral-fecal route, or inhalation of droplets. | • Bed rest, antipyretics, and analgesics are ordered, as needed.<br>• Ocular infections may require corticosteroid therapy and supervision by an ophthalmologist.<br>• Hospitalization is required for infants with pneumonia and in epidemic keratoconjunctivitis to prevent blindness. |

| NAME<br>(other names) | ETIOLOGY | TREATMENT |
|---|---|---|
| Adrenogenital syndrome | Syndrome that may be inherited as an autosomal recessive trait or acquired (tumor) resulting in dysfunctional biosynthesis of adrenocortical steroids. | • Simple virilizing form is corrected by daily administration of cortisone or hydrocortisone. Dosage is modified according to urine 17-ketosteroid levels.<br>• Salt-losing forms require immediate I.V. sodium chloride and glucose, I.M. desoxycorticosterone, and I.V. hydrocortisone. Long-term mineralocorticoid and glucocorticoid replacement is needed. |
| Albinism | Rare, inherited defect in melanin metabolism of the skin or eyes resulting in hypopigmentation. Visual acuity as well as tolerance to sunlight may be impaired. Skin cancer and deafness may result with other forms. | • Glasses with tinted lenses and cosmetic measures provide supportive treatment.<br>• Sunblocks, dark glasses, and clothing can protect against solar radiation.<br>• Visual defects are corrected. |
| Alpha$_1$-antitrypsin deficiency | Autosomal recessive inherited disorder resulting in emphysema and liver dysfunction problems. | • Enzyme replacement therapy is given weekly.<br>• Smoking cessation and asthma control are promoted to prevent Infection and lung problems.<br>• Vaccination against hepatitis B is given prophylactically.<br>• Liver and lung function are monitored. |
| Alport's syndrome | Hereditary nephritis characterized by recurrent gross or microscopic hematuria. It is associated with deafness, albuminuria, and progressive azotemia. | • Antihypertensives and antibiotics used for hypertension and respiratory or urinary tract infections.<br>• Hearing aids and corrective eyewear are employed.<br>• Dialysis or kidney transplantation may be required for end-stage renal failure. |
| Alveolar hydatid disease (echino-coccosis) | Infection due to *Echinococcus multilocularis,* a microscopic tapeworm found in mammals that causes parasitic tumors in the liver and, less often, in other organs. | • Surgery is the common form of treatment, although removal of the cyst isn't usually 100% effective. |
| Amebiasis (amebic dysentery) | Infection with *Entamoeba histolytica* producing no symptoms to fulminant dysentery, with sudden high fever and diffuse abdominal tenderness; can spread to other organs, including the brain. Milder chronic form lasts < 4 weeks. | • Metronidazole, emetine, iodoquinol, and chloroquine are used to treat amebiasis, depending on the site of infection. |

| NAME (other names) | ETIOLOGY | TREATMENT |
|---|---|---|
| Amenorrhea | Abnormal absence or suppression of menstruation resulting from absence of a uterus; endometrial damage; ovarian, adrenal, or pituitary tumors; emotional disorders; psychopharmacotherapy; malnutrition; intense exercise; or prolonged use of oral contraceptives. | • Appropriate hormone replacement is given to reestablish menstruation.<br>• Treatment not related to hormone deficiency depends on the cause. |
| Amyloidosis | A chronic disease resulting in the accumulation of an abnormal fibrillar scleroprotein, which infiltrates body organs and soft tissues, resulting in permanent and usually life-threatening organ damage. | • Kidney transplantation used for renal failure, although new organ may also develop amyloidosis.<br>• If the heart is affected, prophylactic antiarrhythmics are given.<br>• In end-stage GI involvement, total parenteral nutrition is used as needed for malnutrition. |
| Anal fissure | A laceration or crack in the lining of the anus that extends to the circular muscle caused by constipation or straining; also may be related to frequent or diarrheal stools. | • Stool softeners, bulking agents, high-fiber diets, sitz baths, and topical anesthetics used p.r.n.<br>• Surgery used for chronic cases (may cause some incontinence). |
| Anal stricture (anal stenosis or contracture) | Develops when the lumen of the anus decreases and stenosis prevents dilation of the sphincter and defecation. It can result from scarring after surgery, inflammation, laxative abuse, surgical trauma, or congenital abnormality. | • Conservative treatment includes laxatives, suppositories, and enemas.<br>• A dilator is used daily.<br>• Anoplasty or excision of eschar employed with lateral internal sphincterotomy. |
| Angiofibroma, juvenile | Highly vascular nasopharyngeal tumor made up of fibrous tissue with thin-walled blood vessels that may grow to completely fill the nasopharynx, nose, paranasal sinuses, and the orbit. | • Surgery or cryosurgical techniques after embolization decreases vascularization. |
| Anthrax (*Bacillus anthracis*) | Acute infectious disease transmitted by skin contact, inhalation, or ingestion of spores; presents as itching and then a vesicle, which blackens over 2 to 6 days. Inhaled form may result in severe respiratory problems and shock. Intestinal forms result in acute inflammation with varied GI symptoms. | • Microbial therapy includes such drugs as erythromycin, tetracycline, and chloramphenicol.<br>• Vaccination is recommended for people who work with imported animal hides, furs, wool, and animal hair (especially goat). |

| NAME (other names) | ETIOLOGY | TREATMENT |
|---|---|---|
| Ataxia-telangiectasia | Inherited disorder leading to severe central nervous system involvement, telangiectasis, and immunodeficiencies, with onset between ages 2 and 9. | • No treatment is available to halt progression.<br>• Early detection and aggressive antibiotic therapy for infections are important.<br>• Immune globulin infusion is used in immunoglobulin G–deficient patients. |
| Atrial septal defect | An opening between the left and right atria that allows shunting of blood between the chambers with unknown causation. The child may be asymptomatic or have severe symptoms. | • Large defects may require immediate surgery with sutures or a patch graft. Surgery may be delayed until preschool or early school age if asymptomatic. |
| *Blastocystis hominis* infection (blastocystosis) | Parasitic infection resulting in watery or loose stools, diarrhea, abdominal pain, anal itching, weight loss, and flatus; conversely, no symptoms may be present. | • Drug therapy includes ketoconazole or itraconazole.<br>• Amphotericin B is required for severe disease. |
| Blood transfusion reaction | Immune-mediated reaction after I.V. administration of blood components with severity ranging from mild (fever and urticaria) to life-threatening (acute renal failure, hypotension, or shock). | • Transfusion is discontinued; vital signs are closely monitored.<br>• I.V. fluids, oxygen, epinephrine, diphenhydramine, corticosteroids, and antihypotensive agents are given; antipyretics ordered p.r.n.<br>• Confirmation of blood compatibility required. |
| Brainerd diarrhea | Acute onset of watery, explosive diarrhea that lasts for 4 weeks or longer with causative agent unknown. | • There is no known cure.<br>• Symptomatic relief is achieved with opioid antimotility drugs such as loperamide. |
| Brucellosis (undulant fever, Malta fever, or Bang's disease) | Acute febrile infection (fever, chills, sweating, fatigue, headache, backache, enlarged lymph nodes) with hepatosplenomegaly, weight loss, and abscess and granuloma formation in subcutaneous tissues, lymph nodes, liver, and spleen. Transmitted by consumption of unpasteurized dairy products or undercooked meat. | • Bed rest is ordered in the febrile phase.<br>• Combination antibiotic therapy (doxycycline plus gentamycin or rifampin) is used until the fever is gone.<br>• Severe cases require I.V. corticosteroids for 3 days followed by oral dosing. |

| NAME (other names) | ETIOLOGY | TREATMENT |
|---|---|---|
| *Campylobacter* infection | Infectious disease caused by bacteria *Campylobacter* resulting in diarrhea, cramping, abdominal pain, and fever 2 to 5 days after exposure and lasting 1 week. | • No specific treatment exists.<br>• Patients are encouraged to drink fluids.<br>• Severe cases may require erythromycin or fluoroquinolone. |
| Cancer of the vulva | Specific cause is unknown, but cancer usually begins with vulval pruritus, bleeding, or a small mass. Less common indications include a mass in the groin and abnormal urination or defecation. | • Radical or simple vulvectomy used, depending on stage; laser therapy for some small lesions.<br>• Palliative radiation used if surgery is precluded due to extensive metastasis, age, or poor health. |
| Celiac disease (idiopathic steatorrhea, nontropical sprue, gluten enteropathy, and celiac sprue) | Poor food absorption and gluten intolerance due to environmental and genetic factors. Recurrent diarrhea, steatorrhea, abdominal distension, and anorexia, resulting in malnutrition. Hematologic (anemia), musculoskeletal (from vitamin D deficiency), neurologic, dermatologic, and endocrine systems are affected. | • Gluten (wheat, rye, barley, and oat products) should be excluded from the patient's diet for life.<br>• Supplements may be given to correct deficiencies. |
| Chancroid | Painful genital ulcers and inguinal adenitis from sexual transmission of *Haemophilus ducreyi.* Papules appear at the site of entry or on the tongue, lip, breast, or navel. | • Azithromycin or ceftriaxone in a single dose or erythromycin taken q.i.d. for 7 days.<br>• Aspiration of fluid-filled nodes helps prevent spread of infection. |
| Chédiak-Higashi syndrome | Rare genetic disorder characterized by granulocytes' inability to respond to chemotactic factors and fight infection. Presents with recurrent bacterial infections of skin, subcutaneous tissues, and lungs; thrombocytopenia, neutropenia, hepatosplenomegaly; partial albinism; photophobia; and progressive polyneuropathy. | • Provide meticulous skin care.<br>• Early detection and treatment of infections improve the prognosis.<br>• High doses of vitamin C are helpful in some children. |
| Cholera (Asiatic cholera or epidemic cholera) | Acute GI infection caused by the bacillus *Vibrio cholerae,* producing profuse diarrhea, vomiting, massive fluid and electrolyte loss, possibly hypovolemic shock, metabolic acidosis, and death. | • For hypovolemia, I.V. isotonic saline solution is given alternating with isotonic sodium bicarbonate or sodium lactate.<br>• Potassium replacement helps restore electrolyte balance. |

| NAME (other names) | ETIOLOGY | TREATMENT |
|---|---|---|
| Chronic mucocutaneous candidiasis | Inherited defect in cell-mediated (T-cell) immune responses leading to recurrent infections with *Candida albicans* and potential for autoimmune-mediated endocrinopathies. Onset usually in early childhood with chronic candidal infections; endocrinopathies include hypoparathyroidism (and severe hypocalcemia), hypothyroidism, Addison's disease, diabetes, pernicious anemia; and hepatitis. | • Topical or oral antifungal agents (miconazole, nystatin, fluconazole) control chronic infection.<br>• Therapy for endocrinopathy is organ-directed, depending on the system affected. |
| Coarctation of the aorta | Narrowing of the aorta below the left subclavian artery with prognosis depending on the severity of associated cardiac anomalies. Children exhibit cardiac symptoms (tachypnea, dyspnea, pulmonary edema, tachycardia, failure to thrive, cardiomegaly, hepatomegaly). Adolescents may have dyspnea, claudication, headaches, epistaxis, and hypertension. | • Infants with heart failure are treated medically with digoxin, diuretics, oxygen, and sedatives.<br>• If medical management fails, corrective surgery is necessary. |
| Colorado tick fever | A benign infection from the bite of a wood tick infected with *Dermacentor andersoni*. Fever begins abruptly after a 3- to 6-day incubation; severe aching of the back, arms, and legs; lethargy; headache with eye movement; photophobia; abdominal pain; nausea; and vomiting. | • Remove tick and keep for identification.<br>• Administer tetanus-diphtheria booster.<br>• Monitor fluid and electrolyte balance.<br>• Antipyretics are given to reduce fever. |
| Congenital anomalies of the ureter, bladder, and urethra | Birth defect that may produce signs of urinary tract infections (flank pain, chills, decreased urine output, recurrent infections). | • Once the diagnosis is confirmed, surgery is performed p.r.n. |
| Conversion disorder | A disorder that allows a patient to resolve a psychological conflict through the loss of a specific physical function, such as paralysis or blindness. | • Psychotherapy, family therapy, relaxation therapy, behavioral therapy, or hypnosis may be used alone or in combination. |

| NAME<br>(other names) | ETIOLOGY | TREATMENT |
|---|---|---|
| Creutzfeldt-Jakob disease (CJD, bovine spongiform encephalopathy) | Neurologic disorder of cattle caused by a slow viral infection of the central nervous system and passed on to humans, resulting in neurologic abnormalities (ataxia, dementia, myoclonus). | • Provide symptomatic relief; there is no treatment. |
| Cri du chat syndrome (cat's cry syndrome, 5p-syndrome, and partial 5p monosomy syndrome) | A rare congenital disorder characterized by a catlike cry in infancy and severe mental and physical retardation. Many infants don't live past their first year; some may live to adulthood. | • Other congenital problems (heart and eye defects) need to be evaluated and treated.<br>• Emphasize education, training in self-care, and socialization. Social services should be utilized and custodial arrangements usually are required. |
| Cryptosporidiosis | Watery diarrhea, stomach cramps, upset stomach, and slight fever caused by a one-celled parasite, *Cryptosporidium parvum*. | • There is no cure, but paromomycin may reduce symptoms.<br>• Reverse dehydration is used. |
| Cutaneous larva migrans (creeping eruption) | Skin reaction to infestation by nematodes (hookworms or roundworms) that usually infect dogs and cats; passed on by contact with infected soil or sand. Tunnel-like lesions appear on areas that come in contact with the ground. | • Thiabendazole is administered orally, but topical form may also be effective with occlusion.<br>• Lesions clear in 1 to 2 weeks. |
| Cyclosporiasis | Watery diarrhea with frequent explosive bowel movements, anorexia, weight loss, bloating, flatus, cramps, nausea, vomiting, low-grade fever, myalgias, and fatigue. It is caused by the parasite *Cyclospora cayetanensis* and may last a few days to a month. | • Co-trimoxazole is the treatment of choice.<br>• Patient is advised to rest and drink plenty of fluids.<br>• Monitor for relapse. |
| Cystinuria | Autosomal recessive disorder resulting from an inborn error of amino acid transport in the kidneys and intestine that allows excessive urinary excretion of cystine and other dibasic amino acids; resulting in recurrent cystine renal calculi. | • No effective treatment is available.<br>• Increase fluid intake to 3 L/day.<br>• Sodium bicarbonate and an alkaline-ash diet (high in vegetables and fruit, low in protein) help alkalinize the urine.<br>• Penicillamine is used to increase cystine solubility.<br>• Calculi are removed surgically.<br>• Prevent and treat urinary tract infections. |

| NAME (other names) | ETIOLOGY | TREATMENT |
|---|---|---|
| Dacryocystitis | Common infection of the lacrimal sac resulting from obstruction (dacryostenosis) of the nasolacrimal duct. Acute form mostly caused by *Staphylococcus* aureus or, occasionally, beta-hemolytic streptococci. Chronic form caused by *Streptococcus pneumonia* or sometimes a fungus, such as *Actinomyces* or *Candida albicans*. | • Therapy includes warm compresses, topical polymyxin/trimethoprim eyedrops, systemic amoxicillin and, occasionally, incision and drainage. • I.V. antibiotics such as cefazolin are used for the acutely ill. • Dacryocystorhinostomy performed for chronic cases. |
| Decompression sickness (the bends) | Painful condition resulting from too-rapid change from a high-pressure to a low-pressure environment, such as that encountered by scuba divers and pilots. Deep and constant joint and muscle pain, transitory neurologic disturbances, respiratory distress and, possibly, shock can occur. | • Interventions include recompression in a hyperbaric chamber and oxygen administration. • Supportive measures include fluid replacement to correct hypovolemic shock and, sometimes, corticosteroids to reduce risk of spinal edema. |
| Depersonalization disorder | Recurrent episodes of detachment in which self-awareness is temporarily altered or lost in the entire body or only in a limb. Causation is usually severe stress. | • Psychotherapy and reality-based coping strategies may be helpful. |
| Developmental dysplasia of the hip (DDH) | Abnormality of the hip joint present from birth; it can occur as an unstable hip dysplasia, subluxation, or complete or incomplete dislocation. The cause is unknown, but it is more common after breech delivery and in large neonates and twins. Abnormal acetabular development and permanent disability can occur. | • In infants less than 3 months old, gentle manipulation is followed by brace application to maintain flexed abduction for 3 months. • In infants older than 3 months old, bilateral traction (Bryant's) for 2 to 3 weeks reduces dislocation. Closed manipulation under anesthesia and spica cast may be used for 6 months if needed. • For ages 2 to 5, skeletal traction and subcutaneous adductor tenotomy is used; after age 5, treatment is usually unsuccessful. |
| *Dientamoeba fragilis* infection | Loose stools, diarrhea, and abdominal cramping caused by contact with or ingestion of stool, food, or water infected with the parasite *Dientamoeba fragilis*. | • Infection can be prevented by prudent hand washing. • Antimicrobial agents are available to treat *Dientamoeba fragilis*. |

| NAME (other names) | ETIOLOGY | TREATMENT |
|---|---|---|
| DiGeorge's syndrome (congenital thymic hypoplasia or aplasia) | Fetal thymus fails to develop, leading to partial or total absence of T lymphocytes and cell-mediated immunity; may be linked with maternal alcoholism and fetal alcohol syndrome. Increased susceptibility to infections; hypoparathyroidism and cardiac anomalies may also occur. | • Early development of life-threatening hypocalcemia is treated immediately with I.V. 10% calcium gluconate infusion.<br>• Fetal thymic transplantation may be required to restore normal cell-mediated immunity. |
| Diphtheria | Acute, highly contagious toxin-mediated infection due to *Corynebacterium diphtheriae* and transmitted by droplets from asymptomatic carriers. Thick, patchy, grayish green membrane over mucous membranes occurs with sore throat and rasping cough, leading to airway obstruction. | • Diphtheria antitoxin may be administered I.M. or I.V.<br>• Penicillin or erythromycin is administered to treat the infection.<br>• Tracheostomy is performed if airway obstruction occurs. |
| Dissociative amnesia | Sudden inability to recall important personal information that can't be explained by ordinary forgetfulness; usually caused by severe psychological stress. | • Psychotherapy is necessary. |
| Dissociative fugue | Wandering or traveling while mentally blocking out a traumatic event. A different personality may be assumed and later can't recall what happened. It may be related to dissociative identity disorder, narcissistic personality disorder, and sleepwalking. | • Psychotherapy is necessary. |
| Dissociative identity disorder (multiple personality disorder) | Existence of two or more distinct, fully integrated personalities in the same person. Cause is unknown but some type of abuse may have been experienced. | • Psychotherapy may be helpful. |
| Dysfunctional uterine bleeding (DUB) | Abnormal endometrial bleeding without recognizable organic lesions, due to hormonal imbalance or elevated estrogen levels. | • Rule out other causes.<br>• Estrogen-progesterone therapy controls endometrial growth and establishes a normal menstrual cycle.<br>• Dilatation and curettage may be necessary. |

| NAME (other names) | ETIOLOGY | TREATMENT |
|---|---|---|
| Dysmenorrhea | Painful menstruation that can occur as a primary disorder or secondary to an underlying gynecologic disorder such as endometriosis, cervical stenosis, uterine leiomyomas, uterine malposition, pelvic inflammatory disease, pelvic tumors, or adenomyosis. Contributing factors to primary form include hormonal imbalances and psychogenic factors. Pain may result from increased prostaglandin secretion, which intensifies uterine contractions. | • Symptomatic measures include analgesics, prostaglandin inhibitors to decrease uterine contractions, (infrequently) narcotics, and heat applied to the abdomen. <br>• In primary dysmenorrhea, sex steroids may be administered. <br>• Because persistently severe dysmenorrhea may have a psychogenic cause, psychological counseling may be helpful. <br>• Treatment of secondary dysmenorrhea may include surgery if conservative treatment fails. |
| Dysparenuria | Intercourse-associated genital pain. Physical causes include intact hymen; deformities or lesions of the introitus or vagina; uteral retroversion; scar tissue; acute or chronic genitourinary infections (especially chlamydia); and disorders of the surrounding viscera (including residual effects of pelvic inflammatory or adnexal disease); endometriosis; masses; insufficient lubrication, radiation damage; and allergic reactions to contraceptives. Psychological causes include fear of pain, injury, pregnancy, or of injury to the fetus; recollection of a painful experience; guilt about sex; fatigue. | • Treatments for physical causes include creams and water-soluble gels for lubrication, appropriate medications for infections, excision of hymenal scars, gentle stretching of painful scars at the vaginal opening, and change in coital position to reduce pain on deep penetration. <br>• Treatments for psychological causes may include sensate focus exercises or education about methods of contraception or about sexual activity during pregnancy. |
| Ear canal tumors, benign (keloids, osteomas, sebaceous cysts) | Benign ear tumor is usually asymptomatic unless infected. If the tumor grows, hearing loss and sensation of pressure may occur. Cause depends on type of tumor. | • Surgical removal of tumor. <br>• Steroid injections and surgery may be needed for keloids. <br>• Antibiotics are used before surgery for sebaceous cysts. |
| Ectopic pregnancy | Implantation of fertilized ovum outside the uterine cavity, caused by retardation of ovum passage by endosalpingitis, diverticula, tumors, scar tissue, or transmigration of the ovum. Implantation in the fallopian tube may cause rupture, resulting in hemorrhage, shock, and peritonitis. | • Laparoscopy and laparotomy, oophorectomy, or hysterectomy may be performed. <br>• Supportive measures include transfusion for hypovolemia, I.V. antibiotics for sepsis, and supplemental iron. |

| NAME (other names) | ETIOLOGY | TREATMENT |
|---|---|---|
| Enterobiasis (pinworm, seatworm, or threadworm infection; oxyuriasis) | Benign intestinal infection due to the nematode *Enterobias vermicularis*. Adult worms live in the intestine; females migrate to the perianal region to deposit ova, causing intense perianal pruritus. Can spread by *direct transmission* (hands transferring infective eggs from anus to mouth) or by *indirect transmission* (coming in contact with contaminated articles). | • Drug therapy with pyrantel, piperazine, mebendazole, or albendazole destroys these parasites.<br>• Effective eradication requires simultaneous treatment of family members and, in institutions, other patients.<br>• Treatment should be repeated after 2 weeks. |
| Epidermolysis bullosa (EB) | Blisters occur in response to normally harmless heat and friction and may result in scarring with disfigurement. Prognosis depends on severity. May be inherited as an autosomal dominant or recessive disorder and cause multiple complications because skin and mucous membranes are affected. | • Recessive dystrophic forms may be helped with phenytoin.<br>• Corticosteroids and retinoids may help other forms.<br>• Supportive treatment includes protection of the skin.<br>• Diet therapy helps combat malnutrition and promote healing. |
| Erectile disorder (impotence) | Male's inability to attain or maintain penile erection sufficient to complete intercourse; caused by psychogenic and organic factors. | • If the cause is psychogenic, refer the patient for psychotherapy.<br>• If the cause is organic, the underlying pathology is treated. |
| Erythroblastosis fetalis | Hemolytic disease of the fetus and newborn stemming from an incompatibility of fetal and maternal blood and resulting in maternal antibody activity against fetal red cells. | • Intrauterine-intraperitoneal transfusion is performed p.r.n.<br>• Delivery is planned for 2 to 4 weeks before term.<br>• Exchange blood transfusion is performed p.r.n.<br>• Albumin infusion is used to reduce risk of hyperbilirubinemia.<br>• Phototherapy is used to reduce bilirubin levels. |
| Exophthalmos (proptosis) | Unilateral or bilateral bulging or protrusion of the eyeballs or their forward displacement caused by Graves' disease, hemorrhage, varicosities, thrombosis and edema, infection, tumors, or parasitic cysts. | • Treatment is cause-dependent; Graves' disease is treated with antithyroid drugs or surgery, corticosteroids. Trauma requires cold compresses for 24 hours followed by warm compresses and prophylactic antibiotics; infection requires antibiotics; orbital tumors require surgery. |

| NAME (other names) | ETIOLOGY | TREATMENT |
|---|---|---|
| Fallopian tube cancer | Cancer that is usually produces a palpable mass, vague abdominal or pelvic complaints, bloating, or pain in the early stages. Over time, excessive menstrual bleeding may occur. Causes appear to be linked with nulliparity and infertility; more than half of the patients have never given birth. | • Total abdominal hysterectomy, bilateral salpingo-oophorectomy, or omentectomy is performed, followed by chemotherapy.<br>• The patient receives external radiation for 5 to 6 weeks. |
| Fanconi's syndrome (de Toni-Fanconi syndrome) | Hereditary renal disorder producing malfunctions of the proximal renal tubules, leading to electrolyte losses and, eventually, retarded growth and development and rickets. | • Symptomatic treatment may be given to replace the patient's specific deficiencies. |
| Fever, relapsing (tick, fowl-nest, cabin, or vagabond fever or bilious typhoid) | An acute infectious disease caused by spirochetes of the genus *Borrelia* transmitted by lice or ticks; presents with recurring high fever, prostration, headache, severe myalgia, arthralgia, diarrhea, vomiting, coughing, eye or chest pain, splenomegaly, hepatomegaly, lymphadenopathy, and macular rash. | • Doxycycline or erythromycin is given for 4 to 5 days, except during a severe febrile attack because it may cause Jarisch-Herxheimer reaction.<br>• Symptomatic treatment is given; for example, parenteral fluids and electrolytes. |
| Galactorrhea (hyperprolactinemia) | Inappropriate breast milk secretion, usually occurring after discontinuation of breast-feeding or abortion; due to increased prolactin secretion from the anterior pituitary or idiopathic causes. | • Depending on the cause, precipitating factor may be avoided or bromocriptine, oral estrogens, and progestins may be administered. |
| Galactosemia | Genetic multisystem disorder of galactose metabolism that causes cataracts, liver damage, and mental retardation; occurs as an autosomal recessive defect. Usually presents in children as milk intolerance, splenomegaly, proteinuria, and galactosuria. | • Elimination of galactose and lactose from the diet causes reversal of symptoms. |

| NAME<br>(other names) | ETIOLOGY | TREATMENT |
|---|---|---|
| Gas gangrene | Life-threatening local infection with an anaerobe of the *Clostridium* species. Occurs after crushing trauma or surgery in tissues devitalized by compromised arterial circulation. Causes severe localized pain, edema, and discoloration; crepitation (disease hallmark); bullae; and necrosis from subcutaneous release of carbon dioxide and hydrogen, which forms gas bubbles. Causes death in 20% of cases. | • Patient is carefully observed for signs of myositis and cellulitis and given *immediate* treatment if these appear and, in myositis, *immediate* surgical excision of all affected tissue and necrotic muscle.<br>• I.V. administration of high-dose penicillin, adequate debridement, and hyperbaric oxygenation are included. |
| Gaucher's disease | Genetic enzyme deficiency that causes abnormal accumulation of glucocerebrosides in reticuloendothelial cells. Signs include hepatosplenomegaly and bone lesions. | • Long-term therapy includes I.V. replacement of the missing enzyme every 2 weeks.<br>• Gene transfer therapy is under investigation. |
| Gender identity disorder | Persistent feelings of gender discomfort and dissatisfaction due to a combination of predisposing factors (chromosomal anomaly, hormonal imbalance, impaired parent-child bonding, and child-rearing practices). | • Refer patient for psychotherapy to resolve conflict.<br>• Provide supportive care, as needed. |
| Genital warts (venereal warts, condylomata acuminata) | Painless, pedunculated, cauliflower-like papillomas caused by infection with strains of human papilloma virus (HPV). Transmitted through sexual contact and exacerbated by perspiration, poor hygiene, and pregnancy. After 1- to 6-month incubation, warts develop on moist surfaces: in men, on the frenum, coronal sulcus, within the urethral meatus and, less commonly, on the penile shaft; in women, on the vulva and on vaginal and cervical walls. | • Warts often resolve spontaneously, but relapse is common because there is no cure.<br>• A topical drug, such as trichloroacetic acid 85% or podophyllum resin, is applied weekly.<br>• Warts larger than 1″ (2.5 cm) are generally removed by laser, cryosurgery, or electrocautery.<br>• Screen for other sexually transmitted diseases. |

| NAME (other names) | ETIOLOGY | TREATMENT |
|---|---|---|
| Genitourinary infections, non-specific | A group of sexually transmitted infections (including urethritis in men and vaginitis, cervicitis, and PID in women) with similar manifestations that are linked to an organism that may be sexually transmitted. Chlamydia and gonorrhea are most common, followed by *Ureaplasma urealyticum, Mycoplasma genitalium,* and others. Less common causes include preexisting strictures or neoplasms. In females, infections may be caused by a thin vaginal epithelium that can predispose prepubertal and postmenopausal females to vaginitis. | • Prognosis is good if both partners are treated simultaneously. <br> • For both sexes, therapy consists of a single 1-g dose of azithromycin plus a single dose of ofloxacin 400 mg P.O. <br> • For females, treatment may also include application of a sulfa vaginal cream. |
| Giardiasis (*Giardia* enteritis, lambliasis) | Small-bowel infection caused by the protozoan *Giardia lamblia,* which results in mucosal destruction, inflammation, and irritation. Causes chronic GI complaints, such as cramps and pale, loose, greasy, malodorous, frequent stools (up to 10 daily) with nausea, fatigue, and weight loss. | • Giardiasis responds readily to a 10-day course of metronidazole or a 7-day course of quinacrine and oral furazolidone. <br> • Severe diarrhea may require parenteral fluid replacement to prevent dehydration if oral fluid intake is inadequate. |
| Globoid cell leukodystrophy | Caused by deficiency of galacto-cerebrosidase, resulting in progressive CNS deterioration. | • Stem-cell transplantation helps in some cases. |
| Goodpasture's syndrome | Autoantibodies directed against alveolar and glomerular basement membrane leading to immune-mediated inflammation of lung and kidney tissues; symptoms include anemia, cough, dyspnea, hemoptysis, hemorrhage, and glomerulonephritis. | • Corticosteroids and immunosuppressants are used to suppress inflammation and antibody overproduction. <br> • Plasmapheresis is used to remove excessive antibody in the acute setting. |
| Hallux valgus | Lateral deviation of the great toe at the metatarsophalangeal joint, with medial enlargement of the first metatarsal head and painful bunion formation. May be congenital or familial, but is usually acquired from degenerative arthritis or prolonged pressure on the foot, especially from narrow-toed, high-heeled shoes. | • In the early stage, proper shoes and good foot care — such as felt pads to protect the bunion, devices to separate the toes at night, and a supportive pad and exercises to strengthen the metatarsal arch — may eliminate the need for bunionectomy. |

| NAME (other names) | ETIOLOGY | TREATMENT |
|---|---|---|
| Hand, foot, and mouth disease (HFMD) | Common disease of infants and children characterized by fever, mouth sores, and a rash with blisters on the hands and soles; caused by coxsackievirus A16. | • Treatment is symptomatic only because disease is self-limiting. |
| Hereditary fructose intolerance | Inability to metabolize fructose with symptoms of intolerance that can lead to failure to thrive, dehydration, seizures, coma, and anemia. | • Fructose and sucrose (cane sugar or table sugar) are excluded from the diet. Avoid fruits that contain fructose and vegetables that contain sucrose, such as sugar beets, sweet potatoes, and peas. |
| Hereditary hemorrhagic telangiectasia (Rendu-Osler-Weber disease) | Inherited vascular disorder in which venules and capillaries dilate to form fragile masses of thin, convoluted vessels, resulting in an abnormal tendency to hemorrhage. | • Control hemorrhage by applying pressure and topical hemostatic agents, cauterization, and blood transfusion p.r.n.<br>• Protect the patient from trauma and unnecessary bleeding.<br>• Give an iron supplement. |
| Hermansky-Pudlak syndrome | Genetic form of rare albinism that causes impaired vision, bleeding tendency, and lung, bowel, and kidney problems. | • Symptomatic treatment aims to reduce fever and prevent seizures and dehydration. |
| Herpangina | Acute infection caused by group A coxsackieviruses transmitted by the fecal-oral route, resulting in sore throat, pain on swallowing, headache, and fever that persist for 1 to 4 days and may cause seizures, anorexia, vomiting, malaise, diarrhea, and pain. Grayish white papulovesicles appear on the soft palate. | • Symptomatic treatment emphasizes measures to prevent seizures (such as antipyretics and and tepid sponge baths), fluids to prevent dehydration, and bed rest.<br>• Careful hand washing and sanitary disposal of excretions are required, but not isolation or hospitalization. |
| Hirschsprung's disease (congenital megacolon, congenital aganglionic megacolon) | Potentially life-threatening congenital large-bowel disorder characterized by the absence or marked reduction of parasympathetic ganglion cells in a segment of the colorectal wall. This narrowing impairs intestinal motility and causes severe, intractable constipation leading to partial or complete colonic obstruction. With prompt treatment, the prognosis is good; without it, an infant with obstruction may die within 24 hours from severe diarrhea and hypovolemic shock due to enterocilitis. | • Surgical treatment involves pulling the normal ganglionic segment through to the anus. Such corrective surgery is usually delayed until the infant is at least 10 months old and better able to withstand it.<br>• Management before surgery consists of daily colonic saline lavage to empty the bowel.<br>• If the neonate's bowel is totally obstructed, a temporary colostomy or ileostomy is necessary to decompress the colon. |

| NAME (other names) | ETIOLOGY | TREATMENT |
| --- | --- | --- |
| Hirsutism | Excessive growth of hair in women and children, typically in an adult male distribution pattern, possibly stemming from a hereditary trait or endocrine abnormalities. | • Hormonal therapy stops further hair loss but doesn't reverse hair presence.<br>• For the hereditary form, eliminate unwanted hair by plucking, bleaching, shaving, or electrolysis.<br>• For the secondary form, treat the underlying abnormality.<br>• Ovulation induction may be needed to achieve pregnancy. |
| Histoplasmosis (Ohio Valley disease, Central Mississippi Valley disease, Appalachian Mountain disease, Darling's disease) | Fungal infection caused by *Histoplasma capsulatum*, which is found in the feces of birds and bats or in contaminated soil. Transmitted by inhalation or invasion of spores through a break in skin integrity. Incubation period is 5 to 18 days, although chronic pulmonary histoplasmosis may progress slowly for many years. | • Treatment consists of antifungal therapy and surgery.<br>• Supportive care usually includes oxygen for respiratory distress, glucocorticoids for adrenal insufficiency, and perenteral fluids for dysphagia due to oral or laryngeal ulcerations. |
| Hookworm disease (uncinariasis) | Intestinal infection caused by *Ancylostoma duodenale* or *Necator americanus*. Sandy soil, high humidity, warm climate, and bare feet favor transmission. Transmitted to humans through direct skin penetration (usually in the foot) by hookworm larvae in soil contaminated with feces that contain the hookworm ova. | • An anthelmintic, such as mebendazole or pyrantel, eradicates the infection.<br>• An iron supplement is administered to correct anemia.<br>• Stool examinations are repeated in 2 weeks, with retreatment p.r.n. |
| Human papillomavirus (HPV) | Usually sexually transmitted, this virus causes plantar warts, which can increase the risk of cervical cancer. | • Warts are treated with podophyllin in tincture of benzoin, trichloroacetic acid, or liquid nitrogen. |
| Hydatidiform mole | Uncommon chorionic tumor of the placenta that seems to follow death of the embryo and loss of fetal circulation. | • Uterus is evacuated by dilatation and curettage or abdominal hysterectomy.<br>• Supportive treatment is given for postoperative hypovolemia and anemia. |
| Hyperbilirubinemia (neonatal jaundice) | Result of hemolysis in the newborn; marked by elevated serum bilirubin levels and mild jaundice. | • Treatment includes phototherapy, exchange transfusions, and albumin infusion. |

| NAME (other names) | ETIOLOGY | TREATMENT |
|---|---|---|
| Hyperemesis gravidarum | Severe and unremitting nausea and vomiting that persist after the first trimester, resulting in weight loss, malnutrition, dehydration, and acid-base disturbances; causation is unknown. | • Patient is hospitalized to correct electrolyte imbalances and starvation.<br>• Diet is progressive, as tolerated. |
| Hypervitaminoses A and D | Excessive accumulation of vitamin A or D in children from accidental or misguided overdosage by parents. | • Withhold vitamin supplements.<br>• Glucocorticoids are given to control hypercalcemia and prevent renal damage in hypervitaminosis D; diuretics are used for severe hypercalcemia. |
| Hypochondriasis | The unrealistic misinterpretation of the severity and significance of physical signs or sensations as abnormal and preoccupation with the fear of having a serious disease, which persists despite medical reassurance to the contrary. Unlinked to any cause, although stress increases the risk. Frequently develops in people who have experienced an organic disease or have a relative who has experienced one. | • The goal is to help the patient lead a productive life, despite distressing symptoms and fears. Outpatient psychotherapy with behavior modification is the first line of treatment.<br>• Symptoms must be evaluated to rule out medical causes first.<br>• Routine psychiatric appointments, regardless of new symptoms, help as part of psychotherapy. |
| Hypogonadism | Decreased androgen production in males that may cause infertility, erectile dysfunction and, in young males, inhibit development of secondary sex characteristics. Primary form results from faulty development or mechanical damage. Secondary form (hypogonadotropic) results from a pituitary hormone abnormality. | • Depending on the underlying cause, treatment consists of hormonal replacement with testosterone for primary hypogonadism and for secondary hypogonadism if fertility isn't an issue.<br>• If fertility is desired, human chorionic gonadotropin is given for secondary hypogonadism. |
| IgA deficiency, selective (Janeway type 3 dysgammaglobulinemia) | The most common genetic immunoglobin deficiency. Possibly related to autoimmune disorders because many patients with such disorders are also IgA-deficient. Transient IgA deficiency may occur secondary to certain medications. | • The disorder has no known cure. Treatment aims to control symptoms of associated diseases, such as respiratory and GI infections. |

| NAME (other names) | ETIOLOGY | TREATMENT |
|---|---|---|
| Iodine deficiency | Insufficient iodine due to inadequate intake or thyroid dysfunction; complications range from dental caries to cretinism. | • Iodine supplements (potassium iodide [SSKI]) are administered to correct deficiency.<br>• Increase iodine intake with iodized table salt and iodine-rich foods. |
| Klinefelter's syndrome | Genetic abnormality that affects males resulting from extra X chromosome; apparent at puberty with testes failing to mature and degenerative testicular changes resulting in infertility. | • Severe gynecomastia may necessitate mastectomy.<br>• Drug therapy includes administration of supplemental testosterone.<br>• Psychological and genetic counseling are necessary. |
| Labor, premature (preterm labor) | Onset of rhythmic uterine contractions that produce cervical change after fetal viability but before fetal maturity. Possibly caused by premature rupture of the membranes (30% to 50% of premature labors), preeclampsia, chronic hypertensive vascular disease, hydramnios, multiple pregnancy, placenta previa, abruptio placentae, incompetent cervix, abdominal surgery, trauma, structural anomalies of the uterus, infections (such as rubella or toxoplasmosis), congenital adrenal hyperplasia, and fetal death. Other provocative factors include fetal stimulation, oxytocin sensitivity, myometrial oxygen deficiency, and genetic defect in the mother. | • Bed rest and, when indicated, drug therapy are used to suppress premature labor when tests show immature fetal pulmonary development, cervical dilation of less than 1½″ (4 cm), and the absence of factors that contraindicate continuation of pregnancy.<br>• Drug therapy may employ beta-adrenergic stimulants or magnesium sulfate.<br>• Treatment and delivery require an intensive team effort focusing on continuous assessment of the infant's health through fetal monitoring; avoidance of amniotomy, if possible, to prevent cord prolapse or damage to the infant's temder skull; maintenance of adequate hydration through I.V. fluids; and avoidance of sedatives and narcotics that might harm the infant. |
| Lassa fever | Epidemic hemorrhagic fever caused by the Lassa virus; transmitted to humans by contact with infected rodent urine, feces, and saliva. Fever persists for 2 to 3 weeks with exudative pharyngitis, oral ulcers, lymphadenopathy and swelling of the face and neck, purpura, conjunctivitis, and bradycardia. Shock and peripheral vascular collapse can occur. | • Strict isolation is imposed for at least 3 weeks.<br>• Drug therapy includes antiviral (I.V. ribavirin), I.V. colloids for shock, analgesics for pain, and antipyretics for fever.<br>• Immune plasma from patients who have recovered from Lassa fever is infused. |

| NAME<br>(other names) | ETIOLOGY | TREATMENT |
| --- | --- | --- |
| Latex allergy | Hypersensitivity reaction to products that contain natural latex, which is derived from the sap of a rubber tree; causes local dermatitis to anaphylactic reaction. | • Prevent exposure to natural latex.<br>• Before and after surgery or other invasive procedures, administer prednisone, diphenhydramine, and cimetidine.<br>• Provide supportive treatment during a reaction. |
| Legg-Calvé-Perthes disease | Ischemic necrosis leading to eventual flattening of the head of the femur due to vascular interruption; occurs in stages. | • Patient is on bed rest for 1 to 2 weeks.<br>• Bilateral split counterpoised traction with application of a hip abduction splint or cast is used. Braces may remain in place for 6 to 18 months.<br>• Young child in early stages may need surgery with a spica cast for 2 months postoperatively. |
| Leprosy (Hansen's disease) | Chronic, systemic infection with progressive cutaneous lesions caused by *Mycobacterium leprae*; attacks the peripheral nervous system. | • Drug regimen includes antimicrobial therapy with sulfones (dapsone) or rifampin in combination with clofazimine or ethionamide.<br>• Provide supportive care. |
| Lichen planus | Benign, pruritic skin eruption producing scaling, purple papules with white lines or spots that usually resolve in 2 to 3 years; cause unknown. | • Relieve itching with topical steroids and other symptoms with systemic corticosteroids. |
| Listeriosis | Febrile infection caused by the gram-positive bacillus *Listeria monocytogenes*. It's transmitted in utero, by inhalation, or by ingestion of contaminated food or fomites. | • I.V. antibiotics are given for 3 to 6 weeks. |

| NAME (other names) | ETIOLOGY | TREATMENT |
|---|---|---|
| Magnesium imbalance (hypomagnesemia, hypermagnesemia) | Magnesium deficiency (hypomagnesemia) or excess (hypermagnesemia). Deficiency usually results from impaired absorption, as in malabsorption syndrome, chronic diarrhea, chronic alcoholism, severe dehydration and diabetic acidosis, or after bowel resection. Hypermagnesemia may result from chronic renal insufficiency or overuse of magnesium-containing drugs. | • Therapy aims to identify and correct the underlying cause.<br>• For hypomagnesemia, daily magnesium supplements are given I.V. or P.O.<br>• For hypermagnesemia, therapy includes increased fluid intake and loop diuretics, such as furosemide, when renal function is impaired; a magnesium antagonist, such as calcium gluconate, for temporary relief of symptoms in an emergency; and peritoneal dialysis or hemodialysis if renal function fails or excess magnesium can't be eliminated. |
| Malaria | Acute infectious disease caused by protozoa of the genus *Plasmodium*, which are transmitted by the bite of female *Anopheles* mosquitoes. *P. vivax*, and *P. malariae*, and *P. ovale* cause the chronic carrier state; *P. falciparum* causes the most severe and only life-threatening form of malaria. | • All forms of malaria except *P. falciparum* are best treated with chloroquine.<br>• *P. falciparum* requires oral quinine, pyrimethamine, and a sulfonamide.<br>• The only drug effective against the hepatic stage of the disease that is available in the United States is primaquine phosphate. |
| Marfan syndrome | Rare inherited, degenerative generalized disease of the connective tissue that causes ocular, skeletal, and cardiovascular anomalies. | • Treatment is aimed at relieving the symptoms, such as surgical repair of aneurysms and ocular deformities.<br>• Steroids and sex hormones are given to induce precocious puberty and early epiphyseal closure to prevent abnormal adult height. |
| Mastoiditis | Bacterial infection and inflammation of the air cells of the mastoid antrum resulting in dull ache and tenderness in the area of the mastoid process, low-grade fever, headache, and thick, purulent drainage. Meningitis, facial paralysis, brain abscess, and suppurative labyrinthitis may occur. | • Intense antibiotic therapy is administered parenterally.<br>• Myringotomy is performed if bone damage is minimal.<br>• Mastoidectomy is performed if the mastoid is chronically inflamed. |

| NAME (other names) | ETIOLOGY | TREATMENT |
|---|---|---|
| Medullary sponge kidney | Inherited disorder, possibly where collecting ducts in renal pyramids dilate and cavities, clefts, and cysts form, producing complications of calcium oxylate stones and infections. | • Supportive care focuses on preventing or treating complications caused by stones and infection. Includes increasing fluid intake and monitoring renal function. <br> • Surgery may be required to remove stones during acute obstruction. Nephrectomy is required if serious, uncontrollable infection or hemorrhage occur. |
| Melasma (chloasma or mask of pregnancy) | Patchy, hypermelanotic skin disorder that may result due to increased hormonal levels associated with pregnancy, ovarian cancer, or the use of oral contraceptives. | • Bleaching agents containing 4% hydroquinone are applied. <br> • Exposure to sunlight is avoided. <br> • Sunscreen is applied. <br> • Oral contraceptives are discontinued. <br> • Concomitant use of tretinoin cream (Retin A) may be helpful. |
| Mental retardation | Mental disorder defined by the American Association on Mental Retardation as "significantly subaverage general intellectual function existing concurrently with deficits in adaptive behavior manifesting itself during the developmental period (before age 18)." A specific cause is identifiable in only about 25% of mentally retarded people; of these, only 10% are potentially curable. Significant predisposing factors in the remaining 75% include deficient prenatal or perinatal care, inadequate nutrition, poor social environment, and poor child-rearing practices. | • Effective management requires an interdisciplinary team approach that aims to develop the patient's strengths and social adaptive skills. <br> • For children, individualized special education and training, ideally beginning in infancy, can optimize quality of life. |
| Motion sickness | Loss of equilibrium associated with nausea and vomiting that result from irregular or rhythmic movements or from the sensation of motion. May follow excessive stimulation of the labyrinthine receptors of the inner ear by certain motions, such as those experienced in a car, boat, plane, or swing. May also be caused by confusion in the cerebellum from conflicting sensory input; for example, a visual stimulus (such as a moving horizon) conflicts with labyrinthine perception. | • The best treatment is removal of the stimulus. <br> • If removal isn't possible, the patient will benefit from lying down, closing his eyes, and trying to sleep. <br> • Antiemetics may prevent or relieve symptoms. |

| NAME (other names) | ETIOLOGY | TREATMENT |
|---|---|---|
| Mycosis fungoides (malignant cutaneous reticulosis and granuloma fungoides) | Rare, chronic malignant T-cell lymphoma of unknown cause originating in the reticuloendothelial system of the skin; eventually affects lymph nodes and internal organs. | • Treatment depends on stage and progression of symptoms.<br>• Topical, intralesional, or systemic corticosteroids or mechlorethamine is administered.<br>• Other treatments include phototherapy, methoxsalen administration, photochemotherapy, and radiation therapy. |
| Neurofibromatosis | Group of inherited developmental disorders of the nervous system, muscles, bones, and skin that cause formation of multiple, pedunculated, soft tumors and café-au-lait spots. | • Intracerebral or intraspinal tumors are removed and kyphoscoliosis is corrected.<br>• Disfiguring or disabling growths are treated with cosmetic surgery. |
| Nocardiosis | Bacterial infection caused by gram-positive species of the genus *Nocardia* and transmitted by inhalation; causes cough, mucopurulent sputum, high fever, chills, night sweats, anorexia, malaise, and weight loss. | • Co-trimoxazole or high doses of sulfonamides are given for 12 to 18 months.<br>• Abscesses are surgically drained and necrotic tissue is excised.<br>• Bed rest and supportive treatment are ordered. |
| Nystagmus | Involuntary oscillations of one or (more commonly) both eyeballs, usually rhythmic as well as horizontal, vertical, rotary, or mixed. They may be transient or sustained and may occur spontaneously or on deviation or fixation of the eyes. The most common type, jerk nystagmus, results from excessive stimulation of the vestibular apparatus or from lesions of the brainstem or cerebellum. It occurs in acute inflammatory or destructive labyrinthitis, Ménière's disease, multiple sclerosis, optic nerve atrophy, albinism, cerebrovascular accident, any brain inflammation, or congenital neurologic disorders, or drugs and alcohol. | • The goal is to correct the underlying cause, if possible.<br>• Eyeglasses can correct visual disturbances such as astigmatism.<br>• Positioning the head to steady the gaze in one direction often helps the patient see better. |

| NAME (other names) | ETIOLOGY | TREATMENT |
|---|---|---|
| Obesity | Excess of body fat — body mass index (BMI) >27-28 — resulting from excessive calorie intake and inadequate expenditure of energy. Explanatory theories include hypothalamic dysfunction of hunger and satiety centers, genetic predisposition, abnormal absorption of nutrients, impaired action of GI and growth hormones and of hormonal regulators such as insulin and hypothyroidism. | • The patient must increase his activity level while reducing daily calorie intake through a balanced, low-calorie diet that reduces fat and sugar intake.<br>• Treatment may include hypnosis, behavior modification techniques, and psychotherapy.<br>• Amphetamines, amphetamine congeners, and the new drug sibutramine may be used temporarily to enhance compliance by suppressing appetite and creating a feeling of well-being.<br>• Morbid obesity (BMI >40) may be treated surgically with gastric bypass. |
| Optic atrophy | Degeneration of the optic nerve developing spontaneously or after inflammation or edema of the nerve head. | • Underlying cause is corrected to prevent further vision loss.<br>• Steroids are given to decrease inflammation and swelling. |
| Orbital cellulitis | Acute infection of the orbital tissues and eyelids that can spread to the cavernous sinus or meninges; produces unilateral eyelid edema, hyperemia, reddened eyelids, and matted lashes. | • Amoxicillin, cefaclor, or cephalexin is given orally to fight infection.<br>• Supportive therapy includes administration of fluids, application of warm moist compresses, and bed rest. |
| Ornithosis (psittacosis or parrot fever) | Caused by *Chlamydia psittaci* and transmitted by infected birds by way of inhalation of dust from droppings; results in chills, low-grade fever increasing to high fever, headache, myalgia, sore throat, cough, abdominal distention and tenderness, nausea, vomiting, and macular rash. | • Tetracycline therapy continues for 2 weeks after temperature returns to normal. |
| Osteogenesis imperfecta (brittle bones) | Hereditary disease of bones and connective tissue that may cause varying degrees of skeletal fragility (recurring fractures), thin skin, blue sclerae, poor teeth, hypermobility of joints, and progressive deafness; fatal if congenital form is present within the first few days of life. | • Prevent deformities with traction, immobilization, or both.<br>• Aid normal development and rehabilitation.<br>• Perform supportive measures such as monitoring the patient's circulatory, motor, and sensory abilities, encouraging walking, and teaching preventive measures to avoid fractures and other complications. |

| NAME<br>(other names) | ETIOLOGY | TREATMENT |
|---|---|---|
| Parainfluenza | Group of respiratory illnesses caused by paramyxoviruses that affect the upper and lower respiratory tracts; transmitted by direct contact or inhalation of airborne droplets. | • Treatment regimen include bed rest, antipyretics for fever, analgesics for pain, and antitussives for cough. |
| Paraphilias | Dependence on unusual behaviors or fantasies to achieve sexual excitement, such as exhibitionism, fetishism, frotteurism, pedophilia, sexual masochism, sexual sadism, transvestic fetishism, and voyeurism. | • Treatment is mandatory when the patient's sexual preferences result in socially unacceptable, harmful, or criminal behavior.<br>• Depending on the paraphilia, treatment may include psychotherapy, behavior therapy, surgery, or pharmacotherapy. |
| Patent ductus arteriosus (PDA) | Fetal blood vessel that connects the pulmonary artery to the descending aorta remains open after birth, creating a left-to-right shunt of blood from the aorta to the pulmonary artery; recirculation occurs. Patient may be asymptomatic or show signs of pulmonary vascular disease later in life. Infants may have heart failure and respiratory distress if the PDA is large. | • Asymptomatic infants require no immediate treatment; those with heart failure require fluid restriction, diuretics, and digitalis glycosides.<br>• If medical treatment is unsuccessful, surgery is performed to ligate the ductus. |
| Penile cancer | Malignant, ulcerative or papillary (wartlike, nodular) lesions, which may become quite large before spreading beyond the penis, potentially destroying the glans prepuce and invading the corpora. Generally associated with poor personal hygiene and phimosis in uncircumcised men, although the exact cause is unknown. | • Depending on the stage of progression, treatment includes surgical resection of the primary tumor and, possibly, chemotherapy and radiation.<br>• Invasive tumors require partial penectomy (unless contraindicated because of the patient's young age); tumors of the base of the penile shaft require total penectomy and inguinal node dissection.<br>• Radiation therapy may improve treatment effectiveness after resection of lcoalized lesions without metastasis; it may also reduce the size of lymph nodes before nodal resection.<br>• Bleomycin and methotrexate are generally used in chemotherapy but aren't very effective. |

| NAME (other names) | ETIOLOGY | TREATMENT |
| --- | --- | --- |
| Phosphorus imbalance (hypophosphatemia, hyperphosphatemia) | Hypophosphatemia usually results from inadequate dietary intake, often related to malnutrition from a prolonged metabolic state or chronic alcoholism. It may also stem from intestinal malabsorption, chronic diarrhea, hyperparathyroidism, hypomagnesemia, deficiency of vitamin D, chronic use of antacids containing aluminum hydroxide, renal tubular defects, and diabetic acidosis. Hyperphosphatemia generally occurs secondary to hypocalcemia, excess of vitamin D, hypoparathyroidism, or renal failure. It may also result from overuse of laxatives containing phosphates or phosphate enemas. | • The treatment goal for phosphorus imbalance is to correct the underlying cause. <br> • In the acute phase, replace phosphorus through a high-phosphorus diet and administration of phosphate salt tablets or I.V. potassium phosphate. <br> • Hyperphosphatemia is rarely clinically significant. |
| Photosensitivity reaction | Skin eruption that can be a toxic or an allergic response to light alone or to light and chemicals. Erythema, papules, vesicles, urticaria, and eczematous lesions occur on exposed areas. | • Topical steroids are given to reduce inflammation. <br> • Antihistamines are given to relieve itching. <br> • Using sunscreen, wearing protective clothing, and minimizing exposure to sunlight is helpful. |
| Pilonidal disease | Coccygeal cyst forms in the intergluteal cleft on the posterior surface of the lower sacrum, often becoming infected or developing a fistula; may be congenital or caused by irritation from exercise, heat, perspiration, or constrictive clothing. | • Abscesses are incised and drained, protruding hairs are extracted, and sitz baths are ordered. <br> • Entire affected area is excised if infections persist. |
| Pityriasis rosea | Acute, self-limiting, inflammatory skin disease producing a patch, followed by an eruption of papulosquamous lesions; cause is unknown. | • Emollients, oatmeal baths, antihistamines, and occasionally exposure to UV light or sunlight to relieve pruritis. <br> • Systemic corticosteroids to relieve severe inflammation. |

| NAME (other names) | ETIOLOGY | TREATMENT |
| --- | --- | --- |
| Plague (black death, bubonic plague, septicemic plague, pneumonic plague) | Acute infection caused by *Yersinia pestis* and transmitted through the bite of a flea from infected rodents. Mild infection occurs with painful, inflamed buboes and hemorrhagic areas that become necrotic; may present dramatically with sudden high fever, myalgia, delirium, prostration, restlessness, toxemia, and staggering gait. | • Treatment includes large doses of streptomycin; other effective drugs include gentamycin, doxycycline, and chloramphenicol. <br> • Glucocorticoids are given to combat life-threatening toxemia and shock; diazepam is given to relieve restlessness. <br> • Heparin is given for disseminated intravascular coagulation. <br> • Provide supportive therapy for fever, shock, and seizures. |
| Platelet function disorders | Inherited or acquired disorders that cause defects in platelet adhesion or procoagulation activity; result in sudden appearance of petechiae or purpura or excessive bruising and bleeding of the nose and gums. More serious signs of bleeding, such as external or internal hemorrhage, can also occur. | • Platelet replacement is administered for inherited platelet disorders. <br> • Acquired platelet function disorders respond to treating the underlying disease or discontinuing damaging drug therapy. <br> • Plasmapheresis controls bleeding. |
| Poisoning | Inhalation, ingestion, or injection of, or skin contamination with, any harmful substance. In children, accidental poisoning usually involves ingestion of salicylates, acetaminophen, cleaning agents, insecticides, paints, or cosmetics. In adults, common workplace poisonings involve companies that use chlorine, carbon dioxide, hydrogen sulfide, nitrogen dioxide, and ammonia, and those that ignore safety standards. Other causes in adults involve improper cooking, canning, and storage of food; ingestion of, or skin contamination from, plants; and drug overdose. | • Treatment includes emergency resuscitation and support, prevention of further poison absorption, continuing supportive or symptomatic care and, when possible, administration of a special antidote. <br> • If barbiturate, glutethimide, or tranquilizer poisoning causes hypothermia, a hyperthermia blanket may be used to control the patient's temperature. |
| Poliomyelitis (polio, infantile paralysis) | An acute communicable disease caused by the poliovirus and ranging in severity from inapparent infection to fatal paralytic illness. Three antigenically distinct serotypes — types I, II, and III poliovirus — all cause poliomyelitis and are transmitted by direct contact with infected oropharyngeal secretions or stools. | • Supportive treatment includes analgesics and perhaps moist heat applications to ease headache, back, and leg spasms and pain. <br> • Bed rest is necessary until extreme discomfort subsides. <br> • Paralytic polio requires long-term rehabilitation using physical therapy, braces, corrective shoes and, in some cases orthopedic surgery. |

| NAME (other names) | ETIOLOGY | TREATMENT |
|---|---|---|
| Polymyalgia rheumatica | An inflammatory syndrome characterized by significant stiffness and dull aching pain of the proximal muscle groups, weight loss, malaise, and fever. Its cause is unknown, but it predominantly involves whites, tends to run in families, and is possibly associated with HLA-DR4 antigens, all of which suggest a possible genetic predisposition. | • Corticosteroids, such as prednisone or prednisolone, are the treatment of choice. |
| Polymyositis and dermatomyositis | Immune-mediated inflammation and subsequent damage to striated muscle leading to progressive muscle weakness. Insidious onset of slowly progressive, often painless muscle weakness of proximal arms and legs; also may have associated symptoms. | • High doses of corticosteroids are used to suppress inflammation.<br>• Use of immunosuppressants, such as methotrexate or azathioprine, may allow shorter course of steroids.<br>• Low-impact exercise and range-of-motion exercises prevent contractures. |
| Postmenopausal bleeding | Bleeding from the reproductive tract that occurs 1 year or more after cessation of menses; may be caused by hormonal changes, atrophic vaginitis, aging, cancer, adenomatous hyperplasia, or atypical adenomatous hyperplasia. | • Control of massive hemorrhage is seldom necessary except in advanced cancer.<br>• Dilatation and curettage relieve bleeding.<br>• Diagnose and treat underlying cause.<br>• Estrogen creams and suppositories are ordered for deficiencies.<br>• Hysterectomy is performed for repeated episodes of bleeding. |
| Precocious puberty in females | Onset of pubertal changes, such as breast development, pubic and axillary hair development, and menarche, before age 9; results from early development and activation of the endocrine glands without corresponding abnormality or from pathologic causes. | • Medroxyprogesterone reduces the secretion of gonadotropins and prevents menstruation.<br>• Treat the underlying cause (adrenogenital syndrome, abdominal tumors, choriocarcinomas, hypothyroidism, drug ingestion).<br>• No treatment is necessary for precocious thelarche and pubarche. |
| Precocious puberty in males | Sexual maturation before age 10 caused by idiopathic (constitutional) or cerebral (neurogenic) changes. | • Idiopathic causes generally require no medical treatment.<br>• Neurogenic causes require treatment of underlying pathology. |

| NAME<br>(other names) | ETIOLOGY | TREATMENT |
| --- | --- | --- |
| Premeno-<br>pausal bleed-<br>ing, abnormal | Bleeding that deviates from the normal menstrual cycle before menopause; may be caused by oligomenorrhea, polymenorrhea, menorrhagia, hypomenorrhea, cryptomenorrhea, or metrorrhagia. | • Treatment depends on the type of bleeding abnormality and its cause. |
| Pruritus ani | Perianal itching that worsens at night and wakes the patient; also occurs after bowel movement and during stress. Multiple factors contribute to the condition (over-cleaning, trauma, poor hygiene, food sensitivity, sensitivity to toilet paper or other environmental things, medications, and excessive sweating). | • Eliminate underlying cause.<br>• Educate patient regarding anal hygiene. |
| Ptosis | Drooping of the upper eyelid that may be congenital or acquired, unilateral or bilateral, constant or intermittent. Congenital form (usually unilateral) is transmitted as an autosomal dominant trait or results from a congenital anomaly in which the levator muscles of the eyelid fail to develop. Acquired ptosis may result from age; nutritional factors, such as hyperemesis gravidarum; or mechanical factors that make the eyelid heavy, such as swelling, edema, ior an extra fatty fold. Additional causes include myogenic factors, such as muscular dystrophy or myasthenia gravis, and neurogenic factors. | • Slight ptosis that doesn't produce deformity or loss of vision requires no treatment.<br>• Severe ptosis that interferes with vision or is cosmetically undesirable usually necessitates resection of the weak levator muscles.<br>• Effective treatment also requires treatment of the underlying cause, if possible. |
| Puerperal infection | Inflammation of the birth canal during the postpartum period or after abortion; caused by streptococci, coagulase-negative staphylococci, *Clostridium perfringens*, *Bacteroides fragilis*, and *Escherichia coli*. | • I.V. broad-spectrum antibiotics are ordered to combat infection.<br>• Supportive therapy includes analgesics, anticoagulants, antiemetics, and bed rest.<br>• Thrombophlebitis and hypovolemia are resolved. |

| NAME (other names) | ETIOLOGY | TREATMENT |
|---|---|---|
| Rectal polyps | Mass lesions that result from unrestrained cell growth in the upper epithelium and protrude into the intestinal lumen. Varying in appearance, they include common polypoid adenomas, villous adenomas, polyposis syndromes, juvenile polyps, and focal polypoid hyperplasia. Predisposing factors include heredity, age, infection, and diet. | • Specific treatment varies according to type and size of the polyps and their location in the colon.<br>• Common polypoid adenomas less than 1 cm in size require polypectomy, frequently by fulguration (destruction by high-frequency electricity) during endoscopy. For common polypoid adenomas over 4 cm and all invasive villous adenomas, treatment usually consists of abdominoperineal resection or low anterior resection. Transanal excision is performed to remove an adenoma from the rectum.<br>• Depending on large-bowel involvement, hereditary polyposis necessitate restorative proctolectomy, ileoanal anastomosis with temporary ileostomy.<br>• Focal polypoid hyperplasia can be obliterated by a biopsy. |
| Rectal prolapse | Circumferential protrusion of one or more layers of the rectum through the anus caused by straining or conditions that affect the pelvic floor or rectum. The patient may also have a feeling of rectal fullness, bloody diarrhea, and pain. | • Treat the underlying cause and eliminate predisposing factors (straining, coughing, nutritional disorders).<br>• Surgical repair is performed in severe or chronic cases. |
| Reiter's syndrome | Self-limiting syndrome associated with polyarthritis (dominant feature), urethritis, balanitis, conjunctivitis, and mucocutaneous lesions. The cause is unknown, but most cases follow venereal or enteric infection. Because 75% to 85% of patients test positive for the human leukocyte antigen B27, genetic susceptibility is likely. | • No specific treatment exists, but anti-inflammatory agents (the primary treatment) can be given to relieve discomfort and fever.<br>• Steroids may be used for persistent skin lesions; gold therapy, sulfasalazine, methotrexate, or azathioprine for bony erosions.<br>• Physical therapy includes range-of-motion and strengthening exercises and the use of padded or supportive shoes to prevent contractures and foot deformities.<br>• Testing for HIV is also indicated. |

| NAME (other names) | ETIOLOGY | TREATMENT |
|---|---|---|
| Renovascular hypertension | Rise in systemic blood pressure resulting from atherosclerosis or stenosis of the renal arteries. Primary causes in 95% of patients are atherosclerosis (especially in older men) and fibroplasia of the renal artery wall layers. Other causes include arteritis, renal artery anomalies, embolism, trauma, a tumor, and a dissecting aneurysm. | • Surgery, the treatment of choice, is performed to restore adequate circulation and to control severe hypertension or severely impaired renal function by renal artery bypass, endarterectomy, arterioplasty or, as a last resort, nephrectomy.<br>• Renal artery dilation by balloon catheter is used in selected cases to correct renal artery stenosis without the risks and morbidity of surgery.<br>• Symptomatic measures include antihypertensives, diuretics, and a sodium-restricted diet. |
| Retinitis pigmentosa | Genetically induced progressive destruction of the retinal rods resulting in visual field constriction, cataracts, edema, atrophic maculopathy, and blindness. | • No cure exists.<br>• Vitamin A supplementation is given to slow degeneration. |
| Rocky Mountain spotted fever | Febrile rash producing illness caused by *Rickettsia rickettsii* and transmitted by a tick bite. Fever, excruciating headache, nausea, vomiting, and aching occur along with a thick white tongue coating that turns brown; a rash covering the entire body of eruptions follows flushing of the skin. Vascular collapse and death can occur. | • Remove the tick.<br>• Administer antibiotics, such as chloramphenicol and tetracycline, until 3 days after the fever subsides.<br>• Provide supportive and symptomatic treatment. |
| Rosacea | Chronic skin eruption with flushing and dilation of the small blood vessels in the face, papules and pustules, dilated follicles, and thickened bulbous skin on the nose; cause is unknown but may be aggravated by anything that produces flushing of the skin. | • Oral tetracycline is given for acneiform component.<br>• Apply topical metronidazole gel.<br>• Avoid factors that aggravate the condition. |
| Schistosomiasis (bilharziasis) | Infection caused by blood flukes transmitted by contact with water contaminated with *Schistosoma* larvae; symptoms include rash at site of cercariae penetration, fever, myalgia, and cough with later signs of hepatomegaly, splenomegaly, and lymphadenopathy and complications of flaccid paralysis, seizures, and skin abscesses. | • Administer praziquantel and recheck patient in 3 to 10 months.<br>• Provide supportive treatment of symptoms. |

| NAME (other names) | ETIOLOGY | TREATMENT |
|---|---|---|
| Scleroderma (progressive systemic sclerosis) | A diffuse connective tissue disease characterized by inflammatory and then degenerative and fibrotic changes in skin, blood vessels, synovial membranes, skeletal muscles, and internal organs (especially the esophagus, intestinal tract, thyroid, heart, lungs, and kidneys). Occurs in distinctive forms: limited systemic sclerosis, a benign subtype called CREST syndrome, diffuse systemic sclerosis, localized scleroderma, and linear scleroderma. The cause is unknown. | • Currently, no cure exists.<br>• Use of immunosuppressants, such as cyclosporine or chlorambucil, is a common palliative measure to preserve normal body functions and minimize complications. D-penicillamine may be helpful.<br>• Blood platelet levels need to be monitored throughout drug therapy.<br>• Other treatments vary according to symptoms. Experimental treatments include methotrexate, interferon-alpha, interferon-gamma, and FK-506. |
| Septal perforation and deviation | Perforated septum is a hole between the two nasal passages caused by traumatic irritation, cauterization from repeated epistaxis, or other causes and resulting in a whistle on inspiration, rhinitis, epistaxis, and discharge. Deviated septum is a shift from the midline caused by normal development or trauma and resulting in midline deflecting to one side, shortness of breath, discharge, sinusitis, infections, headache, and epistaxis. | • Perforation treatment includes decongestants, local application of lanolin or petroleum jelly (to prevent ulcers and crusting), and antibiotics.<br>• Perforation may be closed surgically.<br>• Deviation treatment is symptomatic and includes analgesics, decongestants, vasoconstrictors, packing, and cauterization.<br>• Deviation may also be treated surgically. |
| Shigellosis (bacillary dysentery) | Acute intestinal infection caused by the bacteria *Shigella* resulting in high fever, acute self-limiting diarrhea with tenesmus, and electrolyte imbalances; transmitted by the fecal-oral route through objects or contaminated food or water. | • Low-residue diet is ordered.<br>• Fluids and electrolytes are replaced by I.V. therapy.<br>• Ampicillin, tetracycline, or cotrimoxazole is given in severe cases. |
| Sporotrichosis | Chronic disease caused by the fungus *Sporothrix schenckii* and resulting in cutaneous, lymphatic (skin lesions on hands or fingers), pulmonary, or disseminated (multifocal lesions that spread) forms. | • Saturated solution of potassium iodide is applied to cutaneous lesions for 1 to 2 months.<br>• Lesions are excised and drained.<br>• Disseminated forms require I.V. amphotericin B.<br>• Cavitary pulmonary lesions may require surgery. |

| NAME (other names) | ETIOLOGY | TREATMENT |
|---|---|---|
| Strongyloidiasis (threadworm infection) | Parasitic intestinal infection caused by the helminth *Strongyloides stercoralis;* transmitted through contaminated soil, and resulting in swelling and pruritus at the site of penetration; as larvae migrate to the lungs, pulmonary signs develop; intestinal infection and malnutrition can occur, resulting in perforation. | • Thiabendazole, albendazole, or ivermectin is given for 2 to 3 days.<br>• Supportive treatment includes protein replacement, blood transfusions, and I.V. fluids. |
| Stye (hordeolum) | Staphylococcal infection that causes an abscess in the follicle of an eyelash, resulting in redness, swelling, and pain. | • Apply warm compresses.<br>• Don't squeeze the stye.<br>• Antibiotic ointment may be used. |
| Taeniasis (tapeworm disease, cestodiasis) | A parasitic intestinal infestation by *Taenia saginata* (beef tapeworm), *Taenia solium* (pork tapeworm), *Diphyllobothrium latum* (fish tapeworm), or *Hymenolepis nana* (dwarf tapeworm). Usually a chronic, benign intestinal disease; however, infestation with *T. solium* may cause dangerous systemic and central nervous system symptoms if larvae invade the brain and striated muscle of vital organs. *T. saginata*, *T. solium*, and *D. latum* are transmitted to humans by ingestion of (respectively) beef, pork, or fish containing tapeworm cysts. *H. nana* (dwarf tapeworm) is transmitted direct from person to person and requires no intermediate host. | • Niclosamide offers a cure in up to 95% of patients. Another anthelmintic agent, praziquantel, may also be effective.<br>• After drug treatment, all types of tapeworm infestation require a follow-up laboratory examination of stool specimens during the next 3 to 5 weeks to check for any remaining ova or worm segments. |
| Tetralogy of Fallot | Combination of four cardiac defects (ventricular septal defect, pulmonary stenosis, right ventricular hypertrophy, and dextroposition of the aorta with overriding of the ventricular septal defect). Symptoms include cyanosis evident several months after birth or sooner with any exertion (crying, straining, infection, fever), squatting when short of breath, and signs of poor oxygenation. | • Prevent or treat complications.<br>• Relieve cyanosis, and anticipate palliative or corrective surgery.<br>• Oxygen and morphine are given to improve oxygenation.<br>• Propranolol may prevent blue spells.<br>• Surgery is performed on infants with potentially fatal hypoxic spells. |

| NAME<br>(other names) | ETIOLOGY | TREATMENT |
|---|---|---|
| Thalassemia | Three hereditary hemolytic anemias characterized by defective synthesis in the polypeptide chains necessary for hemoglobin (Hb) production. Thalasemia major and thalassemia intermedia result from homozygous inheritance, and thalassemia minor from heterozygous inheritance, of the partially dominant autosomal gene responsible for this trait. | For thalassemia major:<br>• Treatment is essentially supportive, such as appropriate antibiotics given promptly for infection.<br>• Folic acid supplements help maintain folic acid levels in the face of increased demand.<br>• Transfusions of packed RBCs raise Hb levels, but must be used judiciously to minimize iron overload.<br>• Splenectomy and bone marrow transplantation have been tried, but their effectiveness hasn't been confirmed.<br>• Thalassemia intermedia and thalassemia minor usually don't require treatment. |
| Throat abscess | Either peritonsillar (quinsy) abscess that forms in the connective tissue space between the tonsil capsule and constrictor muscle of the pharynx or retropharyngeal abscess that forms between the posterior pharyngeal wall and prevertebral fascia. Peritonsillar abscess is a complication of acute tonsillitis, usually after streptococcal or staphylococcal infection. Acute retropharyngeal abscess results from infection in the retropharyngeal lymph glands, which may follow an upper respiratory tract bacterial infection. Chronic retropharyngeal abscess may result from tuberculosis of the cervical spine (Pott's disease). | • For early-stage peritonsillar abscess, large doses of a broad-spectrum antibiotic are given.<br>• For late-stage peritonsillar abscess with cellulitis of the tonsillar space, primary treatment is incision and drainage under a local anesthetic, followed by antibiotic therapy for 7 to 10 days.<br>• For both stages of peritonsillar abscess, tonsillectomy, is recommended after several episodes. It must be scheduled at least 1 month after acute infection.<br>• In acute retropharyngeal abscess, primary treatment is incision and drainage through the pharyngeal wall.<br>• In chronic retropharyngeal abscess, drainage is performed through an external incision behind the sternomastoid muscle. |
| Tinea versicolor | Chronic, superficial fungal infection producing a multicolored rash or macular or raised scaly lesions, commonly on the upper trunk and caused by *Pityrosporum orbiculare*. | • Treat with selenium sulfide lotion or topical antifungals, such as imidazole cream. |

| NAME (other names) | ETIOLOGY | TREATMENT |
| --- | --- | --- |
| Torticollis (wryneck) | Congenital or acquired neck deformity in which the sternocleidomastoid neck muscles are spastic or shortened, causing bending of the head to the affected side and rotation of the chin to the opposite side. Possible causes of the congenital form include malposition of the head in utero, prenatal injury, fibroma, interruption of blood supply, or fibrotic rupture of the sternocleidomastoid muscle, with hematoma and scar formation. In the three forms of acquired torticollis, the acute form results from muscular damage caused by inflammatory diseases, such as myositis, lymphadenitis, and tuberculosis, and from cervical spinal injuries that produce scar tissue contracture. The spasmodic form results from rhythmic muscle spasms caused by an organic central nervous system disorder. The hysterical form results from psychogenic inability to control neck muscles. | For congenital torticollis: <br>• Passive neck stretching and proper positioning during sleep for an infant and active stretching exercises for an older child help stretch the shortened muscle. <br>• Surgical correction involves sectioning the sternocleidomastoid muscle. <br>For acquired torticollis: <br>• Treatment aims to correct the underlying cause. <br>• In the acute form, application of heat, cervical traction, and gentle massage may help relieve pain. <br>• In the spasmodic and hysterical forms, stretching exercises and a neck brace may relieve symptoms. <br>• Treatment of elderly patients may include administration of levodopa-carbodopa, carbamazepine, and haloperidol. |
| Toxic epidermal necrolysis | Rare, severe skin disorder causing epidermal erythema, superficial necrosis, and skin erosions. Mortality is high among debilitated and elderly people; most cases result from a strong drug reaction. | • Treatment is performed at a burn center or in the intensive care unit because allografts and xenografts may be advised. <br>• Fluid replacement is administered I.V. <br>• Antibiotics are given for secondary infections. |
| Toxocariasis (ocular larva migrans, visceral larva migrans) | Infection caused by parasitic roundworms in dogs and cats spread by the fecal-oral route and resulting in eye infections that can cause blindness or visceral (rare) symptoms with swelling of body organs or central nervous system. | • Infection is treated with mebendazole or albendazole. <br>• Prevention measures include treating animals and thorough hand washing. |
| Tracheo-esophageal fistula and esophageal atresia | Developmental anomaly characterized by abnormal connection between the trachea and esophagus causing coughing, cyanosis, and aspiration of fluid as the newborn tries to swallow. | • Emergency surgical correction depends on the type of fistula that is present. <br>• Supportive therapy includes I.V. and antibiotic therapy until surgery is performed. |

| NAME (other names) | ETIOLOGY | TREATMENT |
|---|---|---|
| Trachoma | Infection by *Chlamydia trachomatis* that affects the eye but can also localize in the urethra; may cause permanent damage to the cornea and conjunctiva. | • Topical or systemic antibiotic therapy with tetracycline, erythromycin, or doxycycline is given for 3 to 4 weeks.<br>• Surgical correction is necessary if severe entropion occurs. |
| Transposition of the great arteries | Congenital heart defect in which the great arteries are reversed and the newborn develops cyanosis and tachypnea that worsens with crying; murmurs and other symptoms also occur. | • Atrial balloon septostomy is performed during cardiac catheterization.<br>• Defect is corrected surgically. |
| Trichinosis (trichiniasis, trichinellosis) | An infection caused by larvae of the intestinal roundworm *Trichinella spiralis*. Transmission is through ingestion of uncooked or undercooked meat, expecially pork or bear meat, that contains *T. spiralis* cysts. | • Mebendazole eliminates trichinosis.<br>• Corticosteroids are used for heart or central nervous system involvement, but they extend the parasite elimination time. |
| Trichomoniasis | Protozoal infection of the lower genitourinary tract producing gray or greenish yellow discharge that can be frothy, malodorous, and profuse. Itching, redness, swelling, tenderness, dyspareunia, dysuria, urinary frequency, postcoital spotting, menorrhagia, or dysmenorrhea can also occur. In males, mild to severe urethritis with dysuria and frequency can occur. | • A single 2-g dose of metronidazole is given to all sexual partners.<br>• Screen for other sexually transmitted diseases. |
| Trisomy 13 syndrome (Patau's syndrome) | Multiple malformation syndrome with brain and facial abnormalities as well as major cardiac, GI, and limb malformations. Most fetuses are aborted spontaneously and few live beyond age 5 years. | • Provide supportive care. |
| Undescended testes (cryptorchidism) | Congenital disorder of one or both testes that fail to descend into the scrotum; detectable on palpation. | • Disorder is corrected surgically. |

| NAME (other names) | ETIOLOGY | TREATMENT |
|---|---|---|
| Urticaria and angioedema | Urticaria (hives) is an episodic, usually self-limited skin reaction characterized by local dermal wheals surrounded by an erythematous flare. Angioedema is a subcutaneous and dermal eruption that produces deeper, larger wheals (usually on the hands, feet, lips, eyelids, and genitals) and a more diffuse swelling of loose subcutaneous tisue. May be caused by allergic reactions, such as to drugs, foods, insect stings and, occasionally, inhalant allergens (animal danders, cosmetics) that provoke an immunoglobulin E- (IgE-) mediated response to protein allergens. However, certain drugs may cause urticaria without an IgE response. Nonallergic causes include external physical stimuli, such as cold (usually in younf adults), heat, water, and sunlight. | • Treatment aims to prevent or limit contact with triggering factors or, if impossible, to desensitize the patient to them and to relieve symptoms.<br>• After removal of the stimulus, urticaria usually subsides in a few days. However, drug reactions may persist as long as the drug is in the bloodstream. |
| Uveitis | Inflammation of one uveal tract producing moderate to severe eye pain, severe ciliary injection, photophobia, tearing, a small nonreactive pupil, and blurred vision; results from allergy, infection, chemicals, trauma, surgery, or systemic diseases or may be idiopathic. | • Underlying cause is diagnosed and treated.<br>• Topical cycloplegic and topical corticosteroids are given.<br>• Oral systemic corticosteroids are given in severe cases.<br>• Provide supportive therapy. |
| Vaginal cancer | Usually a squamous cell carcinoma, but occasionally a melanoma, sarcoma, or adenocarcinoma, varying in severity according to its location and effect on lymphatic drainage. Clear-cell adenocarcinoma has an increased incidence in young women whose mothers took diethylstibestrol. Otherwise, the cause is unknown. | • Topical chemotherapy with fluorouracil and laser surgery can be used in stages 0 and I to preserve the normal parts of the vagina.<br>• Radiation or surgery in the early stages varies with the size depth and location of the lesion and the patient's desire to maintain a functional vagina.<br>• Radiation therapy is the preferred treatment for advanced vaginal cancer. Most patients need preliminary external radiation treatment to shrink the tumor before internal radiation can begin.<br>• Surgery is usually recommended only in late-stage cancer, when the tumor is so extensive that exenteration is needed. |

| NAME (other names) | ETIOLOGY | TREATMENT |
|---|---|---|
| Vaginismus | Involuntary spastic constriction of the lower vaginal muscles with pain on insertion of any object into the vagina; cause may be physical or psychological. | • Maladaptive muscle constriction is eliminated with dilators.<br>• Psychotherapy may be indicated. |
| Variola (smallpox) | Acute, highly contagious disease transmitted by respiratory droplets and caused by poxvirus variola; produces chills, high fever, headache, malaise, and sore throat, with lesions on the mucous membranes and then the skin; may lead to coma. | • Hospitalization is necessary with strict isolation.<br>• Antimicrobial therapy is implemented.<br>• Symptomatic treatment includes antipruritics, pain medication, and nutritional support. |
| Velopharyngeal insufficiency | Failure of the velopharyngeal sphincter to close properly during speech, giving the voice a hypernasal quality and permitting nasal emission; unintelligible speech occurs. | • Corrective surgery eliminates palate abnormalities. |
| Ventricular septal defect (VSD) | Congenital anomaly causing an opening in the septum between the ventricles, allowing blood to shunt between the left and right ventricles; depending on the anomaly's size, spontaneous closure may occur (if small); if closure doesn't occur, biventricular heart failure and cyanosis occurs. | • Large defects usually require early surgical correction using patch grafts before heart failure and irreversible pulmonary vascular disease develop.<br>• Small defects may be closed surgically with a simple suture closure.<br>• Supportive therapy is implemented until surgery occurs. |
| Vesicoureteral reflux | Urine flows from the bladder back into the ureters and eventually into the renal pelvis or the parenchyma due to congenital anomalies; results in signs and symptoms of urinary tract infection. | • Antibiotic therapy is given to prevent pyelonephritis and renal dysfunction.<br>• Normal valve effect is created surgically. |
| *Vibrio vulnificus* septicemia | Vomiting, diarrhea, and abdominal pain from eating contaminated seafood (GI illness, fever, or shock) or an open wound that is exposed to seawater (wound infection); in immunocompromised individuals, it can lead to liver disease, septic shock, and blistering skin lesion. | • Drug therapy includes doxycycline or a third-generation cephalosporin (ceftazidime). |

| NAME (other names) | ETIOLOGY | TREATMENT |
|---|---|---|
| Vitamin A deficiency | Inadequate daily intake of vitamin A; malabsorption, massive urinary excretion, or decreased storage or transport results in a deficiency, resulting in night blindness (nyctalopia), xerophthalmia, drying of the conjunctivas, gray plaques, and blindness. | • Vitamin A supplements are administered to correct the deficiency.<br>• Therapy for the underlying problem is implemented.<br>• Symptoms are managed with supportive treatment. |
| Vitamin B deficiency | Malabsorption or organic causes may result in deficiency that produces thiamine deficiency (polyneuritis, Wernicke's encephalopathy, Korsakoff's psychosis, beriberi), riboflavin deficiency (cheilosis, sore throat, glossitis, eye symptoms), niacin deficiency (fatigue, anorexia, muscle weakness, headache, skin eruptions), pyridoxine deficiency (cheilosis, glossitis, abdominal pain, vomiting, seizures) or cobalamin deficiency (pernicious anemia). | • Diet and supplementary vitamins correct or prevent vitamin B deficiency. |
| Vitamin C deficiency (ascorbic acid deficiency or scurvy) | Diet lacking in foods rich in vitamin C, destruction of vitamin C in foods, excessive ingestion of vitamin C during pregnancy, or marginal intake of vitamin C during periods of physiologic stress can result in deficiency. Features include capillary fragility, follicular hyperkeratosis, anemia, anorexia, joint pain, psychological disturbances, swollen or bleeding gums, loose teeth, poor wound healing, and fractures. | • Diet and supplementary vitamins correct or prevent vitamin C deficiency. |
| Vitamin D deficiency (rickets) | Failure of normal bone calcification occurs due to the deficiency, resulting in bone malformations and poorly developed muscles; causes include inherited impairment or reabsorption of phosphate, conditions that lower absorption of fat-soluble vitamins, liver or kidney disease, and malfunctioning parathyroid gland. | • Massive oral doses of vitamin D or cod liver oil are given for osteomalacia and rickets, unless the cause is malabsorption.<br>• Drug therapy includes 25-hydroxycholecalciferol; 1,25-dihydroxycholecalciferol; or a synthetic analogue of active vitamin D for rickets refractory to vitamin D or for rickets accompanied by liver or kidney disease. |

| NAME<br>(other names) | ETIOLOGY | TREATMENT |
|---|---|---|
| Vitamin E deficiency (tocopherol deficiency) | Infants who consume formulas high in polyunsaturated fatty acids that are fortified with iron but not vitamin E or individuals whose diets are high in polyunsaturated fatty acids or who have malabsorption problems may develop vitamin E deficiency. Edema and skin lesions occur in infants, and muscle weakness or intermittent claudication occurs in adults. | • Vitamin E is replaced with a water-soluble supplement, either orally or parenterally. |
| Vitamin K deficiency | Common among newborns; also caused by prolonged use of some drugs, decreased flow of bile, malabsorption, chronic liver disease, and cystic fibrosis. Abnormal bleeding occurs with prolonged prothrombin time. | • Vitamin K is replaced. |
| Warts (verrucae) | Common benign viral infections of the skin and adjacent mucous membranes caused by human papillomavirus; results in formation of rough, elevated lesion that may be flat or moist, depending on the type and its location. | • Treatment varies according to location, size, number, pain level, history of therapy, age of the patient, and compliance with treatment.<br>• Treatment modalities include electrodesiccation and curettage, cryotherapy, acid therapy, 25% podophyllin with tincture of benzoin for genital warts, and laser therapy. |
| Whooping cough (pertussis) | Contagious respiratory infection caused by *Bordetella pertussis* and transmitted by direct inhalation of contaminated droplets; produces tenacious mucus with varying stages of the disease, progressing with a characteristic cough and fever to choking and fatalities. | • Supportive therapy, often given in an intensive care unit, includes fluid and electrolyte replacement, nutrition, codeine (for cough), oxygen, and antibiotics to shorten period of comunicability and prevent secondary infection. |

| NAME (other names) | ETIOLOGY | TREATMENT |
|---|---|---|
| Wilson's disease (hepatolenticular degeneration) | Rare, inherited metabolic disorder characterized by excessive copper retention in the liver, brain, kidneys, and corneas. Kayser-Fleischer rings of the eye are produced, and deposits may lead to tissue necrosis and fibrosis. | • Treatment with pyridoxine in conjunction with D-penicillamine, a copper-chelating agent that mobilizes copper from the tissues and promotes its excretion in the urine, is lifelong.<br>• Trientine may also be used; oral zinc acetate promotes fecal copper excretion and may be used as maintenance.<br>• Copper-containing foods should be avoided.<br>• Patient and family should receive genetic counseling. |
| Wiskott-Aldrich syndrome (immunodeficiency with eczema and thrombocytopenia) | X-linked recessive inherited disease characterized by defective B- and T-cell functions (increased susceptibility to infections) and metabolic defects in platelet synthesis (thrombocytopenia). Male infants develop early bleeding complications (bloody stools, petechia, and purpura) and by 6 months develop recurrent systemic infections; by age 1 year, eczema develops, leading to scratching and skin infections; high susceptibility to neoplastic diseases, such as lymphoma and leukemia, occurs. Average life span is 4 years. | • Bleeding is controlled with platelet transfusions.<br>• Prophylactic or early aggressive therapy with antibiotics is indicated for infections.<br>• Topical steroids help control eczema symptoms.<br>• Bone marrow transplantation may be effective in some patients. |
| X-linked infantile hypogammaglobulinemia (Bruton's agammaglobulinemia) | Inherited deficiency or absence of B cells leading to defective humoral immune responses and depressed production of all five immunoglobulin types (IgG, IgE, IgA, IgM, IgD); affects males, who develop recurrent bacterial infections, dental caries, polyarthritis, and malabsorption disorders. | • Prophylactic or early aggressive antibiotic therapy is indicated to control infections.<br>• Stress the importance of careful hygiene, such as cleaning cuts and scrapes thoroughly.<br>• Immune globulin injections are given to maintain IgG levels, although fresh frozen plasma may be needed to supply IgA and IgM. |

| NAME (other names) | ETIOLOGY | TREATMENT |
| --- | --- | --- |
| Zinc deficiency | Deficiency may produce hepatosplenomegaly, sparse hair growth, soft and misshapen nails, poor wound healing, anorexia, taste and odor changes, severe iron deficiency anemia, bone deformities and, if chronic, hypogonadism, dwarfism, and hyperpigmentation; may be due to dietary causes, blood loss, or corticosteroid therapy. | • Underlying cause of the deficiency is diagnosed and treated.<br>• Zinc supplementation is given, as needed. |

# SELECTED REFERENCES

## General

Beare, P.G., and Myers, J.L. *Adult Health Nursing,* 3rd ed. St. Louis: Mosby–Year Book, Inc., 1998.

Brashers, V.L. *Clinical Applications of Pathophysiology.* St. Louis: Mosby–Year Book, Inc., 1998.

Burrell, L.O., et al. *Adult Nursing: Acute and Community Care,* 2nd ed. Stamford, Conn.: Appleton & Lange, 1997.

Buttaro, T.M., et al. *Primary Care: A Collaborative Practice.* St. Louis: Mosby–Year Book, Inc., 1999.

Dambro, M.R., and Griffith, J.A. *Griffith's 5- Minute Clinical Consult.* Philadelphia: Lippincott Williams & Wilkins, 1999.

Goldlist, B.J. *Appleton & Lange's Review of Internal Medicine,* 2nd ed. Stamford, Conn.: Appleton & Lange, 1998.

Ignatavicius, D.D., et al. *Medical-Surgical Nursing Across the Health Care Continuum,* 3rd ed. Philadelphia: W.B. Saunders Co., 1999.

*Physician's Drug Handbook*, 7th ed. Springhouse, Pa.: Springhouse Corporation, 1997.

*Professional Guide To Diagnostic Tests*, 2nd. ed. Springhouse, Pa.: Springhouse Corporation, 1998.

*Professional Guide to Diseases,* 6th ed. Springhouse, Pa.: Springhouse Corporation, 1998.

Tierney, L.M., et al. *Current Medical Diagnosis and Treatment,* 37th ed. Stamford, Conn.: Appleton & Lange, 1998.

White, L., and Duncan, G. *Medical-Surgical Nursing: An Integrated Approach.* Albany, N.Y.: Delmar Publishers, 1998.

## Cardiovascular disorders

Brunwald, E., ed. *Heart Disease: A Textbook of Cardiovascular Medicine,* 5th ed. Philadelphia: W.B. Saunders Co., 1997.

Chulay, M., et al. *Critical Care Nursing.* Stamford, Conn.: Appleton & Lange, 1997.

Davies, M.J. *Atlas of Coronary Artery Disease.* Philadelphia: Lippincott Williams & Wilkins, 1998.

Fahey, V.A. *Vascular Nursing,* 3rd ed. Philadelphia: W.B. Saunders Co., 1999.

Jaraith, N. *Coronary Heart Disease and Risk Factor Management: A Nursing Perspective.* Philadelphia: W.B. Saunders Co., 1999.

Julian, D., et al. *Cardiology,* 7th ed. Philadelphia: W. B. Saunders Co., 1999.

Kushiwaha, S., et al. "Restrictive Cardiomyopathy," *New England Journal of Medicine* 336:267, 1997.

Lee, R.T., and Braunwald, E. *Atlas of Cardiac Imaging.* Philadelphia: W.B. Saunders Co., 1998.

Otto, C.M. *Valvular Heart Disease.* Philadelphia: W. B. Saunders Co., 1999.

Pashkow, F., and Dafoe, W. *Clinical Cardiac Rehabilitation*, 2nd ed. Philadelphia: Lippincott Williams & Wilkins, 1998.

Perloff, J.K., and Child, J.S. *Congenital Heart Disease In Adults.* Philadelphia: W.B. Saunders Co., 1998.

Rose, E.A. and Stevenson, L.W. *Management of End-Stage Heart Disease.* Philadelphia: Lippincott Williams & Wilkins, 1998.

"Sixth Report of the Joint National Committee on Prevention, Detection, Evaluation, and Treatment of High Blood Pressure," *Archives of Internal Medicine* 157:2413-46, 1997.

Spirigo, P., et al. "The Management of Hypertrophic Cardiomyopathy," *New England Journal of Medicine* 336:775, 1997.

U.S. Department of Health and Human Services. *Heart Failure: Evaluation and Care of Patients with Left-Ventricular Systolic Dysfunction.* Clinical Practice Guideline #11, June 1994.

**Ear, nose, and throat disorders**

Ballenger, J., and Snow, J., Jr. *Otorhinolaryngology: Head and Neck Surgery,* 15th ed. Philadelphia: Lippincott Williams & Wilkins, 1996.

Cummings, C.W., et al. *Otolaryngology: Head and Neck Surgery,* 3rd ed., vols. 1-4. St. Louis: Mosby–Year Book, Inc., 1998.

Fonesca, R., et.al. *Oral and Maxillofacial Trauma,* 2nd ed., vols. 1 and 2. Philadelphia: W.B. Saunders Co., 1997.

Gates, G. *Current Therapy in Otolaryngology: Head And Neck Surgery,* 6th ed. St. Louis: Mosby–Year Book, Inc., 1998.

Hawke, W., et al. *Diagnostic Handbook of Otorhinolaryngology.* St. Louis: Mosby–Year Book, Inc., 1997.

Hay, W., Jr., et al. *Current Pediatric Diagnosis and Treatment,* 13th ed. Stamford, Conn.: Appleton & Lange, 1997.

Hickey, J. *The Clinical Practice of Neurological and Neurosurgical Nursing,* Philadelphia: Lippincott Williams & Wilkins, 1997.

Schaefer, S.T. *Rhinology and Sinus Disease: A Problem-Oriented Approach.* St. Louis: Mosby–Year Book, Inc., 1998.

**Endocrine disorders**

Bardin, W.W. *Current Therapy on Endocrinology and Metabolism,* 6th ed. St. Louis: Mosby–Year Book, Inc., 1997.

Greenspan, F.S., and Strewler, G.J. *Basic and Clinical Endocrinology,* 5th ed. Stamford, Conn.: Appleton & Lange, 1997.

Porte, D. and Sherwin, R.S. *Ellen & Rifkin's Diabetes Mellitus: Theory and Practice,* 5th ed. Stamford, Conn: Appleton & Lange, 1997.

"Report of the Expert Committee on the Diagnosis and Classification of Diabetes Mellitus," *Diabetes Care,* vol. 21, supplement 1, D5-D20, January 1998.

Wiegman, M.E., ed. *Disease of the Pituitary: Diagnosis and Treatment.* Totowa, N.J.: Humana Press, 1997.

Wilson, J., and Williams, R.H., eds. *Williams Textbook of Endocrinology.* Philadelphia: W.B. Saunders Co., 1998.

**Eye disorders**

Arffa, R.C. *Grayson's Diseases of the Cornea,* 4th ed. St. Louis: Mosby–Year Book, Inc., 1998.

Ford, S., and Marsh, R. *CD-Atlas of Ophthalmology, Hybrid.* St. Louis: Mosby–Year Book, Inc., 1998.

Klein, M.L. "Age Related Macular Degeneration," in *Current Ocular Therapy.* Edited by Fraunfeltes, F.T., and Roy, F. Philadelphia: W.B. Saunders Co., 1995.

Reinecke, R.D. "Nystagmus Questions and Answers," *Journal of Ophthalmic X-ray and Technology* 17(5):183-87, 1998.

Rhee, D.J., and Deramo, V.A. *The Wills Eye Hospital Drug Guide.* Philadelphia: Lippincott Williams & Wilkins, 1998.

Vaughn, D., et al. *General Ophthalmology,* 15th ed. Stamford, Conn.: Appleton & Lange, 1998.

*Wills Eye Manual Office and Emergency Diagnosis and Treatment of Eye Diseases.* Philadelphia: Lippincott Williams & Wilkins, 1998.

**Gastrointestinal disorders**

Alexander, J.M. "Viral Hepatitis: Primary Care Diagnosis and Management," *Nurse Practitioner* 23(10):13-43, October 1998.

Aspinall R.J., and Taylor-Robinson, S.D. *Mosby's Color Atlas and Text of Gastroenterology.* St. Louis: Mosby–Year Book, Inc., 1999.

Chandrasoma, P.T. *Gastrointestinal Pathology.* Stamford, Conn.: Appleton & Lange, 1998.

Corman, M.L., ed. *Colon and Rectal Surgery,* 4th ed. Philadelphia: Lippincott Williams & Wilkins, 1998.

Galperin C., and Gershwin M. "Immunopathogenesis of Gastrointestinal and Hepatobiliary Diseases," *JAMA* 278(22):1946-55, December 10, 1997.

Greenfield, L.J., et al., eds. *Surgery: Scientific Principles and Practice,* 2nd ed. Philadelphia: Lippincott Williams & Wilkins, 1997.

Lillemoe, K.D, and Yeo, C.J. "Management of Complications of Pancreatitis," *Current Problems in Surgery* 1: 1-98, January 1998.

Nicholls, R.J., and Bozois, R., eds. *Surgery of the Colon and Rectum.* New York: Churchill Livingstone, Inc., 1997.

**Genetic disorders**

Baraitser, M., and Winter, R.M. *Color Atlas of Congenital Malformation Syndromes.* St. Louis: Mosby–Year Book, Inc., 1996.

Jorde, L.B., et al. *Medical Genetics,* 2nd ed. St. Louis: Mosby–Year Book, Inc., 1998.

Lyons Jones, K. *Smith's Recognizable Patterns of Human Malformations,* 5th ed. Phildelphia: W.B. Saunders Co., 1997.

**Hematologic disorders**

McKance, K.L., and Huether, S.E. *Pathophysiology: The Biologic Basis for Disease in Adults and Children,* 3rd ed. St. Louis: Mosby–Year Book, Inc., 1997.

Lee, G.R., and Wintrobe, MM. *Wintrobe's Clinical Hematology,* 10th ed. Philadelphia: Lippincott Williams & Wilkins, 1998.

**Infectious disorders**

*APIC Infection Control and Applied Epidemiology, Principles and Practice.* St. Louis: Mosby–Year Book, Inc.,1996.

Bartlett, J.G. *1998 Pocket Book of Infectious Disease Therapy.* Philadelphia: Lippincott Williams & Wilkins, 1998.

Bowden, R.A., et al. *Transplant Infections.* Philadephia: Lippincott Williams & Wilkins, 1998.

Connor, D.H., et al. *Pathology of Infectious Diseases.* Stamford, Conn.: Appleton & Lange, 1997.

Cunha, B.A. *Infectious Disease Pearls.* St. Louis: Mosby–Year Book, Inc., 1998.

Books, G.F., et al. *Medical Microbiology,* 21st ed. Stamford, Conn.: Appleton & Lange, 1998.

Gorbach, S.L., et al. *Infectious Diseases,* 2nd ed. Phildadelphia: W. B. Saunders Co., 1998.

Long, S.S., et al. *Principles and Practice of Pediatric Infectious Diseases.* Philadelphia: W.B. Saunders Co., 1997.

Richman, D.D., et al. *Clinical Virology.* Philadelphia: W.B. Saunders Co., 1997.

Zeibig, E.A. *Clinical Parasitology: A Practical Approach.* Philadelphia: W.B. Saunders Co., 1997.

**Immunologic disorders**

Baum, J., et al. "Fibromyalgia Syndrome in Children and Adolescents: Clinical Features at Presentation and Status at Follow-Up," *Pediatrics* 101 (3, part 1):377-82, March 1998.

Brostoff, J., et al. *Immunology Case Studies.* St. Louis: Mosby–Year Book, Inc., 1998.

Carpenter, C.C., et al. "Antiretroviral Therapy for HIV Infection in 1998: Updated Recommendations of the International AIDS Society-USA Panel," *JAMA* 280(1):78-86, July 1998.

Clauw, D.J., and Chrousos, G.P. "Chronic Pain and Fatigue Syndromes: Overlapping Clinical and Neuroendocrine Features and Potential Pathogenic Mechanisms," *Neuroimmunomodulation* 4(3):134-53, May-June 1997.

Dasgupta, B., et al. "An Initially Double-Blind Controlled 96-Week Trial of Depot Methylprednisolone against Oral Prednisone in the Treatment of Polymyalgia Rheumatica," *British Journal of Rheumatology* 37(2):189-95, February 1998.

Garzino-Demo, A., et al. "Chemokine Receptors and Chemokines in HIV Infection," *Journal of Clinical Immunology* 18(4):243-55, July 1998.

Gliniecki, C.M. "Management of Latex Reactions in the Occupational Setting,"*AAOHN J* 46(2):82-93, February 1998.

Griep, E.N., et al. "Function of the Hypothalamic-Pituitary-Adrenal Axis in Patients with Fibromyalgia and Low Back Pain," *Journal of Rheumatology* 25(7):1374-81, July 1998.

Hochberg, M.C. "Updating the American College of Rheumatology Revised Criteria for Classification of Systemic Lupus Erythematosus," *Arthritis and Rheum* 40(9):1725, September 1997.

Janeway, C., and Travers, P., eds. *Immunobiology: The Immune System In Health and Disease,* 3rd ed. New York: Garland Publishing Inc., 1997.

Kirton, C., et al. *HIV/AIDS Nursing Handbook.* St. Louis: Mosby–Year Book, Inc., 1999.

Klippel, J., and Dieppe, P., eds. *Rheumatology,* 2nd ed. St. Louis: Mosby–Year Book, Inc., 1998.

Klippel, J.H., et al, eds. *Primer on the Rheumatic Diseases.* Atlanta: Arthritis Foundation, 1997.

Schmidt, W.A., et al. "Color Duplex Ultrasonography in the Diagnosis of Temporal Arteritis," *New England Journal of Medicine* 337(19):1336-1342, November 6, 1997.

Sprott, H., et al. "Pain Treatment of Fibromyalgia by Acupuncture," *Rheumatology Int* 18(1):35-36, 1998.

Stites, D.P., et al. *Medical Immunology,* 9th ed. Stamford, Conn.: Appleton & Lange, 1997.

VanBushkirk, A., et al. "Transplantation Immunology," *JAMA* 278(22):1993-99, December 1997.

**Musculoskeletal disorders**

Bluemke, D.A., et al. "CT and MRI Evaluation of Musculoskeletal Infection," *Critical Reviews in Diagnostic Imaging* 38(6):535-68, December 1997.

Fu, F.H. *An Atlas of Shoulder Surgery.* Stamford, Conn.: Appleton & Lange, 1998.

Nordin, M., et al. *Musculoskeletal Disorders in the Workplace: Principles and Practice.* St. Louis: Mosby–Year Book, Inc., 1997.

Schoen, D.C.H. *An Illustrated Guide to Orthopaedic Nursing.* Philadelphia: Lippincott Williams & Wilkins, 1999.

Tachdjian, M.O. *Clinical Pediatric Orthopedics.* Stamford, Conn.: Appleton & Lange, 1997.

Wall, E.J. "Childhood Osteomyelitis and Septic Arthritis," *Current Opinion in Pediatrics* 10(1): 73-76, February 1998.

**Neurologic disorders**

Bratina, P., et al. "Pathophysiology and Mechanisms of Acute Ischemic Stroke," *Journal of Neuroscience Nursing* 29(6):351-60, December 1997.

Corey-Bloom, J., and David, R.B., eds. *Adult Neurology,* 4th ed. St. Louis: Mosby–Year Book, Inc., 1998.

Folstein, M.F. "Mini Mental State: A Practical Method for Grading the Cognitive State of Patients for the Clinician," *Journal of Psychological Research* 12(3):189-98, November 1975.

Herring, B., and Wood, P. "Dysphagia: A Screening Tool for Stroke Patients," *Journal of Neuroscience Nursing* 29(5):325-29, October 1997.

Hickey, J. *The Clinical Practice of Neurological and Neurosurgical Nursing.* Philadelphia: Lippincott Williams & Wilkins, 1997.

Leppik, I.L.O., "Contemporary Diagnosis and Management of the Patient with Epilepsy," in *Handbooks in Health Care,* 3rd ed. Newtown, Pa.: Associates in Medical Marketing, 1997.

Lisis, S. "Pathophysiology and Management of Idiopathic Parkinson's Disease," *Journal of Neuroscience Nursing* 29(1):24-31, February 1997.

Logemann, J., "Screening, Diagnosis and Management of Neurological Dysphagia," *Seminars in Neurology* 16(4): 319-27, December 1996.

Nance, M.A., and Sanders, G. "Characteristics of Individuals with Huntington's Disease in Long-Term Care,"*Movement Disorders* 11(5):542-48, September 1996.

Ross, R.T. *How to Examine the Nervous System,* 3rd ed. Stamford, Conn.: Appleton & Lange, 1998.

Sanders, M., and Cummings, J. "Huntington's Disease," *Psychiatric Clinics of North America* 20(4):791-807, December 1997.

Simon, R.P., et al. *Clinical Neurology,* 4th ed. Stamford, Conn.: Appleton & Lange, 1999.

Spilker, J., et al. "Using the NIH Stroke Scale to Assess Stroke Patients," *Journal of Neuroscience Nursing* 29(6): 384-92, December 1997.

Trapp, B., et al. "Axonal Transection in the Lesion of MS," *New England Journal of Medicine* 338(5):278-85, January 1998.

Uiha, R. "Medical Treatment of Essential Tremor and Parkinson's Disease," *Geriatrics* 53:46-57, May 1998.

Uiha, R. "Tremor: How to Determine if the Patient Has Parkinson's Disease," *Geriatrics* 53:30-36, May 1998.

## Obstetric & gynecologic disorders

Carr, B.R., and Blackwell, R.E. *Textbook of Reproductive Medicine,* 2nd ed. Stamford, Conn.: Appleton & Lange, 1998.

Cunningham, F.G., et al., eds. *Williams Obstetrics,* 20th ed. Stamford, Conn.: Appleton & Lange, 1997.

Goff, B. *Atlas of Clinical Gynecology.* Stamford, Conn.: Appleton & Lange, 1998.

Mishell, D.R., et al. *Comprehensive Gynecology: CD Online.* St. Louis: Mosby–Year Book, Inc., 1998.

Novak, J.C., and Broom, B.L. *Ingall's and Salerno's Maternal and Child Health Nursing*, 9th ed. St. Louis: Mosby–Year Book, Inc., 1999.

Ryan, K.J., et al. *Kistner's Gynecology and Women's Health,* 7th ed. St. Louis: Mosby–Year Book, Inc., 1999.

Sherwen, L.N., et al. *Maternity Nursing: Care of the Childbearing Family,* 3rd ed. Stamford, Conn.: Appleton & Lange, 1999.

Youngkin, E.Q., and Davis, M.S. *Women's Health: A Primary Clinical Guide,* 2nd. ed. Stamford, Conn.: Appleton & Lange, 1998.

## Respiratory disorders

Brody, J.S. *The Lung: Molecular Basis of Disease.* Philadelphia: W.B. Saunders Co., 1998.

Dunne, P.J., and McInturff, S.L. *Respiratory Home Care: The Essentials.* Philadelphia: F.A. Davis Co., 1998.

Fink, J.B., and Hunt, G.E. *Clinical Practice in Respiratory Care.* Philadelphia: Lippincott Williams & Wilkins, 1998.

Fraser, R.S., et al. *Fraser and Pare's Diagnosis of Diseases of the Chest,* 4th ed. Philadelphia: W.B. Saunders Co., 1999.

Groenwald, S.L., et al. *Comprehensive Cancer Nursing Review,* 4th ed. Sudbury, Mass.: Jones & Bartlett Pubs., Inc., 1998.

Kumar, A., et al. " Clinical and Personality Profiles and Survival in Patients with COPD," *Chest* 11(1):95, January 1997.

"New Guidelines Are Out for Nosocomial Pneumonia," *The Brown University Long-Term Care Quality Advisor.* 9(9):2, May 12, 1997.

Orenstein, D.M. *Cystic Fibrosis: A Guide for the Patient and Family,* 2nd ed. Philadelphia: Lippincott Williams & Wilkins, 1997.

Sarosi, G.A., and Davies, S.F., eds. *Fungal Diseases of the Lung,* 3rd ed. Philadelphia: Lippincott Williams & Wilkins, 1998.

Thompson, J.M., et al. *Mosby's Clinical Nursing.* 4th ed. St. Louis: Mosby–Year Book, Inc., 1997.

Weinberger, S.E. *Principles of Pulmonary Medicine,* 3rd ed. Philadelphia: W.B. Saunders Co., 1998.

"What's New for Clinicians: Pneumonia. New Prediction Model Proves Promising," *AHCPR* Pub. No. 97-R003, January 1997.

## Traumatic disorders

Carrico, C.J., et al. *Operative Trauma Management: An Atlas.* Stamford, Conn.: Appleton & Lange, 1998.

Goldfrank, L.R., et al. *Goldfrank's Toxicologic Emergencies,* 6th ed. Stamford, Conn.: Appleton & Lange, 1998.

Harwood-Nuss, A., ed. *The Clinical Practice of Emergency Medicine,* 2nd ed. Philadelphia: Lippincott Williams & Wilkins, 1996.

Newberry, L., ed. *Sheehy's Emergency Nursing: Principles and Practice,* 4th ed. St. Louis: Mosby–Year Book, Inc., 1998.

Rosen, P., ed. *Emergency Medicine Concepts and Clinical Practice,* 4th ed. St. Louis: Mosby–Year Book, Inc., 1998.

Sullivan, W.G. "Trauma to the Face," in *Management of Trauma: Pitfalls and Practice,* 2nd ed. Edited by Wilson, R.F., and Walt, A.J. Philadelphia: Lippincott Williams & Wilkins, 1996.

Wald, D.A. "Burn Management: Systematic Patient Evaluation, Fluid Resuscitation and Wound Management," *Emergency Medicine Reports* 19(5): 45-52, March 2, 1998.

# INDEX

t refers to table; i refers to an illustration

t refers to table; i refers to an illustration

t refers to table; i refers to an illustration

t refers to table; i refers to an illustration

t refers to table; i refers to an illustration